Y0-CPB-594

*Orban's*

# PERIODONTICS

*a concept—theory and practice*

# *Orban's*

# PERIODONTICS

## *a concept—theory and practice*

---


**DANIEL A. GRANT, D.D.S.**
San Diego, California
University of Southern California School of Medicine,
Los Angeles, California

**IRVING B. STERN, D.D.S.**
University of Washington School of Dentistry,
Seattle, Washington

**FRANK G. EVERETT, D.M.D., M.D., M.S.**
University of Oregon Dental School,
Portland, Oregon



FOURTH EDITION

With 1089 illustrations, including two color plates

SAINT LOUIS

**THE C. V. MOSBY COMPANY**

1972

FOURTH EDITION



*Printed in the United States of America*

*International Standard Book Number 0-8016-1960-2*

*Library of Congress Catalog Card Number 75-189276*

*Distributed in Great Britain by Henry Kimpton, London*

*Front cover: Periodontium in health (marmoset)*
*Back cover: Periodontium in disease (marmoset)*

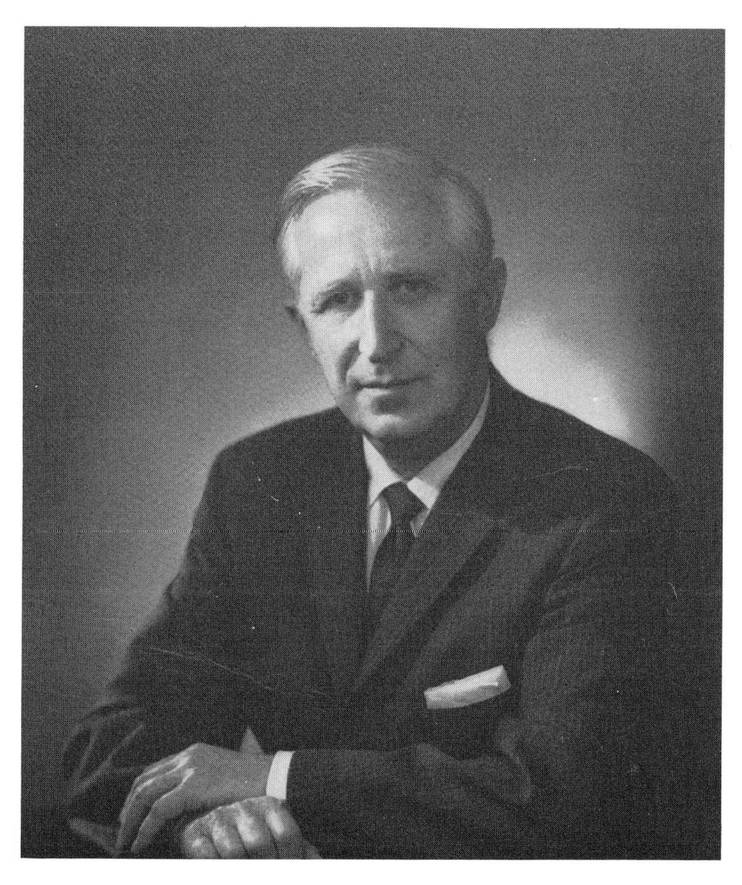

*To*

**BALINT ORBAN**

1899-1960

A clinician of consummate skill; a researcher of an incomparable power of observation and an unprejudiced intellect in interpretation; a teacher of inspiring genius and unstinting generosity; a human being of empathy and humility

The harmonious cooperation of all beings arose,
not from the orders of a superior authority external to themselves,
but from the fact that they were all parts in a hierarchy of wholes forming a cosmic pattern,
and what they obeyed were the internal dictates of their own natures.

**Chung Tzu**
(3rd Century B.C.)

# Preface

This is a *learning* textbook. It is written for the undergraduate dental student and for the general practitioner.

*Credibility* and *readability* are the design of this work. Simplicity in language has been our objective, and the organization of chapters is intended to provide a cohesiveness to learning material. The marginal notes serve as a programmed guide for the reader.

The goal of this book is to supply the reader with the knowledge necessary to treat periodontal disease as an integral part of the practice of dentistry.

The effective treatment of periodontal ailments requires that the dentist be well grounded in basic biologic principles and that the prevention and treatment of periodontal disease be practiced as a part of general dentistry. The general dental treatment of the everyday patient has periodontal considerations, even when extractions and prosthodontia are involved. Periodontal treatment can succeed only when associated restorative treatment is performed, and the converse is also true. Dentitions can be preserved and the well-being of the patient promoted, only when complete treatment is given. The ability to integrate all phases of dental treatment must be mastered by the general dentist, even in those cases in which the cooperation of the specialist is enlisted.

Periodontics, interrelated as it is with all parts of dental practice, and with obvious relationships to basic science, is the part of dentistry that can best be used to promote a unified approach to dental treatment. This concept embraces an integration of periodontics, general practice, and biologic principles in a clinical approach called *complete therapy*.

**Daniel A. Grant**

**Irving B. Stern**

**Frank G. Everett**

# Acknowledgments

When this book was conceived some 18 years ago, we realized that with the explosion of knowledge in our times, a continuing challenge would be present: how to weigh what is currently popular with its validity. Demonstrably, what is modish is not necessarily enduring. The recent literature is filled with therapies once popular and since discarded or shelved as unimportant, with biologic interpretations once accepted and now rejected, with experiments once cited and since refuted. Since prominent objectives of this book were readability and credibility, their fulfillment has exacted a demanding discipline. The vast scope of periodontics has required help of other workers in periodontology. This text is the result of our efforts with the assistance of other workers in the areas indicated. The contributions of the workers listed herein are gratefully acknowledged.

The orientation of this text to the dental student was pursued throughout the writing. Undergraduate students were asked to review material in an effort to make the text simple and understandable. The opinion of general practitioners and specialists was also sought. Dr. Harvey Stallard reviewed the chapter on treatment of periodontal trauma. The chapter on the periodontal flap evolved from a workshop on teaching by Dr. Grant with periodontists at the University of Nebraska College of Dentistry, Dr. Gerald Tussing, Dr. Kent Powers, Dr. William Hollander, Dr. Joseph Keene, and Dr. Mansoor Jabro; and their participation is appreciated.

We wish to thank our co-workers, listed next, whose contributions and critical reviews helped to promote the success of earlier editions. Despite inevitable change, evidence of their efforts may be found in the current work. Our gratitude is hereby expressed to Alvin D. Aisenberg, D.D.S., Charles R. Amen, D.D.S., Ernest L. Banks, D.D.S., Richard E. Bradley, D.D.S., M.S., Martin Cattoni, D.D.S., M.S.D., Marco Droppelmann, D.D.S., Peter D. Ferrigno, D.D.S., Calvin L. Foss, D.D.S., Harold E. Grupe, Sr., D.D.S., Alvin C. Hileman, D.M.D., M.S., Gerald P. Ivancie, D.D.S., M.S., John A. Kollar, Jr., D.D.S., Harold P. Kreski, D.D.S, Sydney Levine, M.D.S., J. H. Manhold, D.M.D., M.A., Nicholas R. Marfino, D.D.S., M.S., Gerald A. Mitchell, D.D.S., Claude L. Nabers, D.D.S., M.S.D., Delbert P. Nachazel, D.D.S., Timothy O'Leary, D.D.S., Gilbert Parfitt, D.M.D., Jacoby T. Rothner, D.D.S., E. M. Schaffer, D.D.S., M.S.D., Harry Sicher, M.D., Leo M. Sreebny, D.D.S., Ph.D., Richard Stallard, D.D.S., Ph.D., James C. Steiner, D.D.S., M.S., J. R. Trott, D.D.S., B.D.S., D. E. Van Scotter, D.D.S., M.S., Frank M. Wentz, D.D.S., Ph.D., M.S., John R. Wilson, D.D.S., Helmut A. Zander, D.D.S., M.S., and Jack D. Zwemer, D.D.S., Ph.D., M.S.

## Contributors

**Paul N. Baer, D.D.S.**
State University of New York
School of Dentistry
Stony Brook, New York

**Sol Bernick, Ph.D.**
University of Southern California
School of Medicine
Los Angeles, California

**Surindar N. Bhaskar, D.D.S., Ph.D.**
Armed Forces Institute of Oral Pathology
Washington, D. C.

**C. Kenneth Collings, D.D.S., M.A.**
Baylor College of Dentistry
Dallas, Texas

**Howard R. Creamer, Ph.D.**
University of Oregon Dental School
Portland, Oregon

**R. D. Emslie, B.D.S., M.S., F.D.S.(Eng.)**
Department of Preventive Dentistry
Guy's Hospital
London, England

**Cyril Enwonwu, Sc.D., M.D.S., B.D.S.**
University of Washington School of Dentistry
Seattle, Washington

**Robert T. Ferris, D.D.S., Ph.D.**
Orlando, Florida

**C. Mahlon Fraleigh, D.D.S., M.S.D.**
University of Iowa College of Dentistry
Iowa City, Iowa

**Anthony Gargiulo, D.D.S., M.S.**
Loyola University School of Dentistry
Maywood, Illinois

**O. M. Gupta B.D.S., M.S., M.S.D., Dr.P.H.**
University of Pittsburgh School of
Dental Medicine
Pittsburgh, Pennsylvania

**Walter B. Hall, D.D.S., M.S.D.**
University of the Pacific School of Dentistry
San Francisco, California

**Stanley P. Hazen, D.D.S., M.S.**
The University of Connecticut
School of Dental Medicine
Farmington, Connecticut

**William H. Hiatt, D.D.S.**
University of Colorado School of Dentistry
Denver, Colorado

**Herbert B. Laffitte, D.D.S.**
University of Oregon Dental School
Portland, Oregon

**Jan Lindhe, L.D.S., Odont. D.**
Göteborgs Universitet
Faculty of Odontology
Göteborg, Sweden

**Irwin Mandel, D.D.S.**
Columbia University School of Dental
and Oral Surgery
New York, New York

**Edward H. Montgomery, Ph.D.**
University of Texas Dental Branch
Houston, Texas

**Melvin Morris, D.D.S.**
Columbia University School of Dental
and Oral Surgery
New York, New York

**Ernest H. Moser, Jr., D.D.S.**
University of the Pacific School of Dentistry
San Francisco, California

**Richard C. Oliver, D.D.S., M.S.D.**
Loma Linda University School of Dentistry
Loma Linda, California

**Richard B. Parker, Ph.D.**
University of Oregon Dental School
Portland, Oregon

**Billy M. Pennel, D.D.S. M.S.**
Medical College of Georgia School of Dentistry
Augusta, Georgia

**Peter D. Roberson, D.D.S., M.S.**
Loyola University School of Dentistry
Maywood, Illinois

**Robert G. Schallhorn, D.D.S., M.S.D.**
University of Colorado School of Dentistry
Denver, Colorado

**Hubert E. Schroeder, Dr.med.dent.**
Zahnärztliches Institut der Universität
Zurich, Switzerland

**Stanley R. Suit, D.D.S., M.S.**
Case Western Reserve University School of Dentistry
Cleveland, Ohio

**Else Theilade, D.D.S.**
Royal Dental College
Aarhus, Denmark

**Jorgen Theilade, D.D.S., B.Sc.D., M.S.**
Royal Dental College
Aarhus, Denmark

**Gerald J. Tussing, D.D.S., M.S.D.**
University of Nebraska College of Dentistry
Lincoln, Nebraska

**Malbern N. Wilderman, D.D.S., M.S.**
Louisiana State University School of Dentistry
New Orleans, Louisiana

**Wellesley H. Wright, D.D.S., M.S.**
University of Oregon Dental School
Portland, Oregon

The chapter on saliva was the work of Dr. Irwin Mandel. Dr. Cyril Enwonwu wrote the chapter on nutrition. Dr. Else Theilade was principally responsible for microbiology with assistance from Dr. Richard Parker. Dr. Jorgen Theilade was largely responsible for the chapter on dental deposits, as were Dr. Howard Creamer and Dr. Edward Montgomery for the chapter on inflammation. Dr. Paul Baer was heavily involved with periodontosis. Dr. Melvin Morris was responsible for the revision and amplification of the sections on wound healing. Dr. O. M. Gupta wrote on epidemiology. Dr. Jan Lindhe contributed the material on chemical plaque control.

Dr. Stanley Suit thoroughly reviewed the chapter on the treatment of periodontal trauma. Drafts were received from Dr. Surindar Bhaskar and Dr. Robert Ferris on inflammation, from Dr. Gerald Tussing on examination, and from Dr. Richard Oliver on treatment planning.

Dr. Walter Hall contributed material on mucogingival surgery, as did Dr. John Nabers. Dr. Anthony Gargiulo contributed material on periodontal trauma and the dimensions of the dentogingival junction. Dr. Malbern Wilderman and Dr. Wellesley Wright contributed material on wound healing, Dr. William Hiatt and Dr. Robert Schallhorn on bone grafts, Dr. Ernest Moser on oral hygiene, Dr. Hubert Schroeder on plaque, Dr. Stephen Clark on ultrasonic instrumentation, and Dr. Sol Bernick for one cover illustration. Dr. Peter Roberson did the indexing. Other contributors reviewed material and offered valued suggestions.

We express our appreciation for the contributions that have so enhanced and added to our own work. In all areas the final wording and the concepts expressed herein are our responsibility.

So very important, we wish to acknowledge the sacrifices made by our wives and families, whose understanding made this work possible.

D. A. G.
I. B. S.
F. G. E.

# Contents

## Part VI
## Elements of therapeutic judgment



## Part VII
## Conditions requiring immediate treatment



## Part VIII
## Therapy



## Part IX
## Traumatic periodontal diseases and their treatment



## Part X
## The treated case

# Color plates

PART I

# The periodontium and periodontal disease

CHAPTER ONE

# Periodontal health and disease



The purpose of this text is to teach the prevention and cure of periodontal disease. Throughout the text the clinical principles will be coupled with basic science. Understanding the biology of the supporting tissues of the teeth makes for a more meaningful application of therapeutic practices and leads to greater success in the treatment of periodontal diseases.

The teeth are supported by the alveolar processes of the maxilla and mandible. Bundles of collagen fibers course between and insert into the cementum and the alveolar bone to hold the teeth in place. The teeth are surrounded by the periodontal tissues (Greek *peri,* "around"; *odont-,* "tooth"), which provide the support that is essential to function. The gingiva covers the alveolar bone and surrounds the neck of each tooth. The ability to chew normally with one's own teeth depends in part on the health of the periodontium.

*Pocket*

Many diseases affect the health of the periodontium and may lead to a loss of alveolar bone and the loosening of teeth. The gingival attachment to the tooth may move apically while the gingiva seemingly remains in place or becomes enlarged. This results in a loose sleeve of diseased gingiva lying against the tooth. The space between this detached gingiva and the tooth is called a pocket.

*Periodontal disease*

The ultimate result of pocket formation, bone loss, and tooth mobility is the loss of a tooth or teeth. Such periodontal disease is found in all people, in all nations. In the United States more than half the people over 40 years of age have lost at least one tooth because of this disease. In fact, 20 million adults have lost all their teeth, and periodontal disease is believed to be the chief cause of this loss.[1-3] The disease process is chronic (slow and progressive in developing) and may very well have been present in these people in their youth, but the signs were not evident to them.

## PROBLEM OF PREVENTION AND TREATMENT

At this point the statement should be made that periodontal disease is preventable and controllable to a large degree. The disease is most easily treated and with best results in its early stages. Since the dentist's professional obligation is to keep the teeth in health and to prevent their loss, his knowledge of periodontal disease and its prevention and treatment are of paramount concern to him and to the patients he treats. In fact, without such knowledge a dentist cannot be considered fully competent.

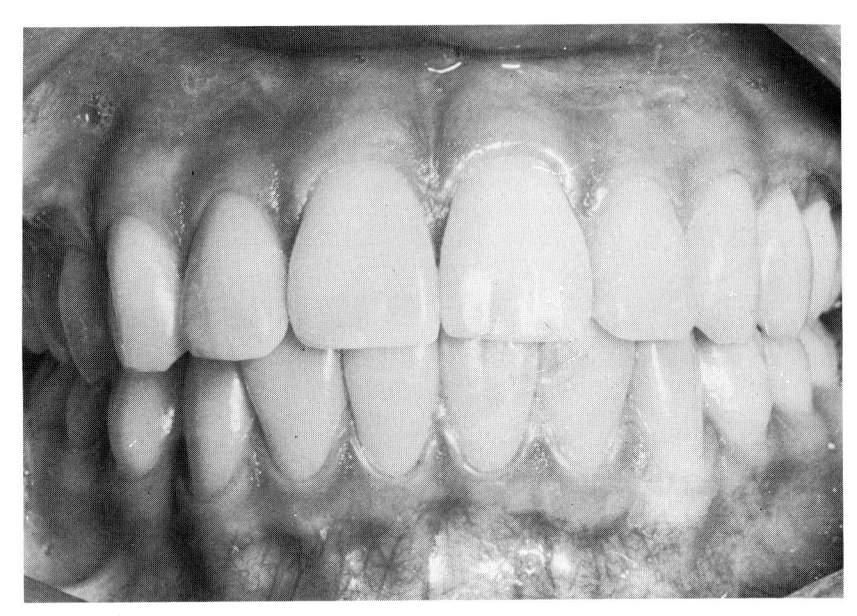

**Fig. 1-1.** Surface characteristics of the clinically normal gingiva. (Courtesy A. L. Ogilvie, Seattle.)

The various diseases of the periodontium are collectively termed *periodontal disease*. Their treatment is referred to as *periodontal therapy*. The clinical science that deals with the periodontium in health and disease is called *periodontology*. The practice of this discipline is *periodontics*.

Before any further consideration of periodontal disease and its treatment, we should agree that the ability to recognize the healthy periodontium is essential, as is also the ability to discern the minute and gross changes that accompany periodontal disease. The dentist who cannot recognize periodontal disease cannot proceed to treat it. Such a shortcoming in the dentist is detrimental to the patient, who may ultimately suffer tooth loss. The patient's need for complete mouth care will not be realized and the dentist will not fulfill his function.

## ORAL MUCOSA—GINGIVA

Fundamentally the oral mucosa may be classified into three different types[4]: the gingiva and the covering of the hard palate (*masticatory* mucosa), the dorsum of the tongue (*specialized* mucosa), and the remainder of the oral mucous membrane (*lining* mucosa).

### Surface characteristics

*Normal gingiva*

The gingiva (masticatory mucosa) is that part of the oral mucous membrane attached to the teeth and the alveolar processes of the jaws (Fig. 1-1). Normal clinical features of the gingiva include the following:

1. *Color.* The color of normal gingiva is pale pink but may vary according to degree of vascularity, epithelial keratinization, pigmentation, and thickness of the epithelium.
2. *Papillary contour.* Papillae should fill the interproximal spaces to the contact point. With increasing age the papillae and other parts of the gingiva may atrophy slightly (together with the underlying alveolar crest). A

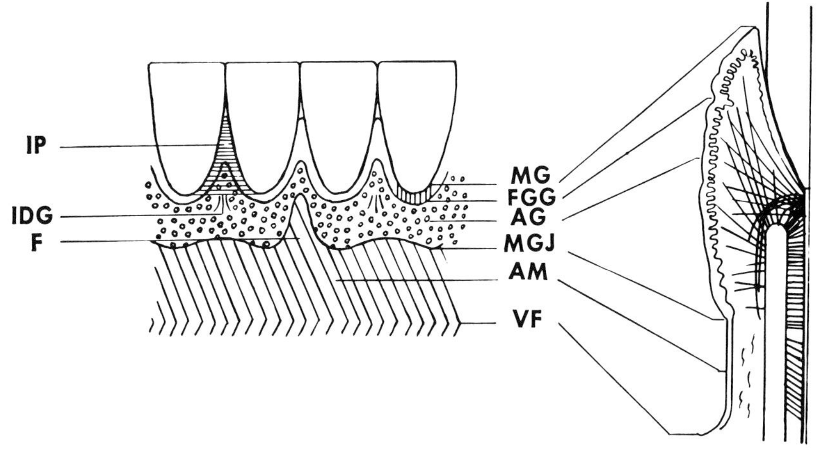


**Fig. 1-2.** Diagrammatic illustration of surface characteristics of the clinically normal gingiva. *IP,* Interdental papilla; *IDG,* interdental grooves; *F,* frenum; *MG,* marginal gingiva; *FGG,* free gingival groove; *AG,* attached gingiva; *MGJ,* mucogingival junction; *AM,* alveolar mucosa; *VF,* vestibular fornix.

more blunt rather than pointed contour may therefore also be considered as normal for older persons.

3. *Marginal contour.* The gingiva should slope coronally to end in a thin edge. Mesiodistally the gingival margins should be scalloped in form.
4. *Texture.* Stippling is generally present to varying degrees on vestibular surfaces of the attached gingiva. This type of surface has been described as "orange peel" in appearance.
5. *Consistency.* The gingiva should be firm and the attached part tightly anchored to the teeth and underlying alveolar bone.
6. *Sulcus.* The sulcus is the space between the free gingiva and the tooth. It is minimal in depth (approximately 1 mm. in health). A normal sulcus should not exceed 3 mm. in depth.

## Morphologic divisions

The gingiva is divided into (1) the attached,[5] (2) the free or marginal (Fig. 1-2), and (3) the papillary[5] gingivae. It is subject to pressure and impacts during mastication, and its structure is adapted to meet these events.[11]

***Attached gingiva and mucogingival junction***

The attached gingiva is demarcated from the loosely anchored and movable alveolar mucosa by a recognizable line, the mucogingival junction (Fig. 1-2). This line of demarcation between the gingiva and the alveolar mucosa occurs on the outer (vestibular)* surfaces of both jaws. A similar line may occur on the inner (oral)* surface of the mandible between the mucosa and the floor of the mouth. There often is no clear dividing line on the palate because the mucosa of the

*The term *vestibular* is used to describe those surfaces that face the vestibule, thus eliminating the need of differentiating between buccal and labial. This tends to simplify descriptions and coincides with proper anatomic usage. The vestibular cavity is bounded anterolaterally by the mucous membranes of the lips and cheeks and internally by the teeth and gingiva. Vestibular would therefore apply to any tooth surface facing the vestibular cavity. Similarly the term *oral* describes the palatal and lingual. The oral cavity proper is bounded anterolaterally by the teeth and gingiva, superiorly by the soft and hard palate, inferiorly by the tongue and mucous membranes of the floor of the mouth, and posteriorly by the pillars of the fauces, the opening into the oral pharynx.

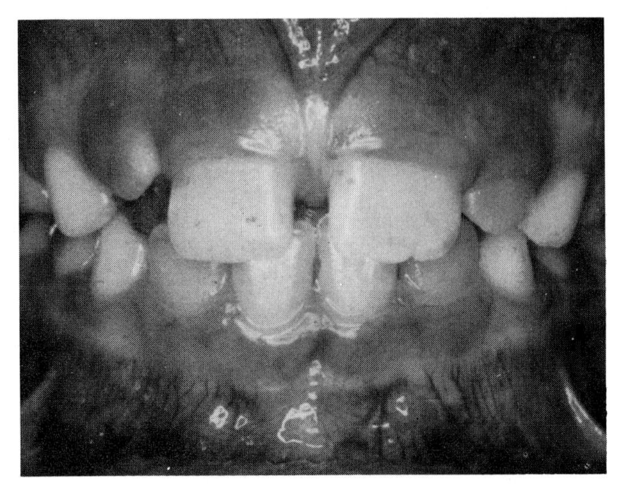

**Fig. 1-3.** Mixed dentition in an 8-year-old boy. Gingival color is pale pink. During eruption the gingival margins (see maxillary central incisors) are thicker. Crowns of the central and lateral incisors are not fully exposed. Where teeth are in proximal contact, the papillae fill the interdental spaces. (Courtesy M. Droppelmann, Valparaiso, Chile.)

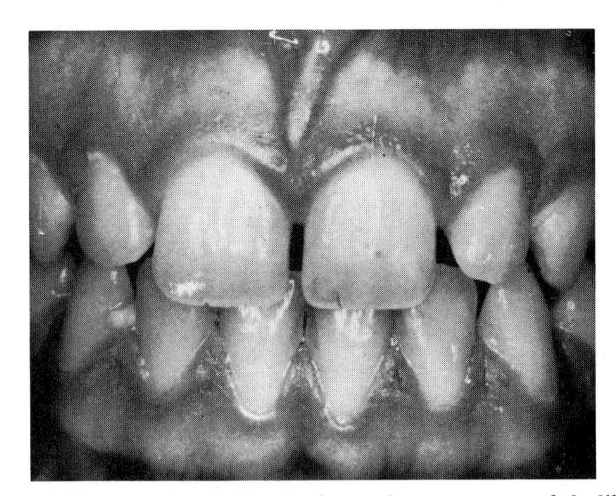

**Fig. 1-4.** At the age of 14 years, the gingiva begins to become more adult like in appearance. The maxillary gingival margins are rolled as passive exposure of the crown proceeds. Gingival color is pale pink.

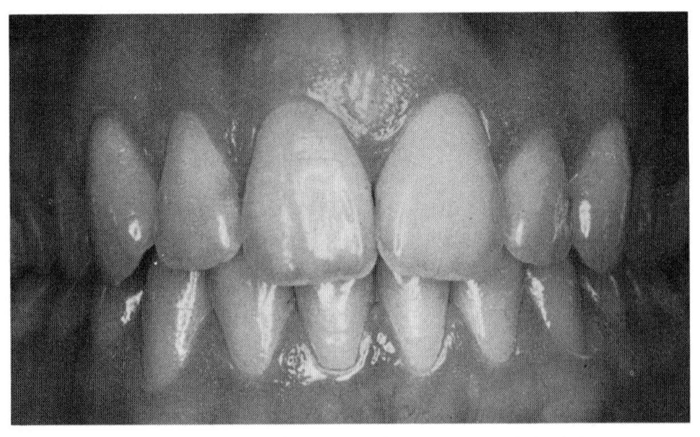

**Fig. 1-5.** Gingival tissues of a 20-year-old girl.

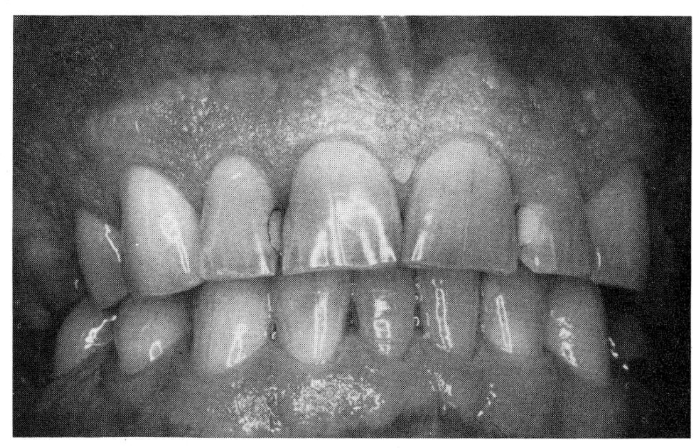

**Fig. 1-6.** Gingival tissues of a 44-year-old man.

hard palate is keratinized and firmly attached to bone and is therefore immovable. The mucogingival junction, although clinically and anatomically evident, is subject to considerable variation in shape and position.

***Width of the attached gingiva***

The attached gingiva is bounded by the mucogingival junction and by the line of free gingival grooves. This zone varies in width between individuals and in different areas of the same mouth. It is usually widest about the anterior teeth, where it may be as much as or more than 4 mm. It is narrower in the premolar region. In the mandibular second and third molar region it is sometimes 1 mm. in width or may even be nonexistent. The zone of attached gingiva is generally wider in the maxilla than in the mandible.

Figs. 1-3 to 1-10 are presented to demonstrate the range of normal gingival width at various ages.

Fig. 1-5 is of a 20-year-old girl. The gingival form is ideal. The gingiva is knife-edged, and festooning is regular. The zone of attached gingiva is delicate in texture, and the mucogingival line is not strongly delineated.

Fig. 1-6 is of a 44-year-old man. The form is similar to that of the previous patient. However, the degree of keratinization and the amount of stippling are more pronounced.

Fig. 1-7, *A*, is of a 46-year-old woman. The photograph is 14 years old, but the appearance of the gingiva cannot be distinguished from that in a more recent photograph taken at age 60 (Fig. 1-7, *B*).

Fig. 1-8 is of a 75-year-old patient. The degree of difference between the tissues of this and younger patients is not great.

Fig. 1-9 is of a 47-year-old patient. Note the slight festooning about the teeth and the saddle form of the edentulous space. There is a faint pigmentation in the attached gingiva of the anterior teeth.

Fig. 1-10 is of a 21-year-old Negro. All the characteristics of ideal form are present. The zone of attached gingiva is made more apparent by the generalized pigmentation of this zone.

***Stippling***

The surface of the attached gingiva is characterized by an orange peel–like appearance called stippling (Fig. 1-12). The stippling may be fine or coarse and may vary in different individuals; it may also vary according to age and sex.[6,7] In girls the stippling is finer than it is in boys. It is normally absent in some locations (e.g., the molar area). In addition to stippling, the epithelial surface may contain scattered minute protuberances that contribute to its texture.[7]

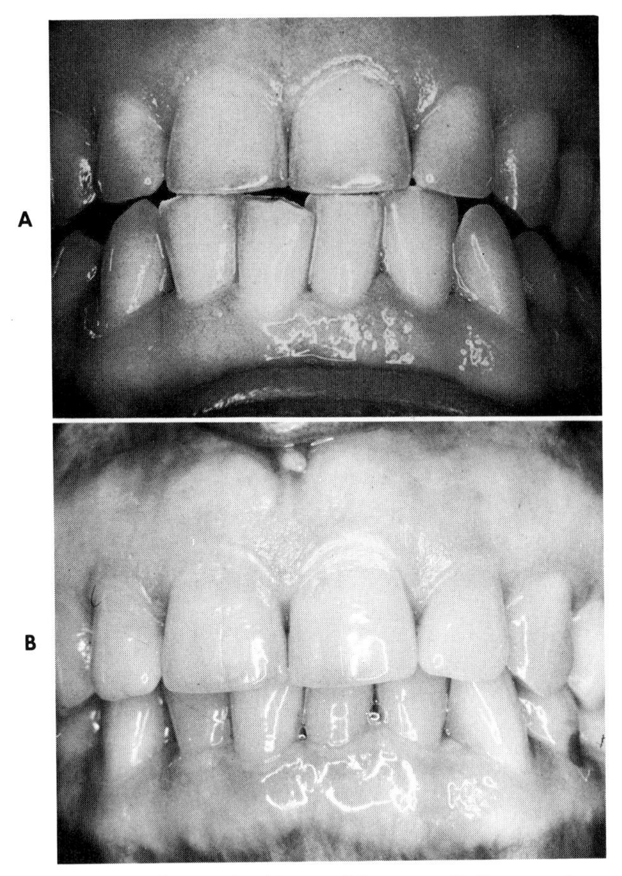


**Fig. 1-7. A,** Gingival tissues of a 46-year-old woman. **B,** Same patient at age 60.

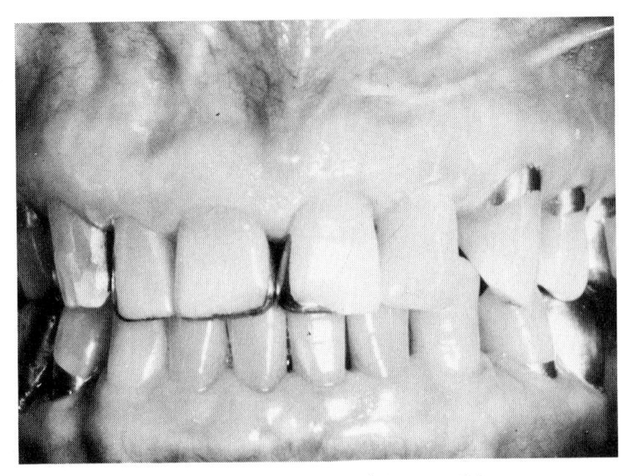

**Fig. 1-8.** Gingival tissues of a 75-year-old woman.

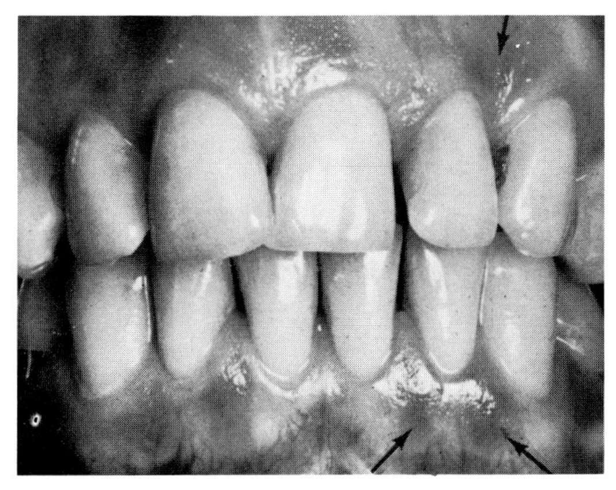

**Fig. 1-9.** Gingiva of a 47-year-old woman. Arrows point to pigmented areas.

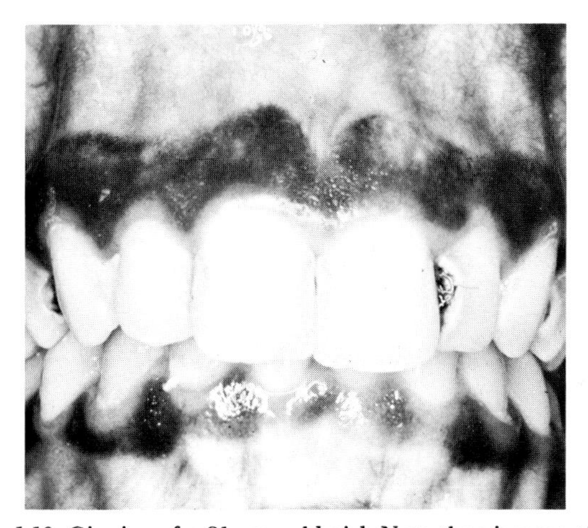

**Fig. 1-10.** Gingiva of a 21-year-old girl. Note the pigmentation.

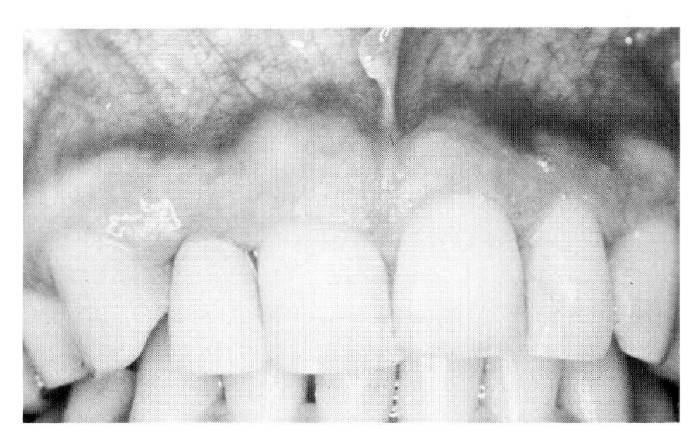

**Fig. 1-11.** Maxillary right central incisor is extruded. Left incisor is vestibular (labial) to it. When viewed from the oral aspect, the gingival margin of the right incisor is attached further coronally. This difference in height of attachment is due to the difference in position of teeth in the arch.

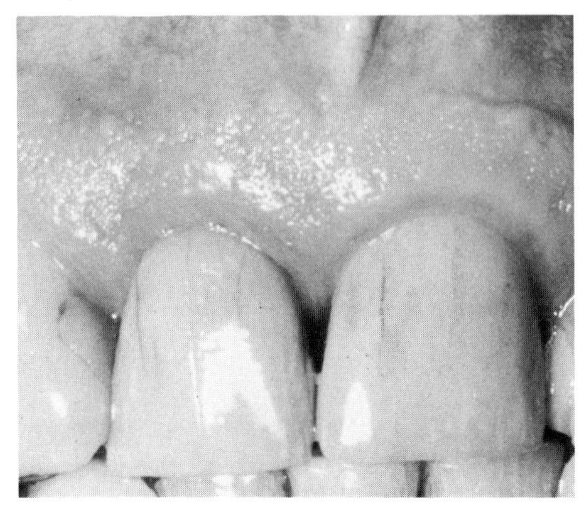

**Fig. 1-12.** Stippling (depressed points) of the attached gingiva.

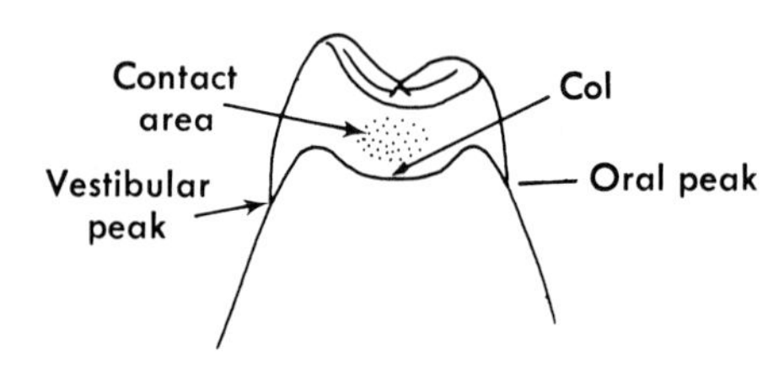


**Fig. 1-13.** Diagrammatic representation of the interdental papilla showing the col and peaks.

***Free gingiva***

The free or marginal gingiva is the unattached sleevelike coronal portion of the gingiva that encircles the tooth to form the gingival sulcus.

***Gingival sulcus***

The gingival sulcus is the space between the unattached, free gingiva and the tooth. Its depth in health is minimal, arbitrarily set at 3 mm. or less.

***Free gingival groove***

The bottom of the gingival sulcus is often marked on the outer surface of the gingiva by a fine groove running parallel to the gingival margin—the free gingival groove (*FGG* in Fig. 1-2). This groove is also the line of demarcation between the free gingiva and the firmly anchored attached gingiva.

***Papillary gingiva***

The gingival tissue that extends interdentally is formed into gingival papillae, which are of special clinical importance and pathologic significance since they are an early and accurate indicator of periodontal disease.[10] In the anterior portion of the mouth, the papillae form a single pyramidal structure. The papillae of the posterior teeth are wedge shaped, with the form of a sagging pup tent. The walls of the "tent" contact the proximal tooth surfaces, and the crest fits snugly under the contact areas of adjoining teeth (Fig. 1-13).

***Col***

This sagging pup tent shape, with the slope rising to two peaks, is referred to as a col.[8,9] Thus the interdental papillae of the posterior teeth may appear triangular in shape when viewed from the lateral aspect but concave when viewed from the proximal aspect. As the gingiva recedes with aging, the oral and vestibular peaks may fall and the interdental papillae may then slope in a coronal direction to form a single arclike crest. In cases of diastema, however, the interdental tissue does not form a crest but rather a blunt ridge or sometimes a concave

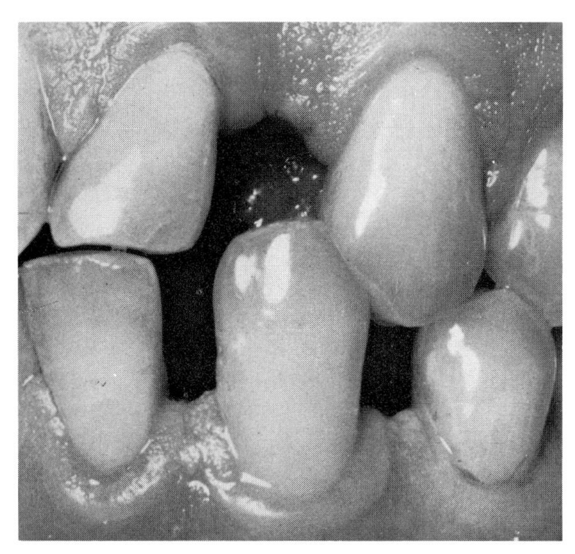

**Fig. 1-14.** Saddlelike appearance of the interdental tissue in a diastema. Free gingiva surrounds the tooth like a collar.

surface[5] (Fig. 1-14). Then the free gingiva of adjacent teeth forms only the mesial and distal margins of the interdental space.

***Alveolar mucosa***

The alveolar mucosa differs from the attached gingiva in structure, function, and color. The attached gingiva is firmly adherent to the underlying bone and is immovable, whereas the alveolar mucosa is loosely connected and movable.

***Color***

Pigmentation of the gingiva occurs frequently in Negroes,[12] Orientals, and Indians and is also seen in whites of Mediterranean ancestry. It may be general or localized and regularly or irregularly distributed. It may vary from faint to intense, but it is normal and should not be confused with the changes that accompany periodontal disease.

This pigmentation ranges from light brown to black. The exact hue is a matter of individual variation. Since the epithelium is translucent, the color depends on the vascularity and thickness of the subjacent connective tissue, which may be altered by the degree of keratinization of the epithelium.

There is no change in coloration between the attached and the free gingivae. The lining mucosa of the cheek and lips, the vestibular fornix, and the alveolar mucosa are different in coloration. This is because the epithelium is thin and nonkeratinized at these sites so that the underlying tissue gives them a reddish or faintly bluish hue.

***Contour and demarcation***

In addition to variations in color, there are variations in papillary and marginal contour, texture, and consistency of normal gingival tissues, as is apparant from Figs. 1-3 to 1-11 and 1-14. Further, there are differences in the width and demarcation of the zone of attached gingiva. The position and prominence of the frenum and muscle attachments are also subject to individual variation.

Variations in gingival contour, thickness, and height are dependent on the following positional factors: presence of diastemas (Figs. 1-8 and 1-14), degree of eruption (Figs. 1-3, 1-5, and 1-14), missing teeth, and positioning of the teeth in the arch. In such instances rotation, overlapping, and labial or lingual (vestibular or oral) placement of teeth (Figs. 1-7 and 1-11) will influence the relation between the dentoenamel junction and the gingival margin. Viewed from the vestibular aspect, teeth that are more prominent (in vestibular version) tend to have a lower gingival margin. Conversely, if the tooth is in oral version, the gingival margin tends to be high and the gingiva is usually thick over such teeth. Similar relationships hold when teeth are viewed from the oral aspect (Fig. 1-11). The position of the tooth in the arch influences the thickness and form of the alveolar bone over the root. The thickness of the alveolar bone plays an important role in determining gingival form.

One must be able to look at a patient's gingiva and dentition and understand how these various factors influence normal gingival form. Further, and perhaps more important, one must also be able to detect the earliest changes produced by periodontal disease. Treatment is always more successful and accomplished with more ease when it is instituted early. In such instances treatment tends to be interceptive. In the later stages of disease, treatment must of necessity be curative. Interceptive and preventive treatment is preferred to curative treatment. There is an old tenet in medicine that the best treatment is the least treatment that will restore health.

## PAPILLAE AS EARLY INDICATORS OF DISEASE

To be able to detect the early changes in periodontal disease, one must recognize the following symptoms in the interdental papillae:

1. Redness
2. Tendency to bleed easily
3. Tenderness
4. Sponginess
5. Very slight swelling

All these symptoms are present in the patient shown in Plate 1, *A*. One papilla is red and bleeding (lower arrow). If these signs are ignored, the condition will deteriorate. Edema and inflammation will extend from the interdental papilla to the marginal gingiva.

In Plate 1, *B,* changes in color are evident in the papillae, and inflammatory enlargement is obliterating the stippling. The gingivitis involves the marginal gingiva as well as the papillae.

In Plate 1, *C,* a hyperplastic inflammatory change is evident. The papilla denoted by the arrows has extended laterally onto the tooth surface and has become blunted. The disease process has extended deeper into the interdental tissues and is now termed periodontitis.

Were the disease to continue, the interdental papillae might be destroyed and the vessels of the inflamed area would become more prominent because they dilate in the areas of inflammation (Plate 1, *D*).

In some instances in which the gingiva is heavy and well stippled, these changes tend to be concealed; yet in Plate 1, *E,* edema has caused a loss of stippling over the incisors despite the heaviness of the gingiva. In addition, frank pus is exuding from the pocket over the oral aspect of the canine.

Such cases are rather insidious since they are not as evident to the untrained eye as the disease seen in the patient in Plate 1, *F;* something is obviously wrong in this patient.

Any inflammatory change shows itself in the vascular supply of the gingiva. How and why are these inflammatory changes so evident clinically? First, the epithelium is translucent. Second, the gingiva has a rich and extensive blood supply. The capillaries form a plexus extending throughout the gingiva and

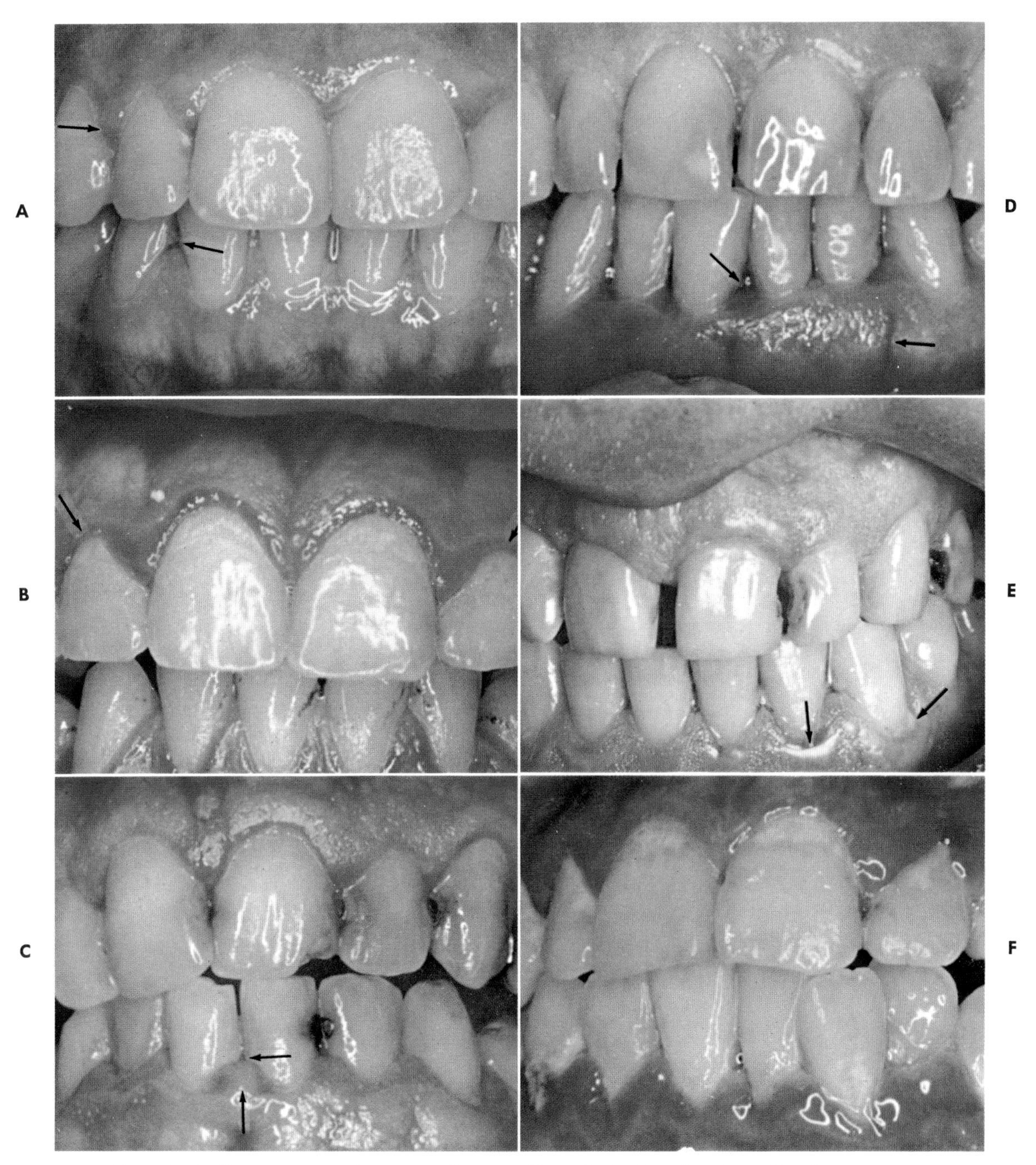


**Plate 1. A,** Upper arrow points to a slight swelling of the interdental papilla. Lower arrow points to bleeding papilla. **B,** Inflammation of papillary and marginal gingivae is noted by arrows. Papillae are hyperplastic and stippling is obliterated. **C,** Hyperplasia of papilla is noted by arrows. The papilla has become blunted. **D,** Continued inflammation has led to a loss of papillary tissue (arrows). The vessels have become enlarged and are obvious (injected) (arrow). **E,** In the presence of denser tissue, these inflammatory changes tend to be concealed. Stippling persists, although loss of stippling may be evident when pockets exist (left arrow) and exudation occurs (right arrow). **F,** Generalized inflammation showing change in color, loss of stippling, edema, and hyperplasia.

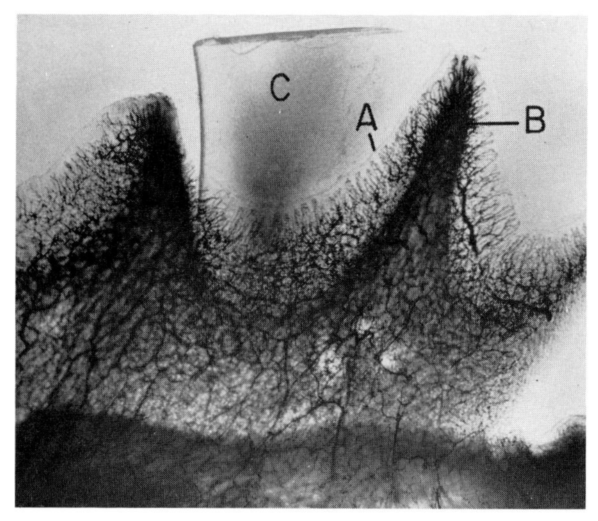


**Fig. 1-15.** Dog gingiva perfused with india ink showing distribution of blood vessels. *A,* Marginal gingiva; *B,* interdental papilla; *C,* tooth. Note that the tooth, a canine, is still evident in this preparation. (Courtesy D. A. Rolfs, University of Washington School of Dentistry, Seattle.)

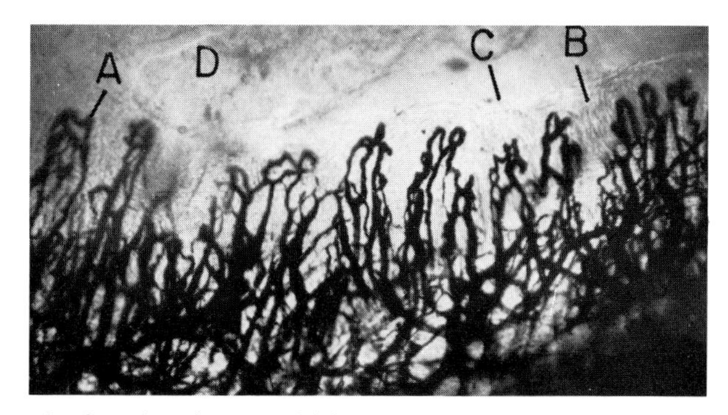


**Fig. 1-16.** Same animal as in Fig. 1-15, higher magnification. *A,* Capillary loops pass toward the epithelium; *B,* epithelium extends between connective tissue papillae; *C,* free margin of the gingiva; *D,* tooth surface. (Courtesy D. A. Rolfs, University of Washington School of Dentistry, Seattle.)

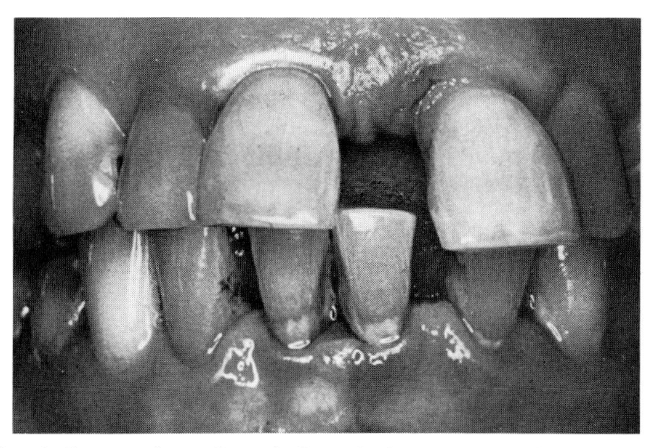

**Fig. 1-17.** Progressive inflammation of periodontal tissues. Deposits are evident on the tooth surface. The teeth have migrated, and diastemas are evident.

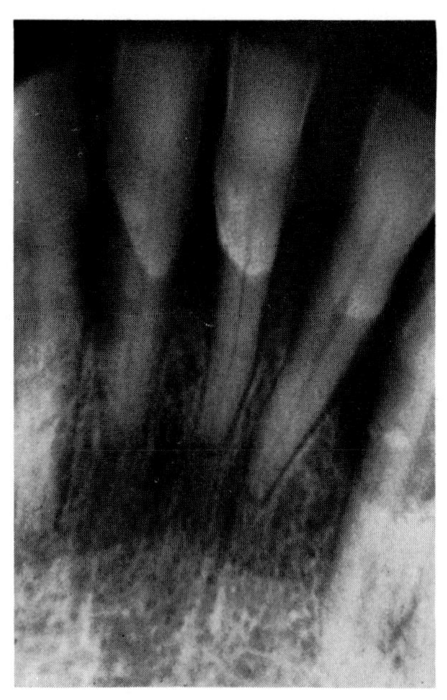

**Fig. 1-18.** Roentgenogram of the mandibular teeth shown in Fig. 1-17. Note the loss of bone and the deposits of calculus.

passing into the free gingiva (Figs. 1-15 and 1-16), where it forms capillary loops subjacent to the epithelium.[13] In inflammatory conditions the permeability of these vessels is increased and a perivascular exudate follows.

With time these changes are reflected by progression of the inflammation into the underlying tissues of the periodontium. This is accompanied by loss of bone, which becomes evident in roentgenograms. In the final stages the tooth may be lost (Figs. 1-17 and 1-18).

**CHAPTER 1**

**References**

1. Allen, E. F.: Statistical study of the primary causes of extraction, J. Dent. Res. **23**:453, 1944.
2. Brekhus, P. J.: Dental disease and its relation to the loss of human teeth, J. Amer. Dent. Ass. **16**:2237, 1929.
3. Research explores pyorrhea and other gum diseases—periodontal disease, Public Health Service Publication no. 1482, Health Information Series no. 133, Washington, D. C., 1966, U. S. Government Printing Office.
4. Orban, R., and Sicher, H.: The oral mucosa, J. Dent. Educ. **10**:94, 1946.
5. Orban, B.: Clinical and histologic study of the surface characteristics of the gingiva, Oral Surg. **1**:827, 1948.
6. Wentz, F. M., Maier, A. W., and Orban, B.: Age changes and sex differences in the clinically "normal" gingiva, J. Periodont. **23**:13, 1952.
7. Rosenberg, H. M., and Massler, M.: Gingival stippling in young adult males, J. Periodont. **38**:473, 1967.
8. Cohen, B.: Comparative studies in periodontal disease, Proc. Roy. Soc. Med. **53**:275, 1960.
9. Kohl, J. T., and Zander, H. A.: Morphology of interdental gingival tissues, Oral Surg. **14**:287, 1961.
10. Massler, M., Schour, I., and Chopra, B.: Occurrence of gingivitis in suburban Chicago school children, J. Periodont. **21**:146, 1950.
11. Baer, P. N.: The relation of the physical character of the diet to the periodontium and periodontal disease, Oral Med. **9**:839, 1956.
12. Dummett, C. O., and Barens, G.: Oromucosal pigmentation; updated review, J. Periodont. **42**:726, 1971.

13. Egelberg, J.: The blood vessels of the dento-gingival junction, J. Periodont. Res. **1**:163, 1966.
14. Cattoni, M.: Correlation of oral histology and periodontics, J. Dent. Educ. **30**:22, 1966.

#### Additional suggested readings

Bowers, G. M.: A study of the width of attached gingiva, J. Periodont. **34**:201, 1963.

Holm, O., Krakau, C. E., Lindhe, J., and others: A photogrammetric method for the assessment of the volume changes of the gingival margin, Odont. Rev. **18**:7, 1967.

Stoner, J. E., and Prophet, A. S.: Early periodontal disease in children and young adults, Dent. Pract. **20**:173, 1970.

Wilcox, C. E., and Everett, F. G.: Friction on the teeth and the gingiva during mastication, J. Amer. Dent. Ass. **66**:513, 1963.

CHAPTER TWO

# Periodontium—gingiva, dentogingival junction



*Periodontium*[1] is a term that refers to the functional unit of tissues supporting the tooth. The tooth and periodontium together are called the dentoperiodontal unit. The tissues of the periodontium include the gingiva, the dentogingival junction, the periodontal ligament, the cementum, and the alveolar process. They are biologically interdependent. The harmonious relationship between the different parts of the periodontium is maintained under normal conditions despite the constant changes that take place in periodontal tissues throughout life.

These changes may be seen on gross anatomic, microscopic, ultramicroscopic, and biochemical levels. It must be understood that tissue changes are mediated by cellular activity. Cellular and tissue morphology and physiology change constantly as the cells adapt to and function under normal conditions. Pathologic changes in cellular and tissue metabolism and in cellular environment also alter the morphology and function of the cells. These changes may appear as the clinical and microscopic signs of periodontal disease.

## GINGIVA

The gross morphology of the gingiva has been described in Chapter 1. The gingiva is made up of the attached, the free or marginal, and the papillary gingivae. It joins the alveolar mucosa at the mucogingival junction.

### Histology

Histologically a clear-cut boundary between the attached gingiva and the alveolar mucosa cannot always be found. There is a gradual change that takes place in the epithelial ridges; they become progressively shorter from gingiva to alveolar mucosa (Fig. 2-1).

*Mucogingival junction*

Transitional characteristics are visible at the mucogingival junction. The elastic tissue fibers are more numerous and thicker in the alveolar mucosa. They gradually decrease in size and quantity at the mucogingival junction. Elastic fibers are rarely demonstrated in the attached gingiva.

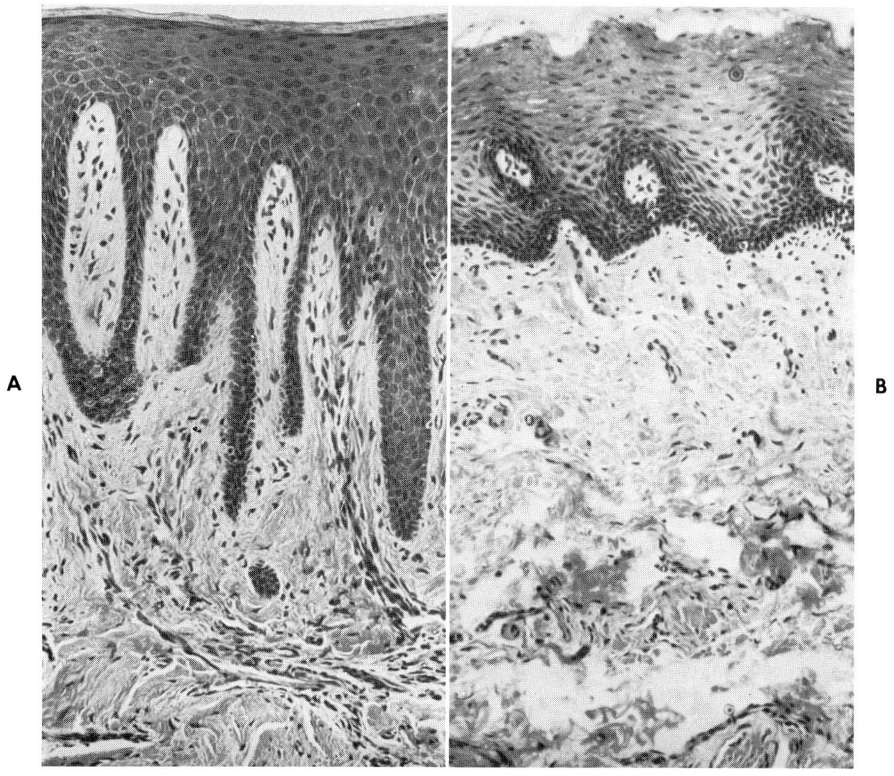


**Fig. 2-1.** Differences between gingiva, **A**, and alveolar mucosa, **B**. The surface of the gingival epithelium is keratinized, whereas that of the alveolar mucosa is not. Epithelial ridges and connective tissue papillae of the gingiva are long as compared with those of the alveolar mucosa. (Courtesy G. P. Ivancie, Denver.)

***Free gingival groove***

The free gingival groove delimits the attached gingiva coronally. Histologically this groove sometimes corresponds to a heavy epithelial ridge (Fig. 2-2). The free gingival groove and the epithelial ridge are caused, it is thought, by functional impacts on the free gingiva. These impacts fold the movable, free part back on the attached and immovable zone.[2]

***Stippling***

The surface of the attached gingiva is characterized by the presence of stippling.[2,3] The stipple is the epithelial depression (Fig. 2-3) and is believed to be the result of bundles of collagen fibers that enter the connective tissue papillae. The degree of stippling and density of the connective tissue varies in different individuals, although in girls the connective tissue is more finely textured. With increasing age there is a tendency for the collagen bundles and the stippling to become more coarse. This is true of both sexes, although with the menopause the gingiva of some women may again become finely textured.

***Connective tissue***

The lamina propria of the gingiva consists of dense connective tissue poor in elastic fibers. Collagen fibers arranged in prominent bundles arise from the cervical area of the cementum (free gingival group of periodontal ligament fibers) and also from the periosteal surface of the alveolar process (Fig. 2-4). They interlace with fiber bundles coursing in various directions.

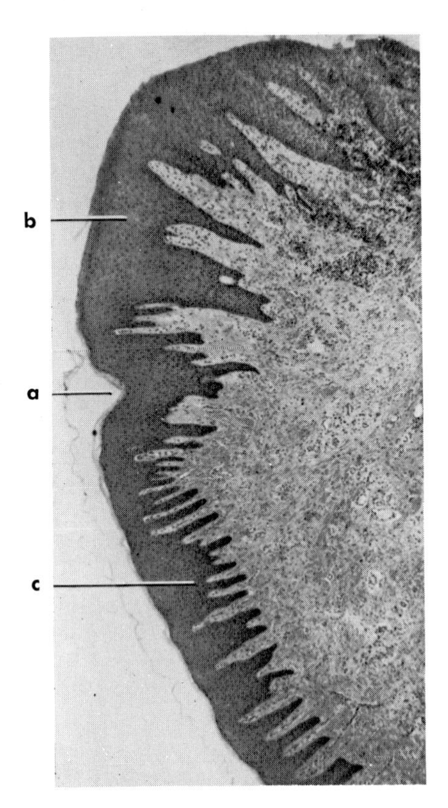


**Fig. 2-2.** Biopsy specimen of gingiva showing free gingival groove, *a*, and corresponding heavy epithelial ridge. *b*, Free gingiva; *c*, attached gingiva.

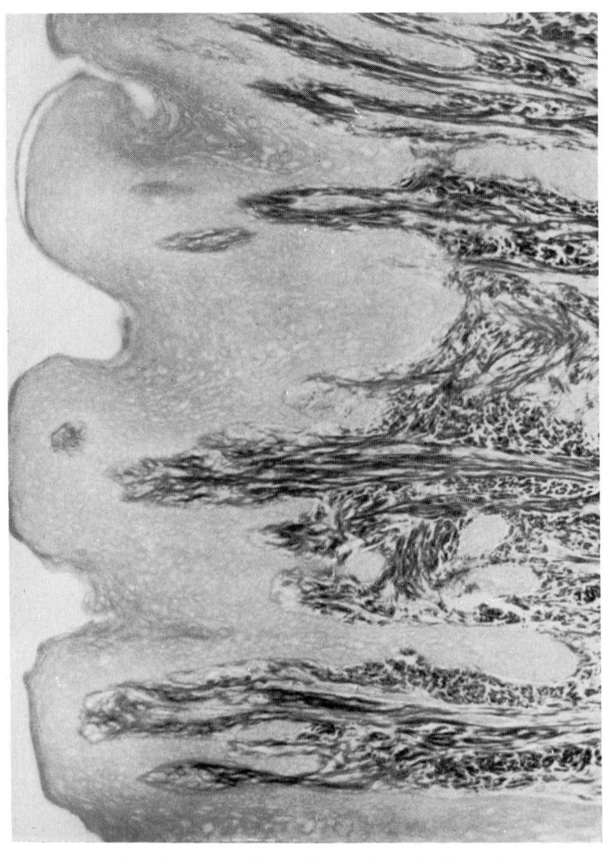

**Fig. 2-3.** Gingival specimen showing stippling. Note the relation of the connective tissue fiber bundles to the stippled surface. (Mallory stain.)

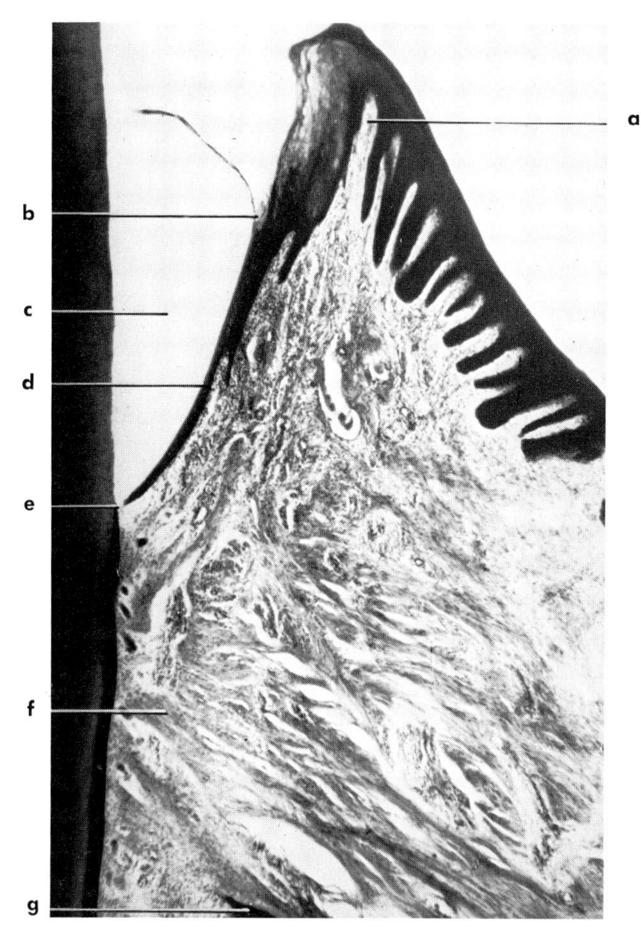


**Fig. 2-4.** Dentogingival junction. Epithelium of the gingival sulcus continues into the attachment (junctional) epithelium, which forms the epithelial attachment. The connective tissue attachment of the cementum and alveolar crest is the bond that holds the gingiva to the tooth. *a,* Free gingiva; *b,* bottom of the gingival sulcus; *c,* enamel space; *d,* attachment epithelium; *e,* cementoenamel junction; *f,* connective tissue attachment of the gingiva; *g,* alveolar crest.

## Functional fiber orientation

In addition to the preceding histologic features of the gingiva, there are structural and functional characteristics.

***Fibers***

The gingival fibers are arranged functionally in the following groups[4] (Fig. 2-5):

1. *Dentogingival group.* The fibers of this group extend from the cementum apical to the epithelial attachment and course laterally and coronally into the lamina propria of the gingiva (Fig. 2-5, *A* and *B*).
2. *Alveologingival group.* The fibers of this small group arise from the alveolar crest and insert coronally into the lamina propria (Figs. 2-5, *C,* and 2-8).
3. *Circular group.* This small group of fibers encircles the teeth[5] (Fig. 2-5, D).
4. *Accessory groups.* A group of prominent horizontal fibers that extend interproximally between adjacent teeth is called *transseptal* fibers (Fig. 2-5,

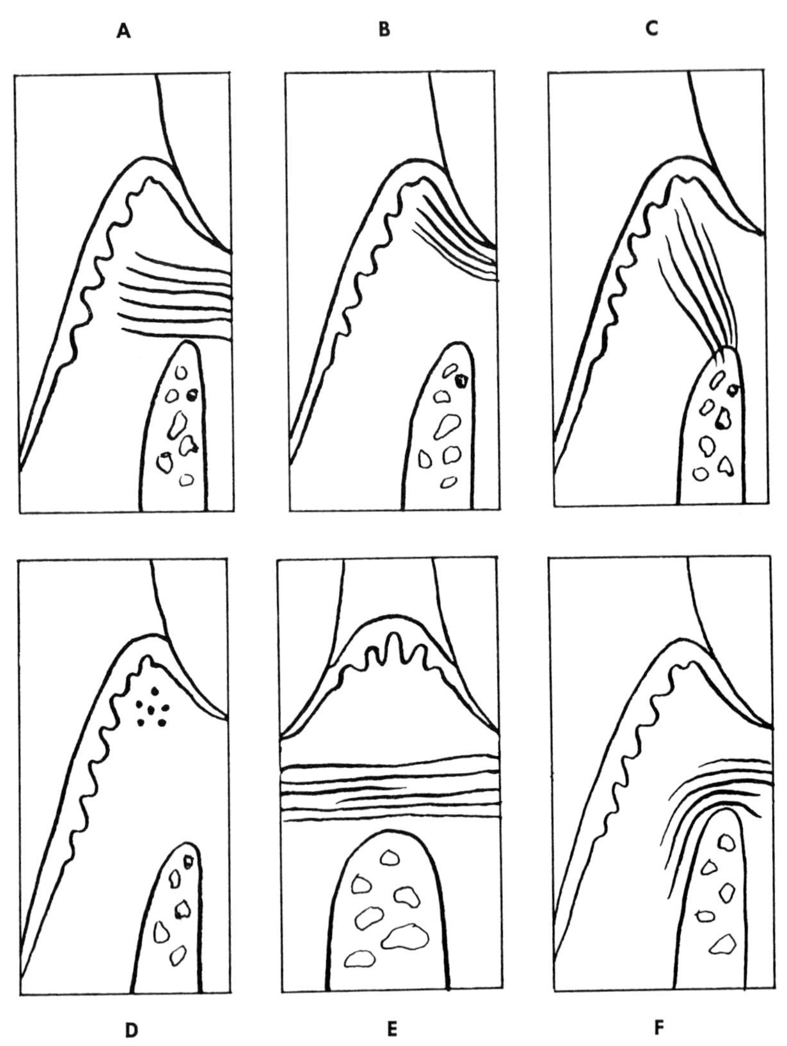


**Fig. 2-5.** Diagram of the connective tissue fiber groups in the region of the dentogingival junction. **A** and **B,** Dentogingival fibers. **C,** Alveologingival fibers. **D,** Circular fibers. **E,** Transseptal fibers. **F,** Dentoperiosteal fibers. (Modified from Erausquin, J.: Histologia dentaria humana, Buenos Aires, 1953, Progrental.)

*E*). On the oral and vestibular surfaces of the jaws, a fiber group, called *dentoperiosteal* fibers,[6] extends from the periosteum of the alveolar bone to the tooth (Fig. 2-5, *F*).

***Gingival and interdental ligaments***

The dentogingival, alveologingival, and circular fibers may be called the gingival ligament, whereas the transseptal fibers comprise the interdental ligament. The fibers that extend from the alveolar bone to the tooth form the alveolodental (periodontal) ligament,[7] which will be discussed in Chapter 3. The bundles of fibers take their names from the differences in their course, but in actuality the various fiber bundles form a continuum (i.e., they are contiguous and form a functional unit) (Figs. 2-6 and 2-7). All these fibers are interspersed with other fibers that are smaller and finer, the subepithelial and the interfibrillar reticulin fibers of the gingiva.[8]

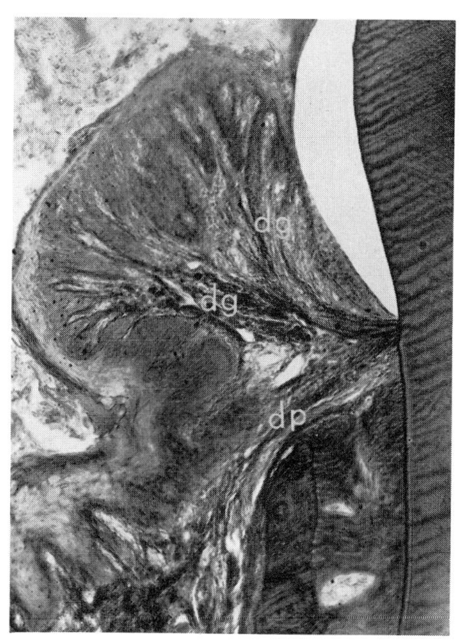


**Fig. 2-6.** Section through marmoset gingiva showing the dentogingival, *dg,* and dentoperiosteal, *dp,* fibers. (Courtesy S. Bernick, University of Southern California School of Medicine, Los Angeles.)

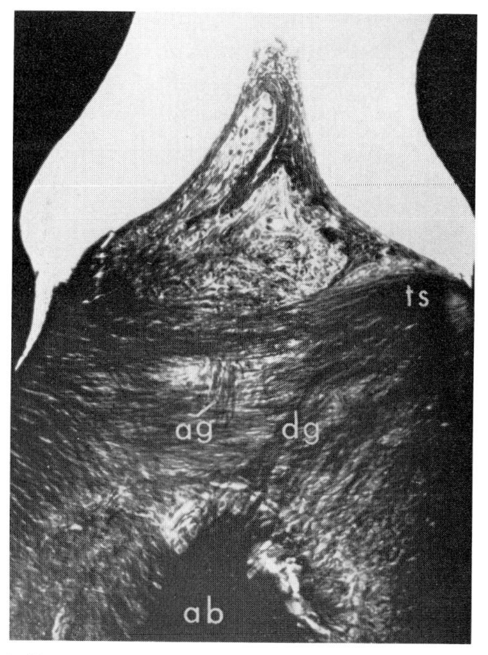


**Fig. 2-7.** Alveologingival fibers, *ag,* in rat gingiva. Alveolar bone, *ab,* and dentogingival, *dg,* and transseptal, *ts,* fibers are also evident. (Courtesy F. Morgan, University of Washington School of Dentistry, Seattle.)

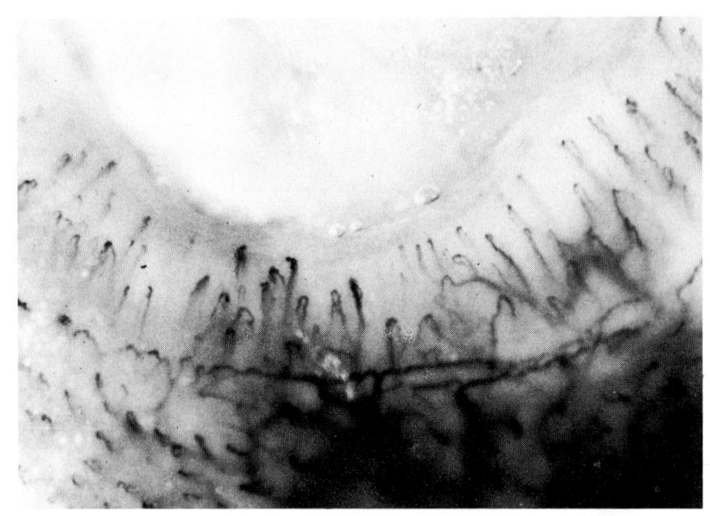

**Fig. 2-8.** Capillary loops of the clinically healthy human gingival margin. (Vital capillary microscopic picture; ×40.) (From Franke, J.: Fortschr. Kiefer- Gesichtschir. **9**:225, 1964.)

***Blood supply***

Numerous connective tissue papillae interdigitate with the epithelium. Capillaries of the gingiva may be observed in the papillary layer,[9] where they form terminal loops (Fig. 2-8). These capillaries arise from the interdental alveolar arteries that traverse intra-alveolar canals (nutrient canals)[10] and perforate the alveolar crest in the interdental spaces. They enter the gingiva, supplying the interdental papillae and the adjacent areas of the vestibular and oral gingivae (Figs. 1-15, 1-16, and 2-4, *A*). Another vascular supply of the gingiva comes from the periosteal vessels arising from the lingual, buccinator, mental, and palatine arteries. The terminal vessels of both sources anastomose. Veins and lymph vessels course in association with the arteries. Vascular distribution is important in the pathogenesis of inflammatory periodontal disease.

***Sensory nerve structures***

The following sensory nerve structures have been described[11]: nonmedullated fibers, which extend from the connective tissue into the epithelium, and, less frequently, specialized nerve endings[12] in the papillary layer of the lamina propria, including Meissner corpuscles and Krause corpuscles.[13]

There is no clearly demarcated submucosa in the gingiva. Periosteum, submucosa, and lamina propria seem to blend into one firm layer of connective tissue.

In the connective tissue adjacent to the base of the gingival sulcus, some infiltration of chronic inflammatory cells is always found. The presence of plasma cells, lymphocytes, and histiocytes usually is interpreted as a part of a defense mechanism against the products of bacterial activity even in the clinically normal sulcus (Fig. 2-4).

***Alveolar mucosa***

The lamina propria of the gingiva is thick and consists of dense connective tissue, whereas the submucosa of the alveolar mucous membrane is a loosely textured connective tissue. It contains glands that are lacking in the gingiva. The elastic fibers are more numerous in the alveolar mucosa and gradually decrease in size and quantity until they disappear in the attached gingiva. The epithelium of the attached gingiva is usually keratinized (cornified) or parakeratinized; epithelial ridges are prominent. The epithelium of the alveolar mucosa is not

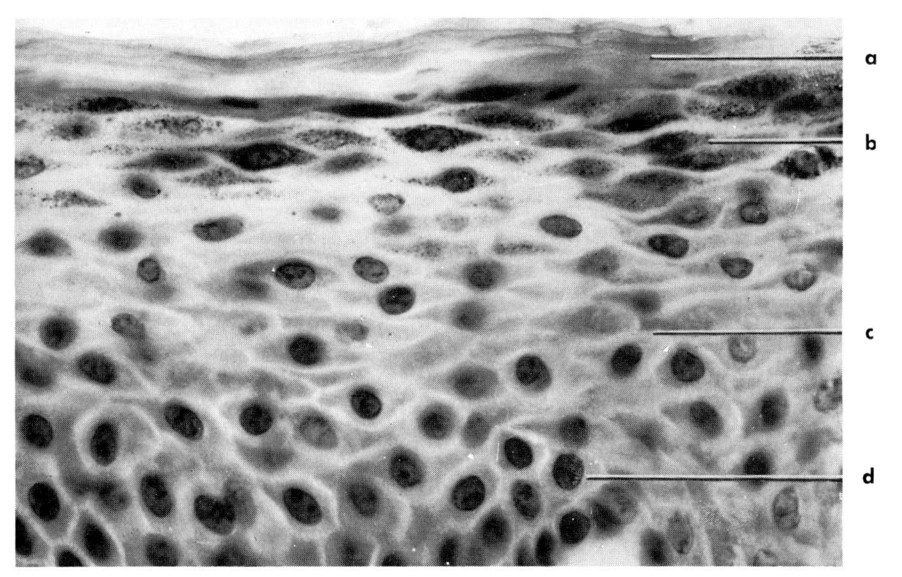


**Fig. 2-9.** Keratinization of the normal gingiva. Keratinized layer, *a,* lacks cellular structure. *b,* Well-developed granular layer; *c,* prickle cell layer; *d,* basal cell layer.

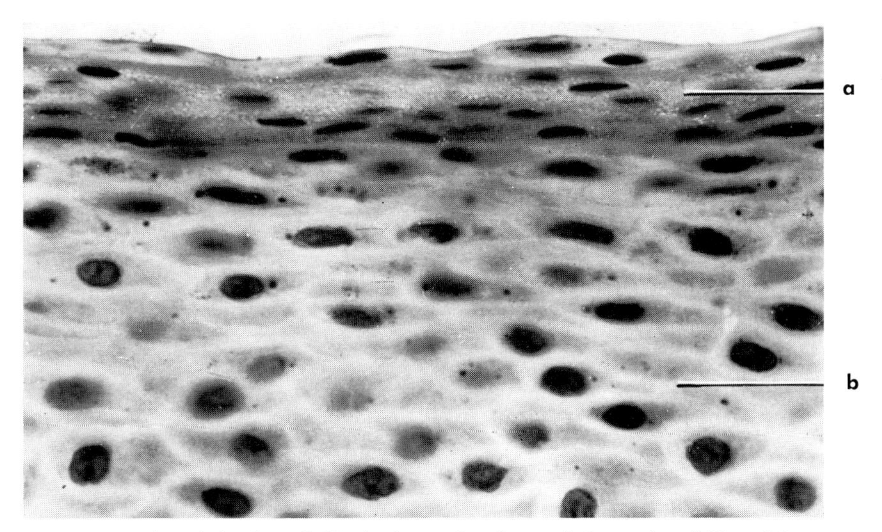


**Fig. 2-10.** Parakeratinization of the gingiva. *a,* Parakeratotic layer; *b,* prickle cell layer.

keratinized, and the epithelial ridges and connective tissue papillae are insignificant or absent (Fig. 2-1).

## Epithelium

The attached gingiva and the outer surface of the free gingiva may be covered by a keratinized,[14,15] stratified squamous epithelium. This epithelium consists of a stratum basale, a stratum spinosum, a stratum granulosum, and a stratum corneum. These terms are synonymous with the basal layer, the prickle cell layer, the granular layer, and the cornified layer (Fig. 2-9).

Mitosis occurs in the stratum basale and possibly in the lower portion of the spinous layer. This region constitutes the stratum germinativum.

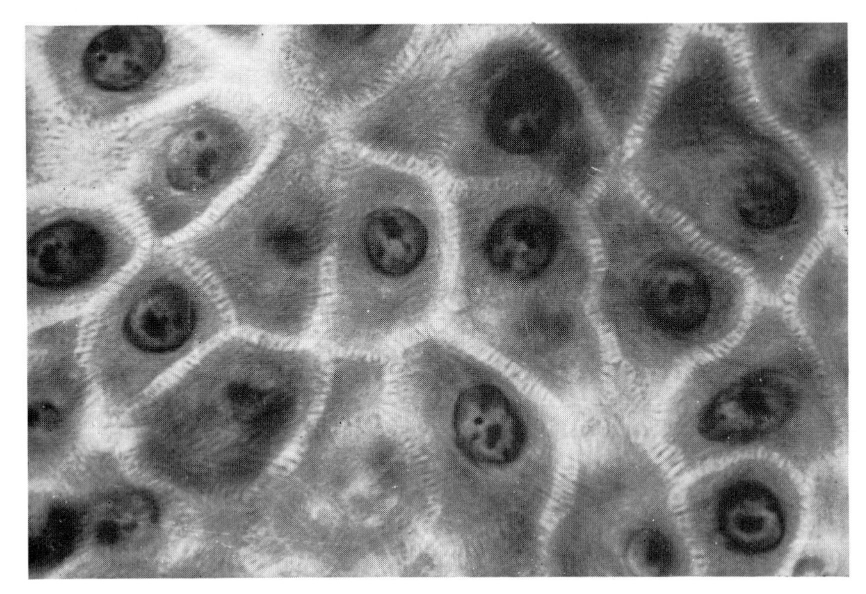

**Fig. 2-11.** High magnification of the prickle cell layer of human gingival epithelium showing intercellular bridges and tonofibrils.

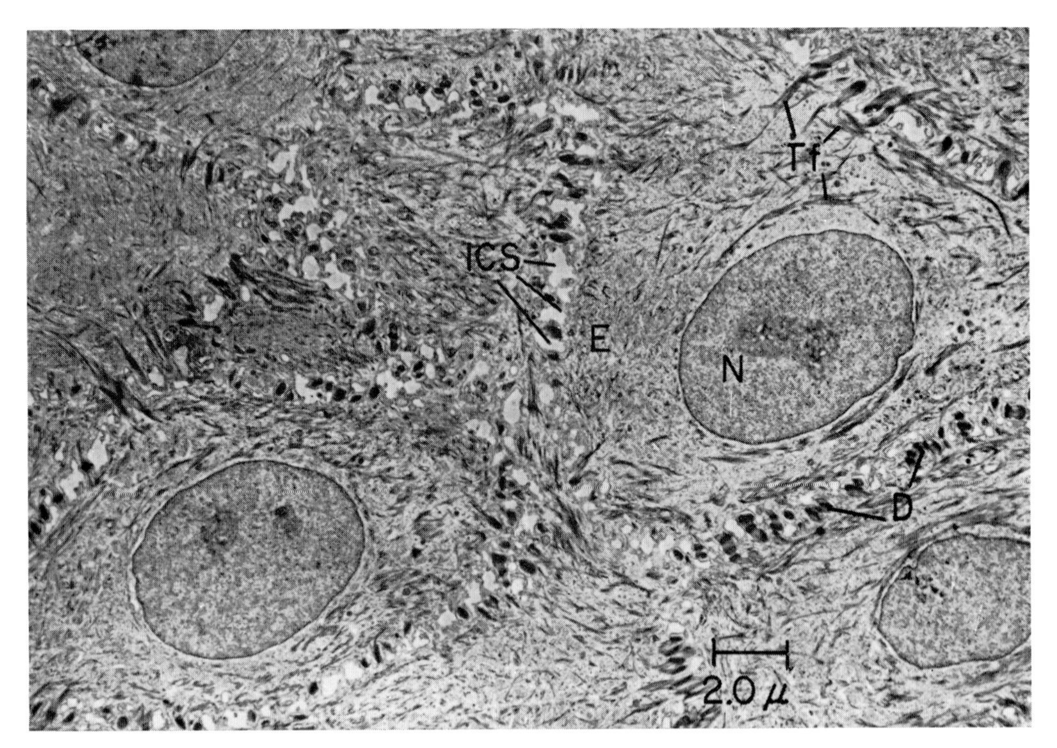


**Fig. 2-12.** Electron micrograph of prickle cells of human gingiva. Portions of epithelial cells, *E,* are evident separated by intercellular space, *ICS.* Several nuclei, *N,* are evident. Tonofilaments, *Tf,* are present in the cytoplasm and extend toward desmosomes, *D,* located at the periphery of the cells. (×6000.)

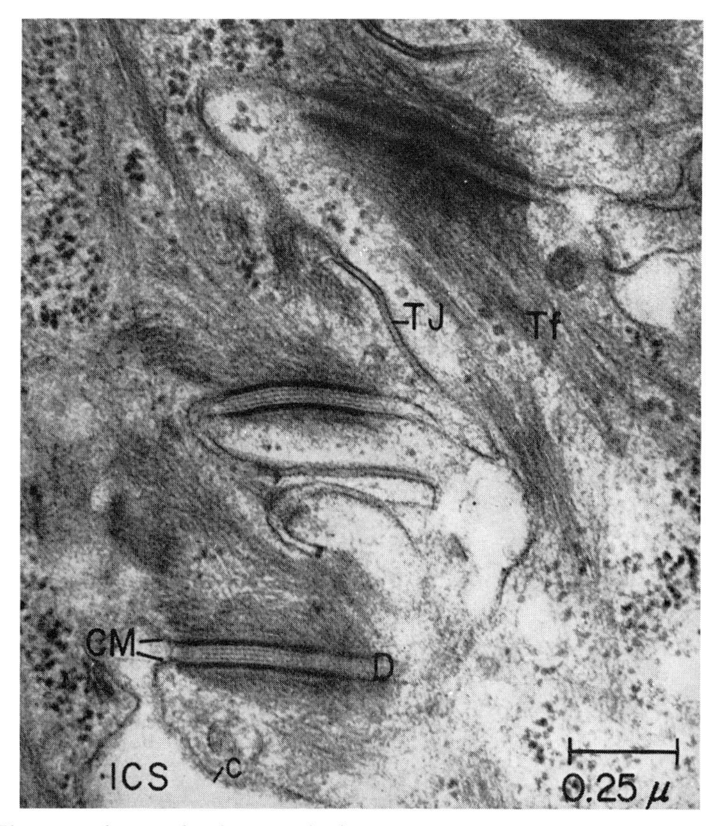


**Fig. 2-13.** Electron micrograph of a rat cheek. Section shows three desmosomes, *D*. Note the various light and dark layers of the desmosome. Some desmosomal components are continuous with the adjacent cell membrane, *CM*. Note also the intercellular space, *ICS*, and the coating, *c*, on the cell membrane there. Tonofilaments, *Tf*, are seen coursing toward the attachment plaques. Another type of cell junction, the tight junction, *TJ*, is also evident. (From Stern, I. B.: Periodontics **3**:224, 1967.)

The surface of the gingival epithelium may often be parakeratinized. Where parakeratinization exists, nucleated cells reach the surface and a stratum granulosum is generally absent (Fig. 2-10).

On the basis of light microscopy, it appears that the epithelial cells are joined by intercellular bridges (Fig. 2-11). Tonofibrils appear to course from cell to cell across the intercellular bridges. Electron microscopic studies have shown that the so-called intercellular bridges are desmosomes, which serve to attach adjacent cells to each other (Fig. 2-12). The desmosomes are composed of adjacent cell membranes and a pair of densities (attachment plaques) as well as intervening extracellular structures[16] (Figs. 2-13 and 2-14).

Under the electron microscope tonofibrils are seen to be composed of bundles of tonofilaments (Fig. 2-14). These bundles course through the cell toward the attachment plaques. They do not cross over into adjacent cells. The tonofilament network contained in several cells attached by desmosomes appears to make up a supporting system for the epithelium (cytoskeleton).

***Pedicles***

Viewed in the light microscope the basal surface of the basal cells is formed into fingerlike projections (pedicles) (Fig. 2-15) that appear to be attached to the basement membrane. The basement membrane is a PAS-positive zone containing reticular fibers[16] (Fig. 2-16).

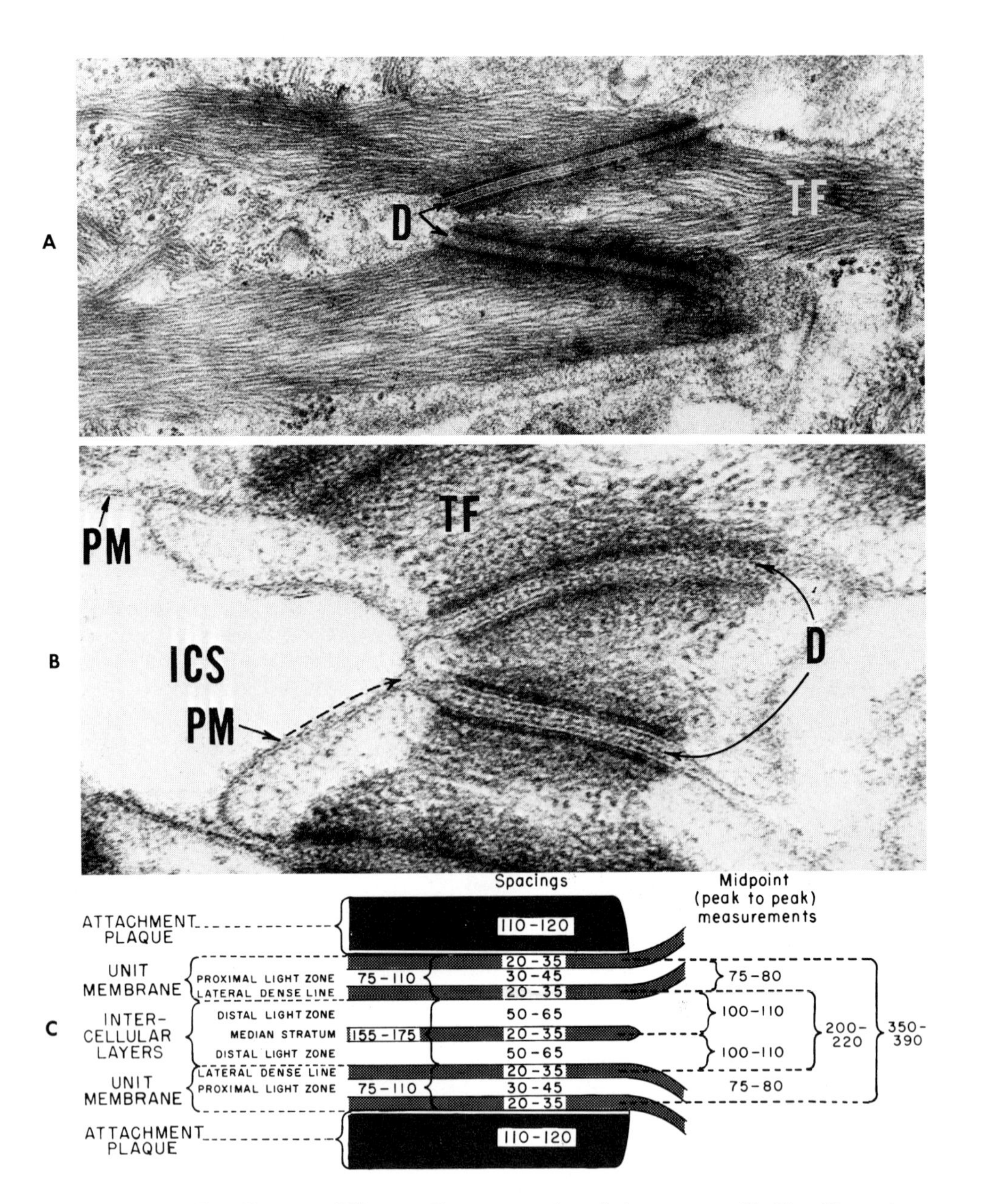


**Fig. 2-14. A,** Tonofilaments, *TF,* extending to a series of desmosomes, *D.* Tonofilaments are sectioned in the long axis (human gingiva). **B,** Higher magnification of two desmosomes, *D,* showing structure. Tonofilaments, *TF,* are cross-sectioned. Intercellular space, *ICS,* is bounded by adjacent cell membranes, *PM,* whose unit membrane is clearly evident (dashed arrow). Unit membranes form part of the structure of the desmosome. **C,** Diagrammatic cross-sectioned representation of a desmosome and dimensions of the various components.

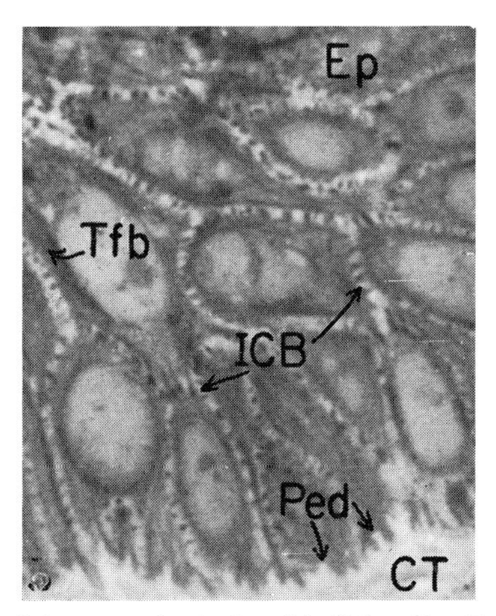


**Fig. 2-15.** Photomicrograph of human gingival epithelial cells, *Ep*. Pedicles, *Ped*, are present at the base of the basal cells and extend toward connective tissue, *CT*. Tonofibrils, *Tfb*, are evident both in the cells and apparently coursing across intercellular bridges, *ICB*. (×1400.) (From Stern, I. B.: Periodontics 3:224, 1967.)

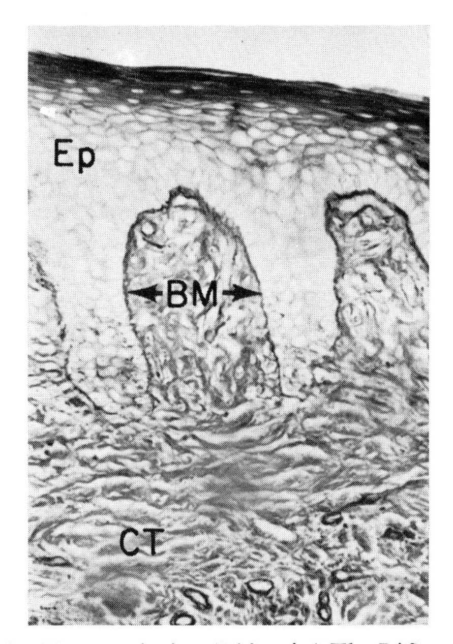


**Fig. 2-16.** Photomicrograph of human gingiva. (PAS stain.) The PAS-positive basement membrane appears as a dense line at the epithelial–connective tissue junction. Note that the blood vessels in the lamina propria also have a PAS-positive basement membrane. *Ep*, Epithelial cells; *CT*, connective tissue; *BM*, basement membrane. (×160.) (From Stern, I. B.: Periodontics 3:224, 1967.)

Remember that basement membranes seen in the optical and electron microscopes are different structures. The electron microscopic basement membrane (basal lamina) lies at the junction of epithelial cells and connective tissue. Its dimensions are such that it cannot be seen by light microscopy. Electron microscopic examination shows that the epithelial basal surface is also attached to the basal lamina by hemidesmosomes[16] (Fig. 2-17). The hemidesmosome consists of a single attachment plaque and associated extracellular structure (Fig. 2-18).

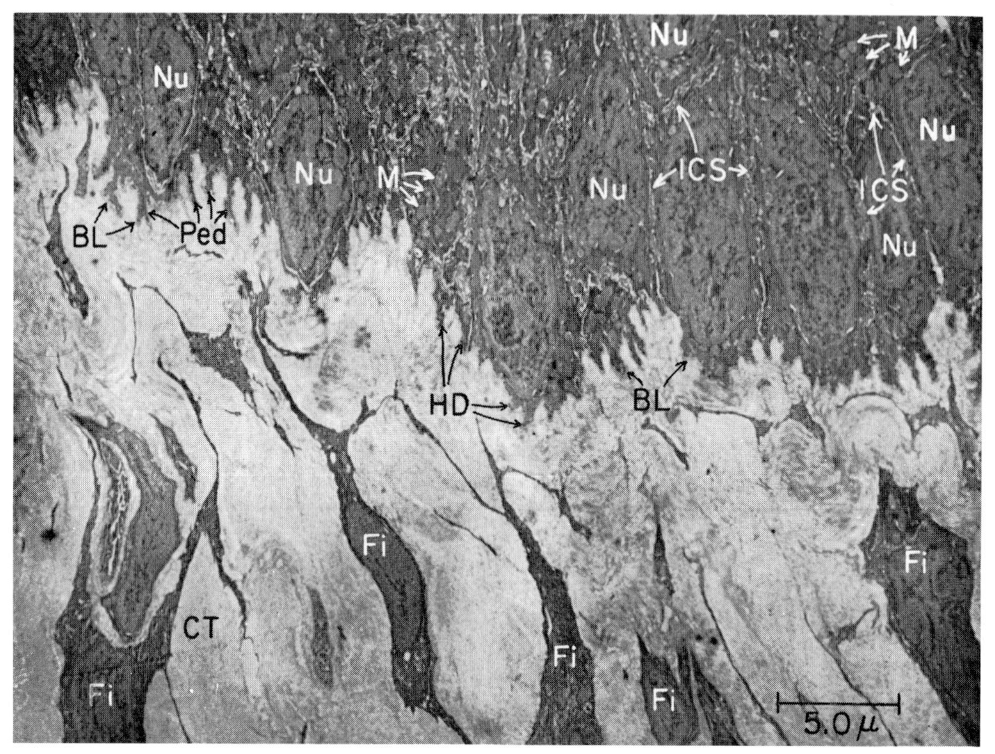


**Fig. 2-17.** Electron micrograph of rat gingiva. Several basal cells are apparent with pedicles, *Ped,* extending toward the connective tissue, *CT,* but separated from it by the basement lamina, *BL,* which is barely visible. Fibroblasts, *Fi,* may be noted within the connective tissue. Epithelial cells contain a prominent nucleus, *Nu,* and are demarcated from the adjacent cells by the lighter appearance of the intercellular spaces, *ICS.* Small, round, light areas in the epithelial cells are mitochondria, *M.* Pedicles, *Ped,* in this electron micrograph are of a much smaller dimension than the larger undulations of the basal cell surface outlined by arrows at *HD.* These, in turn, are smaller than the ridges shown in Fig. 2-15. (From Stern, I. B.: Periodontics 3:224, 1965.)

***Keratinization***

The gingival epithelium may also be incompletely parakeratinized or nonkeratinized.[14] Often the same mouth may contain two or more variants. However, when the stratum corneum is well developed, there is a prominent stratum granulosum (Fig. 2-9) because of the presence of keratohyalin granules.

***Keratohyalin granules***

As the cell approaches the stratum corneum, the tonofilaments tend to become more dense. They are often seen associated with keratohyalin granules of the stratum granulosum. Sometimes dense networks of filaments are evident. The keratohyalin granules disappear as the stratum corneum is formed. The cells of the cornified layer are composed of closely packed filaments developed from the tonofilaments presumably coated with the protein of the keratohyalin granule.[17] Such cells are termed squames.

***Squames***

Squames are continuously shed from the surface while new cells are formed in the stratum germinativum. During migration to the surface and progressive maturation, the cells gradually flatten. The flattened cornified cell covers a greater surface area than did the basal cell from which it developed (Fig. 2-19). Epithelial cells that ultimately keratinize are called keratinoctyes.

***Other cell types***

Some cell types, such as lymphocytes, plasma cells, and polymorphonuclear leukocytes (PMN), are common transients in the gingival epithelium. Others,

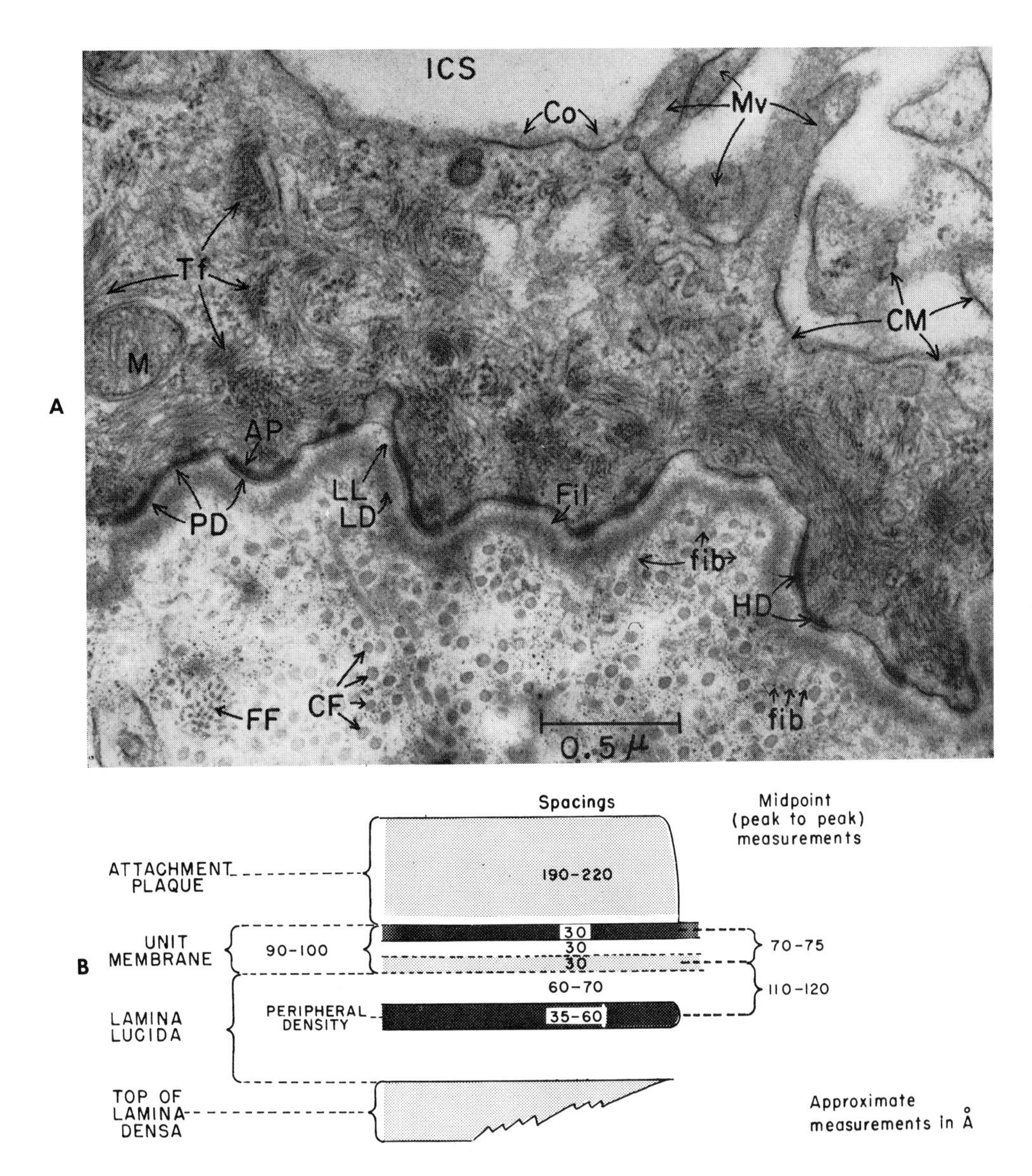


**Fig. 2-18. A,** Electron micrograph of human gingiva. This is a portion of a basal cell showing the basal plasma membrane and also the hemidesmosomes, *HD.* Lamina lucida, *LL,* and lamina densa, *D,* are components of the basement membrane. Collagen fibrils, *CF,* may be seen cut in cross section in the connective tissue. There are also fine fibrils, *FF,* present as a grouping. Other special or anchoring fibrils, *fib,* may be seen inserting into the connective tissue side of the lamina densa. The area of the intercellular space, *ICS,* is evident above the epithelial cell. Microvilli, *Mv,* and coating, *Co,* on the plasma membrane, *CM,* are present there. Fine unlabeled specks seen in the connective tissue are artifacts produced during staining. **B,** Approximate dimensions of a hemidesmosome. (**A** from Stern, I. B.: Periodontics 3:224, 1965.)

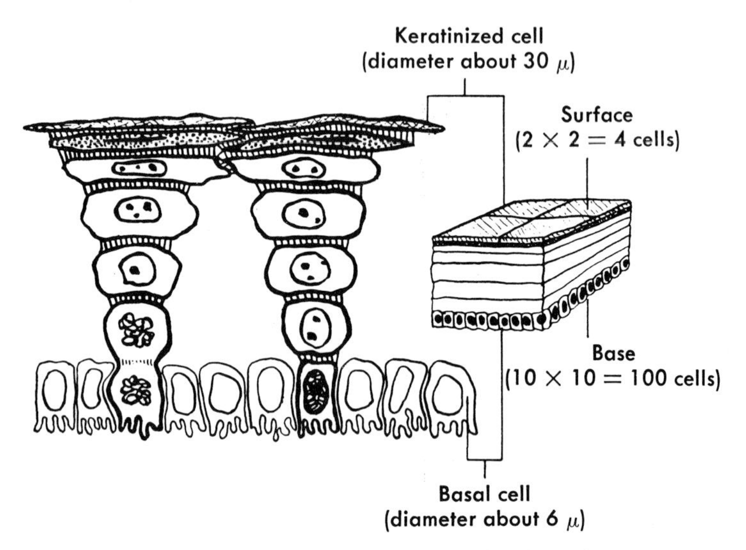


**Fig. 2-19.** Diagram of epithelial cell size in the stratum basale and stratum corneum. About four cornified cells may cover 100 basal cells in area. Since one cell should desquamate for each cell formed, there are no fewer cells in the stratum corneum. They have simply become flattened and compacted one cell above the other. (From Mehregan, A. H., and Pincus, H.: Cancer **17**:609, 1964.)

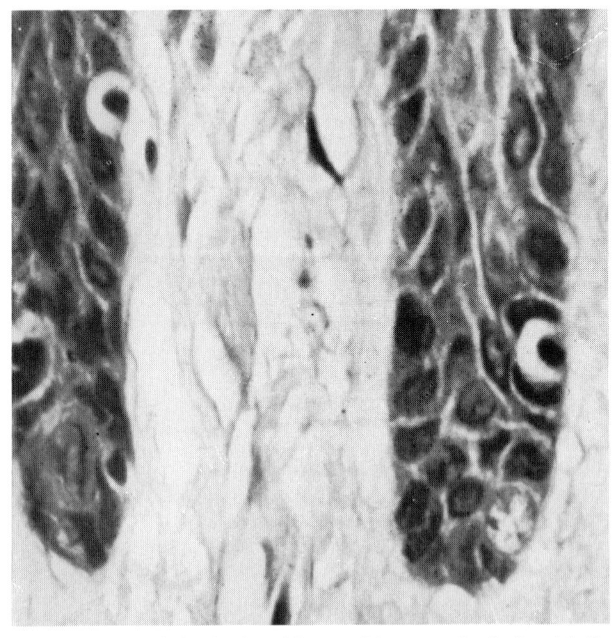

**Fig. 2-20.** Clear cells in the basal layer of human gingival epithelium.

such as the dendritic cells (also known as clear cells,[18] Langerhans cells, and melanocytes) (Fig. 2-20), appear to be permanent residents. Langerhans cells stain with gold chloride and are of unknown function. The melanocytes stain with a special method (dopa reaction). They form the melanin granules (melanosomes) and transfer these into the basal cells, which then become pigmented. The epidermal tissues of all persons contain similar numbers of melanocytes, which are apparently not equally functional. When functional melanocytes occur in the gingiva, the gingiva is pigmented regardless of race.[19] Only the epithelial cells possess desmosomes. The other cell types mentioned in this paragraph do not.

*Gingival sulcus*

The gingival sulcus is the space between the free gingiva and the tooth. It is formed by the invagination of the gingival epithelium and extends from the free margin of the gingiva down to the point where the epithelium adjoins the tooth surface (Fig. 2-4).

*Sulcular epithelium*

The sulcular epithelium differs from the outer gingival epithelium. It is not keratinized, lacks epithelial ridges, and is thinner.[20,21] These differences may be of clinical significance. The sulcular epithelium is assumed to be more vulnerable to irritation. Bacterial toxins may be able to pass through it into the subjacent connective tissue. Conversely, fluids may be able to pass from the connective tissue through the sulcular epithelium into the sulcus.[22-25]

## DENTOGINGIVAL JUNCTION

*Attachment (junctional) epithelium*

The sulcular epithelium is continuous with the epithelium that abuts on the tooth surface. The basal cells of these two epithelia lie side by side on a basement membrane common to both epithelia (Fig. 2-4).

The epithelium that abuts on the tooth surface is the attachment (or junctional) epithelium. Like the sulcular epithelium, it is thin and unkeratinized and lacks epithelial ridges. Capillaries course close to the attachment epithelium and may form connective tissue invaginations, which bring the blood supply into more intimate contact with the epithelium.[26]

Ordinarily the skin forms a continuum broken only by the hair, nails, glandular orifices, and body openings. Except for the body openings, the integrity of the skin is maintained and constitutes a defensive barrier. The oral mucosa is much the same. Here only glandular orifices and the teeth pass through the epithelium. The cells of the gland ducts lie alongside the cells of the oral epithelium and are joined to them. The teeth differ from hair and nails in that they are mineralized. Accordingly we might anticipate that the cells of the junctional epithelium would have a special mode of attachment to the teeth. Actually the dentogingival attachment is a functional unit consisting of (1) the fibrous attachment of the lamina propria to the cementum and (2) the attachment epithelium. Each has a different function.

The connective tissue is able to withstand mechanical stresses. The dentogingival fibers (Fig. 2-5, *A* and *B*) extend from the cementum and fan out into the gingiva. This attachment is reinforced by the other fibers of the gingiva (Fig. 2-5, *C* to *F*), which provide firmness and strength. The connective tissue also contains the circulatory supply.

*Epithelial attachment*

The attachment epithelium, in a broad sense, provides a seal at the base of the sulcus against the penetration of chemical and bacterial substances. It was first called the epithelial attachment by Gottlieb.[27] For reasons that will become obvious, the term epithelial attachment or junctional epithelial attachment is preferred for the precise zone of junction between the attachment epithelium and the tooth surface. Then *epithelial attachment* can also be used to discuss the mode and mechanism of attachment.

According to Gottlieb the ameloblasts form a fibrillar (keratinous) product on their tooth-contacting surfaces that connects the gingival epithelium to the tooth.[27] Gottlieb and others thought of the epithelial attachment as a persistence of the primary union between the ameloblasts and the developing enamel rods. This union was believed to persist after formation and maturation of the enamel and after regression of the ameloblasts into a reduced enamel epithelium. Later an opinion was expressed that tonofibrils of the enamel epithelium provided the structural basis for this kind of attachment.[28]

***Epithelial cuff***

Waerhaug, on the other hand, denied that there was an epithelial attachment.[29] He indicated that if the gingiva were peeled back from the tooth surface and then replaced it would immediately adhere again. In essence, he first viewed the zone of the epithelial attachment as an actual space and in later writings as a potential space. The epithelial cells were believed to be held to the tooth surface by the forces of adhesion. Consequently, he referred to the attachment epithelium as the epithelial cuff.

***Ultrastructure of the epithelial attachment***

The ultrastructural nature of the epithelial attachment to the tooth surface has been demonstrated by Stern[30-32] in rodents and by Listgarten[33,34] and Schroeder[35] in humans. Both reduced ameloblasts and gingival epithelial cells have been shown to form an electron microscopic basement membrane on enamel and cementum. Hemidesmosomes of these cells attach to the basal lamina in the same manner as does any basal cell. Thus there is an epithelial attachment. It is submicroscopic, approximately 400 Å wide, and formed by the attachment epithelium. Its exact biochemical nature is unknown, but some of its constituents have been grossly identified.[36,37] Apparently these constituents are produced by the epithelium.[38] The adhesive forces in this zone are molecular in nature and act across a distance smaller than 400 Å.[39]

***Changing position of the dentogingival junction***

To more fully understand the attachment of the gingiva to the tooth, we must appreciate the changing positional relationship of the gingiva to the tooth. The surface of the enamel, after its formation and calcification are completed, is covered by the reduced enamel epithelium. This epithelium is in organic union with the enamel surface (Fig. 4-20, *A*). During eruption of the tooth, the reduced enamel epithelium comes in contact with the epithelium of the oral mucous membrane, and the two epithelial tissues join (*B*). When the tip of the enamel emerges from the mucous membrane, the reduced epithelium attaches to almost the entire enamel (*C*). However, as the tooth erupts, the epithelium separates from the surface of the enamel, gradually exposing more and more of the crown (*D*).

***Ameloblast attachment epithelium***

At first the attachment epithelium is composed of ameloblasts.[27,40] After this initial phase of eruption, the composition and the relation of the attachment epithelium to the tooth may remain unchanged for several years. It is not unusual to find ameloblasts at the base of the col[41,42] (Fig. 2-21).

The attachment epithelium is long at first but becomes progressively shorter.[43] Before the gingival sulcus reaches the cementoenamel junction, the connective tissue attachment degenerates at the apical end of the attachment epithelium. The epithelium then proliferates along the surface of the cementum (Fig. 4-20, *E*). The downgrowth of the epithelium along the cementum would be impossible in the presence of intact connective tissue fibers. The events that provoke

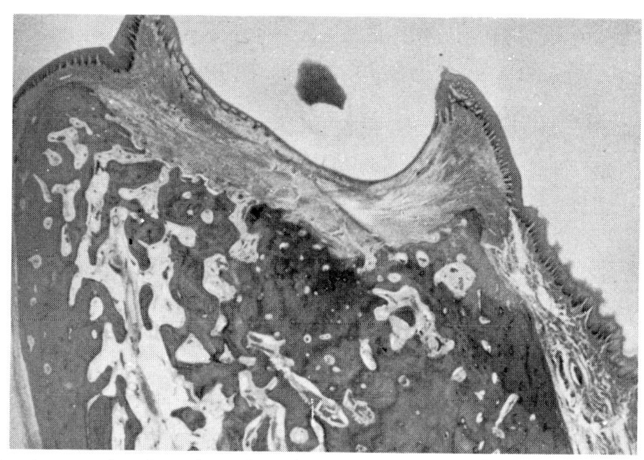

**Fig. 2-21.** Photomicrograph of an interdental papilla demonstrating the col with its oral and vestibular peaks. The epithelium at the base of the col may be made up of ameloblasts, which are gradually replaced by oral epithelium present at the peaks. The dense zone of connective tissue fibers running from peak to peak has been termed the interpapillary ligament. (Courtesy R. Stallard, Boston.)

the loss of the fibers are not yet clear. The fibers may disappear because of toxic influences from the gingival sulcus, enzymatic action of the epithelium,[44] or loss of cementum vitality[45] or possibly because of the presence of tissue collagenases.[46]

*Passive exposure*

As the epithelium separates from the tooth surface, the apical end of the attachment epithelium gradually moves onto the cementum. The bottom of the sulcus, which was first located on enamel, moves progressively to the cemento-enamel junction. Then it continues in an apical direction beyond that point (Fig. 4-20, *F*). Thus the attachment may move from the enamel to the cementum with advancing age. This changing relationship has been termed passive exposure of the tooth. It appears as a gradual recession of the gingival margin with an increased exposure of the clinical crown.

*Cuticles*

In the classical concept there are two cuticles, the primary and the secondary. Before the tooth is fully erupted, the attachment of ameloblasts to the enamel is mediated by the primary enamel cuticle. This cuticle is believed to be the last substance formed by the ameloblasts.

When the ameloblasts are replaced by oral epithelium, a second cuticle is formed. On the enamel it covers the primary enamel cuticle and is called the secondary enamel cuticle. On the cementum it is the only cuticle and it is referred to as the cemental cuticle. The secondary enamel cuticle and the cemental cuticle together constitute the dental cuticle.

Research has demonstrated the presence of mucopolysaccharides in the cuticle.[37,47,48] However, the composition of the cuticle is controversial.[49] Some authors claim that the cuticle is a cementum-like substance.[33,50] Others claim that it is derived from denatured hemoglobin[51] or from salivary mucins.[52] The primary and secondary cuticles of light microscopy are not identifiable as such under the electron microscope.[33,34] There the cuticles appear differently, are of undetermined origin, and may not correspond with those seen under the light microscope. They have been tentatively labeled cuticles A and B. Cuticle A is most likely an afibrillar cementum.[35] The epithelial attachment (electron micro-

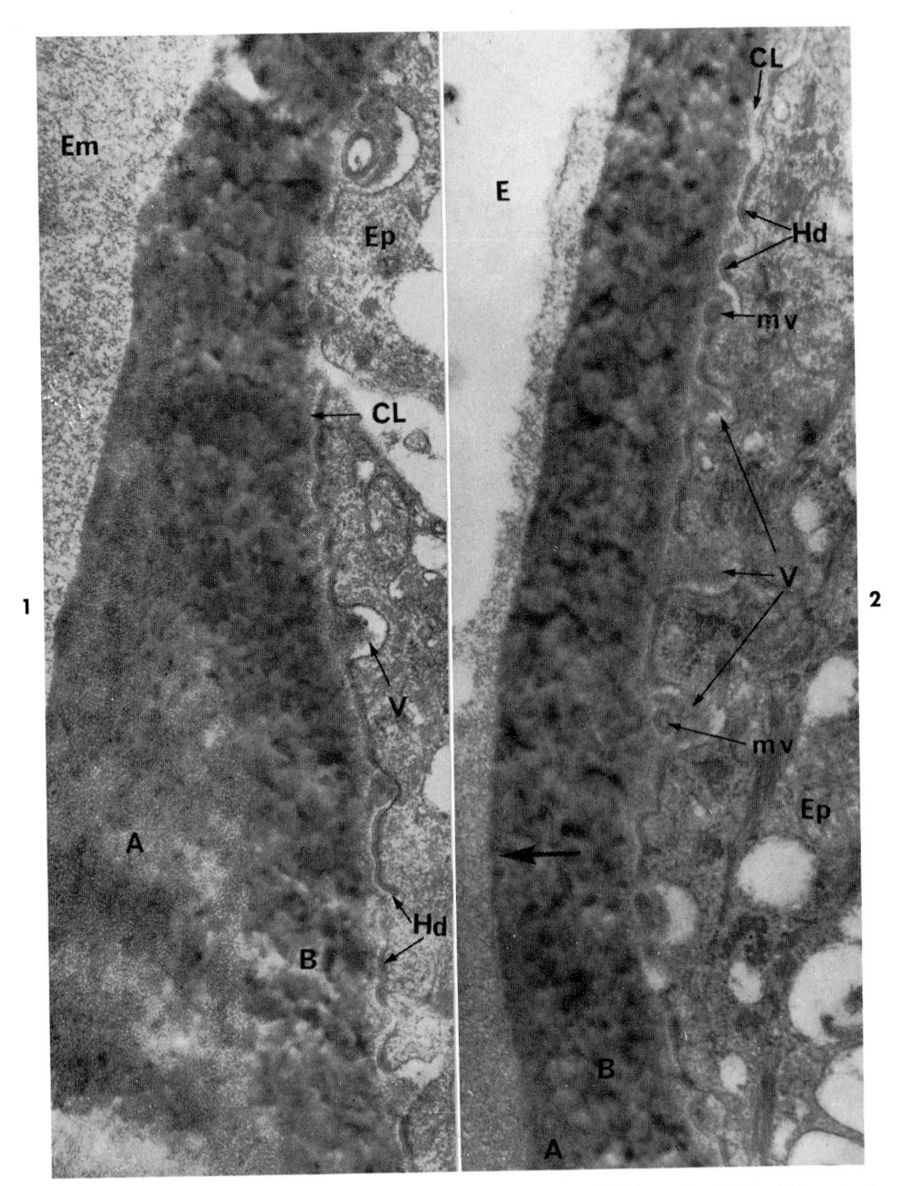


**Fig. 2-22.** Mandibular first deciduous molars of two 5-year-old boys. **1,** Epithelial attachment to type B cuticle, *B,* lies over the type A cuticle, *A,* covering the enamel matrix, *Em.* Structure resembling a discharging vacuole, *V,* can be seen to contain a granular material similar to that of the basement lamina, *CL.* (×37,000.) **2,** Section just coronal to **1** showing the end of type A cuticle (heavy arrow). The type B cuticle continues coronally in direct apposition to the enamel, *E. mv,* Microvilli; *Hd,* hemidesmosome; *Ep,* cells of the attachment epithelium; *CL,* basement lamina (adjacent to tooth); *E,* enamel space. (×39,000.) (From Listgarten, M. A.: Amer. J. Anat. **119:**147, 1966.)

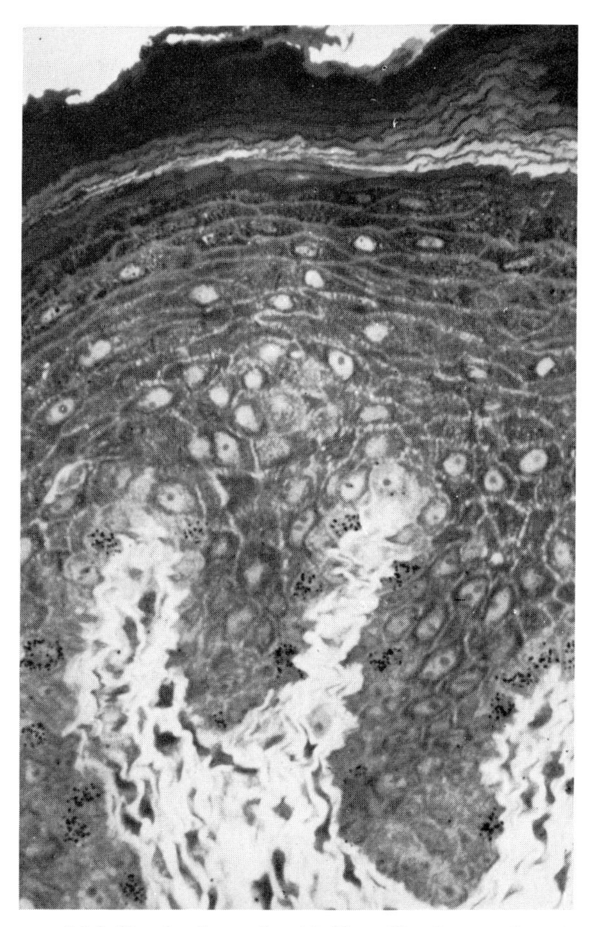

**Fig. 2-23.** Arrangement of labeling in the oral epithelium 30 minutes after the administration of tritiated thymidine. Grains are localized over the nuclei in the stratum basale. (From Anderson, G. S., and Stern, I. B.: Periodontics 4:115, 1966.)

scopic system of hemidesmosomes and basement membrane–like structure) may be formed directly on the tooth surface, but it also can form an attachment to the cuticles (Fig. 2-22).

## Junctional (attachment) epithelium

Perhaps the most significant fact about the epithelial attachment is that it resembles an electron microscopic basal lamina and the cells of the attachment are fastened to this structure by hemidesmosomes. Hemidesmosomes are organelles that are found in viable basal cells.

*Mitosis and labeling of the attachment epithelium*

Can it be that the cells adjacent to the tooth are basal cells? Mitotic figures have been observed in such cells.[53,54] When tritiated thymidine is administered to experimental animals, those cells about to undergo DNA synthesis pick up radioactive thymidine. The radioactivity can be detected in histologic sections by the use of photographic emulsion (Fig. 2-23). After the administration of the tritiated thymidine, labeled cells are found in the attachment epithelium adjacent to the tooth.[55-58]

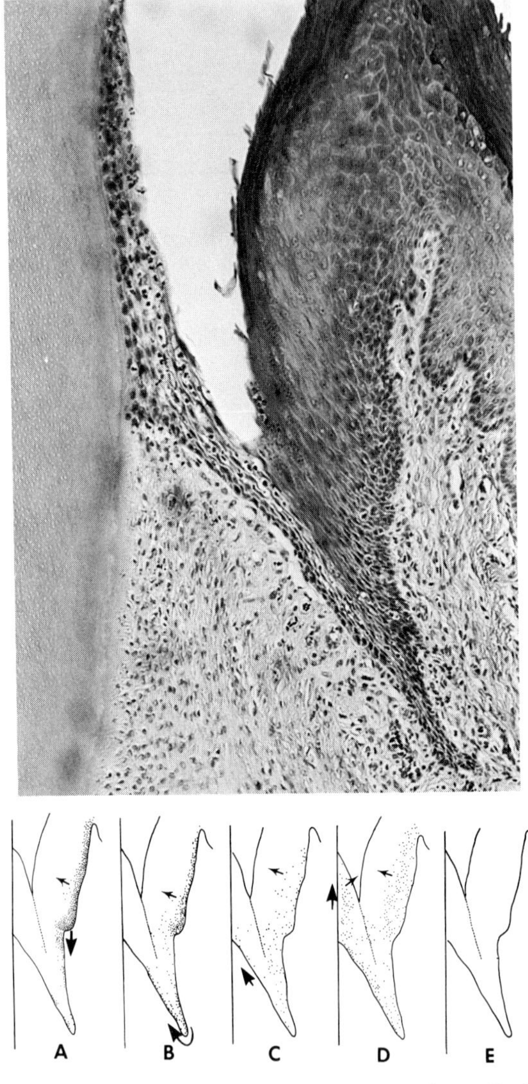


**Fig. 2-24.** Composite of labeled cells and their positions, **A,** ½ hour, **B,** 6 hours, **C,** 24 hours, **D,** 72 hours, and, **E,** 144 hours after the administration of tritiated thymidine to rats. The diagram of the morphology of the attachment epithelium and adjacent tissues is representative of the gingiva on the cemental (oral) surface of the continuously growing rat incisor. Large arrows indicate migration of the attachment (junctional) epithelium toward and along the tooth surface. Small arrows indicate migration of cells toward the sulcus. (From Anderson, G. S., and Stern, I. B.: Periodontics **4:**115, 1966.)

***Lateral migration of the attachment epithelium***

In the case of the attachment epithelium of rat gingiva, the cells are not labeled by the tritiated thymidine at first; yet in 12 hours many labeled cells are found next to the tooth.[59,60] These cells do not seem to divide. How does this phenomenon occur? There is a site adjacent to the attachment epithelium that is very active mitotically. Cells labeled at this site are capable of migrating. Although cells normally migrate toward the surface of the oral epithelium, in the attachment epithelium they migrate toward the tooth surface and then toward the bottom of the sulcus[59,60] (Fig. 2-24).

When cells leave the stratum germinativum, they have become specialized and can no longer divide. For instance, in the oral epithelium the cells may specialize to form the keratinized surface cells. In the attachment epithelium they become specialized for attachment. They synthesize the epithelial attachment and then migrate over it, their attachment maintained by the hemidesmosomes.

***Transit time of the attachment epithelium***

The time it takes for labeled cells to migrate and desquamate (transit time) is less than 144 hours for the continuously growing incisor of rodents[56,59] (Fig. 2-24). The transit time for primate attachment epithelium is in the vicinity of 72 to 120 hours.[57] We can assume, then, that the transit time in man would be much the same.

***Maintenance of the epithelial attachment during migration***

The question might be asked, how can the cells be attached to the tooth if they are actively migrating? The same mechanism is present at the epidermal–connective tissue junction. The epithelial cells are affixed to the connective tissue by means of the electron microscopic basal lamina, yet they can detach and migrate toward the surface. Similarly in healing wounds the epithelial cells form a basal lamina on the connective tissue and migrate over it to epithelize the wound. At no time is the epithelium loose from the connective tissue. The two issues are in intimate connection. Picture the epithelial attachment as the basement membrane of the attachment (junctional) epithelium. It turns about the most apical cell and extends up along the tooth surface. The cells can then migrate along this basement membrane. The hemidesmosomes hold the cells to this structure so that the strength of the attachment is not diminished despite the migration. Similarly the physical integrity of the attachment is maintained during the stages of passive exposure by this same biologic mechanism.

***Gingival fluid***

Another matter of intense interest, but requiring further study, is that of the gingival fluid. When bacteria or particulate matter are introduced into the sulcus, they soon disappear from the sulcus as if flushed out by a flow of fluid.[24,61-63] Fluorescein administered intravenously or by mouth is soon detected in the sulcus.[25,61,64] This is also true of radioactively labeled diiodofluorescein or human serum albumin[65,66] and of tetracycline.[67] The reverse flow of carbon particles through the sulcular epithelium into the connective tissue has also been demonstrated.

This sulcular circulation may have clinical significance. At one time if calculus was found below the gingival margin, it was called serumal calculus. On the other hand, if it was found above the gingival margin, it was termed salivary calculus. The names reflected the supposed source (serum or saliva) of the mineral salts that contributed to the formation of the calculus. This question has now been reopened since intravenously injected fluorescein can be detected in plaque and calculus.[64]

The fluid outflow contains various substances that may be of immunologic significance and may have antimicrobial activity.[69-72] This area also requires further investigation.

The sulcular fluid must originate in the vasculature adjacent to the sulcus.[73-79] The mechanism of fluid production may be physiologic or pathologic.[74] The rate of flow increases with inflammation.[64,73,79-84] Methods of fluid collection are crude and may provoke inflammation. Still, no matter the source and nature of the sulcular circulation, it exists in disease. The question as to whether it exists in health is unresolved.

Those who believe in the existence of an adherent epithelial cuff and deny

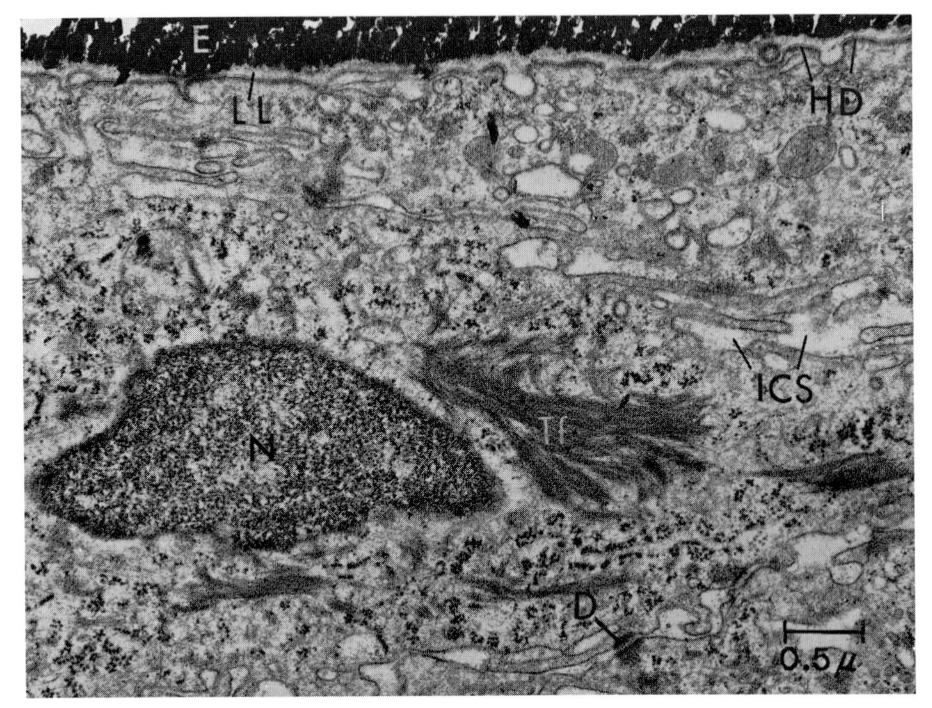


**Fig. 2-25.** Electron micrograph of cells of the attachment epithelium of a rat incisor adjacent to the enamel, *E.* Hemidesmosomes, *HD,* abut on and attach to the lamina lucida, *LL.* The lamina densa is fully calcified and cannot be demonstrated in this calcified specimen. The lamina lucida is approximately 400 Å wide. Note that the intercellular space, *ICS,* is wider than the lamina lucida. Cells are attached to each other by desmosomes, *D. N* represents the nucleus; *Tf,* a bundle of tonofilaments.

organic attachment feel that the fluid passes through the potential space between the cuff and the tooth. There are alternative pathways, however.[65,82] Electron microscopic examination of the epithelial attachment reveals a structure of such narrow diameter (~ 400Å) as to make sulcular circulation unlikely. The intercellular spaces of the cells of the attachment epithelium are much larger and better suited to support the sulcular circulation. In that case the fluid might pass into the sulcus via the intercellular spaces rather than through the epithelial attachment (Figs. 2-25 and 2-26).

***Leukocytes in the sulcular epithelium and saliva***

An interstitial pathway would permit the passage of leukocytes. Leukocytes have been observed in histologic sections of the sulcular and attachment epithelia[85] as well as in the gingival epithelium.[86] These cells move between the epithelial cells and pass through the epithelial surface. When they are detected in the saliva, they are termed salivary corpuscles[87] or salivary leukocytes.[88-90] They can be harvested by the millions from the saliva in a matter of minutes. The main portal of entry into the mouth is the sulcus[88,89]; also the number of salivary leukocytes in the edentulous mouth is low.[91-93] These salivary leukocytes most likely elaborate the enzymes that facilitate their passage through the sulcular epithelium,[94] and they may be the source of some of the proteins, including the immunochemical substances found in the sulcular fluid, since most of the studies on this subject have been made of whole (crude) rather than pure sulcular fluid.

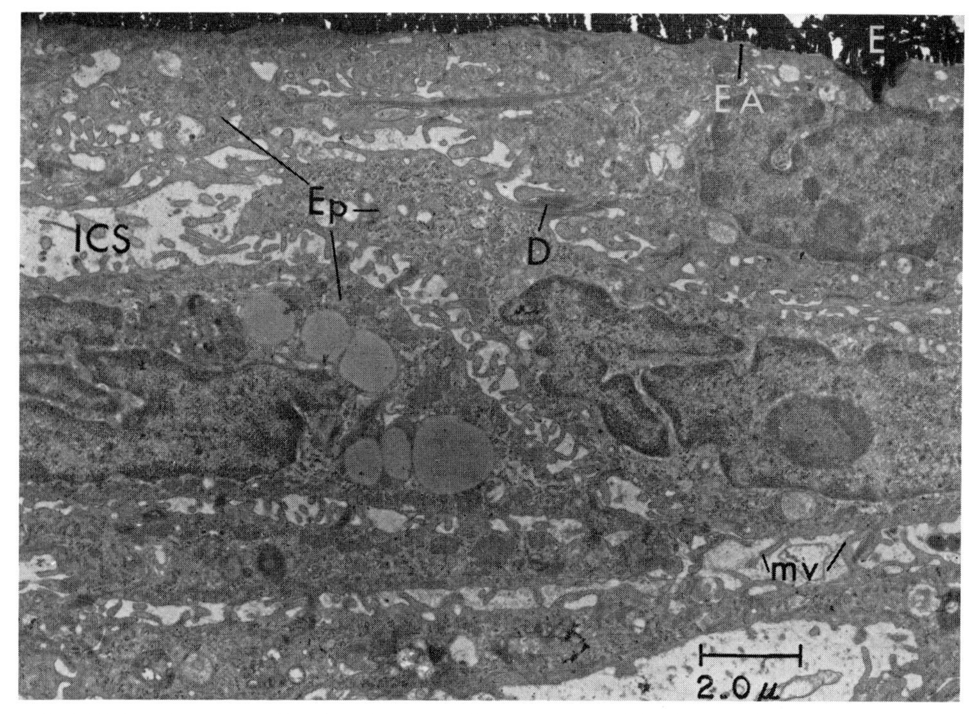


**Fig. 2-26.** At a lower magnification the epithelial attachment, *EA,* is barely visible adjacent to the enamel, *E.* Note how much larger the intercellular space, *ICS,* is between the cells of the attachment epithelium, *Ep.* These cells are attached to each other by desmosomes, *D.* Microvilli, *mv,* extend into the intercellular space.

The thesis that gingival fluid is of significance in the etiology of periodontal disease has been presented. Gingival fluid may also, however, represent a defense mechanism.

## FORMATION OF GINGIVAL SULCUS AND JUNCTIONAL EPITHELIUM

As the erupting tooth approaches the oral cavity, the reduced enamel epithelium and the oral epithelium meet and join. As the tooth erupts into occlusion, the gingiva surrounding the tooth gradually recedes, exposing more and more of the clinical crown.

The gingiva is not attached to the tooth all the way up to its margin but forms a small cuff or marginal invagination, known as the gingival sulcus. The bottom of the sulcus seems to move apically with age.

Gottlieb believed that the base of the sulcus was at the junction of the reduced enamel epithelium and the oral epithelium. The dimension of the attachment epithelium, he felt, was more or less constant so that, as the sulcus migrated apically by a peeling-off process, the attachment epithelium migrated apically, maintaining this dimension.[27] Becks, on the other hand, felt that the reduced enamel epithelium was completely destroyed by the age of 20 to 30 years and that the sulcus formed by a migration of the oral epithelium around and past the reduced enamel epithelium, making a new attachment.[95]

Basal cells can ordinarily form a new junctional epithelium and then migrate along the attachment. The attachment and junctional epithelia are continuous and share a common basal lamina, part of which becomes the epi-

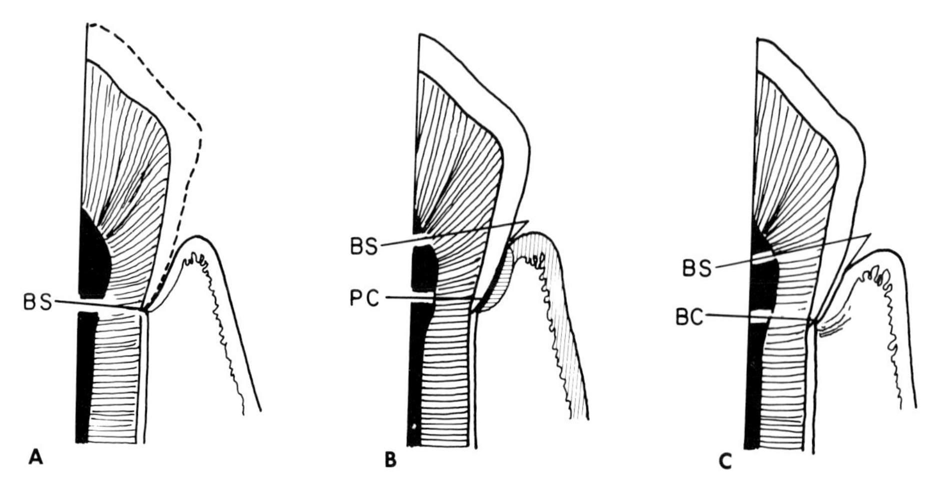


**Fig. 2-27.** Concepts of the formation and relative depth of the gingival sulcus. **A,** Diagram of Black's concept of the attachment and base of the sulcus, *BS,* at the cementoenamel junction. The existence of a decalcified enamel space led to the belief that the gingival sulcus continued without interruption to the cervical line. **B,** Diagram of Gottlieb's and Orban's concepts of the reduced enamel epithelium in organic attachment with the enamel by means of the primary cuticle. The sulcus is merely a shallow groove whose bottom, *BS,* is at the point of separation of the attachment from the tooth. **C,** Diagram of Waerhaug's recent concept of the gingival cuff, which adheres to but is separable from the tooth surface. It is a potential space. The bottom of the cuff, *BC,* is at the cementoenamel junction. The sulcus and cuff are continuous. According to this belief, the bottom of the gingival sulcus does not occur at *BS* but at *BC.*

thelial attachment. Which cells differentiate to form attachment epithelium and which differentiate to form sulcular epithelium? There does not seem to be any definite relationship between the stage of tooth eruption and the downgrowth of cells in fetal rhesus monkeys.[96] The base of the sulcus does not appear to be a point of weakened resistance.[59,96] The primary cuticle and the reduced ameloblasts at first provide an organic attachment that is later replaced by a secondary cuticle and a junctional epithelium capable of self-repair.

The sulcus was once believed to extend from the gingival margin to the cementoenamel junction (Fig. 2-27, *A*). This belief stemmed from the observation of decalcified specimens in which there was always a decalcified enamel space extending to the cementum.[97] The epithelium was thought to contact the young tooth only at the cementoenamel junction.[97] The concept of a broad adhesion of the epithelium to the tooth occurred to Gottlieb primarly as a result of his observations of the behavior of the dental cuticle in such decalcified histologic sections. In young teeth he found the cuticle adhering to junctional epithelium from the cementoenamel junction to a point considerably further coronally. From there, in a coronal direction, he found the cuticle floating unsupported by epithelium (Fig. 2-4). The free-floating coronal part of the cuticle was always coated with a bacterial deposit. Such deposits were not found over the cuticle in its more apical, attached part. Primarily on the basis of these findings, Gottlieb stated that the bottom of the sulcus was located where the cuticle began floating freely in his specimen.[98]

Gottlieb showed that there was an organic attachment between the reduced ameloblasts and the enamel through the primary cuticle.[27] He showed the sulcus to be a shallow groove whose bottom is at the coronal end of the attachment

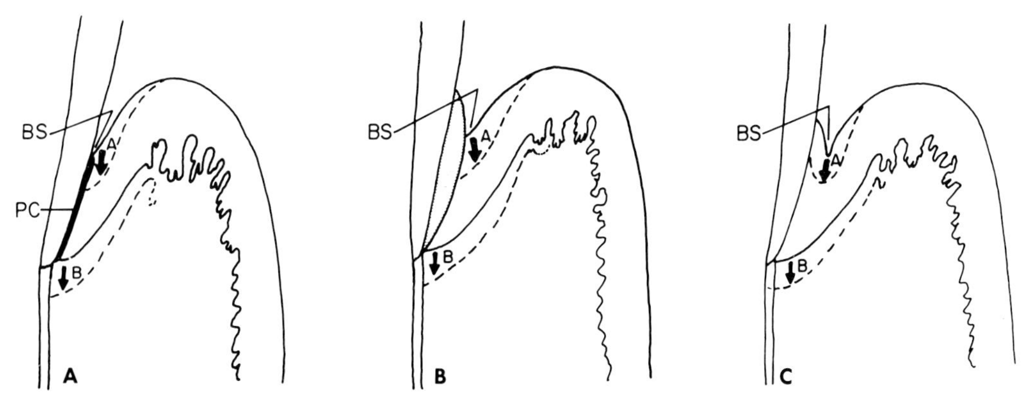


**Fig. 2-28.** Concepts of the mechanism of deepening of the sulcus—recession. **A,** Degeneration or peeling off of cells at point *A,* which is the bottom of the sulcus, *BS,* followed by migration apically of cells at point *B* (Gottlieb and Orban). (*A* refers to deepening of sulcus; *B* to apical migration of the junctional epithelium.) **B,** Becks, Skillen, and Baume conceived of the bottom of the sulcus, *BS,* as forming at the line of fusion between the reduced enamel epithelium (crosshatching) and the gingival epithelium. Progressive degeneration of the reduced enamel epithelium at *A* leads to a deepening of the sulcus and a migration of the junctional epithelium laterally past the reduced enamel epithelium. This is accompanied by an apical migration at point *B.* **C,** Weski's and Euler's concepts were of a split or tear in the attachment epithelium. The split formed the bottom of the sulcus, *BS,* and led to its deepening at point *A.* This was accompanied by an apical migration at point *B.*

(Fig. 2-27, *B*). More recently an alternative concept proposed that there is no organic attachment, merely an agglutination or adherence of cells to the tooth, which is separated from a cuff of epithelium by a potential space (Fig. 2-27, *C*). This view differs from the first in that it visualizes the cuff as being in direct contact with but not attached to the tooth and, in addition, adhering to the tooth but being separable by the lightest of forces.[29]

The entire matter has been settled by the observations of an attachment of ameloblasts to the enamel by hemidesmosomes and of attachment (junctional) epithelium to the tooth by a similar mechanism.[16,30-34]

## Mechanism

How does the attachment migrate apically and how does a pocket form? Gottlieb and Orban felt that the sulcus migrated apically by a peeling-off process due to alteration in the surface of enamel or to the death or degeneration of epithelial cells at the base of the sulcus (Fig. 2-28, *A*). Becks,[95] Baume,[98] and Skillen[99] believed that a line of fusion existed between the oral and the reduced enamel epithelia and that this line constituted a locus minoris resistentiae. The oral epithelium migrated around and past the slowly degenerating reduced enamel epithelium and ultimately replaced it (Fig. 2-28, *B*). Others have contended that the deepening of the sulcus is due to a tear in the attachment epithelium[100,101] (Fig. 2-28, *C*). All these views visualize the apical migration of the base of the sulcus as primary to the migration of the attachment.

Research has shown that the reduced ameloblasts do not divide; on the other hand, basal cells adjacent to the tooth do divide and then migrate up

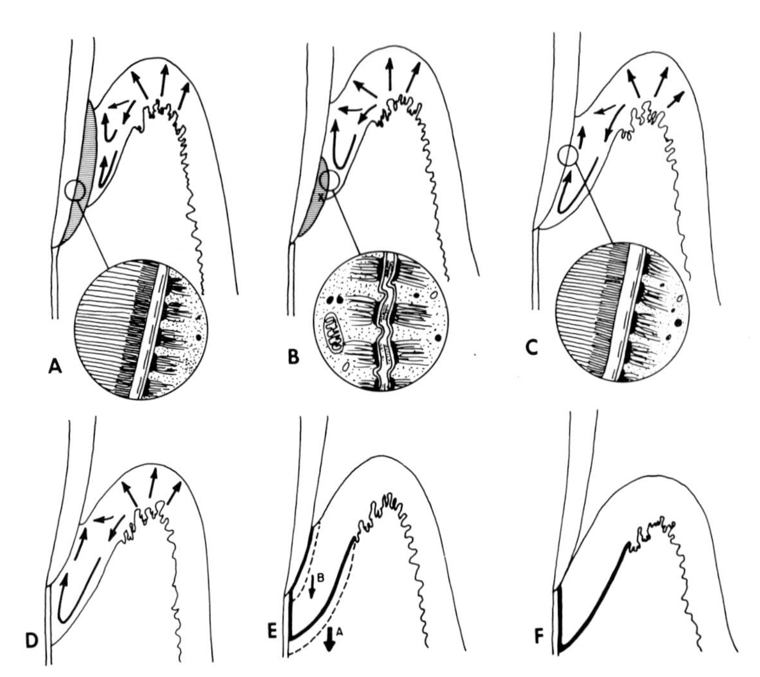


**Fig. 2-29.** Current concepts of the dynamics of migration of the junctional epithelium. **A,** The primary junctional epithelium consists of reduced ameloblasts attached by hemidesmosomes to the lamina lucida of an electron microscopic basement membrane–like structure. The gingival epithelial cells migrate either to the gingival surface and keratinize or (as shown by arrows) toward the reduced enamel epithelium, to which they attach. **B,** The primary junctional epithelium gradually degenerates and is replaced by the secondary junctional epithelium. Cells of the two tissues are joined by desmosomes and by tight junctions. At the point of fusion of the two tissues, X, mitotic activity is increased. Here the cells of the outer enamel epithelium and possibly the stratum intermedium join the cells of the gingival epithelium in forming a locus of proliferation. **C,** With the complete degeneration of the primary attachment epithelium, the secondary attachment epithelium contacts the enamel and the attachment occurs by the same mechanism as shown in **A. D,** In time the secondary junctional epithelium may be found attaching to both the enamel and the cementum. How did this apical migration occur? **E,** The secondary junctional epithelium renews itself in a matter of days, as does the gingival epithelium. Cells migrate in the pathways denoted by the arrows in **D.** The cells of the junctional epithelium travel along the electron microscopic basement membrane–like structure, which forms the epithelial attachment (shown by heavy line). When the basal cells at *A* migrate apically, they form a new attachment. Junctional cells at *B* may also migrate apically with either the resultant deepening of the sulcus or the progressive exposure of the clinical crown (recession). **F,** When the junctional epithelium has completely migrated into the cementum, the attachment is mediated by the lamina lucida and by hemidesmosomes, as it was on the enamel.

and along the tooth, desquamating in 4 to 6 days. They seem to migrate from a locus of proliferation in the basal layer at the junction of the oral and the attachment epithelia[59,96] (Fig. 2-24). While the reduced ameloblasts are still present, the cells of the oral epithelium join them by forming desmosomes. Gradually the reduced enamel epithelium is lost and the cells of the oral epithelium contact the tooth surface, there forming hemidesmosomes and a lamina lucida, by means of which the cells attach themselves to the tooth. The apical migration of the sulcus may not be due to a degeneration of *superficial* cells at the base of the sulcus since the attachment is formed by *basal* cells (Fig. 2-29). Sim-

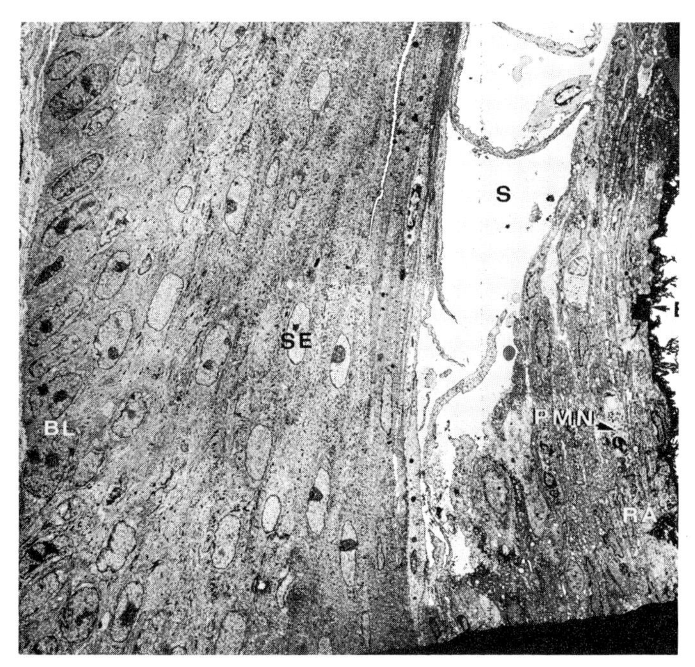


**Fig. 2-30.** Vestibular sulcus of the erupting rat incisor. Reduced ameloblasts, *RA,* are adjacent to the enamel, *E,* and crystals are still present. Cells of the sulcular epithelium, *SE,* form at the basal layer, *BL,* and migrate out toward the sulcus. Desquamating cells of both the sulcular epithelium and the reduced ameloblasts are visible in the sulcus, *S.* Intercellular spaces of the reduced ameloblasts are wider than those of the sulcular epithelium. Some polymorphonuclear leukocytes, *PMN,* are seen in the primary attachment epithelium.

ilarly, since enamel epithelium and its attachment (primary attachment) are replaced by the oral epithelium and its attachment (secondary attachment) in a relatively short time (4½ months in a newborn rhesus monkey),[96] the so-called locus minoris resistentiae may not be the mechanism of sulcus deepening. The concept of pocket formation produced by the deepening of splits also may not be accurate since splits are superficial and the attachment is formed by the basal cells, which are located more deeply. The weak link in the biologic seal afforded by the epithelium of the dentogingival junction may be in the basal cell layer. Perhaps the entrance through the sulcular wall of substances toxic or inflammatory to the tissues influences the ability of the basal cells to synthesize DNA or undergo mitosis and otherwise interferes with cellular physiology of these cells, which form a dynamic rather than a static attachment.

The foregoing observations are supported by Fig. 2-30, which is from a continuously erupting rat incisor. The oral epithelium is distinct from the reduced ameloblasts, yet the two types of cells join by their desmosomes. Ameloblasts are carried up by the erupting tooth and form the primary attachment. Cells of the oral epithelium migrate to form new desmosomal junctions with the ameloblasts. Desquamating cells are visible in the sulcus. The evidence for migration is supported by data of autoradiographic and histologic studies (Fig. 2-24). It is also supported by studies of sulcus formation during tooth eruption.[96]

As the erupting tooth closely approaches the oral cavity, the *reduced ameloblasts* over the cusp tips show signs of cell death. At the same time mitotic figures and premitotic uptake of $^{3}$H-thymidine are seen in the basal cells of

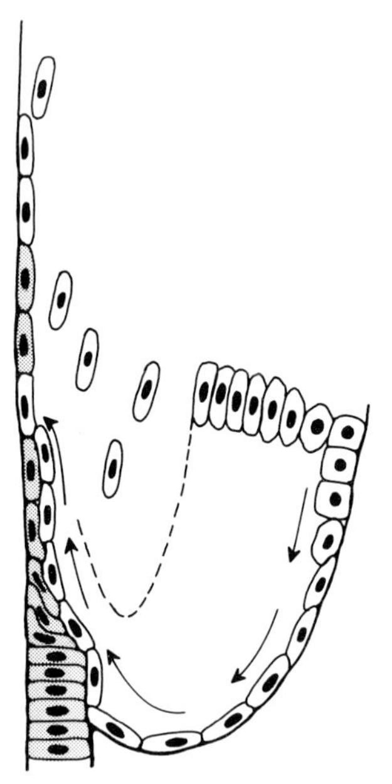

**Fig. 2-31.** Schematic representation of the alteration of columnar ameloblasts into flat cells coating the surface of the enamel (stippled cells). These are gradually replaced by the migrating cells of the basal layer of the gingival epithelium. They are at first cuboidal and later become flat. The bottom of the gingival sulcus is represented by the broken line. Cells desquamating from the sulcular wall and from the tooth surface are shown in the sulcus. (Adapted from Wolf, J.: Deutsch. Zahn- Mund- Kieferheilk. **43**:106, 1964.)

the *oral epithelium* and the cells of the *outer enamel epithelium*. The two proliferating tissues send strands toward each other. Ultimately they meet and form a solid core of cells above the tooth. The surface cells desquamate and the core comes out like a plug, allowing the cusp tip to enter the oral cavity. As the tooth continues to erupt, the cells of the outer enamel epithelium and the basal layer of the adjacent gingival epithelium continue to proliferate down the sides of the tooth. By the time the tooth reaches functional occlusion, the enamel may be one quarter exposed and the proliferating cells may have replaced some of the reduced enamel epithelium. At this time the rate of replacement becomes slower but nevertheless is continuous. There is a similar labeling index for the basal layers of the attachment epithelium (secondary attachment) of both erupting and adult teeth of the rhesus monkey. In rhesus monkeys, after eruption of the deciduous and permanent teeth, the attachment epithelium may reach the cementoenamel junction[96] and the sulcus moves apically with age. There seems to be some arrest of this movement at the cementoenamel junction, and the length of the attachment and the primary cuticles may become temporarily reduced. The sulcus extends coronally from the highest point of the attachment epithelium (Fig. 4-24). When the secondary attachment reaches the cementum, it functions precisely as it did on the enamel (Fig. 2-29).

The epithelial barrier is thus at different ages constituted of reduced ameloblasts, cells that have migrated from the point where the gingival epithelium has fused with the outer enamel epithelium, or migrating gingival epithelial cells. The reduced ameloblasts constitute the primary junctional epithelium. Except for those instances in which continuously erupting teeth are present

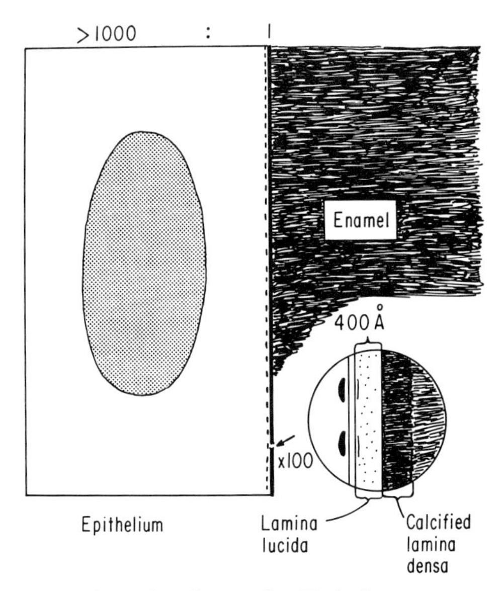


**Fig. 2-32.** Schematic representation of a flattened cell (primary or secondary attachment epithelium). The ratio of the cell width to the area of attachment is greater than 1000 to 1. Assuming a cell width of 10 $\mu$, one could not resolve the attachment in the light microscope since it would be below the level of resolution (i.e., 0.2 $\mu$). However, if this area is viewed in the electron microscope at an additional magnification (100,000×) (area at arrow enlarged in inset), the hemidesmosomes can be resolved. The lamina lucida is approximately 400 Å, and the lamina densa appears to be fully calcified. It is seen only in decalcified specimens. In any event, whether the attachment is formed by the ameloblasts or is derived from the basal layer of the gingival epithelium, its structural size and morphology are the same.

(i.e., incisors of rodents), the primary junctional epithelium is replaced by the secondary junctional epithelium whose origin has already been explained.

The columnar ameloblasts reduce in size and gradually become cuboidal. They then turn and align themselves parallel with the tooth surface (Fig. 2-31). After eruption the basal layer of gingival cells migrates up over the ameloblasts. These cells are at first cuboidal and later turn to lie parallel to the basal lamina and the tooth surface. As the cells of the primary junctional epithelium are lost, they are replaced by the cells of the secondary junctional epithelium.

Whether the attachment is formed by the primary or the secondary attachment (junctional) epithelium, the morphology is the same. It consists of what appears to be the lamina lucida of the electron microscopic basement membrane. The width of the lamina lucida is about 400 Å. The lamina densa is not visible and appears to be calcified. The junctional epithelial cells most likely form this structure. Their hemidesmosomes abut on it and attach to it (Fig. 2-32).

The cells of the primary attachment epithelium do not migrate. They appear to have a fixed position relative to the enamel. However, in continuously erupting teeth, such as the rat incisor, the ameloblasts are carried up with the erupting tooth and are ultimately desquamated. They thus have a shorter life cycle than the ameloblasts of human teeth.

The cells of the secondary junctional epithelium migrate laterally to the tooth surface and tend to creep up the side of the tooth, leaving a cleft between the sulcular wall and themselves. This cleft was first perceived by James and

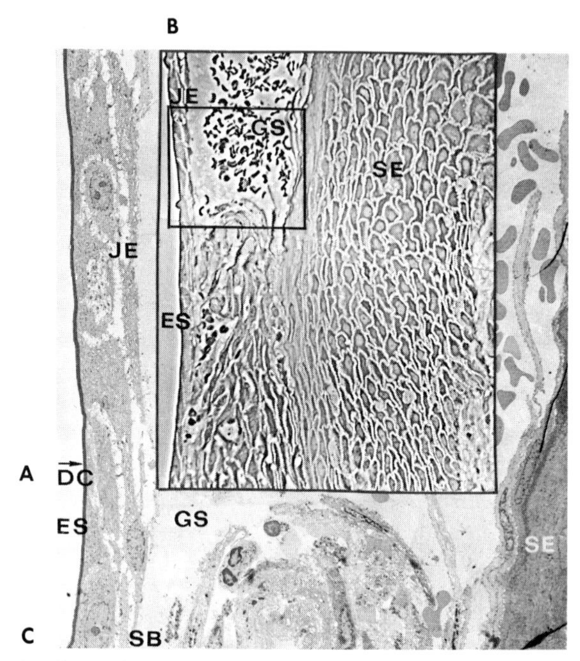


**Fig. 2-33.** Gingival sulcus. Electron micrograph of a serial section of the area outlined in **B.** The gingival suclus, *GS,* contains erythrocytes as a result of surgical hemorrhage. The bottom of the sulcus, *SB,* is formed primarily by the free surface of the junctional epithelium, *JE.* On the tooth side the sulcus is lined by junctional epithelial cells attached to a well-defined dental cuticle, *DC,* which lines the enamel space, *ES.* The sulcular epithelium, *SE,* which lines the lateral aspect of the sulcus, is composed of flattended epithelial cells with relatively small intercellular spaces. This epithelium is cytologically similar to oral epithelium but differs from the loosely knit junctional epithelium. (From Schroeder, H. E., and Listgarten, M. A.: Fine structure of the developing epithelial attachment of human teeth, Basel, 1971, S. Karger, AG., vol. 2.)

Counsell, who called the remnant of cells attached to the tooth surface a tag.[104] The cleft has recently been demonstrated by Schroeder and Listgarten, using electron microscopy (Fig. 2-33); and it remarkably resembles the migration in the rat incisor, in which the secondary junctional epithelium joins the reduced ameloblasts to form the primary attachment epithelium[35] (Fig. 2-30).

**CHAPTER 2**

**References**

1. Weski, O.: Die chronisch-marginale Entzündungen des Alveolarfortsatzes mit besonderer Berücksichtigung der Alveolarpyorrhoe, Vjschr. Zahnheilk. **37:**1, 1921.
2. Orban, B.: Clinical and histologic study of the surface characteristics of the gingiva, Oral Surg. **1:**827, 1948.
3. Rosenberg, H. M., and Massler, M.: Gingival stippling in young adult males, J. Periodont. **38:**473, 1967.
4. Erausquin, J.: Histologia dentaria humana, Buenos Aires, 1953, Progrental.
5. Arnim, S. S., and Hagerman, D. A.: The connective tissue fibers of the marginal gingiva, J. Amer. Dent. Ass. **47:**271, 1953.
6. Goldman, H. M.: Topography and role of the gingival fibers, J. Dent. Res. **30:**331, 1951.
7. Sicher, H., and Bhaskar, S. N., editors: Orban's oral histology and embryology, ed. 7, St. Louis, 1972, The C. V. Mosby Co.

8. Melcher, A. H.: The architecture of human gingival reticulin, Arch. Oral Biol. 9:111, 1964.
9. Keller, G. J., and Cohen, D. W.: India ink perfusions of the vascular plexus of oral tissues, Oral Surg. 8:539, 1955.
10. Hirschfeld, I.: Interdental canals, J. Amer. Dent. Ass. 14:617, 1927.
11. Bernick, S.: Innervation of teeth and periodontium after enzymatic removal of collagenous elements, Oral Surg. 10:323, 1957.
12. De Aprile, E. C., Anderson, D., and Tesorieri, A.: Contribucion al estudio de las formaciones nerviosas terminales en la mucosa gingival. Les parodontopathies, Venice, 1955, L. Salvagno.
13. Gairns, F. W., and Aitchison, J.: A preliminary study of the multiplicity of nerve endings in the human gum, Dent. Record 70:180, 1950.
14. Weiss, M. D., Weinmann, J. P., and Meyer, J.: Degree of keratinization and glycogen content in the uninflamed and inflamed gingiva and alveolar mucosa, J. Periodont. 30:208, 1959.
15. Orban, B.: Hornification of the gums, J. Amer. Dent. Ass. 17:1977, 1930.
16. Stern, I. B.: Electron microscopic observations of oral epithelium. I. Basal cells and the basement membrane, Periodontics 3:224, 1965.
17. Rhodin, J. A. G., and Reith, E. J.: Ultrastructure of keratin in oral mucosa, skin, esophagus, claw, and hair. In Butcher, E. O., and Sognnaes, R. F., editors: Fundamentals of keratinization, Washington, D. C., 1962, A.A.A.S.
18. Barker, D. S.: The dendritic cell system in human gingival epithelium, Arch. Oral Biol. 12:203, 1967.
19. Dummett, C. O.: Oral pigmentation, J. Periodont. 31:356, 1960.
20. Petitet, N. F., and Stern, I. B.: Ultrastructure de l'épithélium gingival humain. In Favard, P., editor: Microscopie électronique, Paris, 1970, Société Française de Microscopie Électronique, vol. 3.
21. Gavin, J. B.: The ultrastructure of the crevicular epithelium of cat gingiva, Amer. J. Anat. 123:283, 1968.
22. Franke, J.: Die Entzündung des Zahnfleischsaumes, Fortschr. Kiefer- Gesichtschir. 9:225, 1964.
23. Waerhaug, J., and Steen, E.: The presence or absence of bacteria in gingival pockets and the reaction in healthy pockets to certain pure cultures, Odont. T. 60:1, 1952.
24. Harvey, P. M.: Elimination of extraneous material from the gingival crevice, J. Periodont. 23:231, 1962.
25. Brill, N., and Krasse, B.: The passage of tissue fluid into the clinically healthy gingival pocket, Acta Odont. Scand. 16:233, 1958.
26. Emslie, R. D., and Weinmann, J. P.: The architectural pattern of the boundary between epithelium and connective tissue of the gingiva in the Rhesus monkey, Anat. Rec. 105:35, 1949.
27. Gottlieb, B.: Der Epithelansatz am Zähne, Deutsch. Mschr. Zahnheilk. 39:142, 1921.
28. Baume, L. J.: Observations concerning the histogenesis of the epithelial attachment, J. Periodont. 23:71, 1952.
29. Waerhaug, J.: The gingival pocket, Odont. T., vol. 60, supp., 1952.
30. Stern, I. B.: The fine structure of the ameloblast-enamel junction in rat incisors; epithelial attachment and cuticular membrane. In Breese, S. S., editor: Electron microscopy, New York, 1962, Academic Press Inc.
31. Stern, I. B.: Electron microscopic observations of the dento-gingival attachment in rat incisors, I.A.D.R. 41:96, 1963. Abstract.
32. Grant, D., Stern, I. B., and Everett, F. G.: Orban's periodontics, ed. 2, St. Louis, 1963, The C. V. Mosby Co.
33. Listgarten, M. A.: Phase-contrast and electron microscopic study of the junction between reduced enamel epithelium and enamel in unerupted human teeth, Arch. Oral Biol. 11:999, 1966.
34. Listgarten, M. A.: Electron microscopic study of the gingivodental junction of man, Amer. J. Anat. 119:147, 1966.
35. Schroeder, H. E., and Listgarten, M. A.: The fine structure of the developing epithelial attachment of human teeth, Basel, 1971, S. Karger, AG.
36. Griffin, C. I., and Gee, E. J.: Some observations on the epithelial attachment and enamel maturation in human incisors, Aust. Dent. J. 8:221, 1963.
37. Toto, P. D., and Sicher, H.: The epithelial attachment, Periodontics 2:154, 1964.

38. Stallard, R. E., Diab, M. A., and Zander, H. A.: The attaching substance between enamel and epithelium—a product of the epithelial cells, J. Periodont. **36**:139, 1965.
39. Schultz-Haudt, S. D., Waerhaug, J., From S. H., and Attramadal, A.: On the nature of contact between the gingival epithelium and the tooth surface, Periodontics **1**:103, 1963.
40. Baume, L. J.: The structure of the epithelial attachment revealed by phase contrast microscopy, J. Periodont. **24**:99, 1953.
41. Cohen, B.: Morphologic factors in the pathogenesis of periodontal disease, Brit. Dent. J. **107**:31, 1959.
42. Cohen, B.: A study of the periodontal epithelium, Brit. Dent. J. **112**:55, 1962.
43. Gargiulo, A. W., Wentz, F. M., and Orban, B. J.: Dimensions and relations of the dentogingival junction in humans, J. Periodont. **32**:261, 1961.
44. Weinmann, J. P., Svoboda, J. F., and Woods, P. W.: Hereditary disturbances of enamel formation and calcification, J. Amer. Dent. Ass. **32**:397, 1945.
45. Gottlieb, B.: Biology of the cementum, J. Periodont. **13**:13, 1942.
46. Fullmer, H. M., and Gibson, W.: Collagenolytic activity in gingiva of man, Nature **209**:728, 1966.
47. Wertheimer, J. C., and Fullmer, H. M.: Morphologic and histochemical observations on the human dental cuticle, J. Periodont. **33**:29, 1962.
48. Cimasoni, G., Fiore-Donno, G., and Held, A.-J.: Mucopolysaccharides in human epithelial reattachment, Helv. Odont. Acta **7**:60, 1963.
49. Schüle, H.: Das Schmelzoberhäutchen, Stuttgart, 1962, Georg Thieme Verlag.
50. Levine, P. T., Glimcher, M. J., and Bonar, L. C.: Collagenous layer covering the crown enamel of unerupted permanent human teeth, Science **46**:1676, 1964.
51. Hodson, J. J.: Origin and nature of the cuticula dentis, Nature **209**:990, 1966.
52. Armstrong, W. G.: Amino-acid composition of the acquired pellicle of human tooth enamel, Nature **210**:197, 1966.
53. Hirt, C. M., Hartl, S., and Mühlemann, H. R.: The distribution of mitoses in the epithelium of interdental papillae of the rat molar, J. Periodont. **26**:229, 1955.
54. McHugh, W. D.: Some aspects of the development of gingival epithelium, Periodontics **1**:239, 1963.
55. Greulich, R. C.: Cell proliferation and migration in the epithelial attachment collar of the mouse molar, I.A.D.R. **40**:80, 1962. Abstract.
56. Beagrie, G. S., and Skougaard, M. R.: Observations on the life cycle of the gingival epithelial cells of mice as revealed by autoradiography, Acta Odont. Scand. **20**:15, 1962.
57. Skougaard, M. R., and Beagrie, G. S.: The renewal of gingival epithelium in marmosets (Callithrix jacchus) as determined through autoradiography with thymidine-$H^3$, Acta Odont. Scand. **20**:467, 1962.
58. McHugh, W. D., and Zander, H. A.: Cell division in the periodontium of developing and erupted teeth, Dent. Pract. **15**:451, 1965.
59. Anderson, G. S., and Stern, I. B.: The proliferation and migration of the attachment epithelium on the cemental surface of the rat incisor, Periodontics **4**:115, 1966.
60. Kirschner, H., and Rühl, E.: Autoradiographische Untersuchungen mit $^3H$-Thymidin über die Regeneration des epithelialen Attachments, Deutsch. Zahnaerztl. Z. **24**:816, 1969.
61. Brill, N., and Björn, H.: Passage of tissue fluid into human gingival pockets, Acta Odont. Scand. **17**:11, 1959.
62. Brill, N.: Removal of particles and bacteria from gingival pockets by tissue fluids, Acta Odont. Scand. **17**:431, 1959.
63. Ratcliff, P. A.: Permeability of healthy gingival epithelium by microscopically observable particles, J. Periodont. **37**:291, 1966.
64. Salkind, A., Oshrain, H. I., and Mandel, I. D.: Observations on the gingival pocket fluid, Periodontics **1**:196, 1963.
65. Browne, R. M.: Some observations on the fluid flow from the gingival crevice, Dent. Pract. **14**:470. 1964.
66. Brown-Grant, K., and Browne, R. M.: The gingival fluid of the labial aspect of the upper incisors in the rabbit, Arch. Oral Biol. **11**:455, 1966.
67. Bader, H. I., and Goldhaber, P.: The passage of intravenously administered tetracycline in the gingival sulcus of dogs, J. Oral Ther. **2**:324, 1966.
68. Fine, D. H., and others: The penetration of human gingival sulcular tissue by carbon particles, Arch. Oral Biol. **14**:1117, 1969.
69. Brill, N., and Brönnestam, R.: Immunoelectrophoretic study of tissue fluid from gingival pockets, Acta Odont. Scand. **18**:95, 1960.

70. Brandtzaeg, P., and Mann, W. V., Jr.: A comparative study of the lysozyme activity of human gingival pocket fluid, serum and saliva, Acta Odont. Scand. **22**:441, 1964.
71. Brandtzaeg, P.: Immunochemical comparison of proteins in human gingival pocket fluid, serum and saliva, Arch. Oral Biol. **10**:795, 1965.
72. Cowley, G. C.: Fluorescence studies of crevicular fluid, J. Dent. Res., vol. 45, supp., p. 655, 1966.
73. Löe, H., and Holm-Pedersen, P.: Absence and presence of fluid from normal and inflamed gingivae, Periodontics **3**:171, 1965.
74. Weinstein, E., and others: Studies of gingival fluid, J. Periodont. **5**:161, 1967.
75. Egelberg, J.: The blood vessels of the dento-gingival junction, J. Periodont. Res. **1**:163, 1966.
76. Egelberg, J.: Permeability of the dento-gingival blood vessels. I. Application of the vascular labelling and gingival fluid measurements, J. Periodont. Res. **1**:180, 1966.
77. Egelberg, J.: Permeability of the dento-gingival blood vessels. II. Clinically healthy gingivae, J. Periodont. Res. **1**:276, 1966.
78. Egelberg, J.: Permeability of the dento-gingival blood vessels. III. Chronically inflamed gingivae, J. Periodont. Res. **1**:287, 1966.
79. Egelberg, J.: Permeability of the dento-gingival blood vessels. IV. Effect of histamine on vessels in clinically healthy and chronically inflamed gingivae, J. Periodont. Res. **1**:297, 1966.
80. Mann, W. V., Jr.: The correlation of gingivitis, pocket depth and exudate from the gingival crevice, J. Periodont. **34**:79, 1963.
81. Egelberg, J.: Gingival exudate measurements of evaluation of inflammatory changes of the gingivae, Odont. Rev. **15**:381, 1964.
82. Löe, H.: Physiologic aspects of the gingival pocket, an experimental study, Acta Odont. Scand. **19**:387, 1961.
83. Klinkhamer, J. M., and Zimmerman, S.: The function and reliability of the orogranulocytic migratory rate as a measure of oral health, J. Dent. Res. **48**:709, 1969.
84. Skougaard, M. R., Bay, I., and Klinkhamer, J. M.: Correlation between gingivitis and orogranulocytic migratory rate, J. Dent. Res. **48**:716, 1969.
85. Grant, D. A., and Orban, B.: Leukocytes in the epithelial attachment, J. Periodont. **31**:87, 1960.
86. Cattoni, M.: Lymphocytes in the epithelium of the healthy gingiva, J. Dent. Res. **30**:627, 1951.
87. Rovelstad, G. H.: Salivary corpuscle activity, J. Amer. Dent. Ass. **68**:50, 1964.
88. Wright, D. E.: The source and rate of entry of leukocytes in the human mouth, Arch. Oral Biol. **9**:321, 1964.
89. Sharry, J. J., and Krasse, B.: Observations on the origin of salivary leukocytes, Acta Odont. Scand. **18**:347, 1960.
90. Klinkhamer, J. M.: Human oral leukocytes, Periodontics **1**:109, 1963.
91. Klein, H.: Cellular elements in the saliva of infants before and after eruption of teeth, J. Dent. Res. **41**:1017, 1962.
92. Wright, D. E.: Leucocytes in the saliva of infants, Brit. Dent. J. **110**:50, 1961.
93. Calonius, P. E. B.: The leukocyte count in saliva, Oral Surg. **11**:43, 1958.
94. Thilander, H.: The effect of leukocytic enzyme activity on the structure of the gingival pocket epithelium in man, Acta Odont. Scand. **21**:431, 1963.
95. Becks, H.: Normal and pathologic pocket formation, J. Amer. Dent. Ass. **16**:2167, 1929.
96. Engler, W. O., and others: Development of epithelial attachment and gingival sulcus in Rhesus monkeys, J. Periodont. **36**:44, 1965.
97. Black, G. V.: Special dental pathology, Chicago, 1915, Medico-Dental Publishing Co.
98. Baume, L. J.: Observations concerning the histogenesis of the epithelial attachment, J. Periodont. **23**:71, 1952.
99. Skillen, W. G.: The morphology of the gingiva of the rat molar, J. Amer. Dent. Ass. **17**:645, 1930.
100. Weski, O.: Roentgenologisch-anatomische Studien aus dem Gebiete der Kieferpathologie, Vjschr. Zahnheilk. **28**:1, 1922.
101. Euler, H.: Der Epithelansatz in neuere Beleuchtung, Vjschr. Zahnheilk. **29**:103, 1923.
102. Hunt, A. M., and Paynter, K. J.: The role of the stratum intermedium in the development of the guinea pig molar. A study of cell differentiation and migration using tritiated thymidine, Arch. Oral Biol. **8**:65, 1963.
103. Wolf, J.: Der gingivodentale Verschlussapparat im Bereich des Schmeltzes, Deutsch. Zahn- Mund- Kieferheilk. **43**:106, 1964.

104. James, W. W., and Counsell, A.: Histological investigation into "so-called pyorrhoea alveolaris," Brit. Dent. J. **48**:1237, 1927.

105. Wolf, J.: Der gingivodentale Verschlussapparat im Bereich des Zements, Deutsch. Zahn-Mund- Kieferheilk. **47**:177, 1966.

**Additional suggested reading**

Forsslund, G.: The structure and function of the capillary system in the gingiva of man, Acta Odont. Scand., vol. 17, supp. 26, 1959.

Frank, R. M., and Cimasoni, G.: Ultrastructure de l'épithélium cliniquement normal du sillon et de la jonction gingivo-dentaire, Z. Zellforsch. **109**:356, 1970.

Haim, G.: Elektronenmikroskopische Untersuchungen des normalen Epithels Mundschleimhaut, Munich, 1964, Carl Hanser Verlag.

Listgarten, M.: Changing concepts about the dento-epithelial junction, J. Canad. Dent. Ass. **36**: 70, 1970.

McDougall, W. A.: Pathways of penetration and effects of horseradish peroxidase in rat molar gingiva, Arch. Oral Biol. **15**:621, 1970.

Schroeder, H. E., and Theilade, J.: Electron microscopy of normal human gingival epithelium, J. Periodont. Res. **1**:93, 1966.

Smith, C. J.: Gingival epithelium. In Melcher, A. H., and Bowen, W. H., editors: Biology of the periodontium, New York, 1969, Academic Press, Inc.

Squier, C. A., and Meyer, J.: Current concepts of the histology of oral mucosa, Springfield, Ill., 1971, Charles C Thomas, Publisher.

Thilander, H., and Hugoson, A.: The border zone tooth-enamel and epithelium after periodontal treatment: an experimental electron microscopic study in the cat, Acta Odont. Scand. **28**:147, 1970.

CHAPTER THREE

# Periodontium—periodontal ligament, cementum, alveolar process



## PERIODONTAL LIGAMENT

The periodontal ligament is a dense connective tissue attaching the tooth to the alveolar bone. Its primary function is to support the tooth in the alveolus and to maintain the physiologic relation between the cementum and the bone. It also has nutritive, defensive, and sensory (mechanoreceptive) properties.

### Histogenesis

*Development*

The organization and function of the periodontal ligament can be better understood by following its histologic development. The periodontal ligament develops from connective tissue elements during embryonic life. Prior to the eruption of the primary teeth and the permanent molars (teeth without predecessors), a recognizable ligament is formed. Secondary succedaneous teeth develop a ligament after they erupt into the oral cavity[1,2] (Fig. 3-1). The formation of the ligament may be illustrated in four sequential steps:

1. Short, brushlike, closely spaced cemental fibers extend from the cementum. A few isolated alveolar fibers extend from the alveolar wall. Between these two groups of fibers are loose collagenous fibers that align themselves parallel to the long axis of the tooth. These fibers make up about seven eighths of the ligament's width (Fig. 3-2, *A*).
2. The alveolar fibers increase in size and number. They become longer and splay out (arborize) at their ends. The alveolar fibers are more widely separated than the cemental fibers (Fig. 3-2, *B*).
3. The alveolar and cemental fibers continue to lengthen and appear to join (Fig. 3-2, *C*).
4. When the tooth becomes functional, the fiber bundles increase in width and are apparently continuous between bone and cementum (Figs. 3-2, *D*, and 3-3).

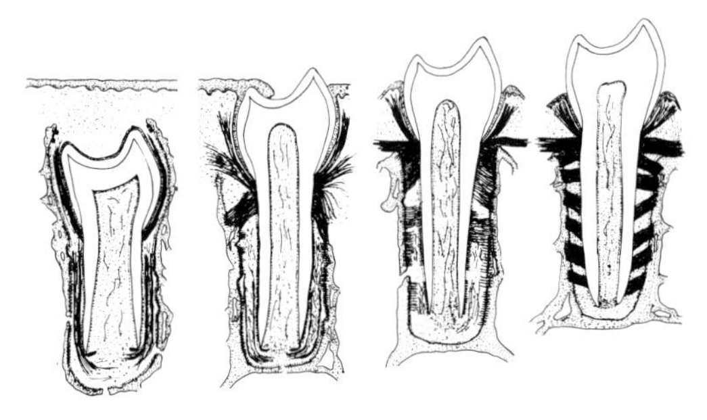

**Fig. 3-1.** Diagrammatic representation of the periodontal ligament of a premolar (a secondary tooth) prior to and during eruption. These stages differ in a permanent molar (which is not a succedaneous tooth) in that the permanent molar has well-defined fibers in the pre-eruptive stages. (From Grant, D. A., and Bernick, S.: J. Periodont. **43**:17, 1972.)

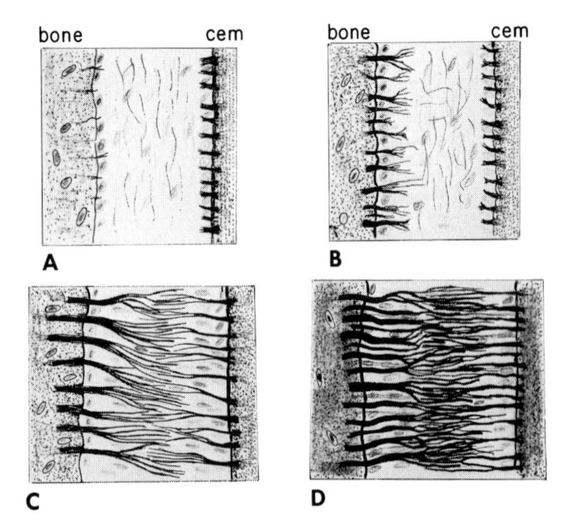


**Fig. 3-2.** Diagrammatic representation of the formation of periodontal ligament fibers during eruption. Although the chronology differs, the sequence of principal periodontal fiber formation is the same for teeth with and without predecessors. In each the developmental pattern occurs as follows: **A,** Fibers first emanate from cementum. These are short and closely spaced. The osteoblast-lined alveolar bone shows no fiber extrusions or only a rare isolated fiber. The greatest part of the periodontal ligament space is occupied by collagenous elements similar in appearance to those of the dental sac. **B,** Fibers, thicker and more widely spaced than those from cementum, emerge from bone to extend briefly toward the tooth and then splay out (arborize) at their ends. The central three fourths of the periodontal ligament space is occupied by loosely structured collagenous elements. **C,** Alveolar fibers extend into the central zone to join lengthening cemental fibers and to obliterate the intermediate plexus. **D,** With occlusal function the principal fibers become classically organized, thicker, and apparently continuous between bone and cementum. (From Grant, D. A., and Bernick, S.: J. Periodont. **43**:17, 1972.)

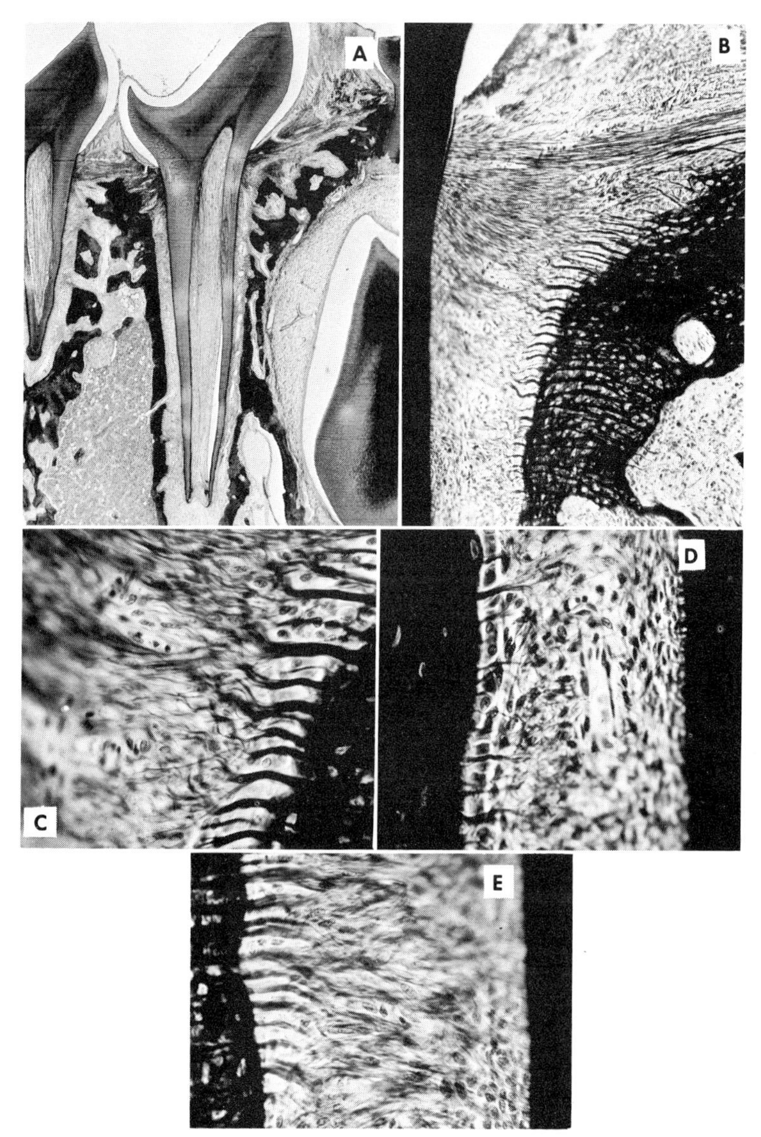

**Fig. 3-3. A,** Squirrel monkey premolars during eruption. At the stage of first occlusal contact, these secondary teeth show only dentogingival, alveolar crest, and horizontal fibers as organized groups. The remainder of the ligament is in a formative stage. **B,** Higher magnification of the alveolar crest of a premolar shows that fiber formation is evident at the cementoenamel junction but is less so apically. In the special region the cemental and alveolar fibers have yet to join. **C,** Higher magnification still shows the thick alveolar fibers at the osseous crest. Alveolar fibers become arborized and then extend toward the cemental fibers. **D,** Midroot, thick, widely spaced alveolar fibers are separated from the fine closely spaced cemental fibers by loosely organized collagen fibers. **E,** With function the principal fibers become thickened and appear to extend between cementum and bone in an uninterrupted fashion. (Overlapping of fibers is due to thickness of this celloidin section.) (From Grant, D. A., and Bernick, S.: J. Periodont. **42:**17, 1972.)

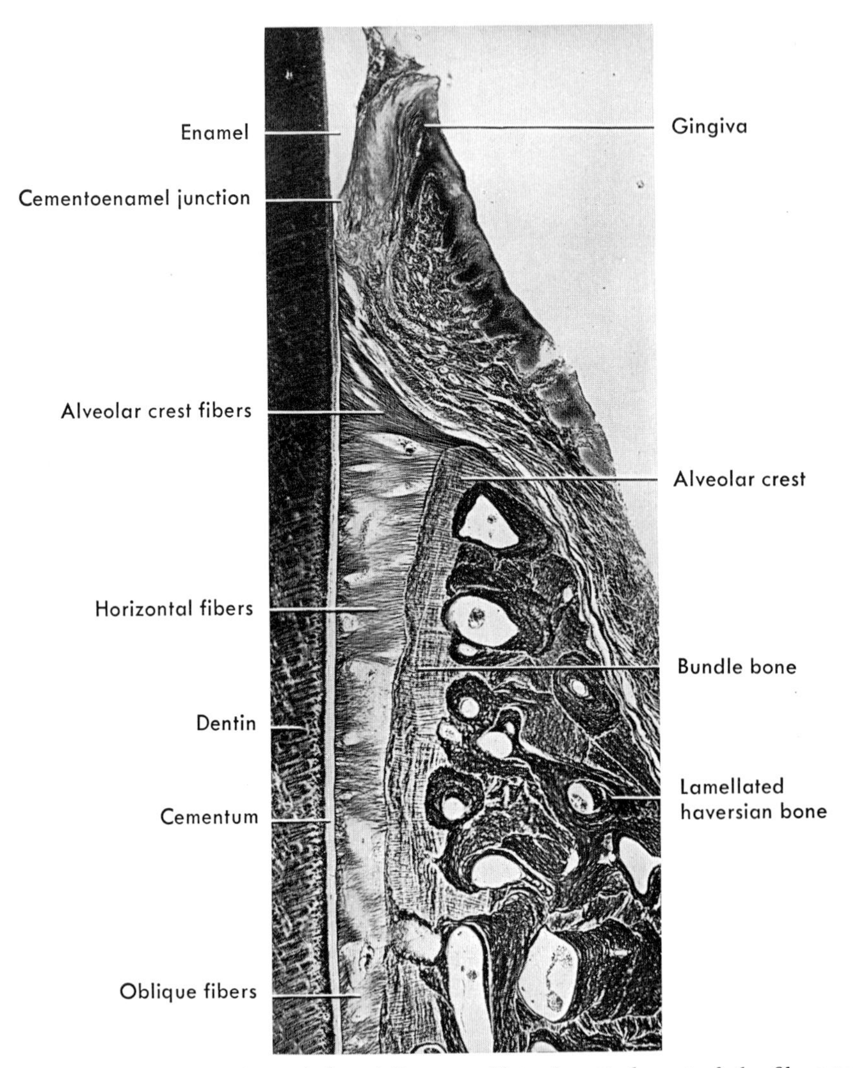


**Fig. 3-4.** Principal fibers of the periodontal ligament. Note the attachment of the fibers to the bone on one side and to the cementum on the other. Bundle bone with Sharpey's fibers is evident.

*Intermediate plexus*

The concept of an intermediate plexus arose from the observation of an apparent meeting of the alveolar and cemental fibers near the center of the ligament. Sicher and Orban believed that a splicing and unsplicing in the region of the intermediate plexus permitted the rearrangement of fibers during eruptive and migratory tooth movements.[3-5]

Once the tooth has erupted into clinical occlusion, however, such an intermediate plexus is no longer demonstrable. The principal fiber bundles become thickened and apparently continuous.[1,6,7]

## Organization and function

*Principal fibers*

The periodontal ligament contains collagen fibers, which are inserted on one side in the cementum and on the other side in the alveolar bone (Fig. 3-3). These

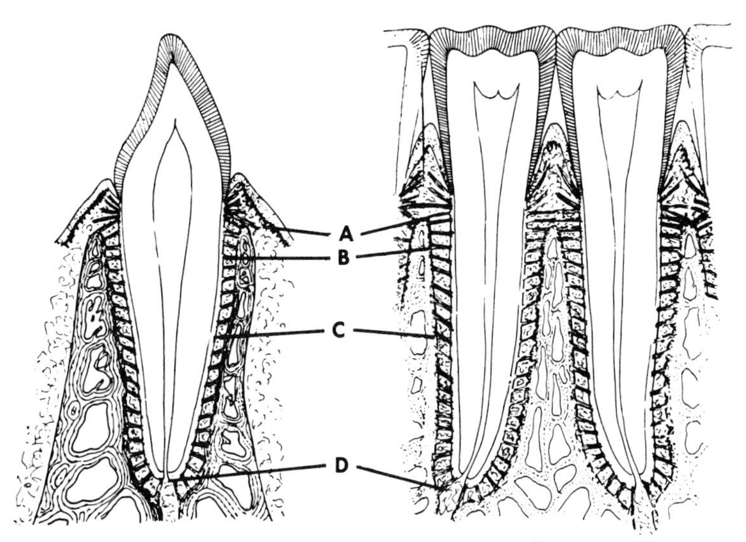


**Fig. 3-5.** Diagram of the principal fiber groups of the periodontal ligament: *A,* Alveolar crest fibers; *B,* horizontal fibers; *C,* oblique fibers; *D,* apical fibers. The oblique fibers are the largest group, followed in order by the apical, horizontal, and alveolar crest groups. (Adapted from Schour, I.: Noyes' oral histology and embryology, ed. 8, Philadelphia, 1960, Lea & Febiger.)

fibers are organized into groups called the principal fiber bundles, which can be distinguished by their prevalent direction[8] (Figs. 3-4 and 3-5):

1. *Alveolar crest group.* The fiber bundles of this group radiate from the crest of the alveolar process and are attached to the cervical part of the cementum.
2. *Horizontal group.* The bundles of this group run at right angles to the long axis of the tooth, from the cementum to the bone.
3. *Oblique group.* The bundles run obliquely and are attached in the cementum somewhat apical from their attachment to the bone. These fiber bundles are most numerous and constitute the main support of the tooth against masticatory forces.
4. *Apical group.* The bundles are irregularly arranged and radiate from the apical region of the root to the surrounding bone (Figs. 3-5 and 3-6).
5. *Interradicular group.* This group courses over the crest of the interradicular septum in the furcations of multirooted teeth, connecting the roots and are commonly called transseptal fibers.

Although the principal fiber bundles run from the cementum to the bone, their direction is not just radial. The paths of the various groups can be somewhat tangential[9] and may cross each other[10-13] (Fig. 3-3, *E*). In this manner the fibers seem to reinforce one another and to be better suited for supporting the tooth (Fig. 3-7).

The arrangement and direction of the fiber bundles are related to the stage of eruption and the height of the alveolar crest[2,10] (Fig. 3-2). The course of the bundles and of the individual collagen fibrils, which are submicroscopic, is wavy[14] (Fig. 3-7).

***Sharpey's fibers***

The ends of the collagen fibers embedded in the cementum and the bone are called Sharpey's fibers[15] (Figs. 3-4 and 3-7).

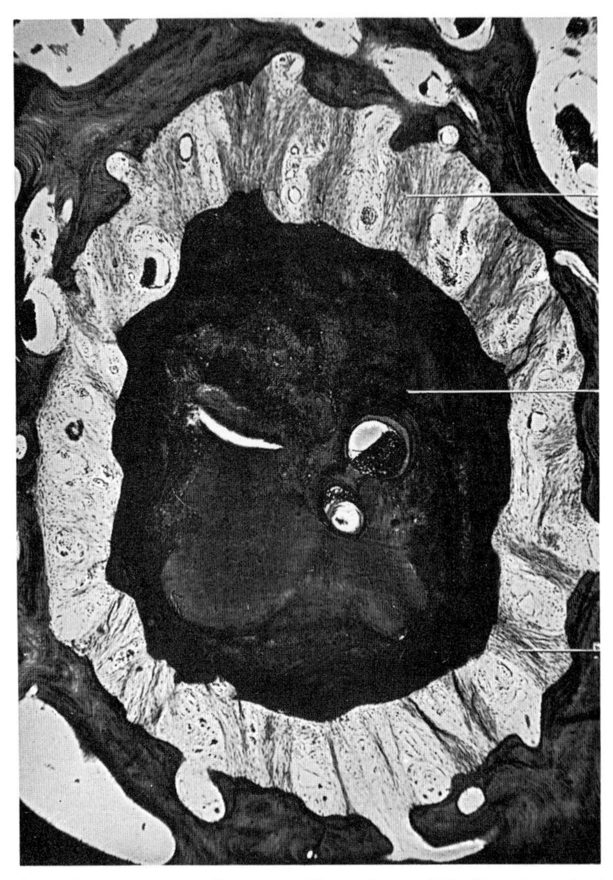

Fig. 3-6. Cross section of a root near the apex. Note the radial direction of the principal fibers in the horizontal plane. Some course tangentially and interweave at different levels, making for stronger support. (From Orban, B.: Dental histology and embryology, ed. 2, Philadelphia, 1929, P. Blakiston's Son & Co.; used by permission of McGraw-Hill Book Co.)

***Influence of function***

The width of the periodontal ligament varies with the age of the person and with the functional demands made on the tooth.[16] The number and thickness of the periodontal fiber bundles also vary according to functional demand.[16,17] In a tooth in functional occlusion, the periodontal ligament is about 0.25 ± 0.1 mm. wide. It is narrowest at the center of the alveolus and widest at the margin and the apex. Thus it possesses an hourglass shape.

In between the fiber bundles are fibroblasts, and adjacent to the cementum and bone are cementoblasts and osteoblasts respectively. Blood vessels and nerves are present in the ligament. These are surrounded by looser, unorganized connective tissue fibers known as the indifferent fibers.

***Collagenolysis and collagen synthesis***

The connective tissue cells of the periodontium synthesize collagen[18,19] (Fig. 3-8). They also possess collagenolytic activity and are, in addition, able to resorb bone and cementum. They are thus able to replace fibers of the ligament. The synthesis of collagen occurs at a very rapid rate in the periodontal tissues[14,20] and takes place throughout the periodontium. The synthetic and lytic activities permit the tooth to adapt by positional change to such demands as eruption, growth, wear, and various functional factors.[21] The periodontium re-

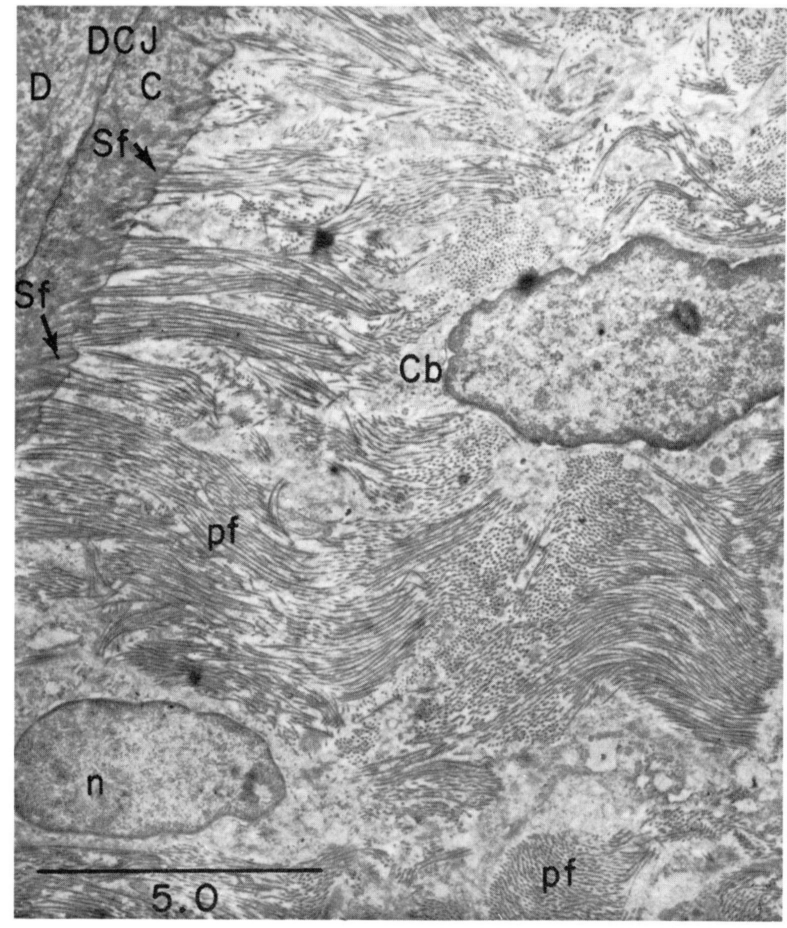


**Fig. 3-7.** Electron micrograph of periodontal fibrils, *pf*, of a rat shown inserting into cementum, *C*. Note the wavy course of the fibrils. Two cementoblasts are evident, *Cb*, as are their nuclei, *n*. *D* indicates the dentin; *DCJ*, the dentinocemental junction; *Sf*, Sharpey's fibrils (so called because they are the ends of the submicroscopic periodontal fibrils embedded in cementum). (From Stern, I. B.: Amer. J. Anat. 115:377, 1964.)

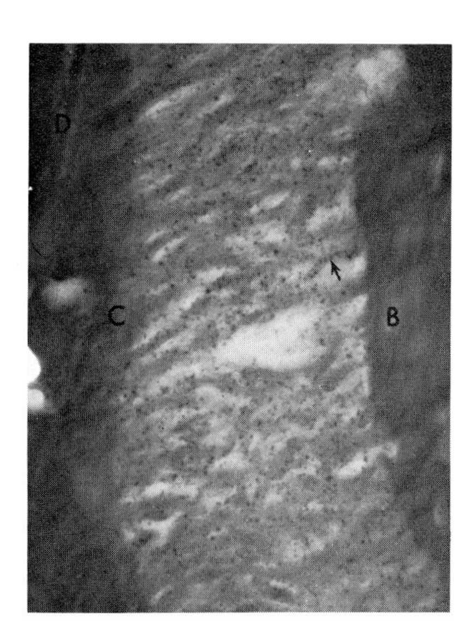


**Fig. 3-8.** Radioautograph of periodontal ligament of a rat molar. The section is stained with Van Gieson's stain, which demonstrates fibers but not cells. This animal was injected with tritiated proline. Silver grains represent sites at which the tritiated proline was incorporated. Proline is a collagen precursor. Thus this micrograph demonstrates proline uptake and hence new collagen synthesis throughout the ligament. *B*, Bone; *C*, cementum; *D*, dentin. (Courtesy R. Stallard, Boston.)

sponds in a similar fashion to damage. Structural changes induced by changes in function or because of periodontitis will be discussed in Chapters 12 and 33.

The concept of the intermediate plexus and its role in mediating eruptive and migratory tooth movements has been mentioned. Since radioisotopic studies suggest that new fibrils may be incorporated into preexisting fibers or form new fibers and since the synthesis and lysis of collagen within the periodontal ligament can occur rapidly, it may be unnecessary to postulate a mechanical arrangement such as a persisting intermediate plexus to explain the movement of teeth.[6,7,10,12-14]

***Oxytalan fibers***

In addition to the principal and the indifferent fibers, the periodontal ligament contains oxytalan fibers.[22-27] These course at right angles to the principal fibers; nevertheless, they anchor in cementum and bone.[28] They may be elastic, for they resemble elastin on the ultrastructural level. In fact, elastin has been reported in the periodontal ligament.[29] The fibers are of unknown function, and their existence as a separate entity is controversial.

***Epithelial rests***

The loose connective tissue between the fiber bundles of the periodontal ligament also has embedded epithelial structures. These are found close to the surface of the cementum and are called Malassez's epithelial rests. They are remnants of Hertwig's epithelial root sheath. The epithelial aggregates are really continuous and form a latticelike network around the root.[30,31] These cells may have a special function; they are viable and metabolically active[32-36] and have been reported to be more numerous in youngsters than in adults.[37-39] Evidence has been presented to indicate that this network of rests may be continuous with the reduced enamel epithelium before eruption and with the attachment epithelium after eruption.[40,41]

## Vascularization and innervation

The blood supply to the periodontal ligament comes from the branches of the alveolar arteries that penetrate the alveolar septa via nutrient canals. These may be seen in roentgenograms of the lower anterior teeth (Fig. 3-9). Some branches may extend from the pulpal vessels before they enter the tooth;

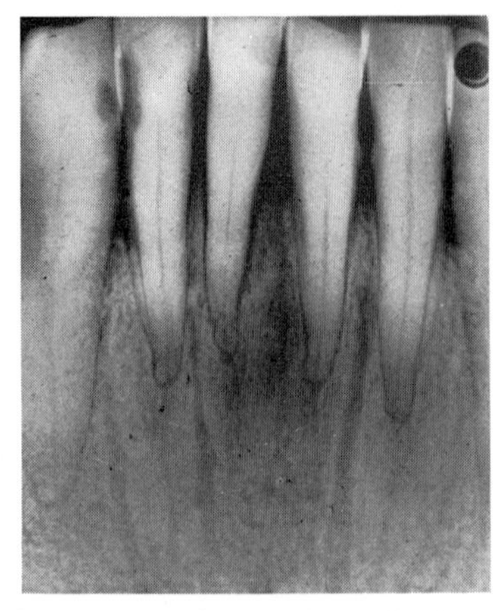

**Fig. 3-9.** Roentgenogram showing the vascular canals in the interdental alveolar septa. In this instance there has been some bone loss.

other branches may come down into the ligament from the gingiva. The circulation of the periodontal ligament will be discussed in greater detail in the section on alveolar bone.

Mechanoreceptive nerve impulses originate in the periodontal ligament and influence the functioning of the muscles of mastication. These impulses are of great importance in coordinating the movements of the masticatory muscles[42-44] and also in providing feedback mechanisms that prevent too forceful a closure of the jaws with consequent damage to the periodontium.

## CEMENTUM

### Function

Cementum is a specialized, calcified connective tissue that covers the surface of the anatomic root of the tooth. Its main function is to attach the fibers of the periodontal ligament to the surface of the tooth (Figs. 3-3, *D* and *E*, 3-4, and 3-7).

Gottlieb has suggested that continuous cementum apposition is necessary for the maintenance of a healthy periodontium.[45]

### Formation

The cementum begins to form during the early stages of root formation. Hertwig's epithelial root sheath is perforated by precementoblasts, which differ morphologically from the other fibroblasts of the periodontal ligament.[46] These cells come to lie adjacent to the dentin and lay down the first layer of cementum (primary cementum).[47-49] At this stage they have become functional cementoblasts. Formation of cementum continues by the deposition of successive layers of cementum.

The width of cementum of healthy teeth increases throughout life. This increase in width is greatest at the apex of the root and least at the most coronal regions of the cementum.[50] In general, cementum apposition increases in a straight-line relationship with age in healthy teeth. The cementum of periodontally diseased teeth, on the other hand, does not increase equally.[51] Moreover, resorption seems to occur with more frequency in periodontally involved teeth.[52]

### Primary and secondary cementum

Cementum may be classified as primary or secondary. Initial cementogenesis is completed when the root becomes fully formed and Hertwig's sheath has been expended. The initially deposited or primary cementum is acellular and is relatively afibrillar although it does contain fine fibers extending radially from the dentin to the surface.[14] Subsequent progressive depositions of cementum over the primary layer are referred to as secondary cementum (Fig. 3-10). These depositions may form one or more strata. Secondary cementum may be cellular or acellular; and it contains numerous embedded collagen fibers,[14] thus resembling fibrous bundle bone.

Whether the cementum is cellular or acellular does not seem to have significance, except that the cellular type forms where the cementum is thickest. Secondary *cellular* cementum is formed primarily at the apical third of the root whereas *acellular* cementum is formed in the coronal two thirds.

***Cementoid***

The surface of the secondary cementum is covered by the most recently formed layer that is as yet uncalcified (cementoid) (Fig. 3-11). When this layer calcifies, it in turn is covered by a newly formed cementoid layer.

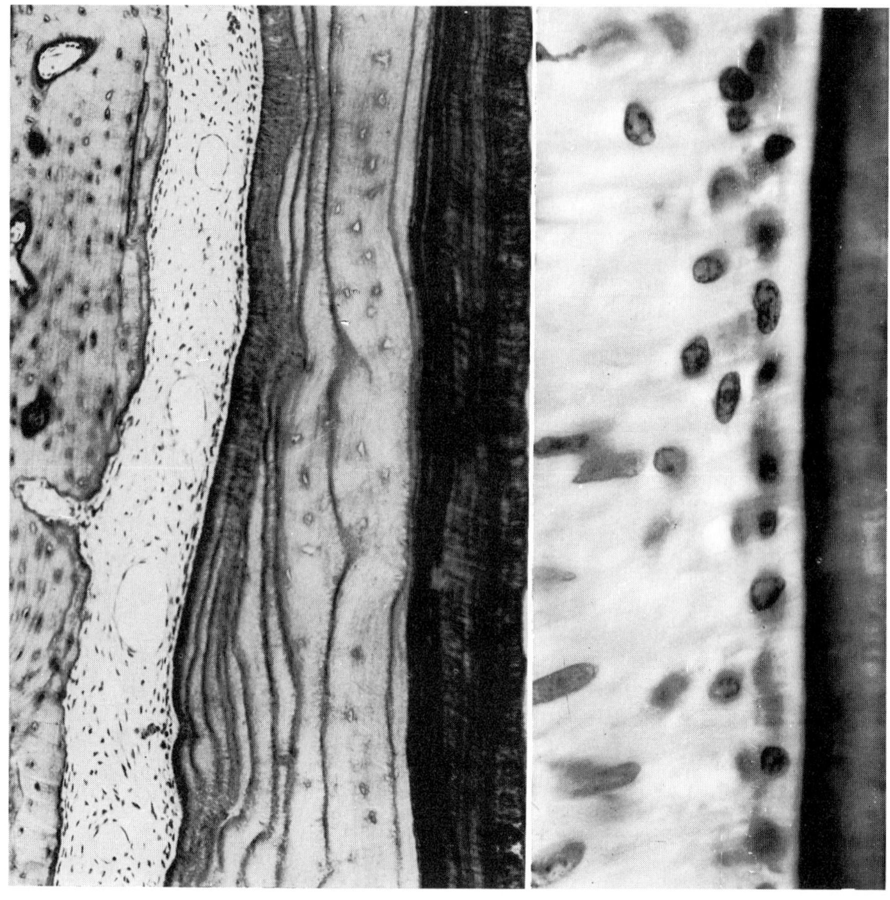

Fig. 3-10 Fig. 3-11

**Fig. 3-10.** Secondary cellular cementum in this micrograph is sandwiched between a base and an outer coat of acellular cementum. It has a lamellar arrangement like that of bundle bone. **Fig. 3-11.** Cementoblasts on the surface of uncalcified cementum (cementoid).

***Exposed cementum***

If vital secondary cementum is resorbed or nicked in surgical procedures, the defect is repaired by the deposition of new cementum. This cannot occur where pockets are present or where the gingiva has receded and the cementum is exposed. Cementum that has become exposed, forming part of the clinical crown, is often completely removed in the course of scaling or root planing.

***Cementocytes***

If the secondary cementum is cellular, it contains cementocytes, which lie in lacunae (Fig. 3-10) much like osteocytes in bone. This cementum thus resembles bone in many respects. Like bone it consists of collagen fibers and hydroxyapatite. Resorption does not occur to any significant extent under normal conditions.[53-55] It forms by intermittent yet continuous deposition of new layers.[50] This main difference between cementum and bone is of extreme importance in understanding alterations in tooth position.

***Cementum resorption***

One may say in comparing the two tissues that cementum, unlike bone, is relatively spared from resorption[55]; yet cementocytes do have cementolytic capability, and in this respect they resemble osteocytes and periosteal cells, which have osteolytic activity.[14,46,56]

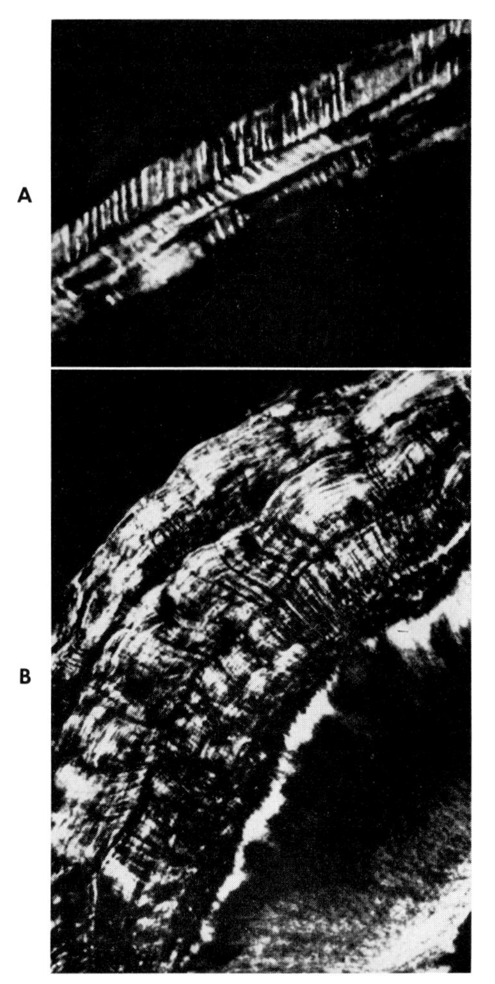


**Fig. 3-12. A,** Individual strata of the cementum are clearly demarcated by the difference in the angular course of the Sharpey's fibers. **B,** Three layers of parallel fibered cellular cementum are shown. The radially coursing Sharpey's fibers are also obvious, as are the differences of their angulations in the various strata. (Courtesy A. Faller and P. Schmid, Fribourg.)

Bélanger used $^3$H-thymidine as a marker for cementoctyes of rat molar cementum. Labeled cells migrated from the surface to the dentinocemental border within 3 days, indicating that cementum may have a rapid turnover rate comparable to that of trabecular bone.[56]

***Sharpey's fibers in cementum***

As has been pointed out, the collagen fiber bundles of the periodontal ligament enter cementum and bone. Their embedded portions are called Sharpey's fibers. Their path is best observed by polarization microscopy[57-61] (Fig. 3-12) or electron microscopy.[14,46,47,56,62]

On the basis of such studies, parallel bundles of fibers may be seen in cementum, differing slightly in their course in each stratum. The conclusion drawn is that the difference in paths marks a different eruptive or migrational position of the tooth (Figs. 3-12 and 3-13). It has been suggested that the collagen fibers function best in supporting the tooth when they extend at approximately right angles from the tooth surface. Shifting of tooth position may provoke the depo-

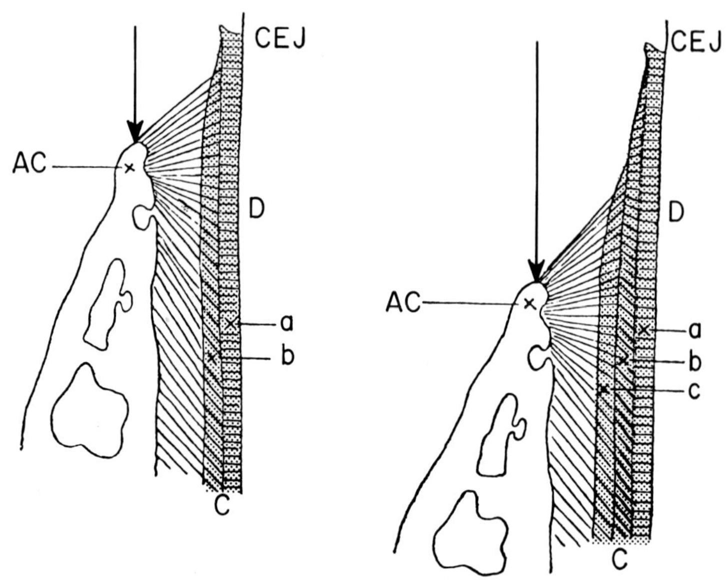


**Fig. 3-13.** Diagrammatic representation of cementum deposition after changes in tooth position caused by eruptive movement. The course of Sharpey's fibers in the cementum is dependent on their course in the prior tooth positions. Labels *a, b,* and *c* represent successive layers of cementum, *C; AC* is the alveolar crest; *D,* the dentin; *CEJ,* the cementoenamel junction. As the tooth erupts (arrows indicating the degree of eruption from *x*), the course of the fibers in strata *a* and *b* is unchanged and a new stratum of cementum, *c,* is laid down to embed Sharpey's fibers in the cementum according to the new position of the tooth. The same type of alteration occurs when the tooth position shifts in a horizontal plane.[57] (Modified from Egli, A. R.: Schweiz. Mschr. Zahnheilk. **56**:23, 1946.)

sition of a new stratum of secondary cementum to embed the fibers at the appropriate angle. The paths of the embedded fibers in the different strata of secondary cementum seem to bear this contention out[57,58] (Fig. 3-12).

***Cemental projections***

On a grosser level the surface of cementum is seen to contain projections.[63-64] These projections may be formed as a result of functional pull transmitted via collagen fiber bundles. Much finer projections can be visualized by means of transmission electron microscopy[14,46,47,56,62] (Fig. 3-14) and scanning electron microscopy[65,66] (Fig. 3-15).

Rodent incisor cementum is perforated by individual or small bundles of periodontal fibrils[14,47] (Fig. 3-14). Human cementum has a much more dense arrangement of perforating (Sharpey's) fibers.[13] It also has an intrinsic collagenous fiber matrix.[46] The projecting Sharpey's fibers are believed to be mineralized,[65] but they may have unmineralized cores.[15,62] Regardless of the degree of calcification, the continuity of Sharpey's fibers and the periodontal ligament is of paramount concern since it serves to take up functional stresses and may be altered during eruptive and migrational tooth movement.

The number and diameter (density) of Sharpey's fibers vary with the functional status and health of a tooth[17] (Fig. 3-16). The mean diameter of a Sharpey's fiber bundle in a normal functioning tooth is approximately 4 $\mu$.[17]

***Cementum matrix***

Cemental or matrix collagen is fully calcified except for a narrow zone near the dentocemental junction.[67] This zone is 10 to 50 $\mu$ wide and is reported to be partially calcified. Some demineralization occurs in the cementum subjacent to

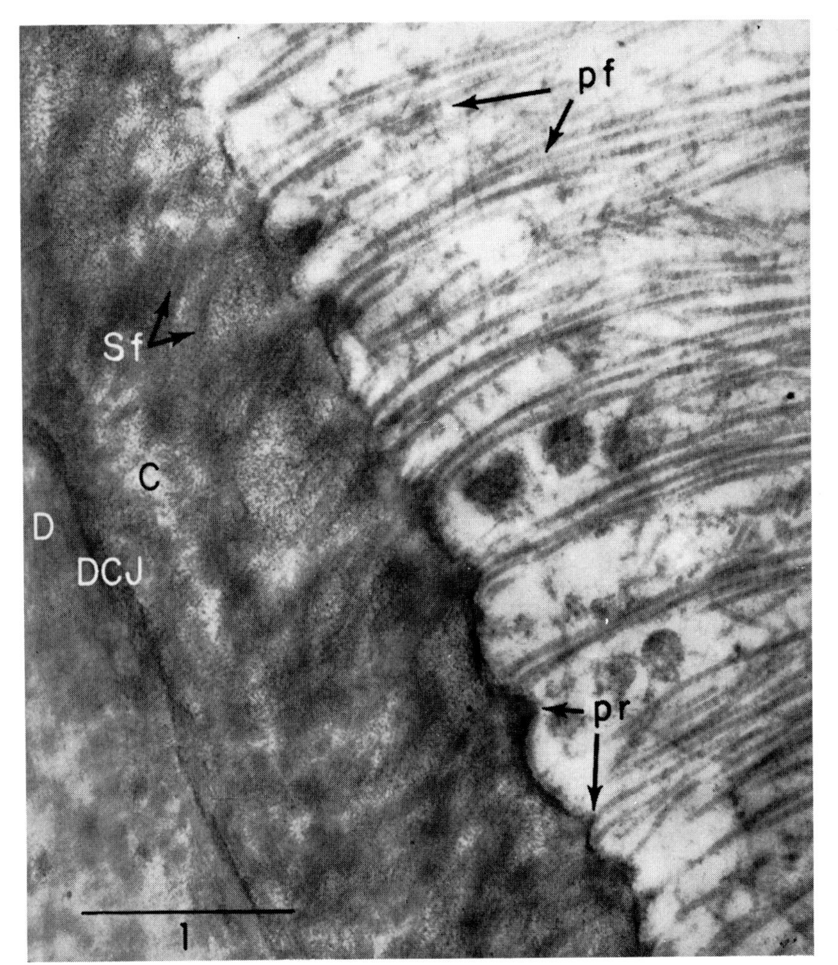


**Fig. 3-14.** Electron micrograph of a rat incisor. Periodontal fibrils, *pf*, are shown inserting into cementum, *C*, where they continue as Sharpey's fibrils, *Sf*. The dentin, *D*, and the dentinocemental junction, *DCJ*, are evident. Collagen fibrils show characteristic banding. Projections of the cementum, *pr*, form about the collagen fibrils. (From Stern, I. B.: Amer. J. Anat. 115:377, 1964.)

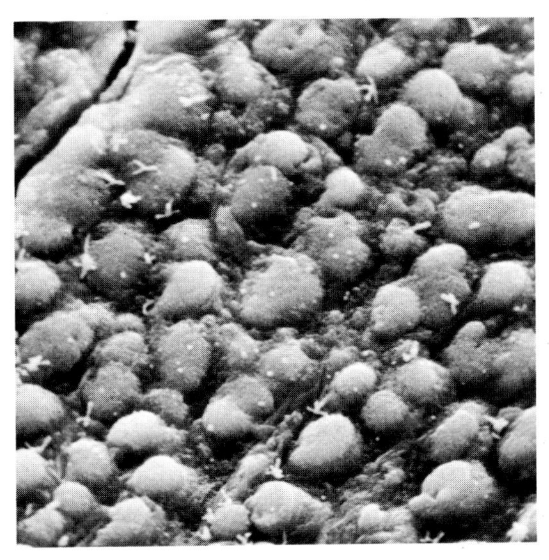

**Fig. 3-15.** Scanning electron microscopic view of human cemental surface. (Courtesy M. Landay, Philadelphia.)

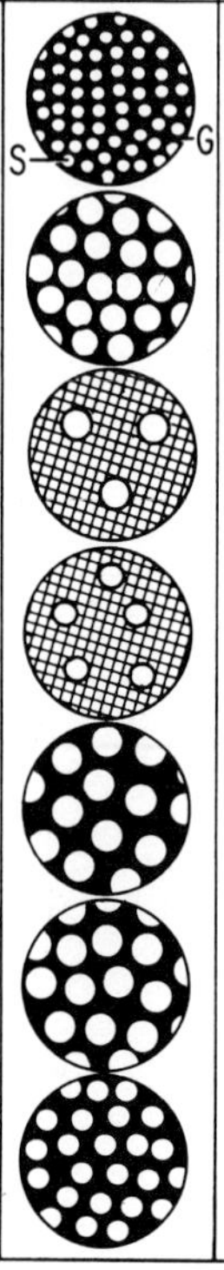

| Functional stage | Tangential section | Density / 1000 $\mu^2$ mean ± SD | Diameter, $\mu$ mean ±SD |
|---|---|---|---|
| Pre-eruptive and eruptive | S G | 53.4 ± 13.5 | 3.0 ± 0.02 |
| Normal functioning | | 28.0 ± 3.2 | 4.0 ± 0.3 |
| Completely embedded | | 2.1 ± 5.3 | 4.1 ± 0.3 |
| Excessive destruction of crown | | 5.5 ± 0.4 | 3.8 ± 0.4 |
| Fixed bridge abutment | | 21.3 ± 5.2 | 4.6 ± 0.6 |
| Remov. part. dent. abut. | | 17.0 ± 0.6 | 4.6 ± 0.6 |
| Excessive bone loss | | 20.0 ± 8.1 | 3.8 ± 0.03 |

**Fig. 3-16.** Density and diameter of Sharpey's fibers in the superficial layers of cementum. (Modified from Akiyoshi, M., and Inoue, M.: Bull. Tokyo Med. Dent. Univ. **10**:41, 1963.)

the pocket in the course of periodontal disease,[68] which may conceivably predispose to cemental caries.

Matrix collagen bundles are finer than Sharpey's fiber bundles (i.e., 2.46 versus 4 $\mu$).[17,69] In addition, cementum matrix fibers differ from osseous matrix fibers in size.[69]

There may be similar differences in the size of Sharpey's fiber bundles in cementum and bone[2,19] (Fig. 3-3, *E*). Moreover, there appears to be some biochemical difference between the two, which suggests that Sharpey's fibers in cementum are calcified whereas those in bone are not.[19]

## ALVEOLAR PROCESS

***Alveolar bone proper and supporting bone***

The alveolar process is that part of the maxilla or mandible forming and supporting the teeth. As a result of functional adaptation, two parts of the alveolar process may be distinguished, the alveolar bone proper and the supporting bone. The alveolar bone proper consists of a thin lamella of bone surrounding the root. Fibers of the periodontal ligament are attached to it (Fig. 3-17). The supporting bone surrounds the alveolar bone proper and acts as a support in its function. Supporting bone consists of (1) the compact cortical plates of the vestibular and oral surfaces of the alveolar processes and (2) the spongy bone found between these cortical plates and the alveolar bone proper.

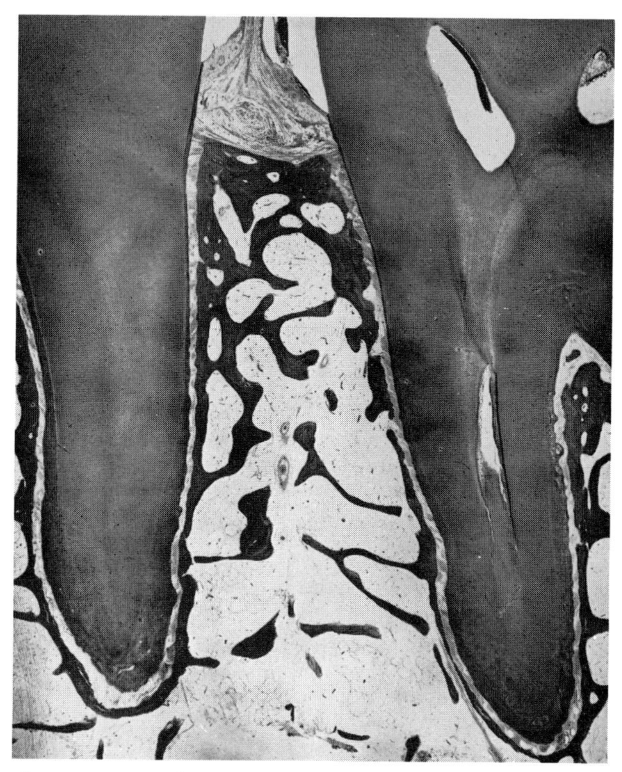

**Fig. 3-17.** Alveolar bone proper and the supporting (cancellous) bone form the alveolar process.

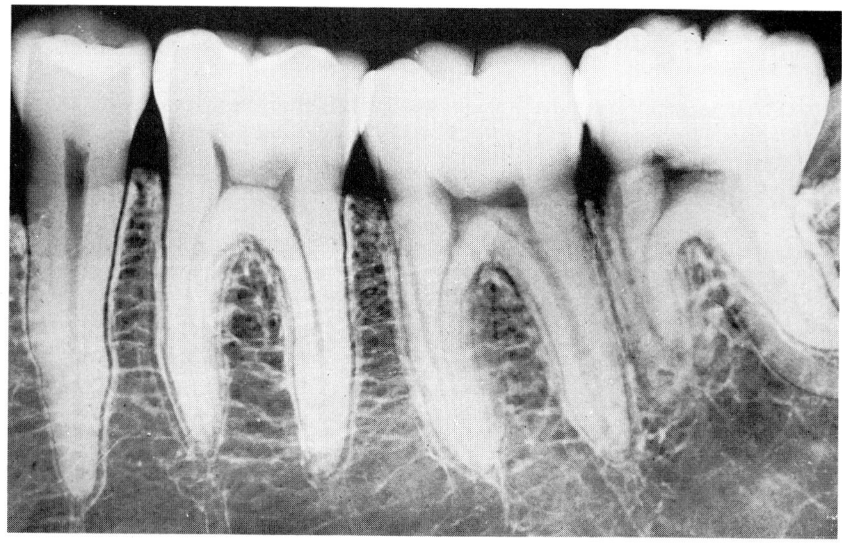

**Fig. 3-18.** Alveolar bone proper appears in the roentgenogram as a compact layer (lamina dura). The supporting bone is cancellous.

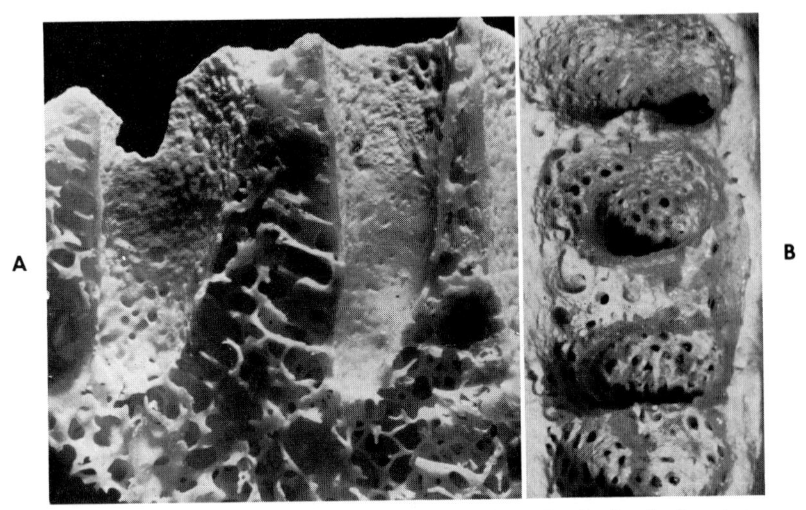


**Fig. 3-19. A,** Section of the alveolar bone of a human jaw. **B,** Occlusal view into two molar sockets. The wall of the tooth sockets (alveolar bone proper) is perforated, forming a cribriform plate. (**A** from the collection of J. B. Weinmann.)

*Lamina dura and cribriform plate*

In roentgenograms the alveolar bone proper (inner wall of the socket) appears as an opaque line called the lamina dura (Fig. 3-18). The alveolar bone proper is perforated by many openings through which the blood vessels and nerves of the periodontal ligament pass (Fig. 3-19). It is also called the cribriform plate because of these perforations.

The shape of the alveolar crest, under normal conditions, depends on the contour of the enamel of adjacent teeth (Fig. 3-20, *A*), the relative positions of the adjacent cementoenamel junctions (*B*), the degree of eruption of the teeth (*B*), the vertical positioning of the teeth (*C*), and the orovestibular width of the teeth[70] (*D*). In general, the bone about each tooth follows the contour of the cervical line.

## Function

The alveolar bone proper adapts itself to the functional demands of the teeth in a dynamic manner. It is formed for the express purpose of supporting the teeth, and after extraction it has a tendency to be reduced, as does the supporting bone.

## Anatomy

*Roentgenograms*

Roentgenograms of cross sections of the alveolar process (Fig. 3-21) show its cortical and cancellous portions. The cortical plates are generally thicker in the mandible. The cortical plates and the cancellous bone are also generally thicker on the oral aspects of the mandible and the maxilla, but there is individual variation.[71]

Anteriorly, along the vestibular aspect of the alveolar arch, is the depression of the incisive fossa, bordered distally by the cuspid eminences. Here the bone is thin and there may be little or no cancellous bone. Posteriorly, in the premolar and molar regions, the bone is thicker and cancellous bone separates the cortical plate from the alveolar bone proper.

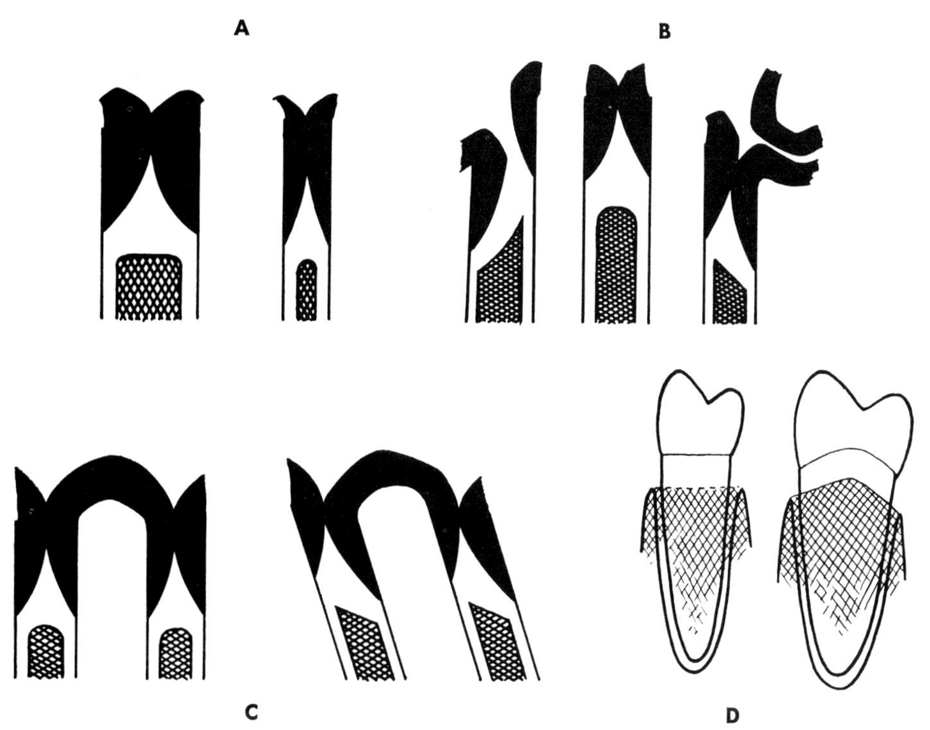


**Fig. 3-20.** Diagrammatic illustration of the variations in shape of the interdental alveolar crest, depending on the following anatomic features: **A,** Contour of the enamel and width of the interdental space. **B,** State of eruption. **C,** Position of the teeth. **D,** Shape of the cementoenamel junction and orovestibular width of the tooth.

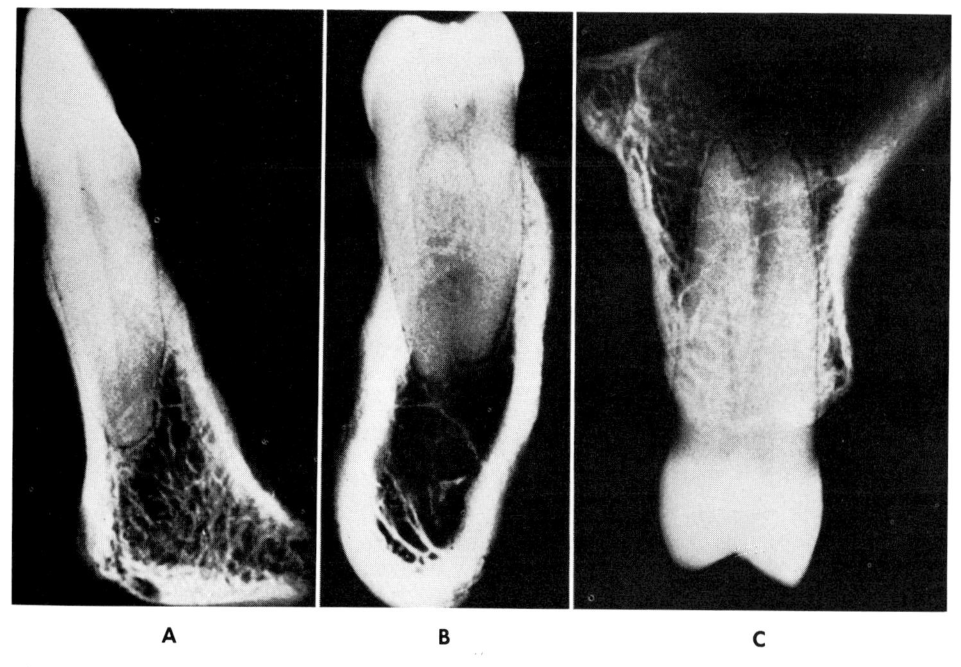


**Fig. 3-21. A,** Mandibular incisor. **B,** Mandibular molar. **C,** Maxillary premolar. (Courtesy J. Easley, Seattle.)

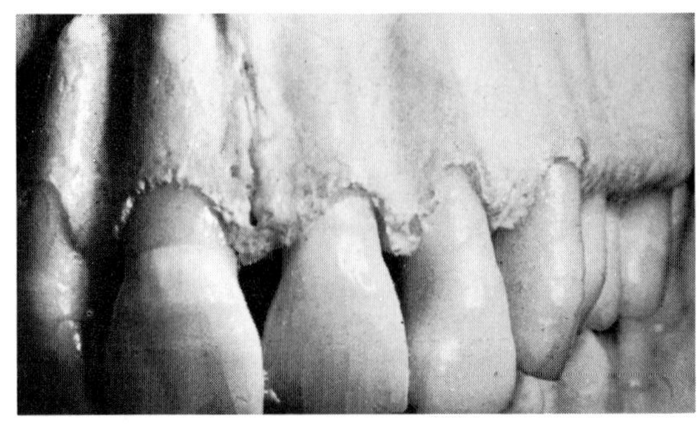

**Fig. 3-22.** Dried maxillary prominences over the roots and depressions between the roots. Note that these do not exist in the posterior region where the alveolar process is thick. (Courtesy J. Easley, Seattle.)

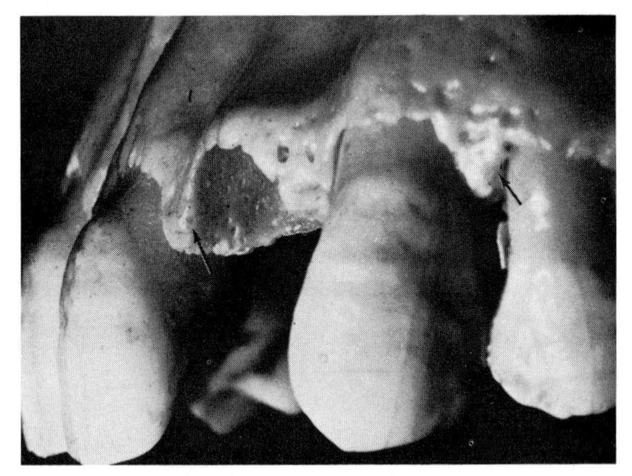

**Fig. 3-23.** Rounded margin of alveolar process (arrows). Note the fine edge on the vestibular surface of the canine. (Courtesy J. Easley, Seattle.)

***Thickness of the alveolar process***

Since the teeth are responsible for the alveolar process, its general form and shape follow the arrangement of the dentition. In addition, the thickness of the alveolar process has a direct bearing on external form.[72] When the alveolar process is thin, there are prominences over the roots and interdental depressions between the roots (Fig. 3-22). When the processes are thick, these prominences and depressions are lacking (Fig. 3-22).

***Alveolar crest***

The margin of the alveolar process is normally rounded or beaded (Fig. 3-23, arrows). However, occasionally the bone margin ends in a fine sharp edge. This occurs only when the bone is extremely thin, for example, on the vestibular surface of the canines (Fig. 3-23).

***Dehiscences and fenestrations***

Dehiscences and fenestrations are common defects in the alveolar process.[73-75] An alveolar dehiscence is a dipping of the crestal bone margin exposing an abnormal amount of root surface.[71,76-79] The defect may be wide and irregular and extend to the middle of the root or even farther (Fig. 3-24).

The alveolar fenestration is a circumscribed hole in the cortical plate over the root and does not communicate with the crestal margin (Fig. 3-24). It varies

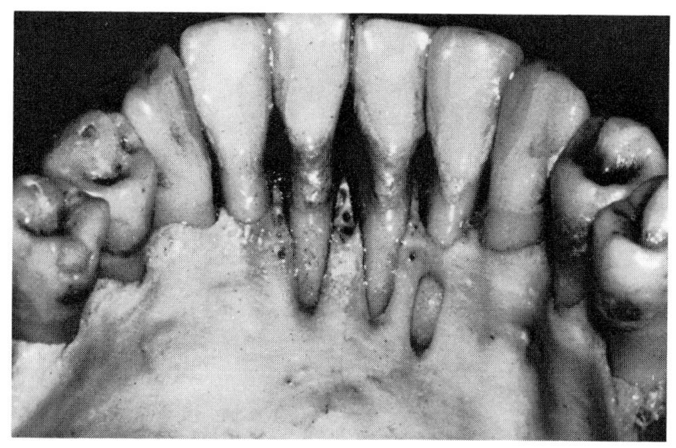

**Fig. 3-24.** Note the dehiscences and fenestration on the vestibular surface of the mandibular incisors. (Courtesy D. Keene, Daytona Beach.)

in size and can be located anywhere along the surface. These irregularities are sometimes found in the alveolus prior to tooth eruption and may represent variations in bone form as well as pathologic resorption.

*Tooth position and osseous form*

The variations of alveolar bone form about malpositioned teeth are so specific that one can predict the shape of the bone by noting the position of the tooth. When a tooth is prominent, the bone on the side of prominence will be thin and will be thick on the opposite side.

A variation of this condition arises when a tooth (e.g., a premolar) has rotated 90 degrees. In such a case the oral and vestibular aspects of the alveolar process will be relatively thick since the tooth is narrow mesiodistally.

Another form change that accompanies tooth malposition is the level of the crestal margin. Where a tooth is prominent, the margin will be located apical to its otherwise normal position. On the opposite side of the tooth, the margin will be in a more coronal position. When a tooth is in supraversion (extruded), the alveolar process may be more coronal than the processes of adjacent teeth.

*Contour of the lateral bone margin*

The contour of the crestal margin of the process is often described as scalloped, yet this is not always the case. The marginal contour varies with the shape of the root.[76] When a root surface is flat, the alveolar border is straight or flat. When the root surface is convex, the border is scalloped. If the root surface is concave, the bone margin may arch coronally. When the bone is thin, the scalloping is accentuated; and when the bone is thick, the scalloping is reduced.

*Form of the interdental septum*

The form of the interdental septum follows the alignment of adjacent cementoenamel junctions. In the posterior part of the mouth, the septa are relatively flat when viewed from the vestibule toward the oral cavity. The septa form peaks primarily in the anterior portion of the mouth. In general, the septa of the posterior teeth are thicker and possess more cancellous bone than the septa of the anterior teeth.

*Furcation defect*

When the bone in the interradicular area of a multirooted tooth is resorbed, it is called a bifurcation or trifurcation defect. These furcation defects are of importance in diagnosis and prognosis, and their treatment will be discussed in the section on furcation involvement.[80-83]

*Enamel projections*

Sometimes these furca defects are associated with enamel projections at the cementoenamel junction.[84-86]

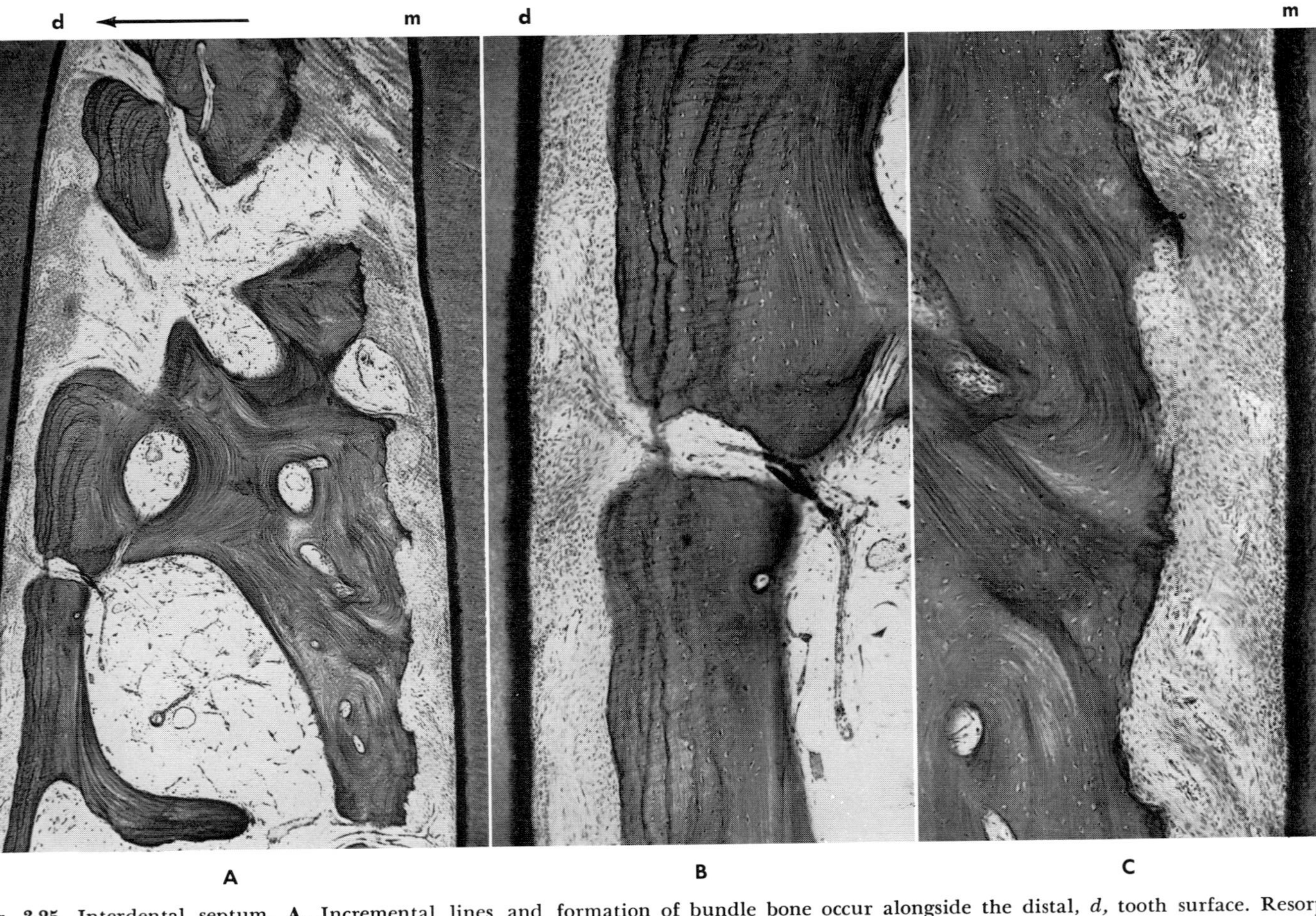


**Fig. 3-25.** Interdental septum. **A,** Incremental lines and formation of bundle bone occur alongside the distal, *d*, tooth surface. Resorption of lamellated bone has taken place alongside the mesial, *m*, surface of the adjacent tooth. This indicates the mesial direction of tooth drift (in the direction of the arrow). **B,** Higher magnification of the distal surface of the alveolar septum. **C,** Higher magnification of the mesial surface.

*Structure, function, and physiologic tooth migration*

The structure of alveolar bone proper varies, on different sides of the tooth, with different functional demands. Under physiologic conditions teeth migrate continuously in a mesial direction toward the midline. This is called physiologic mesial drift.[87] The migration leads to a resorption of the inner wall of the alveolus on the mesial side of the tooth and the formation of new bone on the distal surface. The resorption may be the result of mild compression of the periodontal ligament by the migrating tooth. New bone formation is caused by tension on the periodontal fibers on the distal surface (Fig. 3-25). The bone that is formed here is known as bundle bone because of the presence of Sharpey's fibers, which are fibers of the periodontal ligament embedded in the newly formed bone lamellae on the side of tension. The physiologic migration of teeth occurs both mesially and occlusally. This latter eruptive movement influences the structure of the alveolus, causing bone formation at both the alveolar fundus and the alveolar crest.

Physiologic tooth migration probably continues into old age. The alveolar bone adapts and reconstructs itself continuously. Pathologic changes occur when this process of adaptation is disturbed. Changes in function must result in a tissue response. (This will be discussed further in Chapter 36.)

The supporting bone also adapts itself to functional requirements. Bone is resorbed if functional requirements are reduced, and additional bone is formed if functional influences demand it. The loss of occlusal function will lead to a disuse atrophy of the supporting bone. Increased functional demands will produce denser bone (more bone per unit volume). On the other hand, demands beyond the physiologic tolerance of bone tissue will result in damage. The bone of the alveolar process is in a constant state of flux. It is influenced primarily by functional stimuli and also by systemic factors.

*Bone cells*

The changes in the bone structure are brought about by the activity of osteoblasts, which are capable of laying down new bone. Osteoclasts in the typical Howship's lacunae are capable of resorbing bone.

There are osteocytes within lacunae in the bone. Their long processes pass within canaliculi. These cells are capable of both osteoblastic and osteolytic activity.

*Haversian system*

Bone may be laid down in concentric lamellae about a central blood vessel. Such an arrangement is termed a haversian system. In a three-dimensional reconstruction the lamellae arranged circumferentially about the course of a vessel form a cylindric osteone.

Bone is covered by periosteum. The osteoblasts are arranged on the surface of the bone and may be separated from the bone by a layer of osteoid (uncalcified bone matrix). The alveolar process, which is not arranged in haversian systems, may be arranged as lamellar bundle bone (as in the alveolar bone proper). Bundle bone may be coarsely or finely woven.[87]

Bone consists of collagen fibers, ground substance, and hydroxyapatite crystals. When the bone is remodeled, the portion that is resorbed is completely lysed, both matrix and crystals, and the new bone consists of newly synthesized collagen and crystals.[89]

## Vitality of the bone

The blood supply to the alveolar bone comes from branches of the alveolar artery. The periosteal vessels run over the oral and vestibular plates of bone and contribute to the circulatory supply of the gingiva and the periodontal lig-

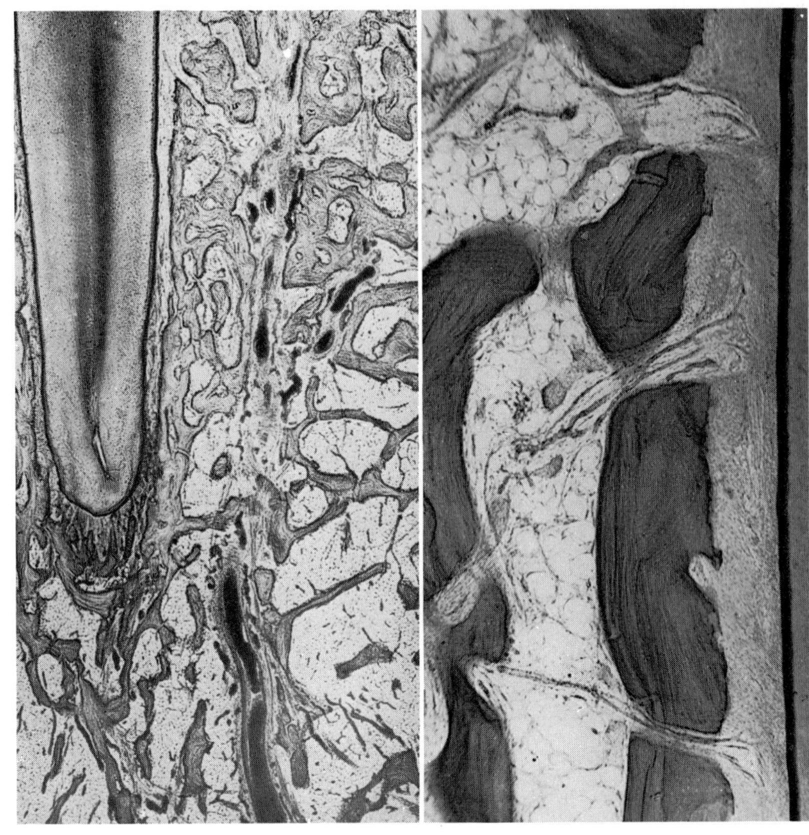

**Fig. 3-26** **Fig. 3-27**

**Fig. 3-26.** Histologic section showing vascular canals entering the interdental alveolar septum. (From Harndt, E.: Paradentitis und Paradentose, Munich, 1950, Carl Hanser Verlag.)
**Fig. 3-27.** Blood vessels enter the periodontal ligament through openings in the alveolar bone.

ament. The major supply comes from the alveolar vessels that pass up the center of the alveolar septum (Fig. 3-26), sending branches laterally from the marrow spaces, and via canals through the cribriform plate to the periodontal ligament[90] (Fig. 3-27). The interdental vessel passes upward to supply the septum and the interdental papilla. In the periodontal ligament the vessels generally take a longitudinal course[91] (Fig. 3-28). The physiology and pathology of the vascular supply to the periodontium are of major importance to the understanding and therapy of periodontal pathology.

Recent studies suggest that in rodent molars periodontal fibers pass completely through the alveolar septal bone to insert into the cementum of the adjacent teeth.[15,92] The tooth and its investing tissues (periodontal ligament, bone, cementum) constitute a developmental and functional entity.[93] Rates of turnover of periodontal ligament and cementum are surprisingly rapid.[18,19,46] The rate of alveolar bone remodeling also seems to be more rapid than that of other bones.[94] The organization into cementum, periodontal ligament, and alveolar bone appears to be a matter of inductive organizational influences since ankylosis rarely occurs. The suggestion has been made that the periodontal liga-

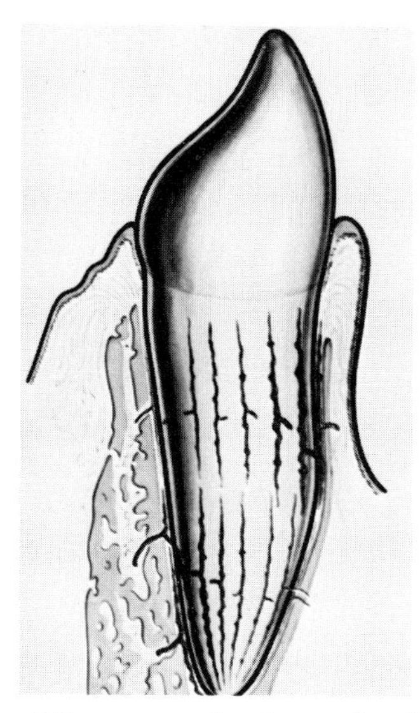

**Fig. 3-28.** Vessels in the periodontal ligament tend to have a longitudinal course. (From Fröhlich, E.: Deutsch. Zahnaerztl. Z. **19:**153, 1964.)

ment possesses some inhibitory quality in this regard.[95] Certainly the periodontal ligament, cementum, and alveolar bone comprise a structure with a function and biology unique among the ligaments and joints of the body.

**CHAPTER 3**

**References**


1. Grant, D. A., and Bernick, S.: The formation of the periodontal ligament, J. Periodont. **43:** 17, 1972.
2. Grant, D. A., and others: Studies on the biology of the periodontium of marmosets. XI. A comparative study of the development of the periodontal ligament in teeth with and without predecessors, J. Periodont. **43:**162, 1972.
3. Sicher, H.: Bau und Funktion des Fixationsapparates der Meerschweinchenmolaren, Z. Stomat. **21:**580, 1923.
4. Sicher, H.: The principal fibers of the periodontal membrane, Bur **55:**2, 1954.
5. Sicher, H., and Bhaskar, S. N., editors: Orban's oral histology and embryology, ed. 7, St. Louis, 1972, The C. V. Mosby Co.
6. Zwarych, P. D., and Quigley, M. B.: The intermediate plexus of the periodontal ligament: history and further observations, J. Dent. Res. **44:**383, 1965.
7. Ciancio, S. C., Neiders, M. E., and Hazen, S. P.: The principal fibers of the periodontal ligament, Periodontics **5:**76, 1967.
8. Black, G. V.: Special dental pathology, Chicago, 1915, Medico-Dental Publishing Co.
9. Erausquin, J.: Histologia dentaria humana, Buenos Aires, 1953, Progrental.
10. Levy, B. M., and Bernick, S.: Studies on the biology of the periodontium of marmosets. II. Development and organization of the periodontal ligament of deciduous teeth in marmosets (Callithrix jacchus), J. Dent. Res. **47:**27, 1968.
11. Wetzel, W.: Zur funktionellen Struktur des Parodontiums einiger Säuger, Stoma **20:**91, 1967.
12. Zampighi, G.: The arrangement of bundles of collagen fibers in rat normal periodontal ligament. Electron microscopic study, J. Microscop. **7:**1081, 1968.
13. Bevelander, G., and Nakahara, H.: The fine structure of the human peridental ligament, Anat. Rec. **162:**313, 1968.
14. Stern, I. B.: An electron microscopic study of the cementum, Sharpey's fibers and periodontal ligament in the rat incisor, Amer. J. Anat. **115:**377, 1964.
15. Quigley, M. B.: Perforating (Sharpey's) fibers of the periodontal ligament and bone, Alabama J. Med. Sci. **7:**336, 1970.

16. Coolidge, E. D.: The thickness of the human periodontal membrane, J. Amer. Dent. Ass. **24**:1260, 1937.
17. Akiyoshi, M., and Inoue, M.: On the functional structure of cementum, Bull. Tokyo Med. Dent. Univ. **10**:41, 1963.
18. Carneiro, J., and Fava de Moraes, F.: Radioautographic visualization of collagen metabolism in the periodontal tissues of the mouse, Arch. Oral Biol. **10**:833, 1965.
19. Anderson, A. A.: The protein matrices of the teeth and periodontium in hamsters. A tritiated proline study, J. Dent. Res. **46**:67, 1967.
20. Fullmer, H. M., and others: The origin of collagenase in periodontal tissues of man, J. Dent. Res. **48**:686, 1969.
21. Kraw, A. G., and Enlow, D. H.: Continuous attachment of the periodontal membrane, Amer. J. Anat. **120**:133, 1967.
22. Fullmer, H. M., and Lillie, R. D.: The oxytalan fiber. A previously undescribed connective tissue fiber, J. Histochem. Cytochem. **6**:425, 1958.
23. Fullmer, H. M.: A critique of normal connective tissues of the periodontium and some alterations with periodontal disease, J. Dent. Res. vol. 41, supp., 1962.
24. Rannie, I.: Observations on the oxytalan fibre of the periodontal membrane. European Orthodontic Society report, 39th Congress, 1963.
25. Kohl, J., and Zander, H. A.: Fibres conjunctives oxytalan dans le tissue gingival interdentaire, Parodontologie **1**:23, 1962.
26. Fullmer, H. M.: Histochemical studies of the periodontium, J. Dent. Res. **45**:469, 1966.
27. Griffin, C. J., and Harris, R.: The fine structure of the developing human periodontium, Arch. Oral Biol. **12**:971, 1967.
28. Goggins, J. F.: The distribution of oxytalan connective tissue fibers in periodontal ligaments of deciduous teeth, Periodontics **4**:182, 1966.
29. Haim, J., and Baumgärtel, R.: Altersveränderungen im Periodont (Desmodont), Deutsch. Zahnaerztl. Z. **23**:340, 1968.
30. Von Brunn, A.: Ueber die Ausdehnung des Schmelzorganes und seine Bedeutung für die Zahnbildung, Arch. Mikrosk. Anat. **29**:367, 1887.
31. Orban, B.: The epithelial network in the periodontal membrane, J. Amer. Dent. Ass. **44**: 632, 1952.
32. Valderhaug, J. P., and Nylen, M. U.: Function of epithelial rests as suggested by their ultrastructure, J. Periodont. Res. **1**:69, 1966.
33. Trowbridge, H. O., and Shibata, F.: Mitotic activity in epithelial rests of Malassez, Periodontics **5**:109, 1967.
34. Ten Cate, A. R.: The histochemical demonstration of specific oxidative enzymes and glycogen in the epithelial cell rests of Malassez, Arch. Oral Biol. **10**:207, 1965.
35. Grupe, H. E., Jr., Ten Cate, A. R., and Zander, H. A.: A histochemical and radiobiologic study of *in vitro* and *in vivo* human epithelial cell rest proliferation, Arch. Oral Biol. **12**: 1321, 1967.
36. Kvam, E., and Gilhuus-Moe, O.: Uptake of $^{3}$H-thymidine by an epithelial rest in the periodontal membrane. A preliminary report, Acta Odont. Scand. **28**:143, 1970.
37. Reitan, K.: Behavior of Malassez' epithelial rests during orthodontic tooth movement, Acta Odont. Scand. **19**:443, 1961.
38. Simpson, H. E.: The degeneration of the rests of Malassez with age as observed by the apoxestic technique, J. Periodont. **36**:288, 1965.
39. Reeve, C. M., and Wentz, F. M.: The prevalence, morphology and distribution of epithelial rests in the human periodontal ligament, Oral Surg. **15**:785, 1962.
40. Grant, D. A., and Bernick, S.: A possible continuity between epithelial rests and epithelial attachment in miniature swine, J. Periodont. **40**:87, 1969.
41. Diab, M. A., Stallard, R. E., and Zander, H. A.: The life cycle of the epithelial elements of the developing molar, Oral Surg. **22**:241, 1966.
42. Sicher, H.: Biologic significance of the hinge axis determination, J. Prosth. Dent. **6**:616, 1956.
43. Ramfjord, S. P., and Ash, M. M.: Occlusion, ed. 2, Philadelphia, 1971, W. B. Saunders Co.
44. Bernick, S., and Levy, B. M.: Studies on the biology of the periodontium of marmosets. IV. Innervation of the periodontal ligament, J. Dent. Res. **47**:1158, 1968.
45. Gottlieb, B.: A new concept of periodontoclasia, J. Periodont. **17**:7, 1946.
46. Jande, S. S., and Bélanger, L. F.: Fine structural study of rat molar cementum, Anat. Rec. **167**:439, 1970.

47. Selvig, K. A.: Electron microscopy of Hertwig's epithelial sheath and of early dentin and cementum formation in the mouse incisor, Acta Odont. Scand. **21**:175, 1963.
48. Shibata, F., and Stern, I. B.: Hertwig's epithelial sheath in the rat incisor: histologic study, J. Periodont. Res. **2**:227, 1967.
49. Freeman, E., and Ten Cate, A. R.: Development of the periodontium: an electron microscopic study, J. Periodont. **42**:387, 1971.
50. Zander, H. A., and Hürzeler, B.: Continuous cementum apposition, J. Dent. Res. **37**:1035, 1958.
51. Hürzeler, B., and Zander, H. A.: Cementum apposition in periodontally diseased teeth, Helv. Odont. Acta **3**:1, 1959.
52. Harvey, B. L. C., and Zander, H. A.: Root surface resorption of periodontally diseased teeth, Oral Surg. **12**:1439, 1959.
53. Kronfeld, R.: Spielt die Qualität der Hartsubstanzen bei der Resorption eine Rolle? Z. Stomat. **25**:1099, 1927.
54. Henry, J. L., and Weinmann, J. P.: The pattern of resorption and repair of human cementum, J. Amer. Dent. Ass. **42**:270, 1951.
55. Kerr, D. A.: The cementum: its role in periodontal health and disease, J. Periodont. **32**: 183, 1961.
56. Bélanger, L. F.: Resorption of cementum by cementocyte activity (cementolysis), Calcif. Tissue Res. **2**:229, 1968.
57. Gustafson, A. G., and Persson, P. A.: The relationship between the direction of Sharpey's fibers and the deposition of cementum, Odont. T. **65**:457, 1957.
58. Egli, A. R.: Ueber die Struktur des Faserzementes, Schweiz. Mschr. Zahnheilk. **56**:23, 1946.
59. Faller, A.: Ueber den Vergleich der Faserstrukturen im Zement normal durchgebrochener und retinierter menschlicher Zähne, Verh. Anat. Ges. **56**:120, 1959.
60. Schmidt, W. J., and Keil, A.: Die gesunden und die erkrankten Zahngewebe des Menschen und der Wirbeltiere im Polarisationsmikroskop, Munich, 1958, Carl Hanser Verlag.
61. Schmid, P.: Polarisationsmikroskopische Untersuchungen über den Faserverlauf des Zahnzementes des Menschen, Z. Zellforsch. **36**:319, 1951.
62. Selvig, K. A.: The fine structure of human cementum, Acta Odont. Scand. **23**:423, 1965.
63. Heuser, H.: Wird die Zementoberfläche des menschlichen Zahnes durch Funktion gestaltet? Deutsch. Zahnaerztl. Z. **17**:861, 1961.
64. Benson, B.: The surface of cementum, J. Periodont. **30**:126, 1959.
65. Boyde, A., and Jones, S. J.: Scanning electron microscopy of cementum and Sharpey fibre bone, Z. Zellforsch. **92**:536, 1968.
66. Landay, M.: J. Periodont. (In press.)
67. Röckert, H.: Röntgenspektrografiska studier av tänder, Odont. T. **6**:500, 1955.
68. Selvig, K. A.: Ultrastructural changes in cementum and adjacent connective tissue in periodontal disease, Acta Odont. Scand. **24**:459, 1966.
69. Giansanti, J. S.: The pattern and width of collagen bundles in bone and cementum, Oral Surg. **30**:508, 1970.
70. Ritchey, B., and Orban, B.: The crests of the interdental alveolar septa, J. Periodont. **24**:75, 1953.
71. Parfitt, G. J.: An investigation of the normal variations in alveolar bone trabeculation, Oral Surg. **15**:1453, 1962.
72. Easley, J. R.: Methods of determining alveolar osseous form, J. Periodont. **38**:112, 1967.
73. Stahl, S. S., Cantor, M., and Zwig, E.: Fenestrations of the labial alveolar plate in human skulls, Periodontics **1**:99, 1963.
74. Elliott, J. R., and Bowers, G. M.: Alveolar dehiscence and fenestrations, Periodontics **1**:245, 1963.
75. Caffesse, R. G., Barletta, B. O., and Carranza, F. A.: Defectos oseos en la tabla vestibular superior de maxilares humanos, Rev. Asoc. Odont. Argent. **52**:238, 1963.
76. Nabers, C. L., Spear, G. R., and Beckham, L. C.: Alveolar dehiscence, Texas Dent. J. **78**:4, 1959.
77. Hirschfeld, I.: A study of skulls in the American Museum of Natural History in relation to periodontal disease, J. Dent. Res. **5**:241, 1923.
78. Larato, D. C.: Alveolar plate fenestrations and dehiscences of the human skull, Oral Surg. **29**:816, 1970.
79. Larato, D. C.: Periodontal defects in the juvenile skull, J. Periodont. **41**:473, 1970.
80. Heins, P. J., and Canter, S. R.: The furca involvement: a classification of bony deformities, Periodontics **6**:84, 1968.

81. Everett, F. G., and others: The intermediate bifurcational ridge: a study of the morphology of the lower first molar, J. Dent. Res. 37:162, 1958.
82. Everett, F. G.: Bifurcation involvement, Oregon Dent. J. 28:2, June 1959.
83. Larato, D. C.: Furcation involvements: incidence and distribution, J. Periodont. 41:499, 1970.
84. Masters, D. H., and Hoskins, S. W.: Projections of the cervical enamel in molar furcations, J. Periodont. 35:49, 1964.
85. Grewe, J. M., Meskin, L. H., and Miller, T.: Cervical enamel projections, location and extent, with associated periodontal implications, J. Periodont. 36:460, 1965.
86. Leib, A. M., Berdon, J. K., and Sabes, W. R.: Furcation involvements correlated with enamel projections from the cementoenamel junction, J. Periodont. 38:330, 1967.
87. Stein, G., and Weinmann, J.: Die physiologische Wanderung der Zähne, Z. Stomat. 23:733, 1925.
88. Pritchard, J. J.: General anatomy and histology of bone. In Bourne, G. H., editor: The biochemistry and physiology of bone, New York, 1956, Academic Press Inc.
89. Weinmann, J. P., and Sicher, H.: Bone and bones, fundamentals of bone biology, ed. 2, St. Louis, 1955, The C. V. Mosby Co.
90. Harndt, E.: Paradentitis und Paradentose, Munich, 1950, Carl Hanser Verlag.
91. Fröhlich, E.: Die Bedeutung der peripheren Durchblutung des Parodontiums für die Entstehung und Therapie der Zahnbetterkrankungen, Forum Parodontologicum, Deutsch. Zahnaerztl. Z. 19:154, 1964.
92. Cohn, S. A.: A new look at the orientation of cementoalveolar fibers of the mouse periodontium, Anat. Rec. 166:292, 1970.
93. Baume, L. J.: Tooth and investing bone: a developmental entity, Oral Surg. 9:736, 1956.
94. Baumhammers, A., Stallard, R. E., and Zander, H. A.: Remodeling of alveolar bone, J. Periodont. 36:439, 1965.
95. Melcher, A. H.: Repair of wounds in the periodontium of the rat. Influence of periodontal ligament on osteogenesis, Arch. Oral Biol. 15:1183, 1970.

**Additional suggested reading**

Melcher, A. H., and Bowen, W. H., editors: Biology of the periodontium, New York, 1969, Academic Press, Inc.

CHAPTER FOUR

# Periodontium of ageing humans



A progression of clinical changes in the periodontium from young to old was shown in Chapter 1. The periodontal tissues in health were discussed in Chapters 2 and 3. Chapter 4 is concerned with what occurs in the periodontal tissues in old age.

*Definition*

Senescence includes any changes in the adult organism that occur with time. Such changes may be intrinsic and chronologically related, or they may be extrinsic and attributable to the environment. Unfortunately the distinction between the physiologic time-related changes and the environmental pathologic changes is often unclear.[1]

## RELATION TO FUNCTION AND DISEASE

It is important to recognize age changes in the periodontium since these may affect function. Also the opinion has been stated that age changes may prepare the way for a pathologic state.[2] This latter hypothesis may be correlated with the evidence of increasing tooth loss[3] and of increasing periodontal disease with advancing age.[4]

Age changes affect the following periodontal tissues:

1. Vasculature
2. Periodontal ligament
3. Cementum
4. Alveolar bone
5. Gingiva and alveolar mucosa

### Vasculature

*Arteriosclerosis*

Arteriosclerosis is a frequent finding in ageing humans.[5,6] It may be seen in large muscular vessels (Fig. 4-1), vessels in the alveolar bone (Fig. 4-2), and vessels in the periodontal ligament (Figs. 4-3 and 4-4). The relationship of this vascular pathology to other changes in the periodontium is inconclusive. The relative ischemia that arteriosclerosis may produce in periodontal tissues because of a reduction in blood flow has been hypothesized as predisposing these tissues

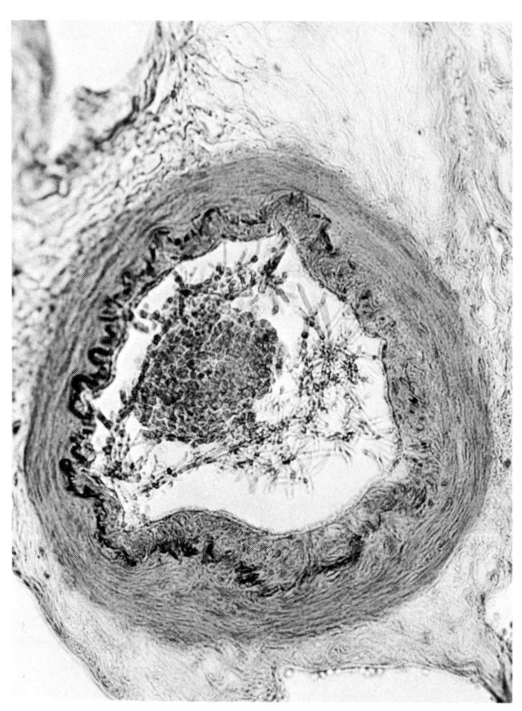

**Fig. 4-1.** Alveolar artery from a 76-year-old man showing changes characteristic of arteriosclerosis, including intimal thickening with cellular and fibrous proliferation. (From Grant, D. A., and Bernick, S.: J. Periodont. **41**:170, 1970.)

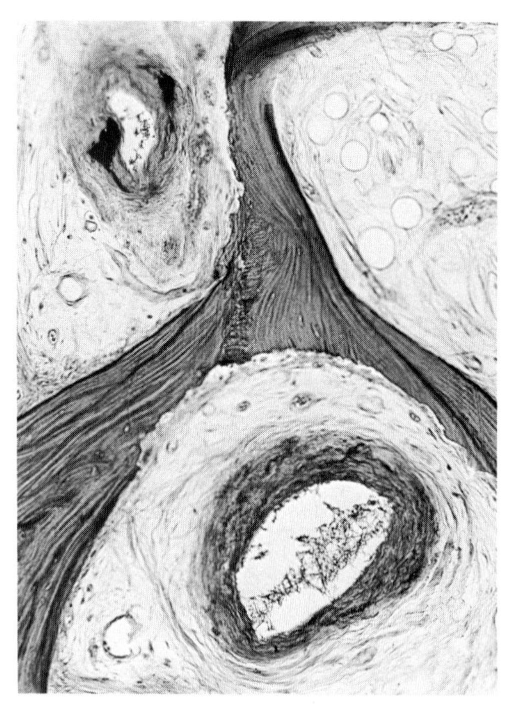

**Fig. 4-2.** Subdivision of the alveolar artery in the spongiosa around the mandibular first molar showing a thickening of the vessel wall and a narrowed and plaque-lined lumen. Superiorly a smaller vessel shows extensive calcification of the lateral and superior portions of the vessel (72-year-old man). (From Grant, D. A., and Bernick, S.: J. Periodont. **41**:170, 1970.)

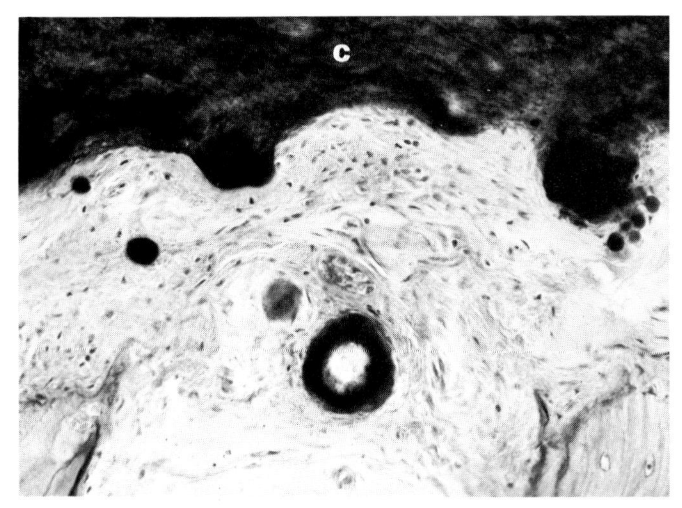


**Fig. 4-3.** In a periodontal ligament arteriole from a 76-year-old man, the calcification has involved all three layers of the vessel. *c,* Cementum. (From Grant, D. A., and Bernick, S.: J. Periodont. **41**:170, 1970.)

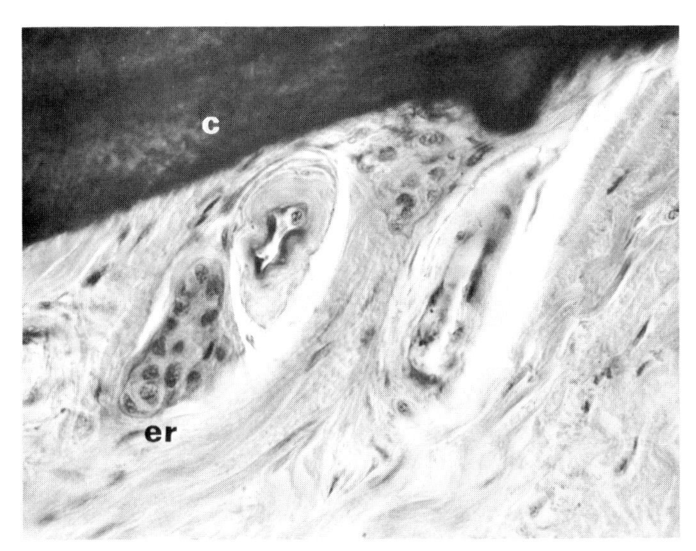


**Fig. 4-4.** Arteriole in the periodontal ligament of a mandibular premolar in a 76-year-old man. The vessel exhibits concentric lamination, giving it an onionskin appearance. *c,* Cementum; *er,* epithelial rest. (From Grant, D. A., and Bernick, S.: J. Periodont. **41**:170, 1970.)

to disease[7] or provoking other changes such as fibrosis, loss of cellularity, and focal calcification.[8]

***Loss of ground substance***

The reduced arterial flow may be related to changes that have been observed elsewhere in the body and in experimental animals. For instance, the loss of ground substance may be due to a reduced supply of oxygen associated with arterial flow.[9] Also basement membranes have been reported to be thicker in old persons and markedly distinguished from the surrounding ground substance.[10]

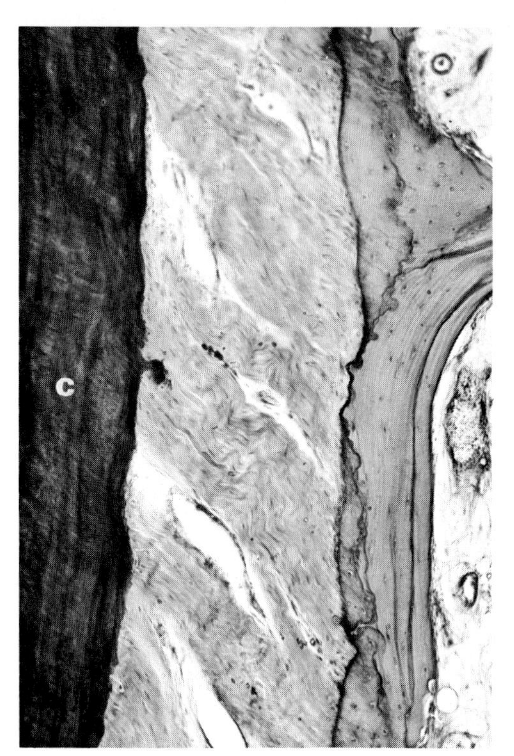


**Fig. 4-5.** Principal fibers are thick and show reduced cellularity. They are strongly PAS positive. The spaces between the fiber bundles are reduced in size. The cementum, *c*, is also thick. (From Grant, D. A., and Bernick, S.: J. Periodont. In press.)

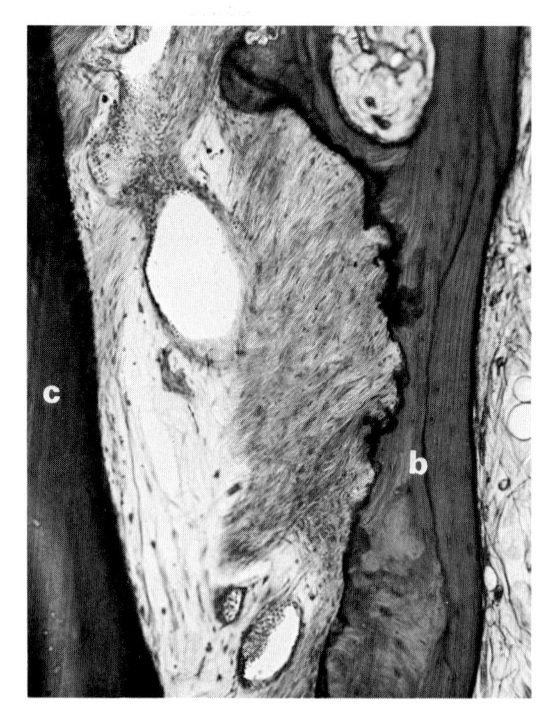


**Fig. 4-6.** Few osteoblasts and cementoblasts are seen bordering bone and tooth. A lessened cellularity of the principal fibers is also evident. *c*, Cementum; *b*, alveolar bone. (From Grant, D. A., and Bernick, S.: J. Periodont. In press.)

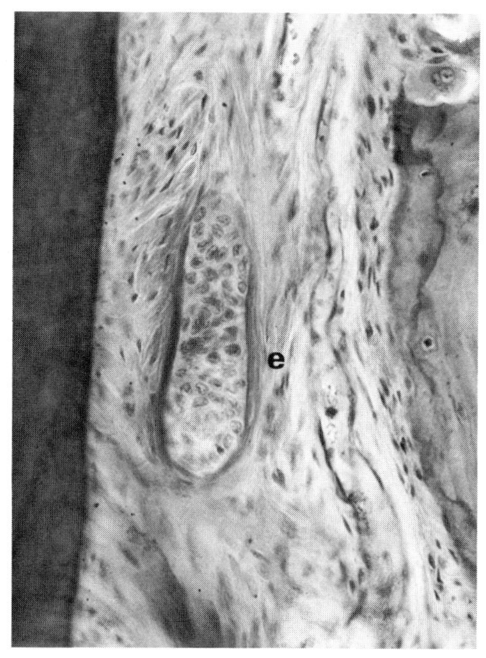


**Fig. 4-13.** Enlarged epithelial rest, *e,* situated midway in the periodontal ligament with a thick PAS-positive basement membrane. (From Grant, D. A., and Bernick, S.: J. Periodont. In press.)

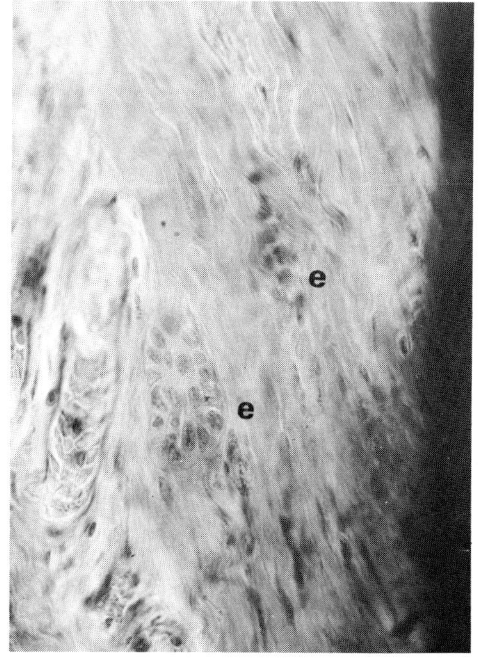


**Fig. 4-14.** Degeneration of epithelial rests, *e,* and hyalinization of principal fibers in an ageing human. (From Grant, D. A., and Bernick, S.: J. Periodont. In press.)

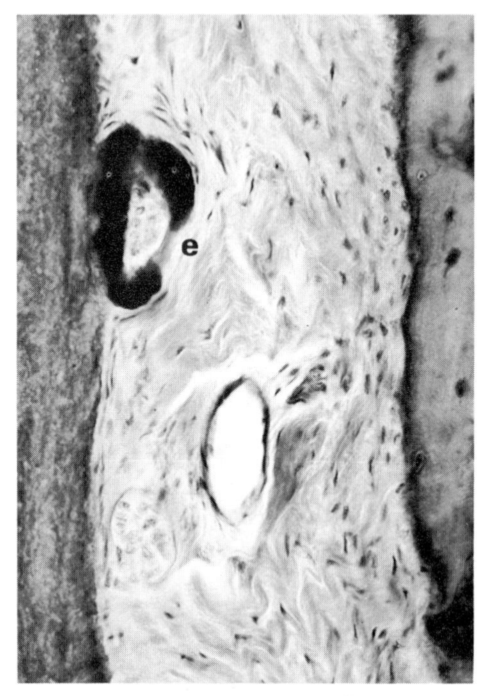


**Fig. 4-15.** Calcification of an epithelial rest, *e,* in a 55-year-old man. (From Grant, D. A., and Bernick, S.: J. Periodont. In press.)

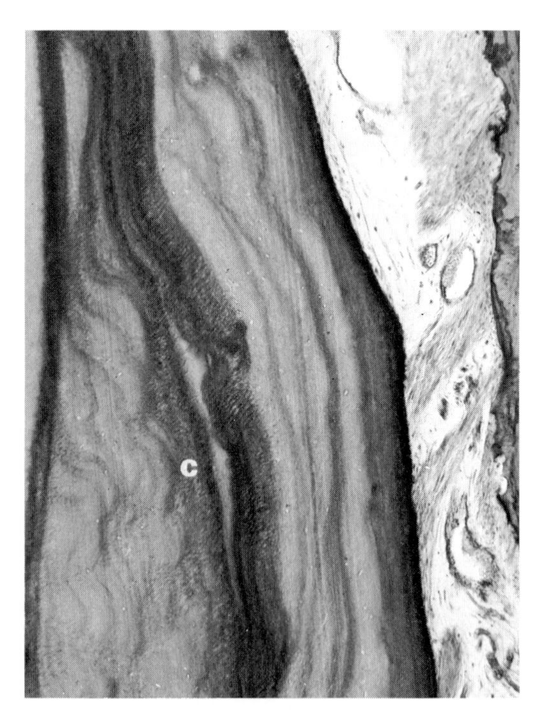


**Fig. 4-16.** Midroot area of a premolar showing the thick layers of cementum, *c,* as a result of continuous apposition in a 92-year-old woman. (From Grant, D. A., and Bernick, S.: J. Periodont. In press.)

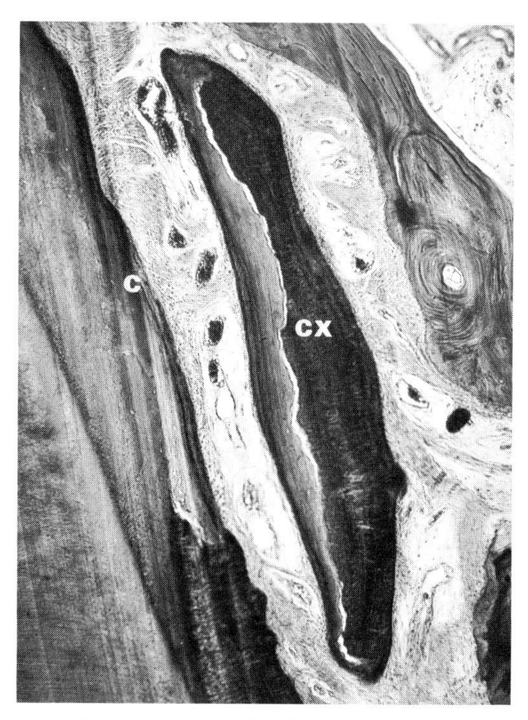


**Fig. 4-17.** A large fragment of cementum, *cx,* has been torn from the tooth and now forms a part of the alveolar bone proper. Bone has been deposited on the fragment. *c,* Cementum. Note that a periodontal ligament remains between the detached fragment of cementum and the bone. A second periodontal ligament has formed between the secondary cementum on the tooth surface and the bundle bone deposited on the detached cementum fragment. (From Grant, D. A., and Bernick, S.: J. Periodont. In press.)

There are indications that cemental deposition slows in old age.[8] In addition, the attachment of cementum to dentin may be weakened. The frequent cemental tears seen in specimens of ageing humans (Fig. 4-17) may be related to age changes in the ground substance of cementum, to reduced vascular supply, or to thickened and less extensible ligament fibers embedded in the cementum.[8]

Spurring of cementum is sometimes the result of the fusion of calcospheroid bodies near cementum or of the calcification of epithelial rest aggregates[8] (Fig. 4-15).

## Alveolar bone

Alveolar bone also shows age changes (Figs. 4-6, 4-11, 4-15, and 4-18). The alveolar bone proper has a darkly stained margin, which may be interpreted as an ageing characteristic of bone.

***Physiologic migration***

Little evidence of continued bone apposition is present in old age. In view of this, physiologic tooth migration may be slowed or even halted in old age.[8] (See discussion on physiologic tooth migration in Chapters 3 and 36.)

***Attrition of tooth substance***

Attrition of tooth substance on occlusal and incisal surfaces and at the contact points is a well-recognized characteristic of ageing.

Wear on occluding tooth surfaces can be related to use (as occurs in chewing), occupational wear (as in Eskimos who soften leather with their teeth), or parafunctional habits (as in bruxism). The attrition may be slow or rapid. The

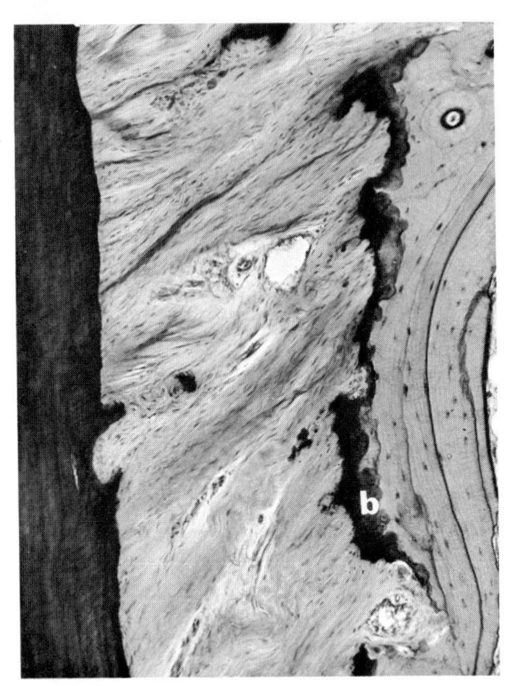


**Fig. 4-18.** The margin of the alveolar bone proper, *b,* of an ageing human is darkly stained, possibly a concomitant of ageing. Physiologic tooth migration appears to be slowed or even halted. (From Grant, D. A., and Bernick, S.: J. Periodont. In press.)

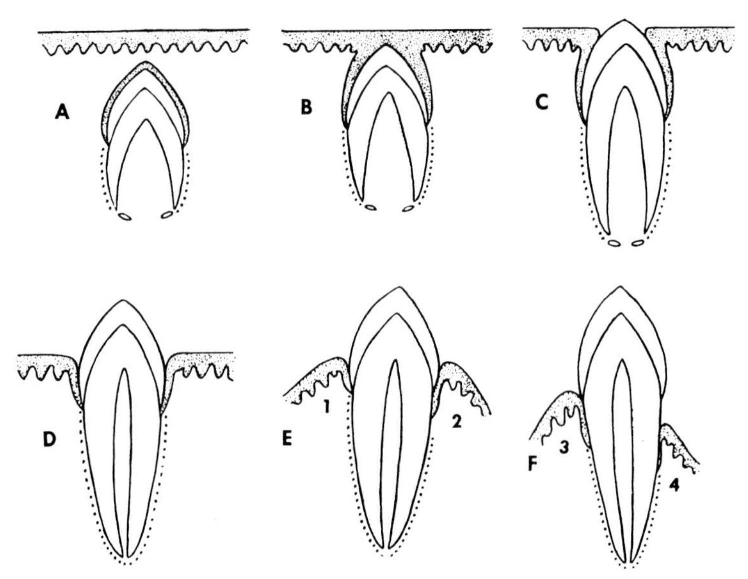


**Fig. 4-19.** Diagram of the development and changing position of the gingival attachment to the surface of the tooth. **A,** Erupting tooth is below the epithelium of the oral mucous membrane. The enamel is covered by reduced enamel epithelium. **B,** Reduced enamel epithelium and epithelium of the oral mucous membrane come into contact. **C,** Tip of the enamel erupts through the epithelium. No connective tissue is exposed. The epithelium is attached to the enamel, and there is no break in continuity. **D,** Tooth erupts into occlusion. The epithelium is still attached to the enamel. Apical end of the attachment epithelium is at the cementoenamel junction. **E** and **F,** Changing position of the dentogingival junction is demonstrated: *1,* Bottom of the gingival sulcus is on the enamel, and the apical end of the attachment epithelium is at the cementoenamel junction; *2,* bottom of the sulcus is still on the enamel, but the apical end of the attachment has shifted to the cementum. *3,* Bottom of the sulcus is at the cementoenamel junction, and the apical end of the attachment has moved onto the cementum; *4,* entire attachment epithelium has shifted apically. The bottom of the sulcus is on the cementum, and part of the root surface is exposed.

loss of tooth substance is of extrinsic origin and is related to the environment; and since time is a factor, it is also chronologically related to senescence.

Attrition of contact points and contact planes occurs with ageing. It is the result of the slight vertical movement imparted to teeth during function. This movement is permitted by the periodontal ligament.

Vertical (interocclusal) dimension and arch continuity are usually maintained into old age, since wear is compensated for by bone apposition on distal surfaces and at the fundus of the sockets. Continuous apposition of cementum also helps to compensate for such wear. If continuous apposition of bone is slowed or even halted (as in senescence), such compensation for attrition does not occur. In concert with atrophy of musculature, a decreased vertical facial height may result (closed bite).[8]

The vascularity of bone appears to be diminished.[8] Moreover, the continuous remodeling of the alveolar bone that occurred throughout earlier life may alter the blood supply by changing the vascular pathways.[8]

*Osteoporosis*

Osteoporosis has been reported in ageing, particularly in the alveolar bone of postmenopausal women; but the decrease in the trabeculation of alveolar bone sometimes seen roentgenographically is more often related to loss of function (extraction of an opposing tooth).

### Gingiva and alveolar mucosa

The gingiva is reported to be increasingly fibrotic in old age, and the amount of surface keratinization is said to be decreased.[11] Elastoid degeneration is reported in the collagen fibers of the alveolar mucosa. Arteriosclerotic vessels have been described.[6]

## RELATION TO COLLAGEN CHANGES IN OTHER TISSUES

As might be anticipated, the age changes that can be seen in cellular, fibrillar, calcified, and ground substance components of the periodontium are similar to those that have been described in connective tissues elsewhere in the body.

The changes in periodontal tissues correlate well with age changes in collagen. Clausen,[23] Verzar,[24] Gross,[25] and Milch[26] have summarized these; and all agree that there is an increase in the thickness of collagen fibrils and that the chemical and physical properties of collagen are altered. There is (1) an increase in the tensile strength of collagen fibers, (2) an increase in thermal contraction, (3) a decrease in extensibility, (4) a reduction in the amount of soluble collagen, (5) a decrease in water content, and (6) an increased resistance to proteolytic enzymes. Some of these changes may be related to the loss of acid mucopolysaccharide and water as well as to increased cross linkages.

## DENTOGINGIVAL JUNCTION

*Changing position of the dentogingival junction (active and passive tooth exposure)*

Most attention in ageing changes has been focused on the apical migration of attachment (junctional) epithelium. Whether this is a physiologic or a pathologic event is controversial.[19,20] However, the relationship of the gingival attachment and the surface of the tooth changes during life, rapidly at the time of eruption and slowly after the tooth has erupted into occlusion. The surface of the enamel, after formation and calcification, is covered by the reduced enamel epithelium (Fig. 4-19, *A*). When the tooth emerges into the oral cavity, the reduced enamel epithelium unites with the oral epithelium (*B*). At the time that the cusp emerges into the oral cavity, most of the enamel surface of the rapidly erupted tooth is covered by soft tissue, which progressively separates from the

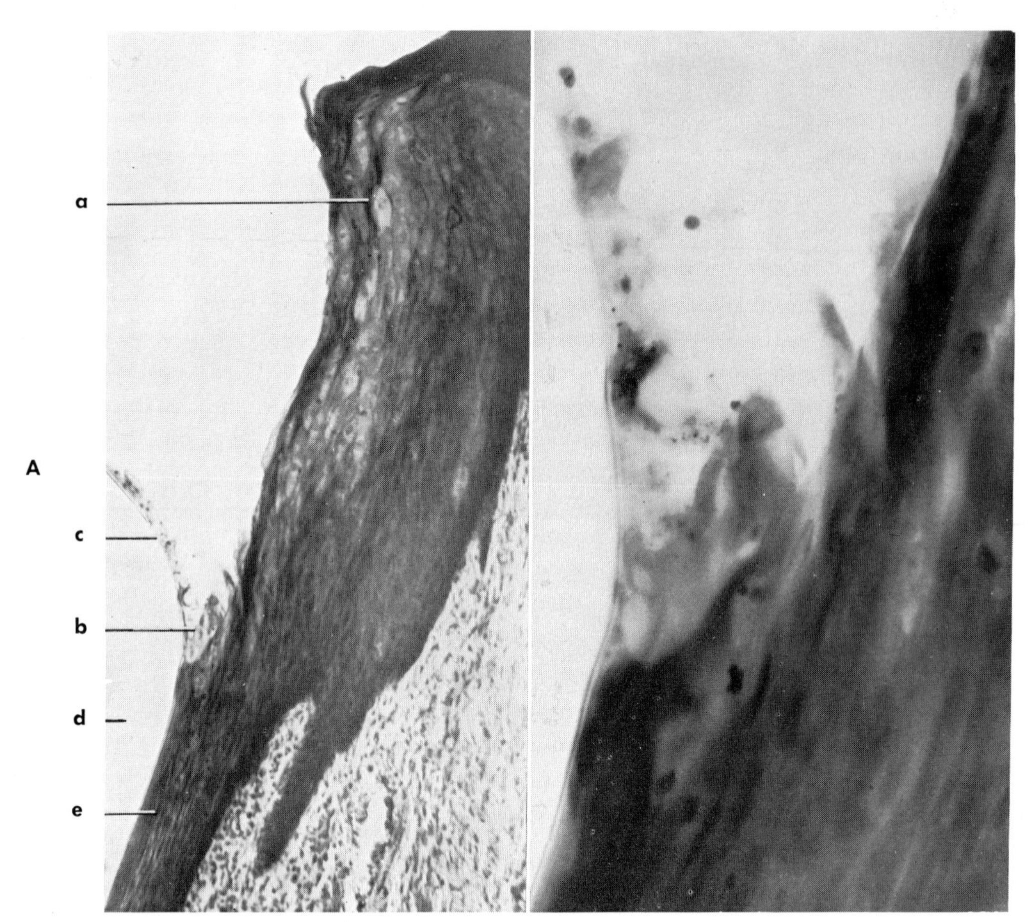


**Fig. 4-20. A,** High magnification of, *a,* gingival margin and, *b,* bottom of gingival sulcus. The enamel cuticle, *c,* appears detached because the enamel, *d,* was lost in decalcification. *e,* Attachment epithelium. **B,** Higher magnification of the bottom of the gingival sulcus. Note the degenerated and desquamating epithelial cells.

tooth, gradually exposing more of the crown (*D*). After occlusal contact the relationship between the gingival attachment and the tooth may remain relatively unchanged for years in the absence of pathology. The foregoing changes may be considered developmental. However, a gradual separation of epithelium from the crown and a proliferation of junctional (attachment) epithelium have been noted with age. These phenomena, separation and proliferation, may be due to inflammation; or they may be a natural ageing process.[21,22]

The area is exposed to bacterial flora. What follows is progressive separation of epithelium from the tooth surface (Fig. 4-20). At the same time events must take place in the connective tissues that permit a proliferation of attachment (junctional) epithelium. Four stages have been described in this process, as shown in Figs. 4-21 to 4-24.

It is important to know the positions of the component parts of the dentogingival junction in all phases of eruption. The importance of these relationships becomes more evident when one considers the influence of periodontal disease on the rate of exposure. The analysis presented in Table 4-1 describes some

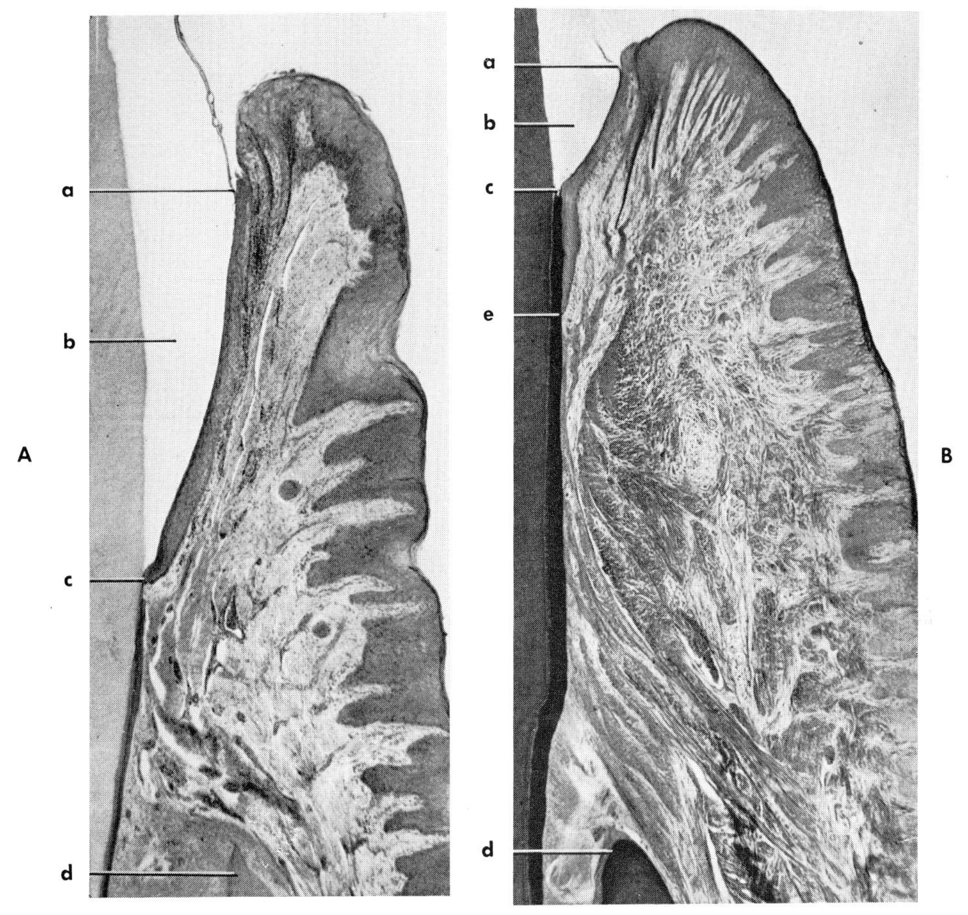


**Fig. 4-21. A,** Attachment epithelium on the enamel (first stage in passive tooth exposure). Apical end of the attachment is at the cementoenamel junction. **B,** Attachment epithelium on enamel and cementum (second stage in passive tooth exposure). Apical end of the attachment has proliferated along the cementum. *a,* Bottom of the gingival sulcus; *b,* enamel; *c,* cementoenamel junction; *d,* alveolar crest; *e,* apical end of the attachment epithelium at the cementoenamel junction.

of the proportionate relationships that exist among the components of the dentogingival junction during the four stages, or phases, of passive exposure.

However, one must always keep in mind that passive exposure is a dynamic sequential process. In actuality there are no clear-cut stages. For instance, the third stage (in which the coronal end of the attachment epithelium and the cementoenamel junction coincide) is a transient stage and is only rarely seen in histologic preparations. Therefore an attachment to either enamel or cementum must exist as well as a progression from one to the other. The position of the attachment epithelium is generally related to the health of the periodontium and also to the tissue to which it is attached.

Early in phase I the length of attachment epithelium is 1.35 mm., decreasing in phase IV to 0.71 mm. This represents a significant diminution. The length of the attachment shortens with chronologic age.

On the other hand, the connective tissue component of the gingival attach-

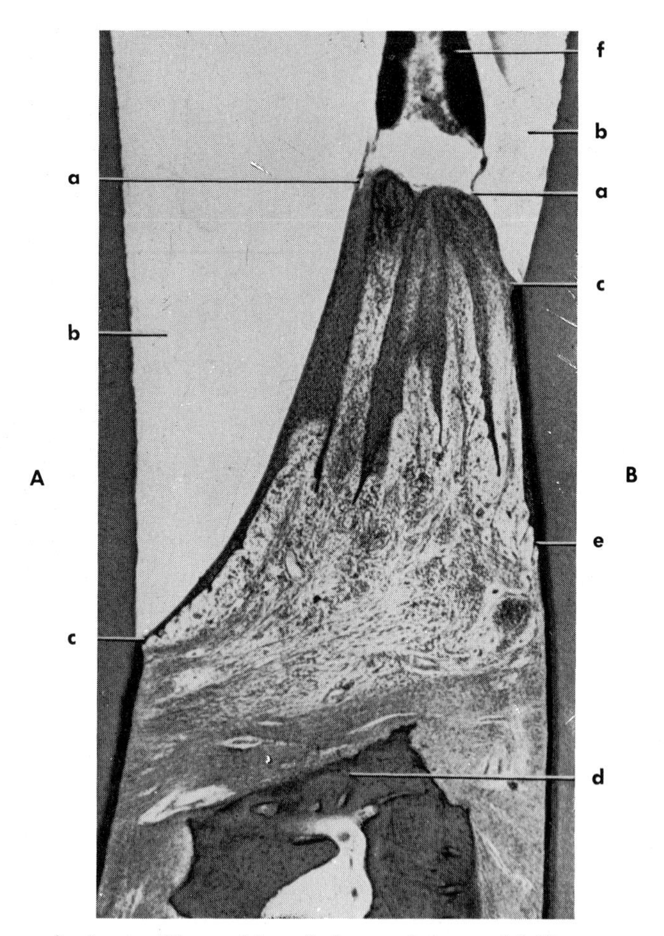


**Fig. 4-22.** Interproximal area. The position of the attachment epithelium on tooth **A** indicates the first stage of passive tooth exposure. Attachment epithelium on tooth **B** is in the second stage of passive tooth exposure (bottom of the sulcus on enamel, apical end of the epithelium on cementum). Note the difference in the degree of eruption of teeth **A** and **B** as indicated by the location of the cementoenamel junctions. *a,* Bottom of the sulcus; *b,* enamel; *c,* cementoenamel junction; *d,* alveolar crest; *e,* apical end of the attachment epithelium; *f,* calculus.

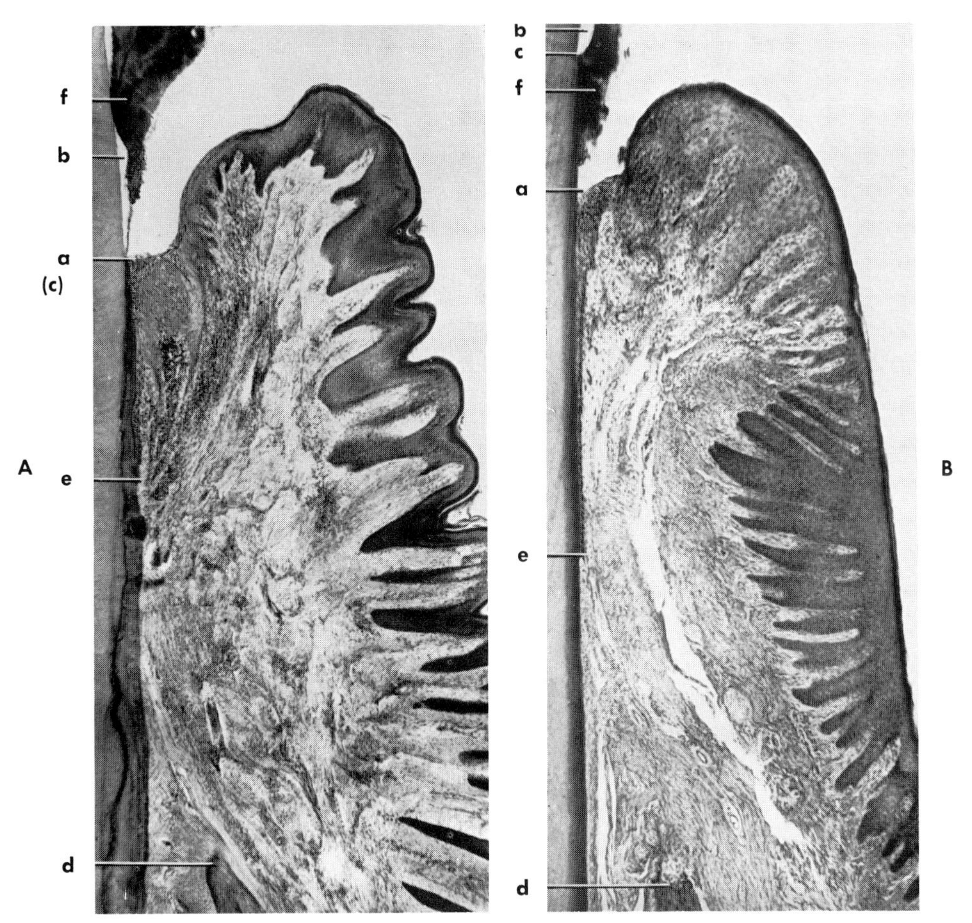


**Fig. 4-23. A,** Attachment epithelium on the cementum. The bottom of the pocket, *a,* is located at the cementoenamel junction (third stage of passive tooth exposure). **B,** Attachment epithelium on the cementum. Part of the root surface is exposed (fourth stage of passive tooth exposure). *a,* Bottom of the gingival sulcus; *b,* enamel; *c,* cementoenamel junction; *d,* alveolar crest; *e,* apical end of the attachment epithelium; *f,* calculus.

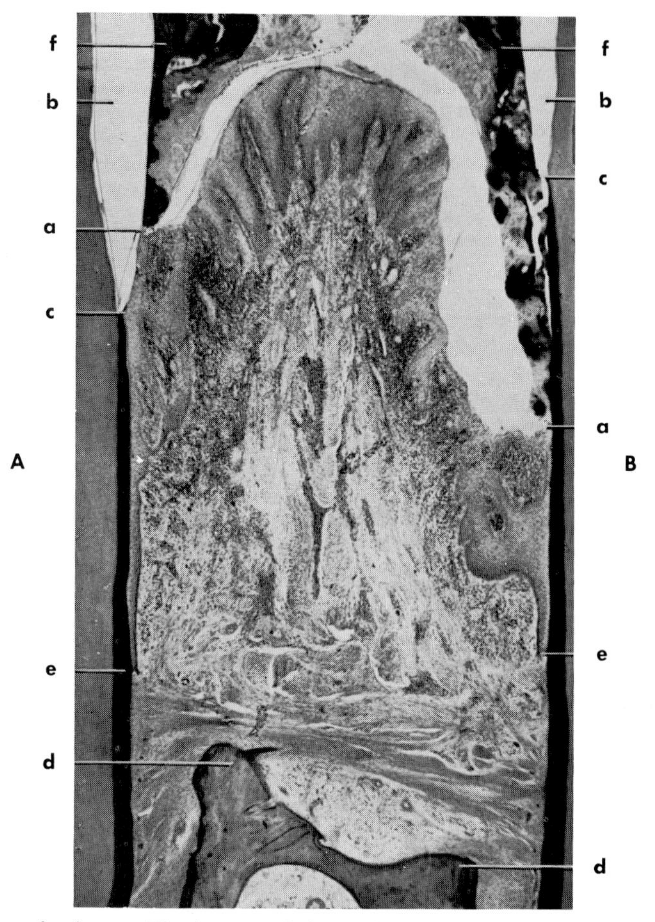


**Fig. 4-24.** Interproximal area. The bottom of the pocket on tooth **A** is located on the enamel; the apical end of the epithelium is on the cementum (second stage of passive tooth exposure). On tooth **B** the bottom of the pocket is on the cementum (fourth stage of passive exposure). *a,* Bottom of the pocket; *b,* enamel; *c,* cementoenamel junction; *d,* alveolar crest; *e,* apical end of the attachment epithelium; *f,* calculus.

ment appears to be rather constant through the stages of passive exposure. The distance between the apical end of the attachment and the alveolar bone crest is about 1 mm. (Figs. 4-21 and 4-24). This represents the amount of connective tissue attachment at the dentogingival junction. In health there is always some distance between the alveolar bone and the base of the attachment epithelium. The apical shift of the dentogingival junction from stage to stage is responsible for the passive exposure of the tooth. *This shift involves the detachment of the attachment epithelium and its apical migration, the dissolution of some gingival collagen fibers, and the atrophy of the alveolar crest or bone destruction.*

## SUMMARY

Physiologic and chronologic age may or may not coincide, but ageing is a demonstrated entity. There are morphologic changes in the periodontium that are a part of this "winding-down process." Periodontal fibers are thicker, and their staining characteristics are different. Calcifications and degeneration are apparent in fibers and epithelial rests. The remodeling of bone is slowed. Ce-

**Table 4-1.** Dimensions of the components of the dentogingival junction in man related to the four stages of passive exposure*

| Measurement | Phase averages (mm.) I | II | III | IV | Total averages (mm.) |
|---|---|---|---|---|---|
| Sulcus depth | 0.80 | 0.61 | 0.61 | 0.76 | 0.69 |
| Attached epithelium | 1.35 | 1.10 | 0.74 | 0.71 | 0.97 |
| Apical point of epithelial attachment below cementoenamel junction | 0.00 | 0.43 | 0.74 | 1.41 | |
| Bottom of sulcus from cementoenamel junction | +1.35 | +0.68 | 0.00 | −1.14 | |
| Cementoenamel junction to alveolar bone | 1.08 | 1.55 | 1.71 | 2.81 | |
| Deepest point of epithelial attachment to alveolar bone | 1.08 | 1.07 | 1.06 | 1.06 | 1.07 |

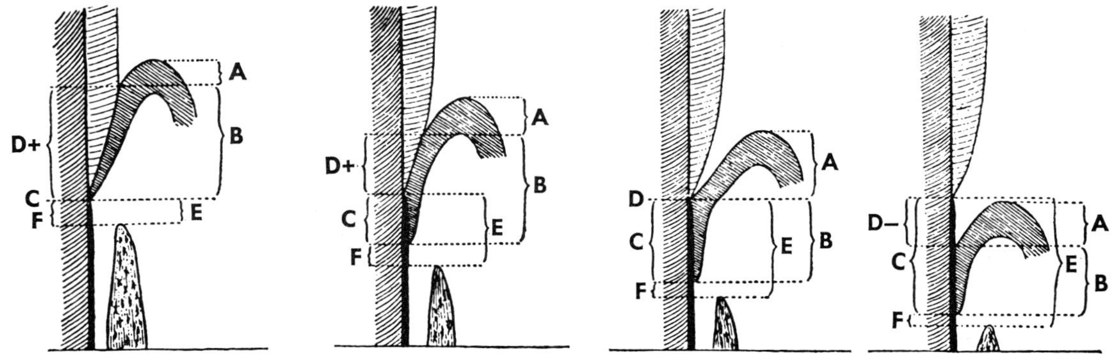

*From Gargiulo, A., Wentz, F. M., and Orban, B.: Dimensions and relation of the dentogingival junction in humans, J. Periodont. **32**:261, 1961.

mentum is thicker, but with an apparent greater susceptibility to injury. Periodontal structures, when injured, are not always repaired by a restoration of the injured part. Cartilage may form in the periodontal ligament. Sometimes the ligament becomes calcified and ankylosis results. Arteriosclerosis is ubiquitous, and a decreased blood supply may be a causative factor in these changes. Whether or not age changes increase the susceptibility to periodontal disease is an important but unanswered question.

**CHAPTER 4**

**References**


1. Grant, D. A., and Bernick, S.: Age changes as seen in human specimens, I.A.D.R. abstract no. 291, 1969.
2. Bernier, J. L.: The role of organ systems and of age in periodontal disease, J. Periodont. **29**:247, 1958.
3. Andrews, G., and Krogh, H. W.: Permanent tooth mortality, Dent. Progr. **1**:130, 1960.
4. Bossert, W. A., and Marks, H. H.: Prevalence and characteristics of periodontal disease in 12,800 persons under periodic dental treatment, J. Amer. Dent. Ass. **52**:429, 1956.
5. Grant, D. A., and Bernick, S.: Arteriosclerosis in periodontal vessels of ageing humans, J. Periodont. **41**:170, 1970.
6. Stahl, S. S., and Fox, L. M.: Histological changes of the oral mucosa associated with certain chronic diseases, Oral Surg. **6**:339, 1953.
7. Doyle, J. L., Hollander, W., Goldman, H. M., and Rubin, M. P.: Experimental arteriosclerosis and the periodontium, J. Periodont. **40**:350, 1969.
8. Grant, D. A., and Bernick, S.: The periodontium of ageing humans, J. Periodont. (In press.)
9. Oliver, J.: Anatomic changes of normal senescence. In Stieglitz, E. J., editor: Geriatric medicine, Philadelphia, 1954, J. B. Lippincott Co.
10. Chvapil, M.: Connective tissues. In Shack, E. D., editor: Perspectives in experimental gerontology, Springfield, Ill., 1966, Charles C Thomas, Publisher.
11. Wentz, F. M., Maier, A. W., and Orban, B.: Age changes and sex differences in the clinically normal gingiva, J. Periodont. **23**:13, 1952.
12. Klingsberg, J., and Butcher, E. O.: Comparative histology of age changes in oral tissues of rat, hamster and monkey, J. Dent. Res. **39**:158, 1960.
13. Flieder, D. E.: Cytochemistry of human oral mucosa, J. Dent. Res. **41**:112, 1962.
14. Jensen, J. L., and Toto, P. D.: Radioactive labelling of the periodontal ligament in ageing rats, J. Dent. Res. **47**:149, 1968.
15. Toto, P. D., and Borg, M.: Effect of age changes on the premitotic index in the periodontium of mice, J. Dent. Res. **47**:40, 1968.
16. Götze, W.: Ueber Altersveränderungen des Parodontiums, Deutsch. Zahnaerztl. Z. **20**:465, 1965.

16a. Everett, F. G., and Bruckner, R. J.: Cartilage in the periodontal ligament space, J. Periodont. **41**:165, 1970.

17. Reeve, C. M., and Wentz, F. M.: The prevalence, morphology and distribution of epithelial rests in the human periodontal ligament, Oral Surg. **15**:785, 1962.
18. Zander, H. A., and Hürzeler, B.: Continuous cementum apposition, J. Dent. Res. **37**:1035, 1958.
19. Orban, B., and Köhler, J.: Die physiologische Zahnfleischtasche, Epithelansatz und Epitheltiefenwucherung, Z. Stomat. **22**:353, 1924.
20. Häupl, K., and Lang, F.: Die marginale Paradentitis, Berlin, 1927, Hermann Meusser.
21. Gargiulo, A., Wentz, F. M., and Orban, B.: Dimension and relations of the dentogingival junction in humans, J. Periodont. **32**:261, 1961.
22. Ten Cate, A. R.: Development of the periodontium. In Melcher, A. H., and Bowen, W. H., editors: Biology of the periodontium, New York, 1969, Academic Press, Inc.
23. Clausen, B.: Ageing of connective tissues. In Asboe-Hansen, G., editor: Hormones and connective tissue, Baltimore, 1966, The Williams & Wilkins Co.
24. Verzar, F.: Ageing of the collagen fibers. In Hall, D. A., editor: International review of connective tissue research, New York, 1964, Academic Press, Inc., vol. 2.
25. Gross, J.: Ageing of connective tissue, the extracellular components. In Bourne, G. H., editor: Structural aspects of ageing, New York, 1961, Hafner Publishing Co., Inc.
26. Milch, R. A.: Aging of connective tissues. In Shack, E. D., editor: Perspectives in experimental gerontology, Springfield, Ill., 1966, Charles C Thomas, Publisher.

PART II

# The oral environment

CHAPTER FIVE

# Saliva



Saliva bathes the oral tissues and may reasonably be assumed to have significance in the health status of the oral environment. The salivary contribution to the digestive process is primarily preparative and gastronomic; the formation of the food bolus allows for more efficient mastication and swallowing; and the maintenance of a proper fluid environment provides for optimal functioning of the taste buds.

The most important attributes of the salivary secretions are protective in nature—helping to maintain the integrity of the teeth, tongue, and mucous membranes of the oral and oropharyngeal areas. The critical importance of saliva in this regard becomes most readily apparent when malfunction of the salivary glands (due to obstruction, drug effects, irradiation, nerve damage, or disease) results in dry mouth or xerostomia. The mucosa becomes dry, rough, and sticky; it bleeds readily and is subject to infection. The tongue becomes red, smooth, slimy, and hypersensitive to irritation and loses taste acuity. In the edentulous patient dentures become extremely difficult to manage. When teeth are present, there is a heavy accumulation of plaque, materia alba, and debris; caries progresses rapidly and extensively; periodontal disease is markedly exacerbated. In mouth breathing, which may be the result of habit, adenoids, deviated nasal septum, sinusitis, allergies, or incomplete lip closure, there is also a drying of the gingiva, which may produce a gingivitis characterized by a shiny erythematous surface with rolled gingival margins. In adolescents this condition may result in a hyperplastic gingival response.

For these and other reasons the secretion and composition of saliva are of direct concern to the dentist.

## CHARACTERISTICS OF SALIVA

Whole saliva—the fluid collected by expectoration—is in reality a mixture of variable composition containing contributions from the major salivary glands (parotid, submaxillary, sublingual) and the minor salivary glands (minor sublingual, labial, buccal, glossopalatine, palatine, lingual) as well as from bacterial, cellular, and food debris and in some instances gingival fluid.

Total salivary fluid produced during a 24-hour period is 1000 to 1500 ml. About 90% of this fluid is derived from the parotid and submaxillary glands (in roughly equal amounts), about 5% from the sublingual, and up to 5% from the minor salivary glands. Since the flow rate of the major salivary glands is less than 0.05 ml./min./gland at rest with no external stimulation and 0.5 ml./min./gland (or greater) with stimulation, it is apparent that 80% to 90% of the daily production of saliva is the result of stimulation—mainly gustatory and masticatory associated with eating. During most of the day and all night, salivary flow is minimal.

## Secretion

*Mechanism*

Salivary secretion is controlled by a salivary center in the medulla composed of the superior and the inferior salivary nuclei. Stimulation of flow is generated mainly by unconditioned reflex stimulation, primarily gustatory (via taste buds) and masticatory (via proprioceptors in the periodontal ligament and the muscles of mastication). Olfactory stimuli, oral pain and irritation, and pharyngeal irritation can also induce stimulation. Conditioned reflexes as well as emotional and psychic factors have also been shown to affect salivary flow rate.[1]

*Pharmacologic agents*

A major factor affecting salivary secretion, especially in older persons, is the large number of pharmacologic agents that can reduce salivary flow. Many drugs list "dry mouth" as a common side effect. Such complaints as dry mouth, taste aberrations, and rampant cervical and root caries are often due to the effect of pharmacologic agents on salivary flow. Common examples are barbiturates, antihistamines, atropinelike agents, dibutoline (Dibuline), chlorpromazine (Thorazine), and other tranquilizers.

## Composition

*Electrolytes*

Table 5-1 lists the concentration of parotid and submaxillary components for which there are quantitative data. Plasma values are included for comparison. In general, the parotid concentration is somewhat higher than the submaxillary concentration. The main exception is calcium—submaxillary calcium being nearly twice parotid calcium.

*Nonelectrolytes*

Glucose is present in very low concentration in saliva; it becomes elevated in diabetes but still appears at about 1% of blood concentration. Lipids and amino acids are also present in very low concentrations in saliva.

*pH*

Saliva is slightly acidic prior to secretion into the oral cavity; it becomes slightly alkaline on excretion from the gland due to a loss of $CO_2$ (carbonic acid in solution). Since bircarbonate concentration increases with increasing flow rate, salivary pH becomes elevated at high flow rates:

*Proteins*

Compared to that in blood, the concentration of proteins in saliva is extremely low.[2] Table 5-2 presents a summary of the proteins of parotid and submaxillary saliva that have been identified to date.[2-6]

The major component of parotid saliva is amylase, which is present in a number of molecular forms known as isoenzymes.[3-5] Amylase activity in the submaxillary gland is only about 20% that in the parotid. There is virtually no amylase in sublingual or minor salivary gland secretions since these glands are almost exclusively mucous (with no serous cells).

*Glycoproteins*

The viscous quality of whole saliva is attributed to salivary mucin. Although mucoid substances have been isolated from extracts of animal salivary glands, there are minimal data on human secretions. It would appear that salivary mucin is a mixture of many glycoproteins, some common to all the salivary glands and some produced exclusively by the submaxillary, sublingual, or minor

**Table 5-1.** Salivary composition in normal adults

| | Mean values | | |
|---|---|---|---|
| Flow rate (ml./min./gland) | Parotid 0.7 | Submaxillary 0.6 | Plasma |
| **mEq./L.** | | | |
| Potassium ($K^+$) | 20 | 17 | 4 |
| Sodium ($Na^+$) | 23 | 21 | 140 |
| Chloride ($Cl^-$) | 23 | 20 | 105 |
| Bicarbonate ($HCO_3^-$) | 20 | 18 | 27 |
| Calcium ($Ca^{++}$) | 2 | 3.6 | 5 |
| Magnesium ($Mg^{+++}$) | 0.2 | 0.2 | 2 |
| Phosphorous ($HPO_4^=$) | 6 | 4.5 | 2 |
| **Mg.%** | | | |
| Urea | 15 | 7 | 25 |
| Ammonia | 0.3 | 0.2 | |
| Uric acid | 3 | 2 | 4 |
| Glucose | <1 | <1 | 80 |
| Total lipid | 2.8 | 2 | 500 |
| Cholesterol | <1 | — | 160 |
| Fatty acids | 1 | — | 300 |
| Amino acids | 1.5 | — | 50 |
| Total proteins | 250 | 150 | 7% |
| **pH** | 6.8 - 7.2 | | 7.35 |

**Table 5-2.** Proteins of parotid and submaxillary saliva*

| | Parotid | Submaxillary |
|---|---|---|
| 1. | Amylase (high) | Amylase (low) |
| | Glycoproteins | Glycoproteins |
| | Cationic (high) | Cationic (low) |
| | Anionic (low) | Anionic (high) |
| | Secretory piece, lactoferrin | Secretory piece, lactoferrin |
| | | Blood group substance |
| | Secretory IgA (immunoglobulin A) | |
| 2. | Lysozyme (low to moderate) | Lysozyme (high) |
| | Phosphatases, esterases, lactoperoxidase, kallikrein | Ribonucleases (low) |
| | Ribonucleases (moderate) | |
| | Lactic acid dehydrogenases | |
| 3. | Albumin, immunoglobulins G and M, lipoprotein, traces of other serum proteins (orosomucoid, ceruloplasmin, etc.) | |

*Modified from Ellison,[2] Caldwell and Pigman,[3] Meyer and Lamberts,[4] Mandel,[5] and Steiner and Keller.[6]

1. Produced in acinar cells.
2. Produced in nonacinar regions of the salivary glands or origin unknown.
3. Leakage from plasma.

salivary glands. These glycoproteins are of two types: (1) cationic (positively charged) and nonviscous in nature, which have an unusual amino acid composition, differentiating them from the material formed by purely mucous cells,[7] and (2) anionic (negatively charged), which appear to be rather heterogeneous, with molecular weights that may approach several million.

Acinar cells of both the parotid and the submaxillary gland produce a small glycoprotein (about 50,000 molecular weight) known as secretory piece, which, together with immunoglobulin A (one of the gamma globulins), forms a specific structural entity, the secretory IgA, produced in exocrine glands for activity on mucous membrane surfaces.[8] The cells also produce small amounts of lactoferrin, an iron-binding protein.

The submaxillary and the sublingual glands produce blood group substance, the glycoprotein responsible for blood type. In secretions of blood group substance, the blood type (e.g., ABO) can be determined in a drop of saliva.

***Secretory IgA***

The secretory immunoglobulin (IgA) found in saliva is produced in plasma cells in the connective tissue of the glands, especially around the intralobular ducts. It travels between the acinar cells, joins with the secretory piece (probably in the intercellular area), and enters the salivary secretion as a dimer joined (and probably stabilized) by the secretory piece. Secretory IgA possesses the ability to neutralize viruses and can act as an antibody to bacterial antigens and probably food antigens. It is relatively resistant to proteolytic enzymes and hence can survive in the oral cavity and the gastrointestinal tract.[8]

***Lysozyme***

The antibacterial enzyme lysozyme is found in both parotid and submaxillary secretions. It is formed (or concentrated) in basal cells in the striated ducts.[9] Lysozyme is a muramidase; that is, it splits bacterial cell walls in the glycopeptide region containing muramic acid. It may act in concert with other antibacterial systems in saliva (IgA) as a general scavenger of susceptible bacterial cell walls.

***Lactoperoxidase***

Another important component of the salivary antibacterial system is the enzyme lactoperoxidase. This enzyme, in concert with hydrogen peroxide and thiocyanate, can affect lactobacilli and cariogenic streptococci.[12] A similar system exists in mother's milk and is considered to be part of the early defense mechanism of the newborn. Comparable peroxidase activity (myeloperoxidase) is part of the antibacterial weaponry of the leukocyte.

***Formed elements***

Saliva contains epithelial cells from the oral mucosa as well as leukocytes (salivary corpuscles) from the gingival sulcus.[10-11]

***Other proteins***

A considerable number of other enzymes have been identified in both parotid and submaxillary saliva. These include acid and alkaline phosphatases, nonspecific esterases, ribonucleases, and kallikrein. The enzyme lactic acid dehydrogenase (LDH) has been found in parotid saliva but not in submaxillary saliva.

Serum proteins can be identified in saliva by immunologic techniques. They are present in low concentration and appear to enter the secretion by "leakage." Only albumin is present at any appreciable level (about 1 mg.%). In salivary gland disease in which ductal integrity is altered (e.g., parotitis or Sjögren's disease), albumin levels are markedly elevated.[13] The finding that IgG is present in saliva in much lower amounts than IgA supports the observation that the salivary IgA is produced in the gland. In blood the IgG-to-IgA ratio is about 10:1; in saliva it is the reverse.

## ROLE OF SALIVA IN ORAL HEALTH

The inorganic and organic components of saliva endow the secretions with considerable protective potential:

1. *Lubrication and protection.* The glycoproteins and mucoids produced by the major and minor salivary glands form a protective coating for the mucous membrane. This coating is a barrier against irritants acting directly on the membrane. It is also a barrier against (a) proteolytic and hydrolytic enzymes produced in the plaque, (b) potential carcinogens (smoking, chemicals, etc.), and (c) desiccation (mouth breathing). The mucoid layer may be considered comparable in some respects to gastric mucin, which protects the stomach from the hydrochloric acid produced therein.
2. *Mechanical cleansing.* The physical flow of saliva acts as a "backward tide" to remove food and cellular and bacterial debris for elimination via the alimentary tract. The rate of clearance may be an important deterrent against plaque formation and may help to reduce the incidence of caries and inflammatory gingival disease.
3. *Buffering action.* Primarily because of its bicarbonate content and secondarily because of phosphate and amphoteric proteins, saliva has considerable buffer capacity. This protective function occurs in the plaque, directed against acidogenic microorganisms, and occasionally on the mucous membrane surface, where acids from foods or regurgitation are involved.
4. *Maintenance of tooth integrity.* Saliva functions to maintain the integrity of the tooth in a number of ways: (a) it provides minerals for post-eruptive maturation; (b) it contains calcium and phosphate, which enter plaque and act to prevent tooth dissolution (solubility product principle); (c) it causes a film of glycoprotein on teeth, which reduces wear due to attrition and abrasion.
5. *Antibacterial activity.* Saliva contains a number of components that can by themselves or in concert marshal an impressive defense against bacterial and viral invasion.[14] Greatest interest is now focused on secretory IgA, which has been demonstrated to be effective against a number of viruses and bacteria.[8] The manner in which IgA operates in the mouth against plaque organisms is the subject of considerable research. Coating of oral streptococci by IgA has been demonstrated.[15] Since IgA does not fix complement (which in turn sets in motion a complex defense mechanism), the manner by which it exerts an antibacterial effect remains to be established.

Lysozyme (as mentioned) breaks up cell walls of susceptible bacteria. Evidence is accumulating that it has a more general scavenger function than has heretofore been considered.[14]

Several antilactobacilli systems have been studied in saliva.[16] The lactoperoxidase–thiocyanate–hydrogen perioxide system has received greatest attention. Evidence also exists that the antibacterial activity can involve potentially cariogenic streptococci as well.[12]

Lactoferrin, by binding iron, can interfere with the metabolism of a number of organisms that are iron dependent.

## SALIVA AND ORAL DISEASE

The role of saliva in oral disease is most apparent when salivary flow is markedly reduced. Where salivary flow is relatively normal, saliva is of greatest interest to the dentist in three areas: plaque deposition, calculus formation, and (perhaps to a lesser extent) dental caries.

### Plaque deposition

Saliva influences supragingival plaque deposition and activity in a variety of ways. It is involved in the first step of plaque formation—deposition of a pellicle (or cuticle)—which is a four-stage process: (1) bathing of the tooth surfaces by salivary fluids, which contain numerous protein constituents, (2) selective adsorption of certain glycoproteins, including a high-molecular weight material called the agglutinating substance,[17] (3) loss of solubility of the adsorbed proteins by surface denaturation and acid precipitation, (4) alteration of the glycoproteins by enzymes from bacteria and the oral secretions.

The pellicle then becomes colonized by bacteria, and the true bacterial plaque forms. Saliva continues to provide agglutinating substance and other proteins for bacterial intercellular adhesion to the intercellular matrix. Salivary proteins and carbohydrates serve as a substrate for metabolic activity of the bacteria. Salivary calcium, phosphorus, magnesium, sodium, and potassium become part of the gel-like interstices of the plaque and influence mineralization and demineralization, cell adhesion, and diffusion of bacterial products. Buffer components from saliva affect plaque pH. Salivary urea and ammonia have a profound effect on bacterial activity and final plaque pH.[18]

### Calculus formation

The mineral components of supragingival calculus are derived almost exclusively from the salivary fluids. Calculus deposition is most rapid and heaviest opposite the orifices of the salivary glands. Parotid and submaxillary saliva is usually saturated in relation to brushite and hydroxyapatite (the major minerals of calculus), and hence saliva is considered a metastable solution; calcium and phosphorous concentrations in saliva are not, per se, the most critical factors in determining individual susceptibility. Elevations in salivary proteins and urea content are very important.[19] Where calcium or phosphorous is unusually high, however, a supersaturation may exist; and these persons are unusually prone to heavy calculus formation. Children with cystic fibrosis or asthma are examples of this situation.[20] Some normal children and adults may also exhibit unusually high salivary calcium concentration, mostly in the submaxillary secretion.

Examination of the salivary proteins that may play a role in plaque mineralization indicates that esterase, pyrophosphatase, and possibly acid phosphatase may be involved.[21] Persons who are heavy calculus formers have higher levels of salivary glycoproteins than noncalculus formers, and perhaps even glycoproteins not found in noncalculus formers.[22]

### Dental caries

A voluminous literature attests to the interest in the relationship between salivary flow, physical properties, composition, and dental caries. Such factors as flow rate, viscosity, buffer capacity, and protein, calcium, phosphorous, chloride, urea, and ammonia content as well as a variety of antibacterial factors have been considered. With the exception of the effect of marked reduction in flow rate, none of the parameters examined have been found to be unequivocally related to caries activity or incidence, although some recent work suggests that salivary IgA may be involved.

## SALIVA AND SYSTEMIC DISEASE

There is a rapidly expanding body of data on the value of salivary examination in the diagnosis of systemic disease and the monitoring of abnormal substances via saliva. In such diseases as cystic fibrosis, asthma, several forms of hypertension, and diseases of the adrenal cortex, saliva has been shown to be abnormal. In toxicity due to overdose of digitalis, salivary examination can be diagnostic. Excess of mercury in the body can be monitored via saliva. Many other substances are now being studied.[23]

The dentist, by examining salivary flow rate and composition, may render valuable help to total health care.

## SUMMARY

Saliva is a complex secretion that plays a major role in general and oral health and disease. It lubricates and protects the structures of the mouth and influences the nature of the oral microbial flora and even the chemical composition of the teeth. Saliva plays a role in the formation of plaque and calculus and is therefore intimately related to caries and periodontal disease. It is also deeply involved in the resistance of the body to these diseases.

**CHAPTER 5**

**References**

1. Burgen, A. S. V., and Emmelin, N. G.: Physiology of the salivary glands, Baltimore, 1961, The Williams & Wilkins Co.
2. Ellison, S. A.: Proteins and glycoproteins of saliva. In Code, C. F., editor: Handbook of physiology. Section 6, Alimentary canal, Baltimore, 1967, The Williams & Wilkins Co.
3. Caldwell, R. C., and Pigman, W.: Disc electrophoresis of human saliva in polyacrylamide gel, Arch. Biochem. **110**:91, 1965.
4. Meyer, T. S., and Lamberts, B. L.: Zone electrophoresis of human parotid saliva in acrylamide gel, Nature **205**:1215, 1965.
5. Mandel, I. D.: Electrophoretic studies of saliva, J. Dent. Res. **45**:634, 1966.
6. Steiner, J. C., and Keller, P.: An electrophoretic analysis of the protein components of human parotid saliva, Arch. Oral Biol. **13**:1213, 1968.
7. Mandel, I. D., Thompson, R. H., Jr., and Ellison, S. A.: Studies on the mucoproteins of human parotid saliva, Arch. Oral Biol. **10**:499, 1965.
8. Tomasi, T. B., Jr., and Bienenstock, J.: Secretory immunoglobulins, Advances Immun. **9**:1, 1968.
9. Kraus, F. W., and Mestecky, J.: Immunohistochemical localization of amylase, lysozyme and immunoglobulins in the human parotid gland, **16**:781, 1971.
10. Orban, B., and Weinman, J. P.: The cellular elements of saliva, J. Amer. Dent. Ass. **26**:2008, 1939.
11. Klinkhamer, J. M.: Quantitative evaluation of gingivitis and periodontal disease. II. The mobile mucous phase of oral secretions, Periodontics **6**:253, 1968.
12. Morrison, M., and Steele, W. F.: Lactoperoxidase, the peroxidase in the salivary gland. In Person, P., editor: Biology of the mouth, Washington, D. C., 1968, A.A.A.S.
13. Mandel, I. D., Mandel, L., and Baurmash, H.: Salivary studies in parotitis, I.A.D.R. abstract no. 492, 1969.
14. Genco, R. J., Evans, R. I., and Ellison, S. A.: Dental research in microbiology with emphasis on periodontal disease, J. Amer. Dent. Ass. **78**:1016, 1969.
15. Brandtzaeg, P., and Fjellanger, I.: Adsorption of gamma A immunoglobulin onto oral bacteria, J. Bact. **96**:242, 1968.
16. Dogon, I. L., and Amdur, B. H.: Further characterization of an antibacterial factor in human parotid secretions active against Lactobacillus casei, Arch. Oral Biol. **10**:605, 1965.
17. Hay, D. I., Gibbons, R. J., and Spinell, D. M.: Characteristics of some high molecular weight constituents with bacterial aggregating activity from whole saliva and dental plaque, Caries Res. **5**:111, 1971.
18. Biswas, S. D., and Kleinberg, I.: Effect of urea concentration on its utilization, on the pH

and the formation of ammonia and carbon dioxide in a human salivary sediment system, Arch. Oral Biol. **16**:759, 1971.

19. Mandel, I. D., and Thompson, R. H., Jr.: The chemistry of parotid and submaxillary saliva in heavy calculus formers and non-formers, J. Periodont. **38**:310, 1967.
20. Wotman, S., Mandel, I. D., Mercadante, J., and Goldman, R.: Calculus in normal children and children with cystic fibrosis, I.A.D.R. abstract no. 63, 1970.
21. Draus, F. J., Tarbet, W. J., and Miklos, F. L.: Salivary enzymes and calculus formation, J. Periodont. Res. **3**:232, 1968.
22. Ericson, T.: Salivary glycoproteins, Acta Odont. Scand. **26**:3, 1968.
23. Wotman, S., and Mandel, I. D.: Salivary indicators of systemic disease, Postgrad. Med. (In press.)

CHAPTER SIX

# Microbiology and periodontal disease



*Indigenous microbiota*

The human body supports, both in it and on it, diverse but characteristic populations that are indigenous to a given body site (e.g., skin, bowel, mouth). These populations are frequently termed indigenous microbiota.

*Transients*

In addition, microorganisms from the surroundings appear in the mouth without being able to establish themselves permanently. Most of these transients appear to have no influence on the host. Transient pathogens may also inhabit the mouth during times of disease but later are forced out when host resistance prevails. It is obvious that in an intimate association as exists between bacteria and tissue of the oral epithelium, both factors, the microbial activity and the host response, are interrelated.

## THE MICROBIOTA

### Location

The oral microbiota grows on the surfaces of teeth and mucous membranes, to which it adheres. The main sites of this microbial colonization are the gingival sulcus, the smooth surfaces and fissures of the crown, and the dorsum of the tongue. The indigenous microbiota constitutes a normal part of the oral environment and seemingly has no adverse effects on the host as long as the host-parasite relationship is in balance. On the other hand, the same normal flora may cause periodontal disease if the general resistance of the host or the local resistance of the gingival tissues is reduced. Usually, however, chronic inflammatory periodontal disease develops because of the effects of massed populations of microorganisms in the gingival sulcus.[1]

*Salivary microbiota*

Saliva flowing from the ducts passes over the tooth and mucosal surfaces colonized by bacteria. Thus saliva becomes heavily contaminated with microorganisms and their products before leaving the oral cavity. Since the microflora of saliva is dependent on the input of organisms from the oral surfaces, it shows great variation in number and composition even in the same individual at different times.[2] The salivary microbiota is also strongly influenced by such factors as the presence or absence of teeth and the effectiveness of oral hygiene procedures. Bacterial counts of saliva are therefore not representative of a given oral site (i.e., the dental plaque or the gingiva) since we do not know the sources from which the individual microorganisms were derived.

### Acquisition

The acquisition of an oral microbiota starts at birth.[3] Among the great variety of microorganisms entering the mouth of the infant, only certain species become established (i.e., those that are suited for growth in the oral environment). It seems logical then to assume that such microorganisms are to a large extent derived from the oral flora of the mother; but organisms from the skin, food, air, and clothing may also appear as transients.

During the first few months after birth, the oral microbiota is dominated by streptococci and contains small and variable numbers of staphylococci, lactobacilli, *Neisseria, Veillonella,* and *Candida.*[3] This early microbiota of the edentulous mouth is mainly facultative (aerotolerant); however, the presence of the strictly anaerobic *Veillonella* suggests that facultative organisms create an anaerobic environment. As the teeth erupt, microorganisms also colonize the teeth, mainly the fissures and the gingival sulcus region. The sulcular ecosystems become highly anaerobic; and new bacterial groups, including *Bacteroides, Fusobacterium, Leptothrix, Selenomonas,* and spirochetes, are found. *Bacteroides melaninogenicus* and spirochetes, however, are only occasionally detected in preschool children and appear to increase in number according to the age of the individual.[4]

## SOFT DENTAL DEPOSITS

Dental deposits acquired after eruption of the teeth may be classified as (1) acquired pellicle, (2) stains, (3) dental plaque, (4) dental calculus, (5) materia alba, and (6) food debris.[5]

### Acquired pellicle

The acquired pellicle (acquired or exogenous cuticle) is a thin membrane (0.1 to 0.5 $\mu$ thick) that is acellular and essentially bacteria free.[6] It consists of salivary proteins adsorbed to the enamel or cementum and is reformed in minutes if removed by polishing of the teeth. Pellicle is also formed on appliances and even plastic strips inserted around the teeth for study purposes.

### Stains

Dental stains occurring as adherent deposits constitute an aesthetic problem. Some of the extrinsic stains are acellular pellicles discolored by food pigments or by tobacco tar (e.g., that seen in smokers). Similar stains in children and nonsmokers are believed to be plaque colored by the activity of chromogenic bacteria (brown, black, green, and orange stain).[7] A roughened enamel surface is often found underneath the green stain, and the stain returns rapidly after it is removed unless the enamel surface is highly polished. Metal salts (e.g., silver nitrate), when used as medication, may also cause unsightly stains.

Intrinsic stains fall outside the range of discussion of this book, except for

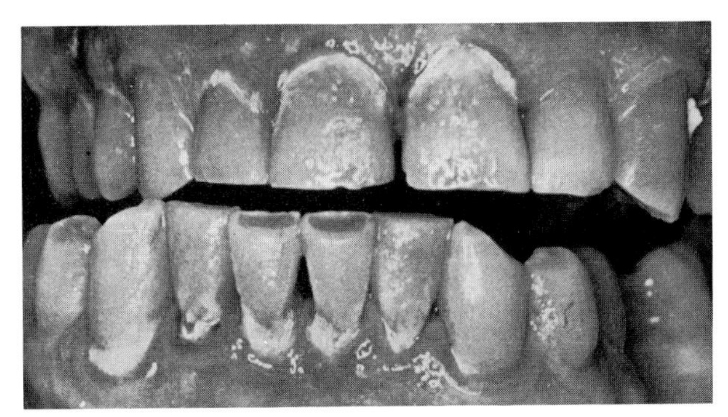

**Fig. 6-1.** Materia alba and dental plaque collected around the cervical area of teeth.

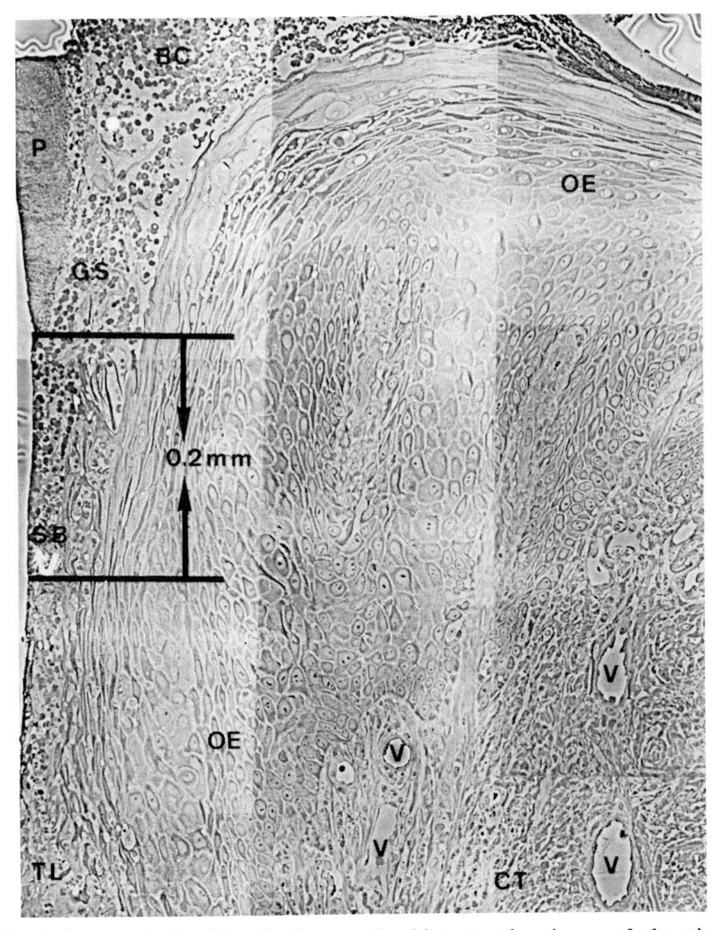


**Fig. 6-2.** The intimate relationship of plaque microbiota to the tissues of the gingival sulcus is evident in this phase contrast photomicrograph. *P,* Plaque; *GS,* gingival sulcus; *SB,* bottom of the sulcus; *SC,* crest of the gingival margin; *OE,* oral epithelium; *CT,* connective tissue; *V,* blood vessels. (Courtesy H. E. Schroeder, Zurich.)

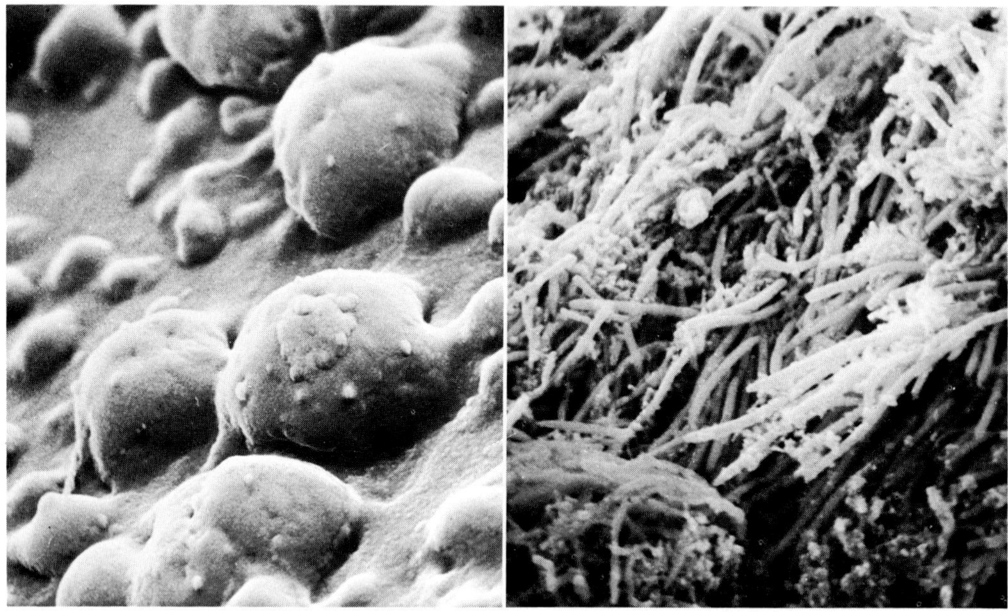

Fig. 6-3 Fig. 6-4

**Fig. 6-3.** Scanning electron micrograph of the surface of an upper central incisor near the sulcus 1 hour after prophylaxis. The formation of these globules is the first indication of plaque. (×12,800.) (From Critchley, P., and Saxton, C. A.: Int. Dent. J. **20:**408, 1970.)
**Fig. 6-4.** Scanning electron micrograph of plaque grown for 4 days. This plaque contains large numbers of filamentous organisms. (×6000.) (Courtesy C. A. Saxton, Isleworth, Middlesex, United Kingdom.)

reasons of differential diagnosis. The most important intrinsic stain is that caused by fluorosis. This discoloration is brownish or opaque whitish and is found to affect the teeth in a symmetric bilateral developmental pattern. The prolonged administration of tetracyclines in children during tooth development can produce a typical symmetric grayish stain. Intrinsic stains in individual teeth may be caused by the loss of vitality of the pulp and decomposition of blood pigments, or they may result from medicaments used in endodontic therapy and filling materials. Congenital or early acquired discoloration of individual teeth can also occur.

## Dental plaque

Dental plaque (Fig. 6-1) consists of soft bacterial deposits firmly adhering to the teeth (Fig. 6-2).[5,6] It can be removed by toothbrushing, but not completely by a water spray, and it reforms rapidly after removal (Fig. 6-3).

Plaque is neither food nor food residue, nor is it just some bacteria from the mouth. In fact, it is a complex, metabolically interconnected, highly organized bacterial system. It consists of dense masses of a large variety of microorganisms embedded in an intermicrobial matrix. In sufficient concentration and with metabolic development, it may disturb the balance of the host-parasite relationship and thereby cause dental caries and periodontal disease. Thus an understanding of dental plaque, its formation, microflora, biochemical activities, and biologic effects on the host is most important.

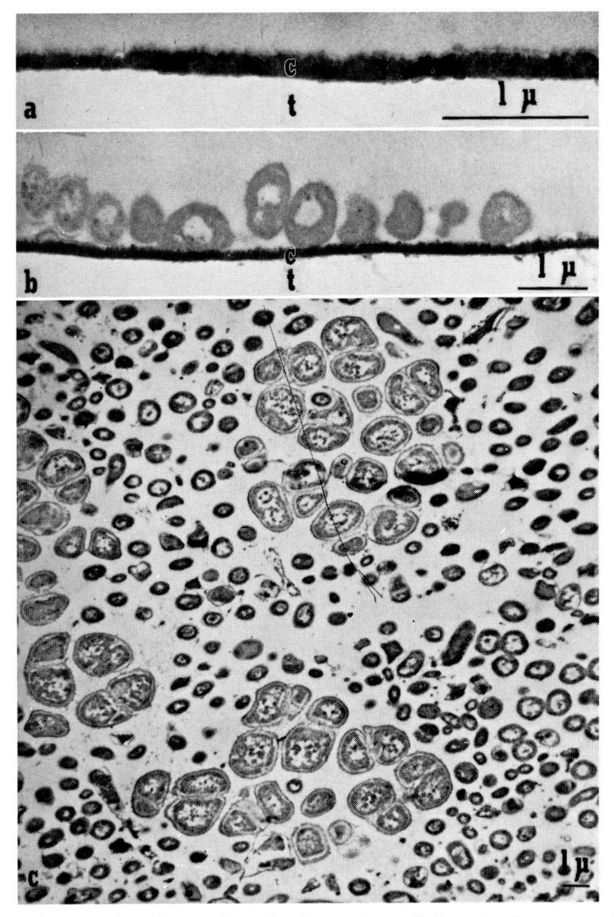


**Fig. 6-5.** Electron micrographs illustrating the formation of dental plaque. **a,** Acquired pellicle, *c,* deposited from salivary proteins. *t,* Space representing tooth surface. (×29,000.) **b,** First microorganisms attached to the acquired membrane, *c. t,* Space representing tooth surface. (×14,500.) **c,** Dental plaque consisting primarily of microorganisms. Note that they seem to proliferate in separate microcolonies. The intermicrobial substance is electron lucent and therefore appears clear. It may be demonstrated by other methods. (×5400.) (Courtesy J. Theilade, Aarhus, Denmark.)

## Dental calculus

Dental calculus appears to be dental plaque that has undergone mineralization.[6] Plaque occurs regularly on the surface of calculus.

## Materia alba

Bacteria and bacterial products mixed with some exfoliated epithelial cells and ingested substances may form loose deposits that can be removed by oral rinse or water spray. Such debris is often termed materia alba (white matter). Although materia alba does not possess the structural organization of plaque, it has been demonstrated to produce tissue-reactive by-products; and it may play a role in contributing to the gingival disease process.

### Food debris

Food debris is recognized as different from both plaque and materia alba.[8] It is merely food retained and decaying in the mouth and is frequently contaminated with bacteria.

## PLAQUE BACTERIA

Plaque formation represents microbial colonization of the surfaces of the clinical crowns (Figs. 6-3 and 6-4). The order of events is not yet fully understood.[9] Salivary proteins have been shown to invite aggregation of several oral bacteria, both in pure cultures and in mixtures.[10,11] Certain oral bacteria are known to stick to surfaces and to each other by means of extracellular polysaccharides. Both glucans[12] (dextranlike polysaccharides) and fructans[13] (levan) are synthesized extracellularly by certain bacteria, using sucrose as a substrate, and these polysaccharides seem to play an important role in plaque dynamics.

On a clean tooth the first step in plaque development is usually the attachment of microorganisms to the acquired salivary pellicle[14] (Fig. 6-5, *a* and *b*). The colonization may start from microorganisms in saliva and those left in microscopic defects in the enamel and the gingival sulcus despite thorough cleansing of the tooth. The second step in plaque formation is a proliferation of the microorganisms on the tooth surface combined with the addition of more

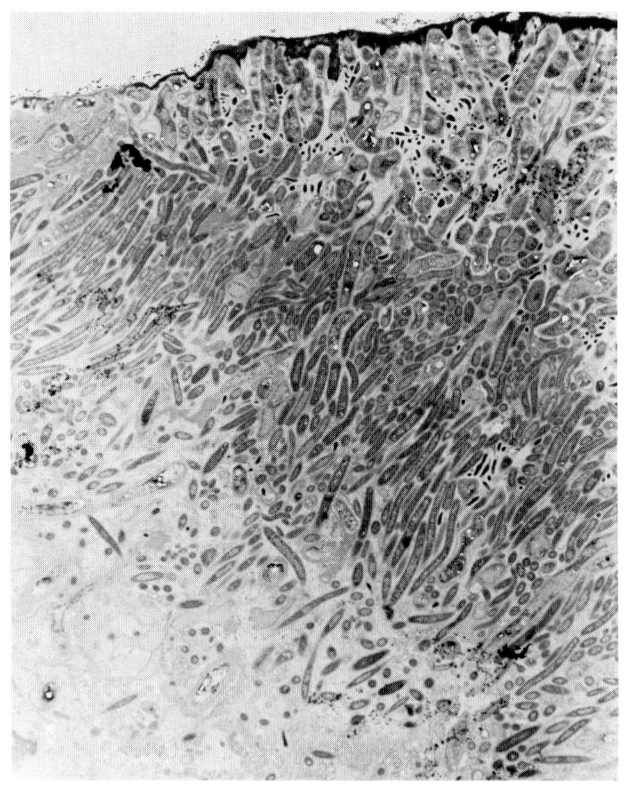

**Fig. 6-6.** Established microbial plaque from the vestibular gingival margin of the maxillary premolar. A deep layer of coccoid and rodlike microorganisms is covered by a superficial layer of filamentous organisms, which are in turn covered by disintegrating polymorphonuclear leukocytes. (×9000.) (Courtesy H. E. Schroeder, Zurich.)

organisms from saliva to those already adhering (Fig. 6-6). If toothbrushing is suspended, small isolated plaque colonies (Fig. 6-7) are formed in 1 to 4 days scattered over the teeth but mainly along the gingival margin. These plaque colonies contain a mixture of various microorganisms. As a third step the plaque colonies fuse in 2 to 5 days to form a continuous deposit. After about 10 days without oral hygiene, the plaque has usually reached its maximum extension and thickness, at which point new depositions counterbalance the amounts worn off by the friction of food and muscle activity. In the early plaque colonies streptococci form a prominent part of the microbiota.[15] Later in the process of plaque development, the microbiota becomes more complex, since the various microbial species proliferate when the environment in the plaque becomes suitable for them. Thus aerotolerant microorganisms proliferate first on the teeth, and these create a low-oxygen tension environment in which anaerobic microorganisms can grow.

## Location

Whereas the acquired pellicle covers all tooth surfaces, plaque is prominent in areas protected against friction from food, tongue, lips, and cheeks. In the gingival sulcus area plaque formation may occur undisturbed by mechanical influences (Fig. 6-8). How far occlusally plaque can remain on the teeth depends on the mechanical forces acting on the individual surfaces. Thus vigorous chew-

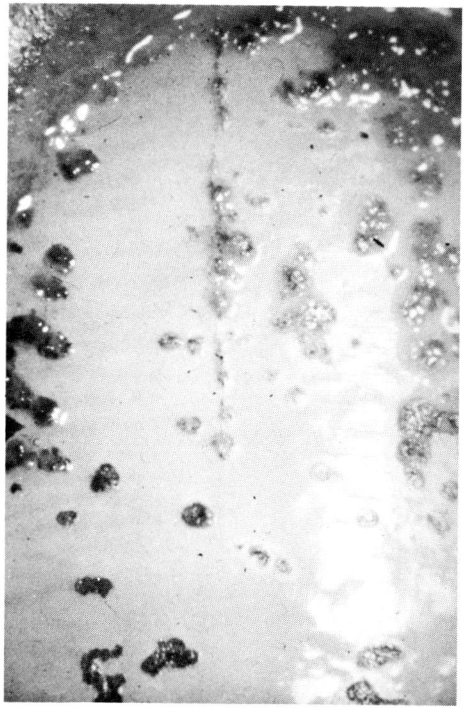

**Fig. 6-7.** Plaque stained with basic fuchsin on a vestibular tooth surface 1 day after cleansing (×30). Note the discrete, small, hemispherical accumulations (plaque colonies). (Courtesy J. Carlsson, Umeå, Sweden.)

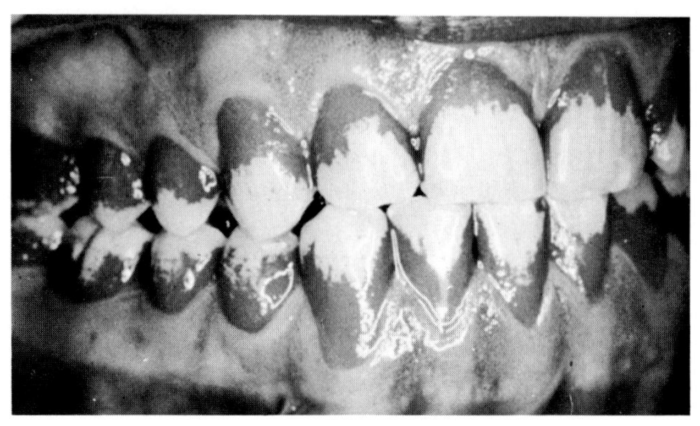

**Fig. 6-8.** Dental plaque formed during 5 days without any oral hygiene. Basic fuchsin is used to demonstrate extension occlusally from the gingival margin.

ing of hard foods (apples, raw carrots) can to a limited extent inhibit the occlusal extension of plaque on buccal and lingual surfaces. It has, however, no inhibiting effect on plaque formation on proximal surfaces and in the gingival sulcus area.[16] The maxillary palatal gingiva is regularly subjected to friction from the tongue and food particles (e.g., fibrous vegetables) and is to a degree self-cleansing; but other areas of the gingiva are not.

## Concentration

*Total microscopic count*

Total counts of microorganisms in dental plaque from the gingival sulcus area have shown the presence of about $10^8$ microorganisms per milligram of plaque. This concentration is similar to that of microorganisms packed together by centrifugation of a liquid culture, which means that the intermicrobial matrix is present in only small amounts compared to the large numbers of microorganisms. The gingival region of a person with periodontal disease may very well harbor 200 mg. of plaque, indicating that an astronomic number of microorganisms are in contact with the gingival tissues.

*Total viable count*

Viable counts performed on gingival sulcus plaque by aerobic and anaerobic culture techniques have averaged about $1.6 \times 10^7$ and $4.1 \times 10^7$ per milligram. Thus with the usual culture techniques only 25% or less of the organisms counted in the microscope are cultivated. This discrepancy is probably due in part to the fact that some microorganisms are dead and in part to difficulties encountered during the dispersing of organisms for tabulating. Also the fact that many organisms do not grow under cultural conditions may contribute to the discrepancy. Anaerobic counts are always much higher than aerobic count, and the major part of the gingival plaque microbiota is composed of obligate anaerobes.

## Cultivation

The microorganisms present in the gingival sulcus area can be identified and classified after cultivation. It is, however, important to realize that not all plaque organisms can be grown with present methods and that they do not always fit into current schemes of classification.

## Gram-stained smears

The complexity of the plaque microbiota can be seen in gram-stained smears, in which gram-positive and gram-negative organisms can be distinguished as well as various morphologic types (cocci, rods, fusiforms, filaments, spirilla, spirochetes).

At this point the statement should be made that the gram reaction is much more than a simple grouping of bacteria based on the retention of one dye or another. Gram-positive bacteria tend to form exotoxins and may be sensitive to penicillin and related antibiotics, whereas gram-negative bacteria form cell-bound toxins (endotoxin) and are usually sensitive to streptomycin and related antibiotics.

In the following discussion we shall consider the relationship of specific bacterial groups as they relate to the indigenous microbiota and to periodontal disease.

***Gram-positive facultative cocci***

The gram-positive facultative cocci belong to the genera *Streptococcus* and *Staphylococcus*. Staphylococci usually comprise no more than 1% to 2% of the gingival sulcus microbiota, whereas streptococci comprise 25% to 30%. One species, *Streptococcus mutans,* produces extracellular glucan from sucrose, by means of which it forms plaque in vitro on glassware and steel wires. When implanted in experimental animals fed a high-sucrose diet, *S. mutans* can produce plaque, dental caries, and possibly periodontal disease.[17] Another species, *Streptococcus sanguis,* also forms extracellular glucan from sucrose and produces plaque in vitro. It is present in large numbers in plaque colonies found during the early phases of plaque formation on human teeth. Different laboratories have reported conflicting results concerning the ability of *S. sanguis* to produce plaque and dental caries in animals. Other species of *Streptococcus* are also present on various oral surfaces. Certain taxonomic groups of streptococci are characteristic on the dorsum of the tongue or in the gingival sulcus or, as noted, on the tooth surface.[1]

***Gram-positive facultative rods***

Gram-positive facultative rods make up less than a fourth the cultivable microbiota of plaque. They comprise members of the genera *Corynebacterium, Nocardia, Actinomyces, Bacterionema,* and *Lactobacillus*. One species, *Actinomyces viscosus (Odontomyces viscosus),* has been shown to form plaque and produce a form of periodontal disease in experimental animals, most notably hamsters.[18]

***Gram-positive anaerobic rods***

Gram-positive anaerobic rods constitute about 20% of the gingival microbiota. They belong to the genera *Corynebacterium, Propionibacterium,* and *Actinomyces*. One species, *Actinomyces naeslundii,* can induce plaque formation and form a periodontal disease in germ-free animals.

***Gram-negative cocci***

Gram-negative anaerobic diplococci belonging to the genus *Veillonella* are numerous in the oral cavity and average more than 10% of the predominant cultivable organisms of gingival plaque, whereas those belonging to the genus *Neisseria* actively colonize the tongue.

***Gram-negative anaerobic rods***

Varying numbers of gram-negative anaerobic rods are present in the gingival sulcus. These belong to the genera *Bacteroides, Fusobacterium, Vibrio, Selenomonas,* and *Leptothrix* (Fig. 21-10). Such groups are notoriously hard to cultivate, and Petri dish counts may underestimate their population severalfold. Gram-negative anaerobic rods may constitute a majority of all genera in the gingival sulcus, especially when there is poor oral hygiene.[9]

Only small numbers of gram-negative facultative rods are present in the gingival plaque microbiota.

***Spirochetes***

Spirochetes constitute a varying percentage of the total flora. In instances of periodontal disease, spirochetes may increase to more than 10% of the total microbiota. Four species, *Treponema denticola, Treponema macrodentium, Treponema oralis,* and *Borrelia vincentii* (Fig. 21-11), can be cultivated by special methods. In addition, one or more species of large spirochetes from the gingival sulcus can be observed by electron microscopy but cannot yet be cultivated. For this reason, in most studies of dental plaque, spirochetes (Fig. 21-12) are assessed by direct microscopy rather than by cultural methods.

### Variation in bacteria

The major groups of microorganisms of dental plaque in the gingival sulcus region appear to be the same in most humans. Detailed studies, however, show considerable variation in microbiota from individual to individual and from site to site in the same person. Certainly much more research is needed in this extremely complex field of dental microbiota.

***The matrix*** As a prerequisite to plaque formation, the microorganisms must adhere to the tooth and pellicle and become glued together in dense masses by an organic matrix, the intermicrobial substance. Part of this intermicrobial substance consists of proteins and glycoproteins derived from saliva and gingival exudate. In the plaque the glycoproteins have lost their carbohydrate components through enzyme action. Carbohydrates freed in this fashion are probably utilized by bacteria.

***Polysaccharides*** Another major plaque component is polysaccharide that is produced extracellularly by numerous species of the microbiota. Important among these extracellular products are dextrans and glucans, polymers of glucose. These sticky substances may be synthesized from dietary sucrose by plaque streptococci. Levans or fructose polymers are also produced by plaque streptococci. In general, the dextrans appear to function as glue to hold streptococci together against the tooth surface whereas the levans constitute an important carbohydrate reserve for the same microorganisms. In the absence of dietary sucrose, a much thinner plaque is formed. However, some plaque is formed even in the absence of any food intake through the mouth. This has been demonstrated in patients fed via a stomach tube.[19]

## PLAQUE AND PERIODONTAL DISEASE

***Epidemiology*** Epidemiologic surveys have shown a direct correlation between the amount of dental plaque as determined by various oral hygiene index scores and the severity of gingivitis.[20]

Investigations have been conducted on human volunteers with excellent oral hygiene and healthy gingiva.[21,22] When all oral hygiene measures were withdrawn, the result was an accumulation of plaque and the development of gingivitis (Fig. 6-9).

Microscopy of gram-stained smears has demonstrated that teeth kept clean by meticulous toothbrushing harbor only a spare flora of gram-positive cocci and rods. When gingival plaque is allowed to accumulate in the absence of oral hygiene, a gradual development of flora may be seen in smears. During the first 1 to 2 days, the gingival sulcus area is colonized by gram-positive cocci and rods. Thereafter a continuous shift to more diverse morphologic forms occurs with increases first in filamentous bacteria, then in vibrios and spirochetes, and finally in gram-negative cocci (Fig. 6-10). A mild gingivitis may be diagnosed clinically after 10 to 21 days without oral hygiene. When oral hygiene procedures are reinstituted to remove plaque, gingivitis subsides in a few days.

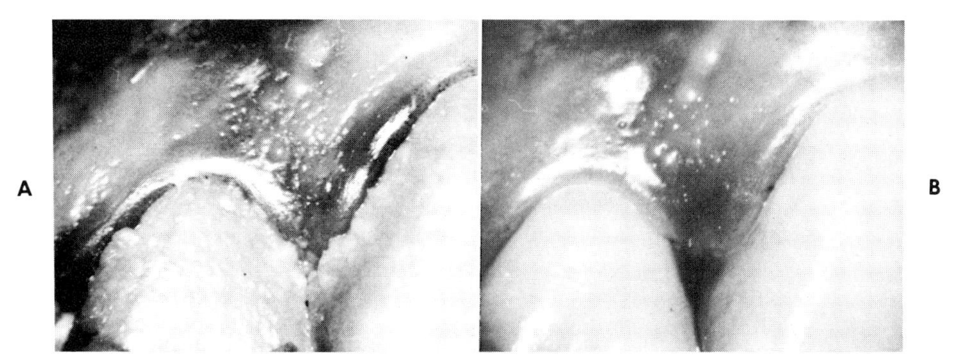


**Fig. 6-9. A,** Dental plaque and gingivitis developed during 21 days without any oral hygiene. Before that, the teeth were clean and the gingiva healthy. **B,** Same area 8 days after resumption of efficient oral hygiene. The teeth are again clean and the gingiva healthy. (Courtesy H. Löe and E. Theilade, Aarhus, Denmark.)

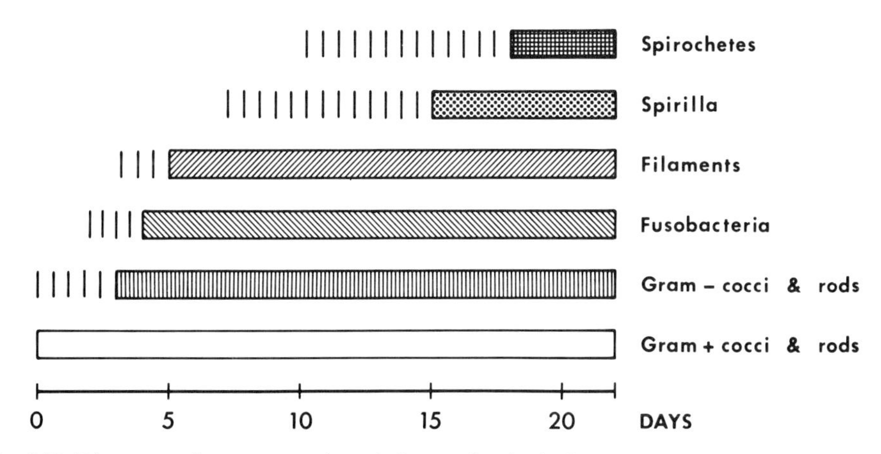


**Fig. 6-10.** Diagrammatic representation of changes in gingival sulcus microbiota during a 22-day period without oral hygiene. At day 0 the teeth were clean and the gingiva healthy. Horizontal bars indicate presence of the organisms in the plaque of all of six persons. Vertical lines indicate presence of the organisms in one or more but not in all six persons. (From Jensen, S. B., Löe, H., Schiøtt, C. R., and Theilade, E.: J. Periodont. Res. 3:284, 1968.)

## Pathogenic potentials of plaque microbiota

Although there is overwhelming evidence that the microorganisms of dental plaque cause periodontal disease, the mechanism of action of these microorganisms remains obscure. The plaque microbiota has pathogenic potential as evidenced by the finding that bite wounds and wounds caused by contaminated dental instruments can cause serious infection.

*Experimental infections*

Pathogenicity of plaque bacteria can be demonstrated experimentally by injecting human gingival microbiota subcutaneously into guinea pigs, thereby causing a mixed infection and abscess formation. The infection can be transmitted from animal to animal by injection of exudate from a lesion. The presence of *Bacteroides melaninogenicus* in the mixture is important for infectivity in this experimental model.[23]

*Lack of invasiveness*

The plaque microbiota seems to lack invasiveness. In the preceding situations microorganisms were brought deep into the tissues through a wound or by injection. In chronic periodontal disease, however, the microorganisms reside mainly outside the tissues. Most investigators studying histologic sections of gingiva have been unable to find microorganisms in the tissues, or they have found microorganisms in only a small percentage of specimens.[24] Histology admittedly is not a very sensitive technique for demonstration of microorganisms in tissue.

Since the microorganisms are situated outside the tissues, they are not removed by phagocytosis. Therefore the irritation of the gingival tissues continues until the plaque is removed by oral hygiene or its activities are inhibited by antibiotics or chemotherapy.

The plaque microbiota is extremely complex, and no species has yet been identifiable as the agent responsible for gingival inflammation. Apparently several of the organisms present produce various irritants (enzymes, cytoxic metabolites, lipopolysaccharide endotoxins, mucopeptides, antigens) all of which may contribute to the inflammatory response.[25] Thus, at least from present knowledge, there may be more than one combination of bacteria with the ability to induce the clinical responses of gingivitis or periodontitis.

## Enzymes

A possible mechanism of destruction of periodontal tissues is the action of enzymes produced by the gingival microbiota on the intercellular substance of sulcular epithelium and the fibers and ground substance of connective tissue. Mucopolysaccharidases, notably hyaluronidase, have been demonstrated in gingival plaque by several investigators. Such enzymes are produced by strains of diphtheroids, streptococci, and possibly other organisms. Proteolytic enzymes are also present.

*Possible action on epithelium*

These enzymes may cause a breakdown of proteins and mucopolysaccharides in the intercellular substance of the sulcular epithelium as well as on the surface of the sulcular epithelium in contact with the tooth. This may open the way for penetration of the various microbial irritants into the gingival corium, which contains mucopolysaccharides, glycoproteins, and collagen fibers. As microbial mucopolysaccharidases, proteases, and collagenase enter the corium, they may contribute directly to tissue destruction or provocation of inflammation. Evaluation of the exact role of microbial enzymes, however, has not been possible because their presence in the tissues has never been demonstrated and because the tissue cells also produce such lytic enzymes.

## Metabolic end products

During metabolism of the plaque microorganisms, carbohydrates, amino acids, and proteins are utilized and a series of metabolic end products accumulate in the plaque. Organic acids produced by fermentation of carbohydrates are essential to caries development. Whether these acids have any effect on the gingiva, however, is unknown. Ammonia is produced in the plaque and has a cytotoxic effect on the epithelium. Hydrogen sulfide is produced by several plaque microorganisms and is present in plaque and gingival exudate. Even small concentrations of hydrogen sulfide in air are known to cause irritation of mucous membranes and skin. Other cytotoxic products are formed by microbial degradation of amino acids.

In spite of such possibilities, the importance of individual microbial metabolites to the etiology of gingivitis cannot be assessed until more is known about the presence and concentration of the metabolites in the gingival sulcus area as well as the concentrations needed to cause tissue damage on prolonged exposure. The metabolites, however, together with other causes are responsible for halitosis.

### Chemotactic factions

Two kinds of chemotactic (white cell–attracting) substances are known to be produced in the gingiva: the first appears to be a small peptide produced by microorganisms; the second is the result of immune reactions with the C5 fragment of complement[31] (Fig. 13-3). Such substances are of interest since the accumulated white cells in the gingival sulcus may be stimulated to rupture, releasing lysosomal and other products that have the capacity to destroy tissue.

### Bacterial antigens

In addition to the direct initiation of the inflammatory response by microbial irritants, periodontal inflammation may be produced indirectly by immunopathologic processes set in action by the penetration of microbial antigens into the tissues. Altogether it seems likely, but it has not been proved, that some immunologic mechanism is related to the tissue responses of periodontal disease.[32,33] A further discussion of the immunologic mechanisms is found in Chapter 13.

The microbiology of necrotizing gingivitis might be discussed in this section; but for learning continuity it is covered in Chapter 21. The subject of plaque control is discussed in Chapters 12 and 25.

## CELL WALL COMPONENTS

Two microbial cell wall components are known to influence mammalian tissue and may be involved in the problems of periodontal disease: the first and most completely studied is lipopolysaccharide endotoxin, which is a constituent of gram-negative microorganisms; the second is the mucopeptide complex of gram-positive bacteria.

### Endotoxin

Endotoxin is a complex lipopolysaccharide with a molecular weight of over 1 million. It is a constituent of the cell walls of all gram-negative bacteria and may be extracted by enzymes, phenol, ether, and other reagents. Injection of this substance into experimental animals may result in fever, necrotic reactions, diarrhea, or even death. Minute amounts in the oral mucosa can cause inflammation and resorption of adjacent bone.

Free endotoxin is known to be produced in dental plaque.[26] The extent to which these molecules penetrate gingival epithelium is in dispute. Free endotoxin has not been shown to penetrate rabbit gingiva totally free of inflammation[27] whereas radioactive endotoxin has been shown to penetrate clinically healthy gingival epithelium of the dog.[28,29] It could easily be absorbed from gingival pockets with ulcerated epithelium and would thereby contribute to existing inflammatory processes once so absorbed.

### Mucopeptide complex

Inflammation may also be provoked by injection of mucopeptides extracted from the cell walls of gram-positive bacteria, such as those occurring in gingival plaque.[30] Neither the possible release nor the penetration of plaque mucopeptide into gingival tissues has been investigated so far.

## OTHER AGENTS

### Viruses

Although bacteria are numerically and clinically the most significant microbial forms found in the gingival sulcus, other infective agents may be present from time to time in the mouth. An example is the herpesvirus, the etiologic agent for herpetic gingivostomatitis and herpes labialis (fever blisters). (See Chapter 18.) The essential character of a virus is that the organism has no metabolic machinery of its own. It lives and reproduces only by redirecting the organized components of a living host cell. Viruses are incredibly small; their size distribution ranges from 10 to 250 m$\mu$, as compared with the dimensions of most bacteria, which exceed 1 $\mu$. They are, in essence, a nucleic acid core (RNA or DNA) enrobed in a protein coat. The coat confers specificity, whereas the nucleic acid core serves as director of the host cell's activities. As a result of their ability to control cell activity, certain viruses have been well established as a cause of a limited group of cancers in animals. It would be reasonable to expect that the same situation might apply in man.

### Protozoa

Only the simplest, unicellular members of the animal kingdom, the protozoa, are found in the mouth. They vary from 2 to almost 80 $\mu$ in length. Most of them are hundreds of thousands of times larger than bacteria. They contain a highly organized internal structure, including a nucleus, vacuoles, and other organelles.

Protozoa are classified by their means of locomotion. They usually subsist on living or dead particulate matter, which they ingest or engulf.

The ameba *Entamoeba gingivalis* can often be demonstrated in suppurative gingival pockets. This organism varies from 6 to 35 $\mu$ in diameter. The nucleus is spherical in shape. At present it is assumed to be a harmless inhabitant of the mouth, although the evidence for this assumption is incomplete.[34] Occasionally also *Trichomonas* is found in the mouth.

### Yeasts and molds

Fungi, including yeast and molds, are simple plant forms and possess no chlorophyll. They are much larger than bacteria. They are nonmotile and multiply asexually, by budding or spore formation. As a plant they cannot ingest particulate matter but absorb dissolved food materials from the appropriate substrate upon which they thrive.

The member of this group most frequently identified in the mouth is *Candida albicans,* which is not uncommon in smears of the gingival sulcus. These organisms appear as round or oval bodies. In infections they may grow predominantly as filamentous forms and may produce a mycelium. Such infections of the mouth and other organs are seen frequently in patients on extended therapy with antibiotics, especially penicillin. In such cases the normal oral microbiologic equilibrium is destroyed when the greater number of mouth bacteria are killed off and *Candida albicans* takes over.

## SUMMARY

The presence of bacteria seems to be indispensable for the production of inflammatory periodontal disease and caries in man. Bacteria colonize the surface of the clinicial crown, especially the protected area of the sulcus, and the resulting matte of organisms is called dental *plaque*. The attachment to the tooth surface is tenacious, and after physical removal, plaque is quickly reformed by colonization of bacterial species in a definite sequence. Many different species and genera are involved. The role of individual bacterial species and their products has not been defined; and indeed the pathogenic effect of a single species may not be specific at all. These microorganisms may damage the periodontium in two different ways: directly, by the production of noxious substances (toxins and enzymes), or indirectly, by inducing possible harmful effects through immune response.

Although dental plaque is not the only cause of periodontal disease, it is of major importance. Further studies of plaque may provide at least a partial solution to the control of this so prevalent condition.

***Koch's postulates***

The abundant literature on the relationship of microorganisms to periodontal disease attests to the major role played by the microbiota in the causation of periodontal disease. Regardless of this evidence, no one species or group of organisms has yet been related causally to the natural course of this disease. The fulfillment of Koch's postulates (as yet unfulfilled) has been and will continue to be the sine qua non of any of the agents of infection. The indictment of one or more microbial species thus awaits this benchmark achievement.

**CHAPTER 6**

**References**

1. Krasse, B.: Oral aggregations of microbes, J. Dent. Res. **42**:521, 1963.
2. Burnett, G. W., and Scherp, H. W.: Oral microbiology and infectious disease, ed. 3, Baltimore, 1968, The Williams & Wilkins Co.
3. McCarthy, C., Snyder, M. L., and Parker, R. B.: The indigenous oral flora of man. I. The newborn to the 1-year-old infant, Arch. Oral Biol. **10**:61, 1965.
4. de Araujo, W. C., and Macdonald. J. B.: Gingival crevice microbiota of preschool children, Arch. Oral Biol. **9**:227, 1964.
5. Dawes, C., Jenkins, G. N., and Tonge, C. H.: The nomenclature of the integuments of the enamel of teeth, Brit. Dent. J. **115**:65, 1963.
6. Theilade, J.: Electron microscopic structure of calculus attachment to smooth surfaces, Acta Odont. Scand. **22**:379, 1964.
7. Bartels, H. A.: A note on chromogenic microorganisms from an orange colored deposit of the teeth, Amer. J. Orthodont. **25**:795, 1939.
8. World Health Organization: Periodontal disease. Report of an Expert Committee on Dental Health, Int. Dent. J. **11**:544, 1961.
9. Parker, R. B.: Paired culture interactions of the oral microbiota, J. Dent. Res. **49**:804, 1970.
10. Gibbons, R. J., and Spinell, D. M.: Salivary-induced aggregation of plaque bacteria. In McHugh, W. D., editor: Dental plaque, Edinburgh, 1970, E & S Livingstone, Ltd.
11. Gibbons, R. J., and Banghart, S. B.: Synthesis of extracellular dextran by cariogenic bacteria and its presence in human dental plaque, Arch. Oral Biol. **12**:11, 1967.
12. Critchley, P., Wood, J. M., Saxton, C. A., and Leach, S. A.: The polymerisation of dietary sugars by dental plaque, Caries Res. **1**:112, 1967.
13. McDougall, W. A.: Studies on the dental plaque. IV. Levans and the dental plaque, Aust. Dent. J. **9**:1, 1964.
14. Theilade, E., and Theilade, J.: Bacteriological and ultrastructural studies of developing dental plaque. In McHugh, W. D., editor: Dental plaque, Edinburgh, 1970, E & S Livingstone, Ltd.
15. Ritz, H. L.: Microbial population shifts in developing human dental plaque, Arch. Oral Biol. **12**:1561, 1967.
16. Wilcox, C. E., and Everett, F. G.: Friction on the teeth and the gingiva during mastication, J. Amer. Dent. Ass. **66**:513, 1963.
17. Gibbons, R. J., Berman, K. S., Knoetter, P., and Kapsimalis, B.: Dental caries and alveolar

bone loss in gnotobiotic rats infected with capsule forming streptococci of human origin, Arch. Oral Biol. **11**:549, 1966.
18. Jordan, H. V., Keyes, P. H., and Lim, S.: Plaque formation and implantation of *Odontomyces viscosus* in hamsters fed different carbohydrates, J. Dent. Res. **48**:824, 1969.
19. Littleton, N. W., McCabe, R. M., and Carter, C. H.: Studies of oral health in persons nourished by stomach tube. II. Acidogenic properties and selected bacterial components of plaque material, Arch. Oral Biol. **12**:601, 1967.
20. Lovdal, A., Arno, A., and Waerhaug, J.: Incidence of clinical manifestations of periodontal disease in light of oral hygiene and calculus formation, J. Amer. Dent. Ass. **56**:21, 1958.
21. Löe, H., Theilade, E., and Jensen, S. B.: Experimental gingivitis in man, J. Periodont. **36**:177, 1965.
22. Theilade, E., Wright, W. H., Jensen, S. B., and Löe, H.: Experimental gingivitis in man. II. A longitudinal and bacteriological investigation, J. Periodont. Res. **1**:1, 1966.
23. Socransky, S. S., and Gibbons, R. J.: Required role of Bacteroides melaninogenicus in mixed anaerobic infections, J. Infect. Dis. **115**:247, 1965.
24. Gibson, W. A., and Shannon, I. L.: Microorganisms in human gingival tissues, Periodontics **2**:119, 1964.
25. Schultz-Haudt, S. D.: Biochemical aspects of periodontal disease, Int. Dent. J. **14**:398, 1964.
26. Parker, R. B., Burbano, E. L., and Gardner, M. K.: Free endotoxin of oral flora, I.A.D.R. abstract no. 198, 1971.
27. Rizzo, A. A.: Absorption of bacterial endotoxin into rabbit gingival pocket tissue, Periodontics **6**:65, 1968.
28. Schwartz, J., Stinson, F. L., and Parker, R. B.: The passage of tritiated bacterial endotoxin across intact gingival crevicular epithelium, J. Periodont. **43**:270, 1972.
29. Montgomery, E. H., Cowan, F. F., Parker, R. B., and Hubbard, G. L.: Kinin release in the progression of endotoxin induced gingival inflammation, I.A.D.R. abstract no. 325, 1971.
30. Schuster, G. S., Hayashi, J. A., and Bahn, A. N.: Toxic properties of the cell wall of gram positive bacteria, J. Bact. **93**:47, 1967.
31. Mergenhagen, S. E., Tempel, T. R., and Snyderman, R.: Immunologic reactions and periodontal inflammation, J. Dent. Res. **49**:256, 1970.
32. Brandtzaeg, P., and Kraus, F. W.: Autoimmunity and periodontal disease, Odont. T. **73**:281, 1965.
33. Ranney, R. R., and Zander, H. A.: Allergic periodontal disease in sensitized squirrel monkeys, J. Periodont. **41**:12, 1970.
34. Gottlieb, S. D., and Miller, L. H.: Entamoeba gingivalis in periodontal disease, J. Periodont. **42**:412, 1971.

**Additional suggested reading**

Björn, H., and Carlsson, J.: Observations on dental plaque morphogenesis, Odont. Rev. **15**:23, 1964.

Conference on Specific Questions Related to Periodontal Diseases: Role of bacteria and role of the host in periodontal diseases, J. Dent. Res., vol. 49, supp., p. 191, 1970.

Critchley, P., and Saxton, C. A.: The metabolism of gingival plaque, Int. Dent. J. **20**:408, 1970.

Hyman, H. M.: The role of microorganisms in periodontal disease, Periodont. Abstr. **15**:106, 1967.

International Conference on Gingivodental Plaque, Int. Dent. J. **20**:351, 1970.

Lindhe, J., and Wicen, P.: The effects on the gingiva of chewing fibrous foods, J. Periodont. Res. **4**:193, 1969.

MacDonald, J. B., and Gibbons, R. J.: The relationship of indigenous bacteria to periodontal disease, J. Dent. Res. **41**:320, 1962.

McHugh, W. D., editor: Dental plaque. Symposium, University of Dundee, Edinburgh, 1970, E & S Livingstone, Ltd.

Schroeder, H. E.: Formation and inhibition of dental calculus, Berne, 1969, Hans Huber Medical Publisher.

CHAPTER SEVEN

# Dental calculus



The role of calcified and uncalcified deposits on teeth as a primary etiologic factor in periodontal disease has been demonstrated repeatedly by epidemiologic, experimental, and clinical research.[1-11] Although dental plaque has been demonstrated to be a major initiating factor in the development of gingivitis, the presence of dental calculus is of equal concern to the therapist. These hard deposits play a role in maintaining and aggravating periodontal disease.[6,7,9,12-14] Soft deposits have already been discussed in detail. This chapter will be concerned with dental calculus.

What is the significance of calculus in periodontal disease? (1) Calculus is rough and irritating to the gingiva. (2) Calculus is permeable and may store toxic products. (3) Calculus is covered by plaque. Therefore calculus may be harmful both physically and chemically. Where it exists in contact with the gingiva, the gingiva is inflamed. Years of experience have shown that the removal of calculus has reduced or eliminated gingival inflammation. Consequently the clinician must be versed in the art of calculus removal and the smoothing of root surfaces by careful instrumentation. The intimate relationship of the calcified deposit to the tooth (Figs. 7-9 and 7-10) must be fully appreciated by the dentist. Of equal importance is the improvement in personal periodontal care by well-presented and repeated toothbrushing instructions. A change in the oral flora subsequent to the improved oral hygiene may also be of significance.

When dental plaque calcifies, the resulting deposit is called dental calculus. These calcified deposits occur as hard, firmly adhering masses on the clinical crowns of teeth. They may also form on dentures and other oral appliances. The surface of dental calculus is always covered with uncalcified plaque. This coating consists of cells, mostly microorganisms of many types, desquamated epithelial cells, and leukocytes that have migrated through the sulcular epithelium, all incorporated into a matrix.

## CLASSIFICATION

With the free gingival margin as a reference, calculus may be classified clinically as supragingival and subgingival. This classification refers to the location

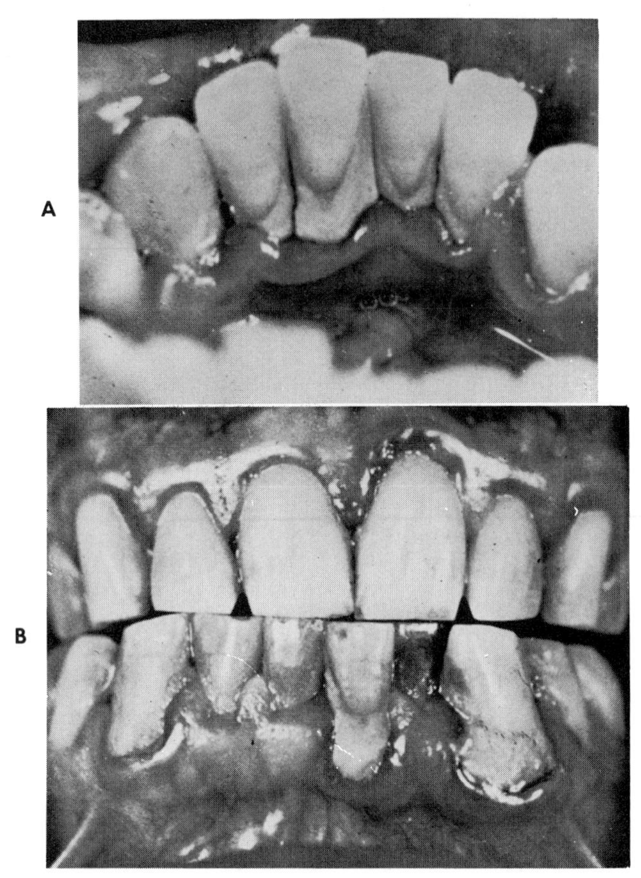


**Fig. 7-1. A,** Supragingival calculus on the oral (lingual) surface of the mandibular anterior teeth. **B,** Large masses of supragingival calculus on the vestibular (labial) surfaces of the mandibular anterior teeth.

of the calculus only at the time of examination because the position of the gingival margin may change.

## Supragingival calculus

Supragingival deposits are usually most abundant opposite the openings of major salivary glands, that is, on the oral surfaces of the lower anterior teeth and the vestibular surfaces of the upper first molars. Most adults acquire varying amounts of supragingival calculus, from a little to a lot. Inadequate oral hygiene, malposition of teeth, rough surfaces, or existing deposits favor the deposition of this material. Supragingival calculus usually is creamy white or yellowish in color (Fig. 7-1) unless it is stained by tobacco or other pigments. The consistency is moderately hard, and recurrence after removal may be rapid.

## Subgingival calculus

Subgingival calculus, unlike the supragingival variety, may not have a preferential location in the mouth and may be found in any periodontal pocket. These deposits are more dense than supragingival calculus. Old subgingival calculus seems to be harder than cementum and dentin.[15] It is usually dark brown to

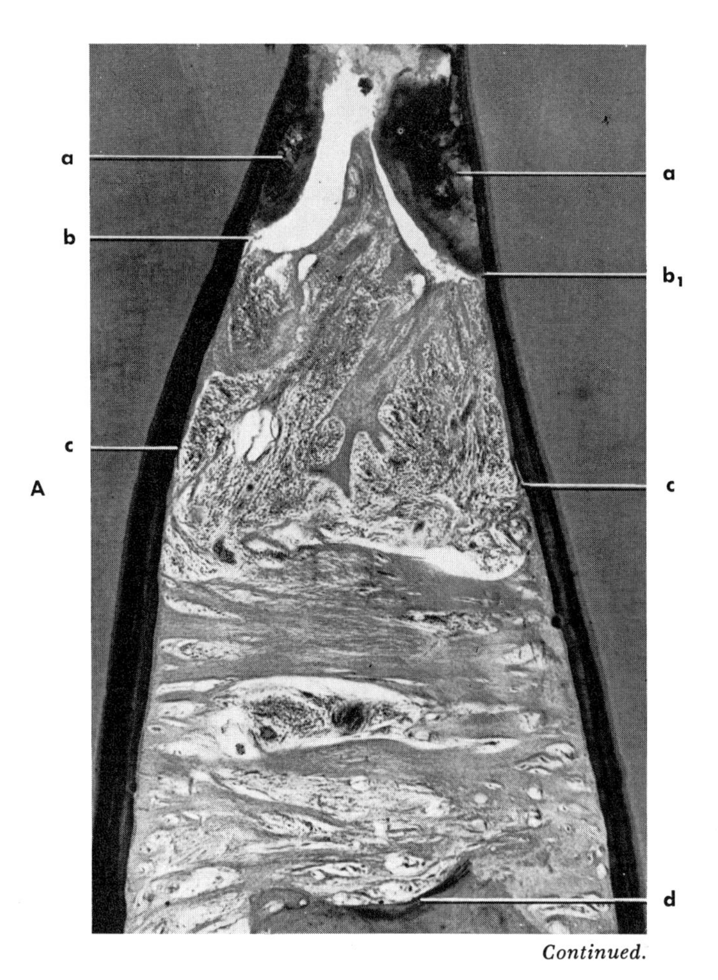


*Continued.*

**Fig. 7-2. A,** Interdental space showing large masses of supragingival and subgingival calculus. The deposits extend to the bottom of the pockets. *a,* Calculus; *b* and $b_1$, bottom of the pocket; *c,* apical end of the epithelial attachment; *d,* alveolar crest.

black and is found as a concretion on the tooth in confines of the gingival sulcus or in a periodontal pocket. The extent of its deposition may indicate approximately the depth of the pocket. The deposits always extend to the base of the pocket. This fact is demonstrated clearly by microscopic study of human autopsy and biopsy specimens[16] (Fig. 7-2). The space often seen in the microscopic specimen between the deposit and the soft tissue wall of the pocket is an artifact caused by shrinkage during the preparation of sections for microscopic observation.

## Similarities and dissimilarities

Supragingival calculus and subgingival calculus, although similar in their histology, chemistry, and microbiology,[17-19] do have slight differences[20-23]; and some of their constituents are probably from different sources. Quite likely supragingival calculus is derived mainly from saliva, whereas subgingival calculus is derived from gingival pocket exudate and possibly also from saliva.[16,19,21,24-28,31-33]

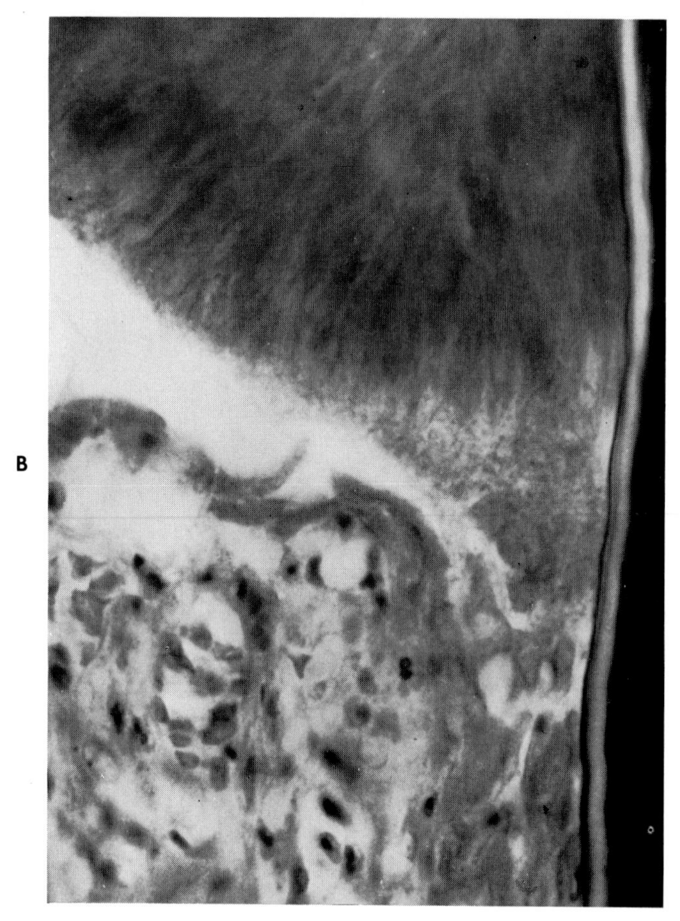


**Fig. 7-2, cont'd. B,** Higher magnification of the bottom of the pocket ($b_1$ in **A**). The unmineralized surface layer of plaque extends to the bottom of the pocket. The pocket epithelium is extremely thin, and the tissues show an infiltration of inflammatory cells.

***Morphology of subgingival calculus***

The following forms of subgingival calcified deposits have been described[29,30]:

1. Crusty, spiny, or nodular deposits (Fig. 7-3, *A*)
2. Ringlike or ledgelike formations encircling the tooth (Fig. 7-3, *B*)
3. Veneer type consisting of a thin, glassy, smooth layer
4. Fingerlike or fernlike extensions toward the bottom of the periodontal pocket (Fig. 7-3, *C* and *D*)
5. Individual islands or spots of calculus

Combinations of these forms may, of course, occur.

As the gingiva recedes, subgingival calcified deposits may become supragingival. Thus subgingival calculus may be covered by the supragingival variety.

***Appearance of calculus in the roentgenogram***

Subgingival calcified deposits are often seen in roentgenograms as irregularly shaped nodules or as ledges (Figs. 7-4 and 7-5). They do not indicate the depth of the pocket because the most apical part of the calculus may not be calcified enough to be roentgenopaque. Supragingival calculus presents a somewhat different view roentgenographically (Fig. 7-6). The presence of calculus can be diagnosed from the roentgenogram, but not the absence because only a profile of the tooth is seen on the film and only well-calcified deposits are readily recog-

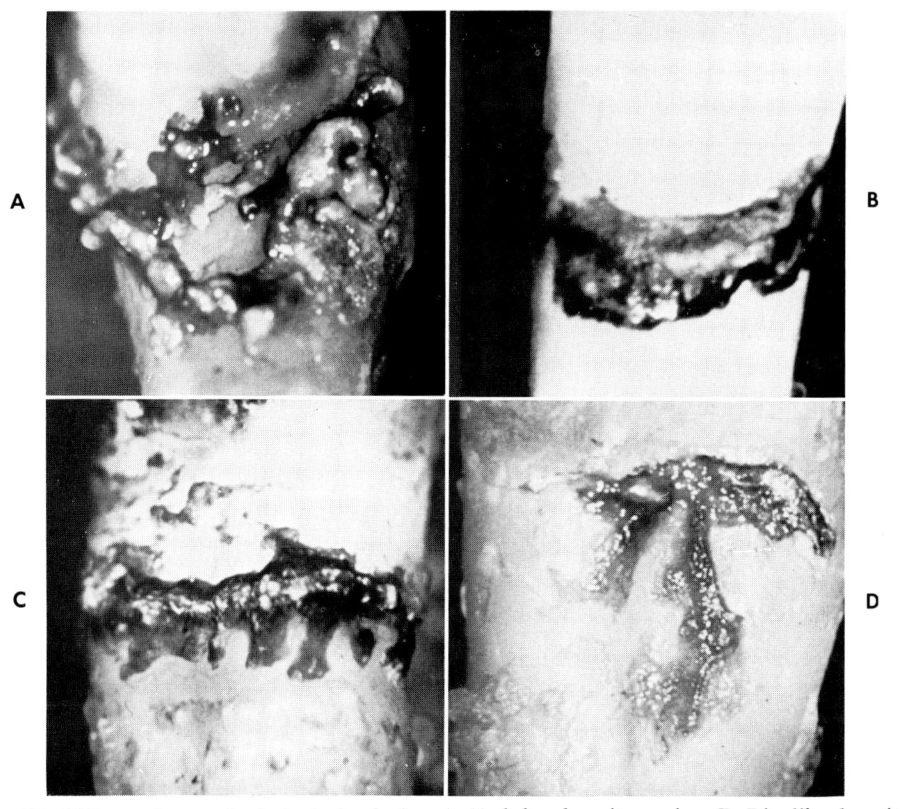


**Fig. 7-3.** Different forms of subgingival calculus. **A,** Nodular deposit on ring. **B,** Ringlike deposit. **C,** Fingerlike deposit on ring. **D,** Fernlike deposit.

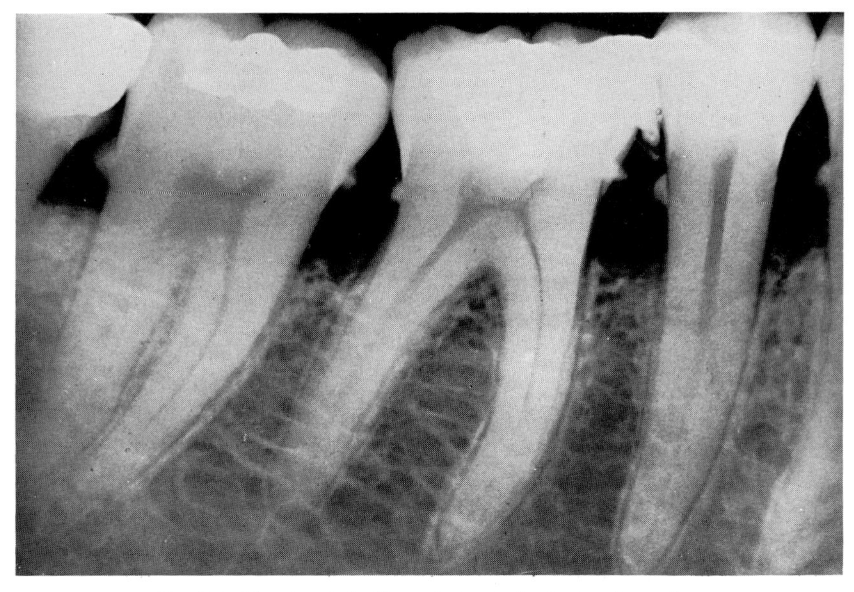

**Fig. 7-4.** Circular, ledgelike subgingival calculus formation.

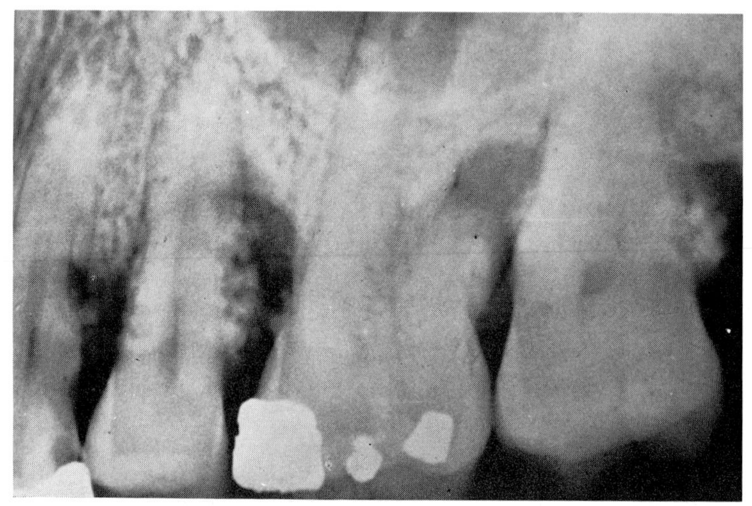

**Fig. 7-5.** Heavy, nodular subgingival calculus deposits. Submarginal calculus may sometimes reach a roentgenopacity exceeding that of the tooth substance; this signifies a thoroughly calcified and probably old deposit.

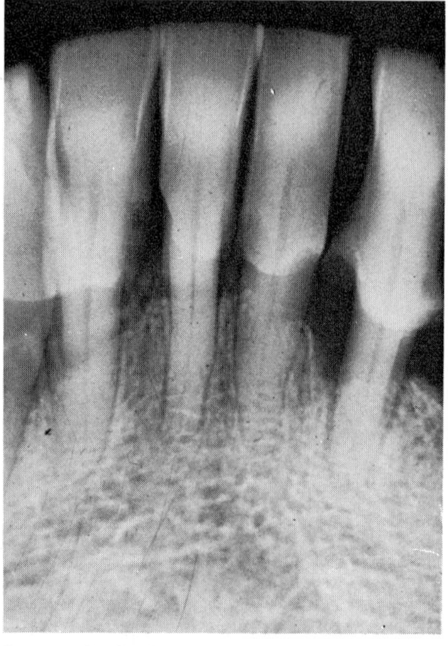

**Fig. 7-6.** Roentgenogram of supragingival calculus, which can be seen forming arcs at the level of the marginal gingiva. The marginal gingiva fits into these arcs.

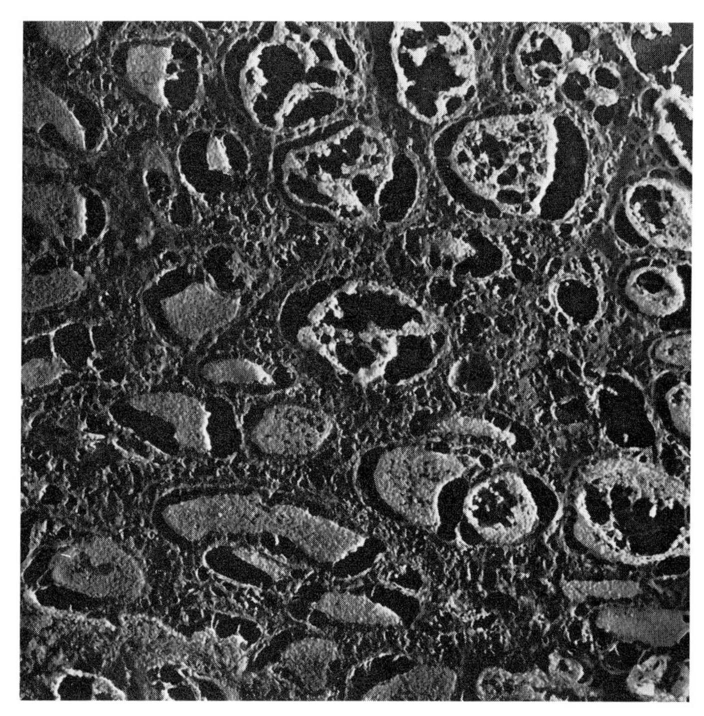

**Fig. 7-7.** Electron micrograph of decalcified calculus. The round ovoid structures are crosscut microorganisms. Note the interbacterial matrix. (×26,000.) (Courtesy J. Theilade, Aarhus, Denmark, M. U. Nylen, Bethesda, and D. B. Scott, Cleveland.)

nizable roentgenographically. Old deposits, particularly of the subgingival type, sometimes have a radiopacity similar to that of tooth structure (Figs. 7-4 and 7-5).

Dental calculus has been studied by many investigators using chemical and physical analytic methodology (histochemistry, polarization microscopy, spectroscopy, and x-ray diffraction[31]). Since calculus is calcified plaque, the composition of its organic fraction[32-36] (Fig. 7-7) corresponds to that of dental plaque, which was mentioned in Chapter 5.

*Organic components*

The organic components consist mainly of calcium and phosphates with small amounts of magnesium and carbonate. Traces of numerous other elements may also be found.[21,37-41]

*Inorganic components*

Most of the inorganic components are present in various types of calcium phosphate crystals. The principal types found are hydroxyapatite ($Ca_{10}[PO_4]_6[OH]_2$), whitlockite ($Ca_{21}[PO_4]_{14}$), octocalcium phosphate ($Ca_8H_2[PO_4]_6{,}6H_2O$), and brushite ($CaHPO_4{\cdot}2H_2O$).[22,23,41] Whereas brushite is the simple secondary calcium phosphate crystal, the other types mentioned have complex crystal lattices.

A compositional analysis of the percentage of inorganic constituents for calculus is surprisingly similar to that of other hard tissues of the body although the sources of the minerals may vary.[17,26]

## FORMATION

The formation of calculus has been elucidated by the examination of deposits of known age collected on plastic strips fastened temporarily to the teeth of per-

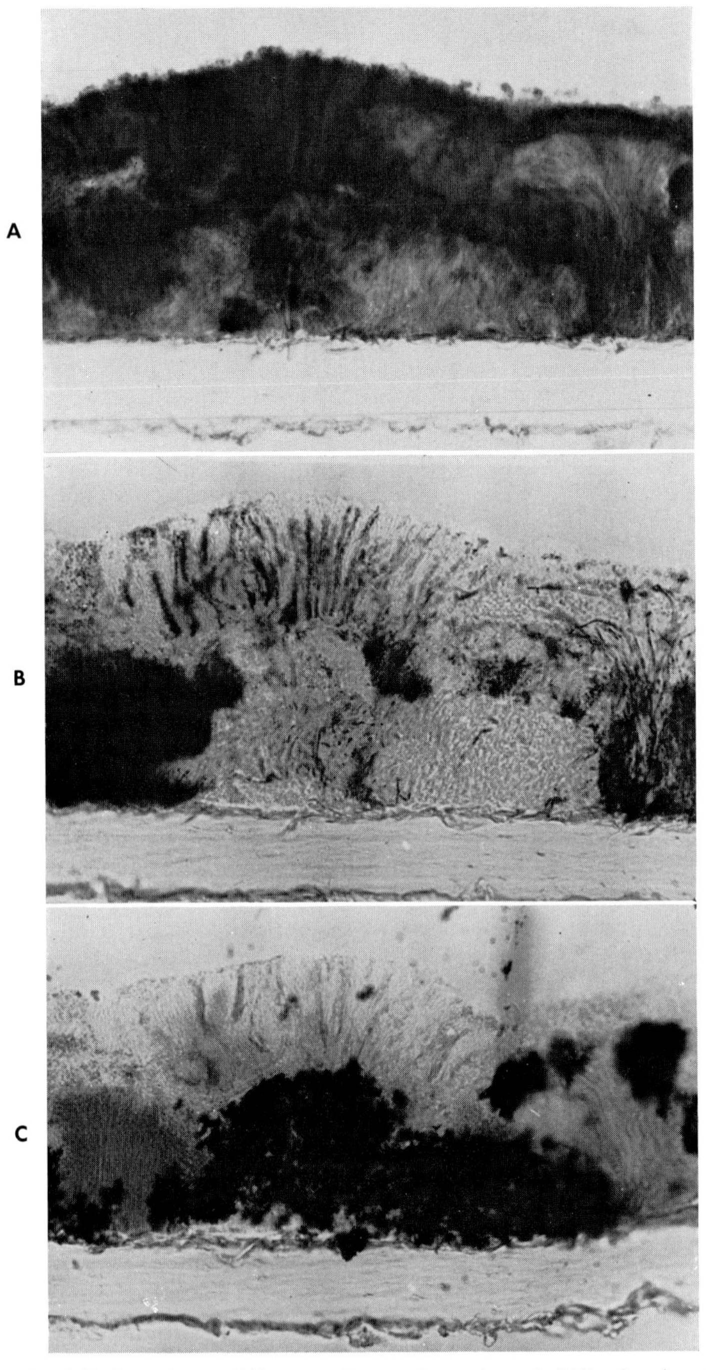


**Fig. 7-8.** Undecalcified specimen. Adjacent microscopic sections (×510) of a 4-week-old deposit show areas of mineralization and nonmineralization that have been stained as follows: **A,** Hematoxylin and eosin stain—note the morphology of the deposit. **B,** Gram stain for bacteria—note the organisms circumscribing the area of mineralization. **C,** von Kossa stain to visualize areas of mineralization—a polyester strip had been ligated to the tooth and was removed after 4 weeks to study calculus deposition. (Courtesy S. P. Hazen, Hartford.)

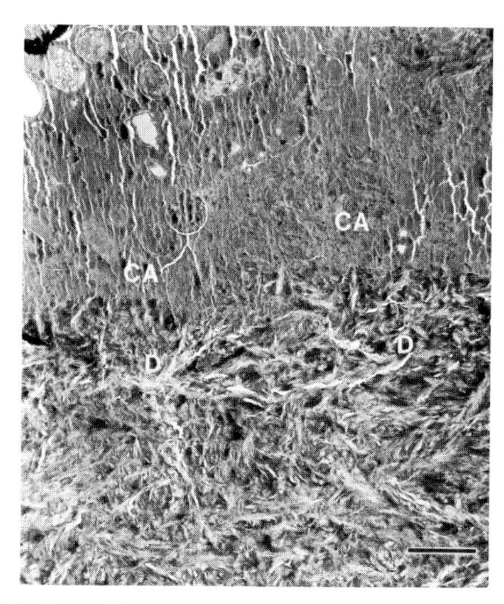


**Fig. 7-9.** Calculus *(CA)* in immediate contact with dentin *(D)* that has become exposed as a result of root planing. Calcified bacteria appear as circular profiles. The concrement contains crystals that are smaller and more densely packed than those of the dentin. The intimate connection between calculus and underlying hard tissue can be appreciated. The calculus-dentin interface cannot be precisely located. (×9000.) (From Selvig, K. A.: J. Periodont. Res. 5:8, 1970.)

sons known to form calculus[42,46] (Fig. 7-8). The formation of calculus can be divided into three phases: (1) the initial attachment of organic material to a solid surface in the oral cavity, (2) the development of the plaque, and (3) the mineralization of the plaque. The first two stages were discussed in Chapter 5.

Understanding the nature of the attachment of well-established calculus is important for the successful removal of calculus during periodontal therapy and for the removal procedure subsequently to benefit the health of the periodontal tissues (Figs. 7-9 and 7-10).

## Mode of attachment

Investigations with the aid of light and electron microscopy have revealed various modes of attachment of calculus to the hard dental tissues, enamel, cementum, and exposed dentin[43,46,47,50-55]: (1) The calculus attachment may be mediated through an organic pellicle or cuticle-like structure. This type of attachment seems to predominate in relation to enamel and is frequently observed when calculus forms on plastic strips; but it occurs only infrequently in relation to cementum. (2) The calculus may be attached directly to the tooth surface through apposition of the organic calculus matrix to the tooth surface. (3) Finally, the attachment may occur by the penetration of the calculus matrix into carious defects and other surface irregularities such as resorption lacunae.

In experiments utilizing plastic strips, the mineralization of the plaque starts when the deposit is from 1 to a few days old (Figs. 7-8 and 7-11, *A* and *B*). Concomitantly with the onset of mineralization, histochemical changes occur in isolated areas in the plaque, usually close to the tooth surface.[44,45,47,48] Similarly, prior to the initiation of mineralization, structural changes of the intermicrobial matrix have been observed in the electron microscope.[41,44,49] It is therefore proposed that the matrix in some way induces the mineralization.

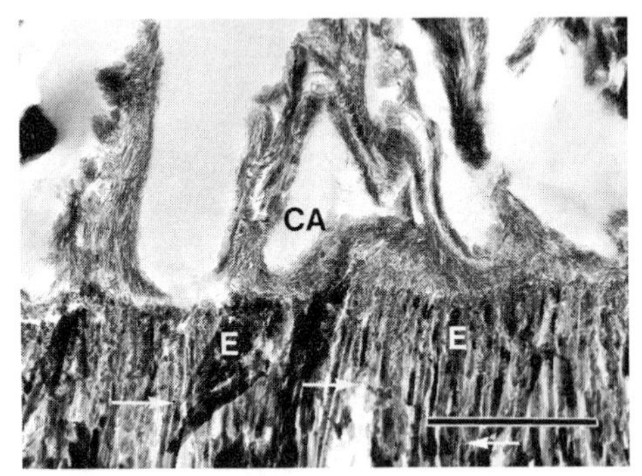


**Fig. 7-10.** Calculus *(CA)* attached to enamel *(E)*. Small crystals, similar to those in the concrement, can be seen between the larger crystals of the enamel to the depth indicated by arrows. (×16,000.) (From Selvig, K. A.: J. Periodont. Res. 5:8, 1970.)

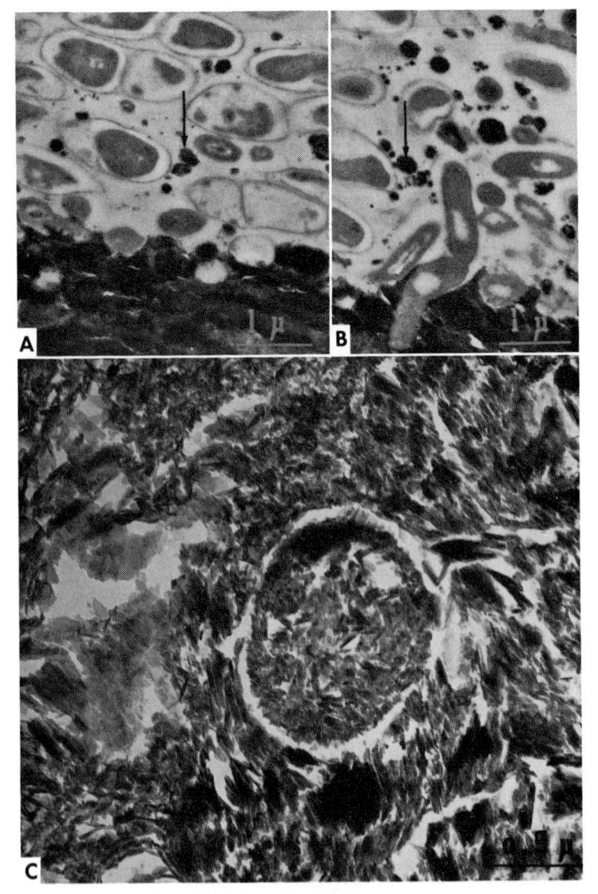


**Fig. 7-11.** Various patterns of intra- and extramicrobial types of mineralization. **A** and **B,** Electron micrographs of calculus from which the organic material has been removed. **C,** Note the crystals of varying form and size outside as well as inside the microorganisms. The round structure in the middle of the illustration represents a cross-sectioned mineralized microorganism. (×43,500.) **D,** Microorganisms permeated with needle-shaped crystals occur in B centers of mineralization. **E,** Microorganisms with destroyed cytoplasm are surrounded by a ring of platelet-shaped crystals oriented along the former cell membrane. (**A** and **B** courtesy J. Theilade, Aarhus, Denmark; **C** courtesy J. Theilade, Aarhus, Denmark, M. U. Nylen, Bethesda, and D. B. Scott, Cleveland; **D** and **E** courtesy H. E. Schroeder, Zurich.)

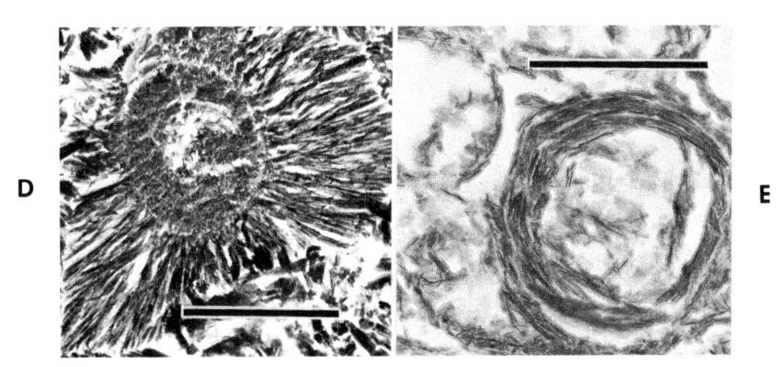


**Fig. 7-11, cont'd.** For legend see opposite page.

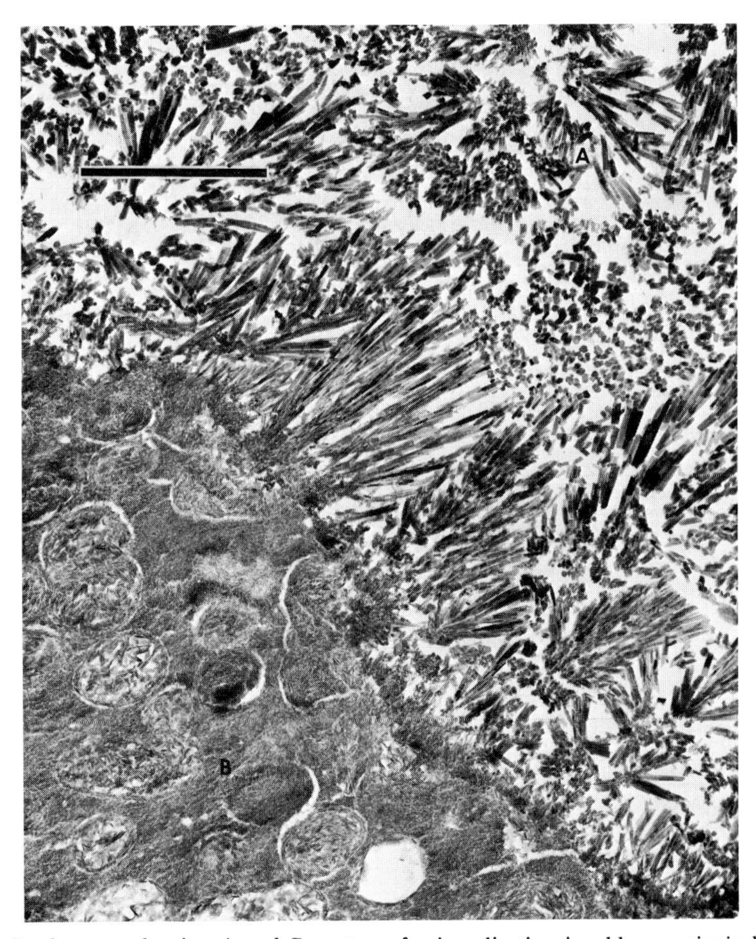


**Fig. 7-12.** Border area showing A and B centers of mineralization in old supragingival calculus (extracted with ethylene diamine). The B center in the right upper part *(A)* consists of hexagonal monocrystal columns (cross sections in black squares, longitudinal aspect in circles), which grow in lanciform bunches. The B center in the lower left is densely packed with small needle-shaped or in part platelet-shaped crystals (arrows) and shows calcified microorganisms *(cm)*. (×31,000.) (From Schroeder, H. E.: Formation and inhibition of dental calculus, Berne, 1971, Hans Huber Medical Publisher.)

## Mineralization

The minerals deposited may be observed in ground sections by the light microscope.[31] Two modes of mineralization, type A and type B centers, can be distinguished. In centers of type A, matrix can be shown to originate from dental plaque. In the rarer centers of type B, no such organic material, either microorganisms or extracellular ground substance, can be demonstrated.[41] In the electron microscope the individual crystals appear as needlelike structures from 5 to 10 $m\mu$ long (Figs. 7-9 and 7-12). In addition, platelike and ribbonlike crystals may be seen. The specific type of calcium phosphate that these crystals represent has not yet been determined.[41]

## Mineralization theories

There is no general agreement on the factors responsible for the deposition of inorganic salts in the bacterial nidus attached to the tooth surface. Various hypotheses have placed emphasis on the following:

1. Metabolism and degeneration of the bacteria in the plaque[18,36,56-58]
2. Loss of $CO_2$ from the saliva at the time of its secretion[17,19,59]
3. Epitaxis[36]

***Bacterial theory***

Evidence for the role of bacteria in the formation of calculus is based on the finding that microorganisms are always associated with dental calculus in man. The adherents to this hypothesis propose that the bacteria through their metabolism produce local changes leading to the deposition of calcium salts.

Evidence against the sole responsibility of bacteria in the formation of calculus is the finding of similar concretions in germ-free animals.[60-64] However, this does not exclude the existence of other mechanisms for calculus deposition in which bacteria do participate.

***$CO_2$ theory***

Saliva in the major salivary ducts is secreted at a high $CO_2$ tension, about 54 to 65 mm. Hg, whereas the $CO_2$ pressure in atmospheric air is only about 0.3 mm. Hg. Saliva emerging from the salivary ducts is believed to give off $CO_2$ to the atmosphere as a result of this large difference in $CO_2$ tension. Since the pH in saliva depends largely on the ratio between bicarbonate and free carbonic acid, the pH in saliva will increase when $CO_2$ escapes. Furthermore, the dissociation of phosphoric acid increases with a rise in alkalinity so that the concentration of less soluble secondary and tertiary phosphate ions increases. This increase in phosphate ions presumably leads to a situation whereby the solubility product of calcium phosphate is exceeded and crystals form. Carbonic anhydrase, present in the saliva, may be one of the biochemical mechanisms of this reaction.[59]

***Epitaxis theory***

According to another hypothesis, calculus formation may be initiated through epitaxis by organic complexes in the matrix. Epitaxis implies crystal formation of a compound (e.g., hydroxyapatite) through induction by another compound not identical with it. The second compound has a special molecular configuration that is similar to the crystal lattice of hydroxyapatite to such an extent that calcium salts precipitate onto it from the metastable solution in saliva. The organic matrix of plaque is assumed to provide sites with molecular configurations capable of inducing an oriented precipitation of hydroxyapatite not requiring the solubility product for hydroxyapatite to be surpassed.[65] Although this hypothesis was first advanced in the 1950's, it has not yet been proved. On the contrary, recent reports point to a more likely seeding of hydroxyapatite by transformation from brushite and octocalcium phosphate.[41]

### Deficiencies in proposed hypotheses

The foregoing theories not only lack qualitative confirmation and demonstration of their quantitative importance but also fail to account for the distribution of calculus in the population and the preferential sites for the deposition of supragingival calculus in the oral cavity. The question remains also why many children[66] and some adults are exempt from calculus deposition.

*Location of calculus*

Dental plaques are almost always found on teeth, yet supragingival calculus forms most extensively near the orifices of the salivary gland ducts.[67,68] The bacterial theory does not explain this location of supragingival calculus, whereas the $CO_2$ theory readily explains it.

*Calculus-free versus calculus-susceptible individuals*

There are few chemical and no bacterial studies in which calculus-immune and calculus-susceptible persons are compared. Saliva from calculus-free and calculus-susceptible individuals has been analyzed for calcium, inorganic phosphate, protein, and pH.[69] The only statistically demonstrable difference was the higher concentration of calcium in the saliva of individuals who form calculus. Rapid calculus formers have more phosphorus and less potassium in the newly formed deposits than the average. Mineralization is followed by an increase in calcium and phosphorus and a decrease in the proportion of potassium.[70] Individuals with a high viscosity of saliva seem to have a lower calculus formation rate than do those with a low viscosity.[41]

### Inhibition with drugs

Prevention or suppression of calculus formation by means of chemicals has often been attempted.[71-81] Complexing drugs such as hexametaphosphate or chelating agents have been recommended for the control of calculus formation.[79] Of the so-called calculus solvents that have been suggested, many are nothing more than dilute (and sometimes not so dilute) acids. Since composition of calculus closely resembles that of the calcified structures of the tooth, destruction of the tooth is inevitable when acids are applied. Of the calculus solvents, both sodium hexametaphosphate and the chelating agents should probably be considered skeptically for similar reasons.[24]

*Antimicrobial agents*

Since the microbial plaque provides the bulk of the organic matrix in calculus, a number of antimicrobial compounds have been tested for their capacity to reduce plaque formation or to inhibit its mineralization.[41,71-80] Enzyme preparations have been employed to liberate the inorganic constituents of calculus by degradation of the organic matrix or to inhibit the formation of the matrix necessary for mineralization.[76-78] These experiments were reviewed in Chapter 5. Very few drugs, however, have been found to be completely effective in preventing calculus formation. In fact, a partial reduction in plaque and calculus formation may not even benefit the state of gingival health. Chemical compounds that appear to be fully effective are not warranted as a preventive or therapeutic measure in practice until their safety for the periodontal structures in particular and the patient in general has been fully established.

## CONCLUSION

Many clinicians have observed that persons who form calculus have less and less trouble from these deposits if they follow a regimen of good oral hygiene and regular recall care. This improvement in oral health seems to be in part the result of improved personal periodontal care, through improved plaque control by repeated toothbrushing and flossing, and in part facilitated by the repeated smoothing of the root surfaces by regular, careful instrumentation. A change in the oral flora subsequent to the improved oral hygiene may also result and be of significance.

Calcification of dental plaque can be demonstrated if the material is left undisturbed in the mouth for as short a time as one day. If the plaque is removed from the teeth everyday by brushing, formation of calculus can be reduced. The safest, most effective, and as yet only practical method for calculus control is still effective oral hygiene and frequent, thorough prophylaxis.

**CHAPTER 7**

**References**


1. Lovdal, A., Arno, A., and Waerhaug, J.: Incidence of clinical manifestations of periodontal disease in light of oral hygiene and calculus formation, J. Amer. Dent. Ass. **56**:21, 1958.
2. Schei, O., Waerhaug, J., Lovdal, A., and Arno, A.: Alveolar bones loss as related to oral hygiene and age, J. Periodont. **30**:7, 1959.
3. Theilade, J., and Schroeder, H. E.: Recent results in dental calculus research, Int. Dent. J. **16**:205, 1966.
4. Löe, H., Theilade, E., and Jensen, S. B.: Experimental gingivitis in man, J. Periodont. **36**:177, 1965.
5. Theilade, E., Wright, W. H., Jensen, S. B., and Löe, H.: Experimental gingivitis in man. II. A longitudinal clinical and bacteriological investigation, J. Periodont. Res. **1**:1, 1966.
6. Russell, A. L.: International nutrition surveys: a summary of preliminary dental findings, J. Dent. Res. **42**:233, 1963.
7. Greene, J. C.: Periodontal disease in India: report of an epidemiological study, J. Dent. Res. **39**:302, 1960.
8. Ramfjord, S. P.: The periodontal status of boys 11 to 17 years old in Bombay, India, J. Periodont. **32**:237, 1961.
9. Baumhammers, A., and Rohrbaugh, E. A.: Permeability of human and rat dental calculus, J. Periodont. **41**:279, 1970.
10. Löe, H.: Epidemiology of periodontal disease. An evaluation of the relative significance of the etiological factors in the light of recent epidemiological research, Odont. T. **71**:479, 1963.
11. Lovdal, A., Arno, A., Schei, O., and Waerhaug, J.: Combined effects of subgingival scaling and controlled oral hygiene on the incidence of gingivitis, Acta Odont. Scand. **19**:537, 1961.
12. Moskow, B. S., Baer, P. N., Hazen, S. P., and Turesky, S. S.: What is the role of subgingival calculus in the etiology and progression of periodontal disease? J. Periodont. **41**:283, 1970.
13. Theilade, J., Lobene, R. R., Mandel, I. D., and Hazen, S.: What is the relationship between bacterial plaque and calculus formation? Periodont. Abstr. **15**:53, 1967.
14. Allen, D. L., and Kerr, D. A.: Tissue response in the guinea pig to sterile and non-sterile calculus, J. Periodont. **36**:121, 1965.
15. Rautiola, C. A., and Craig, R. G.: The microhardness of cementum and underlying dentin of normal teeth and teeth exposed to periodontal disease, J. Periodont. **32**:113, 1961.
16. Orban, B., and Manella, V. B.: A macroscopic and microscopic study of instruments designed for root planing, J. Periodont. **27**:120, 1956.
17. Hodge, H. C., and Leung, S. W.: Calculus formation, J. Periodont **21**:211, 1950.
18. Mandel, I. D.: Calculus formation; the role of bacteria and mucoprotein, Dental Clinics of North America, Philadelphia, November 1960, W. B. Saunders Co.
19. Leung, S. W.: Calculus formation; salivary factors, Dental Clinics of North America, Philadelphia, November 1960, W. B. Saunders Co.
20. Oshrain, H. I., Salkind, A., and Mandel, I. D.: An histologic comparison of supra and subgingival plaque and calculus, J. Periodont. **42**:31, 1971.
21. Little, M. F., and Hazen, S. P.: Dental calculus composition. II. Subgingival calculus: ash, calcium, phosphorus, and sodium, J. Dent. Res. **43**:645, 1964.
22. Rowles, S. L.: The inorganic composition of dental calculus. In Blackwood, H. J. J., editor: Bone and tooth, Proceedings of the First European Symposium (Oxford, 1963), New York, 1964, Pergamon Press, Inc.
23. Lundberg, M., Söremark, R., and Thilander, H.: Analysis of some elements in supra- and subgingival calculus, J. Periodont. Res. **1**:245, 1966.

24. Everett, F. G.: Calculus, J. Dent. Hygienist Ass. **30**:121, 1956.
25. Brill, N., and Krasse, B.: The passage of tissue fluid into the clinically healthy gingival pocket, Acta Odont. Scand. **16**:233, 1958.
26. Waerhaug, J.: The source of mineral salts in subgingival calculus, J. Dent. Res. **34**:563, 1955.
27. Mandel, I. D.: Dental plaque: nature, formation and effects, J. Periodont. **37**:357, 1966.
28. Salkind, A., Oshrain, H. I., and Mandel, I. D.: Observations on gingival pocket fluid, Periodontics **1**:196, 1963.
29. Greene, J. H.: Form, location and classification of subgingival calculus, Amer. J. Orthodont. (Oral Surg. section) **30**:505, 1944.
30. Everett, F. G., and Potter, G. R.: Morphology of submarginal calculus, J. Periodont. **30**:27, 1959.
31. Mathis, H.: Der supragingivale Zahnstein, Deutsch. Zahn- Mund- Kieferheilk. **5**:114, 1938.
32. Little, M. F., Casciani, C., and Lensky, S.: The organic matrix of dental calculus, J. Dent. Res. **40**:753, 1961.
33. Mandel, I. D., Hampar, B., and Ellison, S. A.: Carbohydrate components of supragingival salivary calculus, Proc. Soc. Exp. Biol. Med. **110**:301, 1962.
34. Stanford, J. W.: Analysis of the organic portion of dental calculus, J. Dent. Res. **45**:128, 1966.
35. Little, M. F., Bowman, L. M., and Dirksen, T. R.: The lipids of supragingival calculus, J. Dent. Res. **43**:836, 1964.
36. Mandel, I. D.: Histochemical and biochemical aspects of calculus formation, Periodontics **1**:43, 1963.
37. Little, M. F., Casciani, C. A., and Rowley, J.: Dental calculus composition. I. Supragingival calculus: ash, calcium, phosphorus, sodium, and density, J. Dent. Res. **42**:78, 1963.
38. Kinoshita, S., Schait, A., Schroeder, H. E., and Mühleman, H. R.: Origin of fluoride in early dental calculus, Helv. Odont. Acta **9:141, 1965.**
39. Grøn, P., Van Campen, G. J., and Lindström, I.: Human dental calculus: inorganic chemical and crystallographic composition, Arch. Oral Biol. **12**:829, 1967.
40. Grøn, P., and Van Campen, G. J.: Mineral composition of human dental calculus, Helv. Odont. Acta **11**:71, 1967.
41. Schroeder, H. E.: Formation and inhibition of dental calculus, Berne, 1969, Hans Huber Medical Publisher.
42. Mandel, I. D., Levy, B. M., and Wasserman, B. H.: Histochemistry of calculus formation, J. Periodont. **28**:132, 1957.
43. Theilade, J.: Electron microscopic structure of calculus attachment to smooth surfaces, Acta Odont. Scand. **22**:379, 1964.
44. Zander, H. A., Hazen, S. P., and Scott, D. B.: Mineralization of dental calculus, Proc. Soc. Exp. Biol. Med. **103**:257, 1960.
45. Mühlemann, H. R., and Schneider, U. K.: Early calculus formation, Helv. Odont. Acta **3**:22, 1959.
46. Mühlemann, H. R., and Schroeder, H. E.: Dynamics of supragingival calculus formation, Advances Oral Biol. **1**:175, 1964.
47. Turesky, S., Renstrup, G., and Glickman, I.: Histologic and histochemical observations regarding early calculus formation in children and adults, J. Periodont. **32**:7, 1961.
48. Oshrain, H. I., Salkind, A., and Mandel, I. D.: A method for collection of subgingival plaque and calculus, J. Periodont. **39**:322, 1968.
49. Schroeder, H. E., Lenz, H., and Mühlemann, H. R.: Microstructures and mineralization of early dental calculus, Helv. Odont. Acta **8**:1, 1964.
50. Zander, H. A.: The attachment of calculus to root surfaces, J. Periodont **24**:16, 1953.
51. Voreadis, E. G., and Zander, H. A.: Cuticular calculus attachment, Oral Surg. **11**:1120, 1958.
52. Selvig, K. A.: Attachment of plaque and calculus to tooth surfaces, J. Periodont. Res. **5**:8, 1970.
53. Kopczyk, R. A., and Conroy, C. W.: The attachment of calculus to root planed surfaces, Periodontics **6**:78, 1968.
54. Shroff, F. R.: An observation on the attachment of calculus, Oral Surg. **8**:154, 1955.
55. Moskow, B. S.: Calculus attachment in cemental separations, J. Periodont. **40**:125, 1969.
56. Takazoe, I., Kurahashi, Y., and Takuma, S.: Electron microscopy in intercellular mineralization of oral filamentous microorganisms in vitro, J. Dent. Res. **42**:681, 1963.

57. Rizzo, A. A., Martin, G. R., Scott, D. B., and Mergenhagen, S. E.: Mineralization of bacteria, Science **135**:439, 1962.
58. Rizzo, A. A., Scott, D. B., and Bladen, H. A.: Calcification on oral bacteria, Ann. N. Y. Acad. Sci. **109**:14, 1963.
59. Rapp, G. W.: The biochemistry of oral calculus. I. Conditions predisposing to oral calculus deposition, J. Amer. Dent. Ass. **32**:1368, 1945.
60. Baer, P. N., and Newton, W. L.: The occurrence of periodontal disease in germfree mice, J. Dent. Res. **38**:1238, 1959.
61. Fitzgerald, R. J., and McDaniel, E. G.: Dental calculus in the germfree rat, Arch. Oral Biol. **2**:239, 1960.
62. Glas, J. E., and Krasse, B.: Biophysical studies on dental calculus from germfree and conventional rats, Acta Odont. Scand. **20**:127, 1962.
63. Gustafsson, B. E., and Krasse, B.: Dental calculus in germfree rats, Acta Odont. Scand. **20**:135, 1962.
64. Theilade, J., Fitzgerald, R. J., Scott, D. B., and Nylen, M. U.: Electron microscopic observations of dental calculus in germfree and conventional rats, Arch. Oral Biol. **9**:97, 1964.
65. Glimcher, M. J.: Specificity of the molecular structure of organic matrices in mineralization. In Sognnaes, R. F., editor: Calcification in biological systems, Washington, D.C., 1960, A.A.A.S.
66. Everett, F. G., Tuchler, H., and Lu, K. H.: Occurrence of calculus in grade school children in Portland, Oregon, J. Periodont. **34**:54, 1963.
67. Leung, S. W.: The uneven distribution of calculus in the mouth, J. Periodont. **22**:7, 1951.
68. Everett, F. G.: The uneven distribution of salivary calculus in the mouth, J. Periodont. **27**:50, 1956.
69. Tenenbaum, B., and Karshan, M.: The composition and formation of salivary calculus, J. Periodont. **15**:72, 1944.
70. Mandel, I. D.: Biochemical aspects of calculus formation, J. Periodont. Res. supp. 4, p. 7, 1969.
71. Theilade, J., and Fitzgerald, R. J.: Dental calculus in the rat. Effect of diet and erythromycin, Acta Odont. Scand. **21**:571, 1963.
72. Mitchell, D. F., and Holmes, L. A.: Topical antibiotics control of dentogingival plaque, J. Periodont. **36**:202, 1965.
73. Müller, E., Schroeder, H. E., and Mühlemann, H. R.: The effect of two oral antiseptics on early calculus formation, Helv. Odont. Acta **6**:42, 1962.
74. Dossenbach, W. F., and Mühlemann, H. R.: Effect of penicillin and ricinoleate on early calculus formation, Helv. Odont. Acta **5**:25, 1961.
75. Jensen, A. L.: Use of dehydrated pancreas in oral hygiene, J. Amer. Dent. Ass. **59**:923, 1959.
76. Ennever, J., and Sturzenberger, O. P.: Inhibition of dental calculus formation by use of an enzyme chewing gum, J. Periodont. **32**:331, 1961.
77. Aleece, A. A., and Forscher, B. K.: Calculus reduction with a mucinase dentifrice, J. Periodont. **25**:122, 1954.
78. Löe, H., Mandell, M., Derry, A., and Schiøtt, C. R.: The effect of mouthrinses and topical application of chlorhexidine on calculus formation in man, J. Periodont. Res. **6**:312, 1971.
79. Weinstein, E., and Mandel, I. D.: The present status of anti-calculus agents, J. Oral Ther. **1**:327, 1964.
80. Stallard, R. E., Volpe, A. R., and Orban, J. E.: The effect of an antimicrobial mouth rinse on dental plaque, calculus and gingivitis, J. Periodont. **40**:683, 1969.
81. McNeal, D. R.: Anticalculus agents for the treatment, control, and prevention of periodontal disease, J. Public Health Dent. **29**:138, 1969.

#### Additional suggested reading

Mandel, I. D., and Thompson, R. H.: The chemistry of parotid and submaxillary saliva in heavy calculus formers and non-formers, J. Periodont. **38**:310, 1967.

Mukherjee, S.: Formation and prevention of supragingival calculus, J. Periodont. Res. supp. 2, 1968.

Schaffer, E. M., Schindler, C. W., and McHugh, R. B.: The effect of two ion exchange resins on the inhibition of calculus like deposits in vitro, J. Periodont. **34**:296, 1964.

Stewart, R. T., and Ratcliff, P. A.: The source of components of subgingival plaque and calculus, Periodont. Abstr. **14**:102, 1966.

PART III

# Introduction to periodontal disease

CHAPTER EIGHT

# Classification of periodontal diseases

Although no generally accepted classification for periodontal diseases exists at the present time and there are differences in opinion, a classification is needed and these differences are not insurmountable. A classification must not be a rigid structure; rather it must be adaptable to new knowledge.[1-9] Like a filing cabinet, its function is the logical and systematic separation and organization of knowledge about diseases. Facts need to be filed for future reference. There is no reason for *not* adding to a classification or changing its sequence to simplify it if the changes are based on sound principles and added knowledge.

Periodontal diseases follow the same pattern as diseases of other organs of the body. There are minor differences, however, that have to be recognized and labeled properly. Still the basic pathologic tissue changes are the same as those in other organs. According to the principles of general pathology, there are three major tissue reactions: inflammatory, dystrophic, and neoplastic. Few neoplastic changes are in the therapeutic realm of periodontics, and neoplasms are therefore not covered in this text. Very often the term *periodontal disease* is used to imply a single entity, when in fact the term should be periodontal *diseases.*

Environmental factors, however, dictate the inclusion of another and different category of pathologic reaction in periodontology, trauma. Because of the fact that the periodontium is exposed constantly to occlusal forces, attention must be given to pathologic reactions brought about by these forces. Therefore the third category of pathologic reactions is included, and the morbid condition is known as periodontal trauma.

Periodontal diseases thus may be classified as follows: (1) inflammatory reactions, (2) dystrophic conditions, and (3) traumatic disturbances. Because of insufficient data, periodontosis is placed in a separate category as an entity of unknown etiology.

The three categories—inflammatory, degenerative, and traumatic—are of great importance in periodontics and will be discussed in all their ramifications, including diagnosis, etiology, treatment, and prognosis, in the following chapters.

**Table 8-1.** Classification of periodontal diseases

| Inflammatory | Dystrophic | Traumatic | Unknown etiology |
|---|---|---|---|
| Gingivitis | Atrophic degenerative conditions | Periodontal trauma | Periodontosis |
| Periodontis | Recession | Primary | |
| | Disuse | Secondary | |
| | Gingival hyperplasia | | |


**CHAPTER 8**

**References**

1. Box, H. K.: Periodontal studies, Dent. Items Interest 62:915, 1940.
2. Fish, E. W.: Parodontal disease, ed. 2, London, 1952, Eyre & Spottiswoode, Ltd.

3. Hine, M. K., and Hine, C. L.: Classification and etiology of periodontal disturbances, J. Amer. Dent. Ass. **31**:1297, 1944.
4. Hulin, C.: Nomenclature and classification, Paradentologie **3**:82, 1949.
5. Held, A. J., and Chaput, A.: Les parodontolyses, Paris, 1959, Prelat.
6. Orban, B.: Classification and nomenclature of periodontal diseases, J. Periodont. **13**:88, 1942.
7. Orban, B.: Classification of periodontal disease, Paradentologie **3**:159, 1949.
8. Kantorowicz, A.: Klinische Zahnheilkunde, Berlin, 1924, Hermann Meusser.
9. Weski, O.: Parodontopathien und Parodontosis, Berichte des 9ten internationalen Zahnärzte kongresses der F.D.I., Vienna, 1936, Urban & Schwarzenberg.

CHAPTER NINE

# Etiology



In the study of etiology, we seek to discover those causes or factors that contribute to disease. We are obviously concerned with the causes of periodontal disease, for, if we could eliminate them, we could cure or prevent the disease.

In dealing with illness, we customarily reason from the symptoms to the cause and from the cause to the remedy. This approach has been traditional in teaching. For example, we can picture a physician as having knowledge of some ten or twelve diseases and some fifteen to twenty treatments at his disposal. Each patient would be measured against the list of diseases; and once the physican had selected an appropriate disease, he would prescribe or perform the corresponding treatment.

Can a physician or dentist function with two strengths—one a list of diseases and the other a kit of treatments? No! There is no formula or treatment that can be applied with 100% success all the time. On some occasions he will treat a disease entity in a certain way, and on other occasions the same entity may be so discreetly altered as to require additional or alternate treatment. Moreover, with the expansion of knowledge, the list of diseases may be modified; and with even greater certainty, the methods of treatment will change. The dentist, therefore, must keep up with and be capable of critically evaluating professional advances; and he must also expand those areas of knowledge in which his schooling may have been incomplete. The only basis from which he can proceed with any degree of assurance is from a knowledge of the biology of the tissues that he treats and of the etiology that has caused tissue changes.

The factors that influence the health of the periodontium are broadly classified into those of extrinsic (local) and those of intrinsic (systemic) origin.[1-3] The extrinsic causes include both irritational and functional factors that are associated with mastication, deglutition, and speech. The intrinsic causes are important but are more difficult to demonstrate. At the present time treatment must be directed primarily toward the elimination or correction of extrinsic factors in the absence of demonstrable intrinsic etiology.[4]

## EXTRINSIC FACTORS

*Oral hygiene and calcified and uncalcified deposits*

There is little doubt that neglected or improper oral hygiene is responsible for the largest percentage of gingivitis and periodontitis[5-8] (Fig. 9-1). Dental plaque,[9] bacteria, calculus,[10] materia alba, and food debris collected along gingival margins and in sulci irritate the gingiva and provoke the destructive changes

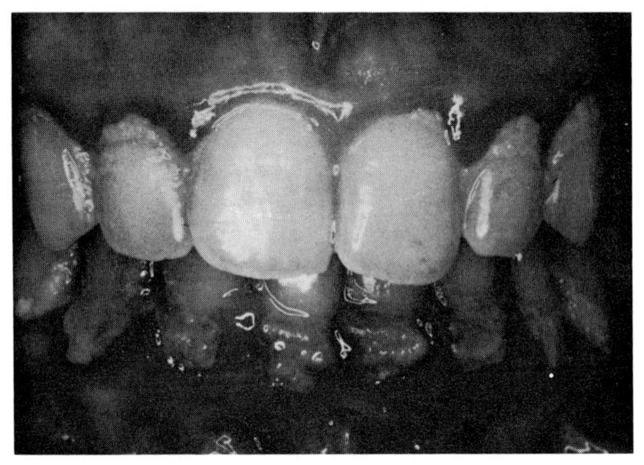

**Fig. 9-1.** Poor oral hygiene and the accumulation of plaque and calcified deposits are evident in a 34-year-old woman.

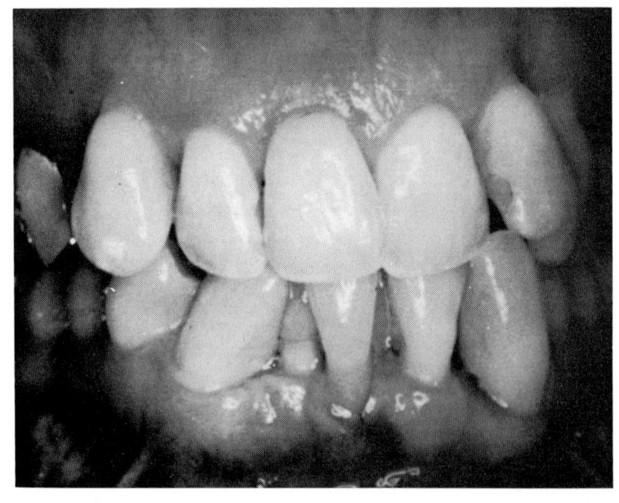

**Fig. 9-2.** Overlapping malposed teeth in a 45-year-old woman encourage plaque retention and food impaction and make good oral hygiene difficult to achieve.

that follow. Bacterial plaque[9,11,12] and calcified deposits are so frequently associated with tooth loss that they may be considered the prime etiologic factors in inflammatory periodontal disease.[13] Whether or not they provoke destruction, they are so common that they are regarded as a part of the oral environment and are discussed in greater detail under that heading. (See Chapter 6.)

***Consistency of diet***

Soft or sticky foods that tend to collect between the teeth and along the gingiva can be a prominent cause of inflammation. Animal experimentation tends to substantiate this clinical observation.[14-16]

***Tooth position and anatomy and food impaction***

Even when the physical consistency of the diet is not soft or sticky, the impaction, impingement, and retention of plaque and food may be encouraged by irregularities of tooth position or inclination. Overlapping, malposed, tilted, or drifted teeth are frequently associated with food impaction or retention (Fig. 9-2). Plunger cusps may force or funnel food into relatively inaccessible embra-

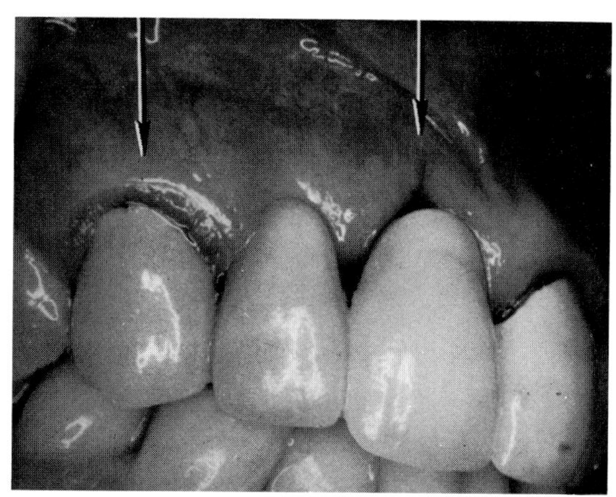

**Fig. 9-3.** Gingival inflammation can be seen above the canine, caused by irritation from jacket crown margins. A gingival cleft is present over the right central incisor possibly caused by irritation from the margin of the jacket crown.

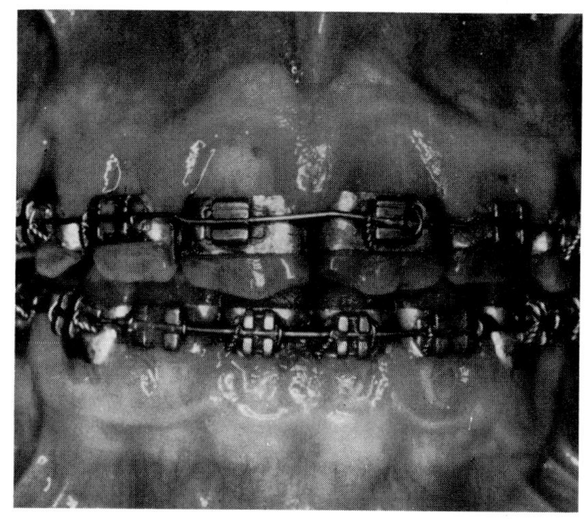

**Fig. 9-4.** Orthodontic appliances can cause irritation to the gingiva and make proper oral hygiene difficult to perform. An inflammatory hyperplasia is evident.

sures. Cavities, poorly designed restorations, or congenital defects such as bell-shaped crowns may also dispose the periodontium to insult.[17]

*Improper dental treatment*

Further irritation may be caused by poor dentistry. Overhanging or deficient margins, improperly designed prostheses, or injuries caused by dental treatment methods can provoke or initiate periodontal disease (Fig. 9-3). There is a direct correlation between surface roughness or marginal irregularities of a tooth and the retention of plaque.

*Orthodontic appliances*

Orthodontic appliances may be irritating or may interfere with the performance of good oral hygiene (Fig. 9-4). Prolonged orthodontic treatment has long been associated with the causation of inflammatory and traumatic periodontal disease.[18]

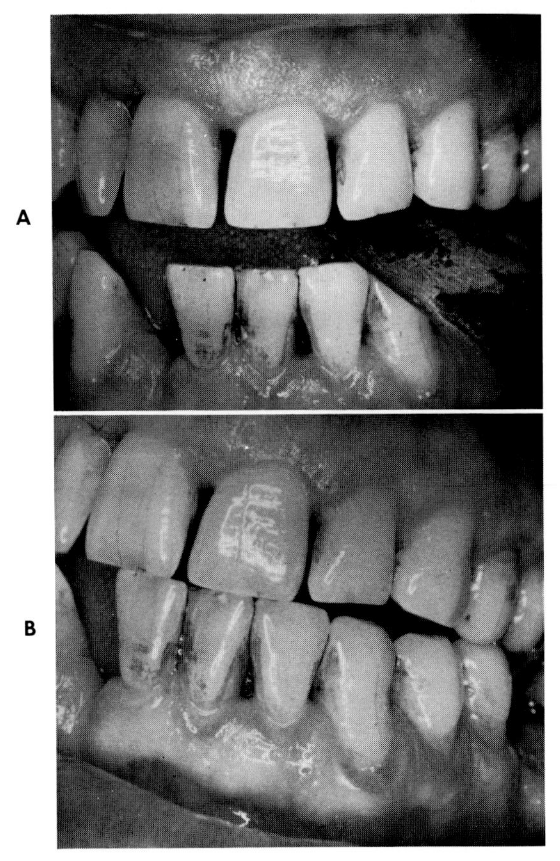


**Fig. 9-5. A,** Habitual grasping of a pipestem has caused an open bite between the maxillary and mandibular teeth. **B,** Plaque was found around the necks of the teeth used to grasp the pipestem. This may have been caused by the altered position of the teeth, interfering with habit patterns in the patient's oral hygiene methods. The depressed teeth were not cleansed as thoroughly as other teeth.

***Habits***

Injurious oral habits (Fig. 9-5) such as biting threads, fingernails, or pencils may contribute to gingivitis, periodontitis, or dystrophic changes. The careless use of home care implements may damage tissues and thus lower resistance to bacterial insult.[8] Tongue thrusting (Fig. 14-13) may cause tooth malposition or gingival recession. Mouth breathing or incomplete lip closure tends to impart a glossy erythematous appearance to the gingiva (Fig. 14-12).

***Function***

Functional and parafunctional factors such as nonocclusion, indolent mastication, clenching, bruxism, and others are frequently incriminated in periodontal pathosis. These will be discussed in greater detail in Chapter 36.

***Anatomy of the soft tissues***

Anatomic factors that may predispose to disease include the inadequacies inherent in the form of soft tissues or in their spatial relations to teeth. High frena or muscle attachments can encourage the collection of debris along gingival margins or impede home dental care. Shallow vestibules or narrow inadequate zones of gingiva may also predispose to disease. Thin, finely textured gingiva may be easily injured during mastication or brushing, and recession of gingival margins may follow.

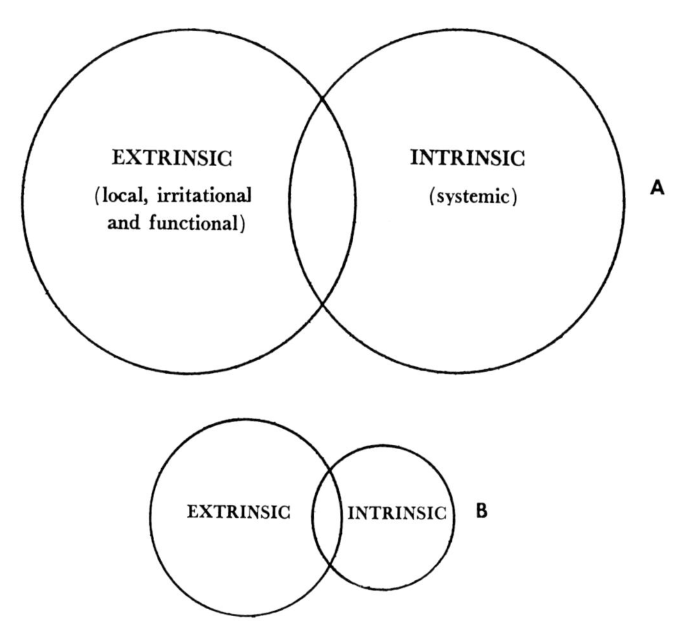


**Fig. 9-6.** An interplay of extrinsic and intrinsic factors can cause periodontal disease or predispose an individual to periodontal disease, **A.** Although we are aware of this overlapping etiology and sometimes consider the extrinsic and intrinsic as equally important, our knowledge of these factors is proportionate to the size of the circles in **B.**

An interplay of etiologic causes includes the extrinsic and the intrinsic factors as shown in Fig. 9-6, *A*. Our knowledge of these factors, however, is proportionate to the size given the circles in Fig. 9-6, *B*.

## INTRINSIC FACTORS

The entire organism shares in the genesis of periodontal disease. There seems to be little argument that what happens elsewhere in the organism affects the oral tissues. However, although periodontal disease can have intrinsic causation, the precise role of intrinsic factors in the production of periodontal disease is largely a matter of opinion. Undoubtedly periodontal disease is an expression of the interplay of extrinsic and intrinsic factors.[19]

### Interplay with extrinsic factors

Clinical expressions of disease may result from a basic insult—physical, chemical, or microbial. The influence of this exogenous insult will be modified by the resistance of the host.[20,21] For example, not all persons are equally susceptible to a communicable disease such as measles, and therefore not all who are exposed to the virus will contract the disease. Similarly, if plaque were the sole cause of periodontal diseases, there would be a total equivalence between plaque and periodontal disease. All patients with plaque would have periodontitis, whereas no patients without plaque would have periodontitis. Although the presence of plaque is usually associated with the presence of inflammation, there are some instances in which plaque is present and no disease occurs and other instances in which disease occurs but little plaque is present. It can therefore be concluded that plaque is not solely responsible for periodontal disease.

More likely there is a collection of different local insults inflicted on a host minimally defective in a number of metabolic processes. For example, plaque and calculus, food impaction, periodontal trauma, and poor oral hygiene may be found in a patient with multiple minor metabolic defects; but because the extrinsic factors are better understood, they are more amenable to treatment and are discussed more fully. This does not imply that intrinsic factors are not operative[22]; rather they are just not equally understood and hence are less amenable to management.

## Detection

There are four major sources that can provide information concerning lowered host resistance: (1) medical history of the patient, (2) examination, (3) clinical tests, and (4) natural history of the disease[23-25] (Chapter 10).

***Medical history of the patient***

Careful interrogation of the patient may yield significant information concerning his present physical status or may provide clues to undetected disease.[26] On occasion the history can be suggestive of a lowered host resistance, even when the specific biologic factor is not revealed. Although there are formalized medical inventory questionnaires, these have shortcomings if used routinely. (See the section on patient interview in Chapter 18.) An interview does not constitute an examination; rather the patient relates his history and symptoms, which may not be completely accurate. However, the manner in which the patient expresses himself may be significant. (See discussion of aspects of dentist-patient relationship in Chapter 17.)

***Examination***

The dentist is handicapped in his total evaluation of the patient's health insofar as he is unable to make and properly interpret a physical examination. There is no reason, however, why he cannot call for competent medical consultation when he believes it necessary. On the other hand, routine medical examination may fail to supply any additional information. When specific positive findings are present, there may be a relationship to the dental status.

When both medical and oral signs of disease are present, important relationships may be demonstrable. Protein-calorie nutritional deficiency has been related to periodontal disease. Gingival bleeding and bruisability may be related; and tooth mobility and ascorbic acid metabolism[27] or carbohydrate metabolism may be associated.[28-32] Clinical experience may indicate that when changes in tissue form, color, consistency, and disposition are present these may be suggestive of intrinsic disturbance even if the examiner cannot demonstrate the specific deficiency.

***Clinical tests***

Although the routine use of medical laboratory tests is rarely productive, such tests are of undisputed value when the examiner is suspicious of specific intrinsic pathology.[31-34] No startling results have been forthcoming when routine clinical tests were made on patients with periodontal disease. This fact may indicate that patients with periodontal disease can be intrinsically well, which would be an oddity, since recent studies indicate that 92% of presumably healthy patients are actually afflicted with disease.[26] Finally, one would presume that when specific intrinsic factors are present and are related to periodontal disease intrinsic medication would cure the disease. This has not been the case. However, when a related intrinsic deficiency has been adequately altered, local treatment was observed to be more effective. Beyond this, except for gingival changes in frank intrinsic diseases such as leukemia, nutritional deficiencies, diabetes,[35] and bone changes in osteodystrophies, little is known about the precise relationship between intrinsic factors and periodontal disease. Much more will undoubtedly be learned by future research.

*Natural history of the disease*

According to Forbus an individual is capable of reacting to noxious influences in one of three ways[36]: (1) by resisting, (2) by submitting, or (3) by effecting an adaptation. This resistance, submission, or adaptability is a basic characteristic of living cells and is governed by many factors. The responses may be affected or altered by the function of the endocrine glands, the autonomic nervous system, or the blood circulation. The equilibrium or stability of these factors is termed *homeostasis.*

## CLASSIFICATION OF EXTRINSIC AND INTRINSIC FACTORS

Although it is likely that intrinsic factors contribute to the production of periodontal disease, it is difficult to evaluate their exact role.[15] Intrinsic causes may be divided into demonstrable and nondemonstrable factors. Some demonstrable diseases have been associated with periodontopathies. These include uncontrolled diabetes, leukemia, frank nutritional deficiencies, endocrine changes in pregnancy and puberty, infectious mononucleosis, stress, cyclic neutropenia, hyperkeratosis palmoplantaris, and hypophosphatasia. Factors of minor metabolic imbalance may not be demonstrable, although they may influence host response to an insult.

Etiology will be discussed throughout the text in case presentations and in discussions of therapy. The causative factors will be amplified, and wherever possible, their specific roles illustrated.

Following is a list of etiologic or complicating factors in periodontal disease:

**Extrinsic (local) factors**

- A. Bacterial
  1. Plaque
  2. Calculus
  3. Enzymes and decomposition products
  4. Materia alba
  5. Food debris
- B. Mechanical
  1. Calculus
  2. Food impaction and retention
     - (a) Open and loose contacts
     - (b) Mobility and spreading teeth
     - (c) Malposed teeth
     - (d) Plunger cusp mechanism
  3. Overhanging margins of restorations, poorly designed or fitting prostheses
  4. Soft or sticky consistency of diet
  5. Mouth breathing, incomplete lip closure
  6. Improper oral hygiene
  7. Injurious habits
  8. Improper dental treatment methods
  9. Accidental trauma
- C. Combined bacterial and mechanical
  1. Calculus
  2. Overhanging margin
- D. Anatomic predisposing
  1. Tooth malalignment, malposition, altered anatomy
  2. High frena or muscle attachments
  3. Shallow vestibule
  4. Functionally insufficient zone of attached gingiva
  5. Very thin, finely textured gingiva or thick, bulbous gingival margins

6. Bony exostoses or ledges, very thin bony plates
7. Unfavorable crown-root ratio

E. Functional
1. Insufficient function
   (a) Nonocclusion
   (b) Indolent mastication
   (c) Muscle paralysis
   (d) Muscle hypotonicity
2. Overfunction and parafunction
   (a) Muscle hypertonicity
   (b) Bruxism
   (c) Clenching and clamping
   (d) Accidental trauma
   (e) Excessive loads on abutment teeth

**Intrinsic (systemic) factors**

A. Demonstrable
1. Endocrine dysfunctions
   (a) Pubertal
   (b) Pregnancy
   (c) Postmenopausal
2. Metabolic and other diseases
   (a) Nutritional deficiency
   (b) Diabetes
   (c) Hyperkeratosis palmoplantaris
   (d) Cyclic neutropenia
   (e) Hypophosphatasia
   (f) Debilitating disease
3. Psychosomatic or emotional disorders
4. Drugs and metallic poisons
   (a) Diphenylhydantoin
   (b) Hematologic effects
   (c) Allergy
   (d) Heavy metals
5. Diet and nutrition

B. Nondemonstrable
1. Poor resistance and repair
2. Nutritional, emotional, metabolic, hormonal deficiencies
   (a) Fatigue
   (b) Stress

**CHAPTER 9**

**References**


1. Stahl, S. S.: The etiology of periodontal disease. In Ramfjord, S. P., Kerr, D. A., and Ash, M., editors: World workshop in periodontics, sec. III, Ann Arbor, Mich., 1966, University of Michigan Press.
2. Gottlieb, B., and Orban, B.: Zahnfleischentzündung und Zahnlockerung, ed. 2, Berlin, 1936, Berlinische Verlagsanstalt.
3. Gottlieb, B., Orban, B., and Diamond, M.: Biology and pathology of the tooth and its supporting mechanism, New York, 1938, The Macmillan Co.
4. Weinmann, J. P.: Periodontitis: etiology, pathology, symptomatology, J. Amer. Dent. Ass. **44**:701, 1952.
5. Berg, M., Burrill, D. Y., and Fosdick, L. S.: Chemical studies in periodontal disease. IV. Putrefaction rate as an index of periodontal disease, J. Dent. Res. **26**:67, 1947.
6. Bernier, J. L.: The role of inflammation in periodontal disease, Oral Surg. **2**:583, 1949.
7. Löe, H., Theilade, E., and Jensen, S. B.: Experimental gingivitis in man, J. Periodont. **36**:177, 1965.
8. Ramfjord, S.: Local factors in periodontal disease, J. Amer. Dent. Ass. **44**:647, 1952.
9. Gibbons, R. J.: Bacterial plaque as a common denominator in dental caries and periodontal disease, American Institute of Oral Biology, annual meeting, 1969.

10. Hazen, S. P., Baer, P. N., Moskow, B. S., and Turesky, S. S.: What is the role of subgingival calculus in the etiology of periodontal disease? J. Periodont. **41**:285, 1970.
11. Ellison, S. A.: Oral bacteria and periodontal disease, J. Dent. Res. **49**:198, 1970.
12. Socransky, S. S.: Relationship of bacteria to the etiology of periodontal disease, J. Dent. Res. **49**:203, 1970.
13. Björby, A., and Löe, H.: The relative significance of different local factors in the initiation and development of periodontal inflammation, J. Periodont. Res. **2**:76, 1967.
14. Mitchell, D. F.: The production of periodontal disease in the hamster as related to diet, coprophagy, and maintenance factors, J. Dent. Res. **29**:732, 1950.
15. Sognnaes, R. F.: Experimental production of periodontal disease in animals fed on a purified nutritionally adequate diet, J. Dent. Res. **26**:475, 1947.
16. King, J. D., and Glover, R. E.: The relative effects of dietary constituents and other factors upon calculus and gingival disease in the ferret, J. Path. Bact. **57**:353, 1945.
17. Romine, E. R.: Relation of operative and prosthetic dentistry to periodontal disease, J. Amer. Dent. Ass. **44**:742, 1952.
18. Morris, M. L.: Orthodontic-periodontic relationship. In Horowitz, S. L., and Hixon, E. H.: The nature of orthodontic diagnosis, St. Louis, 1966, The C. V. Mosby Co.
19. Orban, B.: Symposium on systemic aspects of periodontal disease, J. Periodont. **19**:123, 1948.
20. Cheraskin, E.: Diagnostic stomatology, New York, 1961, Blakiston Division, McGraw-Hill Book Co.
21. Stahl, S. S.: Host resistance and periodontal disease, J. Dent. Res. **49**:248, 1970.
22. Russell, A. L.: International nutrition surveys: a summary of preliminary dental findings, J. Dent. Res. **42**:233, 1963.
23. Thoma, K. H., and Robinson, H. B. G.: Oral and dental diagnosis, ed. 5, Philadelphia, 1960, W. B. Saunders Co.
24. Kerr, D. A., Ash, M. M., Jr., and Millard, H. D.: Oral diagnosis, ed. 3, St. Louis, 1970, The C. V. Mosby Co.
25. Cheraskin, E., and Langley, L. L.: Dynamics of oral diagnosis, ed. 2, New York, 1965, Reinhold Publishing Co.
26. Schenthal, J. E.: Multiphasic screening of the well patient, J.A.M.A. **172**:1, 1960.
27. Karlson, F. A., Jr., Cheraskin, E., and Dunbar, J. B.: Subclinical scurvy and subclinical tooth mobility, J. West. Soc. Periodont. **7**:6, 1959.
28. Cheraskin, E.: Advances in oral medicine related to periodontal disease, Bull. Greater Milwaukee Dent. Ass. **30**:61, 1964.
29. Mosenthal, H. O., and Barry, E.: Criteria for and interpretation of normal glucose tolerance tests, Ann. Intern. Med. **33**:1175, 1950.
30. Shannon, I. L., and Kilgore, W. G.: Fasting and postprandial serum glucose in relation to periodontal status, J. Periodont. Res. **3**:129, 1968.
31. Gottsegen, R.: Dental considerations in diabetes mellitus, Dent. Abstr. **8**:278, 1963.
32. Schallhorn, R. G.: Diabetes mellitus and periodontal disease, Periodont. Abstr. **14**:9, 1966.
33. Elsom, K. A., Schoor, S., Clark, T. W., Elsom, K. O., and Hubbard, J. P.: Periodic health examination: nature and distribution of newly discovered disease in executives, J.A.M.A. **172**:5, 1960.
34. Belting, C. M.: Prevalence of periodontal disease in hospitalized populations, J. Periodont. **38**:302, 1967.
35. Cohen, D. W., and others: Studies on periodontal pattern in diabetes mellitus, J. Periodont. Res., vol. 4, supp., p. 35, 1969.
36. Forbus, W. D.: Reaction to injury, Baltimore, 1943 and 1952, The Williams & Wilkins Co., vols. 1 and 2.

#### Additional suggested reading

Baumhammers, A., and Rohrbaugh, E. A.: Permeability of human and rat dental calculus, J. Periodont. **41**:279, 1970.

Dummett, C. O.: Advances made in determining the local etiology of periodontics, Periodontics **4**:322, 1966.

Egelberg, J.: Local effect of diet on plaque formation and development of gingivitis in dogs, Odont. Rev. **16**:50, 1965.

Frostell, G., and Söder, P.: The proteolytic activity of plaque and its relation to soft tissue pathology, Int. Dent. J. **20**:436, 1970.

Kerr, D. A.: Relations between periodontal disease and systemic disease, J. Dent. Res. **41**:302, 1962.

Lynch, M.: Systemic diseases, J. Periodont. **38**:771, 1967.
Lynch, M., Crowley, M., and Ash, M.: Correlation between plaque and bacterial flora, J. Periodont. **40**:634, 1969.
Nizel, A. F.: The science of nutrition and its application in clinical dentistry, ed. 2, Philadelphia, 1966, W. B. Saunders Co.
Russell, A. L.: Periodontal disease and nutrition, Dent. Abstr. **8**:96, 1963.
Scherp, H. W.: Discussion of bacterial factors in periodontal disease, J. Dent. Res. **41**:327, 1962.
Schroeder, H. E.: The structure and relationship to the hard and soft tissues: electron microscopic interpretation, Int. Dent. J. **20**:353, 1970.
Shaw, J. H.: The relation of nutrition to periodontal disease, J. Dent. Res. **41**:264, 1962.

CHAPTER TEN

# Nature, epidemiology, and prevention of periodontal disease



## NATURE

As previously noted, periodontal diseases may be inflammatory, dystrophic, or traumatic. Moreover, combinations of these conditions often exist in the same mouth. Individually and together they destroy supporting structures of the teeth and are the single greatest cause of tooth loss in adults.

The teeth and periodontium coexist in a potentially hazardous environment. They are constantly bathed by a bacteria-laden saliva, irritated by the impingement and retention of food, exposed to occlusal forces, and in many cases subjected to neglectful oral hygiene. Thus the common causes of periodontal disease are persistent or recurrent, or both. The intrinsic (systemic) factors that may contribute to disease and also influence resistance and repair are as yet poorly understood. Since periodontal disease is widely prevalent, the study of its epidemiology may yield important information on its etiology, diagnosis, treatment, and prevention.

The three basic approaches to the acquisition of knowledge about any disease are clinical observation, laboratory experimentation, and epidemiologic study. In the past, epidemiologic studies have been concerned mainly with the infectious or communicable diseases and their incidence and distribution in population groups. The present concern of epidemiology is shifting toward a study of noncommunicable organic diseases. The concept of a triad of required factors, with an interplay among host, environment, and causative agent, is receiving much attention. Epidemiology thus has become a part of ecology, concerning itself with the mutual relationships and interactions of groups of individuals with their environments—be they animate or inanimate, physical or biologic, social or economic. A complete understanding of the factors involved in the establishment and the course of mass disease in a community is often necessary before the problem can be resolved on an individual basis.

**Table 10-1.** World-wide prevalence of periodontal disease

| Country | Year | Investigator | Population studied | Number examined | Age group (yr.) | Percent with gingivitis | Percent with advanced periodontal disease (alveolar bone loss) |
|---|---|---|---|---|---|---|---|
| United States | 1949 | Massler et al.[3] | Suburban school children of Chicago | 804 | 5-14 | 64.3 | — |
| | 1933 | McCall[9] | Children of New York | 4,600 | 1-14 | 98 | — |
| | 1943 | Brucker[10] | Children of Newark, N. J. | 1,634 | 4-16 | 8.7 | — |
| | 1954 | Marshall-Day et al.[11] | Representative cross section of population of Boston | 332 | 13-22 | 66.2 | 11.3 |
| | | | | 238 | 23-24 | 79.4 | 80.4 |
| | | | | 331 | 35-48 | 86.8 | 98.7 |
| | | | | 286 | 49- | 91.8 | 100.0 |
| | 1957 | Russell[12] | Series of urban populations (white) from 14 cities of six states | 6,682 | 5-9 | 10.7 | 0.1 |
| | | | | 15,922 | 10-14 | 24.5 | 1.0 |
| | | | | 4,031 | 15-19 | 34.3 | 3.0 |
| | | | | 592 | 20-29 | 39.2 | 8.1 |
| | | | | 731 | 30-39 | 33.1 | 20.4 |
| | | | | 510 | 40-49 | 30.6 | 33.1 |
| | | | | 285 | 50-59 | 23.9 | 45.6 |
| | 1960 | Greene[13] | School children of Atlanta | 577 | 11-17 | 92.0 | 0.5 |
| | 1965 | Johnson et al.[14] | National Health Examination Survey—random sample of entire United States (males only) | | 18-24 | 60.6 | 10.3 |
| | | | | | 25-34 | 51.7 | 22.0 |
| | | | | | 35-44 | 48.1 | 29.7 |
| | | | | | 45-54 | 48.1 | 36.9 |
| | | | | | 55-64 | 39.1 | 45.6 |
| | | | | | 65-74 | 36.0 | 58.4 |
| Canada | 1953 | McIntosh[15] | | 398 | 6-11 | — | 74.5 |
| Great Britain | 1925 | Ainsworth and Young[16] | School children of England and Wales | 4,063 | 2-15 | 60.0 | — |

| | | | | | | | |
|---|---|---|---|---|---|---|---|
| | 1944 | King et al.[17] | Evacuees from Gibraltar | 135 | 10-14 | 85.2 | — |
| | 1945 | King[18] | School children of Scotland | 103 | 12-14 | 90.6 | — |
| Virgin Islands | 1950 | Marshall-Day and Shourie[19] | 90% Negro population | 823 | 6-18 | 57.1 | — |
| Sweden | 1937 | Westin[20] | School children | 1,141 | — | 86.5 | — |
| Egypt | 1946 | Dawson[21] | Hospitalized population | 423 | 15-25 | 95.9 | — |
| | | | | 351 | 26-35 | 99.6 | — |
| | | | | 200 | 36- | 100.0 | — |
| India | 1944 | Marshall-Day and Shourie[22] | School children | 613 | 5-15 | 73.7 | 5.7 |
| | | | Policemen | 525 | 21-30 | 27.2 | 62.4 |
| | | | Hospital patients | 996 | 5-60 | 28.5 | 68.6 |
| | 1962 | Gupta[23] | Cross section of population of Kerala | 155 | 11-20 | 73.5 | 16.8 |
| | | | | 275 | 21-30 | 41.1 | 55.6 |
| | | | | 153 | 31-40 | 12.4 | 87.6 |
| | | | | 135 | 41-80 | 5.2 | 94.8 |
| | 1964 | Gupta[24] | Household examination of a cross section of population of Trivandrum | 551 | 5-14 | 71.3 | 0.6 |
| | | | | 536 | 15-29 | 91.1 | 27.2 |
| | | | | 274 | 30-39 | 100.0 | 75.2 |
| | | | | 312 | 41- | 100.0 | 96.9 |
| China | 1929 | Anderson[25] | Male workers | 100 | 15-30 | 90.0 | — |
| Australia | 1938 | Clements and Kirkpatrick[26] | Preschool and school children | 530 | — | 63.0 | — |
| | 1939 | Campbell[27] | Aborigines, all ages | 350 | — | 50.0 | — |

## EPIDEMIOLOGY

Epidemiology is the science concerned with the factors and conditions that determine the occurrence and distribution of health, disease, defects, disability, and death among groups of individuals.[1] The science of epidemiology is also concerned with the determination of the factors that favor the origin and spread of a disease process or a physiologic state in a community. It is further concerned with elaborating ways and means of preventing and controlling the spread of disease with the ultimate aim of complete elimination of the disease.

The principal distinction between epidemiology and clinical practice is that an epidemiologist observes groups of individuals and his observations pertain to the whole group, both the affected and the nonaffected, whereas a clinician concerns himself with the individual patient. The epidemiologist studies mass phenomena in terms of type, extent, and frequency of occurrence in relation to age, sex, race, occupation, heredity, socioeconomic status, etc.

To discover factors and conditions of the origin and spread of a disease process, the epidemiologist must study the three important epidemiologic constants: the *disease agents,* the *environment of the host,* and the *host itself.* The epidemiologist is aware that disease production takes place only when there is an interaction among the agent, the host, and the environment. Once the epidemiologist has thoroughly studied the environmental factors, the disease agents, and the human host factors, he may be able to identify the causes of the disease process and take appropriate measures to intercept these causes to prevent the occurrence of the disease in a community.

***Dental epidemiology***

The methods of epidemiology have been applied in dentistry for finding the causes of dental diseases. In fact, the investigations on mottled enamel or dental fluorosis rank among the classics of epidemiologic studies. Periodontal disease is highly suitable for epidemiologic investigations since it is chronic in nature and there is a latent period between the initiation of the disease process and the appearance of the clinical manifestations.

***Prevalence and incidence***

The first step in an epidemiologic investigation is to discover the prevalence and severity of the disease and the composition of the population affected. The prevalence refers to the number of events or defects in an individual or a population at a specified time. Incidence refers to the number of defects that may occur during a given period of time. The data on prevalence and incidence indicate the extent and severity of the problem. Although data for the prevalence of gingivitis in children vary widely, the results of most studies indicate that a relatively large segment of the child population has gingivitis. The high prevalence of periodontal disease in the adult population has been fairly well established over the entire world, as can be seen from Table 10-1. This information is utilized for searching out the nature and causes of the disease. Developing and testing indices for the measurement of a disease are an essential part of epidemiology. If an index is to be applied for epidemiologic studies, it must be simple and relatively objective. The data obtained by this method must be quantitative and easily reproducible by any trained examiner with the least effort.

### Indices

A number of methods for the measurement and assessment of periodontal disease have been reported in the literature. Some of the more widely accepted are discussed in the succeeding paragraphs.

**Table 10-2.** Criteria for the periodontal index*

| Score | Criteria and scoring for field studies | Additional x-ray criteria followed in clinical test |
|---|---|---|
| 0 | Negative: neither overt inflammation in investing tissues nor loss of function caused by destruction of supporting tissues | Essentially normal radiographic appearance |
| 1 | Mild gingivitis: overt area of inflammation in free gingivae that does not circumscribe tooth | |
| 2 | Gingivitis: inflammation that completely circumscribes tooth, but no apparent break in epithelial attachment | |
| 4 | (Used when radiographs are taken) | Early, notchlike resorption of alveolar crest |
| 6 | Gingivitis with pocket formation: epithelial attachment broken, with pocket (not merely a deepened gingival sulcus caused by swelling in free gingivae); no interference with normal masticatory function; tooth firm in its socket and has not drifted | Horizontal bone loss involving entire alveolar crest, up to half of length of tooth root (distance from apex to cementoenamel junction) |
| 8 | Advanced destruction with loss of masticatory function: tooth loose, may have drifted; dull on percussion with metallic instrument; depressible in its socket | Advanced bone loss, involving more than half of length of tooth root; or definite infrabony pocket with definite widening of periodontal membrane; root resorption or rarefaction at apex |
| | **Rule:** when in doubt, assign the lesser score | |

*Adapted from Russell, A. L.: A system of classification and scoring for prevalence surveys of periodontal disease, J. Dent. Res. **35**:352, 1956.

***Periodontal disease index (Russell)***

In Russell's periodontal disease index[2] the condition of both the gingiva and the bone is estimated individually for each tooth in the mouth. A progressive scale that gives relatively little weight to gingival inflammation and relatively much weight to alveolar bone resorption is used for scoring. The scores from each tooth are added together and the total is divided by the number of teeth present in the mouth. The result gives the periodontal disease index of the patient, which reflects the average status of periodontal disease in a given mouth without reference to the type or etiology of the disease (Table 10-2). The community's score is the arithmetic average of individual scores of persons examined.

***PMA index (Schour and Massler)***

The PMA index[3] is used for recording the prevalence and severity of gingivitis in school children. The presence or absence of gingivitis is noted in each of three areas: the gingival papillae (P), the gingival margin (M), and the attached gingiva (A). Each of these areas is scored according to the presence or absence of inflammation as 1 or 0, respectively. PMA values are totaled separately, added together, and then expressed in one figure (the PMA index). When the values for papillae are between 1 and 4 and those for margins between 0 and 2, the cases are termed mild; if values are 4 to 8 for papillae and 2 to 4 for margins, the cases are called moderate. If values of more than 9 for papillae and more than 4 for margins are assigned, the patients are classified as having severe inflammation. Whenever the attached gingiva is involved, the case is always

Table 10-3. Gingiva-bone count*

| Observation | Score | |
|---|---|---|
| **Gingivitis** | | |
| (one score assigned for each tooth studied and a mean computed for whole mouth) | | |
| Negative | 0 | |
| Mild gingivitis involving free gingiva (margin, papilla, or both) | 1 | |
| Moderate gingivitis (involving both free and attached gingiva) | 2 | |
| Severe gingivitis with hypertrophy and easy hemorrhage | 3 | |
| Maximum | | 3 |
| **Bone loss** | | |
| (one score assigned for each tooth studied visually or by x-ray film, and a mean computed for whole mouth) | | |
| Negative | 0 | |
| Incipient (not greater than 2 mm.) bone loss or notching of alveolar crest | 1 | |
| Bone loss approximating one fourth of root length or pocket formation one side not over one half of root length | 2 | |
| Bone loss approximating one half of root length or pocket formation one side not over three fourths of root length; mobility slight† | 3 | |
| Bone loss approximating three fourths of root length or pocket formation one side to apex; mobility moderate† | 4 | |
| Bone loss complete; mobility marked† | 5 | |
| Maximum | | 5 |
| Maximum GB count per person | | 8 |

*Adapted from Dunning, J. M., and Leach, L. B.: Gingival bone count: a method for epidemiological study of periodontal disease, J. Dent. Res. **39**:506, 1960.

†If mobility varies considerably from that to be expected with the bone loss seen, the score may be altered up or down one point.

considered one of severe inflammation. The index is computed from findings in the anterior ten teeth; it has been found to represent 82% to 85% of the gingival inflammation in the entire mouth. The average PMA for the group is determined by totaling the number of units affected and dividing by the number of cases under study. This method has been found to be relatively useful and gives fairly accurate information on the gingival inflammation status of children.

***Gingiva-bone count index (Dunning and Leach)***

The gingiva-bone count index[4] permits differential recording of both gingival and bone conditions. Subjective measurement of gingivitis is made on an arbitrary scale of 0 to 3 for each tooth, and proportionate measurement of bone loss is made on a 0 to 5 scale. Scores of the entire mouth are then added to obtain the gingiva-bone (or GB) count. This count weighs gingivitis and bone loss on an arbitrary relation of a 3 to 5 basis (Table 10-3).

***Periodontal index (Ramfjord)***

For the periodontal index[5] a thorough clinical examination of the periodontal status of six teeth—maxillary right first molar, left central incisor, left first premolar, mandibular left first molar, right central incisor, and right first premolar—is made. The following factors are evaluated: gingival condition, pocket depth, calculus and plaque deposits, attrition, mobility, and lack of contact. The gingivitis is graded on a numerical scale from 0 to 3, depending on the severity and extent of the inflammation. The pocket depth is measured in millimeters on the mesial, vestibular, distal, and oral aspects of each tooth examined. The pocket depths are measured from the cementoenamel junction as a reference point. A numerical periodontal score is tabulated for each of the examined teeth. If the gingival sulcus in none of the four measured areas extends apically to the cementoenamel junction, the recorded score for gingivitis is the score for periodontal disease for that tooth. If the gingival sulcus in any of the four measured areas extends apically beyond the cementoenamel junction, but not more than 3 mm. in any area, the tooth is assigned a score of 4. When there is periodontal disease, the score for gingivitis for that tooth is disregarded in the final index. If the gingival sulcus in any of the four recorded areas of the tooth extends apically from 3 to 6 mm. beyond the cementoenamel junction, the tooth is assigned a score of 5. If the gingival sulcus extends more than 6 mm. apically beyond the cementoenamel junction in any of the measured areas of the tooth, a score of 6 is given. The scores of individual teeth are added and divided by the number of teeth examined, which yields Ramfjord's periodontal disease index.

***Simplified oral hygiene index (Greene and Vermillion)***

The simplified oral hygiene index[6] (OHI-S) has two components—the plaque or debris index (DI-S) and the calculus index (CI-S). Each of these indices in turn is based on numerical determinations representing the amount of debris or calculus found on six preselected tooth surfaces. The six surfaces examined for the OHI-S are selected from four posterior and two anterior teeth. In the posterior portion of the dentition, the first fully erupted tooth distal to the second premolar, usually the first molar, is examined on each side of each arch. The vestibular surfaces of the selected upper molars and the oral surfaces of the selected lower molars are inspected. In the anterior portion of the mouth, the vestibular surfaces of the upper right and the lower left central incisors are scored. In the absence of either of these anterior teeth, the central incisor on the opposite side of the midline is substituted. Plaque and calculus are graded on a numerical scale from 0 to 3, depending on the severity and extent of the deposits. The debris scores are totaled and divided by the number of surfaces scored for each individual. The score for a group of individuals is obtained by computing the average of the individual scores, which is the DI-S; the same methods are used to obtain the CI-S. The average individual or group DI-S and CI-S scores are combined to obtain the simplified oral hygiene index (OHI-S).

***Plaque index (Silness and Löe)***

There is no universally accepted index for the assessment of plaque. However, such an assessment can be made with the DI-S of Greene and Vermillion as well as the oral hygiene component of Ramfjord's periodontal index. A specific index for scoring plaque has been given by Löe[7] and by Silness and Löe.[8] This method is based on an assessment of the severity and the location of soft debris aggregates in terms of 0, 1, 2, and 3 scores. A plaque score of 0 is given when the gingival area of the tooth surface is free of plaque. The examination is made by passing a probe over the tooth surface into the gingival sulcus. If no soft material adheres to the probe, the area is considered to be 0. A plaque score of 1 is given when plaque cannot be observed in situ but can be observed on the probe after it has been passed over the tooth surface. Disclosing solution may be used for the recognition of this film of plaque. A score of 2 is given when a thin to moderately thick layer of plaque is visible with the unaided eye at the gingival margin. A plaque score of 3 is assigned when there is a heavy accumulation of soft matter whose thickness fills out the niche between the gingival margin and the tooth surface and when the interdental area is stuffed with soft debris. Approximately 1 to 2 mm. of soft material must be observed.

In this system of scoring plaque, the authors place most stress on the thickness of the plaque at the gingival margin area on all the four surfaces of each tooth. They suggest that the plaque index be computed for all surfaces, mesial, distal, oral, and vestibular, of all or selected teeth or for specific areas of all or selected teeth. This index may be utilized for large-scale epidemiologic studies as well as for clinical studies of smaller groups. The assessment of the index requires a light source, gentle drying of the teeth and gingiva, a mirror, and a probe. If optimal conditions and chairside assistance are provided, approximately 5 minutes should be sufficient time to score all the teeth in the oral cavity. The scores of all the four areas of all the teeth can then be added and divided by the number of teeth.

The plaque index has not been utilized by various investigators and thus does not have universal acceptability; rather the debris index of Greene and Vermillion, which includes plaque, has been employed to indicate the severity of plaque deposits.

## PREVENTION

The foregoing review indicates that a large segment of the population of the world is affected by periodontal disease. The periodontal status of people in the United States has been well documented by the recently conducted National Health Survey. The data of this survey indicate that periodontal disease affects 79.1% of the people between the ages of 18 and 24 years, 77.9% of the people between the ages of 35 and 44, and 94.4% between the ages of 65 and 74.[14] Periodontal disease has been reported to be the major cause of tooth loss in the adult population. Approximately 60% to 70% of the teeth lost in the United States after the age of 40 years are lost because of periodontal disease.

***Primary prevention***

Prevention of any disease depends on knowledge of the natural history of the disease, comprising the prepathogenesis and pathogenesis of the disease process. Prevention can be instituted prior to the occurrence of the disease, that is, in the prepathogenesis period. Training in plaque control, periodic oral examination and prophylaxis, and measures to increase the resistance of the periodontal tissues to injury and infection prior to the occurrence of the disease are termed primary prevention.

***Secondary and tertiary prevention***

After the disease process is initiated and recognized, secondary prevention may be accomplished by prompt treatment; and when the disease is in the advanced stages, control can still be achieved by tertiary prevention (corrective therapy). Procedures at the tertiary stage are designed to limit further disability. At later stages rehabilitation plays a preventive role. The aforementioned phases of prevention (primary, secondary, tertiary) are divided into the following five distinct levels by Leavell and Clark[1]: (1) health promotion, (2) specific protection, (3) early diagnosis and prompt treatment, (4) disability limitation, and (5) rehabilitation. Methods for the prevention of periodontal disease at these five levels are given in Table 10-4.

### Application of levels of prevention

Since periodontal disease has a multifactorial etiology, preventive procedures can be applied at several points in the chain of events occurring during the disease process. *Health promotion* aims at improving the tissue resistance by good nutrition, general and oral health education, motivation for maintaining good oral hygiene, and better living conditions. *Specific protection* against peri-

**Table 10-4.** Levels of prevention of periodontal disease

| Primary prevention (prepathogenesis) | | Secondary prevention (pathogenesis) | | Tertiary prevention |
|---|---|---|---|---|
| **Health promotion** | **Specific protection** | **Early diagnosis and prompt treatment** | **Disability limitation** | **Rehabilitation** |
| 1. Health education | 1. Periodic prophylaxis, training in plaque control | 1. Periodic radiographic examination | 1. Treatment of periodontal abscesses | 1. Replacement of lost teeth by suitable appliances for aesthetics and function |
| 2. Patient motivation | 2. Effective oral hygiene procedures: toothbrushing, dental floss, Perioaid, and interdental stimulation to control plaque | 2. Regular oral examination | 2. Root planing, gingival curettage | 2. Periodontal prosthesis, surgical intervention |
| 3. Periodic oral examination | 3. Correction of poor restorative dentistry | 3. Prompt treatment of incipient periodontal lesions, elimination of pockets | 3. Minor or major surgical interventions | 3. Psychotherapy when indicated |
| 4. Oral hygiene instruction | 4. Correction of abnormal habits | 4. Prompt treatment of all periodontal lesions | 4. Splinting procedures | |
| 5. Adequate nutrition | 5. Restoration of gingival and bone morphology | 5. Treatment of other oral lesions contributory to to periodontal disease | 5. Other periodontal treatment procedures | |
| 6. Diet planning | 6. Correction of gross occlusal disharmonies | | 6. Extractions of teeth with poor prognosis | |
| 7. Healthy living conditions | 7. Fluoridation of public water supplies | | | |

odontal disease is achieved by regular and periodic oral prophylaxis and effective and correct oral hygiene procedures. Correction of poor restorative dentistry and gross disharmonies in occlusion, restoration of gingival and bone morphology, and elimination of abnormal oral habits are also specific protective measures to prevent the occurrence of periodontal disease. Some information already exists to indicate that fluoride may help to render alveolar bone resistant to periodontal disease. The fluoridation of communal water supplies, so beneficial in reducing caries incidence, may perhaps be beneficial in preventing periodontal disease.

Once the disease has begun and progressed, *early diagnosis and prompt treatment* should be applied to prevent further progression. At this level of prevention, periodic clinical and radiographic examinations of the oral tissues should be undertaken for the diagnosis of the incipient periodontal lesions. Once these are diagnosed, prompt treatment, if instituted, becomes a sound preventive procedure. If the disease has escaped diagnosis and has thus advanced, *disability limitation* and *rehabilitation* should be instituted. These rehabilitation measures aim at preventing further progression of the disease and disability. At these levels periodontal treatment procedures should be instituted in an attempt to prevent the further progression of the disease. The replacement of lost teeth by suitable prosthesis to reestablish function and aesthetics may be necessary.

To date, the most promising procedure for the prevention of periodontal disease is plaque control. An introduction to plaque control will be found in Chapter 12.

## EPIDEMIOLOGIC CHARACTERISTICS

### Host factors

The data on major host factors—age, sex, and race—are fairly well documented and indicate a definite epidemiologic pattern in this regard. However,

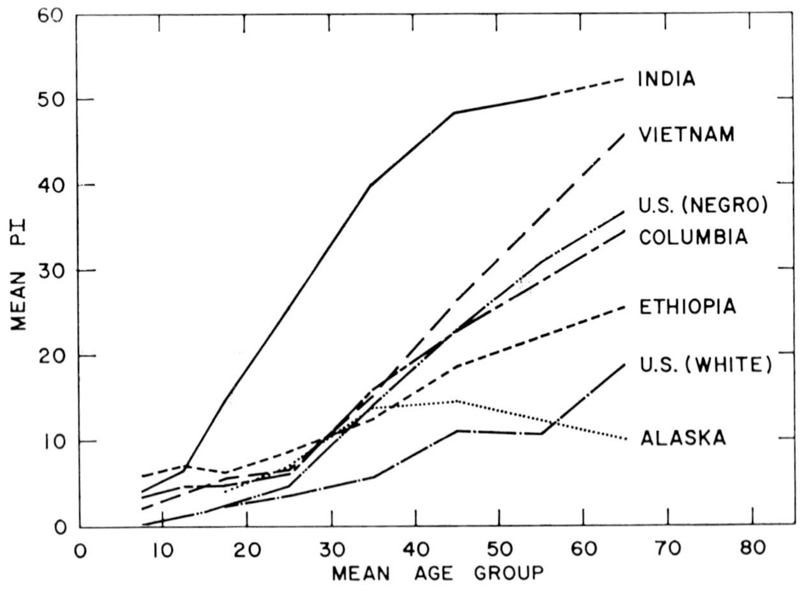


**Fig. 10-1.** Mean periodontal index scores *(PI)* of persons of six countries for various age groups. (Based on data from Gupta[24] and Russell.[32])

other factors are significant too—socioeconomic status, emotion, systemic conditions, intraoral variations, and local irritants.

*Age differences*

Gingivitis usually begins at about 5 years of age and progresses rapidly until puberty; thereafter it declines slightly. The prevalence of gingivitis in the adult population is not fully known since the disease is complicated by the presence of more advanced periodontal disease. The prevalence and severity of periodontal disease have been reported to increase with age.[28] The periodontal scores rise moderately from age 5 to about age 13 years in India and to about age 25 (Negro) and age 35 years (white) in the United States; thereafter the scores rise sharply (Figs. 10-1 and 10-2). The incidence of periodontal disease in the United States at the ages of 18 to 24 years has been reported to be 71%. By the age of 50 years, 85% of the people have periodontal disease; after age 65, 95% have advanced periodontal lesions.[14]

*Sex differences*

Although a general agreement on the sex incidence of periodontal disease does not exist, most studies indicate that women show lower prevalence and severity of periodontal disease than do men. Up to the age of 14, girls appear to have a higher prevalence and greater severity of periodontal disease than do boys[29]; thereafter the incidence is slightly greater in boys and men.[30] Gupta reported lower periodontal scores for females than for males in all age groups[23]; however, there were no statistical differences in age groups except in the 30-to-39-year age bracket. Similar results were reported by Russell[12] and by Marshall-Day and co-workers.[11] In the National Health Examination Survey of the United States, women consistently showed lower periodontal index scores than did men; and the prevalence of periodontal pockets was higher in men than in women.[14]

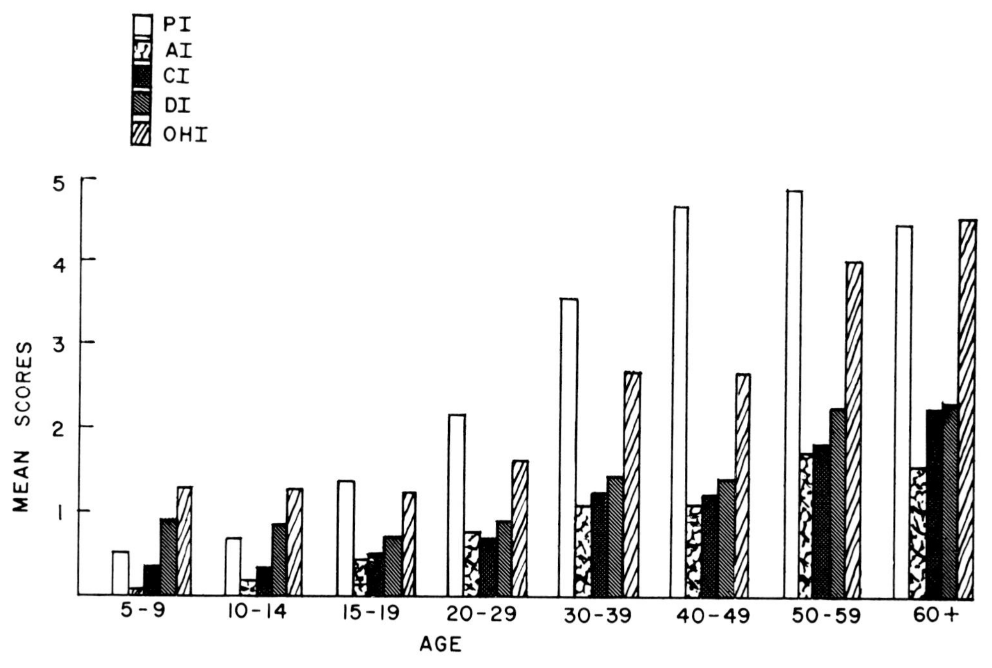


**Fig. 10-2.** Periodontal, *PI*, attrition, *AI*, debris, *DI*, calculus, *CI*, and oral hygiene, *OHI*, indices by age for 1673 persons of Trivandrum, India. (From Gupta, O. P.: J. Dent. Res. 43:876, 1964.)

***Race differences***

Epidemiologic data on race incidence of periodontal disease are not sufficient to indicate conclusively a racial susceptibility; however, studies in the United States do indicate a higher prevalence and severity of periodontal disease in Negroes than in whites. Massler and co-workers[31] reported after examination of 17,079 white and 6975 Negro schoolchildren that Negro children between the ages of 6 and 11 years had significantly higher prevalence and greater severity of gingivitis than did the white children. Negroes were found to have higher prevalence and severity of periodontal disease than were whites in fourteen urban localities of the United States.[12] In the National Health Examination Survey the mean periodontal score for Negro adults was higher than that for white adults, 1.60 as compared with 1.06. The periodontal score for Negroes at ages 20 to 29 years was 0.48, and 13.5% had periodontal pockets whereas the same score for whites was 0.44, and only 8.16% had pockets. The periodontal index increased to 3.65 and 2.35 in Negroes and whites respectively as age increased. Beyond the age of 60 years, 77.7% of Negroes and 53.2% of whites had periodontal disease.[14]

***Socio-economic status***

Epidemiologic data are not sufficient as yet to establish a definite relationship between socioeconomic status and periodontal disease. However, a small number of studies do indicate that persons with a high income level have lower periodontal disease scores.[12] Persons with a higher education level tend to exhibit periodontal disease in milder stages.[32]

Social customs and group habits (e.g., food fads, use of tobacco, betel nut chewing) influence the prevalence and severity of periodontal disease.[24,33] The relationship between the nutritional status of a community and the prevalence and severity of periodontal disease has recently been studied thoroughly in Alaska, Ethiopia, Equador, Montana, Chile, Ceylon, and South Vietnam.[34] These studies did not reveal any strong association between a specific nutrient and periodontal disease when the effects of age and oral hygiene were considered simultaneously. The effect of nutrition on the prevalence and incidence of periodontal disease is discussed in Chapter 11.

***Emotional factors***

Epidemiologic data are not sufficient to implicate the emotional status of communities with periodontal disease. However, studies by Belting and Gupta[35] and by Gupta and Travaglini[36] indicate that persons with mental disorders have significantly higher incidence and severity of periodontal disease than do control groups, regardless of the frequency of toothbrushing and oral hygiene.

***Intrinsic conditions***

Some intrinsic conditions of the host (e.g., pregnancy, diabetes, heavy metal poisoning, anemias, leukemias) have been reported to aggravate the existing periodontal conditions.

***Intraoral variations***

A somewhat definite pattern in the intraoral variation of periodontal disease has been documented. Bossert and Marks found that the upper molars and lower central incisors were the teeth most frequently affected.[37] The least affected teeth were the mandibular premolars and the maxillary canines. Maxillary left molars showed more severe periodontal disease than did the maxillary right molars. Marshall-Day observed the following regions of the oral cavity most commonly affected with periodontal disease (in descending order of frequency): vestibular surfaces of the maxillary anterior and mandibular anterior canine, maxillary and mandibular molar and premolar, and oral surfaces of the maxilla and mandible.[38] The oral surfaces in the mandible were more frequently involved than the oral surfaces in the maxilla in the older age groups. Various studies indicate greater bone resorption interproximally than vestibularly and orally.

Alveolar bone loss in the incisor and molar areas has been reported to be greater than in the canine and premolar areas.

*Extrinsic factors*

The number of extrinsic factors such as calculus, poor restorative dentistry, and oral microorganisms has been shown to influence the initiation and progression of periodontal disease. Of these factors, oral hygiene, calculus, and debris deposits have repeatedly had a positive correlation with the prevalence and severity of periodontal disease. Greene[39] and Gupta[24] found that people with higher oral hygiene scores (poorer oral hygiene) consistently had higher periodontal scores. This relation existed even when the effect of age was eliminated. Other studies also indicate a definite relationship between calculus and poor oral hygiene and periodontal disease.[11,12,14,22]

## Plaque and calculus

One of the major factors in the intiation and progression of periodontal disease is microbial plaque and calculus. Numerous studies have shown that microbial plaque is most likely the direct cause of gingivitis. The process of supragingival plaque and calculus formation entails three phases: (1) the deposition of cuticle or pellicle, (2) bacterial colonization and plaque maturation, and (3) mineralization. All three steps are not essential since bacteria can deposit without a cuticular intermediary[40] and mineralized deposits can occur in germ-free animals.[41] However, the usual process in humans occurs in the three phases. Simultaneous with and soon after the formation of the pellicle, microorganisms start colonizing in it and a thin layer of bacterial plaque is formed in the course of hours. After about 24 hours tooth surfaces exhibit a clinically observable soft deposit at the tooth-gingival margin interface.[42] Plaque formation is relatively independent of the passing of food through the oral cavity. Tube feeding experiments have shown, in fact, that animals given no food by mouth can have microbial plaque deposits.[43] The rate of formation of plaque, however, is influenced by the composition of the diet and the physical and chemical composition of the saliva.[44] Although the exact chemical composition of microbial plaque has not been determined, a specific glycoprotein in the organic plaque pellicle has been found. Basically the pellicle is a salivary derivative, and most of the available evidence points to the fact that its major mechanism may be one of adsorption. Plaque is normally composed of various bacterial and fungal organisms, leukocytes, macrophages, and desquamated epithelial cells contained in a matrix of amorphous ground substance.[45,46] The matrix consists of PAS-positive mucopolysaccharides, sulfhydryls, and disulfides that can provide a protein template for apatite crystal formation.[47] Histochemical studies have also shown that mucopolysaccharides of plaque bind calcium, which suggests that the process of plaque formation may be similar to that of other ectopic calcification such as in renal, bladder, arterial, and urinary deposits.[48-50] The source of mucopolysaccharides for dental plaque formation could be saliva,[51] bacteria,[52-55] a secretion of the epithelial cells,[56] or the fluid flowing from the gingival sulcus.[57] Results from numerous investigations suggest that all components of subgingival calculus may originate in the gingival fluid although few studies suggest the salivary origin of calculus.

Available evidence strongly suggests the hypothesis that fluid from the gingival sulcus is a source of the components of subgingival plaque and calculus. The presence of gingival exudate is well established, and the origin of the exudate appears to be the subepithelial connective tissue, the epithelial cell export of mucopolysaccharides, desquamating epithelial cells, and leukocytes. Gingival fluid always accompanies gingival inflammation, and the flow increases with the degree of inflammation. The exudate contains all the necessary constituents to form plaque and the minerals to calcify into calculus. Some of the components enter into subgingival plaque formation whereas no salivary components have been identified.

### Microorganisms

The influence of microorganisms on human periodontal disease is not clear cut. The oral bacteria in humans with and without periodontal disease are qualitatively similar except that in the former group the total number is increased and there is a slight relative increase in the proportion of spirochetes and gram-negative cocci. However, the data of recent studies show that humans receiving antibiotics for various systemic diseases over a long period of time have fewer and less severe periodontal lesions than do those of control groups. Similar results have been reported in experimental animals by Gupta and his co-workers.[58]

### Fluorides

Recent studies show that the fluoride ion, when ingested at low concentrations, produces bone resistant to periodontal lesions. Experimental animals highly susceptible to periodontal disease, when maintained on fluoridated water, had fewer alveolar bone lesions than their littermate controls.[59] People ingesting naturally fluoridated water routinely have less severe periodontal disease than do those drinking fluoride-free water.[60]

### Geographic differences and environmental factors

Studies utilizing a single method of assessment indicate significant differences in periodontal scores for persons of widely different geographic areas—the United States, Alaska, Colombia, Equador, Ethiopia, India, South Vietnam, and Thailand.[28]

Although studies conducted in various parts of the world indicate widely different prevalence and severity of periodontal disease, the validity of the results is difficult to evaluate because of individual variability, small samples of the population surveyed, and differences in the method of assessment. Studies made by Russell in various parts of the world, however, circumvent these difficulties[28] (Fig. 10-2). They reveal that periodontal disease is more widespread and more destructive among primitive and underdeveloped persons than among those who are culturally more advanced. Nutritional deficiencies were not found to cause the differences in the prevalence of periodontal disease between the underdeveloped and the culturally advanced people. Gingivitis was reported to be prevalent in 23% of the white children between the ages of 6 and 12 years in Boston, 51% in Philadelphia, and 74% in Chicago.[31] In Canada, Brantford showed a 59% prevalence, in Sarnia a 62% prevalence, and in Stratford 77%. Texas children had significantly more severe gingival disease than did Maryland children of the same age, race, socioeconomic group.

The degree of urbanization appears to affect the prevalence and severity of periodontal disease. Gingivitis was reported to be more prevalent in rural areas than in urban areas,[61] but the prevalence and severity of periodontal disease were reported higher in urban than in rural areas of India.[22,62] Similar findings were reported by Gupta,[24] who found higher periodontal scores for the urban than for the rural populations of Kerala, India.

**CHAPTER 10**

**References**

1. Leavell, H. R., and Clark, E. G.: Preventive medicine for the doctor in his community, New York, 1965, McGraw-Hill Book Co.
2. Russell, A. L.: A system of classification and scoring for prevalence surveys of periodontal disease, J. Dent. Res. **35**:350, 1956.
3. Massler, M., Schour, I., and Chopra, B.: Occurrence of gingivitis in suburban Chicago school children, J. Periodont. **21**:146, 1950.
4. Dunning, J. M., and Leach, L. B.: Gingival bone count: a method for epidemiological study of periodontal disease, J. Dent. Res. **39**:506, 1960.
5. Ramfjord, S. P.: Indices for prevalence and incidence of periodontal disease, J. Periodont. **30**:51, 1959.
6. Greene, J. C., and Vermillion, J. R.: The oral hygiene index, J. Amer. Dent. Ass. **61**:172, 1960.
7. Löe, H.: The gingival index, the plaque index, and the retention index systems, J. Periodont. **38**:610, 1967.
8. Silness, J., and Löe, H.: Periodontal disease in pregnancy. II. Correlation between oral hygiene and periodontal condition, Acta Odont. Scand. **22**:121, 1964.
9. McCall, J. O.: The periodontist looks at children's dentistry, J. Amer. Dent. Ass. **20**:1518, 1933.
10. Brucker, M.: Studies of the incidence and cause of dental defects in children. III. Gingivitis, J. Dent. Res. **22**:309, 1943.
11. Marshall-Day, C. D., Stephens, R. G., and Quigley, L. F., Jr.: Periodontal disease: prevalence and incidence, J. Periodont. **26**:185, 1955.
12. Russell, A. L.: Some epidemiological characteristics of periodontal disease in a series of urban populations, J. Periodont. **28**:286, 1957.
13. Greene, J. C.: Periodontal disease in India: report of an epidemiological study, J. Dent. Res. **39**:302, 1960.
14. Johnson, E. S., Kelly, J. E., and Van Kirk, L. E.: Selected dental findings in adults by age, race, and sex: United States—1960-1962, Vital Health Statist. **11**:1, 1965.
15. McIntosh, W. G.: Gingival and periodontal disease in children, J. Canad. Dent. Ass. **20**:12, 1954.
16. Ainsworth, M. J., and Young, M.: Incidence of dental disease in children, Medical Research Council, Special Report Series, no. 97, London, 1925, H. M. Stationery Office.
17. King, J. D., Franklyn, A. B., and Allen, I.: Gingival disease in Gilbraltar evacuee children, Lancet **1**:495, 1944.
18. King, J. D.: Gingival disease in Dundee, Dent. Record **65**:9, 32, 55, 1945.
19. Marshall-Day, C. D., and Shourie, K. L.: Gingival disease in the Virgin Islands, J. Amer. Dent. Ass. **40**:175, 1950.
20. Westin, G. Quoted in Schour, I., and Massler, M.: Gingival disease in post-war Italy (1945). I. Prevalence of gingivitis in various age groups, J. Amer. Dent. Ass. **35**:475, 1947.
21. Dawson, C. E.: Dental defects and periodontal disease in Egypt, 1946-1947, J. Dent. Res. **27**:512, 1948.
22. Marshall-Day, C. D., and Shourie, K. L.: Incidence of periodontal disease in the Punjab, Indian J. Med. Res. **32**:47, 1944.
23. Gupta, O. P.: Epidemiological studies of dental diseases in the state of Kerala. I. Prevalence and severity of periodontal disease, J. All India Dent. Ass. **35**:45, 1962.
24. Gupta, O. P.: An epidemiological study of periodontal disease in Trivandrum, J. Dent. Res. **43**:876, 1964.
25. Anderson, B. G.: Hypertrophic gingivitis among Chinese, Nat. Med. J. China **15**:453, 1929.
26. Clements, F. W., and Kirkpatrick, R. M.: Medical and dental survey of school and preschool children of New South Wales, Aust. Dent. J. **10**:418, 1938.
27. Campbell, T. D.: Food, food values and food habits of the Australian Aborigines in relation to their dental condition, Aust. Dent. J. **43**:1, 1939.
28. Russell, A. L.: World epidemiology and oral health, environmental variables in oral disease. In Kreshover, S. G., and McClure, F. J., editors: Environmental variables in oral disease, Washington, D. C., 1966, A.A.A.S.
29. Parfitt, G. J.: A five year longitudinal study of the gingival condition of a group of children in England, J. Periodont. **28**:26, 1957.
30. Massler, M., and Savara, B. S.: Relation of gingivitis to dental caries and malocclusion in children 14 to 17 years of age, J. Periodont. **22**:87, 1951.

31. Massler, M., Cohen, A., and Schour, I.: Epidemiology of gingivitis in children, J. Amer. Dent. Ass. **45**:319, 1952.
32. Russell, A. L.: A social factor associated with the severity of periodontal disease, J. Dent. Res. **36**:922, 1957.
33. Balendra, W.: The effect of betel chewing on the dental and oral tissues and its possible relationship to buccal carcinoma, Brit. Dent. J. **87**:83, 1949.
34. Russell, A. L.: International nutrition surveys: a summary of preliminary dental findings, J. Dent. Res. **42**:233, 1963.
35. Belting, C. M., and Gupta, O. P.: The influence of psychiatric disturbances on the severity of periodontal disease, J. Periodont. **32**:219, 1961.
36. Gupta, O. P., and Travaglini, E. A.: Effects of neuropsychiatric conditions on the human periodontium, I.A.D.R. abstract, p. 124, 1966.
37. Bossert, W. A., and Marks, H. H.: Prevalence and characteristics of periodontal disease of 12,800 persons under periodic dental observation, J. Amer. Dent. Ass. **52**:429, 1956.
38. Marshall-Day, C. D.: The epidemiology of periodontal disease, J. Periodont. **22**:13, 1951.
39. Greene, J. C.: Oral hygiene and periodontal disease, Amer. J. Public Health **53**:913, 1963.
40. Frank, R. M., and Brendel, A.: Ultrastructure of the approximal dental plaque and the underlying normal and carious enamel, Arch. Oral Biol. **11**:883, 1966.
41. Theilade, J., Fitzgerald, R. J., Scott, D. B., and Nylen, M. U.: Electron microscopic observations of dental calculus in germfree and conventional rats, Arch. Oral Biol. **9**:97, 1964.
42. Schroeder, H. E., and Bambauer, H. V.: Stages of calcium phosphate crystallization during calculus formation, Arch. Oral Biol. **11**:1, 1966.
43. Bowen, W. H.: The monitoring of acid production in dental plaque in monkeys, Brit. Dent. J. **126**:506, 1969.
44. Bowen, W. H., and Cornick, D. E.: The microbiology of gingival-dental plaque—recent findings from primate research, Int. Dent. J. **20**:382, 1970.
45. Baer, P. N., and Burstone, S.: Esterase activity associated with formation of deposits on teeth, Oral Surg. **12**:147, 1959.
46. Glickman, I.: Clinical periodontology, ed. 3, Philadelphia, 1964, W. B. Saunders Co.
47. Turesky, S., Renstrup, G., and Glickman, I.: Histologic and histochemical observations regarding early calculus formation in children and adults, J. Periodont. **32**:7, 1961.
48. Adamson, K. T.: The role of enzyme action in the formation of dental calculus, Aust. J. Exp. Biol. Med. **6**:215, 1929.
49. Leung, S. W.: The uneven distribution of calculus in the mouth, J. Periodont. **22**:7, 1951.
50. Mandel, I. D.: Calculus formation, Dental Clinics of North America, Philadelphia, November 1960, W. B. Saunders Co.
51. Gressly, F.: Experimental calculus formation, Periodontics **1**:53, 1963.
52. Hodge, H. C., and Leung, S. W.: Calculus formation, J. Periodont. **21**:211, 1950.
53. Leung, S. W.: Calculus research 1959: a review, J. Amer. Dent. Ass. **60**:583, 1960.
54. Zander, H. A., Hazen, S. P., and Scott, D. B.: Mineralization of dental calculus, Proc. Soc. Exp. Biol. Med. **103**:257, 1960.
55. Rizzo, A. A., Martin, G. R., Scott, D. B., and Mergenhagen, S. W.: Mineralization of bacteria, Science **135**:439, 1962.
56. Toto, P. D., and Sicher, H.: The epithelial attachment, Periodontics **2**:154, 1964.
57. Weinstein, E., and Mandel, I. D.: The fluid of the gingival sulcus, Periodontics **2**:147, 1964.
58. Gupta, O. P., Auskaps, A. M., and Shaw, J. H.: Periodontal disease in the rice rat. IV. The beneficial effects of penicillin and streptomycin on the incidence of periodontal disease in the rice rat, Oral Surg. **10**:1169, 1957.
59. Auskaps, A. M., Gupta, O. P., and Shaw, J. H.: Periodontal disease in the rice rat. III. Survey of dietary influences, J. Nutr. **63**:325, 1957.
60. Englander, H. R., Kesel, R. G., and Gupta, O. P.: The Aurora-Rockford, Ill., study. II. Effects of natural fluoride on the periodontal health of adults, Amer. J. Public Health **53**: 1233, 1963.
61. Benjamin, E. M., Russell, A. L., and Smiley, R. D.: Periodontal disease in rural children of 25 Indiana counties, J. Periodont. **28**:294, 1957.
62. Mehta, F. S., Baretto, M. A., Raut, R. B., Sanjana, M. K., and Shourie, K. L.: The incidence of periodontal disease amongst Indian adults, J. All India Dent. Ass. **26**:4, 1953.

**Additional suggested reading**

Baume, L. J.: Limitations of simplified indexes in prevalence studies of periodontal disease, Int. Dent. J. **18**:570, 1968.

Greene, J. C.: Epidemiologic research 1964-1967, J. Amer. Dent. Ass. **76**:1350, 1968.

Kelly, J. E., and Engel, A.: Selected examination findings related to periodontal disease among adults, United States—1960-1962, Vital Health Statist. **11**:1, 1969.

Lindhe, J., Lundgren, D., and Nyman, S.: Considerations on prevention of periodontal disease, Periodont. Abstr. **18**:50, 1970.

Orban, J. E., Stallard, R. E., and Bandt, C. L.: An evaluation of indexes for periodontal health, J. Amer. Dent. Ass. **81**:683, 1970.

Ramfjord, S. P., Emslie, R. D., Greene, J. C., and others: Epidemiologic studies of periodontal diseases, Parodont. Acad. Rev. **2**:109, 1968.

Russell, A. L.: The periodontal index, J. Periodont. **38**:585, 602, 1967.

Ship, I. I., Cohen, D. W., and Laster, L.: A study of gingival, periodontal and oral hygiene examination methods in a single population, J. Periodont. **38**:638, 1967.

CHAPTER ELEVEN

# Nutrition and periodontal disease



Years ago periodontists were divided into two camps: the localists and the generalists. The localists claimed that periodontal disease was due to local irritative and occlusal circumstances. The generalists said that systemic conditions were the immediate cause of periodontal disturbances. The tendency today is to consider systemic (intrinsic) influences of minor importance primarily because of our inability to pinpoint them. We thus have silently convinced ourselves that such influences do not exist or at least are rare and of minor importance. In addition, many generalists who pursued a dietary approach to therapy were food faddists. This, coupled with the fact that inflammatory periodontal disease did not yield to dietary treatment, has tended to discredit the systemic approach. In recent years, however, serious scientists have investigated the role of nutrition in periodontal disease. This chapter is intended to provide some information on the current status of this research.

The first essential of life is the maintenance of the internal environment of the cell, and this is achieved by complex regulatory mechanisms in which food nutrients play a major role. Nutrition is concerned with feeding the animal, and ultimately the cells, thus ensuring not only the optimal development of the tissues but also the adequate functioning and metabolism of the cells.

More than half the world's population is still afflicted with hunger and severe malnutrition. In the subeconomic areas of the world, such factors as illiteracy, overpopulation, low productivity of soil (resulting from inadequate methods of agriculture and animal husbandry), and low levels of industrialization account for the nutritional problems. Unlike such problems in developing countries, where malnutrition constitutes a major public health concern, nutritional problems in the industrialized nations are quite often conditioned malnutrition. This type is secondary to mental, physical, physiologic, and habitual stress and often occurs as a complication of other diseases. Recent studies have, nevertheless, uncovered areas in the United States where nutritional problems approximate situations presently characterizing most of the technically underdeveloped countries.[1] It is therefore essential that any conclusions regarding the pattern and distribution of diseases among various population groups recognize both the role of disease-producing agents and the possible contribution of host factors.

Although the full meaning and implications of tissue resistance are still not adequately clarified, science has long recognized host resistance as an important factor in determining the severity of a disease. Tissue resistance is modified by several factors, among which are physical and emotional stress, nutritional status, and numerous systemic conditions. The course and severity of most infections are exaggerated in malnutrition.[2]

The status of periodontal health can be interrelated with nutrition in several ways: (1) through the growth, development, and metabolic activities of the periodontium, (2) through malnutrition as the potential primary etiologic agent in periodontal disease or the potential modifying etiologic agent to other primary etiologic factors, and (3) through the effect of food quality, quantity, and consistency on the pathogenesis of periodontal lesions. Tissues with a rapid rate of cell renewal, such as the periodontium, are dependent on the ready availability of essential nutrients for the maintenance of their integrity and metabolic activities; and they are therefore most susceptible to the effects of malnutrition.[3-5]

A high prevalence of periodontal disease exists in all age groups in the developing countries.[6-13] There is a strong correlation between periodontal health and socioeconomic status in both the developed and the underdeveloped countries.[14-17] Whether this is because of poor oral hygiene, inadequate diet, or both is not clearly defined. However, nutritional deficiencies in humans are usually multiple and are often complicated by cultural and other environmental factors.

## PROTEINS

### Protein-calorie deficiency syndrome

Protein-calorie malnutrition is by far the most widespread nutritional disorder in underdeveloped countries[18] and is usually complicated by the concurrent deficiencies of other essential nutrients.[2,19-21] It is primarily a disease of infants and young children, with a peak age incidence of 1 to 3 years. Poor lactation, due to maternal malnutrition, and inadequacy of the diets of weaned children are major causative factors.[22,23] Lesions of the buccal mucosa may be observed in this disease.[18,24] Buccal scrapings show typical histologic changes when compared with normal scrapings.[25,26] Significant generalized osteoporosis has been demonstrated,[27] and there is evidence of alveolar bone loss.[28] Epidemiologic studies reveal that children suffering from kwashiorkor show significant differences in their OHI scores and demonstrate more periodontal pathology when compared with children of similar ages drawn from a higher socioeconomic level.[11,17,29] Well-fed Nigerian children enjoy a better state of periodontal health than do their age counterparts in the poor rural areas regardless of local factors.[17] These observations are supported by studies of malnutrition in experimental animals that show degeneration of the connective tissue fibers in the gingiva and periodontal ligament, pronounced osteoporosis of the alveolar bone, and marked retardation in deposition of cementum.[30-35] There is also good evidence that the younger the animal the more profound are the effects of protein malnutrition on the periodontium.[36]

Of particular interest are the severity and age distribution patterns of cer-

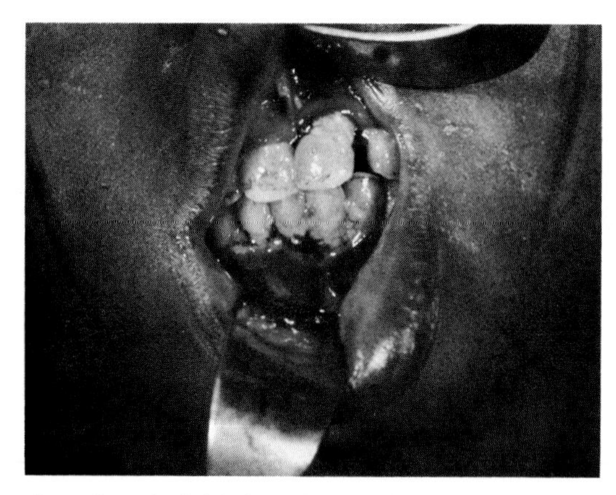

**Fig. 11-1.** Necrotizing ulcerative gingivitis in a 3-year-old Nigerian girl. The typical ulcerations, gingival craters, pseudomembranous slough, and oral debris are seen around the mandibular incisors. (Courtesy C. O. Enwonwu,[11] Seattle.)

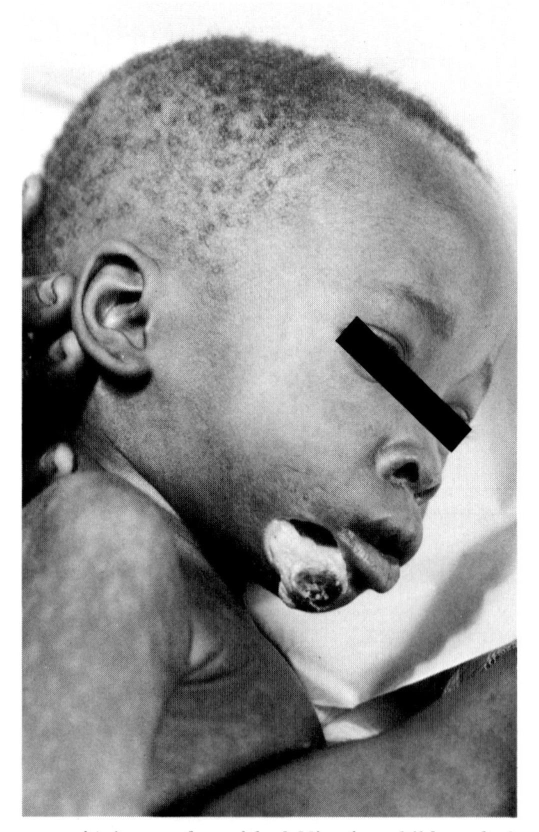

**Fig. 11-2.** Noma (cancrum oris) in a malnourished Nigerian child aged about 4 years. (Courtesy C. O. Enwonwu,[11] Seattle.)

tain oral diseases in protein-calorie–deficient populations. Necrotizing ulcerative gingivitis (NUG) is rarely seen in children in developed countries[37,38] but assumes a different age distribution pattern in poor nations. More than half the cases seen in India are reported in children under 10 years of age.[39,40] Protein-calorie–malnourished children have a higher incidence of NUG than do well-fed age controls in the same country.[8,29,41,42] Fig. 11-1 shows a case of NUG in a 3-year-old Nigerian village child. Examination of children from high and low socioeconomic groups in Nigeria revealed no case of NUG in the former group.[11] In the latter group, drawn from a village with high incidence of protein malnutrition, eighty-seven cases of NUG were observed in a period of 15 months, and all but two were in children 1 to 10 years old. The peak incidence was at 2 to 3 years of age, which corresponded with the immediate post-weaning period. In some cases the NUG extended into adjacent tissues, producing extensive necrosis and destruction of orofacial tissues (Fig. 11-2). This condition, known as noma or cancrum oris, is extremely rare in developed countries except during famines. It is commonly encountered in poor nations[8,43,45] and is closely associated with malnutrition and states of debilitation.[43,45,46] Jelliffe reported fifty-three cases in which the ages of the patients varied from 2 to 5 years.[43] He noted that all had had protein-deficient diets for periods of 6 months to 2 years. On the rare occasion when noma is encountered in developed countries, the patient almost invariably is nutritionally deprived.[47,47a] Thus cancrum oris, essentially a socioeconomic disease, represents an outcome of the synergism between malnutrition and infection.

### Possible mechanisms of protein-calorie malnutrition on oral tissues

Regeneration of the gingival epithelium takes place from the basal layer, and mitosis is a prerequisite. A 20% to 30% decrease in food supply in mice results in a 35% decrease in mitotic activity.[48] Lesions in organs with rapid cell renewal and high protein turnover are characteristic of protein-calorie malnutrition.[49] Histologic findings of such effects on epithelial tissues have been confirmed biochemically and by radioisotopic studies.[50-52] Connective tissue collagen, especially the soluble fraction, is also susceptible to protein deprivation.[53]

In view of the ubiquitous presence of local etiologic factors in periodontal disease, the periodontium is believed to exist in a state of continuous wound healing and repair.[48] Gingival wounds heal rapidly compared to wounds in other parts of the body.[54,56] The healing wound presents a picture of rapid turnover of cells, collagen, and mucopolysaccharides.[57] Not surprisingly therefore this process is susceptible to deficiency of essential nutrients. Deficiency of dietary protein[58,59] or of certain essential amino acids[60-63] causes a decrease in the tensile strength of wounds corresponding to a diminution in both the number of fibroblasts and the amount of collagen formed in the wounds.[57] There is also evidence that the protein-synthesizing capacity of lysine-deficient fibroblasts is reduced, resulting in diminished collagen production.[64]

Protein-calorie malnutrition also impairs normal endocrine balance.[65] This could conceivably affect the health of the periodontium. There is adrenal hyperfunction in protein-calorie–malnourished children[18,66-68] and in experimental animals.[69] Adrenocortical function in such children demonstrates impairment of cortisol catabolism; anabolism is relatively unaffected, resulting in elevated plasma cortisol levels.[70,71] In effect, protein-calorie malnutrition produces stresses that override the normal control mechanisms so that cortisol synthesis remains high in the face of high levels of plasma cortisol. In addition to interference with adrenocortical function, there is impairment in glucose tolerance and insulin sensitivity.[72] The percentage of $\beta$ cells is reduced, and of $\alpha$ cells is increased, in the endocrine pancreas of protein-calorie–deficient pigs.[65] Malnourished pigs also show a reduction in size or a virtual absence of the thymus gland.[65] Against this background of complex structural and functional alterations in the endocrine system, one must evaluate the possible consequences of prolonged protein-calorie malnutrition on the health of the periodontium. Except for the liver, where cortisol and related corticosteroids produce an anabolic effect,[73,74] these hormones are generally catabolic. They evoke myo- and lymphocytolysis and thereby induce a negative nitrogen balance in the body.[75-78] Injection of corticotropin decreases mitotic activity of the human epidermis.[79] This diminished mitosis might also occur in the gingival epithelium of malnourished persons exposed to high levels of circulating steroids. With regard to the connective tissue, corticosteroids may decrease the amount of collagen by retarding its synthesis.[80-84] High levels of adrenocorticosteroids also decrease the synthesis of hyaluronic acid, chondroitin sulfates, and other components of the ground substance.[80] This fact has been confirmed in the rat gingiva.[85] Since some steroids are anti-inflammatory,[80] it is reasonable to assume that adrenocortical hyperfunction might exert deleterious effects on the periodontium. Recent studies demonstrate that daily administration of cortisone acetate to marmosets (*Sanquinus oedipus*) diminishes the inflammatory cell reaction in gingivitis and periodontitis.[86] These findings agree with earlier observations in white mice.[87] Such observations offer an explanation for the high prevalence of NUG in persons under stress[88] and the significant rise in the level of 17-hydrocorticosteroids in patients suffering from periodontal lesions.[89] They also lend some credence to the speculation of Goldhaber and Giddon that adrenocortical hormones may be one of the factors involved in the etiology of NUG.[90] In this regard it is significant to note the production of a noma-like lesion in rats treated with cortisone and exposed to mechanical injury.[91]

The impairment of pancreatic endocrine function that occurs in protein-calorie malnutrition could also affect the structural integrity of the periodontium.[65,92] Increased production of glucagon by the $\alpha$ cells exerts an anti-insulin activity. Insulin apparently plays an important role in the synthesis of mucopolysaccharides.[80] Studies by Löe indicate that even well-controlled diabetics exhibit greater loss of periodontal structure than do comparable nondiabetics.[93]

## CARBOHYDRATES AND FATS

Although studies in various experimental animals indicate that high-carbohydrate diets are conducive to the development of severe periodontal lesions, such experiments are difficult to interpret.[94-97] For instance, it is difficult to separate those effects due to the high carbohydrate content from those attributable to the low protein content of such diets. It is also dangerous to consider the quantity of food in diets in isolation from the composition or quality of the food.[98] Animals eat to satisfy their energy requirements primarily; and in the absence of force-feeding, they will not ingest enough protein from a predominantly carbohydrate diet to meet these requirements. In addition, many of the high-carbohydrate diets employed in such studies are of powdery consistency. This factor introduces a major variable with regard to retention of food particles in the mouth. There is sufficient evidence that ingestion of liquid or powdered food has an adverse effect on the structure and function of the salivary glands,[99-101] attributable to reduced masticatory function,[97] and this could affect the clearance of food particles from the oral cavity.

Changes in the periodontium have also been reported in rats fed either a fat-free[98,99] or a high-fat[98] diet. More detailed, adequately controlled studies are necessary before any meaningful extrapolations of these findings to human periodontal disease can be undertaken.

## VITAMINS

Vitamins are organic substances that the body requires in small amounts for its metabolism. Their absence from diets results in deficiency diseases. The human body cannot make these essential accessory food substances, at least not in sufficient quantity, and therefore it must acquire them in foods. Vitamins form part of the structures of several coenzymes, and they participate in many cellular reactions. The vitamins are generally considered under two major subdivisions: the water-soluble vitamins and the fat-soluble vitamins. The latter are usually found in association with the lipids of natural foods.

### Water-soluble vitamins

*Vitamin C (ascorbic acid)*

Recent work by Hodges indicates that the body stores of ascorbic acid in healthy, well-fed men approximate 1500 mg. and are utilized at an average daily rate of 3% of the existing pool.[105] Three months of dietary deprivation of vitamin C precede marked depletion of the body stores, and at this stage the amount available for daily catabolism is not enough to prevent scurvy.[105] Many of the signs of deficiency may appear during the first month of dietary deprivation. There is still some controversy regarding the human daily dietary requirement of vitamin C. Although 30 mg./day is the recommended intake for normal persons, a daily intake of 10 mg. is believed to be necessary to prevent scurvy in healthy adults.[106] This opinion is supported by the recent observation of Hodges that a daily dose of only 6.5 mg. of ascorbic acid produces remarkable improvement in experimentally induced scurvy in adult males.[105] On the contrary, Berry and Schaefer found a close association between the prevalence of gingival pathology and dietary intake of 15 to 23 mg. of ascorbic acid per day.[107] The situation has recently been further complicated by the report of Pauling, who proposed 2.3 Gm./day for an adult man with energy requirement of 2500 Kcal./day.[108]

The main sources of dietary vitamin C are fresh fruits. Diagnosis of vitamin C deficiency is often based on the plasma ascorbic acid level, and there is good evidence that this test lacks precision.[105] The absence of measurable vitamin C in serum or plasma is compatible with scurvy; but it is not diagnostic, since zero levels have also been reported in persons without any clinical manifestations of scurvy.[105,110] This occurs because plasma vitamin C is labile and varies with the recent dietary intake as well as with other conditions (e.g., infections). Values below 0.2 mg./100 ml. of serum have for a long time been accepted as indicative of marked ascorbic acid deficiency,[111] but recent experimental studies have shown obvious scurvy when serum levels were above 0.2 mg./100 ml.[105]

Among the signs and symptoms often observed in marked ascorbic acid depletion are ocular hemorrhages, Sjögren's syndrome, femoral neuropathy, impaired vascular reactivity or poor responses to stimuli that normally activate the

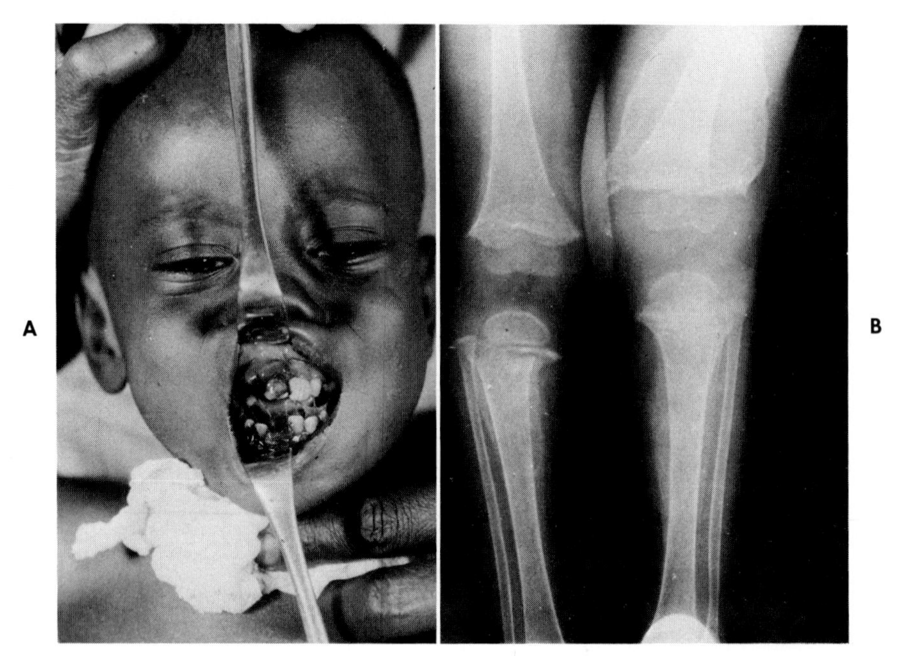


**Fig. 11-3. A,** Oral lesions of scurvy. **B,** Roentgenographic appearance of skeletal alterations in infantile scurvy. Nigerian child aged 3 years. (Courtesy C. O. Enwonwu,[11] Seattle.)

vasomotor adaptive mechanisms, psychologic disturbances, scorbutic arthritis, and gingivitis.

Gingival pathosis is a common classical manifestation of frank scurvy,[112] although some investigators believe that local irritation must be present for acute deficiency of vitamin C to cause gingivitis and periodontitis.[113-115] Among the oral manifestations of scurvy are intense gingival reddening, attributable to engorgement of the underlying blood vessels, and fiery red, smooth, glazed, swollen gingivae devoid of the normal stippling. The gingival lesions usually start in the interdental area and spread to involve the marginal gingivae. Secondary infection of the gingivae occurs quite frequently, resulting in ulceration, necrosis, and sloughing.[112] The gingival lesions of scurvy rarely occur in the absence of teeth.

Fig. 11-3, *A,* demonstrates some of the oral lesions in a case of infantile scurvy in a 3-year-old child observed in western Nigeria. The child had had an attack of measles; and later the mother had noticed the child's inability to stand erect for an appreciable length of time. The knee joints were very tender on examination. The gingiva was hemorrhagic and hypertrophied, the teeth were mobile, and the mandibular right deciduous central incisor had been exfoliated. Roentgenographic examination showed separation of the epiphyses of the femur and tibia of the left knee, together with calcification in the large hematoma around the lower femoral diaphysis (Fig. 11-3, *B*).

Blood examination showed a serum ascorbic acid level of 0.07 mg./100 ml., which was compatible with the diagnosis of scurvy. Treatment with 30 mg. of ascorbic acid daily produced marked remission of the oral lesions in 1 week.

Among the prominent features of scorbutic gingivitis are a periodontal ligament widened by resorption of surrounding bone and a breakdown of collagen fibers in the periodontium.[116]

*Biochemical basis of changes in vitamin C deficiency*

Vitamin C deficiency affects three types of cells: fibroblasts, osteoblasts, and odontoblasts. The cells fail to produce normal collagen, osteoid, and dentin; and the ability of the cells to form epithelial and vascular basement membranes is also restricted.[117] Severe vitamin C deficiency is characterized by hemorrhagic tendencies, impaired wound healing, and osteoporosis.

The principal cell involved in wound healing and repair is the fibroblast; and among the prominent alterations in this cell in vitamin C deficiency are the following: vacuolization of the cisternae of the ergastoplasm with loss of the characteristic configuration of the membrane-bound polyribosomes; increase in the number of free ribosomes; and presence of large numbers of lipid deposits in the cytoplasm.[118,119] These features reflect reduced protein biosynthesis.[120,121] The extracellular space shows fewer collagen bundles although individual fibrils of indeterminate nature are present.[119] Vitamin C may also be involved in the metabolism of mucopolysaccharides.[119,122]

*Niacin (nicotinamide)*

Deficiency of niacin, or of tryptophan (which could be metabolized inefficiently to niacin), is responsible for pellagra. Gingivitis attributable to deficiency of niacin is characterized by extremely painful, wedge-shaped, punched-out ulcers involving the interdental papillae and marginal gingiva.[112] The lesions in the human are necrotic, exudative, and foul smelling. In dogs severe inflammatory changes in the oral mucosa, including the sulcular epithelium, capillary dilatation, and osteoporosis of the alveolar bone have been reported.[123]

*Riboflavin*

Riboflavin is a constituent of the flavoproteins, which are important in tissue oxidation. Deficiency of riboflavin causes glossitis and angular cheilosis, although these lesions are not specific for riboflavin deficiency. Epithelial atrophy is a basic feature, which may very well account for the association of this condition with gingivitis in monkeys.[124,125]

*Folic acid (pteroylglutamic acid)*

The important food sources of folic acid are liver, kidney, yeast, and mushrooms. Folic acid deficiency is characterized by lesions in cells with rapid rate of renewal, which demonstrates the importance of this vitamin in the synthesis of DNA.[126] In folic acid deficiency, there is impairment of keratinization with increased susceptibility to ulceration and secondary infections.[127,128] Severe gingivitis and necrosis of oral and gingival mucosae have been reported in folic acid–deficient monkeys.[112,124,125,129]

*Other water-soluble vitamins*

The relationship of the remaining water-soluble vitamins to periodontal pathology in the human has not been adequately studied.

## Fat-soluble vitamins

*Vitamin A*

Vitamin A occurs in the animal kingdom, especially in marine fish liver oils, liver fat, fat of dairy products, and eggs. The provitamins (carotenoid precursors) are found in green vegetables, carrots, etc. Preformed vitamin A is deposited primarily in the liver and kidneys. In view of this storage, to produce clinical and biochemical manifestations of deficiency, there must be a prolonged period of deprivation.

Deficiency of vitamin A produces marked retardation in growth, alterations in epithelial and nervous tissues, cartilage, and bone, and severe interference with vision and reproduction. Hyperplasia and keratinization in mucous membranes are characteristic features. Evidence is inconclusive for participation of vitamin A depletion in human periodontal disease.[130]

Ingestion of excessive amounts of vitamin A (more than a hundred times required amount) is just as deleterious to health as dietary deprivation of the vitamin. Among the features observed in hypervitaminosis A are mucous dysplasia of epithelium, thickening of skin and suppression of keratinization, bleeding tendency due to prolonged prothrombin time, and increased absorption of bone with loss of chondroitin sulfate.

***Vitamin D*** Vitamin D is represented by a group of steroid alcohols, primarily vitamin $D_2$ (ergocalciferol) and vitamin $D_3$ (cholecalciferol). The latter is believed to be the most potent of the D vitamins, and its relative importance varies with the species of animal under consideration. Among the precursors are ergosterol (provitamin $D_2$) and 7-dehydrocholesterol (provitamin $D_3$). The main food sources of the D vitamins are the liver oils of many fishes. Vitamin D is stored by mammals in small amounts. It influences absorption and excretion of calcium, phosphate, magnesium, and other minerals; and it also plays an important role in the ossification of cartilage. In man and certain animal species severe vitamin D deficiency produces rickets in the young and osteomalacia in the old, and these lesions are characterized by defective mineralization of osteoid.

Information on the role of vitamin D deficiency in human periodontal disease is fragmentary and often contradictory. Feeding young rats a diet that has a high calcium-to-phosphorus ratio but is deficient in vitamin D results in defective calcification of cementum and alveolar bone with hyaline degeneration of connective tissue in some cases.[131-133]

Ingestion of excessive amounts of all forms of vitamin D (hypervitaminosis D) is dangerous, and the characteristic features of the syndrome are hypercalcemia and deposition of calcium phosphate in any matrix containing mucoproteins. The calcinosis is widespread, affecting the kidneys, myocardium, endocrine glands, arteries, gastrointestinal tract, joints, corneae, and several other tissues. Advanced stages of hypervitaminosis D often present with demineralization of bones. Little is known regarding involvement of the human periodontal tissues in this syndrome. Among the outstanding features seen in young rats subjected to hypervitaminosis D were large numbers of enlarged osteocytes engaged in lacunar resorption, enlarged cementocytes with the presence of cementoid, and increased amounts of connective tissue fibers of the periodontium (resulting in an enlargement of the interdental papillae).[133] Calcification of periodontal ligament fibers and ankylosis were noted in rats fed excessive amounts of vitamin D.[133a]

***Vitamin E*** Vitamin E is represented by the compounds known as tocopherols. Vegetable oils are the most important sources of this vitamin. The clinical features of vitamin E deficiency show marked variability in different animal species. The prominent deficiency sign in the human is increased tendency to hemolysis. Vitamin E deficiency is believed to affect the cross-linking of collagen.[122]

***Vitamin K*** The main sources of the naturally occurring K vitamins, which are methylnaphthoquinone derivatives, are green plants and bacteria. Vitamin K is necessary for prevention of the hemorrhagic condition associated with insufficient ability of the blood to coagulate. The defect in coagulation may result from inadequate biosynthesis of proconvertin, prothrombin, and some other plasmatic factors involved in the blood-clotting system. Vitamin K deficiency can be induced by administration of antagonists like coumarin and other related compounds. Avitaminosis K promotes a hemorrhagic diathesis.

## MINERALS

Maintenance of life and optimal health requires the availability of several inorganic elements, of which some (calcium, phosphorus, magnesium) are present in the body in macroquantities and others (iron, copper, cobalt, iodine, sulfur, manganese, zinc, fluorine, sodium, potassium, chlorine) are required in relatively trace amounts.[134] These nutrients participate in essential metabolic processes in the body, functioning in a complex and interrelated manner with one another and with the major food nutrients and the endocrine and enzyme systems. Prolonged ingestion of foods that are imbalanced, deficient, or high in these elements produces physiologic and biochemical defects as well as structural alterations in various tissues and organs, depending on the elements involved.

*Calcium and phosphorus*

There is general agreement that dietary deficiency of phosphorus hardly exists in humans. Nordin is of the opinion that some forms of osteoporosis can be explained on the basis of malabsorption of calcium or dietary lack of the element.[135] The latter view is now adequately substantiated only in experimental animal studies.[133] Among the findings in calcium-deficient young rats and cats are osteoporosis of alveolar bone, reduction in amount of secondary cementum, and reduction in size and number of the periodontal fibers. In rats fed diets deficient in phosphorus, slight rachitic and osteomalacic alterations were observed in the young and adult animals respectively.[133,136,137]

*Magnesium*

Simple, uncomplicated deficiency of magnesium hardly occurs in man but is a frequent complication of protein-calorie malnutrition due to gastrointestinal losses of the ion during chronic diarrhea and vomiting[138] and renal losses after intensive intravenous administration of magnesium-free electrolyte and glucose solutions.[139] Skin and oral lesions have been described in magnesium-deficient rats.[140] In studies of sixty-seven seriously malnourished Nigerian children with orofacial lesions of cancrum oris, Caddell found magnesium-supplemented therapy superior to therapy without magnesium supplementation.[141]

*Iron and other minerals*

Very few studies have been undertaken to establish the role of iron and other elements in the maintenance of good periodontal health. Abnormalities of the mouth such as angular stomatitis and atrophic changes on the dorsum of the tongue and the buccal mucosa have been noted in iron deficiency.[142-144] It is also worthy to note that one of the two enzymes intimately involved with the antimicrobial activities of the phagocytic cell is an iron-containing enzyme called myeloperoxidase.[145] Higashi and co-workers showed that patients with iron deficiency have a deficiency of this enzyme and a consequent decrease in bactericidal activity.[146] The possible effects of such a situation in terms of the defense of the periodontal tissues against plaque microorganisms should not be overlooked.

There are conflicting reports on the role of fluoride in periodontal health.[133] Studies in humans have failed to show a beneficial or detrimental effect of ingested fluoride on periodontal health.[147]

Many essential metabolic functions are carried out by microelements, and thus more information on their relevance to dental health is needed.

## EFFECTS OF PHYSICAL CHARACTERISTICS OF FOOD ON THE PERIODONTIUM

Numerous studies have suggested the importance of food consistency as well as quality in the maintenance of optimal periodontal health. Rats maintained on hard pelleted diets were reported to develop more marked periodontal lesions than those maintained on a soft diet.[148,149] This is in conflict with the ob-

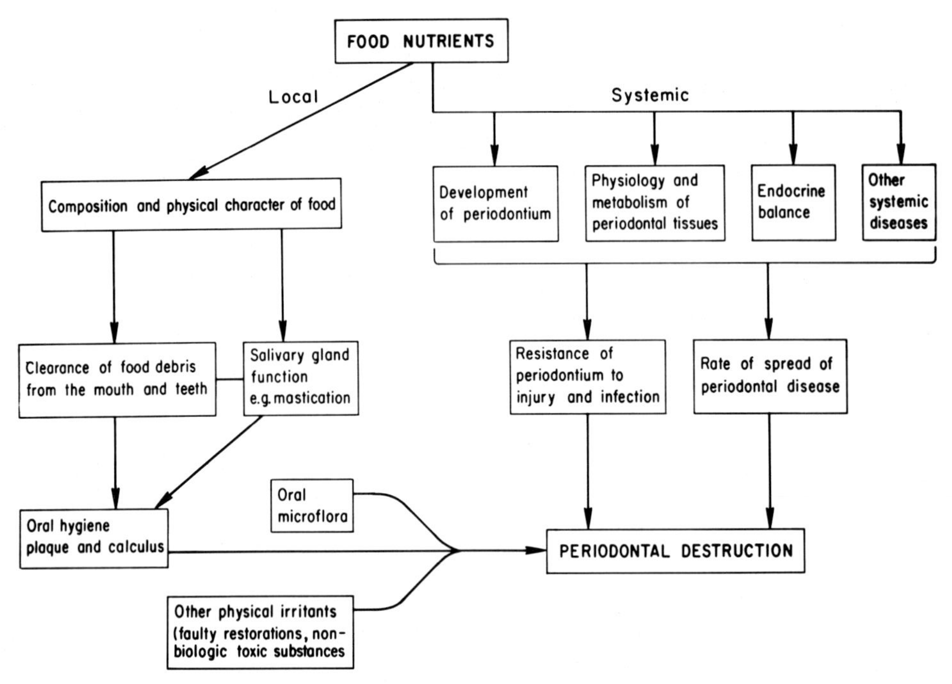


**Fig. 11-4.** Interaction of food nutrients and factors associated with periodontal health and disease states.

servations of other investigators who found that soft diets promoted gingival inflammation.[150-152] Evidence has also been produced for the enhancement of plaque formation by feeding soft diets to dogs.[152] The detrimental effect of soft foods on periodontal health has been confirmed in humans. It would thus seem that foods of hard consistency, in contrast to soft diets, promote mechanical cleansing of the dental tissues. Wilcox and Everett[155] and Lindhe and Wicen,[156] however, question the effectiveness of chewing fibrous foods (apples, carrots) in cleansing the bacterial plaque from the gingival third of the tooth surface. Although it sounds reasonable that hard foods should have a cleansing action,[156a] this may not be the only mechanism by which such diets promote periodontal health. The recent finding of higher proliferative activity in the crestal epithelium and in the fibroblasts of the interradicular septum of pellet-fed rats compared to those in powdered diet–fed animals is significant.[157]

## SUMMARY AND COMMENTARY

The relationship between nutrition and the health of most tissues and organs is a close one, although often difficult to evaluate. As summarized in Fig. 11-4, food nutrients not only control the growth, development, and physiologic activity of periodontal tissues but also dictate the fate of these tissues in the event of infection and injury by influencing their response to the effects of the hostile local factors. Thus studies of the prevalence and severity of periodontal disease, especially in poor population groups, should take a proper ecologic approach, which should recognize not only the local etiologic factors but also the possible contribution of such factors as the nutritional status of the host.

Periodontal disease is insidious in its course. Although local etiologic factors have always been readily amenable to investigation, only recently have major attempts been focused on possible contributions of intrinsic and host factors to the etiology, pathogenesis, and sequelae of periodontal lesions. Plaque microorganisms constitute the single most important local factor that has received the greatest attention of investigators. The oral microbial potential in the causation of periodontal disease was recently reviewed[158]; and Socransky summarized the mechanisms that account for destruction of the periodontium as follows: (1) factors that destroy the intercellular matrix of the epithelium and connective tissues, (2) factors that are toxic to cells or that interfere with the capacity of the cells to maintain the integrity of the periodontium, and (3) factors that lead to inflammation, which eventually leads to destruction of the tissues.[159] The importance of adequate nutrition in the maintenance of good periodontal health or in retarding the rate of the disease process is easily appreciated when food nutrients are evaluated in light of their contribution to the protection of the periodontium against destructive factors.

The presence of microorganisms in the body does not necessarily lead to infections and establishment of disease states. Bacterial penetration of human gingival tissues has been convincingly demonstrated only in necrotizing ulcerative gingivitis although endotoxin can pass through an intact epithelial barrier. Thus plaque organisms exert their effects on the periodontium through other means (e.g., elaboration of toxins, enzymes, and antigens and via endotoxins). Numerous studies already mentioned indicate that in some states of malnutrition, tissue integrity is markedly affected, resulting in increased permeability of mucosal surfaces.[160] This may be a consequence of the interference with normal cellular replacement and repair; and such a situation could create portals of entry for oral bacteria and their products. There is also good evidence that malnutrition produces (1) reduction or absence of mucus and other secretions, (2) accumulations of cellular debris that provide favorable culture media, (3) increased fluid in tissues, and (4) alteration of intercellular substances.[57,118,122] Immune processes are known to be impaired in malnutrition,[161-164] and there is evidence for reduction of phagocytic activity.[145,146,160] Nutritional factors produce intrinsic diseases, induce genetic defects, impair hormonal balance of the host, and adversely affect tissue vascularity and wound repair.

Most investigations of the role of nutrition in periodontal disease have involved acute deficiencies of short duration. For meaningful information we ought to be more concerned with prolonged states of malnutrition. The important role of adequate supply of essential nutrients in the protection against infection and disease is best appreciated if one reflects on the following statement by Spies: "Today germs are not our principal enemy. Our chief medical adversary is a disturbance of the inner balance of the constituents of our tissues, which are built from and maintained by necessary chemicals in the air we breathe, the water we drink, and the food we eat. Our cells are never static, and in time must be replaced in varying degrees by the nutrients obtained from food."* This statement is probably more true of the periodontium than of most organs since periodontal tissues undergo rapid cellular renewal and remodeling, as well as exhibit a high rate of protein biosynthesis.[48,166-169]

*From Spies, T. D.: Some recent advances in nutrition, J.A.M.A. 7:675, 1958.

**CHAPTER 11**

**References**


1. Mayer, J.: White House Conference on Food, Nutrition and Health, final report. Publication no. 0-378-473, Washington, D. C., 1970, United States Government Printing Office.
2. Scrimshaw, N. S.: Ecological factors in nutritional disease, Amer J. Clin. Nutr. **14:**112, 1964.
3. Ramalingaswami, V.: Perspectives in protein malnutrition, Nature **201:**546, 1964.
4. Winick, M., and Noble, A.: Quantitative changes in DNA, RNA and protein during prenatal and postnatal growth in the rat, Develop. Biol. **12:**451, 1965.
5. Winick, M., and Noble, A.: Cellular response in rats during malnutrition at various ages, J. Nutr. **89:**300, 1966.
6. Greene, J. C.: Periodontal disease in India. Report of an epidemiological study, J. Dent. Res. **39:**302, 1960.
7. Ramfjord, S. P.: The periodontal status of boys 11-17 years old in Bombay, India, J. Periodont. **32:**237, 1961.
8. Emslie, R. D.: Cancrum oris, Dent. Pract. **13:**481, 1963.
9. Emslie, R. D.: A dental health survey in the Republic of Sudan, Brit. Dent. J. **120:**167, 1966.
10. Sheiham, A.: The prevalence and severity of periodontal disease in rural Nigerians, Dent. Pract. **17:**51, 1966.
11. Enwonwu, C. O.: Nutrition and dental health: epidemiological study of dental growth and dental diseases in western Nigerian children in relation to socio-economic status. Thesis, M.D.S., Bristol University, England, 1966.
12. The West Indies. Nutrition survey. Report by the Interdepartmental Committee on Nutrition for National Defense, N.I.H., Bethesda, 1961, National Institutes of Health.
13. Nigeria. Nutrition survey. Report by the Office of Internatonal Nutrition, N.I.H., Bethesda, 1967, National Institutes of Health.
14. Mehta, F. S., Sanjana, M. K., Shroff, B. C., and Doctor, R. H.: Prevalence of periodontal (parodontal) disease. 5. Epidemiology in Indian child population in relation to their socio-economic status, Int. Dent. J. **6:**31, 1956.
15. Russell, A. L., and Ayers, P.: Periodontal disease and socio-economic status in Birmingham, Alabama, Amer. J. Public Health **50:**206, 1960.
16. Mobley, E. L., and Smith, S. H.: Some social and economic factors relating to periodontal disease in young Negroes, J. Amer. Dent. Ass. **66:**486, 1963.
17. Enwonwu, C. O., and Edozien, J. C.: Epidemiology of periodontal disease in western Nigerians in relation to socio-economic status, Arch. Oral Biol. **15:**1231, 1970.
18. Scrimshaw, N. S., and Behar, M.: Protein malnutrition in young children, Science **133:**2039, 1961.
19. Viteri, F., Behar, M., and Arroyave, G.: Clinical aspects of protein malnutrition. In Munro, H. N., and Allison, J. B., editors: Mammalian protein metabolism, New York, 1964, Academic Press, Inc.
20. Scrimshaw, N. S., and Waterlow, J. C.: The concept of kwashiorkor from a public health point of view, Bull. WHO **16:**458, 1957.
21. Scrimshaw, N. S.: World-wide importance of protein malnutrition and progress toward its prevention, Amer. J. Public Health **53:**1781, 1963.
22. Platt, B. S.: Infant-feeding practices. Breast feeding and the prevention of infant malnutrition, Proc. Nutr. Soc. **13:**94, 1954.
23. Behar, M., and Scrimshaw, N. S.: Effect of environment on nutritional status, Arch. Environ. Health **5:**257, 1962.
24. Trowell, H. C., Davies, J. N. P., and Dean, R. F. A.: Kwashiorkor, London, 1954, Edward Arnold & Co.
25. Squires, B. T.: Observations upon the oral mucosa of the African, Cent. Afr. J. Med. **4:**104, 1958.
26. Squires, B. T.: Differential staining of buccal epithelial smears as an indicator of poor nutritional status due to protein-calorie deficiency, J. Pediat. **66:**891, 1965.
27. Garn, S. M., Rohmann, C. G., Behar, M., Viteri, F., and Guzman, M. A.: Compact bone deficiency in protein-calorie malnutrition, Science **145:**1444, 1964.
28. Owens, P. D. A.: The effects of undernutrition and rehabilitation on the jaws and teeth of pigs. In McCance, R. A., and Widdowson, E. M., editors: Calorie deficiencies and protein deficiencies, Boston, 1968, Little, Brown & Co.

29. Pindborg, J. J., Bhat, M., and Roed-Petersen, B.: Oral changes in South Indian children with severe protein deficiency, J. Periodont. **38**:218, 1967.
30. Stahl, S. S.: Response of the periodontium to protein-calorie malnutrition, J. Oral Med. **21**:146, 1966.
31. Stahl, S. S.: Host resistance and periodontal disease, J. Dent. Res. vol. 49, supp., p. 248, 1970.
32. Stein, G., and Ziskin, D. E.: The effect of a protein free diet on the teeth and periodontium of the albino rat, J. Dent. Res. **28**:529, 1949.
33. Chawla, T. N., and Glickman, I.: Protein deprivation and the periodontal structures of the albino rat, Oral Surg. **4**:578, 1951.
34. Stahl, S. S., Sandler, H. C., and Cahn, L.: The effects of protein deprivation upon the oral tissues of the rat, and particularly upon periodontal structures under irritation, Oral Surg. **8**:760, 1955.
35. Carranza, F. A., Jr., Cabrini, R. L., Lopez, O. R., and Stahl, S. S.: Histometric analysis of interradicular bone in protein deficient animals, J. Periodont. Res. **4**:292, 1969.
36. Goldman, H. M.: The effects of dietary protein deprivation and of age on the periodontal tissues of the rat and spider monkey, J. Periodont. **25**:87, 1954.
37. Manson, J. D., and Rand, H.: Recurrent Vincent's disease (a survey of 61 cases), Brit. Dent. J. **110**:386, 1961.
38. Skach, M., Zabrodsky, S, and Mrklas, L.: A study of the effect of age and season on the incidence of ulcerative gingivitis, J. Periodont. Res. **5**:187, 1970.
39. Miglani D. C., and Sharma, O. P.: Incidence of acute necrotizing gingivitis and periodontosis among cases seen at the Government Hospital, Madras, J. All India Dent. Ass. **37**:183, 1965.
40. Pindborg, J. J., Bhat, M., Devanath, K. R., Narayana H. R., and Ramachandra, S.: Occurrence of acute necrotizing gingivitis in South Indian children, J. Periodont. **37**:14, 1966.
41. Sheiham, A.: An epidemiological study of oral disease in Nigerians, J. Dent. Res. **44**: 1184, 1965.
42. Malberger, E.: Acute infectious oral necrosis among young children in the Gambia, West Africa, J. Periodont. Res. **2**:154, 1967.
43. Jelliffe, D. B.: Infective gangrene of the mouth (cancrum oris), Pediatrics **9**:544, 1952.
44. Phan-Dinh-Tuan: Noma in Vietnam, Indian J. Pediat. **29**:367, 1962.
45. Tempest, M. N.: Cancrum oris, Brit. J. Surg. **53**:949, 1966.
46. Agnew, R. G.: Cancrum oris, J. Periodont. **18**:22, 1947.
47. Ruben, M. P., and Miller, M.: Noma: its association with nutritional deprivation and physical debilitation. Report of a case, Oral Surg. **18**:167, 1964.
47a. Zinserling, W. D.: Ueber die fusospirochatöse Gangrän und einige verwandte Prozesse vorzugsweise bei Kindern, Jena, 1928, Gustav Fischer.
48. Schultz-Haudt, S. D., and From, S.: Dynamics of periodontal tissues. I. The epithelium, Odont. T. **69**:431, 1961.
49. Deo, M. G., Mathur, M., and Ramalingaswami, V.: Cell regeneration in protein deficiency, Nature **216**:499, 1967.
50. Brown, H. O., Levine, M. L., and Lipkin, M.: Inhibition of intestinal epithelial cell renewal and migration induced by starvation, Amer. J. Physiol. **205**:868, 1963.
51. Munro, H. N., and Goldberg, D. M.: The effect of protein intake on the protein and nucleic acid metabolism of the intestinal mucosal cell. In Munro, H. N., editor: The role of the gastrointestinal tract in protein metabolism, Oxford, 1964, Blackwell Scientific Publications, Ltd.
52. Deo, M. G., and Ramalingaswami, V.: Reaction of the small intestine to induced protein malnutrition in Rhesus monkeys—a study of cell population kinetics in the jejunum, Gastroenterology **49**:150, 1965.
53. Bollet, A. J.: Effect of protein depletion on skin and bone collagen, Mount Sinai J. Med. **37**:445, 1970.
54. Melcher, A. H.: Healing of wounds in the periodontium. In Melcher, A. H., and Bowen, W. H., editors: Biology of the periodontium, New York, 1969, Academic Presss, Inc.
55. Cohen, B.: Clinical applications of studies into the pathogenesis of parodontal disease, Parodontopathies, p. 59, 1963.
56. Mühleman, H. R., Toto, P. D., Sicher, H., and Wentz, F. M.: Healing in the human attached gingiva, Periodontics **2**:106, 1964.
57. Ross, R.: The fibroblast and wound repair, Biol. Rev. **43**:51, 1968.

58. Kobak, M. W., Benditt, E. P., Wissler, R. W., and Steffee, C. H.: The relation of periodontal deficiency to experimental wound healing, Surg. Gynec. Obstet. **85**:751, 1947.
59. Stahl, S. S.: The effect of a protein-free diet on the healing of gingival wounds in rats, Arch. Oral Biol. **7**:551, 1962.
60. Localio, S. A., Morgan, M. E., and Hinton, J. W.: The biological chemistry of wound healing. I. The effect of dl-methionine on the healing of wounds in protein-depleted animals, Surg. Gynec. Obstet. **86**:582, 1948.
61. Williamson, M. B., and Fromm, H. J.: Utilization of sulphur amino acids during healing of experimental wounds, Proc. Soc. Exp. Biol. Med. **83**:329, 1953.
62. Udupa, K. N., Woessner, J. F., and Dunphy, J. E.: The effect of methionine on the production of mucopolysaccharides and collagen in healing wounds of protein-depleted animals, Surg. Gynec. Obstet. **102**:639, 1956.
63. Williamson, M. B.: Protein metabolism during healing of wounds, Clin. Chem. **2**:1, 1956.
64. Stary, H. C., McMillan, G. G., and Weigensberg, B. I.: Wound healing in lysine deficiency, Arch. Path. **82**:280, 1966.
65. Platt, B. S., and Stewart, R. J. C.: Experimental protein-calorie deficiency: histopathological changes in the endocrine glands of pigs, J. Endocr. **38**:121, 1967.
66. Gillman, J., and Gillman, T.: Perspectives in human malnutrition, New York, 1951, Grune & Stratton, Inc.
67. Castellanos, H., and Arroyave, G.: Role of the adrenal cortical system in the response of children to severe protein malnutrition, Amer. J. Clin. Nutr. **9**:186, 1961.
68. Rao, K. S. J., Srikantia, S. G., and Gopalan, C.: Plasma cortisol levels in protein-calorie malnutrition, Arch. Dis. Child. **43**:365, 1968.
69. Durbin, P. A. J., and Heard, C. R. C.: Corticosteroid excretion in experimental protein-calorie deficiency in pigs, Proc. Nutr. Soc. **21**:xxviii, 1962.
70. Alleyne, G. A., and Young, V. H.: Synacthen as a test of adrenocortical reserve in children, Lancet **2**:503, 1966.
71. Alleyne, G. A., and Young, V. H.: Adrenocortical function in children with severe protein-calorie malnutrition, Clin. Sci. **33**:189, 1967.
72. Kahn, E., and Wayburne, S.: Hypoglycaemia in patients suffering from advanced protein malnutrition (kwashiorkor), Proc. Nutr. Soc. **1**:21, 1960.
73. Korner, A.: The role of the adrenal gland in the control of amino acid incorporation into protein of isolated rat liver microsomes, J. Endocr. **21**:177, 1960.
74. Enwonwu, C. O.: Regulation of liver ribosome metabolism: a study of regulation by hormones and diet. Thesis, S. D., Massachusetts Institute of Technology, Cambridge, Mass., 1968.
75. Clark, I.: The effect of cortisone upon protein synthesis, J. Biol. Chem. **200**:69, 1953.
76. Kit, S., and Barron, E. S. G.: The effect of adrenal cortical hormones on the incorporation of $C^{14}$ into the protein of lymphatic cells, Endocrinology **52**:1, 1953.
77. Blecher, M., and White, A.: Effects of various steroids and metabolic inhibitors on the incorporation of glycine-2-$C^{14}$ into total proteins and nucleic acids in normal and malignant lymphocytes *in vitro,* J. Biol. Chem. **233**:1161, 1958.
78. Wool, I. G., and Weinshelbaum, E. I.: Corticosteroids and incorporation of $C^{14}$-phenylalanine into protein of isolated rat diaphragm, Amer. J. Physiol. **198**:1111, 1960.
79. Fisher, L. B., and Maibach, H. I.: The effect of corticosteroids on human epidermal mitotic activity, Arch. Derm. **103**:39, 1971.
80. Dougherty, T. F., and Berliner, D. L.: The effects of hormones on connective tissue cells. In Gould, B. S., editor: Biology of collagen, New York, 1968, Academic Press, Inc., vol. 2.
81. Houck, J. C., and Patel, Y. M.: Proposed mode of action of corticosteroids on the connective tissue, Nature **206**:158, 1965.
82. Kivirikko, K. I.: Hydroxyproline-containing fractions in normal and cortisone-treated chick embryos, Acta Physiol. Scand., vol. 60, supp., p. 219, 1963.
83. Asboe-Hansen, G.: Hormone control of connective tissue, Fed. Proc. **25**:1136, 1966.
84. Gould, B. S.: Collagen biosynthesis. In Gould, B. S., editor: Biology of collagen, New York, 1968, Academic Press. Inc., vol. 2.
85. Kofoed, J. A., and Bozzini, C. E.: The effect of hydrocortisone on the concentration and synthesis of acid mucopolysaccharides in the rat gingiva, J. Periodont. Res. **5**:259, 1970.
86. Dreizen, S., Levy, B. M., and Bernick, S.: Studies on the biology of the periodontium in marmosets. X. Cortisone induces periodontal and skeletal changes in adult cotton top marmosets, J. Periodont. **42**:217, 1971.

87. Glickman, I., Stone, I. C., and Chawla, T. N.: The effect of systemic administration of cortisone upon the periodontium of white mice, J. Periodont. **24**:161, 1953.
88. Goldberg, H., Ambinder, W. J., Cooper, L., and Abrams, L. A.: Emotional status of patients with acute gingivitis, New York Dent. J. **22**:308, 1956.
89. O'Leary, T. J., Shannon, I. L., and Prigmore, J. R.: Clinical and systemic findings in periodontal disease, J. Periodont. **33**:243, 1962.
90. Goldhaber, P., and Giddon, D. B.: Present concepts concerning the etiology of acute necrotizing ulcerative gingivitis, Int. Dent. J. **14**:468, 1964.
91. Selye, H.: Effect of cortisone and somatotrophic hormone upon the development of a noma-like condition in the rat, Oral. Surg. **6**:557, 1953.
92. Baig, H. A., and Edozien, J. C.: Carbohydrate metabolism in kwashiorkor, Lancet **2**:662, 1966.
93. Löe, H.: Endocrinologic influences on periodontal disease. Pregnancy and diabetes mellitus, Alabama J. Med. Sci. **5**:336, 1968.
94. Keyes, P. H., and Likins, R. C.: Plaque formation, periodontal disease, and dental caries in Syrian hamsters, J. Dent. Res. **25**:166, 1946. Abstract.
95. Auskaps, A. M., Gupta, O. P., and Shaw, J. H.: Periodontal disease in the rice rat. III. Survey of dietary influences, J. Nutr. **63**:325, 1957.
96. Shaw, J. H., and Griffiths, D.: Relation of protein, carbohydrate, and fat intake to the periodontal syndrome, J. Dent. Res. **40**:614, 1961.
97. Keyes, P. H., and Jordan, H. V.: Periodontal lesions in the Syrian hamster. III. Findings related to an infective and transmissible component, Arch. Oral Biol. **9**:377, 1964.
98. Food and Agriculture Organization of the United Nations: Calorie requirements, FAO nutritional studies no. 15, Rome, 1957, Food and Agriculture Organization.
99. Hall, H. D., and Schneyer, C. A.: Salivary gland atrophy in rat induced by liquid diet, Proc. Soc. Exp. Biol. Med. **117**:789, 1964.
100. Sreebny, L. M., and Johnson, D. A.: Effect of food consistency and decreased food intake on rat parotid and pancreas, Amer. J. Physiol. **215**:455, 1968.
101. Wilborn, W. H., and Schneyer, C. A.: Ultrastructural changes of rat parotid glands induced by a diet of liquid Metrecal, Z. Zellforsch. **103**:1, 1970.
102. Sreebny, L. M., Johnson, D. A., and Robinovitch, M. R.: Functional regulation of protein synthesis in the rat parotid gland, J. Biol. Chem. **246**:3879, 1971.
103. Rao, S. S., Shourie, K. L., and Shankwalker, G. B.: Effect of dietary fat variations on the periodontium. An experimental study in rats, Periodontics **3**:66, 1965.
104. Prout, R. E. S., and Tring, F. C.: Periodontal changes in the rat induced by a fat-free diet, J. Periodont. Res. **6**:182, 1971.
105. Hodges, R. E: What's new about scurvy? Amer J. Clin. Nutr. **24**:383, 1971.
106. British Medical Research Council: Vitamin C requirements in human adults, Special Report Series of the Medical Research Council, no. 280, London, 1953, H. M. Stationery Office.
107. Berry, F. B., and Schaefer, A.: Nutrition surveys in the Near and Far East. Report of the Interdepartmental Committee on Nutrition for National Defense, N.I.H., Amer. J. Clin. Nutr. **6**:342, 1958.
108. Pauling, L.: Vitamin C and the common cold, San Francisco, 1970, W. H. Freeman & Co.
109. Dogramaci, I.: Scurvy: a survey of 241 cases, New Eng. J. Med. **235**:185, 1946.
110. Vilter, R. W., Woolford, R., and Spies, T. D. S: Severe scurvy: a clinical and hematologic study, J. Lab. Clin. Med. **31**:609, 1946.
111. Pearson, W. N.: Biochemical appraisal of the vitamin nutritional status in man, J.A.M.A. **180**:49, 1962.
112. Dreizen, A.: Oral indications of the deficiency states, Postgrad. Med. **49**:97, 1971.
113. Glickman, I.: Acute vitamin C deficiency and periodontal disease. II. The effect of acute vitamin C deficiency upon the response of the periodontal tissues of the guinea pig to artificially induced inflammation, J. Dent. Res. **27**:201, 1948.
114. Glickman, I.: Nutrition in the prevention and treatment of gingival and periodontal diseases, J. Dent. Med. **19**:179, 1964.
115. El-Ashiry, G. M., Ringsdorf, Jr., W. M., and Cheraskin, E.: Local and systemic influences in periodontal disease. II. Effect of prophylaxis and natural versus synthetic vitamin C upon gingivitis, J. Periodont. **35**:250, 1964.
116. Dreizen, S., Levy, B. M., and Bernick, S.: Studies on the biology of the periodontium of marmosets. VII. The effect of vitamin C deficiency on the marmoset periodontium, J. Periodont. Res. **4**:274, 1969.

117. Priest, R. E.: Formation of epithelial basement membrane is restricted by scurvy in vitro and is stimulated by vitamin C, Nature **225**:744, 1970.
118. Ross, R., and Benditt, E. P.: Wound healing in components of guinea pig skin wounds observed in the electron microscope, J. Biophys. Biochem. Cytol. **11**:677, 1961.
119. Ross, R., and Benditt, E. P.: Wound healing and collagen formation. IV. Distortion of ribosomal patterns of fibroblasts in scurvy, J. Cell. Biol. **22**:365, 1964.
120. Enwonwu, C. O., and Sreebny, L. M.: Experimental protein-calorie malnutrition in rats: biochemical and ultrastructural studies, Exp. Molec. Path. **12**:332, 1970.
121. Enwonwu, C. O., and Sreebny, L. M.: Studies of hepatic lesions in experimental protein-calorie malnutrition in rats and immediate effects of refeeding on an adequate protein diet, J. Nutr. **101**:501, 1971.
122. Gould, B. S.: The role of certain vitamins in collagen formation. In Gould, B. S., editor: Biology of collagen, New York, 1968, Academic Press, Inc., vol. 2.
123. Becks, H., Wainright, W. W., and Morgan, A. F.: Comparative study of oral changes in dogs due to pantothenic acid, nicotinic acid and unknowns of the B vitamin complex, Amer. J. Orthodont. **29**:183, 1943.
124. Topping, N. N., and Fraser, H. F.: Mouth lesions associated with dietary deficiencies in monkeys, Public Health Rep. **54**:416, 1939.
125. Chapman, O. D., and Harris, A. E.: Oral lesions associated with dietary deficiences in monkeys, J. Infect. Dis. **69**:7, 1941.
126. O'Brien, J. A.: The role of the folate coenzymes in cellular division. A review, Cancer Res. **22**:267, 1962.
127. Langston, W. C., Darby, W. J., Shukers, C. F., and Day, P. L: Nutritional cytopenia (vitamin M deficiency) in the monkey, J. Exp. Med. **69**:923, 1938.
128 Shaw, J. H.: The relation of nutrition to periodontal disease, J. Dent. Res. **41**:264, 1962.
129. Dreizen, S., Levy, B. M., and Bernick, S.: Studies on the biology of the periodontium of marmosets. VIII. The effect of folic acid deficiency on the marmoset oral mucosa, J. Dent. Res. **49**:616, 1970.
130. Jolly, M.: Vitamin A deficiency: a review. II, J. Oral Ther. **3**:439, 1967.
131. Oliver, W. M.: The effect of deficiencies of calcium, vitamin D or calcium and vitamin D and or variations in the source of dietary protein on the supporting tissues of the rat molar, J. Periodont. Res. **4**:56, 1969.
132. Ferguson, H. W., and Hertles, R. L.: The effect of vitamin D on the dentine of the incisor teeth and on the alveolar bone of young rats maintained on diets deficient in calcium or phosphorus, Arch. Oral Biol. **9**:447, 1964.
133. Ferguson, H. W.: Effect of nutrition on the periodontium. In Melcher, A. H., and Bowen, W. H., editors: Biology of the periodontium, New York, 1969, Academic Press, Inc.
133a. Bernick, S., Ershoff, B. H., and Lal, J. B.: Effect of hypervitaminosis D on bones and teeth of rats, Int. J. Nutr. Res. **41**:480, 1971.
134. Harris, R. S.: Macrominerals: calcium, phosphorus, magnesium and calcification; iron and micro elements. In Nizel, A. E., editor: The science of nutrition and its application in clinical dentistry, Philadelphia, 1966, W. B. Saunders Co.
135. Nordin, B. E. C.: Osteomalacia, osteoporosis and calcium deficiency, Clin. Orthop. **17**:235, 1960.
136. Ferguson, H. W., and Hertles, R. L.: The effects of diets deficient in calcium or phosphorus in the presence and absence of supplements of vitamin D on the secondary cementum and alevolar bone of young rats, Arch. Oral Biol. **9**:647, 1964.
137. Ferguson, H. W., and Hertles, R. L.: The effect of diets deficient in calcium or phosphorus in the presence and absence of supplements of vitamin D on the incisor teeth and bone of adult rats, Arch. Oral Biol. **11**:1345, 1966.
138. Thorén, L.: Magnesium deficiency in gastrointestinal fluid loss, Acta Chir. Scand., supp. 306, 1963.
139. Flink, E. B., McCollister, R., Prasad, A. S., Melby, J. C., and Doe, R. P.: Evidences for clinical magnesium deficiency, Ann. Intern. Med. **47**:956, 1957.
140. Klein, H., Orent, E. R., and McCollum, E. V.: The effects of magnesium deficiency on the teeth and their supporting structures in rats, Amer. J. Physiol. **112**:256, 1935.
141. Caddell, J. L.: Magnesium in the therapy of orofacial lesions of severe protein-calorie malnutrition, Brit. J. Surg. **56**:826, 1969.
142. Beveridge, B. T., Bannerman, R. M., Evanson, J. M., and Witts, L. J.: Hypochromic anaemia. A retrospective study of follow up of 378 in-patients, Quart. J. Med. **34**:145, 1965.

143. Jacobs, A.: Carbohydrates and sulphur-containing compounds in the anaemic buccal epithelium, J. Clin. Path. **14**:610, 1961.
144. Jacobs, A.: Iron-containing enzymes in the buccal epithelium, Lancet **2**:1331, 1961.
145. Sbarra, A. J., Jacobs, A. A., Strauss, R. R., Paul, B. B., and Mitchell, G. W: The biochemical and antimicrobial activities of phagocytozing cells, Amer. J. Clin. Nutr. **24**:272, 1971.
146. Higashi, O., Sato, U., Takamatsu, H., and Oyama, M.: Mean cellular peroxidase (MCP) of leukocytes in iron deficiency anemia, Tohoku J. Exp. Med. **93**:105, 1967.
147. Russell, A. L., and White, C. L.: In Muhler, J. C., and Hine, M. K., editors: Fluorine and dental health, London, 1960, Staples Press.
148. Cohen, B.: Comparative studies in periodontal disease, Proc. Roy. Soc. Med. **53**:275, 1960.
149. Person, P.: Diet consistency and periodontal disease in old albino rats, J. Periodont. **32**: 308, 1961.
150. Baer, P.: The relation of the physical character of the diet to the periodontium and periodontal disease, Oral Surg. **9**:839, 1956.
151. Stahl, S. S., and Dreizen, S.: The adaptation of the rat periodontium to prolonged feeding of pellet, powder and liquid diets, J. Periodont. **35**:312, 1964.
152. Egelberg, J.: Local effect of diet on plaque formation and development of gingivitis in dogs, Odont. Rev. **16**:31, 1965.
153. Bundgaard-Jorgensen, F.: Kostens betydning for caries-og paradentose-profylaksen, Tandlaegebladet **62**:477, 1958.
154. Bastein, V. G.: Diet, its dynamics and dental disorders, J. Canad. Dent. Ass. **26**:332, 1960.
155. Wilcox, C. E., and Everett, F. G: Friction on the teeth and the gingiva during mastication, J. Amer. Dent. Ass. **66**:513, 1963.
156. Lindhe, J., and Wicen, P. O.: The effects on the gingivae of chewing fibrous foods, J. Periodont. Res. **4**:193, 1969.
156a. Wade, A. B.: Effect on dental plaque of chewing apples, Dent. Pract. **21**:194, 1971.
157. Weiss, R., Stahl, S. S., and Tonna, E. A.: The effects of diets of different physical consistencies on the periodontal proliferative activity in young adult rats, J. Periodont. Res. **4**:296, 1969.
158. Bahn, A. N.: Microbial potential in the etiology of periodontal disease, Periodontics **41**: 603, 1960.
159. Socransky, S. S.: Relationship of bacteria to the etiology of periodontal disease, J. Dent. Res. **49**:203, 1970.
160. Gordon, J. E., and Scrimshaw, N. S.: Infectious disease in the malnourished, Medical Clinics of North America, Philadelphia, November 1970, W. B. Saunders Co.
161. Reddy, V., and Srikantia, S. G.: Antibody response in kwashiorkor, Indian J. Med. Res. **52**:1154, 1964.
162. Brown, R. E., and Katz, M.: Antigenic stimulation in undernourished children, E. Afr. Med. J. **42**:221, 1965.
163. Kumate, R. J.: Desnutrición e immunologia. In Ramos Galvan, R., Mariscal Abascal, C., Viniegra Carreras, A., and Perez Ortiz, B., editors: Desnutrición en el niño, Mexico, D. F., 1969, Impresiones Modernas, S. A.
164. Axelrod, A. E.: Immune processes in vitamin deficiency states, Amer. J. Clin. Nutr. **24**:265, 1971.
165. Spies, T. D.: Some recent advances in nutrition, J.A.M.A. **7**:675, 1958.
166. Stallard, R. E., Diab, M. A., and Zander, H. A.: The attaching substance between enamel and epithelium—a product of the epithelial cells, J. Periodont. **36**:130, 1965.
167. Cutright, D. E., and Bauer, H.: Cell renewal in the oral mucosa and skin of the rat. I. Turnover time, Oral Surg. **23**:249, 1967.
168. Carneiro, J.: Synthesis and turnover of collagen in periodontal tissues. In Leblond, C. P., and Warren, K. B., editors: The use of radioautography in investigating protein synthesis, New York, 1965, Academic Press, Inc.
169. Nelson, R. C., and Jeffray, H.: Protein synthesis, microsomes and polyribosomes in oral tissues, J. Dent. Res. **48**:857, 1969.

**Additional suggested reading**

Clark, J. W., Cheraskin, W. M., and Ringsdorf, W. M.: Diet and the periodontal patient, Springfield, Ill., 1970, Charles C Thomas, Publisher.
Nizel, A. E.: Nutrition in preventive dentistry, Philadelphia, 1972, W. B. Saunders Co.

CHAPTER TWELVE

# Plaque control

**Disclosing agents**
**Plaque index**
**Training the patient**

Bacterial plaque forms continuously. It is a major cause of gingivitis and periodontitis. Regular removal of the dental plaque can help to cure gingivitis and periodontitis and can help to prevent their recurrence.[1,2] Plaque can be removed by the patient who has been trained in the methods of plaque control.

Plaque starts to form at the gingival margin of teeth and builds up over the crown. If it is not eliminated, in about 1 week the crown is literally and completely covered with this soft deposit. Since plaque formation starts at the gingival margin, the microorganisms are in contact with the tooth and the gingiva; and from this location they appear to exert their deleterious influence. On the basis of the preceding information, effective prevention requires the removal of plaque.

A discussion of plaque in greater depth may be found in Chapter 6. The importance of other etiologic factors is discussed in Chapter 8; and the role of the immune response and inflammation is discussed in Chapter 13. At this stage we shall concentrate on establishing a workable program for the prevention and treatment of periodontal inflammation by the regular removal of plaque.

## DISCLOSING AGENTS

***Plaque stains***

Because plaque can be difficult to detect, stains may be applied to make it readily visible.[3] The virtual invisibility of plaque is illustrated in Plate 2, *B* and *E*. After rinsing with an aqueous solution containing 0.3% basic fuchsin, the patient can see with the unaided eye the plaque that coats the tooth surfaces (Plate 2, *C* and *F*).

Obviously the use of stains such as basic fuchsin, bismark brown, or erythrosin can facilitate the patient's efforts at plaque removal. Stains give the patient an objective, that is, the complete removal of plaque from the tooth surfaces. They also give him an effective means of determining whether this objective has been reached, namely, the absence of a red stain on exposed tooth surfaces.

***Disclosing solutions and tablets***

Disclosing solutions and tablets may also be used to make plaque visible. Disclosing solutions (e.g., basic fuchsin 0.3%) impart a bright red color to the plaque, stains, and calcified deposits. They also stain the imperfect margins of plastic fillings and the mucosa of the lips, cheeks, tongue, and floor of the mouth. Because these stains tend to last on mucosal surfaces for several hours, some patients object to the regular use of disclosing solutions. Disclosing tablets, on the other hand, do not impart such a lasting coloration; but they do stain the plaque less brilliantly, making it more difficult to detect.

| TOOTH NO. | 3 | 9 | 12 | |
|---|---|---|---|---|
| FACIAL AND LINGUAL SCORES | F L<br>M<br>G<br>D | F L<br>M<br>G<br>D | F L<br>M<br>G<br>D | RECORD IN CIRCLE THE HIGHEST SCORE FOUND ON ANY ONE TOOTH. |
| TOTAL | | | | |
| FACIAL AND LINGUAL SCORES | F L<br>M<br>G<br>D | F L<br>M<br>G<br>D | F L<br>M<br>G<br>D | |
| TOTAL | | | | |
| TOOTH NO. | 28 | 25 | 19 | |

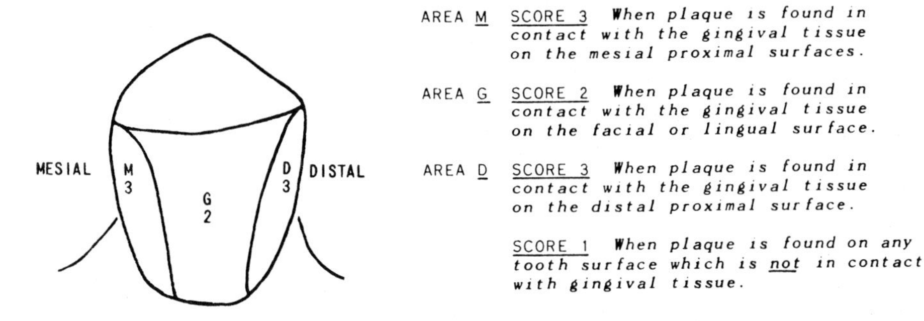


**Fig. 12-1.** Plaque index form useful for recording and for patient education. (Courtesy F. Grossman, U. S. Navy.)

When basic fuchsin is used as a disclosing solution, ten drops are dispensed with an eyedropper into an ounce of water. The patient is asked to rinse vigorously for 30 seconds and to expectorate. He then should rinse with several mouthfuls of water to remove excess stain. The examination may then be made.

When disclosing tablets are used, the patient is instructed to chew the wafer thoroughly, working it into the saliva, and then to swish the fluid vigorously about his mouth for a minute. Care must be taken that the solution reaches all parts of the mouth. If it does not, surfaces of some teeth may not be stained, even when plaque is present. Proper disclosure can be attained by a vigorous pumping action of the cheeks to force the solution between the teeth. After about a minute the mouth may be emptied and rinsed gently with water. Examination should be made immediately. The patient should be encouraged to observe the procedure with a mirror.

## PLAQUE INDEX

At this time it will be valuable to take a plaque index. The score will indicate to the dentist and to the patient the status of the patient's oral hygiene efforts as shown by the plaque that is found on selected surfaces of a number of teeth. At subsequent appointments new indexes can be taken, and comparisons can then be made with earlier indexes to gauge the improvement or lack of improvement in plaque control.

A typical index chart is shown in Fig. 12-1. Originally such oral hygiene indexes were designed for epidemiologic studies. These studies have shown that there is a direct relationship between plaque and gingivitis. Subsequently the oral hygiene index was adapted for office use in preventive periodontics.

Once the index has been taken and explained to the patient, procedures for plaque control may be started. The training methods are described in Chapter 25.

## TRAINING THE PATIENT

The training program should consist of closely spaced visits either daily or every other day. Four or five such visits may be used. At each visit a new plaque index may be taken to illustrate the improvement to the patient.

On recall visits a new index may be taken to assess the status of oral hygiene and to compare with indexes taken at the end of treatment. The plaque index has an important motivational role in the prevention of disease, and it also serves as a record.

In Plate 2, *A* to *C,* a gingivitis around the mandibular right lateral incisor can be seen in a 25-year-old woman who did not brush for 2 weeks while participating in a study on the relationship of plaque to gingival inflammation. In *D* to *F* of this plate, a 26-year-old woman, also participating in the study, showed extensive plaque that literally covered the crowns; however, no gingival inflammation could be detected after 2 weeks.

**CHAPTER 12**

**References**

1. Lightner, L. M., O'Leary, T. J., Drake, R. B., Crump, P. P., and Allen, M. F.: Preventive periodontic treatment procedures: results over 46 months, J. Periodont **42:**555, 1971.
2. Suomi, J. D., Greene, J. C., Vermillion, J. R., Chang, J. J., and Leatherwood, E. C.: The effect of controlled oral hygiene procedures on the progession of periodontal disease in adults: results after two years, J. Periodont. **40:**416, 1969.
3. Arnim, S. S.: The use of disclosing agents for measuring tooth cleanliness, J. Periodont. **34:** 227, 1963.

**Additional suggested reading**

Keyes, P. H., and Sherp, R.: Chemical adjuvants for control and prevention of dental plaque disease, J. Amer. Soc. Prev. Dent. **1:**18, 1971.

O'Leary, T. J., Drake, R. B., and Naylor, J. E.: The plaque control record, J. Periodont. **43:** 38, 1972.

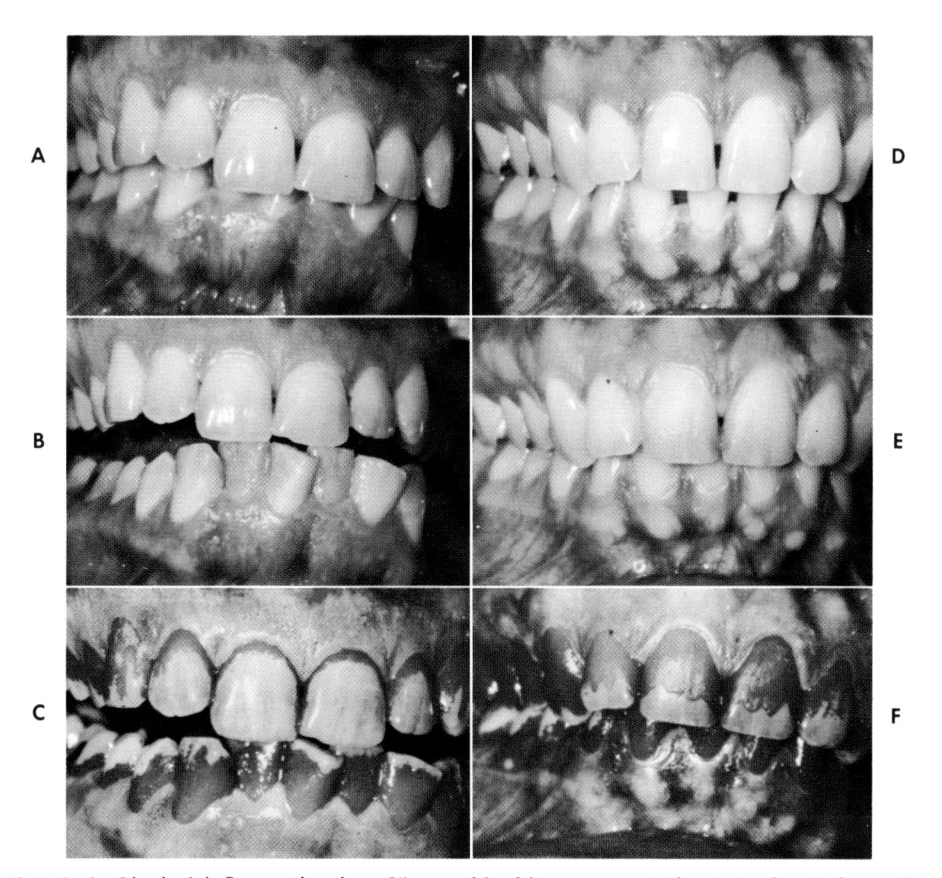


**Plate 2. A,** Gingival inflammation in a 25-year-old white woman at the start of a study on the relationship of oral hygiene and gingival inflammation. **B,** After 2 weeks of no oral hygiene, plaque is visible even without disclosing solution. **C,** Use of a disclosing solution vividly illustrates abundant plaque. **D,** Plaque in a 26-year-old dental assistant at the start of a plaque experiment. **E,** After 14 days without oral hygiene, plaque may be seen on teeth and gingiva. **F,** Rinsing with 0.2% basic fuchsin solution reveals the extent of plaque collected.

PART IV

# Inflammatory periodontal disease

CHAPTER THIRTEEN

# Inflammation



The majority of periodontal diseases are inflammatory, as evidenced by the dense cellular infiltrate in the gingival corium subjacent to the pocket and by the exudate, which contains polymorphonuclear leukocytes and inflammatory serum components, emanating from the pocket. The intimate contact of plaque with the contiguous gingiva makes such inflammation readily understandable. Inflammation soon superimposes itself even in those periodontal diseases that are not primarily inflammatory. For this reason a good understanding of the process is essential.

## CHARACTERISTICS OF INFLAMMATION

*Definition*

Inflammation may be defined as the normal response of living tissue to injury. It is characterized by a specific course of physiologic and biochemical alterations. The inflammatory process brings together all the resources of the body and presents them at the site of injury as a defense against microbial invaders and inanimate noxious substances or stimuli.

*History*

The cardinal signs of inflammation are redness and swelling, with heat and pain (Celsus, 1st century A.D.) and loss of function (Galen, 2nd century A.D.). The changes and processes of inflammation were not well understood until Cohnheim in 1882 gave his classical description of the vascular events that occur in inflammation. Metchnikoff, in another classical work, outlined the cellular events in inflammation and in 1905 gave his description of phagocytosis.

*Gross stages*

The gross stages in the inflammatory process are as follows[1]:

1. Injury to tissues initiating the inflammatory reaction
2. Hyperemia caused by dilatation of capillaries and venules
3. Increased vascular permeability and the accumulation of inflammatory

exudate containing polymorphonuclear leukocytes, macrophages, and lymphocytes
4. Neutralization, dilution, and destruction of the irritant
5. Limiting of the inflammation and circumscribing of the area with young fibrous connective tissue
6. Initiation of repair

Healing and repair are mainly brought about by the response of the connective tissues. One of the first signs of healing is the appearance of macrophages, which digest the precipitated fibrin and engulf debris. Capillaries then invade the area. With these come fibroblasts, which lay down fibrous tissue. Lymphatics follow along the course of the blood vessels. In 3 to 4 weeks, the area is vascularized and maturation of collagen commences.

Cell injury caused by external noxious stimuli provokes inflammation. On the other hand, inflammation induced by the activation of various endogenous systems[2] (e.g., complement) may lead to cellular self-injury. Thus the defense may become more harmful to the body than the noxious stimulus that originated the reaction, reminding one of the saying "God help me against my friends; against my enemies, I know how to defend myself!"

The acute inflammatory event may progress to a chronic inflammatory reaction, resulting in permanent damage to the involved tissues. Chronicity is probably due to extended triggering of the inflammatory response.

How do antigens gain entrance in the region of the periodontium? The gingiva is in close contact with plaque and calculus. Both endotoxins and other foreign proteins probably pervade the clinically normal[3,4] as well as the ulcerated[5] sulcular epithelium. The quantity of endotoxin found in gingival exudate can be correlated with the degree of clinical inflammation.[6] Circulating antibodies against oral organisms have been demonstrated against oral spirochetes[7]; and other plaque organisms have been demonstrated in patients suffering from periodontal disease.[8-12]

In summary, (1) the inflammatory response is a basic defense system of the animal that functions both to dilute and to remove or inactivate the inciting agent (stimulus) as well as to prepare the site for healing; (2) tissue injury is one such stimulus; other stimuli, which in themselves do not directly damage tissue, may lead indirectly to tissue damage through activation of the inflammatory mechanism; (3) regardless of the nature of the stimulus, the symptoms or characteristic events of the inflammatory response are brought about by specific endogenous compounds called mediators.[2]

## HISTOPATHOLOGY AND PHYSIOLOGY OF INFLAMMATION

Depending on the intensity and duration and to some extent the type of tissue insult, the resulting inflammation may range from mild to severe and from acute to chronic. Regardless of these differences, the tissue evidently reacts in a stereotyped manner to any insult or injurious agent. This reaction involves two basic events: vascular alterations and cellular phenomena, in that order.

### Vascular alterations

The initial changes occur in the microcirculation and exhibit three major features: vasodilatation and augmented blood flow, increased vascular permeability, and (somewhat later) emigration of neutrophilic leukocytes. Each of these features is controlled by specific factors, and each appears to be mediated by different endogenous compounds.

*Histology and physiology of the microcirculation in inflammation*

The microcirculation consists of the arterioles and venules and their direct intercommunications, the metarterioles.[13] Capillaries arise from both metarterioles and terminal arterioles. Metarterioles act as shunts or thoroughfare channels leading directly from the arterioles to the venules. The flow of blood through the metarteriolar shunts, in turn, governs capillary blood flow by bypassing the terminal capillary bed. The terminal capillary bed may be open or closed according to functional demands. When increased blood flow is required, for example, in exercise, the terminal capillaries open. Most often the major blood flow is by means of the metarteriolar shunt.

*Precapillary sphincter*

A ring of smooth muscle, the precapillary sphincter, found at the junction of a capillary with a metarteriole, is involved in the local regulation of capillary blood flow. Vasomotion is the local humoral control of blood flow to the tissues past the precapillary sphincters. All vessels are controlled by sympathetic vasoconstrictor tone, although the local tissue cells have final determination in their region through humoral factors. For example, in exercise, accumulation of metabolic products (lactic acid, carbon dioxide, other metabolites) produces a direct relaxation of the smooth muscle of the blood vessels. The precapillary sphincters apparently are the most sensitive to these factors and are thus relaxed to permit increased blood flow to the tissues involved.

Under normal circumstances fluid leaves the vessel at the precapillary end of the terminal vascular bed and enters the interstitial spaces. The decreased luminal pressure in the postcapillary vessels enhances the return of fluid to the vasculature from the interstitial spaces. In inflammation an increase in postcapillary intraluminal pressure causes a shift in equilibrium so that fluid stays out of the vessel and remains in the tissue; the resultant effect is edema or excess interstitial fluid.

Under the electron microscope the walls of the capillaries and venules are made up of a mosaic of flattened endothelial cells. Although these cells are closely adjacent, intercellular junctions of 150 to 200 Å occur between them. A mucoprotein material present in these junctions acts as both an intercellular cement and a differential filter to various materials. The endothelial cells also contain pinocytotic vesicles, which form at both the luminal surface and the surface adjacent to the basement membrane. During the usual physiologic function of the microvasculature, substances leave the vessels by two mechanisms: (1) diffusion of low-molecular weight substances through the intercellular junctions and (2) ferrying of larger molecules across the endothelial cells, via pinocytotic vesicles.

*Alteration of the microcirculation in inflammation*

Although preceded by numerous cellular biochemical changes in the vasculature and connective tissue, the earliest visible alterations in the acute inflammatory reaction involve the microcirculation. First, a transient arteriolar constriction is seen that lasts from 10 seconds to several minutes and is rapidly followed by a prolonged vasodilatation of the arterioles, metarterioles, and venules. Second, capillary sphincters become relaxed and engorgement of the capillaries occurs. Blood flow through the metarterioles at first increases greatly; venular dilatation lags behind arteriolar dilatation, resulting in an increase in hydrostatic pressure in the vascular bed. Endothelial cells in the venules then become spherical, permitting large openings to occur between the cells at the intercellular junctions (increased vascular permeability). Loss of fluid from the vascular compartment occurs primarily through this increased permeability of the venules to plasma proteins and fluid. Leakage of plasma proteins into the interstitial spaces results in a concentration of 1 to 6 gm. of protein per 100 ml. of exudate. The increased hydrostatic pressure also contributes secondarily to the loss of fluid from the vascular compartment. Blood flow, which was at first quickened via the vasodilatation, now becomes sluggish and finally static due to the increased viscosity of the blood resulting from the loss of fluid from the vascular compartment. Some margination of polymorphonuclear (PMN) leukocytes can be seen during this time; but emigration occurs mainly during the prolonged late phase of vascular alterations.[4]

## Cellular phenomena

In the area of injury, the white blood cells stick to the venular walls and diapedesis of white cells occurs (sometimes accompanied by a few red cells) during the prolonged late phase of increased vascular permeability. The first white cells passing between the endothelial cells of the vessels and accumulating in the tissue at the area of injury are the PMN leukocytes. However, all the granulocytic cells as well as the monocytes and platelets emigrate through the vascular wall. PMN leukocytes have the faculty of phagocytosis and also contain a number of proteolytic and other enzymes in organelles called lysosomes. Those bacteria, antigen-antibody complexes, and other substances that attract leukocytes are said to have the faculty of chemotaxis.

*Monocytes*

The emigration of monocytes from the bloodstream apparently begins at about the same time as emigration of the PMN leukocytes. These large, phagocytic, mononuclear cells (15 to 80 $\mu$) move more slowly than the PMN leukocytes. Inflammatory exudates during early stages of the acute inflammatory reaction principally contain PMN leukocytes, whereas exudates obtained from later stages of acute and from chronic inflammation mainly contain the larger mononucleated cells (i.e., macrophages). The same is true for the appearance of these cells in inflamed tissues, which may be explained on the basis of the short life-span of the PMN leukocyte (approximately 6 hours). The PMN is an end cell and does not undergo division. In contrast, the macrophage, which is believed to be capable of undergoing mitosis, has a much longer life-span. The function of the macrophage is phagocytosis of bacteria and cell debris. When PMN cells die, their fragments and contents may be phagocytosed by macrophages. A group of antibodies, the opsonins, attach to the surface of bacteria and aid in the ingestion of these microorganisms by both the PMN's and the macrophages. Once the material is within the leukocyte (either the PMN or the macrophage), it lies in a phagocytotic vesicle. Lysosomal enzymes are discharged into this vesicle to digest the bacteria, etc.[15] However, lysosomal enzymes may be released with the death and lysis of the leukocytes and are capable of enhancing and prolonging the inflammatory reaction.

PMN leukocytes also have the ability to produce a kininlike peptide that may function as an endogenous inflammatory mediator during the late phase of the acute inflammatory reaction. Other released lysosomal enzymes are capable of dissolving proteins and carbohydrates and may be involved in the degeneration of connective tissue at the area of injury. In the Shwartzman reaction* the release

*"If a filtrate of *Bacillus typhosis* is injected into the skin of a rabbit, it produces relatively little reaction. If this is followed 24 hours later by an intravenous challenge with the same bacterial filtrate, a hemorrhagic and often necrotic lesion is produced at the original site of intradermal injection." (From Zweifach, B. W., et al.: The inflammatory process, New York, 1965, Academic Press, Inc., p. 13.)

of lysosomal enzymes is believed to be involved in the production of the hemorrhagic necrotizing reaction.

*Eosinophils*

A cell type frequently seen in inflammation is the eosinophil. This type of cell, which is present in the blood in lesser numbers than the PMN, may function in hypersensitivity reactions.[16]

*Lymphocytes*

The lymphocyte is another cell type that typifies the chronic inflammatory reaction. However, this type may be seen also in connective tissues early in the inflammatory reaction. Lymphocytes are members of a cell series whose essential function is to mediate the immune response. Their presence in the gingival connective tissue near the sulcus implies a local defense against the antigens of the dental plaque. Lymphocytes house immunologic information and may thus be called memory cells; their life-span is in excess of 90 days.

*Plasma cells*

The plasma cell, like the lymphocyte, is typical of chronic inflammation. As a rule, this type is seen in tissues rather than in circulating blood. Plasma cells produce antibodies and are lŏcated in the gingiva near the pocket.

*Mast cells*

The mast cell is also believed to play a vital role in some acute inflammatory reaction. Its function in the production of inflammatory mediators will be discussed in the section on the release and activation of mediators.

*pH*

Changes in intracellular and extracellular pH toward the acidic range and other changes in intracellular metabolic activity appear to be vitally important in the inflammatory reaction. They influence the activity of PMN leukocytes, macrophages, and endogenous compounds acting as inflammatory mediators.

*Fibrinolysis*

During the prolonged late phase of the acute inflammatory reaction, alterations in fibrinolytic activity in the affected tissues and vessels result in sludging and thrombus formation via platelet aggregation and the formation of fibrin. If these alterations are sufficiently severe, ischemia, tissue anoxia, acidosis, and finally necrosis of the involved vessels and tissue ensue.

*Resolution*

If the defense reaction of the tissue in the acute phase of the inflammatory response is successful, the acute inflammation subsides and healing results. The alternative is the production of a chronic inflammatory reaction and possibly permanent tissue damage.

## Lymphatics

Lymphatics play an important part in inflammation. Lymphatic capillaries are blind sacks that differ in their histologic makeup from blood capillaries. They lack a distinct basal lamina, and contiguous cells may be separated by junctions of 1500 to 2000 Å.[17] Lymph capillaries, because of their wide intercellular endothelial spaces, permit the entry of large–molecular weight proteins, blood cells, and macrophages. Lymphatic flow is increased in the presence of inflammation.[18] In cases of severe infection, an inflammation of the large lymphatic vessels may result (lymphangitis). A good knowledge of the topography of the regional lymph glands and their behavior in inflammation (lymphadenitis) is essential for the diagnostician.

## Conclusion

Inflammation is a defense reaction that may be viewed as a prerequisite for tissue repair and healing. Therefore, it should not be completely inhibited. On the other hand, it should be intercepted early enough to prevent its becoming chronic and causing permanent tissue damage.

For example, bone regeneration in an infrabony defect occurs more readily in an acute periodontal abscess than in a chronically inflamed condition.

In conclusion, we may well remember the statement of Billroth, the famous Viennese surgeon of the last century: "The inflammatory reaction like other physiological processes is chemico-physiological; these we never see even with the best microscopes, we merely perceive the result of their action."[19]

## ENDOGENOUS MEDIATORS OF INFLAMMATION

The vascular and cellular events just discussed are in only small measure due to the direct action of the injurious stimulus. In greater part they are due to the release and activation of substances called mediators as a result of sublethal injury. At present, the following groups are thought to be chemical mediators of inflammation[20]:

1. *Vasoactive amines.* Histamine and 5-hydroxytryptamine as well as their natural liberators and enzymes, which inactivate normally occurring vasoconstrictor substances
2. *Proteases.* Plasmin, kallikrein, and various permeability factors
3. *Polypeptides.* Bradykinin, kallidin, other kinin peptides, and other basic and acidic polypeptides
4. *Nucleic acids and derivatives.* Lymph node permeability factor (LNPF)
5. *Lipid-soluble acids.* Lysolecithin, slow-reacting–substance anaphylaxis (SRS-A), and prostaglandins
6. *Lysosome contents.* Lysosomal enzymes, proteases, and other constituents

### Vasoactive amines

Histamine mediates the early phase of the permeability response of the acute inflammatory reaction in man. Histamine is released from cells of the skin by injurious stimuli and by certain immune reactions. The triple response,*[21] occurring from mild injury to the skin, is a classical bit of evidence for the role of histamine in acute inflammation.

Histamine is formed by the action of the enzyme histidine decarboxylase. It is inactivated by the enzyme histaminase. Except for the large quantities of histamine present in the parietal cells of the stomach, the major storage sites for histamine are the mast cells in various tissues and the platelets and basophils in the circulation. Mast cell histamine is released when tissues are damaged. As discussed later in this chapter in the section on the release and activation of mediators, antigen-antibody reactions can also cause release of mast cell histamine and thereby become cytotoxic.

Increased vascular permeability has been shown to occur by a direct action of histamine on the endothelial cells of the venules. In the presence of histamine, gaps appear at the intercellular junctions of the endothelial cells; and vascular leakage of plasma protein and fluid results. Histamine does not cause emigration of leukocytes or produce any of the cellular changes of the inflammatory re-

---

*"Triple response is the reaction that follows a heavy stroke of a sharp edge (such as a ruler edge) across the skin. First there is a dull red line that begins to appear in 20 seconds and is sharply demarcated and corresponds to the line of pressure. This is followed in about 30 seconds by a dull red halo (axon reflex) and, last, after 70 seconds by a wheal that is at first dull red and subsequently becomes pale." (From Zweifach, B. W., et al.: The inflammatory process, New York, 1965, Academic Press, Inc., p. 26.)

action; nor does it seem to be involved in the more prolonged late changes in vascular permeability.

## Protease enzymes and polypeptide products

It has been suggested that the increased proteolysis evident in tissue injury comes about through the activation of normally occurring but inactive proteolytic enzyme (protease) systems.[23] In fact, the acute inflammatory reaction may be described as a sequence of events resulting from the initial release of intracellular and intravascular protease and esterase systems into the extracellular and extravascular compartments. These enzymes then act on various substrates that produce substances mediating the observable aspects of the inflammatory reaction.[24] One of these protease systems, the kallikrein-kinin system, is an excellent candidate for one of the mediators of the prolonged late phase of acute inflammation. Some of the interrelationships and probable means of activation of the kallikrein-kinin system are shown in Fig. 13-1. At least four polypeptides, known as kinins, are produced by kallikreins from various sources.[20,25,26] These are among the most potent compounds known for producing some of the classic signs of acute inflammation. Minute (nanogram) quantities of these compounds can cause vasodilatation, increased capillary permeability, pain, and at higher doses emigration of leukocytes.[27]

There is some evidence that bacterial endotoxins applied to the gingiva activate the kallikrein-kinin system by a presently unknown mechanism.[28,29] Some of the highly active kininase enzymes are inhibited by the slightly acid pH (6.0) attained at inflammatory sites. Therefore the activity of these compounds is likely to be increased by the acidosis present in inflamed tissue. Inhibi-

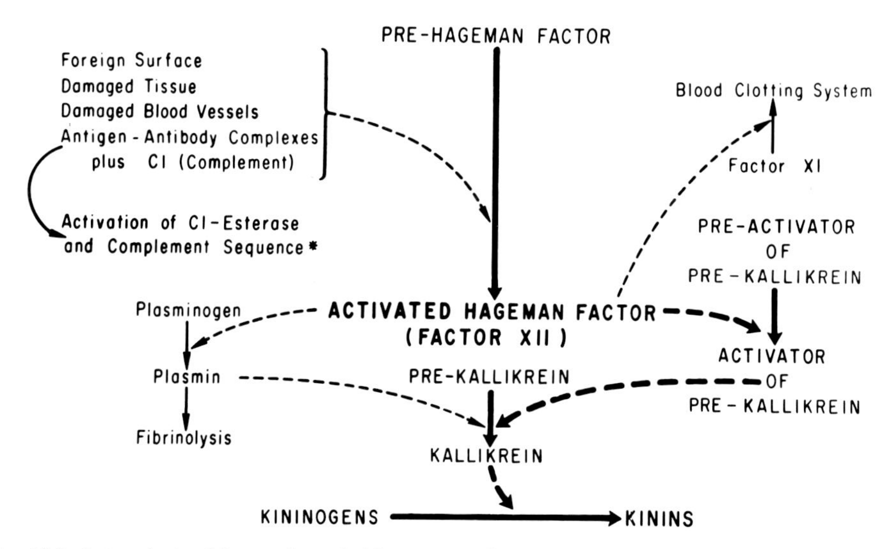


**Fig. 13-1.** Interrelationships and probable means of activation of the kallikrein-kinin system, complement sequence, fibrinolysis, and blood clotting system. Dashed arrows signify activation of or influence on the system indicated by solid arrows. The pathway for kinin formation is shown by heavy dashed and solid arrows. The asterisk (*) refers to Fig. 13-3 (complement sequence). (The term *Hageman factor* refers to a serum protein found originally in the blood of a patient by the name of Hageman. This factor starts the intrinsic clotting mechanism.) (Modified by E. H. Montgomery, Portland, Ore., from Movat, H. Z.: Inflammation, immunity and hypersensitivity, New York, 1971, Harper & Row, Publishers.)

tion of kallikrein activity prevents the vascular permeability increase seen during the late phase of acute inflammation. A number of anti-inflammatory drugs (salicylates, glucocorticosteroids) may exert their antiphlogistic action by preventing the formation of kinin peptides.

### Lysosomal enzymes

Lysosomes are minute cellular vacuoles containing numerous tissue-active substances, among which are proteases and other enzymes. It is currently recognized that lysosomes in PMN leukocytes, macrophages, and possibly other cells are important in producing some of the changes seen in acute inflammation because they release inflammatory mediators.[20] In addition, hydrolytic lysosomal enzymes may cause tissue damage, since they degrade proteins and carbohydrates, and may include collagenase, hyaluronidase, esterases, phosphatases, arylsulfatases, and other enzymes. They appear to be particularly important in causing the inflammatory changes and tissue damage that occur in certain immunologic reactions; and they are probably prerequisite for the tissue damage and necrosis occurring in the Arthus and Shwartzman reactions.

Of interest is the recent finding that lysosomal and extralysosomal fractions of PMN leukocytes contain enzymes for both the formation and the degradation of kinin-like peptides.[20] Thus a mechanism is provided by which the leukocytes emigrating to the inflamed area can contribute to the formation and destruction of inflammatory mediators. Speculatively, such processes may play a role in the perpetuation of inflammation in periodontal disease.[15]

## RELEASE AND ACTIVATION OF MEDIATORS VIA IMMUNE REACTIONS

It has been stated previously that all or some part of the classic components of the inflammatory response (increased vascular permeability, chemotactic response, diapedesis of leukocytes) can be initiated through immune reactions. The inflammatory response thus may be triggered by various types of real and potential insult to the tissues as well as by beneficial (e.g., homografts) or harmless (e.g., ragweed pollen) substances.

The immune potential of man is activated through two major, interconnecting systems: (1) humoral antibody-mediated reactions and (2) cell-mediated reactions.[30] In the one the effector system of the acquired response (defense, or allergic inflammation) is antibody; in the other the effector system is the sensitized lymphocyte.

### Antibody-mediated reactions

***Anaphylactic, formerly termed reagin-dependent, reactions (homocytotropic antibody)***

Homocytotropic antibody has the capacity of becoming fixed or bound to the surfaces of various cells in the species in which it was produced. The cell types to which homocytotropic antibody is known to be fixed are tissue mast cells, blood basophils, and other formed elements of the blood. The ability to become fixed to cell surfaces is controlled through a specific receptor site on the Fc* component of the antibody molecule. Such fixation does not involve the Fab† components. Thus the specific reaction between antigen and antibody may still occur. The class of antibody molecules that function in man as homocytotropic antibody is IgE.‡ These antibodies have also been called skin-fixing antibodies and reagins.

---

*Fraction c, crystallizable.

†Fraction that connects with the antigen.

‡Immunoglobulin E.

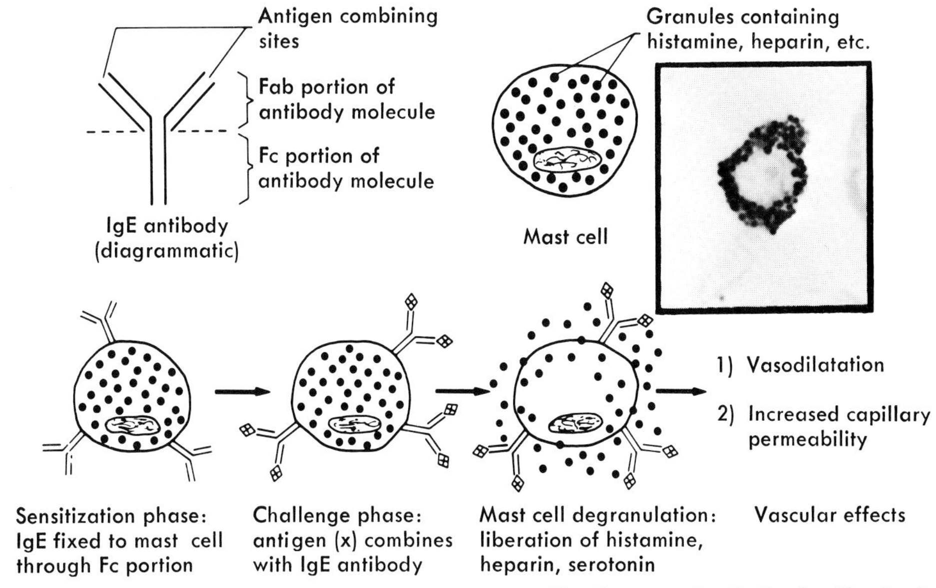


**Fig. 13-2.** Degranulation of mast cells. (Inset: mast cell.) (Courtesy R. T. Ferris, Cleveland, and S. N. Bhaskar, Washington, D. C.).

The reaction of specific antigen with homocytotropic antibody bound to the surfaces of tissue mast cells leads to the degranulation and subsequent destruction of the affected mast cell (Fig. 13-2). Cationic exchange processes in the medium then result in the release of histamine from the freed granules. The finding that gingival mast cells decrease in number in the presence of inflammation should be mentioned.[31,32]

***Complement-fixing antibody (cytotoxic reactions)***

Complement fixation or activation refers to the sequential involvement of the nine components of complement. Complement-dependent cytolysis of susceptible cells requires the involvement of all nine components during these sequential steps. Pharmacologically active split products are released (Fig. 13-3). The term *cytotoxic* means that, as a result of the antigen-antibody reaction, complement is activated (fixed) and the cell is lysed by the action of complement (not by the direct action of the cytotoxic antibody).

Thus, although immunocytolysis may be an important defense mechanism (or allergic reaction) in itself, the activation of the complement sequence by any means results in the formation and release of various products that directly or indirectly mediate phenomena that we classically associate with inflammation: increased vascular permeability, smooth muscle contraction, chemotaxis, and enhanced phagocytosis.

***Arthus reaction***

Arthus demonstrated that repeated injections of horse serum into the skin of a rabbit could ultimately produce a hemorrhagic and necrotic reaction. He noted, as had others, that at first there was the rapid development of a wheal with erythema but that this reaction subsided quickly. He found after each succeeding injection that the reaction became more intense until finally the necrotic lesion noted above was produced. The intensity of this reaction, which has come to be known as the Arthus phenomenon, is related to the level of circulating antibody.[22] The phenomenon demonstrates how an immune reaction can

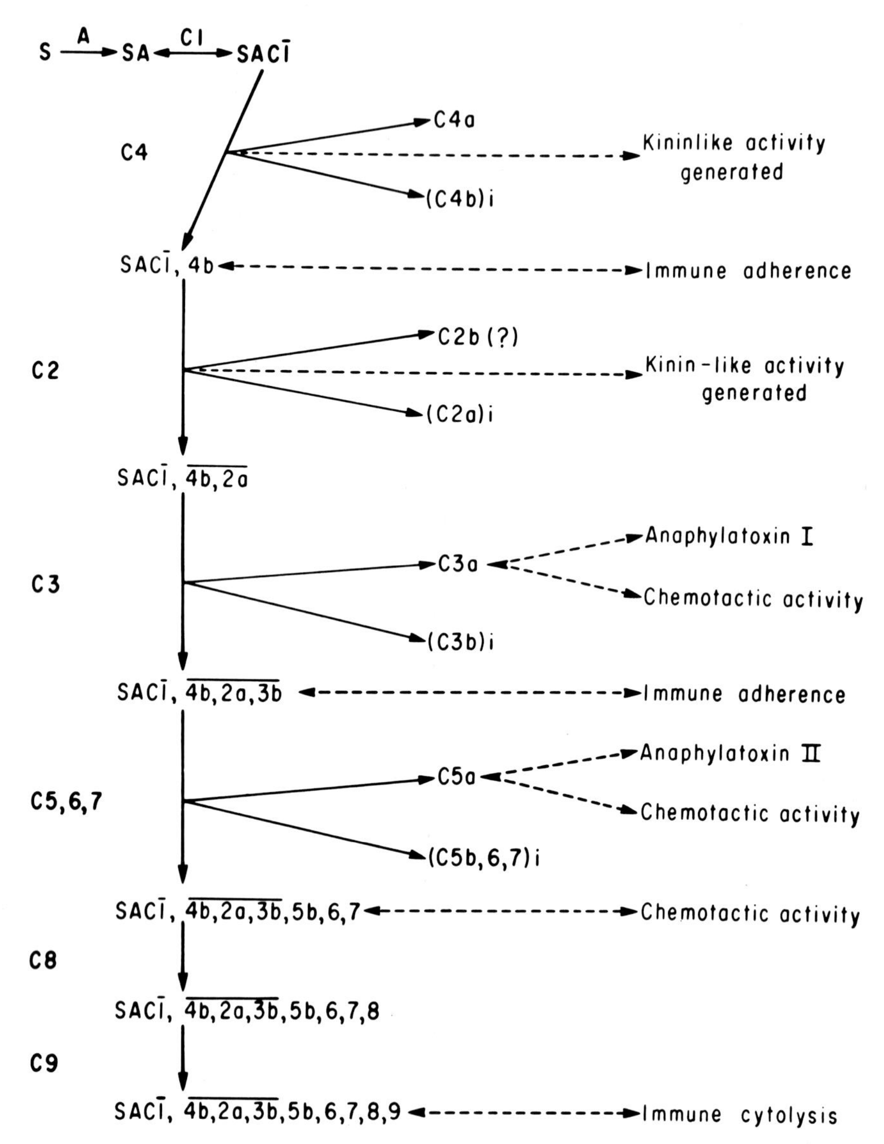


**Fig. 13-3.** Sequential steps of complement-dependent immune cytolysis and the generation of pharmacologically active products. *S,* Determinant site; *A,* antibody; *C,* complement; *C1, C2,* complement component 1, 2, etc.; *a, b,* reaction products; *i* inactive product. (The bar above signifies an activated product; the broken bar with arrowheads the physiologic effect of the compound.) (Arranged from data presented in various publications by H. R. Creamer, Portland, Ore.)

engender an inflammatory response and cause local tissue destruction. The precipitation of a soluble antigen (e.g., foreign albumin) by complement-fixing antibody in the walls of venules leads to the activation of complement, the subsequent chemotactic attraction of PMN's, and the destruction of tissue due to activities of the PMN's. Arthus reactions have been observed in the oral cavity of experimental animals.[33]

## Cell-mediated reactions (delayed-type hypersensitivity)

The term *cell-mediated* is reserved for those immune reactions in which the effector mechanism or trigger is a mononuclear cell antibody (especially the small lymphocyte) as differentiated from the previously discussed humoral or cell-fixed homocytotropic antibody. It encompasses such phenomena as bacterial allergy (e.g., tuberculin sensitivity), contact allergy (poison ivy), and transplantation immunity (allograft and isograft rejections).

The small lymphocyte response may involve a number of molecular mediators, including a macrophage inhibitor factor, a macrophage chemotactic factor, a lymphotoxin, and other physiologically reactive substances.[34]

The possibility of delayed-type hypersensitivity in aphthous stomatitis has been studied. Oppenheim and Francis believe that the prominence of lymphocytic infiltration in periodontal disease suggests the probability that delayed hypersensitivity reactions may play a role in this disease.[35]

## Conclusion

The immune responses serve only in part to neutralize antigens. They must be seen as acquired capacities of the animal directed toward triggering the inflammatory responses. A mechanism that activates and completes the essentially nonspecific inflammatory response, but does so in terms of immunologic specificity, is readily acceptable as a valuable asset for defense of the system; yet equally evident is the fact that clinically significant extrinsic or even intrinsic damage may be a result of such responses.

## SUMMARY

Following is the assumed course of events in inflammatory periodontal disease: Microorganisms from dental plaque release endotoxins and other antigens into the gingival sulcus.[35,36] This antigenic message is delivered to the regional lymph nodes by mobile phagocytes that migrate from the gingival connective tissue to the regional lymph nodes.[37] Immunologically competent cells in the regional lymph nodes undergo transformation to plasma cells that have the capacity to produce antibody to the specific microbial antigen. These antibodies may then combine with antigen in the gingival connective tissue to form immune complexes. The formation of immune complexes then activates the complement system, with the resultant production of vasoactive mediators of the inflammatory response.

The interaction of host and bacterial factors in the development of periodontal inflammation most likely involves the passage of enzymes, metabolic waste products, and chemotactic factors into the gingiva from plaque. This may result in the emigration of cells and cellular products from the gingiva out into the periodontal pocket.

The exact mechanism by which these immunopathologic processes are active has not been fully demonstrated[39]; and therefore this explanation of the causation of periodontal disease remains, though very attractive, only speculation.

The importance of fuller knowledge of the vascular alterations and cellular phenomena in periodontal disease and their causation is evident. The damage to cells by the bacterial products of plaque (cytotoxic substances, enzymes) is one such cause. Tissue damage may also be mediated by the by-products of the antigen-antibody reaction. This mechanism is suggested by the presence of immunoglobulins in the inflammatory exudate, the presence of lymphocytes and plasma cells in the inflamed gingival corium, and the elevation of serum antibody titers to plaque microorganisms in patients with periodontal disease.

**CHAPTER 13**

**References**


1. Bhaskar, S. N.: Synopsis of oral pathology, ed. 3, St. Louis, 1969, The C. V. Mosby Co.
2. Spector, W. G., and Willoughby, D. A.: Chemical mediators. In Zweifach, B. W., Grant, L., and McCluskey, R. T., editors: The inflammatory process, New York, 1965, Academic Press, Inc.
3. Stinson, F. L., Schwartz, J., and Parker, R. B.: Passage of $H_3$ labelled bacterial endotoxin across intact gingival sulcular epithelium, I.A.D.R. abstract no. 324, 1971.
4. Ranney, R. R.: Specific antibody in gingiva and submandibular nodes of monkeys with allergic periodontal diseases, J. Periodont. Res. **5**:1, 1970.
5. Rizzo, A. A.: Histologic and immunologic evaluation of antigen penetration into oral tissues after topical application, J. Periodont. **41**:210, 1970.
6. Simon, B. I., Goldman, H. M., Ruben, M. P., and Baker, E.: The role of endotoxin in periodontal disease. I, J. Periodont. **40**:695, 1969; II, J. Periodont. **41**:81, 1970.
7. Steinberg, A. I.: Evidence for the presence of circulating antibody to an oral spirochete in the sera of clinic patients, J. Periodont. **41**:213, 1970.
8. Brandtzaeg, P., and Kraus, F. W.: Autoimmunity and periodontal disease, Odont. T. **73**:285, 1965.
9. Nisengard, R. J., Beutner, E. H., and Hazen, S. P.: Immunologic studies of periodontal disease. IV, Bacterial hypersensitivity and periodontal disease, J. Periodont. **39**:329, 1968.
10. Nisengard, R. J., and Beutner, E. H.: Relation of immediate hypersensitivity to periodontitis in animals and man, J. Periodont. **41**:223, 1970.
11. Nisengard, R. J., and Beutner, E. H.: Immunologic studies of periodontal disease. V, Type antibodies and skin test responses to actinomyces and mixed flora, J. Periodont. **41**:149, 1970.
12. Kristofferson, T., and Hofstad, T.: Antibodies in humans to an isolated antigen from oral fusobacteria, J. Periodont. Res. **5**:110, 1970.
13. Zweifach, B. W.: Functional behavior of the microcirculation, Springfield, Ill., 1961, Charles C Thomas, Publisher.
14. Thomas, L., Uhr, J. W., and Grant, L.: Injury, inflammation and immunity, Baltimore, 1964, The Williams & Wilkins Co.
15. Taichman, N. S.: Mediation of inflammation by the polymorphonuclear leukocyte as a sequela of immune reactions, J. Periodont. **41**:228, 1970.
16. Hirsch, J. G.: Neutrophil and eosinophil leucocytes. In Zweifach, B. W., Grant, L., and McCluskey, R. T. editors: The inflammatory process, New York, 1965, Academic Press, Inc.
17. Palay, S. L., and Karlin, L. J.: An electron microscopic study of the intestinal villus, J. Biophys. Biochem. Cytol. **5**:373, 1959.
18. Pullinger, B. H., and Florey, H. W.: Some observations on structure and function of lymphatics, Brit. J. Exp. Path. **16**:49, 1935.
19. Billroth, T.: General surgical pathology and therapeutics, New York, 1883, Appleton.
20. Movat, H. Z.: Inflammation, immunity and hypersensitivity, New York, 1971, Harper & Row, Publishers.
21. Lewis, T.: The blood vessels of the human skin and their responses, London, 1927, Shaw & Sons, Ltd.
22. Zweifach, B. W., Grant, L., and McCluskey, R. T.: The inflammatory process, New York, 1965, Academic Press, Inc.
23. Ungar, G.: The fibrinolytic system and inflammation. In Jasmin, G., and Robert, A., editors: The mechanism of inflammation, Montreal, 1953, Acta, Inc.
24. Houck, J. C.: A personal overview of inflammation. In Forscher, B. K., editor: Chemical biology of inflammation, New York, 1968, Pergamon Press, Inc.
25. Erdös, E. G.: Hypotensive peptides; bradykinin, kallidin, and eledoisin, Advances Pharmacol. **4**:1, 1966.
26. Rocha e Silva, M.: Kinin hormones, Springfield, Ill., 1970, Charles C Thomas, Publisher.
27. Erdös, E. G.: Chemical biology of inflammation, New York, 1968, Pergamon Press, Inc.
28. Montgomery, E. H., Cowan, F. F., Parker, R. B., and Hubbard, G. L.: Kinin release in the progression of endotoxin-induced gingival inflammation, I.A.D.R. abstract no. 325, 1971.

29. Bremner, F. A., Montgomery, E. H., and Ranney, R. R.: Effect of protease inhibitor on endotoxin-induced acute gingivitis, I.A.D.R. abstract no. 326, 1971.
30. Humphrey, J. H., and White, R. G.: Immunology for students of medicine, ed. 3, Philadelphia, 1970, F. A. Davis Co.
31. Shelton, L. E., and Hall, W. B.: Human gingival mast cells; effects on chronic inflammation, J. Periodont. Res. 3:214, 1968.
32. Zachrisson, B. U.: Mast cells of the human gingiva, J. Periodont. Res. 3:136, 1968.
33. Terner, B.: Arthus reaction in the oral cavity of laboratory animals, Periodontics 3:18, 1965.
34. Bloom, B. R., and Glade, P. R.: In vitro methods in cell-mediated immunity, New York, 1971, Academic Press, Inc.
35. Oppenheim, J. J., and Francis, T. C.: The role of delayed hypersensitivity in immunological processes and its relationship to aphthous stomatitis, J. Periodont. 41:205, 1971.
36. Mergenhagen, S. E., Tempel, T. R., and Snyderman, R.: Immunologic reactions and periodontal inflammation, J. Dent. Res. 49:256, 1970.
37. Schultz-Haudt, S. D., and Sölna, J.: Dynamics of the inflammatory reaction, J. Periodont. Res. 1:205, 1966.
38. Berglund, S. E., Rizzo, A. A., and Mergenhagen, S. E.: The immune response in rabbits to bacterial somatic antigens administered via the oral mucosa, Arch. Oral Biol. 14:7, 1969.
39. Bickley, H. C.: A concept of allergy with reference to oral disease, J. Periodont. 41:302, 1970.

#### Additional suggested reading

Conference on the implication of immune reactions in the pathogenesis of periodontal disease, J. Periodont. 41:1, 1970.

Dick, H. M., and Trott, J. R.: The role of inflammation and sensitization on antigen penetration in rabbit gingiva, J. Periodont. 42:796, 1971.

Genco, R. J.: Immunoglobulins and periodontal disease, J. Periodont. 41:196, 1970.

Groat, J. F.: The immune response and periodontal disease, Periodont. Abstr. 19:64, 1971.

Hamp, S. E., and Folke, L. E. A.: The lysosomes and their possible role in periodontal disease, Periodont. Abstr. 17:94, 1969.

Ivanyi, L., and Lehner, T.: Stimulation of lymphocyte transformation by bacterial antigens in patients with periodontal disease, Arch. Oral Biol. 15:1089, 1970.

Ranney, R. R., Immunoglobulin and specific antibody in mild gingivitis, I.A.D.R. abstract no. 330, 1971.

Spector, W. G., and Willoughby, D. A.: The pharmacology of inflammation, New York, 1970, Grune & Stratton, Inc.

Stahl, S. S.: Host resistance and periodontal disease, J. Dent. Res. 49:248, 1970.

Stallard, R. E., Orban, J. E., and Hove, K. A., Clinical significance of the inflammatory process, J. Periodont. 41:620, 1971.

Tempel, T. R., and others: Factors from saliva and oral bacteria, chemotactic for polymorphonuclear leukocytes; their possible role in gingival inflammation, J. Periodont. 41:71, 1971.

Wilton, J. M. A., Ivanyi, L., and Lehner, T.: Cell-mediated immunity and humoral antibodies in acute ulcerative gingivitis, J. Periodont. Res. 6:9, 1971.

CHAPTER FOURTEEN

# Gingivitis



The processes of inflammation are similar whether they occur in the gingiva or in other areas of the body. When one examines the gingiva histologically, however, a mild chronic inflammatory reaction may be seen even in clinically normal gingiva. This may occur because of the ever-present bacterial flora that is found in shallow or deep gingival sulci. The bacteria or their products incite an inflammatory reaction in the connective tissue as a defense mechanism. The change from the clinically normal to the inflamed gingiva may be very gradual in some cases and quite distinct in others. The two conditions, normal gingiva and gingivitis, must be looked on as end points in a spectrum with graduated intermediate steps. Clinically gingivitis is recognized by the usual signs of inflammation—redness, swelling, bleeding, exudate, and (less frequently) pain.

*Definition*

Gingivitis is an inflammation of the gingiva. Microscopically gingivitis may be characterized by the presence of an inflammatory exudate and edema in the gingival lamina propria, some destruction of gingival fibers, and ulceration and proliferation of the sulcular epithelium.

## CLINICAL FEATURES

The outstanding clinical features of gingivitis are changes in tissue color and form and bleeding. The inflammation may be acute or more often chronic, and there may be hyperplasia, ulceration, necrosis, formation of pseudomembranes, and purulent and serous exudation. The lesions may be localized or generalized.

In examining the gingiva, one should always bear in mind a picture of what is "normal" gingiva (Chapter 1). With this guide the extent of the inflammatory reaction (localized or generalized), the distribution of the lesions (affecting the papillary, marginal, or attached gingiva), and the state of the inflammation (acute or chronic) can be readily observed.

The clinical characteristics of gingivitis may be determined by careful evaluation of the inflammatory reaction.[1-3] An acute gingivitis will show a bright red gingiva that is often ulcerated, hemorrhagic, and possibly painful. Pain, ulceration, and hemorrhage may be seen in cases of gingival abscess, Vincent's infection, streptococcal gingivitis, plasmocytosis, or injuries to the gingiva; and they are sometimes encountered in gingivitis in pregnancy, blood dyscrasias, nutritional deficiencies (e.g., vitamin C), and endocrine disturbances.

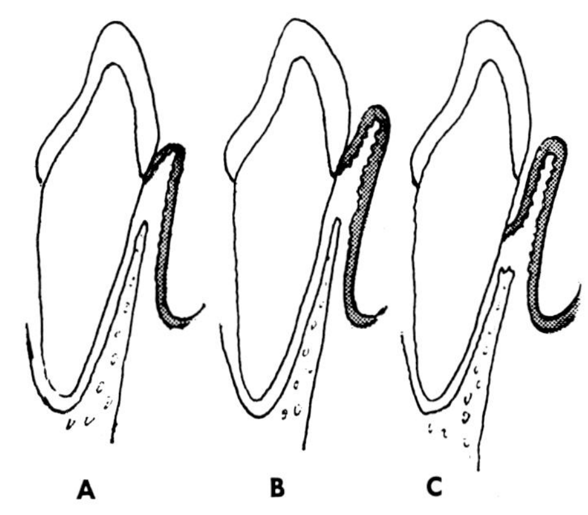


**Fig. 14-1. A,** Normal gingival sulcus. The depth is minimal (1 to 3 mm.) and the sulcular tissues are healthy. **B,** Pseudopocket. The pocket depth is caused by coronal enlargement of the gingiva and not by bone destruction at the crest and subsequent apical proliferation of the attachment epithelium. **C,** Pocket caused by bone destruction, apical proliferation of the attachment epithelium, and separation of the coronal portions of the attachment epithelium from the tooth (periodontitis).

Chronic inflammation often occurs with an overgrowth of tissue. The gingiva is magenta in color; or it may be more fibrous and not as hemorrhagic as in acute inflammation. As a rule it is painless.

Acute inflammation may be superimposed on chronic gingivitis. Such acute episodes are generally caused by extrinsic factors (e.g., food impaction, injuries by toothbrush bristles, fish bones, toothpicks) or by unhygienic conditions of the mouth (e.g., accumulation of plaque). Intrinsic factors may aggravate or modify the inflammation.[4,5] These factors include pregnancy, nutritional deficiencies (e.g., vitamin C), endocrine disturbances, or blood dyscrasias that aggravate or modify the existing inflammatory reaction.

A person's inherited intrinsic response to an injury may modify the reactions. In the final analysis the etiology of a gingivitis is the end result of the interplay of extrinsic and intrinsic factors.

After the state and degree of gingival inflammation have been observed, one may further characterize the gingivitis as hyperplastic (enlarged or overgrown gingiva), ulcerative, necrotic, or pseudomembranous. There may be a purulent exudate. For example, a patient may have a localized, papillary, acute, ulcerative, necrotizing gingivitis. This description means much more than the single term *gingivitis.*

***Pocket***

When the gingival sulcus is deepened because of disease, it is called a pocket (Fig. 14-1, *C*). In gingivitis, increased depth may be caused by a coronal enlargement of the gingival margin because of edema or inflammatory fibrous hyperplasia (pseudopockets), or both (Fig. 14-1 *B*). Regardless of depth, the gingival sulcus is diseased when there are major inflammatory changes in the soft tissue wall. The term *pocket,* which connotes depth, tends to divert attention from incipient lesions such as might occur in gingivitis. A diseased dentogingival junction should be treated and not neglected because the clinical lesion is not spectacular.

***Cytology***

The cellular characteristics of gingival inflammation include plasma cells., lymphocytes, polymorphonuclear (PMN) leukocytes, and some macrophages (Fig.

14-3). The plasma cells normally found in clinically healthy gingiva increase in number in inflammation and become predominant in the characteristic round cell infiltrate. Lesser numbers of lymphocytes are usually found, with some macrophages and mast cells also present. PMN leukocytes have been described as clustered around calculus, bacteria, and debris in the pocket. They are mobilized in ulcerations of pocket epithelium and are teeming with microabscesses. These leukocytes, frequently seen in chronically inflamed connective tissue, are described as moving from vessels toward the pocket.[1]

***Changes in epithelium***

The epithelium lining the pocket, as well as that of the attachment and of the outer gingiva, usually proliferates into the lamina propria. This might be a response to the inflammation. Some epithelial cells may be distended, intercellular spaces may be widened, and PMN leukocytes[1,3] and lymphocytes[2] may infiltrate the pocket epithelium, the attachment (junctional) epithelium,[1] and the oral epithelium. PMN leukocytes may migrate through small ulcerations in the sulcular wall toward plaque, calculus, and bacteria. Engorged, proliferating capillaries may be found in the inflamed lamina propria close to the surface of the pocket (sulcular) epithelium.

***Changes in connective tissue***

The subepithelial connective tissue may be infiltrated by plasma cells and lymphocytes. The infiltrate may be concentrated close to the pocket wall or may be diffusely dispersed throughout the lamina propria. Some destruction of dentogingival fibers may take place, and clusters of inflammatory cells may be found around vessels and between fiber bundles. Where destruction has occurred, the fiber bundles may be replaced by a young, proliferating connective tissue consisting of newly formed capillaries, mesenchymal cells, and inflammatory cells. Some repair may take place concurrent with the inflammatory changes, and some new fiber bundles may be evident.

## Illustrative cases

A few cases of gingivitis with differing etiologies and clinical characteristics are presented in illustration.

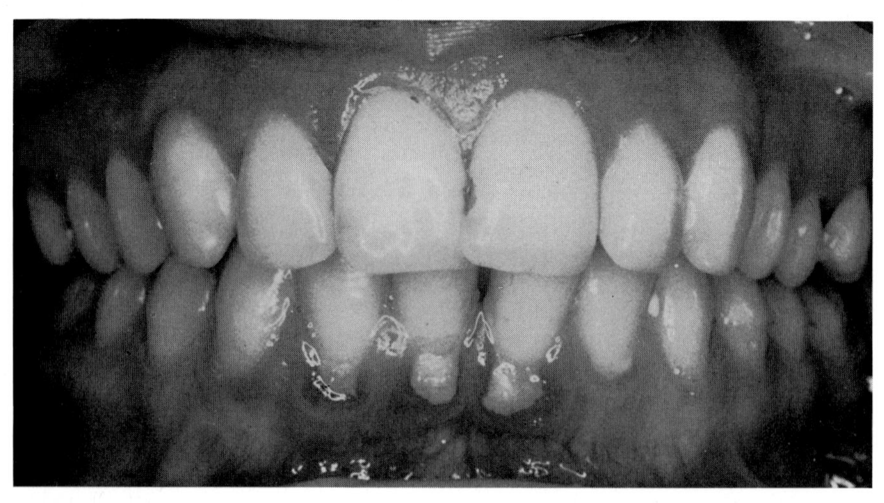

**Fig. 14-2.** Localized acute gingivitis in a 34-year-old white woman. This was an exacerbation of a preexisting chronic gingivitis.

*Acute gingivitis*

A localized acute exacerbation of a chronic gingival inflammation around the mandibular central and lateral incisors can be seen in Fig. 14-2. The inflammation extends from the gingival margins to the alveolar mucosa and appears to involve the latter tissue. The gingiva is receded around the right lateral incisor and the central incisors. Diagnosis was localized acute gingivitis. Compare the clinical characteristics of this inflammation and the character of the tissue response to irritation with the cases that follow. (See Fig. 24-6 for treatment of this patient.)

A biopsy specimen taken from the papilla and margin of the lateral incisor confirmed the diagnosis of a highly acute inflammatory reaction close to the surface, as may be seen in Fig. 14-3, with chronic inflammatory cells, especially plasma cells, in the deeper areas. There are small ulcerations in the sulcular epithelium of the specimen, and the surface epithelium is extremely thin in many areas. Higher magnification (Fig. 14-4) shows dilated blood vessels filled with leukocytes that are migrating from the connective tissue through the epithelium.

The case shown in Fig. 14-5, *A,* is of a 17-year-old girl who complained of bleeding and the unsightly appearance of the gingiva. She was referred for treatment by a dentist who wrote that he had attempted to treat this patient for a year. According to his report he had tried scaling and medication with various drugs, all without success. He suspected a systemic involvement and had the patient undergo medical examination. There were no pertinent findings. He suspected nutritional deficiencies and placed the patient on a balanced diet. This also failed to resolve the inflammation.

On examination the patient was found to have a generalized papillary and marginal inflammation. The attached gingiva was pink and firm but glossy and without stippling. The gingival papillae were soft, and a slightly hemorrhagic and purulent exudate was elicited on pressure. There were moderately deep pockets containing hard, calcified deposits (subgingival sulcus) that were heaviest in the interproximal areas (Fig. 14-5).

The biopsy specimen revealed a chronic inflammatory process with signs of acute gingivitis close to the surface similar to the preceding case but less acute.

*Chronic gingivitis*

A case of localized, papillary, chronic gingivitis is shown in Fig. 14-6, *A*. The papillae were magenta in color, swollen, and glossy. The marginal gingiva was pink and thin. The gingiva was stippled and, except for the papillae, appeared firm with no exudate from shallow pockets. A hard but rather fine subgingival calcareous deposit was present in the interproximal areas. The biopsy specimen revealed a chronic inflammatory process localized adjacent to the pocket. There were large numbers of plasma cells and some lymphocytes present (*B*). The blood vessels were thin, and some areas of necrosis were found in the deeper regions around the plasma cells. The pocket epithelium was characterized by proliferating epithelial ridges and very thin suprapapillary epithelium. The connective tissue papillae were separated from the surface of the pocket by just a few layers of epithelial cells (*C*).

The patient, a man 32 years of age, had been treated for gingivitis with inadequate measures (medication, superficial scaling) for 2 years and thus without beneficial result. The gingiva continued to bleed each time he brushed his teeth or bit into hard food. He changed dentists but was extremely skeptical of his prospects for cure. Three appointments of proper root planing and education in oral hygiene techniques helped to reduce the inflammation (Fig. 14-6, *D*).

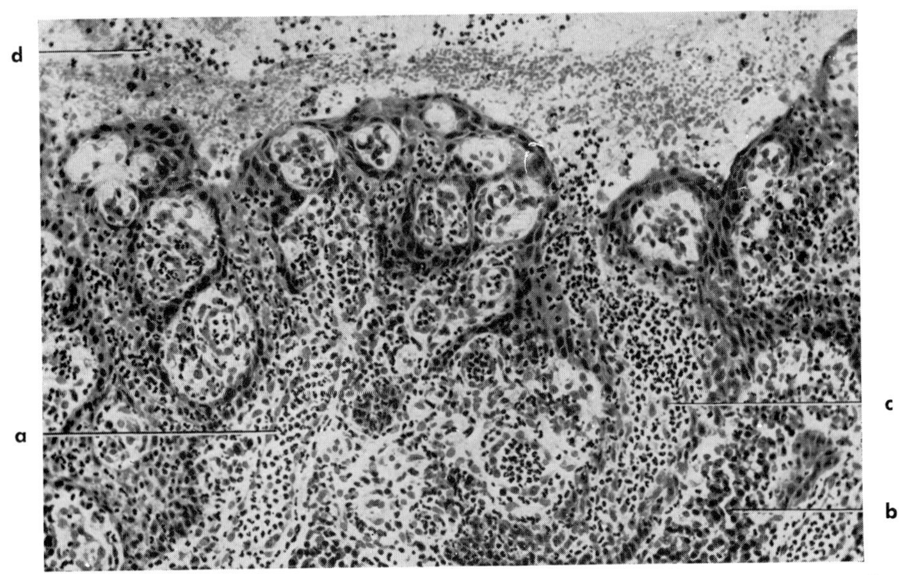


**Fig. 14-3.** Biopsy specimen of gingiva of the patient shown in Fig. 14-2. In the connective tissue, close to the surface, *a,* dilated blood vessels filled with leukocytes are prominent. In the deeper layer plasma cells, *b,* are numerous. The leukocytes migrate through the epithelium, *c,* to the surface, *d.*

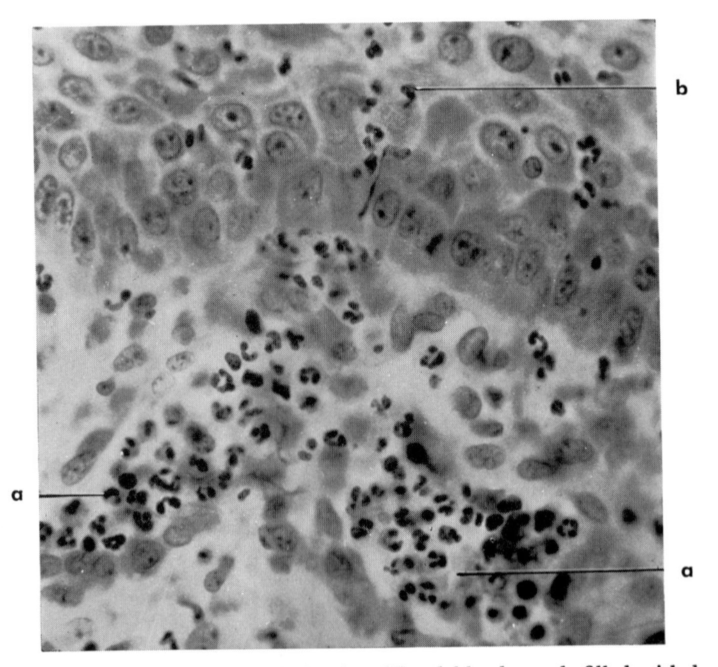


**Fig. 14-4.** High magnification of Fig. 14-3 showing dilated blood vessels filled with leukocytes, *a.* The leukocytes migrate through the epithelium, *b.*

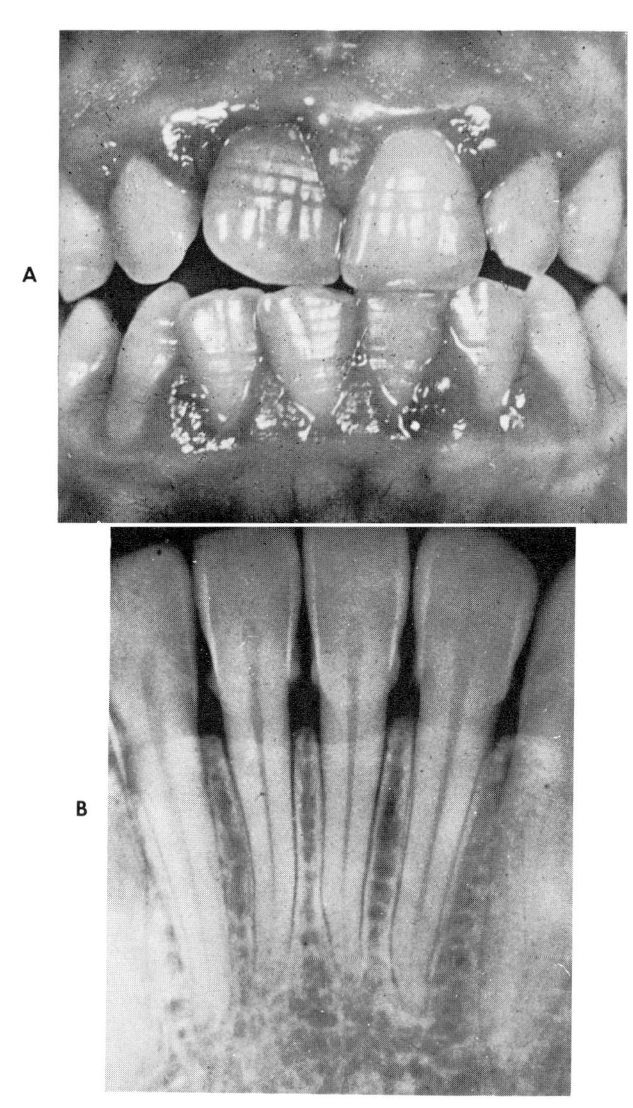


*Continued.*

**Fig. 14-5. A,** Generalized papillary and marginal gingivitis in a 17-year-old girl. The marginal gingiva has become enlarged, contributing to pocket depth (pseudopockets) and distortion of gingival form. **B,** Roentgenogram of the mandibular anterior teeth showing heavy calcified deposits.

The foregoing cases of acute and chronic gingivitis, all successfully treated by local measures, illustrate etiology based primarily on extrinsic factors alone, namely plaque and calculus.

***Gingivitis from trauma to gingiva***

Another extrinsic factor in the etiology of gingivitis may be direct injury to the gingiva by the incisal edges of opposing teeth. This occurs most often on either the vestibular papilla between the mandibular incisors or the oral papilla between the maxillary incisors. A typical case is shown in Fig. 14-7, *A,* in which a highly inflamed papilla can be seen between the two incisors. This papilla was sensitive to touch. As the result of an acute inflammatory process, necrotic margins developed. The imprints of the mandibular incisor teeth were found

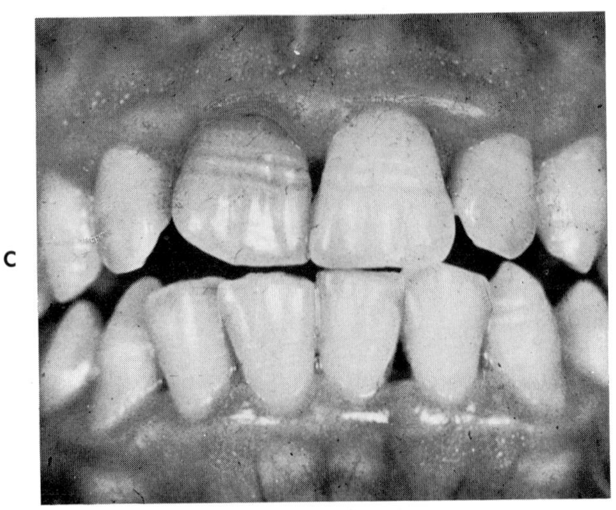


**Fig. 14-5, cont'd. C,** After root planing. Note that resolution of most of the inflammation and elimination of the edema have resulted in some reduction of pocket depth and improvment in gingival form. Residual tissue deformities are caused by some persistent inflammation and hyperplastic gingival enlargement. Tooth malalignment also contributes to tissue deformity in this patient.

on the oral surface (Fig. 14-7, *B*). The swelling started with an injury to the papilla between the maxillary central incisors by a piece of toast. The lower incisors impinged on the injured tissue and aggravated the existing inflammation. The gingiva was edematous and swollen with necrotic margins along the incisors. The teeth were scaled, a periodontal dressing was placed over the injured area, and a palatal bite plane was constructed to prevent further injury. The inflammation was resolved in a few days, and the cause of the secondary injury was eliminated. The mandibular incisors no longer traumatized the palatal gingiva. In such cases the elimination of a deep overbite and the prevention of minor injuries would be a prophylactic measure. Without this treatment, recurrence of the disturbance caused by renewed extrinsic irritation might occur.

***Gingivitis in mouth breathers***

Local treatment sometimes is not sufficient to cure gingival inflammation. This is illustrated in the case shown in Fig. 14-8, a marginal, papillary, hyperplastic gingivitis in an adolescent girl. The exaggerated tissue changes were most pronounced in the anterior vestibular gingiva. The patient was a mouth breather with poor oral hygiene. Local treatment failed to resolve the inflammation until the mouth breathing was corrected by removal of the adenoids.

In most cases local treatment is effective in resolving or reducing the inflammation of gingivitis. A marginal, papillary, hyperplastic gingivitis in a 17-year-old white girl is shown in Fig. 14-9, *A*. The patient was also a mouth breather and had an anterior open bite and poor oral hygiene. Calcified deposits cover the cervical half of the mandibular central incisors, and the hyperplastic, inflamed gingiva has proliferated to bridge and enclose the deposits. The patient had suffered dysmenorrhea since the start of puberty. Acne, which often occurs concurrent with the endocrine adjustment in puberty, was also present. Nothing else in the patient's medical history could be related to the gingival condition.

Treatment consisted of root planing, gingival curettage, oral hygiene instruction, occlusal adjustment, and construction of a mouth screen (for control of the

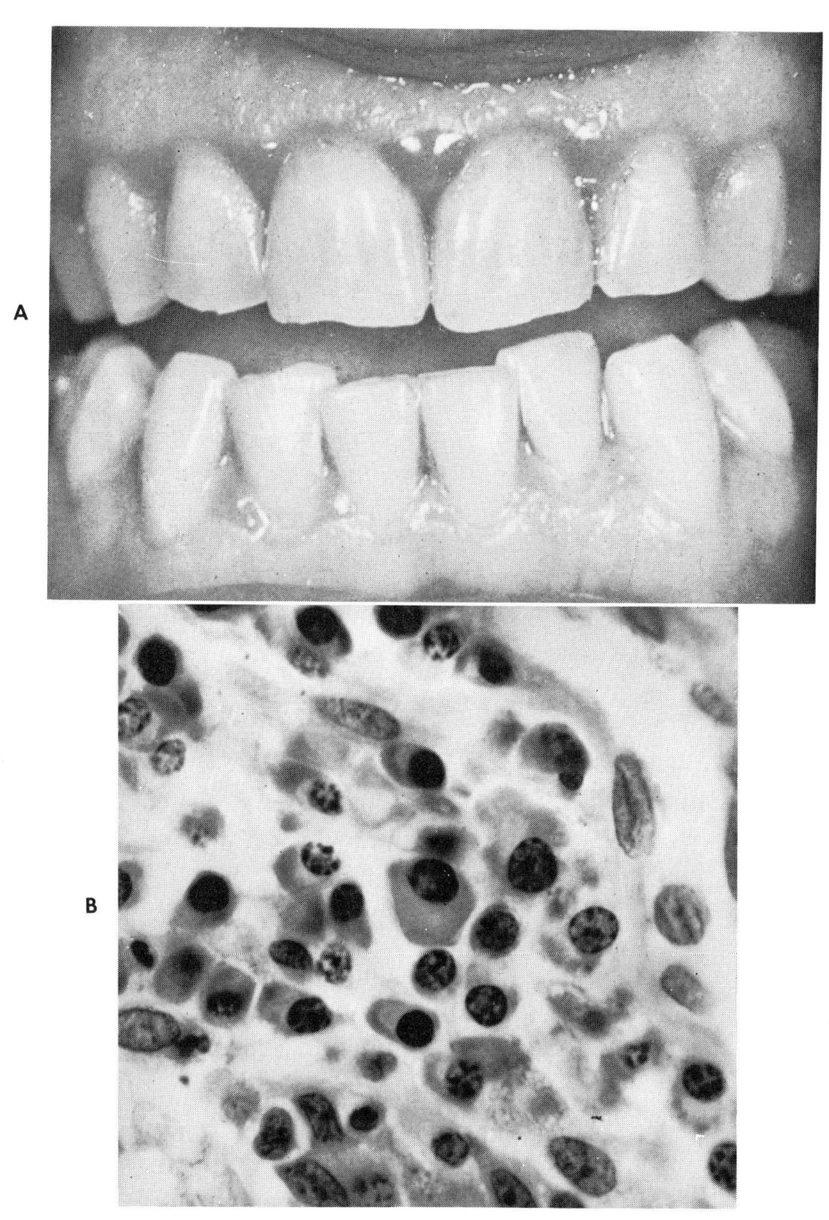


*Continued.*

**Fig. 14-6. A,** Generalized, chronic, papillary gingivitis. The papillae were magenta in color, swollen, and glossy. **B,** Biopsy of the patient. Plasma cells predominate, and the capillaries are thin.

mouth breathing) to be worn during sleep. The result of treatment is seen 6 months later in Fig. 14-9, *B*.

In all cases of gingival hyperplasia in mouth breathers, an attempt should be made, with the help of the otolaryngologist and allergist, to determine the presence of and to remove any obstruction to nasal respiration. Sometimes a case of mouth breathing is encountered in which the nasal and pharyngeal air passages appear clear and the patient still persists in his deleterious habit.[6] Some patients breathe through the mouth during sleep only; others have incomplete

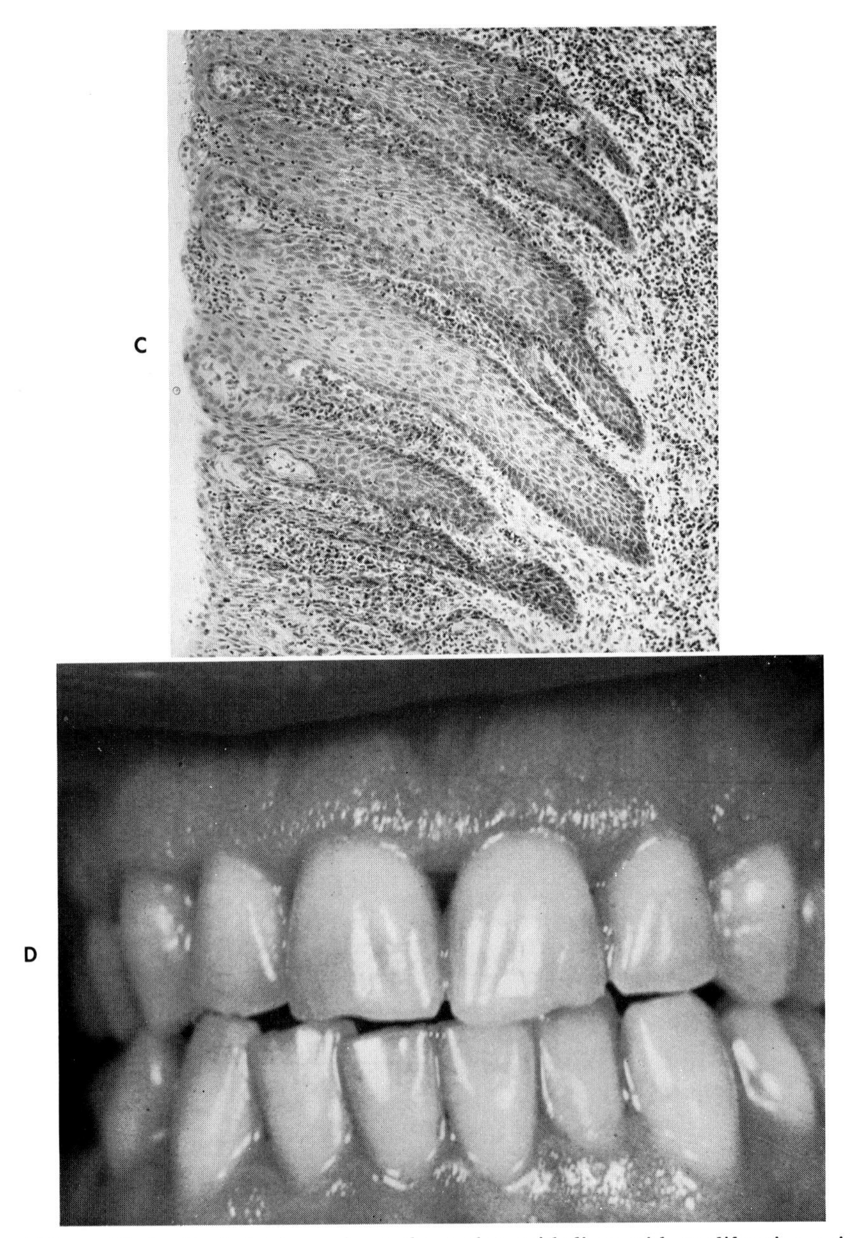


**Fig. 14-6, cont'd. C,** Gingival biopsy shows the pocket epithelium with proliferating epithelial ridges and thin suprapapillary epithelium. Note the dense accumulation of inflammatory cells. **D,** Postoperative condition after three appointments for root planing.

lip closure without mouth breathing. Certain measures may be taken for the treatment of this condition:

1. Application of petroleum jelly to the gingiva before retiring
2. Correction of sleeping position (advise the patient to sleep on his side or, if he can sleep only on his back, to use one or two hard pillows)
3. Construction of a so-called mouth screen resembling a boxer's guard but thinner

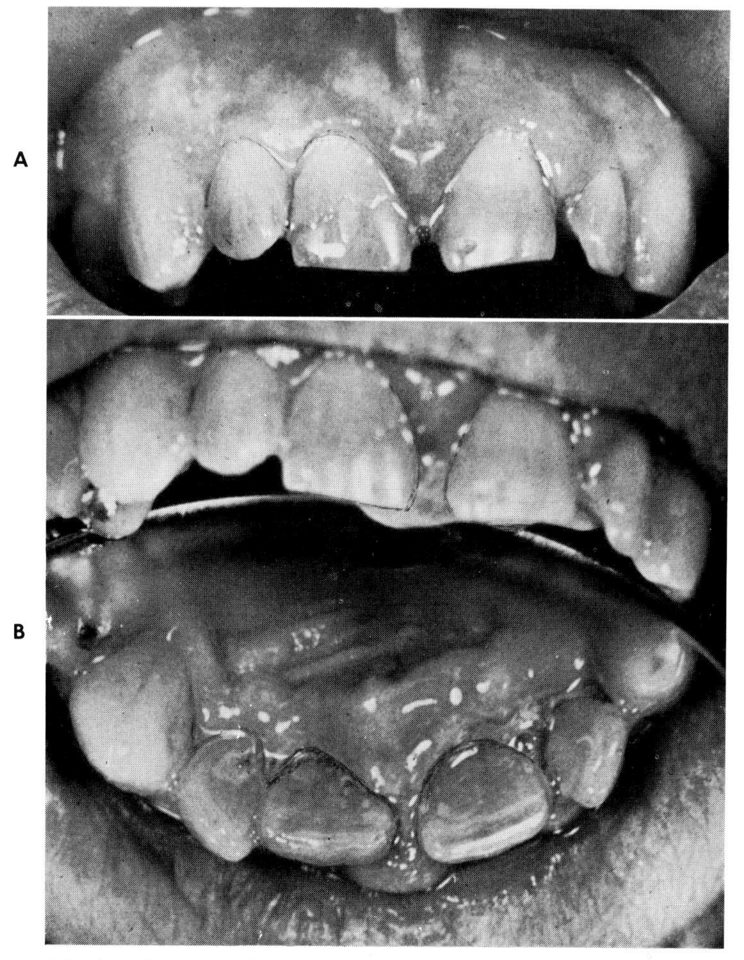


**Fig. 14-7. A,** The interdental papilla between the maxillary central incisors is swollen, edematous, and ulcerated at the tip. The lesion resulted from a direct traumatic injury caused by the mandibular incisors in a deep overbite (traumatic gingivitis). **B,** Oral view of the maxillary incisors. The interdental papilla is swollen and the tip is necrotic because of direct traumatic injury by the mandibular incisors (deep overbite).

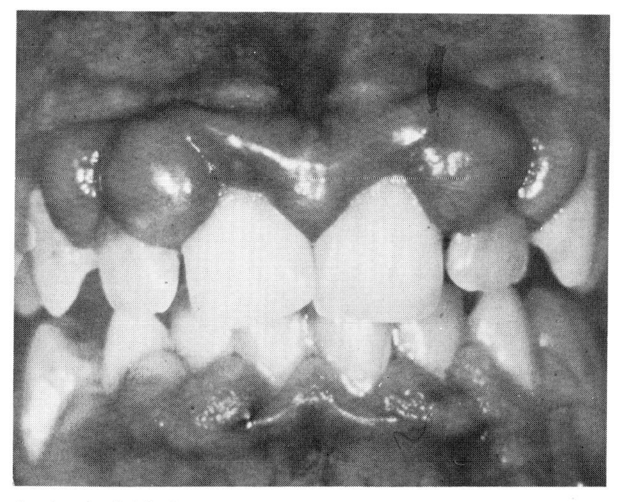

**Fig. 14-8.** Hyperplastic gingivitis in an adolescent girl. Mouth breathing and poor hygiene aggravated the condition. The lip line is clearly indicated by the outline of the hyperplastic tissue.

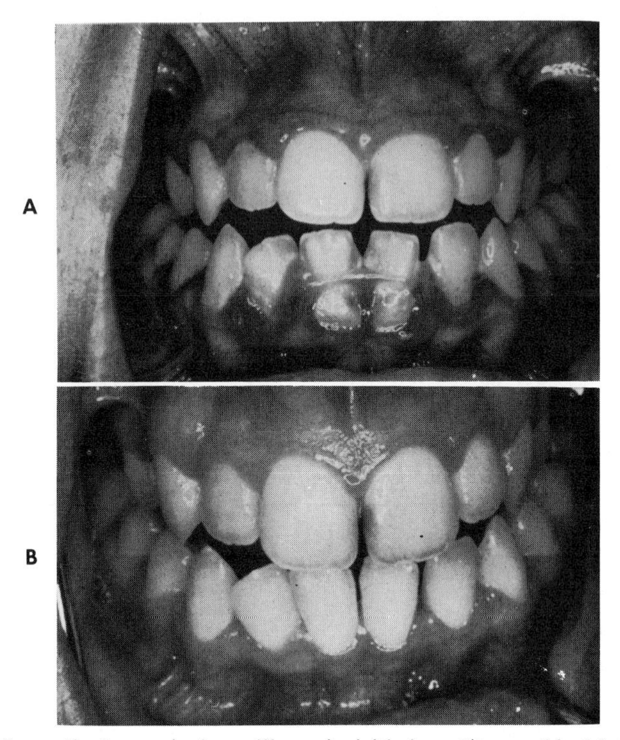


**Fig. 14-9. A,** Generalized, marginal, papillary gingivitis in a 17-year-old girl. Note the calcified deposits on the mandibular incisors. The red, edematous gingiva has proliferated to bridge and enclose the calculus. The teeth are festooned by this soft, friable, edematous tissue. Complete closure is not possible anteriorly because of the effects of a tongue thrust habit. **B,** Six months later. Root planing, gingival curettage, some occlusal adjustment, and the construction of a mouth screen have produced this acceptable result.

A microscopic specimen (Fig. 14-10) of hyperplastic gingivitis shows an increase in the thickness of both the epithelium and the connective tissue. The epithelium appears acanthotic, and the connective tissue shows an increased thickness of the collagen fibers, with large groups of plasma cells accumulating around the blood vessels and between the fibrous elements.

## INTRINSICALLY CONDITIONED GINGIVITIS

***Gingivitis in puberty***

A chronic, marginal, hyperplastic gingivitis in a 15-year-old white girl is shown in Fig. 14-11. The inflammatory changes were first noted at the age of 13, about the time of inception of puberty. Vitamins were prescribed to treat the inflamed, bleeding gingiva. This treatment, along with polishing of the teeth and oral hygiene instruction, was continued for 2 years. The gingival condition became progressively worse, resulting in fibrotic tissue deformities requiring surgical intervention. For the correct treatment of this patient, see Figs. 25-17 to 25-20.

An exaggerated response to irritants is seen frequently during puberty and sometimes before puberty.[7] This may be caused by hormonal changes and may be aggravated by the incomplete exposure of the anatomic crowns. The latter condition sometimes encourages food impingement, where the gingiva lacks the protection of a food-deflecting, cervical, tooth bulge. Both factors may contribute

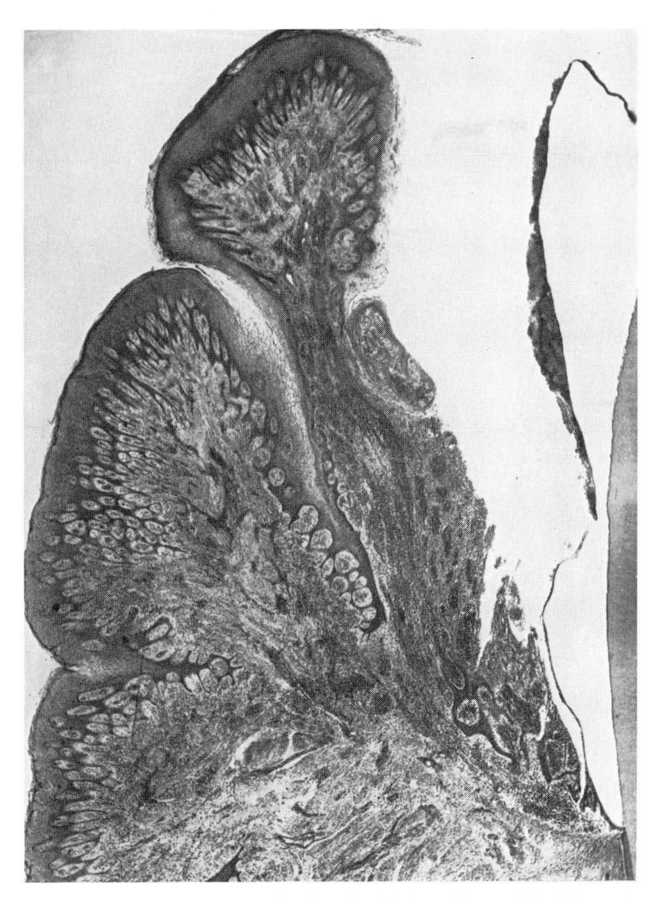

**Fig. 14-10.** Histologic section of hyperplastic gingivitis with epithelial and connective tissue proliferation. (From the collection of B. Gottlieb.)

to the gingivitis so frequently seen during puberty. Many dentists believe that the condition will resolve itself with the culmination of adolescence. In some cases they may be right. Too often, however, chronic, destructive periodontal disease has its inception during puberty or earlier and, if left untreated, becomes progressively worse.

*Gingivitis in children*

Gingivitis in children is not uncommon.[8,9] Oral hygiene practices are often poor. However, the possible cumulative effect of persistent gingival inflammation in children on their adult periodontium has not been assessed.

*Gingivitis in pregnancy*

Intrinsic influences play an important part in the etiology of gingivitis, not as a primary but as a secondary or modifying influence. This becomes evident especially in conditions such as pregnancy,[10,12] in which an endocrine alteration is present. About 50% of all pregnant women may have gingivitis, ranging from mild to severe. Nonpregnant women may also show the same incidence of gingivitis but to a milder degree. During pregnancy gingivitis becomes aggravated by the proliferative tendencies in the tissues. Epithelium, connective tissue, and endothelial cells all show such signs. One of the most characteristic microscopic features of gingivitis during pregnancy is the proliferation of the capillaries, as shown in Fig. 14-12, sometimes combined with ulcerations and sloughing.

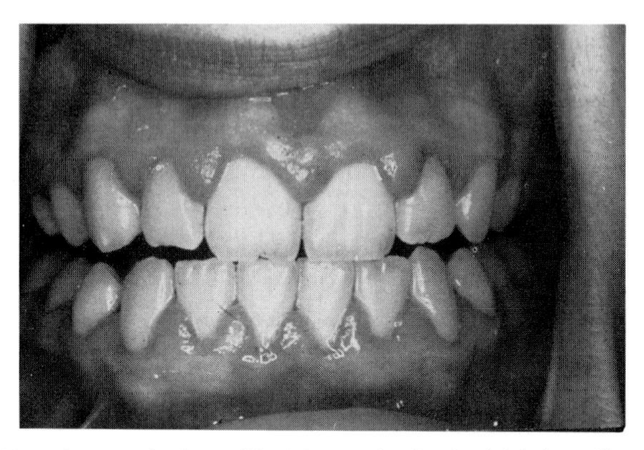

**Fig. 14-11.** Chronic, marginal, papillary hyperplastic gingivitis in a 15-year-old girl.

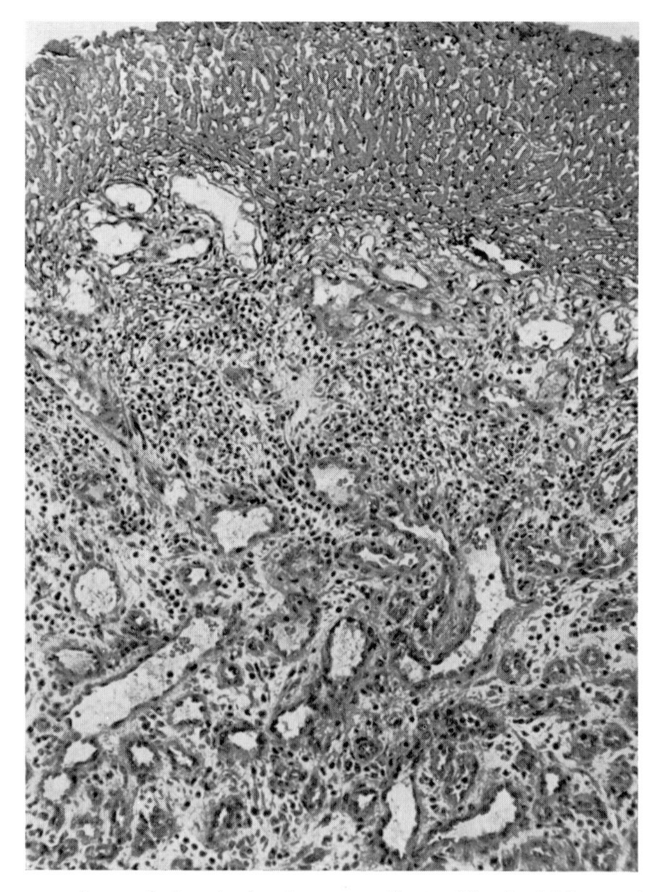

**Fig 14-12.** Biopsy specimen of the gingiva from a patient with gingivitis associated with pregnancy. The microscopic picture resembles that of a pyogenic granuloma.

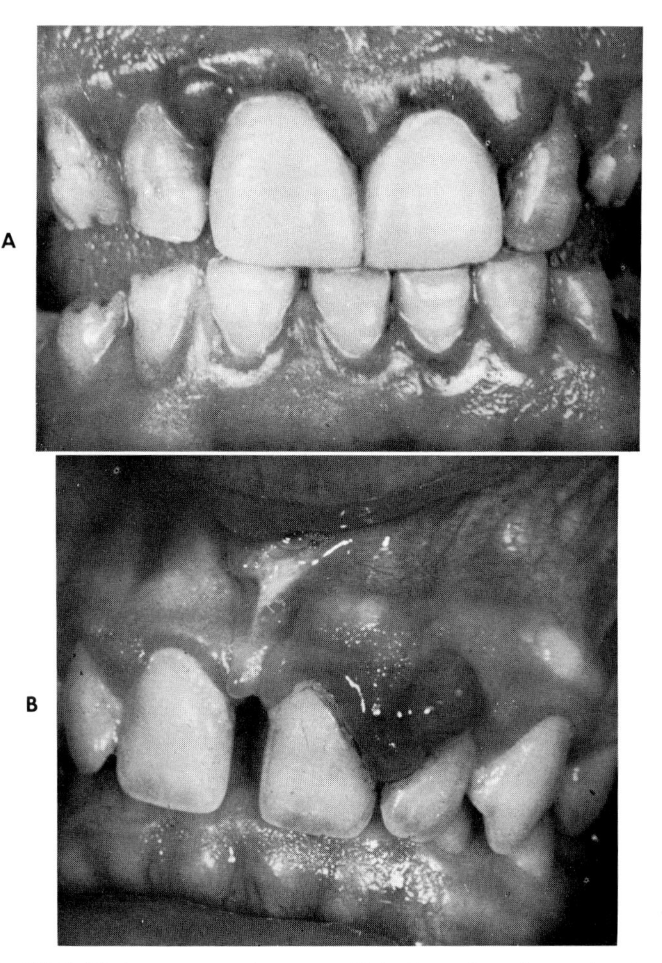


**Fig. 14-13. A,** Gingivitis in a pregnant woman. Note the enlarged prominent papillae and the irregular, fringed gingival margins. **B,** Epulis-like enlargement of the gingiva in a pregnant woman (pregnancy tumor).

In general, the clinical inflammation is confined to the papillae, which are prominent and sharply demarcated from the attached gingiva (Fig. 14-13, *A*). The margins often are irregular and appear fringed. Frequently the hyperplasia in gingivitis during pregnancy is confined to several localized areas. Such gingiva is extremely friable and bleeds on the slightest touch. Individual hyperplastic papillae may become extremely large and then are called pregnancy tumors (Fig. 14-13, *B*). Histologically such tumors are indistinguishable from pyogenic granulomas. Occasionally they cause considerable resorption of the underlying bone. Both pregnancy tumors and the aggravated state of the gingivitis have a tendency to disappear spontaneously after parturition, but they may occur during subsequent pregnancies.[12]

The treatment most often consists of root planing, curettage, and establishing good plaque control and stimulation of the tissues. After parturition a thorough oral examination is desirable to ensure that all manifestations of the inflammation have been resolved without residual tissue damage. Remember that gingivitis in pregnancy will *not* develop if there is no gingival inflammation prior

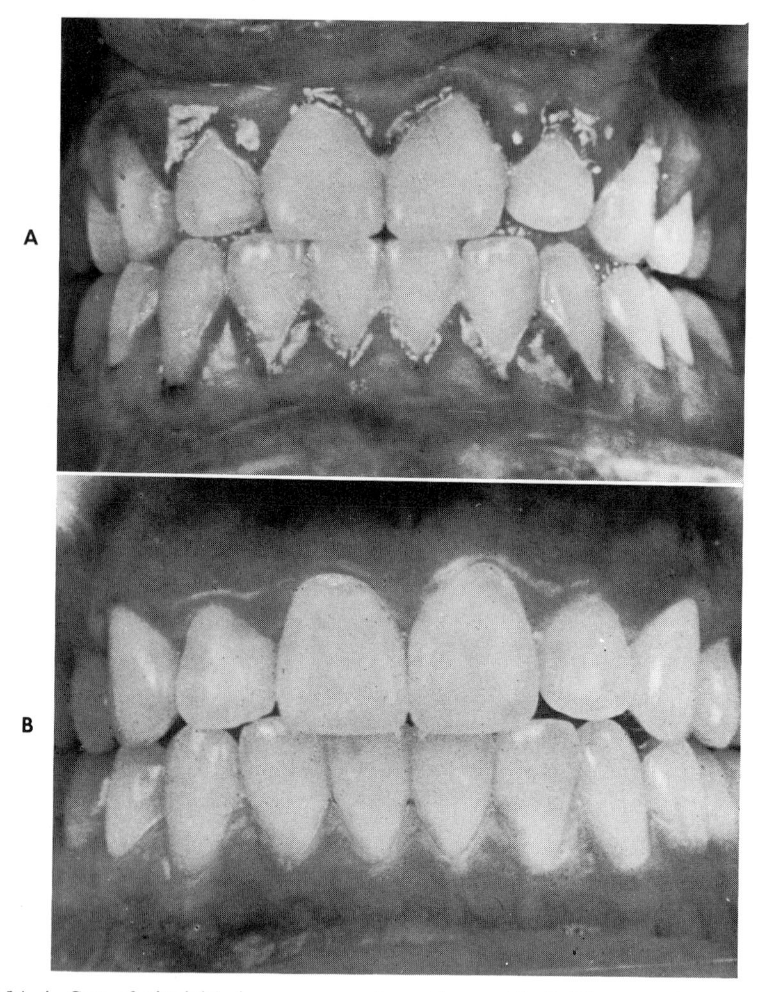


**Fig. 14-14. A,** Case of gingivitis in pregnancy (seventh month). **B,** Therapeutic root planing and oral hygiene led to resolution. (Courtesy J. A. Kollar, Jr., Chicago.)

to or during pregnancy. If the gingivitis is severe and tumor formations and tissue enlargements are present, surgery should be considered. The second trimester is usually the safest time. The eighth month is also considered safe because of a more advantageous endocrine balance.

In some cases of gingivitis during pregnancy, unhygienic conditions are prevalent, as may be seen in Fig. 14-14, *A*. In this patient, root planing eliminated the irritation and was followed by resolution of the inflammation. A healthy gingiva was maintained by proper oral hygiene during the rest of the pregnancy (Fig. 14-14, *B*). The use of oral contraceptives has been implicated sometimes in the production of a gingivitis resembling pregnancy gingivitis.[15]

***Scorbutic gingivitis***

A case of scorbutic gingivitis[13] is shown to illustrate another aspect of intrinsic influence on inflammation of the gingiva.[14] The patient was admitted to the hospital with general symptoms of scurvy, including hemorrhage in the joints, muscles, and skin, and an inability to walk. The gingiva appeared bright red. There was a generalized papillary and marginal gingivitis (Fig. 14-15, *A*),

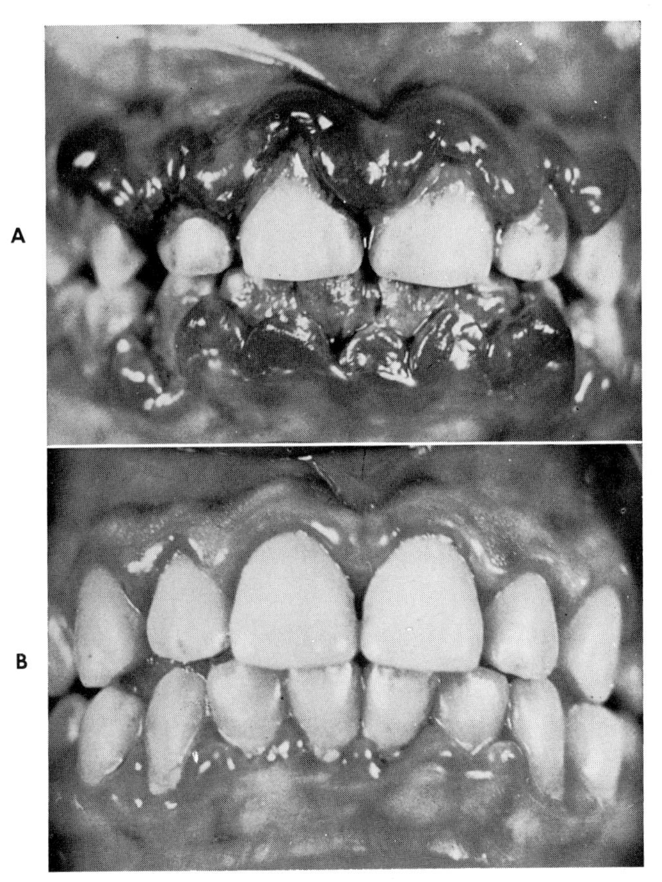


**Fig. 14-15. A,** Scorbutic gingivitis. Note the generalized, marginal, papillary, acute hyperplastic gingivitis. **B,** The improvement after 3 months of vitamin C therapy, without debridement, is evident. A marginal gingivitis is still present as a result of local irritation. It requires additional treatment.

which extended slightly into the attached gingiva. The gingiva was hyperplastic, ulcerative, and hemorrhagic. Initial therapy was limited to a high dosage of vitamin C, 1500 mg. per day for a week. This then was reduced to 500 mg. per day for the next 4 weeks; then 300 mg. per day for a month, and 100 mg. per day thereafter. No local treatment was given during this period of medication. After about 3 months of treatment, the clinical appearance of the gingiva was as shown in Fig. 14-15, *B*. The acuteness of the inflammation had resolved, but a chronic papillary and marginal gingivitis remained. Most likely gingivitis was present prior to the scorbutic symptoms. The residual inflammation required local treatment. Vitamin C therapy eliminated the scorbutic manifestations, but the inflammation caused by local irritation remained.

The microscopic appearance of the tissues (Fig. 14-16) shows a highly edematous, acutely inflamed gingiva with an ulceration of the entire pocket surface. The blood vessels are dilated and microscopic hemorrhages are evident throughout the gingiva. At higher magnification numerous macrophages filled with hemosiderin crystals may be seen. One of the most characteristic features of gingivitis in scurvy is the disappearance of collagen fibers from the connective tissue, as may be seen in Fig. 14-17, *A*. Three months later there is a regenera-

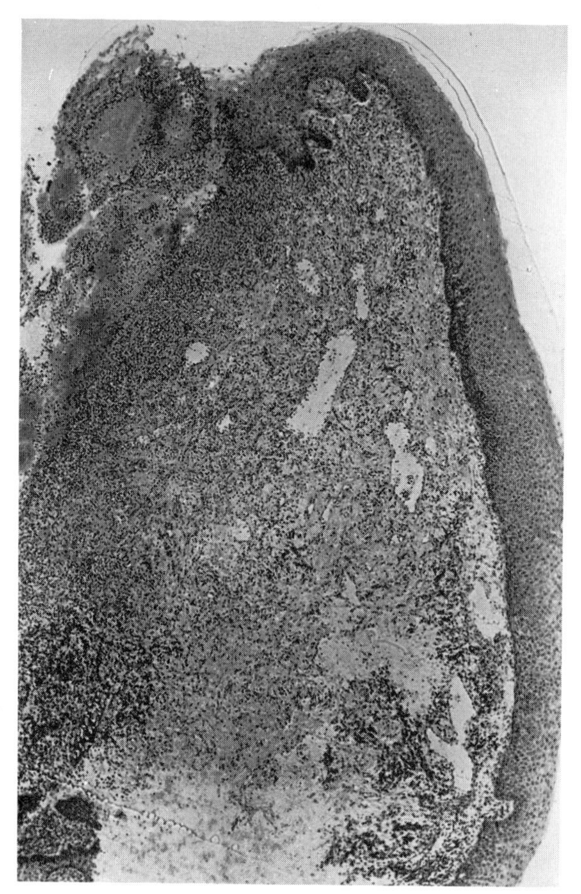

**Fig. 14-16.** Biopsy specimen of the gingiva in the patient with scorbutus shown in Fig. 14-6, *C*. There was acutely inflamed, edematous tissue with almost complete disappearance of collagenous fibers. With appropriate stains, hemosiderin crystals could be seen.

tion of the collagen fibers (Fig. 14-17, *B*). Scorbutic gingivitis is extremely rare and is usually seen in Western civilizations only in hospital practice. This patient did not complain of the gingival condition. His was a severe intrinsic disease of which the oral manifestation was only a local and minor symptom.

In summing up the importance of intrinsic factors in the etiology of gingivitis, the statement must be made that there is no intrinsic factor that, in itself, can initiate a localized oral inflammatory process such as gingivitis. The role that intrinsic factors play is an aggravating and modifying one such as has been demonstrated in pregnancy and scurvy.

The following may be considered contributory intrinsic etiologic factors in gingivitis: pregnancy, puberty, diabetes mellitus, metal poisoning, and nutritional disturbances such as deficiencies in ascorbic acid. There undoubtedly are other factors that have not yet become evident. From the foregoing, it is clear that the periodontal prognosis for patients with intrinsic contributory etiology may have to be more guarded than that for patients with primary extrinsic etiology.

Notwithstanding the presence of intrinsic factors that might require special

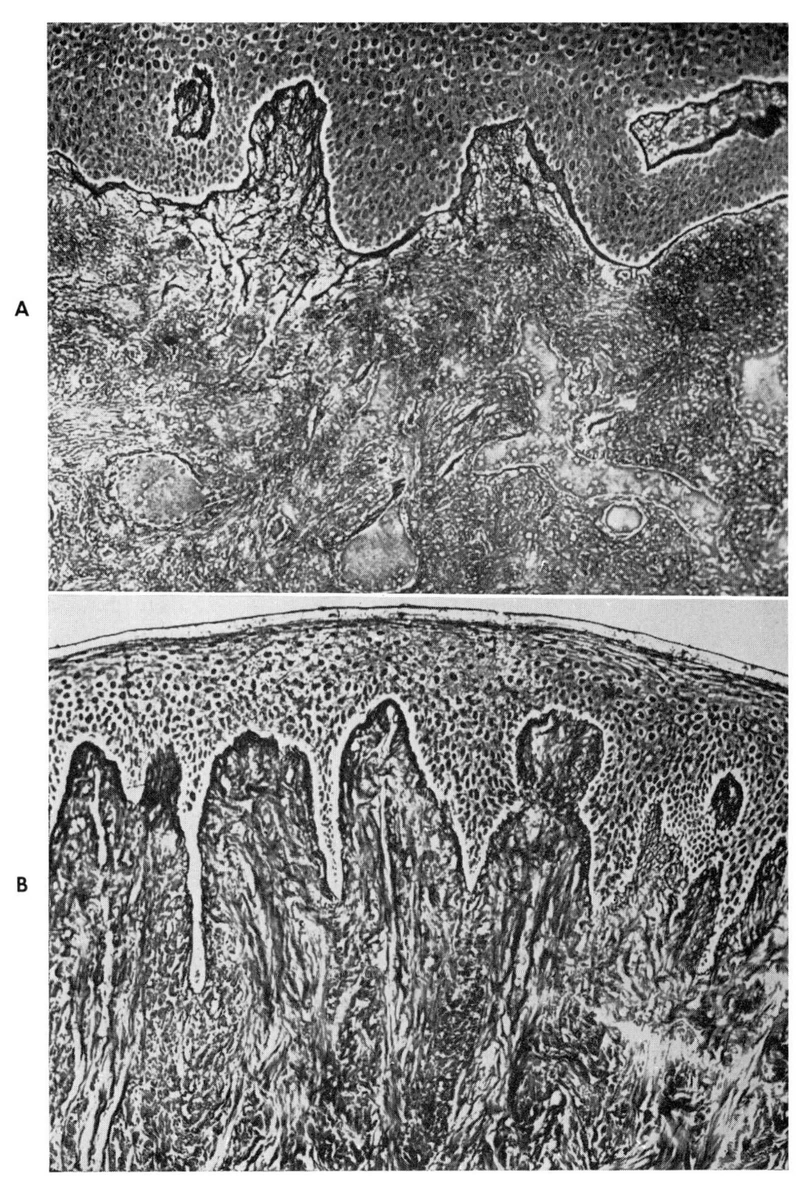


**Fig. 14-17.** Biopsy specimens of the gingiva of the patient with scorbutus shown in Fig. 14-15. (Silver stain.) **A,** After 3 months of vitamin C therapy, regeneration of collagenous fibers has occurred. **B,** The collagenous fibers are replaced by a fine argyrophilic network of fibrils.

measures, treatment of gingivitis requires root planing and good oral hygiene. In some cases, gingival curettage may be necessary; and when hyperplastic gingivitis is present, other periodontal surgery might be indicated (see appropriate sections on treatment in Chapters 24 to 31).

## NECROTIZING ULCERATIVE GINGIVITIS

Although necrotizing ulcerative gingivitis is patently included in the gingivitis category, it may also contribute to periodontitis and be superimposed on periodontitis. Because of its unique clinical characteristics and special treatment, it will be discussed in a separate section on acute conditions requiring immediate treatment (Chapter 18).

## CHRONIC DESQUAMATIVE GINGIVITIS

Chronic desquamative gingivitis is a rare condition involving the papillary, marginal, and attached gingivae. Irregular areas on the entire gingiva are fiery red, smooth, and shiny. Stroking the gingiva with a finger, cotton roll, or blast of air may peel away the surface epithelium, exposing the painful bleeding surface of the connective tissue.[16,17]

In more severe cases the gingiva is covered by multiple raw bleeding areas on a background of intense erythema. These lesions may begin as blisterlike eruptions that break. Subjectively patients complain of a burning sensation aggravated by spices, acid foods, and carbonated beverages. They may experience a salty taste and may suffer spontaneous pain in rare instances.

The pathogenesis of this condition has been ascribed to a disturbance of the metabolism of the ground substance and the basement membrane.[18]

Although chronic desquamative gingivitis most frequently affects menopausal women, it is also seen occasionally in men. In typical desquamative gingivitis (Fig. 14-18) the affected areas of gingiva are bright red, smooth, and shiny. A few patches of relatively normal tissue are interspersed.

Lesions are most often confined to the vestibular gingiva, but occasionally they occur in the alveolar mucosa, the buccal mucosa, or the hard palate around the teeth. Edentulous areas are seldom affected. Periods of spontaneous remissions and exacerbations occur.

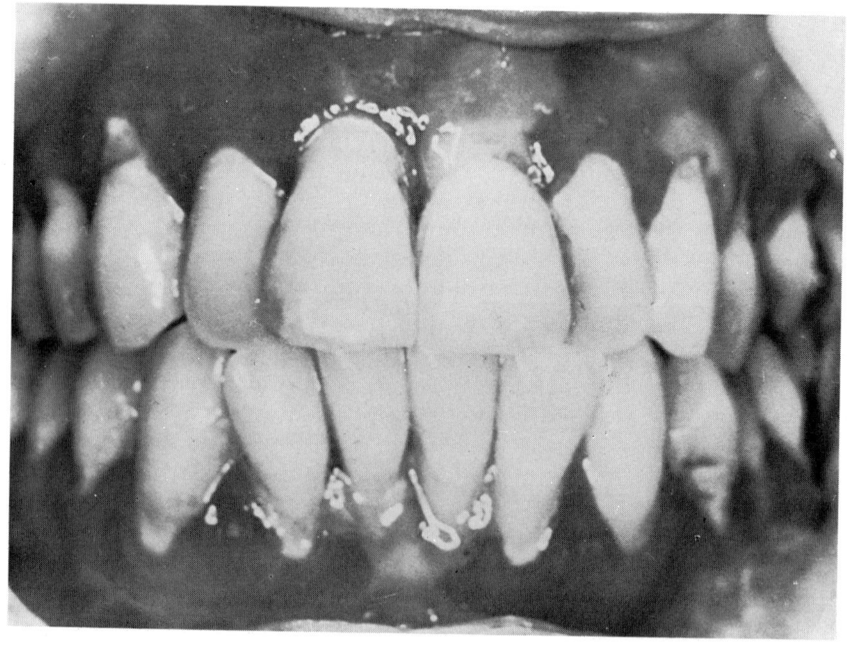

**Fig. 14-18.** Typical case of desquamative gingivitis. The gingiva is smooth, glossy, and fiery red.

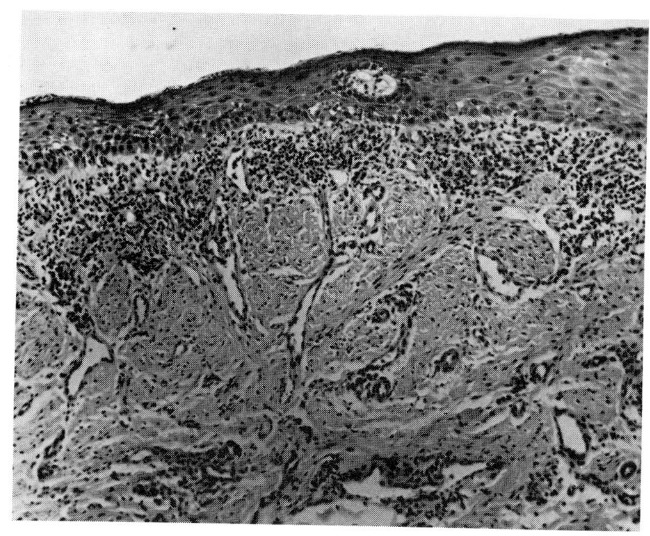

**Fig. 14-19.** Biopsy specimen from a patient with the lichenoid type of desquamative gingivitis. The epithelium is atrophic without keratinization. Connective tissue papillae are missing, and there is severe subepithelial inflammation.

## Differential diagnosis and histopathology

Chronic desquamative gingivitis must be differentiated from acute streptococcal stomatitis, pemphigus vulgaris, and some mycotic infections.

Mainly two forms can be distinguished microscopically: lichenoid and bullous. In the lichenoid form the most characteristic features are atrophy of the epithelium and lack of keratinization.[17] There are no connective tissue papillae; the epithelium–connective tissue border thus appears as a more or less straight line (Fig. 14-19). The epithelium may appear edematous, and the intercellular spaces are widened. The basal cells may show lytic destruction (Fig. 14-20). In the bullous form (Figs. 14-21 and 14-22) splits occur between the epithelium and the connective tissue.[19,20] Combinations of the two forms, lichenoid and bullous, may be seen in the same specimen. The changes are probably caused by depolymerization of the cementing substances and the basement membrane.[18] Electron microscopic studies have shown deficient keratin formation.[21] Because of depolymerization the connective tissue appears washed out (Fig. 14-23). The character of the infiltrate in the connective tissue is mostly chronic inflammatory. Plasma cells, lymphocytes, eosinophilic leukocytes, and macrophages are apparent. Mast cells are plentiful, particularly near the junction of epithelium and lamina propria[22] (Fig. 14-22). The inflammatory reaction in chronic desquamative gingivitis has been suggested as being secondary to the degenerative enzymatic disturbance of the connective tissue ground substance. Clinically, however, inflammation tends to dominate the picture.

## Etiology, treatment, and prognosis

The etiology of chronic desquamative gingivitis is unknown. The conjecture that the disease is associated with disturbances in sex hormones is based on the predominance of occurrence in menopausal women.[16] Most cases of desquamative gingivitis probably represent localized lesions of erosive lichen planus

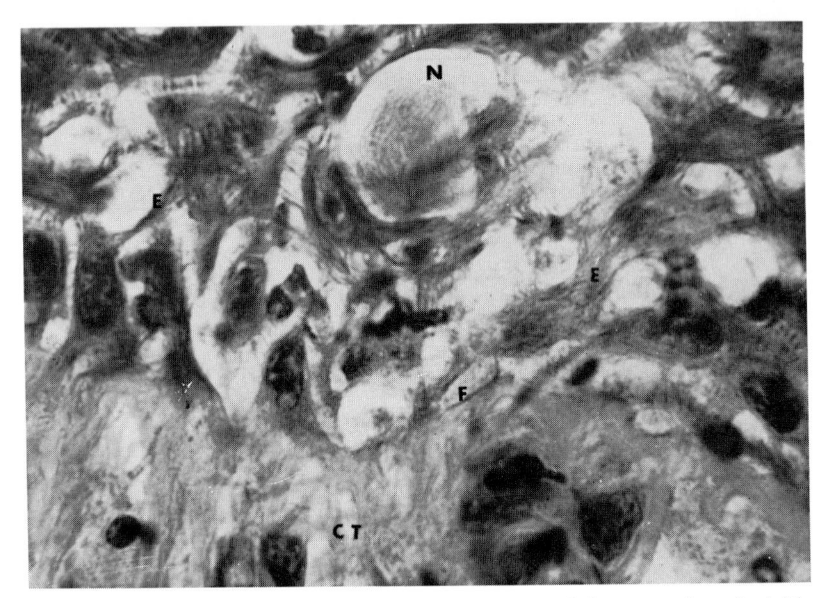


**Fig 14-20.** Lytic destruction of the basal cell area in a case of desquamative gingivitis of the lichenoid type. The pattern of destruction is such that some of the fibrillar elements are often preserved and appear to maintain some connection of the epithelium to the connective tissue. *CT,* Connective tissue; *E,* epithelium; *N,* coagulative necrosis of cellular material; *F,* epithelial fibrillar attachment to the connective tissue. (Trichrome stain; ×600.) (Courtesy J. S. Bennett, Portland, Ore.)

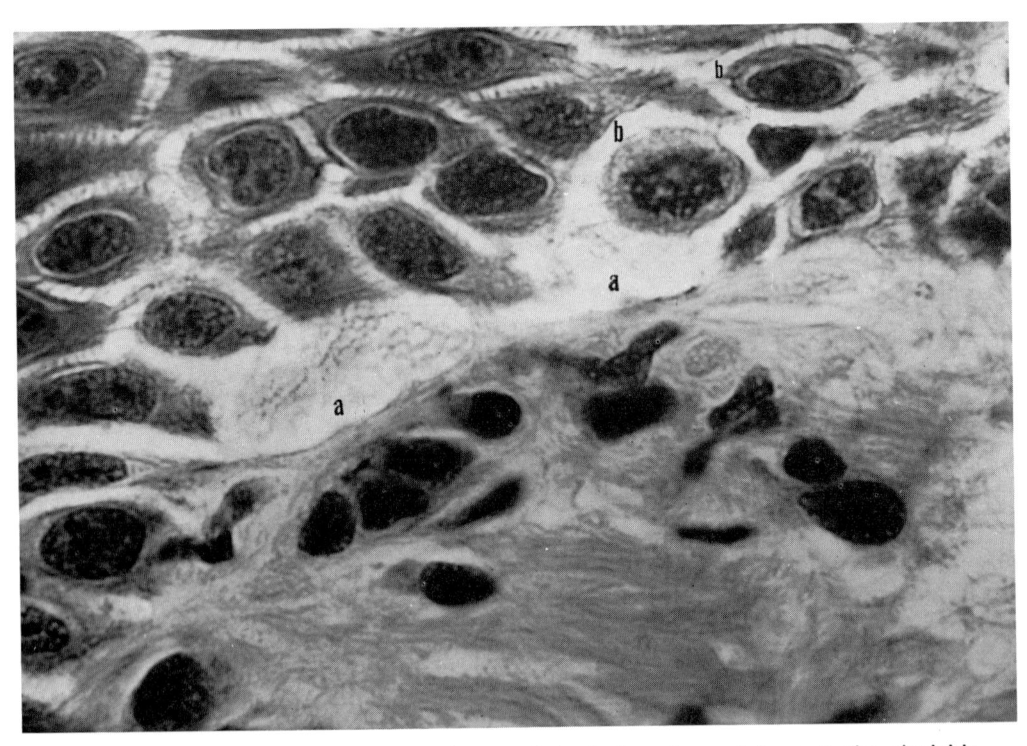


**Fig. 14-21.** Microscopic changes in an early case of the bullous form of desquamative gingivitis. Note, *a,* the separation of the epithelial cells from the lamina propria and, *b,* the destruction of some of the tonofibrils and of intercellular substance. (Trichome stain; ×600.) (Courtesy J. S. Bennett, Portland, Ore.)

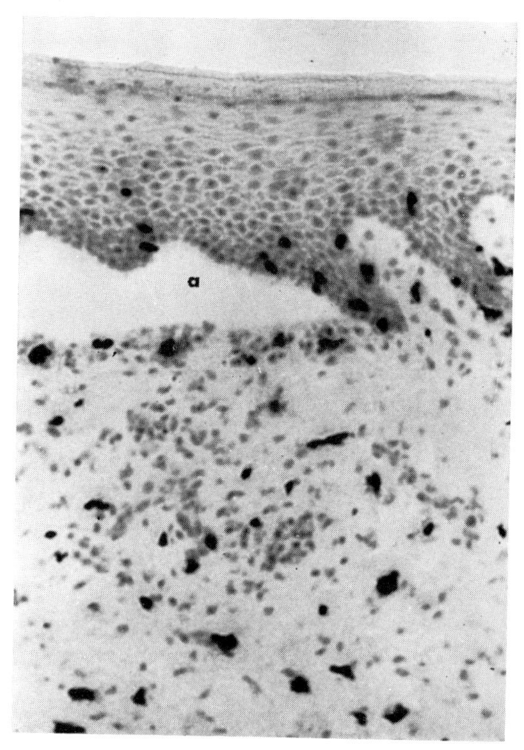


**Fig. 14-22.** Specimen from a case of the bullous form of desquamative gingivitis showing a split at the basement membrane, *a,* and the mast cell stained dark. Mast cells are found in desquamative gingivitis in the entire lamina propria but are most plentiful on both sides of the basement membrane, the connective tissue side, and the side of the epithelium. (Specific mast cell stain.[22]) (Courtesy W. B. Hall, San Francisco.)

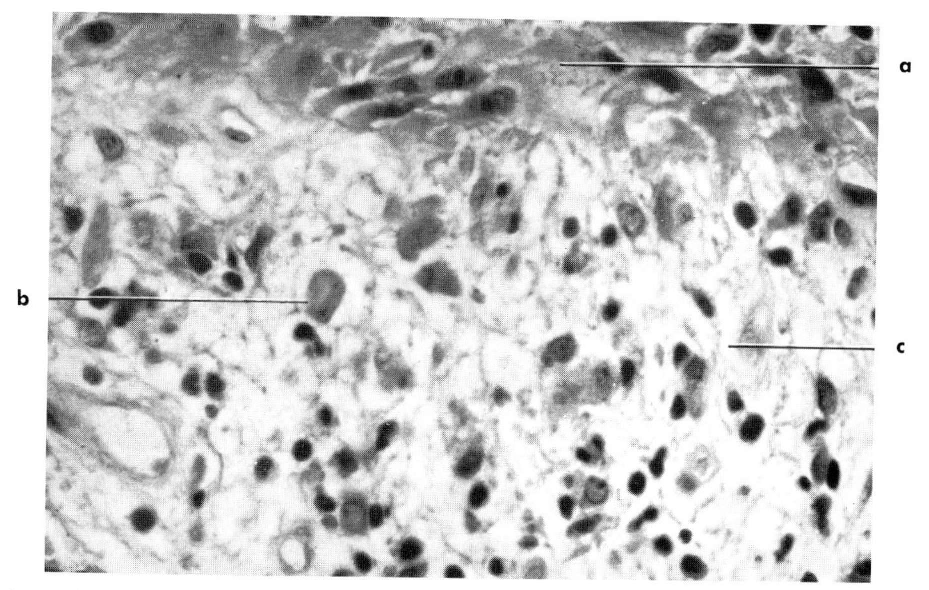


**Fig. 14-23.** Granular appearance of connective tissue ground substance. No basement membrane between the connective tissue and the epithelium, *a,* is apparent. Macrophages, *b,* may be observed in the degenerated connective tissue, *c.*

or of benign mucous membrane pemphigoid.[20,23,24-26] The majority of patients with this disease enjoy good general health. Similar clinical pictures may also be seen occasionally in ordinary gingivitis, after certain medications, in acute monocytic leukemia, in plasmocytosis, and idiopathically.[25]

Treatment of desquamative gingivitis has been a problem from the time that it was first recognized clinically. Most procedures have afforded only temporary relief. The topical application of estrogenic hormones in the form of ointment has brought some temporary improvement in a few cases.[16] Greater improvement has been obtained with topical application of corticoids.[17,27] Corticoid ointment (2.5%) in an adhesive base (Kenalog in Orabase) is recommended. Treatment with this preparation over 6 months and longer is often necessary to obtain clinical and histologic improvement. Excellent oral hygiene is also beneficial. In obstinate and painful cases, and when mastication is difficult, protective plastic devices are employed. They cover the gingiva and retain the medication. Occasionally this disease is confused with necrotizing ulcerative gingivitis. Distinction between the two is important, however, because oxygenating mouthwashes are contraindicated in desquamative gingivitis.

The prognosis for desquamative gingivitis is guarded. Some patients can be kept at least subjectively comfortable by the use of corticoids. Remissions also may occur spontaneously. With such an undefined etiology and course, however, prognosis and treatment are only vague, and the appraisal of therapy difficult.

**CHAPTER 14**

**References**


1. Grant, D. A., and Orban, B.: Leukocytes in the epithelial attachment, J. Periodont. **31**:87, 1960.
2. Cattoni, M.: Lymphocytes in the epithelium of the healthy gingiva, J. Dent. Res. **30**:627, 1951.
3. Attström, R.: Studies on neutrophil polymorphonuclear leukocytes at the dentogingival junction in gingival health and disease, J. Periodont. Res., supp. 8, 1971.
4. Carranza, F. A., Jr.: Systemic factors in periodontal disease, Rev. Asoc. Odont. Argent. **52**:295, 1964.
5. Stahl, S. S.: The etiology of periodontal disease. In Ramfjord, S. P., Kerr, D. A., and Ash, M., editors: World workshop in periodontics, Ann Arbor, Mich., 1966, University of Michigan Press, sect. III.
6. Lite, T., Diucaio, D. J., and Burman, L. R.: Gingival pathosis in mouth breathers, Oral Surg. **8**:382, 1955.
7. Schour, I., and Massler, M.: Prevalence of gingivitis in young adults, J. Dent. Res. **27**:733, 1948.
8. Cohen, M. M.: Recognition of periodontal disease in children, J. Dent. Child. **31**:7, 1964.
9. Parfitt, G. J.: Periodontal diseases in children. In Finn, S. B.: Clinical pedodontics, Philadelphia, 1967, W. B. Saunders Co.
10. Maier, A. W., and Orban, B.: Gingivitis in pregnancy, Oral Surg. **2**:334, 1949.
11. Hugoson, A.: Gingival inflammation and female sex hormones, J. Periodont. Res., supp. 5, 1971.
12. Everett, F. G.: Oral lesions in the female patient, West. J. Surg. Obst. Gyn. **59**:62, 1951.
13. Orban, B., Martin, W. B., and Hehn, R. M.: Histopathologic investigation of a case of scorbutic gingivitis, J. Periodont. **18**:95, 1947.
14. Waerhaug, J.: The role of ascorbic acid in periodontal tissues, J. Dent. Res. **39**:1089, 1960.
15. El-Ashiri, G., and others: Effects of oral contraceptives on the gingiva, J. Periodont. **42**:273, 1971.
16. Ziskin, D. E., and Zegarelli, E. V.: Chronic desquamative gingivitis, Amer. J. Orthodont. (Oral Surg. section) **31**:1, 1945.
17. Foss, C. L., Grupe, H. E., and Orban, B.: Gingivosis, J. Periodont. **24**:207, 1953.
18. Engel, M. B., Ray, H. G., and Orban, B.: The pathogenesis of desquamative gingivitis, J. Dent. Res. **29**:410, 1950.

19. Whitten, J. B.: The fine structure of desquamative gingivitis, J. Periodont. 39:75, 1968.
20. Glickman, I., and Smulow, J. B.: Histopathology and histochemistry of chronic desquamative gingivitis, Oral Surg. 21:325, 1966.
21. Sognnaes, R. F., Weisberger, D., and Allbright, J. T. Pathologic desquamation of oral epithelium examined by electron microscopy and histochemistry, J. Nat. Cancer Inst. 17:329, 1956.
22. Hall, W. B. Staining mast cells in human gingiva, Arch. Oral Biol. 11:1325, 1966.
23. McCarty, F. P., McCarty, P. L., Shklar, G.: Chronic desquamative gingivitis: a reconsideration, Oral Surg. 13:1300, 1960.
24. Nikai, H., Rose, G. G., and Cattoni, M.: Electron microscopic study of chronic desquamative gingivitis, J. Periodont. Res., supp. 6, 1971.
25. McCarthy, P., and Shklar, G.: Diseases of the oral mucosa, New York, 1964, McGraw-Hill Book Co.
26. Laufer, J., and Kuffer, R.: Le lichen plan buccal, Paris, 1970, Masson & Cie.
27. Zegarelli, E. V., Kutscher, A. H., Silvers, H. F., Beube, F. E., Stern, I. B., Berman, C. L., and Herlands, R. E.: Triamcinolone in the treatment of acute and chronic lesions of the oral mucous membranes, Oral Surg. 13:170, 1960.

**Additional suggested reading**

Jonek, J., and others: Aktivität und Verteilung einiger Enzyme in der Mundschleimhaut und in den Speicheldrüsen bei experimenteller akuter Bleivergiftung, Parodont. Acad. Rev. 2:19, 1968.
Lange, D. E.: Zytologische charakteristika der akuten Gingivitis, Deutsch. Zahnaerztl. Z. 27: 273, 1972.
Mühlemann, H. R.: Der marginale Parodontalinfekt, Schweiz. Mschr. Zahnheilk. 80:36, 1970.
Stern, I. B.: Electronmicroscopic observations of desquamative gingivitis, I.A.D.R. abstract no. 602, 1970.

CHAPTER FIFTEEN

# Periodontitis



*Definition*

Periodontitis is an inflammatory disease of the gingiva and the deeper tissues of the periodontium. It is characterized by pocket formation and bone destruction. Periodontitis is considered a direct extension of gingivitis that has advanced and has been neglected. The difference between the two is quantitative rather than qualitative, and in some cases an advanced gingivitis can hardly be distinguished from a beginning periodontitis. Periodontitis is caused primarily by extrinsic irritational factors and may be complicated by intrinsic disease, endocrine disturbances, nutritional deficiencies, periodontal traumatism, or other factors.

## PATHOGENESIS

Whenever the inflammation in the gingiva extends into the deeper supporting tissues[1-3,7] and part of the periodontal ligament has been destroyed, a diagnosis of periodontitis can be made. The characteristic feature in periodontitis is the periodontal pocket.[4] Pocket depth in periodontitis is not caused primarily by enlargement and swelling of the gingival margin but rather by progressive pocket encroachment on the periodontal ligament. This process is always accompanied by resorption of the alveolar crest (Figs. 15-1 and 15-2). The clinical diagnosis of periodontitis is based on gingival inflammation, pocket formation, exudation from these pockets, and alveolar resorption. The condition is usually painless. Mobility may occur early, or be a late symptom; it is sometimes minimal, even after extensive alveolar bone loss.

## CLINICAL FEATURES

The most important clinical features of periodontitis are the periodontal pocket with exudate and the resorption of the alveolar crest.

### Periodontal pocket

The periodontal pocket is bordered on the one side by the surface of the tooth, with its exposed cementum covered by calcareous deposits and plaque, and on the other by the gingiva, which exhibits varying degrees of inflamma-

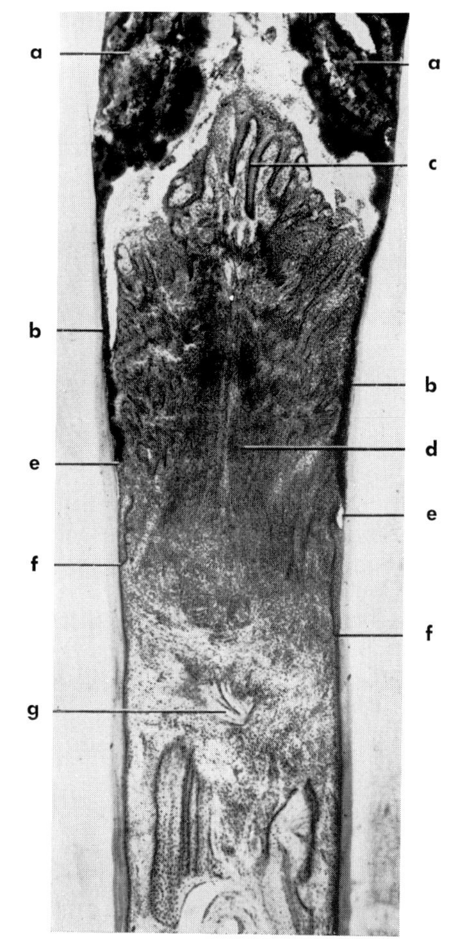


**Fig. 15-1.** Severe inflammation of an interdental papilla extending into the alveolar septum. Heavy calcareous dental deposits extend to the bottom of the pockets. *a,* Supragingival calculus; *b,* subgingival calculus; *c,* gingival papilla; *d,* heavy inflammatory infiltrate; *e,* bottom of the periodontal pocket; *f,* apical end of the epithelial attachment; *g,* alveolar crest. (Courtesy L. R. Cahn, New York.)

tion. The cementum that is coronal to the bottom of the pocket is a necrotic, nonvital tissue. The calcareous deposits consist of an organic matrix impregnated by inorganic salts (Chapter 6). The calcified mass is covered by plaque.

***Pocket epithelium***

The soft tissue side of the pocket is covered by stratified, nonkeratinized squamous epithelium. In inflammation this epithelium is frequently ulcerated. Toxic products from the sulcus (pocket) enter the underlying connective tissue by way of such ulcerations (Fig. 15-3). The connective tissue papillae are frequently long and extend nearly to the surface (Fig. 15-4). Invasion of connective tissue papillae by leukocytes may leave blood vessels covered only by a coagulated exudate (Fig. 15-5). For plaque bacterial products to provoke an inflammatory response, they must either pass through ulcerations into the connective tissue or be able to pass through the intercellular spaces of the pocket and the junctional (attachment) epithelium.

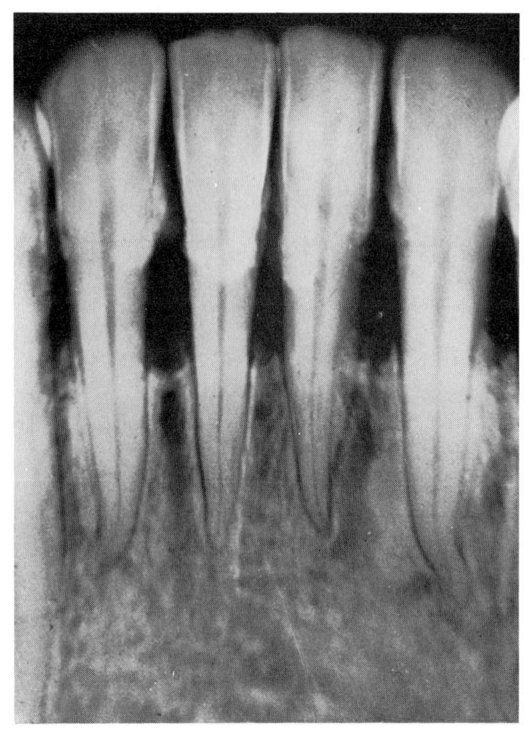

**Fig. 15-2.** Roentgenogram showing cup-shaped alveolar crests and widened nutrient canals in bone. These are indicative of resorption caused by penetration of the inflammation into the deeper tissues.

The outer (oral) surface of the gingival epithelium is characterized by a keratinized surface layer that ends abruptly at the free margin of the gingiva. In severe, chronic inflammation the oral epithelium may become less heavily keratinized.[4]

***Bottom of the pocket***

The apical end of the periodontal pocket (bottom of the pocket) is found at the coronal end of the attachment epithelium. This attachment extends apically from the bottom of the pocket and completely encircles the tooth.

The progression from gingivitis to periodontitis seems to be based on the extension of the inflammatory reaction along vascular channels to the bone. Inflammation is presumed also to spread in the lamina propria to destroy the fiber bundles directly beneath the attachment epithelium. This process may affect the vitality of cementoblasts in this area. These events, together with bone destruction, apical proliferation of the attachment epithelium, and pocket formation, are characteristic of periodontitis.[3,6,7]

***Pathogenesis of the pocket***

The bottom of the pocket is a vulnerable point of the attachment epithelium. At this point, where the epithelium is attached to a calcified structure (cementum), a unique biologic situation exists. If the epithelial cells are damaged or destroyed, the pocket can become deeper. There are deposits, bacteria, toxins, and other irritants in the pocket. These products provoke the inflammatory response.[6]

The irritants lead to inflammation, migration of leukocytes, and exudation into the pocket. The noxious influences remain in the pocket outside the epithelial covering of the body and outside the body defenses. A vicious cycle

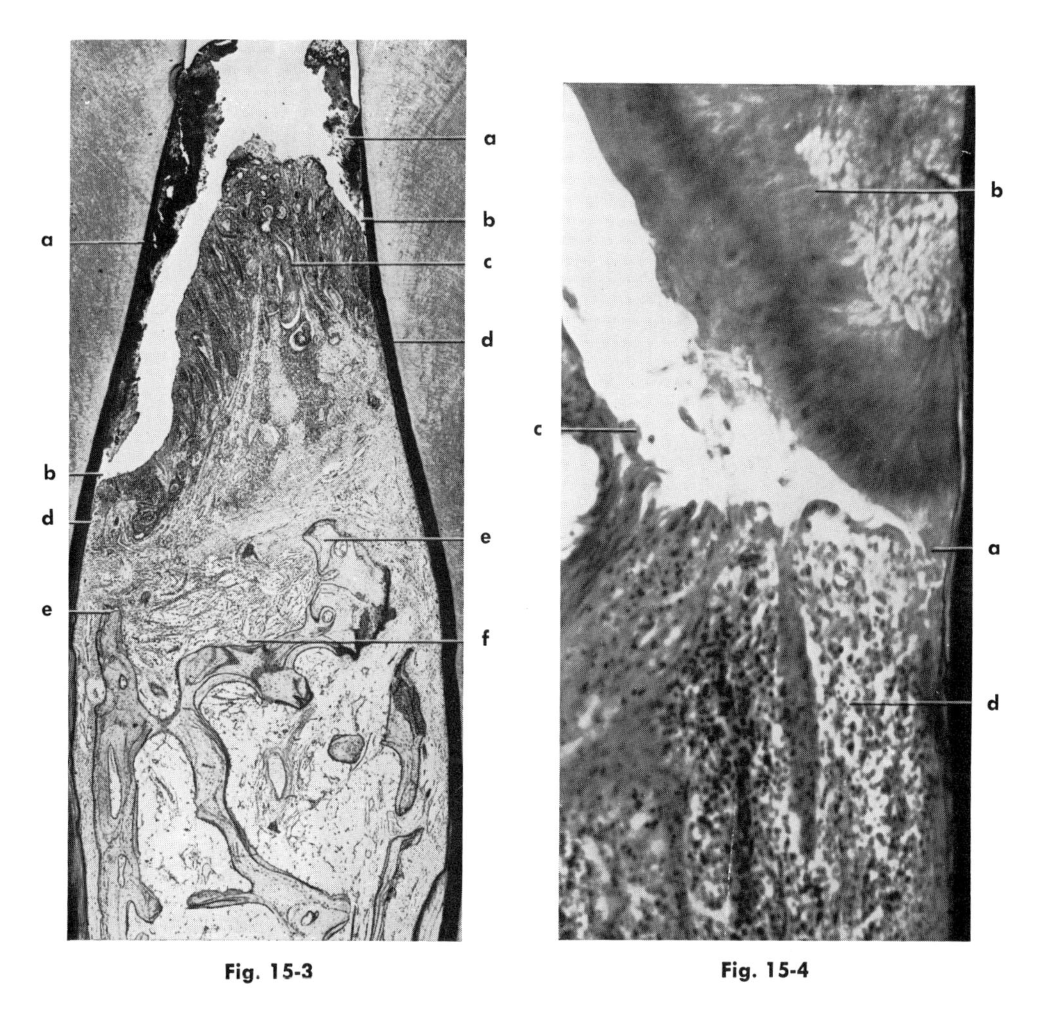


Fig. 15-3

Fig. 15-4

**Fig. 15-3.** Interdental area with inflammation from a periodontal pocket encroaching on the interdental alveolar septum. An osteitis is evident in the alveolar process. Bone is being resorbed. There are ulcerations in the pocket epithelium. *a,* Calculus; *b,* bottom of the periodontal pocket; *c,* highly inflamed gingival papilla; *d,* apical end of the epithelial attachment; *e,* alveolar bone; *f,* cup-shaped form of the alveolar crest.

**Fig. 15-4.** *a,* Bottom of a periodontal pocket. *b,* Dental deposits extend to the bottom of the pocket. The epithelium is thin and ulcerated. Epithelial cells, *c,* are shedding from the surface of the pocket epithelium, and there is severe inflammation, *d,* in the subepithelial connective tissue.

then occurs, resulting in more irritation, further damage to cells bordering the pocket, and an ever-deepening pocket. This deepened pocket again contributes to the cycle. Since the source of irritation remains outside the epithelial covering of the body, the body's defenses are unable to deal effectively with the situation and eliminate the irritants.

***Physiology of the dentogingival junction***

The cells of the attachment (junctional) epithelium, like most other epithelial cells, undergo constant desquamation and are replaced by new cells. The primary function of the attachment (junctional) epithelium is to maintain the epithelial attachment, which forms a protective seal. The sulcular epithelium also has a protective function. It is supported in this function by the defense

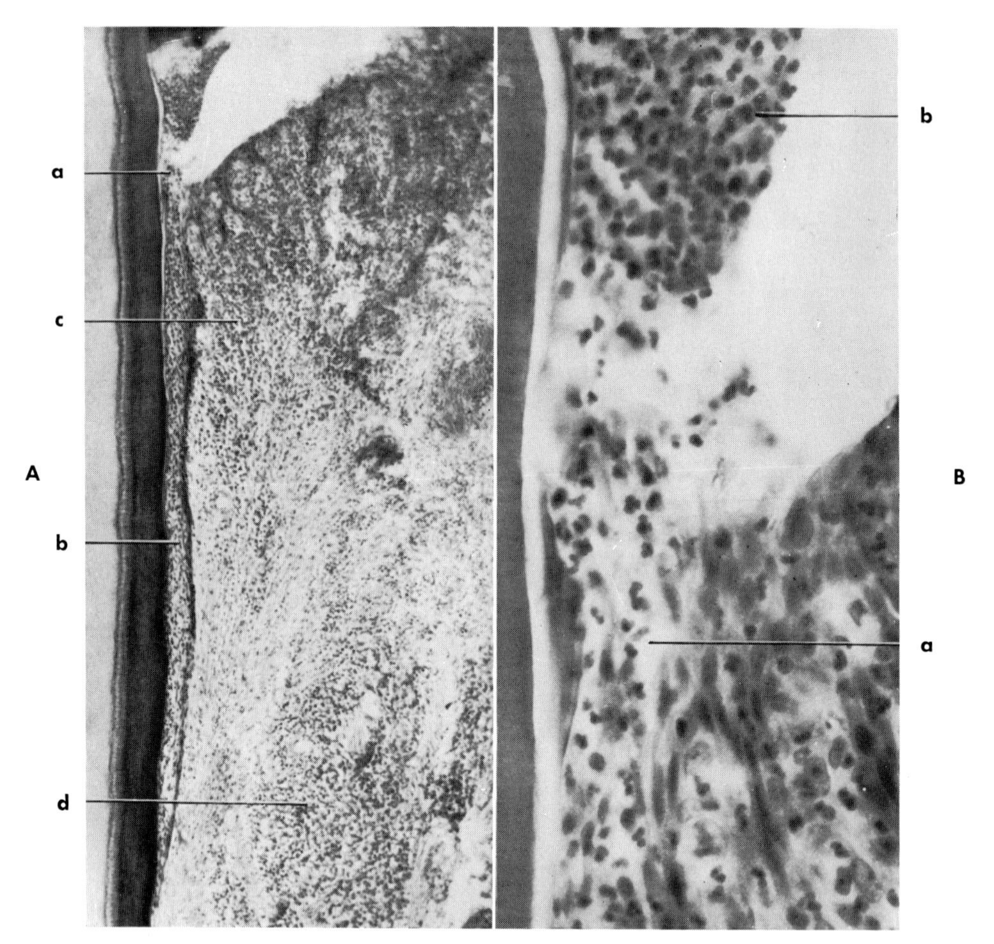


**Fig. 15-5. A,** Pocket area, *a,* and long epithelial attachment, *b,* in a case of periodontitis. Severe inflammation below the bottom of the pocket, *c,* extends to deeper areas, *d.* **B,** Higher magnification of the bottom of the pocket. Polymorphonuclear leukocytes migrate through the epithelium, *a,* into the pocket, forming pus, *b.* Note the dental cuticle on the surface of the tooth.

mechanism of the body, the inflammatory reaction, which is a function of connective tissue. The connective tissue of the gingiva, then, also plays a double role in supporting the epithelium both mechanically and biologically: the mechanical role of the connective tissue is performed by the collagen fibers; the biologic role by the inflammatory reaction of the tissues to irritation.

In periodontitis the mechanical role of the connective tissue is impaired by the inflammatory process. The collagen fibers and the ground substance may be altered enzymatically.[5,8,11] Fluid accumulates where fibrous elements were present. This breakdown of the fibrous tissue causes the gingiva to be loose and flabby. The accompanying edema can produce a glossy appearance on the surface of the tissue as well as loss of stippling. The accompanying stasis and cyanosis produce a dark red to bluish discoloration of the marginal and papillary gingiva. Occasionally, the extent of a pocket can be discerned by the cyanotic outline on the gingiva.

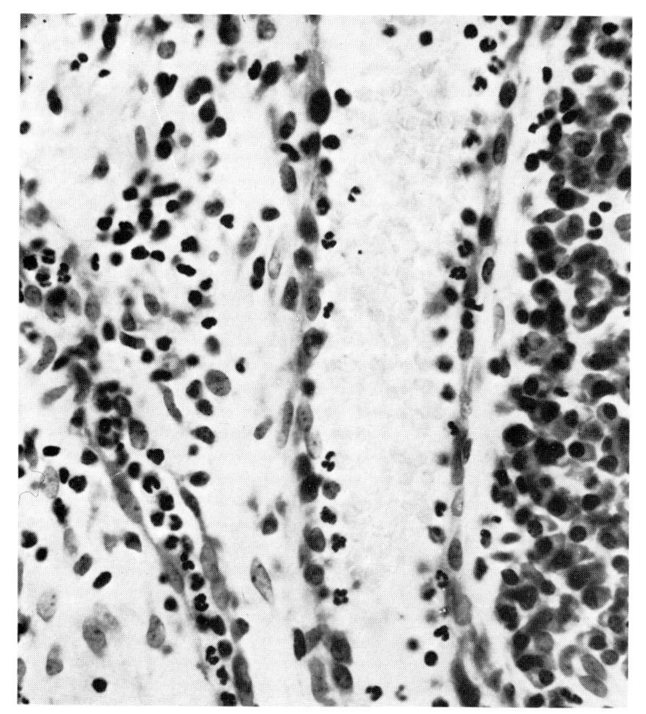

**Fig. 15-6.** Accumulation of polymorphonuclear leukocytes in blood vessels and migrating into the surrounding tissue.

### Resorption of alveolar crest

The process of osteoclastic resorption of the alveolar crest can be intensified by intrinsic factors, which favor breakdown of protein substances such as the ground substance of bone matrix.

In some cases, the inflammatory infiltrate may follow the course of periosteal vessels on the outer alveolar surface. Clinically, this may be seen as a diffuse inflammation of the entire zone of gingiva.

## HISTOPATHOLOGY

The cytologic characteristics of inflammation in periodontitis are typical. Polymorphonuclear leukocytes predominate close to the bottom of the pocket and in ulcerated areas (Fig. 15-5). These cells migrate from dilated blood vessels (Fig. 15-6) in an attempt to protect the tissues from invading organisms by their phagocytic and enzymatic action. The more violent the injury and virulent the bacteria, the greater is the leukocytic migration into the affected tissue area and through the epithelium into the pocket. The presence of pus in a pocket is an indication of this leukocytic activity.

### Gingival abscess

Gingival abscesses may develop because of the rapid migration of leukocytes toward bacteria in the pocket in the absence of sufficient drainage. The abscess develops whenever bacteria enter the connective tissue, which may occur through an injury such as from hard food, a toothpick, or dental manipulation. Except

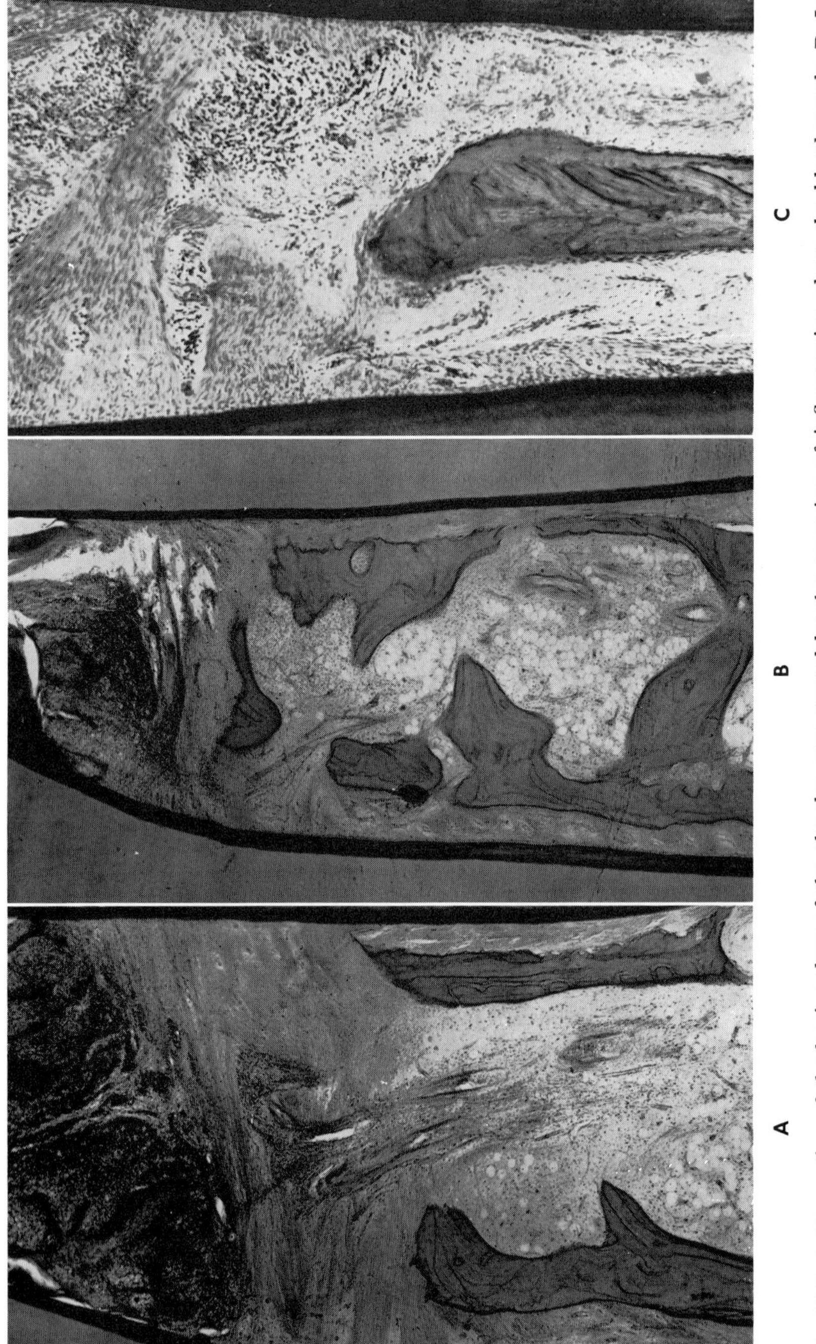


**Fig. 15-7. A,** Resorption of the lamina dura of the alveolar crest caused by the extension of inflammation along the blood vessels. **B,** Intraseptal blood vessels entering the gingiva. Note the Y-shaped configuration of the canals at the crest. **C,** High magnification of a narrow interdental space and a very thin alveolar crest. In this instance the inflammation extends into the periodontal ligament. (From the collection of J. P. Weinmann.)

in cases of necrotizing ulcerative gingivitis, bacteria are rarely present in the connective tissue. When bacteria enter the tissues, as in injury, a barrier is created by the rapid migration of leukocytes, and a blockade is created by thrombosis and development of a fibrinous network around the area.

### Periodontal abscess

In cases of extremely deep pockets, especially of the intra-alveolar (intrabony) type, the abscess may develop in deeper supporting tissues and form a lateral periodontal abscess. This often is caused by impairment of drainage from a deep or tortuous pocket or from a furcation. Plasmocytic and lymphocytic infiltration is the predominant feature of periodontitis in deeper tissue areas (not near the surface of the pocket). The function of plasma and lymphocytes in the inflammatory defense reaction may be production of antibodies. Dense masses of plasma cells in the gingiva may create the impression of a plasma cell tumor. The presence of these cells in periodontitis of long duration probably is an indication of the body's attempt to neutralize the toxic effects of bacteria and the products of tissue breakdown.

## PROGRESS OF INFLAMMATION

When the inflammatory process is of longer duration, it tends to progress deeper. This extension of the inflammatory infiltrate proceeds through the loose connective tissue along vascular pathways and is a characteristic feature of periodontitis. The blood and lymph vessels of the gingiva and periodontal ligament originate from or send branches to the alveolar arteries and penetrate the interdental and interradicular septa (Chapters 1 and 3). These vessels extend into the gingiva and send branches into the periodontal ligament; they also perforate the alveolar bone proper (cribriform plate). If an inflammatory process exists, as in periodontitis, the toxins and the cellular infiltrate follow backward along the course of the accompanying veins and lymph vessels. This fact explains the roentgenographic appearance of the alveolar septa in periodontitis (Fig. 15-2). However, the roentgenographic picture lags behind the biologic process, and changes may not be evident immediately in the roentgenogram.

***Course of the blood vessels and x-ray appearance***

The microscopic as well as roentgenographic appearance of the blood vessels is determined largely by the course of the vessels. If the vessels extend through the top of the alveolar crest, the crest appears cup shaped in periodontitis (Fig. 15-7, *A*). If the vessels branch off before piercing the crest, the resorption may appear Y-shaped (*B*) and the crest appear blurred roentgenographically. If the teeth are close together with only thin septal bone, the inflammatory process may enter the periodontal ligament on one or both sides (*C*) and the coronal part of the septum be completely lost.

***Extension to bone***

The inflammatory reaction extends into the bone marrow spaces following the course of the blood vessels. The toxins and enzymes from the inflammatory process are carried into the bone marrow and other deeper tissue areas along the loose connective tissue that surrounds the blood and lymph vessels. The extension of the inflammatory process into the deeper supporting tissues is, in part at least, responsible for the resorption of the alveolar crest. The increased pressure in the area, the edema and swelling, the active and passive hyperemia, and the enzymatic action are all causes of bone resorption. However, the extension of toxins into the deeper tissues also may be responsible for this resorption.

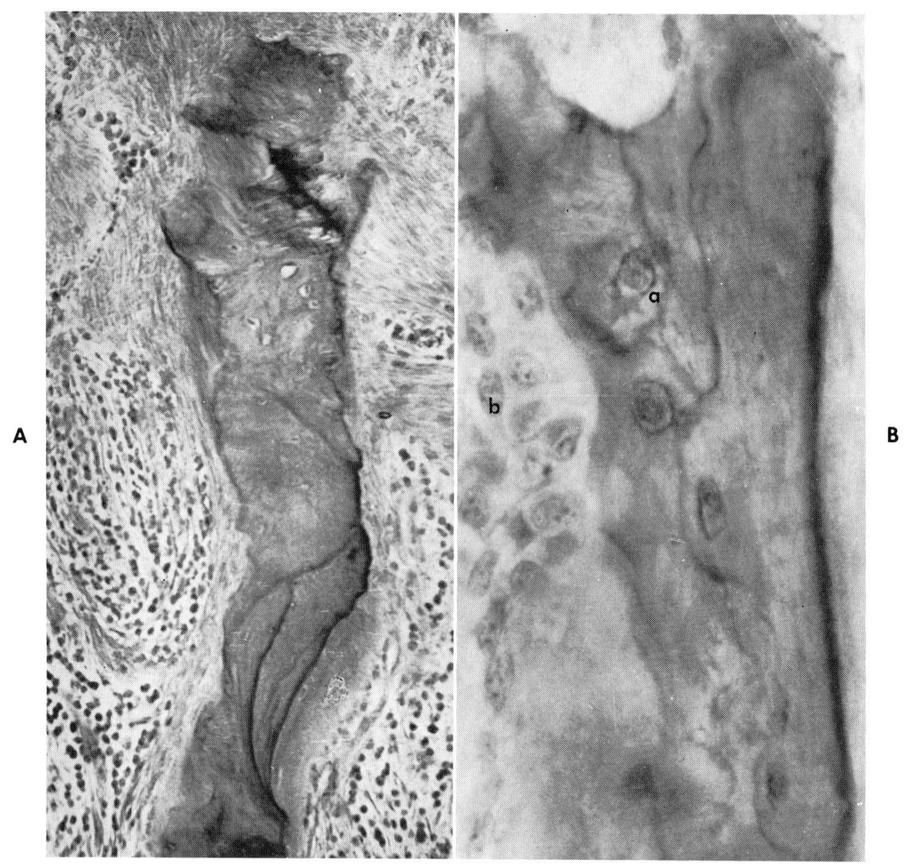


**Fig. 15-8. A,** Bone spicule forming the alveolar crest surrounded by inflammatory cells. Osteocytes are present. New bone formation is in progress in some areas. **B,** High magnification of a bone spicule showing osteocytes, *a,* and osteoblasts, *b.*

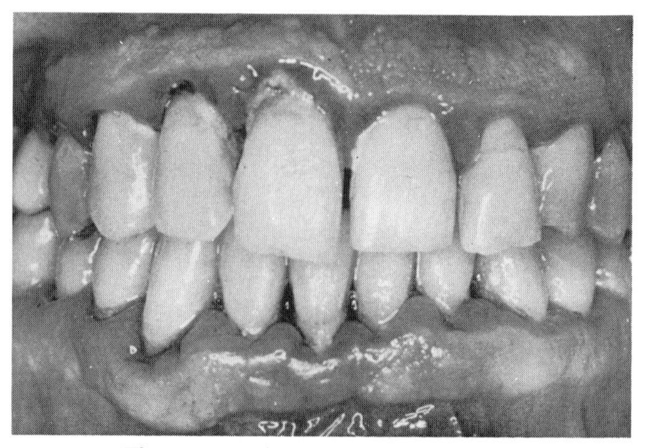

**Fig. 15-9.** Typical case of periodontitis.

*Localized osteitis*

The toxins probably can affect the vitality of the osteocytes. The inflammatory reaction follows the blood vessels into the marrow spaces; and the normal marrow changes into fibrous marrow. From the point of view of the pathologist, this is a localized osteitis. In rare instances it may progress to a localized osteomyelitis with the formation of sequestra. Bone takes a rather passive part, and vital osteocytes can be observed even in very thin bone spicules (Fig. 15-8). Osteoblastic and osteoclastic activity continues. Bone breakdown is an expression of a negative balance in the processes of bone formation and bone resorption.[9,10]

## EXTRINSIC ETIOLOGY

### Irritation

Presumably, extrinsic irritation is the primary etiologic factor in periodontitis. As a typical example, the following case is presented (Fig. 15-9):

The patient was a 46-year-old man with complaints of bleeding gums and some looseness of the teeth. The medical history was noncontributory. The clinical examination revealed a nearly complete dentition. Two teeth had been replaced by a fixed bridge extending from the first premolar to the second molar in the right maxilla. The abutment teeth of the bridge, as well as most of the remaining teeth, showed varying degrees of mobility. The gingiva was severely inflamed–magenta in color, glossy in texture. The papillae were blunted, the gingival margins were swollen, and pockets of 3 to 6 mm. depth with a purulent exudate were present. Large masses of both calcified and uncalcified dental deposits were present, and halitosis could be detected.

The roentgenograms (Fig. 15-10) revealed alveolar bone resorption that was irregular (horizontal and vertical) in form and distribution. The interdental alveolar septa did not show a distinct lamina dura (cortical plate) at the crest. The fuzzy appearance at the crest was interpreted to indicate an active disease process. Clinical and roentgenographic findings indicated a typical advanced periodontitis caused primarily by local irritation.

Another illustrative case of periodontitis is that of a 29-year-old white woman. There were no subjective complaints. The medical history was negative. Clinically some papillae were slightly swollen, indicating irritation (Fig. 15-11). Notwithstanding the nearly normal clincial appearance, examination revealed considerable pocket formation in the molar and premolar regions of both the maxilla and the mandible.

The roentgenograms (Fig. 15-12) showed a rather unusual condition. Typical cup-shaped or fuzzy alveolar crests could be seen in the incisor region and the maxillary molar and premolar regions. In the mandibular premolar regions, however, oblique alveolar crests were present on both sides. Such crestal patterns have been interpreted variously in the literature as an indication of occlusal trauma[12] or of periodontosis. In this patient the oblique inclination of the alveolar crests was caused primarily by the anterior inclination of the teeth and by the relation of the cementoenamel junctions of the approximating teeth.[12] The oblique inclination of the alveolar crests was exaggerated by the existing severe inflammatory process. The diagnosis was periodontitis.

The dentition of a 38-year-old woman with a chronic hyperplastic periodontitis is shown in Fig. 15-13, *A*. The gingiva around the mandibular incisors is enlarged, except near the central incisors, where the large accumulation of calculus has resulted in a destruction of the gingiva and recession of the gingival margins

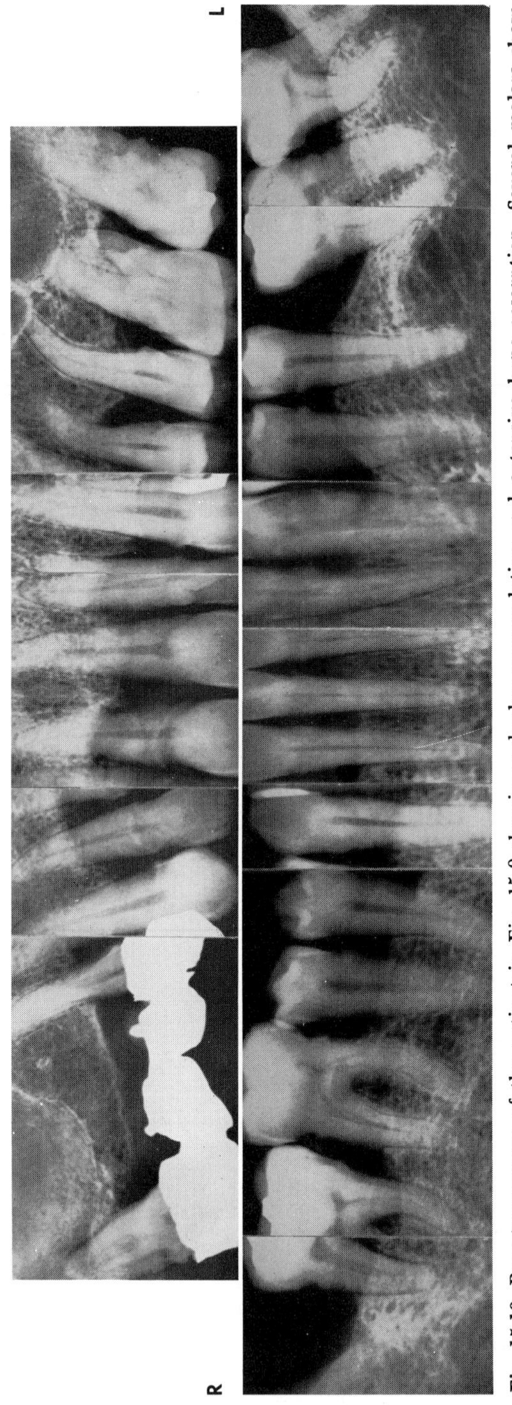


**Fig. 15-10.** Roentgenograms of the patient in Fig. 15-9 showing calculus accumulation and extensive bone resorption. Several molars show furcation involvements. Note the irregularity of the alveolar crests.

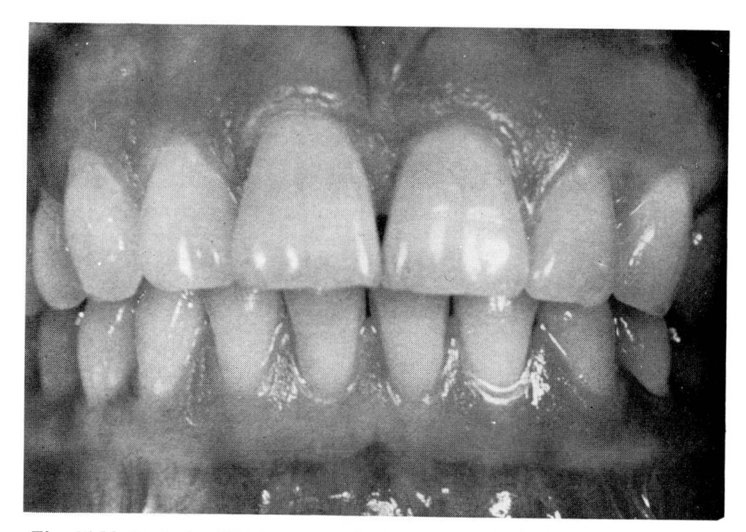

**Fig. 15-11.** Periodontitis in a mouth that appeared clinically fairly normal.

(Fig. 15-13, *B*). The clinical appearance of the enlargement was primarily that of fibrosis with some edema. The maxillary gingival margins were less enlarged and retained a regular mesiodistal scalloped form.

The gingiva was dark red to magenta in color. Probing was painful and elicited easy bleeding. Pockets ranged in depth from 3 to 9 mm. and were distributed irregularly throughout the mouth. Class 2 mobility was present on the right maxillary central incisor and the mandibular central incisors. Some mobility was present elsewhere in the mouth and could be attributed to loss of supporting structure. Missing teeth had not been replaced; and drifting, tilting, and malpositioning of the remaining teeth were evident in some areas. Oral hygiene was noteworthy by its absence. Roentgenograms (Fig. 15-14) showed extensive bone loss that was irregular in form and distribution. The ratio of clinical crown length to root length was unfavorable for the maxillary and mandibular incisors. Poor prognosis was projected for the maxillary right central incisor and the mandibular incisors. The prognosis for the remaining teeth was guarded because of the multiple etiologic factors present. These included irritational factors from calcified and uncalcified deposits, bacteria, food impingement and impaction, secondary traumatism, and poor oral hygiene. Medical history was noncontributory, and clinical laboratory tests revealed no intrinsic influence. For treatment of this patient, see Chapter 33.

### Occlusal trauma

The controversial topic of the role played by occlusal trauma as an aggravating factor in inflammatory periodontal disease is discussed in Chapter 36.

## INTRINSIC ETIOLOGY

Local (extrinsic) factors are of paramount etiologic importance in periodontitis. Irritation by deposits with the ever-present microbial flora is a primary factor in the inflammatory reaction and the deepening of pockets. However, these extrinsic factors do not explain satisfactorily the development of certain forms of periodontitis. There can be no question that systemic (intrinsic) factors

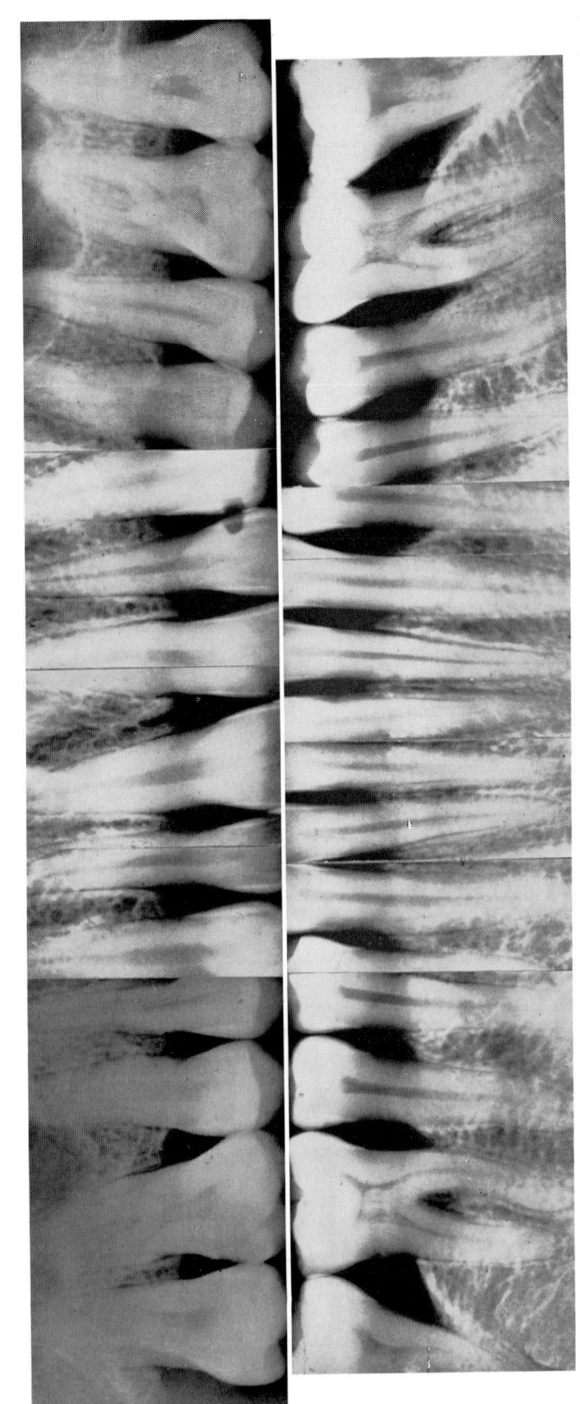

**Fig. 15-12.** Roentgenograms of the patient shown in Fig. 15-11. Note the cup-shaped alveolar crests in the maxilla and the oblique inclination of the alveolar crests in the mandible.

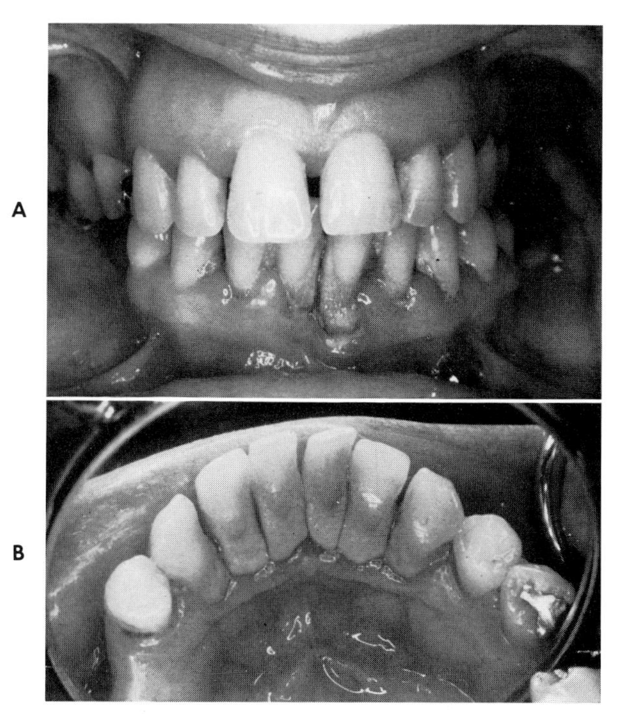


**Fig 15-13. A,** Enlarged gingival margins, recession, and heavy calcified deposits are evident in a 38-year-old white woman. **B,** Heavy deposition of calculus and edematous receded gingival margins can be seen on the oral surface of the mandibular incisors.

play an important role in the development, form, and severity of some cases of this disease. We cannot incriminate any one intrinsic disease or nutritional deficiency that will lead consistently to the development of periodontitis from a persisting gingivitis. Nevertheless, there are diseases that predispose to tissue breakdown and inflammatory reactions.[17,22,23] One example is diabetes.[12-16] Others are tuberculosis, endocrine dysfunction, and nutritional disturbances.

*Congenital organ weakness*

Congenital organ weakness may play a role in the progression from gingivitis to periodontitis. This factor has been discussed in the literature under various titles (resistance, susceptibility, organ weakness, bone factor). What it means is that some individuals are resistant to the deleterious effects of chronic gingival inflammation. Despite persistent plaque and calculus, they exhibit only mild gingival inflammation, little or no pocket depth, and no evident bone loss. Conversely, other individuals show severe destructive changes in the presence of minimal plaque and calculus. Between these extremes is a spectrum of responses that reflect the genetically influenced susceptibility to specific disease-causing agents.

*Allergic reaction*

The exact role of the immune reaction in the causation of periodontitis is not known. There are strong indications, however, that these mechanisms play an important part in the causation and in the attending breakdown.[20,21,24,25] These phenomena have been discussed in Chapter 13.

*Senescence*

Age may also be a determining factor in the incidence of periodontal diseases. The strikingly low incidence of inflammatory periodontal disease in the young child and the increasing incidence in the elderly cannot be ignored. The possible effects of ageing are discussed in Chapter 4.

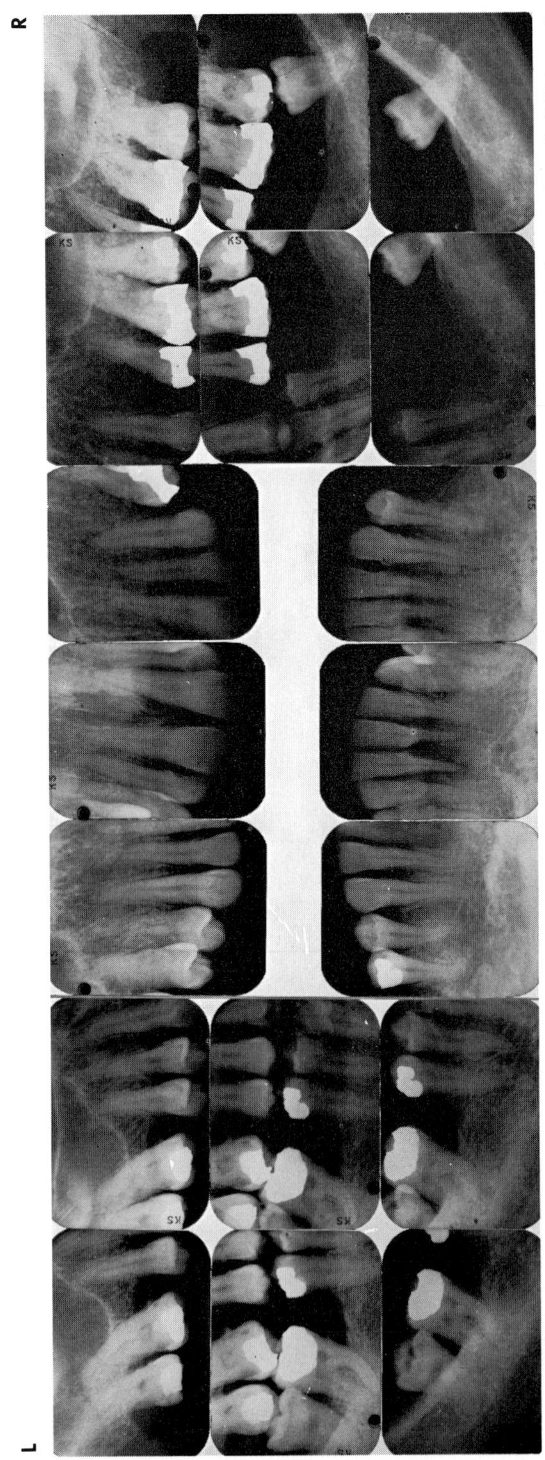


**Fig. 15-14.** Roentgenograms showing extensive bone loss that is irregular in form and generalized in distribution. Missing teeth and drifting of other teeth are evident. Loss of proximal tooth contacts and heavy supragingival subgingival calculus also can be seen.

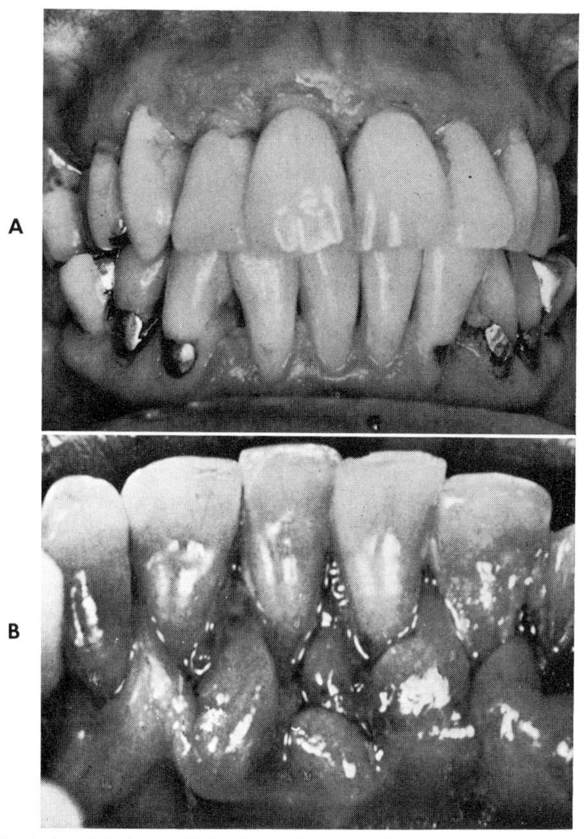


**Fig. 15-15. A,** Periodontitis in a diabetic patient. **B,** Hyperplastic tissue reaction on the oral (lingual) surface of the mandibular incisors in the same patient.

## Diabetes mellitus

Diabetes mellitus is a disturbance of the function of the pancreatic islands of Langerhans and the function of the liver, sometimes combined with a disturbance in the function of other endocrine glands such as the thyroid and the adrenals. It leads to protein breakdown, degenerative processes, lowered resistance to infection, vascular changes, and an increase in the severity of inflammatory reactions. In turn, the increased severity of diabetes when inflammation is present is the result of glucose formed locally at the inflammatory sites from the breakdown of protein and from the liberation of toxic or injurious exudates at these sites. This acts on the liver, raising the level of the blood sugar (glyconeogenesis) and increasing insulin requirements.

The mouth of a diabetic patient with severe periodontitis is shown in Fig. 15-15, *A*. Antibiotics may be necessary in the treatment of such patients. After successful treatment sometimes the patients' requirements for insulin are reduced.

Another case with a diabetic history is that of a patient who was seen after an acute attack of influenza. He had been bedridden with a temperature of 102° F. for 2 weeks. His lower incisors became loose, and a mass of inflammatory tissue developed on the oral surfaces of these teeth[15] (Fig. 15-15, *B*). Roentgenograms showed considerable resorption of bone around the mandibular in-

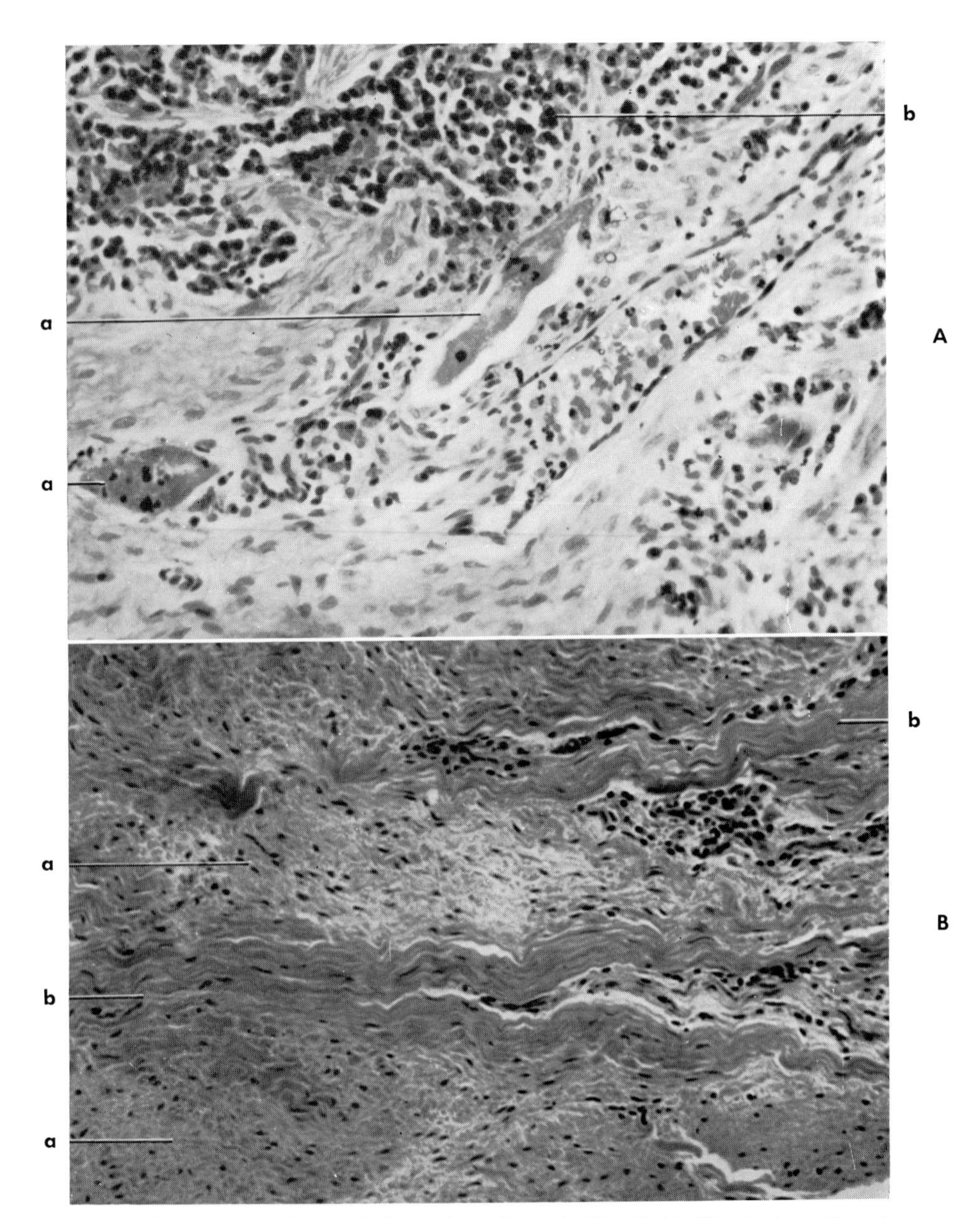


**Fig. 15-16. A,** Biopsy of the gingiva of the patient shown in Fig. 15-15. Histologic section shows, *a,* thrombosis of blood vessels and, *b,* chronic inflammatory infiltration. **B,** Biopsy of the gingiva in a diabetic patient with periodontitis. Degeneration of collagen, *a,* is observed between unchanged collagen fiber bundles, *b.*

cisors. On questioning, the patient revealed that he had had a very mild diabetes for several years. This condition had been controlled by diet. (Often in the course of acute, infectious disease processes, a latent diabetic condition will be activated.) The patient was advised to have a blood sugar determination and urinalysis, which revealed an exacerbation of the diabetic condition.

A biopsy specimen taken from the granulomatous gingiva (Fig. 15-16, *A*) showed thrombosed blood vessels in one area. This is an unusual finding in any gingival biopsy and may be attributed to the diabetic condition. Degeneration of

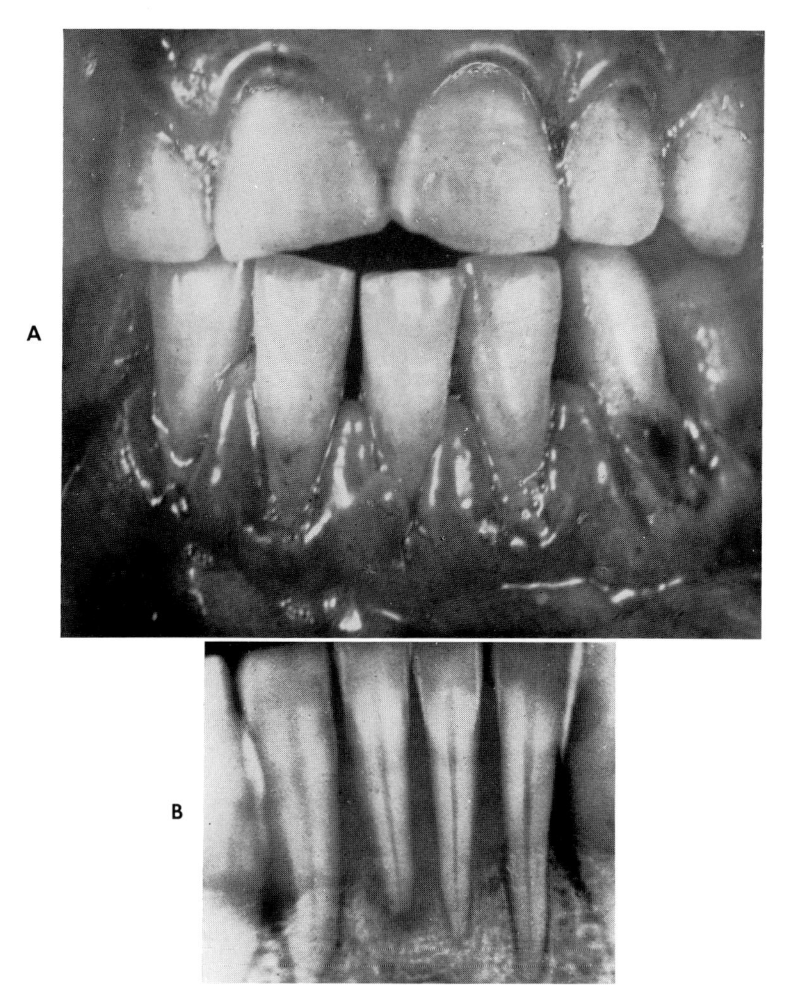


**Fig. 15-17. A,** Tuberculous periodontitis. **B,** Roentgenogram of the same patient showing extensive resorption of bone.

collagen fibers is also seen in biopsies from diabetics (Fig. 15-16, *B*). After the diabetes had been controlled, the influenza cured; and with the extrinsic irritational factors eliminated, the granulomatous masses disappeared.

Investigations conducted on a large number of diabetic patients have not so far shown consistent characteristic histologic changes in the gingiva. Tissue changes found in diabetic patients with periodontitis, however, have appeared to be more severe. The walls of small blood vessels were reported to have become thickened.[15]

In summarizing the role of diabetes in periodontitis, we may note that the diabetes is a severe aggravating factor. There is a lowered tissue resistance brought about by breakdown and diminished synthesis of proteins. Tissue regeneration, in general, is slower and less effective than normal, and the breakdown process is hastened. Diabetes predisposes to infection and thus to periodontitis; and infection in turn worsens the diabetic condition, increasing the need for insulin.

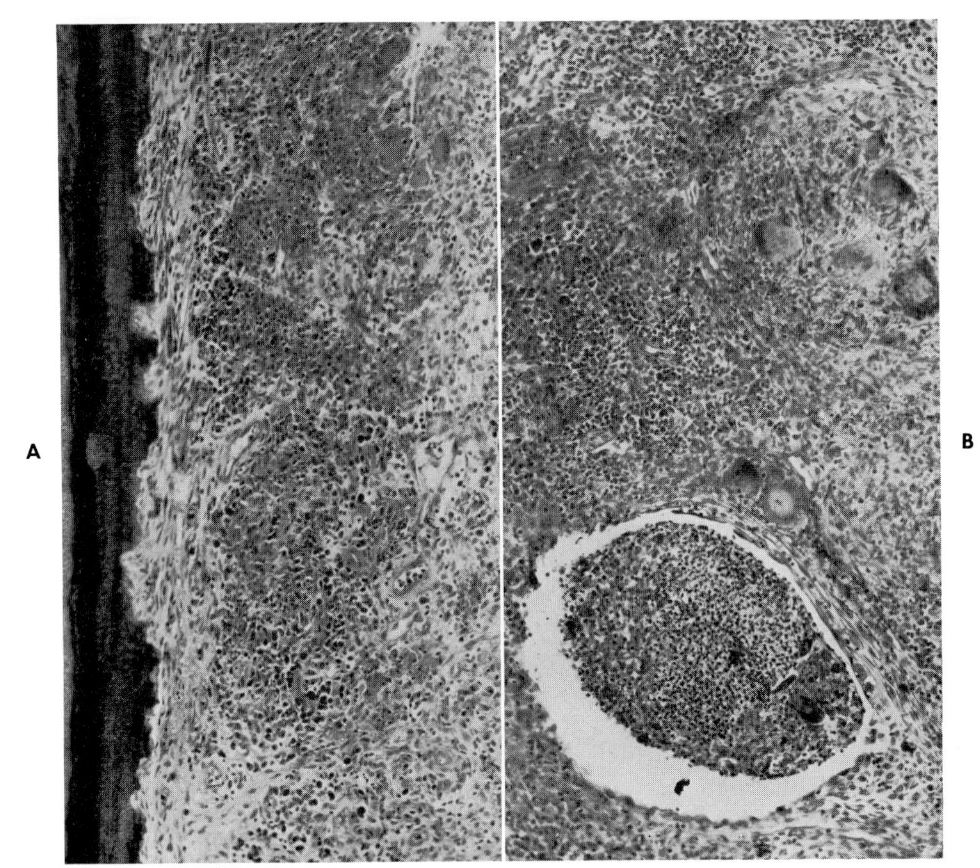


**Fig. 15-18. A,** Biopsy of a tooth and surrounding periodontal tissue of the patient shown in Fig. 15-9. Histologic section shows tuberculous granulation tissue and resorption of the root surface. **B,** Tuberculous granulation tissue with giant cells, epitheloid cells, and lymphocytic infiltration.

## Tuberculosis

Tuberculosis may have periodontal manifestations. A clinical photograph and roentgenograms of a 26-year-old individual with acute, disseminated, miliary tuberculosis and diabetes are shown in Fig. 15-17. The teeth were extremely loose. Numerous yellowish pinhead-sized tubercles could be seen on the mucous membranes, including the gingival margin. Some of the teeth were extracted, and a considerable amount of soft, adherent, granulomatous tissue was removed with them. The microscopic examination of this tissue revealed numerous tubercles in the periodontum (Fig. 15-18). The patient died of tuberculosis meningitis. The periodontal condition can be interpreted in part as the oral manifestation of an intrinsic disease.

## Endocrine dysfunction

Dysfunction of endocrine glands (thyroid, ovaries) or medication (birth control pills) leads to changes in the general metabolic processes and thus can act as an aggravating factor in otherwise extrinsic irritational disturbances.[17]

## Nutritional disturbances

Dietary deficiencies[18,19] and other nutritional disturbances can play a similar role, as can also disturbances of the blood-forming organs (Chapter 11). Anemia can be a contributing factor by leading to lowered resistance to infection. Nutritional disturbances, however, are probably not prominent causes in the production of periodontal disease in the United States or in other advanced countries.[18,19]

**CHAPTER 15**

**References**


1. Weinmann, J. P.: Periodontitis: etiology, pathology, symptomatology, J. Amer. Dent. Ass. **44**:701, 1952.
2. Weinmann, J. P.: Progress of gingival inflammation into the supporting structures of the teeth, J. Periodont. **12**:71, 1941.
3. Toto, P. D., and Gargiulo, A. W.: Epithelial and connective tissue changes in periodontitis, J. Periodont. **41**:587, 1970.
4. Ritchey, B., and Orban, B.: The periodontal pocket, J. Periodont. **23**:199, 1952.
5. Winer, R. A., O'Donnell, L. J., Chauncey, H. H., and McNamara, T. F.: Enzyme activity in periodontal disease, J. Periodont. **41**:449, 1970.
6. Grant, D. A., and Orban, B.: Leukocytes in the epithelial attachment, J. Periodont. **31**:87, 1960.
7. Toto, P. D., Pollock, R. J., and Gargiulo, A. W.: Pathogenesis of periodontitis, Periodontics **2**:197, 1964.
8. Stahl, S. S., Sandler, H., and Suben, E.: Histochemical changes in inflammatory periodontal disease, J. Periodont. **29**:183, 1958.
9. Reichborn-Kjennerud, L.: Dento-alveolar resorption in periodontal disorders. In Sognnaes, R. F.: Mechanisms of hard tissue destruction, Washington, D. C., 1963, A.A.A.S.
10. Sicher, H., and Weinmann, J. P.: Bone and bones, St. Louis, 1955, The C. V. Mosby Co.
11. Hershon, L. E.: Elaboration of hyaluronidase and chondroitin sulphatase by microorganisms inhabiting the gingival sulcus, J. Periodont. **42**:34, 1971.
12. Ritchey, B., and Orban, B.: The crests of the interdental alveolar septa, J. Periodont. **24**:75, 1953.
13. Hirschfeld, I.: Periodontal symptoms associated with diabetes, J. Periodont. **5**:37, 1934.
14. Belting, C. M., Hinniker, J. J., and Dummett, C. O.: Influence of diabetes mellitus on the severity of periodontal disease, J. Periodont. **35**:476, 1964.
15. Ray, H. G., and Orban, B.: The gingival structures in diabetes mellitus, J. Periodont. **21**:85, 1950.
16. Cohen, D. W., and others: Studies on periodontal patterns in diabetes mellitus, J. Periodont. Res., supp. 4, 1969.
17. Burket, L. W.: Oral medicine, ed. 6, Philadelphia, 1971, J. B. Lippincott Co.
18. Nizel, A.: Nutrition in preventive dentistry, Philadelphia, 1972, W. B. Saunders Co.
19. Clark, J. W., Cheraskin, E., and Ringsdorf, W. M.: Diet and the periodontal patient, Springfield, Ill., 1970, Charles C Thomas, Publisher.
20. Ranney, H. H., and Zander, H. A.: Allergic periodontal disease in sensitized monkeys, J. Periodont. **41**:12, 1970.
21. Bickley, H. C.: A concept of allergy with reference to oral disease, J. Periodont. **41**:302, 1970.
22. Stahl, S. S.: The etiology of periodontal disease. In Ramfjord, S. P., Kerr, D. A., and Ash, M., editors: World workshop in periodontics, Ann Arbor, Mich., 1966, University of Michigan Press.
23. Lynch, M.: Systemic diseases, J. Periodont. **38**:771, 1967.
24. Platt, D., Crosby, R. G., and Dalbow, M. H.: Evidence for the presence of immunoglobulins and circulating antibodies in inflamed periodontal tissues, J. Periodont. **41**:215, 1970.
25. Brandtzaeg, P., and Kraus, F. W.: Autoimmunity and periodontal disease, Odont. T. **73**:285, 1965.


**Additional suggested reading**


Akiyoshi, M., and Mori, K.: Marginal periodontitis; a histologic study of the incipient stage, J. Periodont. **38**:45, 1967.

Cohen, B.: Morphological factors in the pathogenesis of periodontal disease, Brit. Dent. J. **107**:31, 1959.

Michel, C.: Étude ultrastructurale de l'os alvéolaire au cours des parodontolyses, Parodontologie **23**:191, 1969.

Riethe, P.: Diagnostik der marginalen Parodontitis, Parodontologie **24**:9, 1970.

Schallhorn, R. G.: Diabetes mellitus and periodontal disease, Periodont. Abstr. **14**:9, 1966.

PART V

# Dystrophic periodontal conditions

CHAPTER SIXTEEN

# Dystrophies and periodontosis



## Dystrophies

*Definition*

Dystrophy is a term used to designate pathologic conditions produced by abnormal tissue nutrition leading to disturbances in cell metabolism and manifested by degeneration, atrophy, or hyperplasia.

### ATROPHIC PERIODONTAL CONDITIONS

Atrophy is a condition in which an organ or its cellular elements become decreased in size after reaching normal maturity. As compared to degeneration, it is more or less a quantitative tissue change (degeneration is a qualitative one). This differentiation is not absolute because atrophy often is accompanied by some degenerative changes.

Atrophy need not necessarily be a pathologic process. It occurs in various stages of life as a result of environmental influences and alterations in body metabolism, and it is a rather common problem in the geriatric patient.

Some of the other causes of atrophy are starvation, disuse, excessive pressure, and toxic and chemical influences. All these factors will cause an alteration in cellular metabolism.

#### Recession of gingiva

The effect of atrophy on the gingiva is often manifested by gingival recession. The gingiva may not show any other sign of pathology. It often is thin and finely textured and may be pale pink with a thin gingival margin and relatively elongated, pointed papillae (Fig. 16-1). The gingival sulci are usually very shallow.

Recession may be generalized or it may be localized (Fig. 16-2) to a single

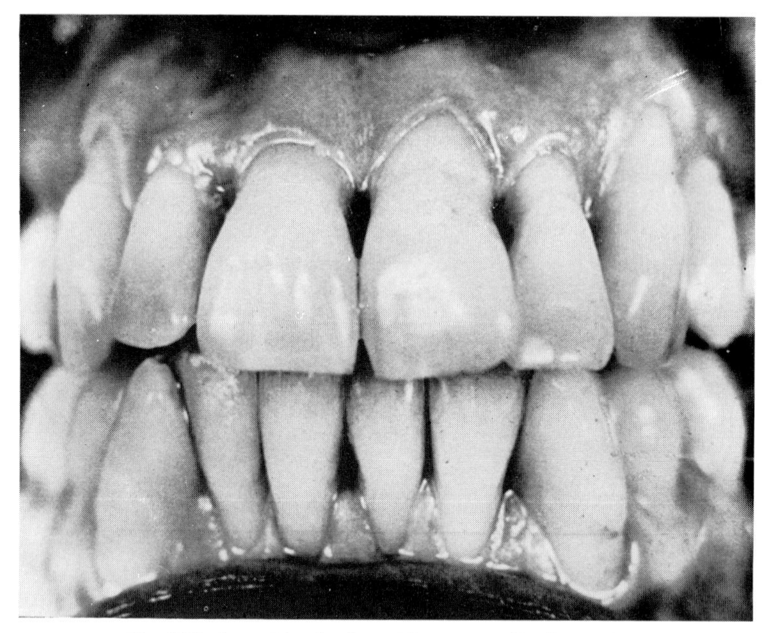

**Fig. 16-1.** Atrophic gingiva with a generalized recession.

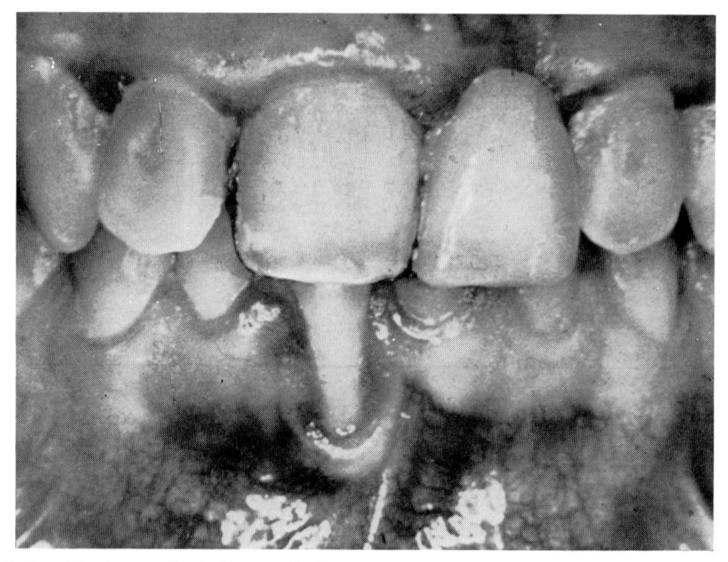

**Fig. 16-2.** Localized recession of a vestibularly (labially) located mandibular central incisor.

tooth or group of teeth. It may be physiologic or an expression of disease. Whether it occurs as a result of ageing is controversial. The intrinsic changes that occur with time cannot easily be separated from those that are the result of pathology.

Gingival recession may be related to certain predisposing anatomic factors. The position of gingival margins is partly determined by the height and thickness of the underlying bone and by tooth alignment. Orally malposed teeth have a thicker and more coronal vestibular alveolar plate than do their properly

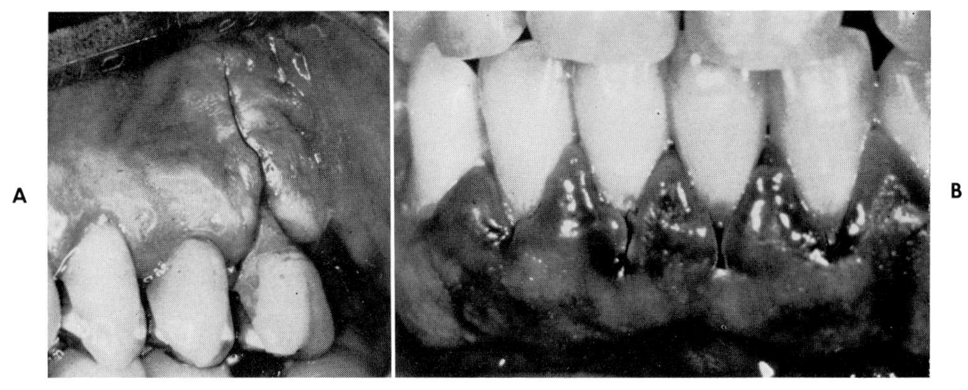


**Fig. 16-3. A,** Extensive cleft on the vestibular surface of a maxillary molar possibly associated with toothbrush injury. **B,** Pseudoclefts on the vestibular surfaces of the mandibular incisors primarily caused by hyperplastic overgrowth of the adjacent tissues.

positioned neighbors.[1,2] Vestibularly malposed teeth (Fig. 16-2) usually have a thinner vestibular alveolar plate and a margin more apically positioned than do adjacent teeth. The gingival margins are thus positioned in accordance with tooth alignment and with bone thickness and height. In cases in which a thin gingiva and thin underlying bone are subjected to traumatism or other irritation, destruction of bone and gingiva may take place and result in a localized or generalized recession of the gingival margins.

*Clefts*

Clefts of the gingiva (Fig. 16-3, *A*) apparently are caused by an uneven atrophy or destruction of the marginal gingiva. They may develop on the oral surface but are most often seen on the vestibular surface. Downgrowth and fusion of long epithelial ridges have been observed in the subepithelial connective tissue. The fusion of such proliferated epithelial ridges with the sulcular epithelium may be responsible for the formation of gingival clefts. Occasionally clefts may be due to faulty brushing (Fones' method) with a hard brush with sharp bristles.[5] Some clefts disappear spontaneously.[3] Pseudoclefts may be formed by overgrowth of adjacent tissue (Fig. 16-3, *B*).

*Etiology*

The etiology of gingival recession, whether localized or generalized, is not always easily determined.[4] The following factors have been incriminated[4-6b]:

1. Toothbrush injury (Fig. 16-3, *A*)
2. Orthodontic forces (Fig. 16-4) that have moved a tooth too far orally or vestibularly (irritation from bands or arch wires)
3. Other extrinsic irritations (chemical, physical, bacterial)
4. Occlusal traumatism
5. Faulty tooth alignment[6]
6. Anatomic abnormalities (thin bony plates, high frenum attachments)
7. Deleterious habits (pressure of foreign objects, fingernails, pencils, hairpins)[5]
8. Clasps and mandibular oral (lingual) denture bars or aprons in partial dentures that have settled
9. Ageing

Repeated and prolonged toothbrush injury is often assumed to lead to atrophic changes in the periodontium and to subsequent recession.[3-6] Fig. 16-5 shows a recession associated with extensive abrasion at the cementoenamel junc-

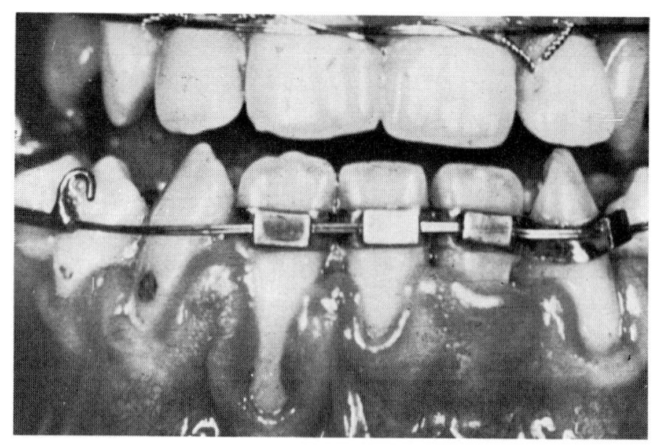

**Fig. 16-4.** Recession of the gingiva brought about during orthodontic therapy when a tooth was moved too rapidly or too far in a labial direction.

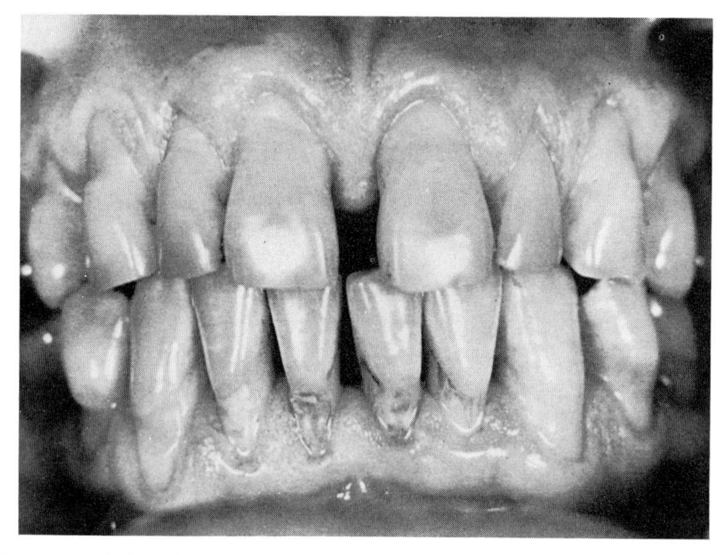

**Fig. 16-5.** Recession of the gingiva and abrasion of the teeth brought about by overly vigorous and incorrect brushing or the use of a brush with sharp, hard bristles.

tion. History revealed vigorous brushing in a horizontal direction with a hard toothbrush. This type of recession is common on the left canines of right-handed persons.

Occlusal traumatism is another factor incriminated in gingival recession and cleft formation. Available evidence tends to indicate that occlusal trauma does not produce recession ordinarily. Further discussion of the effect of occlusal traumatism will be found in Chapter 36.

The case of a young person shown in Fig. 16-6 demonstrates recession, claimed by some to be caused by occlusal traumatism. Several primary teeth were missing. One mandibular incisor was vestibular to the maxillary incisor, and the gingival margin on this tooth was located further apically than on the other teeth. The gingival recession was, in fact, brought about by the vestibular position of this tooth.

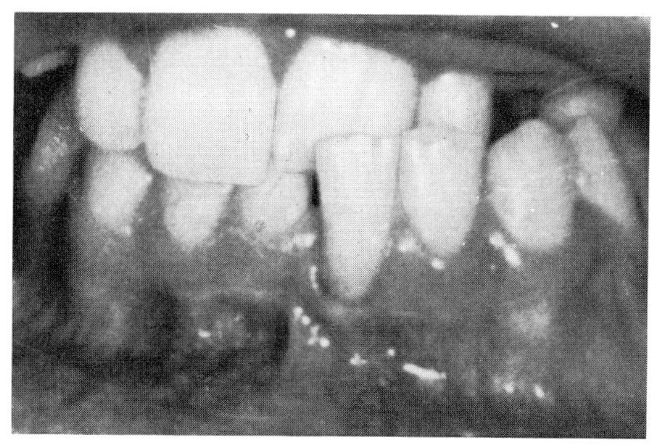

**Fig. 16-6.** Linguoversion of the maxillary incisors and recession of the gingiva of a mandibular central incisor, allegedly caused by occlusal traumatism. (Courtesy J. R. Thompson, Chicago.)

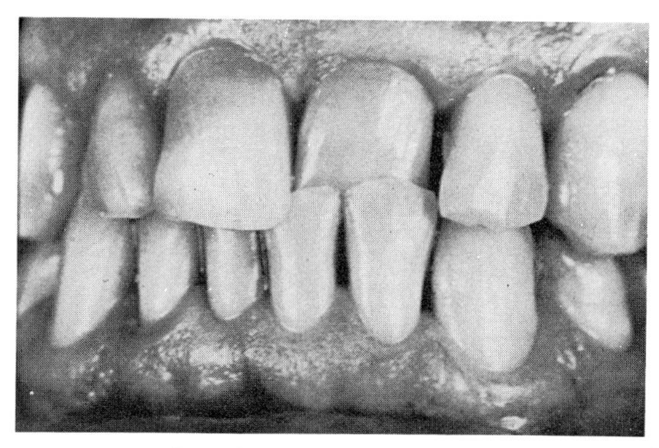

**Fig. 16-7.** Occlusal arrangement of teeth similar to that shown in Fig. 16-6 without recession. (Courtesy H. A. Brayshaw, Denver.)

A seemingly similar occlusal situation without any recession of the gingiva, shown in Fig. 16-7, is of a 20-year-old adult. The incisor in Fig. 16-6, showing some recession, was considerably vestibular to its neighbors, whereas the mandibular incisors in Fig. 16-7 were not so vestibularly malpositioned. In this latter case an adequate thickness of vestibular bone was present and, despite the similarity of the articulative and occlusal situations, no gingival recession occurred. These cases demonstrate the importance of the thickness of the oral and vestibular plates of bone that invest the tooth. Teeth that are malposed toward the oral or toward the vestibular cortical plates tend to have thinner bone in the direction of the malposition. This point is illustrated further in Fig. 16-8. Six anterior teeth are present. The two canines are prominent vestibularly and the gingiva is receded. Two incisors are located more orally and show no recession. The two incisors located vestibularly show recession. The vestibular alveolar plate is thin in the incisor and canine regions. If a tooth becomes inclined vestibularly or orally, the thin alveolar covering bone can easily become resorbed, leaving a bony dehiscence. There is relatively constant spatial relation between the gingival attachment and the alveolar crest in health.[7-9]

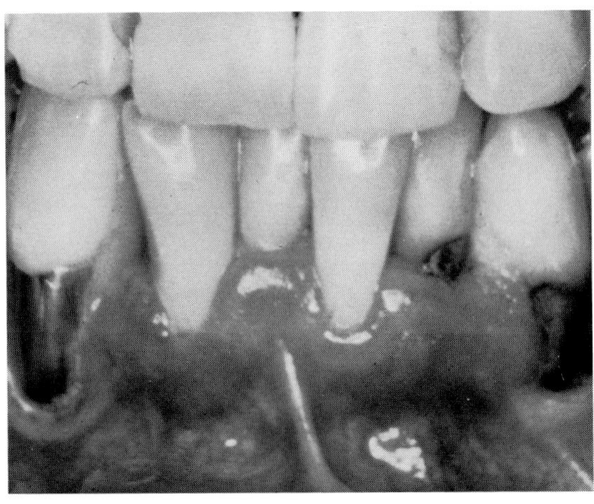

**Fig. 16-8.** Tooth position influences bony anatomy and the position of gingival margins. Teeth that are orally positioned have higher gingival margins (on the vestibular) than do their more vestibularly positioned neighbors.

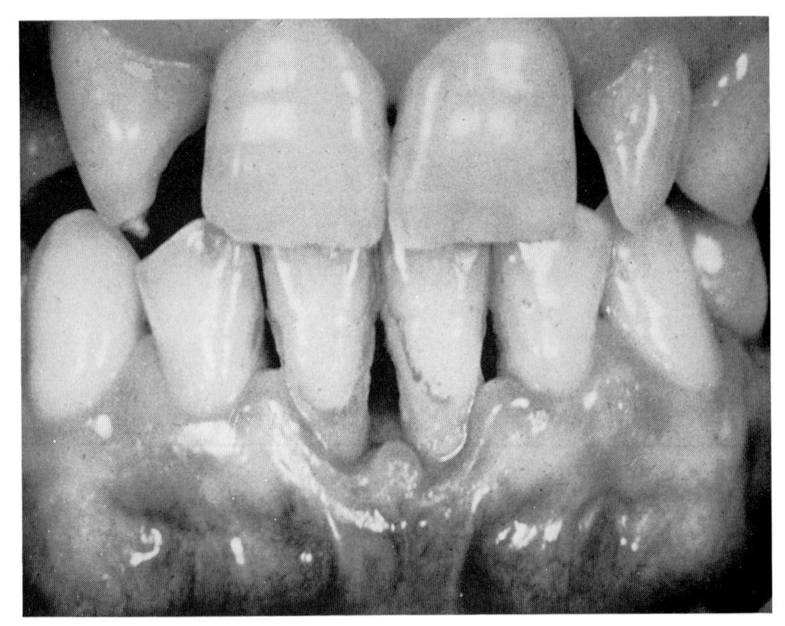

**Fig. 16-9.** Wide vestibular frenum encroaching on the gingival margin and associated with recession.

If the alveolar crest is resorbed, the gingival margin may follow, particularly when the overlying gingiva is thin and finely textured. Contributing extrinsic factors might be injury from brushing or mastication.

Gingival recession may also result from irritation.[10] Some people respond to irritation by recession; some by overgrowth; and some by no change in the position of the gingival margin. A person's response to an irritant may differ according to intrinsic and extrinsic factors. Gingival recession may be caused by

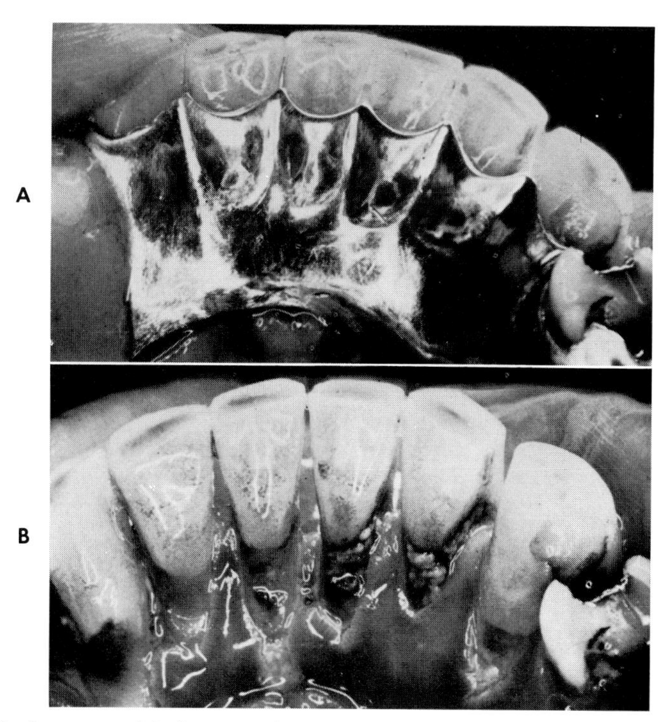


**Fig. 16-10. A,** Lower partial denture with lingual apron from canine to canine. The apron presses against the orogingival margins. **B,** Denture removed. The gingiva has been sheared away by the settling metal apron.

calculus, imperfect margins on dental restorations, clasps, and bars of ill-fitting, removable prostheses. Indicated therapy is to remove the irritants and, when necessary, restore the proper gingival form and tooth-to-tissue relationship.

***Influence of frenum***

The vestibular frenum, as seen in Fig. 16-8, is an anatomic structure that often is blamed for recession of the gingiva, especially on the mandibular central incisors. This factor was not contributory in the patient shown in the illustration. However, a high vestibular frenum might play a part in the recession of the gingiva on some teeth. Such a situation is shown in Fig. 16-9.

Less frequently, considerable recession of the gingiva may be found on the oral surfaces of the teeth. This may occur in the maxillary and occasionally the mandibular incisor area.[11] It may occur with lower partial dentures when a settling lower denture shears away the oral gingiva (Fig. 16-10) or induces a pressure atrophy.

In some instances isolated recession occurs on the oral root of a maxillary molar (Fig. 16-11). Conceivably pressure and friction of the tongue can contribute to atrophy of the gingiva over a prominent root. The bone in this area often is thin, a factor that can predispose to recession of the gingiva.

***Physiologic gingival recession***

Gingival recession may also be an expression of a physiologic process. A gradual recession of the gingival margins has been noted with ageing.[8] This is apparent in older persons who have receded gingival margins, flattened papillae, and widened embrasures in a clinically healthy mouth. Whether ageing is the direct cause of the recession is controversial. This type of recession should be differentiated from the obvious pathologically induced recessions, which tend to be more extensive or locally precipitous.

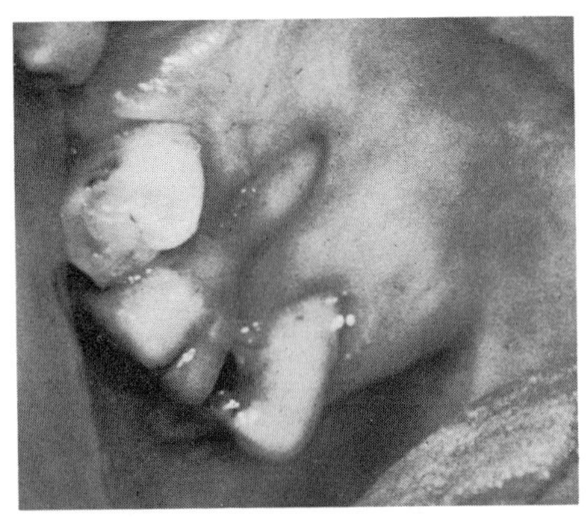

**Fig. 16-11.** Recession on the palatal root of a maxillary molar.

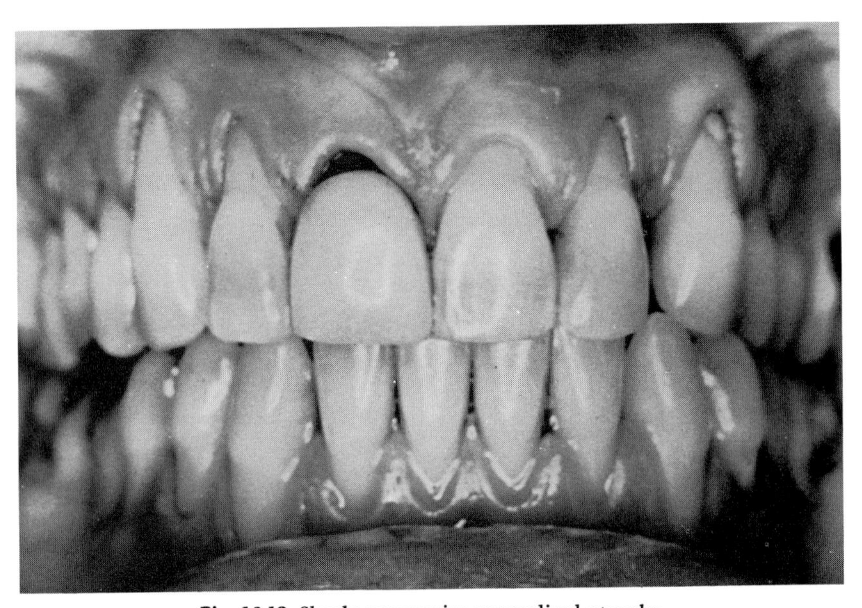

**Fig. 16-12.** Slowly progressive generalized atrophy.

Physiologic gingival recession can be correlated with a decrease in the size of the junctional epithelium,[8,9] which occurs coincident with ageing and probably with an atrophy of alveolar bone. Physiologic bone atrophy may be postulated as an alteration in the delicate balance of continual bone replacement. Theoretically this would involve a decrease in bone replacement rather than an increase in bone destruction. (See discussion of passive exposure in Chapter 4.) Since the distance between the bottom of the junctional epithelium and the alveolar crest remains relatively constant in health, the clinical expression of this process might be gingival recession.

***Outlook*** Some recessions can be arrested; others slowly progress with time despite all measures to arrest them. The patient shown in Fig. 16-12 had been under treatment for about 10 years. The mouth was reasonably clean. Brushing was fairly efficient, careful, and nontraumatic; yet slow progressive recession was evident.

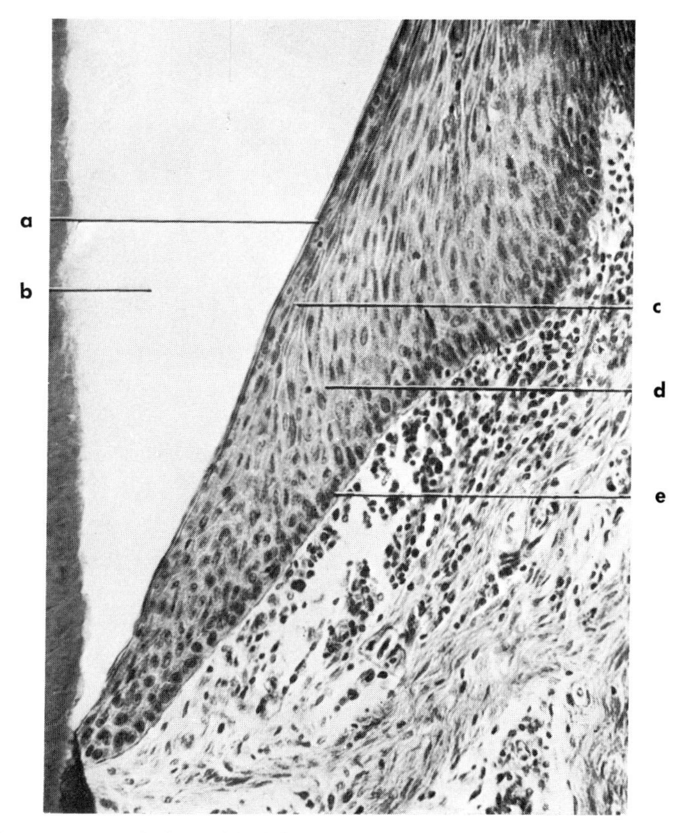


**Fig. 16-13.** Arrangement of the epithelial cells in the junctional epithelium. The innermost layer of cells, *a*, is attached to the surface of the enamel, *b*. The cells are cuboidal in shape. The subjacent layer consists of flattened cells, *c*, running parallel to the surface of the tooth. The central layer, *d*, shows striation possibly brought about by functional stimuli. The basal layer is marked by *e*.

Teeth are rarely lost because of gingival recession alone. Recession may advance during some periods and then slow down and remain stationary for years. In a few cases pockets may complicate the picture and cause tooth loss.

*Therapeutic measures*

The most important therapeutic measure is the institution of proper oral hygiene (correct method of brushing, soft brush with polished rounded bristle tips, dentifrice with the finest scouring agents). No two cases require the same care. The basic principles are (1) meticulous plaque control and (2) frequent careful root planing, both without injury to the gingiva. Restorations may be necessary to create proper deflecting tooth contours for soft tissue protection. Gingival grafts are sometimes used to correct localized defects or to create a new zone of gingiva.

## Periodontal atrophy caused by disuse

*Functional changes*

The periodontal tissues are in functional interdependence with each other. The different tissues react to changes in function by constant adaptation. The free gingival groove at the border of the free and the attached gingivae (Fig. 2-2) may also be an expression of such functional influences.[12] The junctional epithelium shows possibly a functional arrangement in the cells (Fig. 16-13).

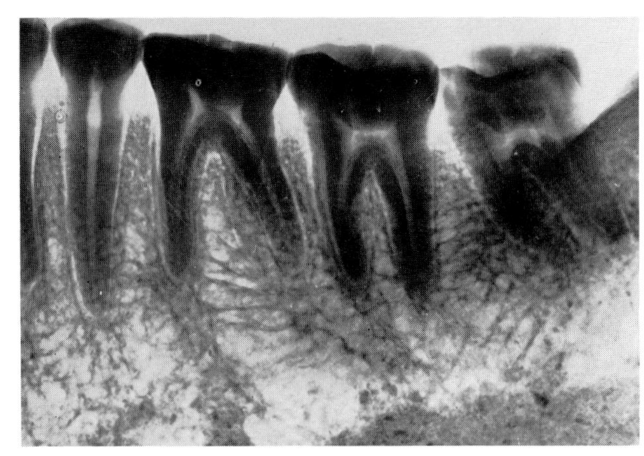

**Fig. 16-14.** Functional arrangement of the bone trabeculae in the cancellous bone of the mandible.

The connective tissue elements of the periodontium—the periodontal ligament, cementum, and alveolar bone—are even more subject to functional influences. Trabeculation in cancellous bone is arranged according to functional stresses,[13] as has been demonstrated often in sections of the head of the femur. The bone trabeculae are arranged to best serve the functional demands to which the bone is exposed. This is true also of the mandible and the maxilla. Fig. 16-14 shows the arrangement of the trabeculae radiating toward the roots as if to form bracing scaffolds or girders. Trabecular patterns also vary from individual to individual.[14] (See discussion on roentgenographic interpretation.)

One can often observe a difference in density of bone on a side of the mandible that is not in occlusal function (Fig. 16-15, *A*) as compared to a side that is in function (Fig. 16-15, *B*). The side that has no occlusal function appears porous, with trabeculae that are thin and sparse and marrow spaces that are wide. The functional side shows more trabeculae that are heavier and have smaller bone marrow spaces.[15]

***Microscopic pathology***

Microscopically disuse atrophy appears as an enlargement of the bone marrow spaces and a disappearance of a large portion of the bone trabeculae. Two maxillary molars are shown in Fig. 16-16. *A* represents a tooth out of function for years, and *B* a tooth in function. The most striking difference is the sparse amount of cancellous bone around one and the good network of bone around the other. In comparison the functioning tooth shows a heavy, short, honeycomb arrangement of the trabeculae. A lamina dura is present around both teeth.

***Osteoporosis***

When osteoporosis develops in disuse atrophy, it takes place by osteoclastic resorption of bone trabeculae in areas of functional inactivity. It involves the entire bone tissue, organic ground substance as well as mineral salts.[16] This fact is important in the diagnosis and treatment of localized osteoporotic areas in the jaw. No amount of medication will benefit if the osteoporosis is caused by lack of function. Proper therapy would be to restore function.

On closer examination of the photographs shown in Fig. 16-16, in higher power, several other differences can be detected between the functioning and the nonfunctioning tooth. Around the functioning tooth the periodontal space is wider and the cementum is thinner than about the nonfunctioning tooth[15] (Fig. 16-17). In addition to these findings, the periodontal ligament is well

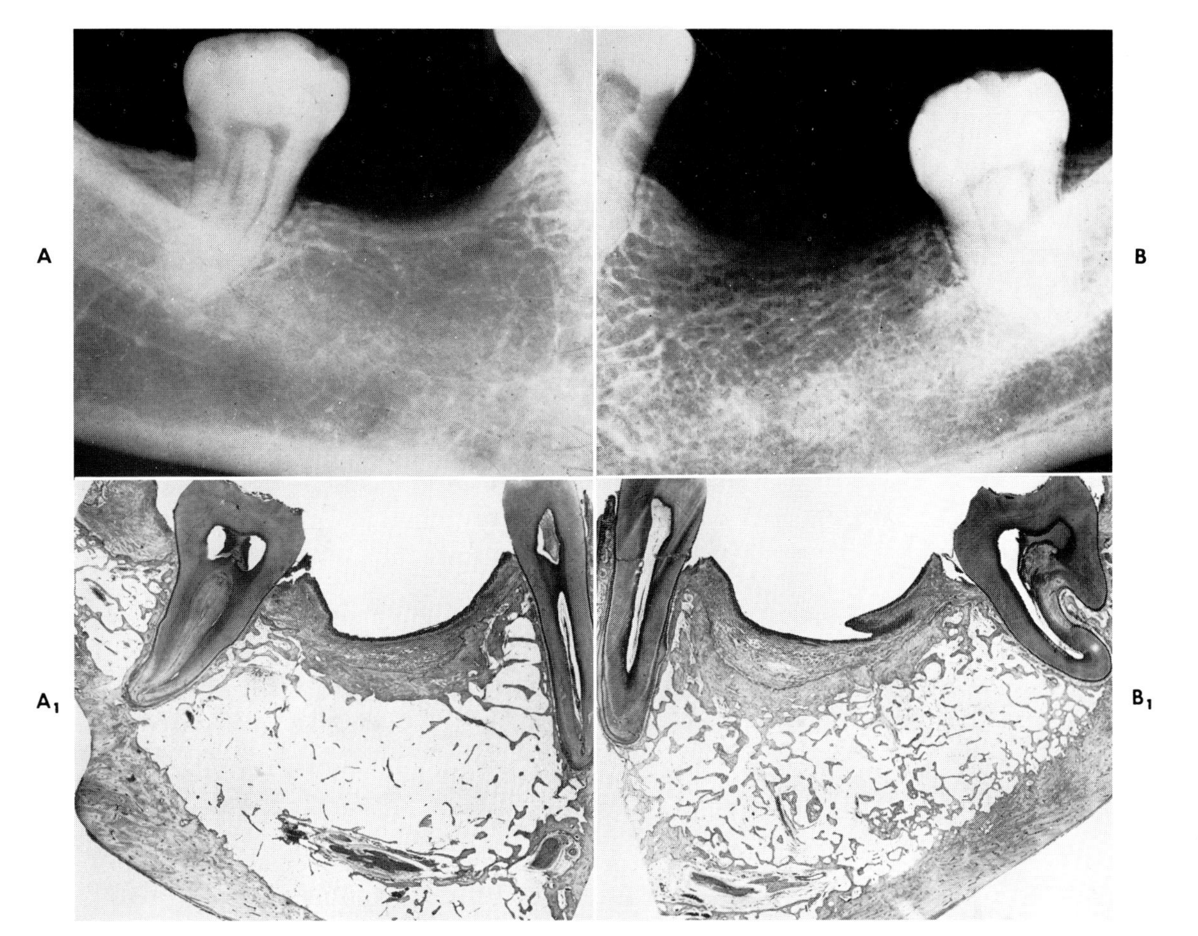


**Fig. 16-15.** Differing density of trabecular arrangement of bone tissue in the mandible as seen in roentgenograms and accompanying microscopic sections. On **A** and **$A_1$**, the side without occlusal function, the bone trabeculae are thin and less densely arranged than those on **B** and **$B_1$**, the side with function. (From the collection of J. P. Weinmann.)

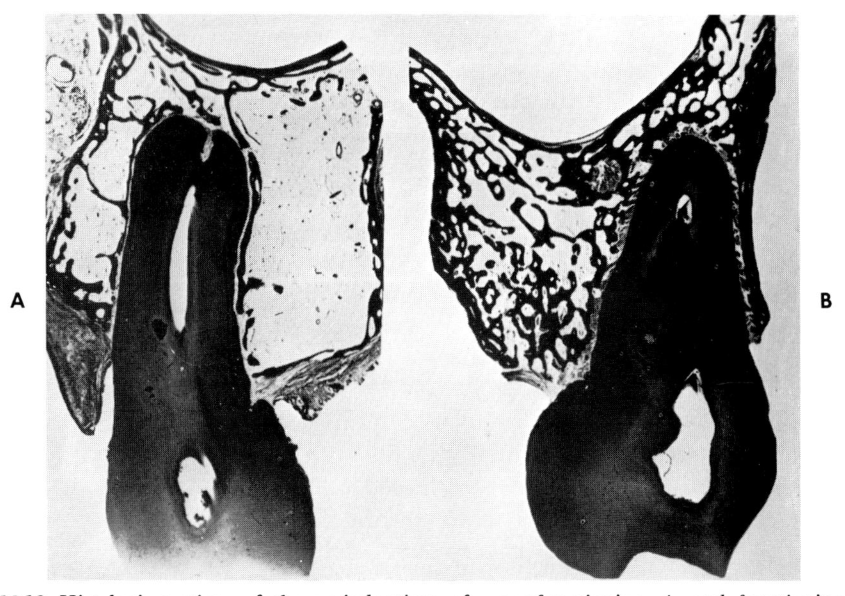


**Fig. 16-16.** Histologic sections of the periodontium of a nonfunctioning, **A,** and functioning, **B,** tooth showing differences in bone trabeculation and width of the periodontal ligament.

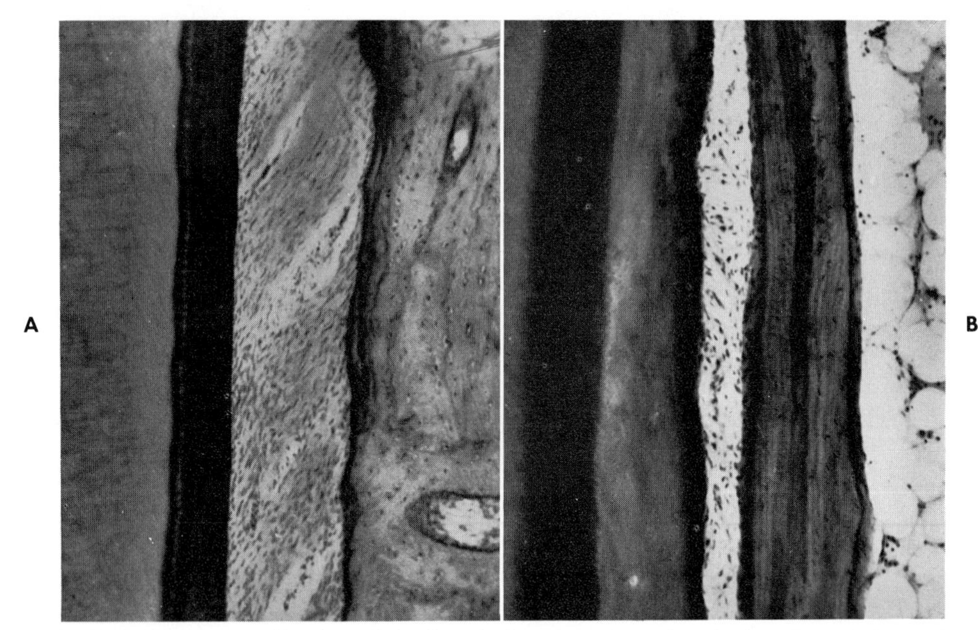


**Fig. 16-17.** Higher magnification of the functioning, **A,** and nonfunctioning, **B,** periodontal ligament. **A,** The periodontal space is wider, the cementum is thinner, and the periodontal ligament is well organized on the side of function. **B,** On the side of disuse, the periodontal space is narrow, cementum is thick, and the periodontal ligament has been replaced by a loose connective tissue. The bone also shows changes caused by the functional influences.

organized in the functioning tooth (*A*). The principal fibers are extended between bone and cementum and enter the hard structures as Sharpey's fibers. In the thin periodontal ligament of the nonfunctioning tooth (*B*), no principal fibers are demonstrable. Only loosely organized connective tissue is present, occupying the periodontal ligament space without any functional orientation. A thick layer of cementum is laid down on the surface of the old cementum, but no fibrous arrangement can be demonstrated in this cementum. The bone is laid down parallel to the surface, layer on layer; and the periodontal side of the lamina dura appears as a thick, dark line, a so-called resting line.

All these changes in the bone, periodontal ligament, and cementum are expressions of a lack of functional stimuli. Such tissues show disuse atrophy.[15-17]

## Prevention

It is obvious that atrophic changes in the periodontium are undesirable; and the aim should be to prevent the development of such pathologic conditions. Prevention consists of replacing missing or lost teeth at the earliest time possible. Replacement of missing teeth in a dentition where teeth have been lost years previously will lead to changes in the functional requirements of the entire dentition. These changes will be radical, especially in those areas that are directly affected—the teeth that are to be used as abutments and teeth that have been without occlusal function.

Can teeth with such atrophic periodontal tissues withstand the stresses that occur during occlusal function? A periodontal ligament, as shown in Fig. 16-17, *B,* without the principal fibers, cannot suddenly support occlusal forces without difficulty. The narrow periodontal space does not permit the necessary movement

**Table 16-1.** Functional changes in supporting tissues of the teeth (tissue adaptation)

| Tooth | Gingiva | Bone | Cementum | Periodontal ligament |
|---|---|---|---|---|
| Functioning | Normal epithelial surface | Well-defined patterns of trabeculation corresponding to functional demands | Thinner cementum | Definite arrangement of principal fiber bundles according to functional demands<br>Width normal, 0.1-0.25 mm. |
| Nonfunctioning | Thinner epithelium, less keratinization | Localized sparse bone trabeculation | Thicker cementum | Principal fiber bundles reduced or absent, loose connective tissue, no functional orientation of fibers<br>Width narrower, 0.06-0.1 mm. |

of a functioning tooth. The periodontal tissues must be rebuilt in accord with the new functional demands. This rebuilding process will not come about without subjective symptoms. The periodontal ligament with its blood vessels and nerve fibers will become compressed, leading to minute hemorrhages. The teeth may become sensitive to percussion or to occlusal use. In due time, by bone resorption, the periodontal space will resume a normal width in response to function. New fibers of the periodontal ligament will be laid down oriented in the direction of the functional force as they are produced, and pain and sensitivity may disappear. According to experience this process may take between 4 and 6 weeks. However, to establish the functional reorientation of the supporting alveolar bone may require considerably more time. New trabeculae have to be formed and oriented in accordance with the altered function. This process might take 3 to 6 months. The dentist who restores function to a tooth that has not been in function for a long time should forewarn the patient of possible temporary discomfort.

All these tissue changes are made possible by the functional adaptability of the periodontium (Table 16-1). This phase of the physiology of the periodontium will be enlarged upon in the chapter dealing with problems of occlusion (Chapter 36).

## HYPERPLASTIC AND HYPERTROPHIC PERIODONTAL CONDITIONS

Hyperplasia is the increase in size of an organ or its parts. It is characterized by an increase in the number of cellular elements of the organ and does not serve a functional purpose. Hyperplasia should be differentiated from hypertrophy, which is an overgrowth resulting from the increase in size of the cellular elements of an organ in response to increased function. The overgrowth (enlargement) of the gingiva is a hyperplasia. There is no gingival hypertrophy. Other structures of the periodontium may experience hypertrophy in response to an increase in functional demand. The cementum may overgrow, with formation of

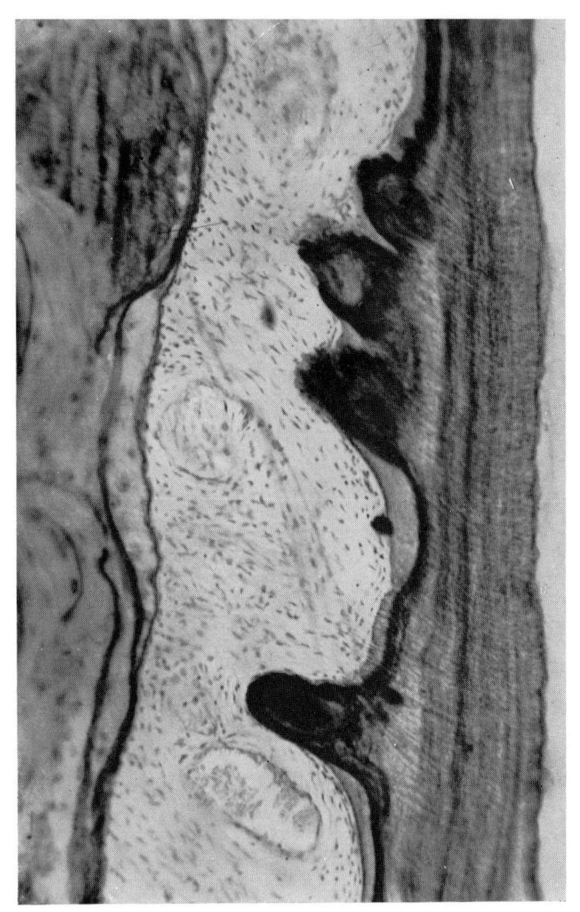

**Fig. 16-18.** Spikelike cemental overgrowth caused by increased function of a tooth (hypertrophy).

spurs, resulting from an increase in function (Fig. 16-18). This may be termed cemental hypertrophy. The periodontal ligament may become elongated by increased function. The supporting alveolar bone may become more heavily trabeculated because of functional stimuli. Microscopically (Fig. 16-19) formation of new bone may be observed surrounding the alveolar bone, increasing its thickness because of increased functional influences. This may be termed periodontal hypertrophy. The choice of the term hypertrophy or hyperplasia will depend on which definition of the word is regarded as more important—the functional or the structural. In other words, any increase in the thickness of cementum may be caused by an increase in the number of its elements (hyperplasia), as in the nonfunctioning tooth (Fig. 16-17), or by increased function (hypertrophy) (Fig. 16-18). (See discussion of cementum in Chapter 3.)

## Gingival hyperplasia

Gingival hyperplasia is an overgrowth caused by an increase in the fibrous tissue elements of the gingiva, a fibrous hyperplasia. It is not an inflammatory condition, although we must realize that hyperplasia and inflammation of the gingiva most often occur concurrently. Both cause gingival enlargement. Only their respective contributions to the gingival enlargement vary.

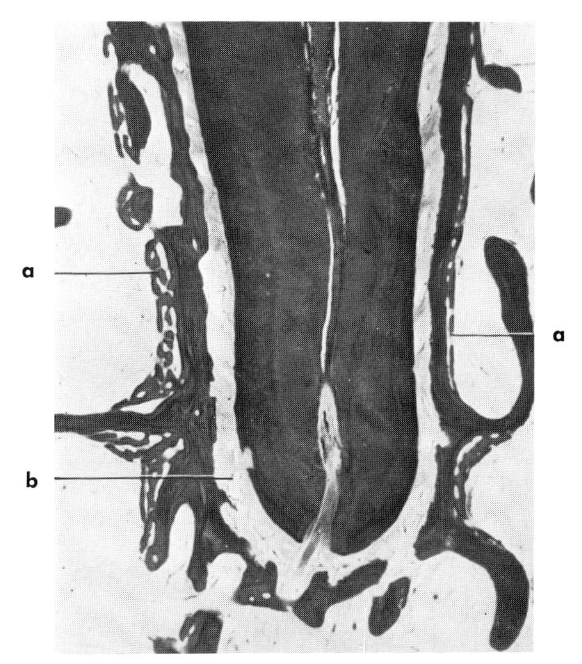


**Fig. 16-19.** Microscopic specimen showing formation of new bone, *a,* around the alveolar bone proper, increasing bone thickness by increased functional demands. Widening of the apical periodontal ligament, *b,* has occurred by bone resorption caused by increased functional influences.

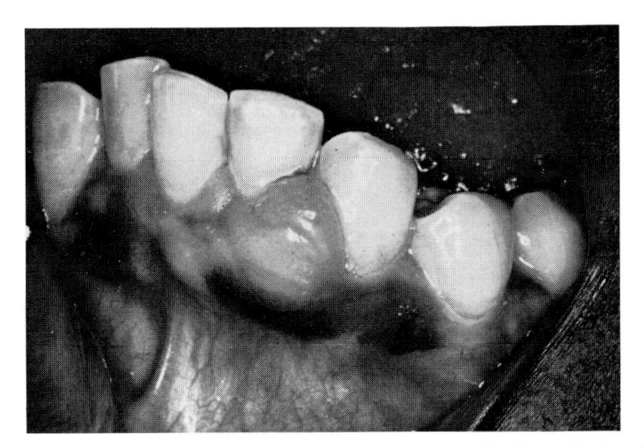

**Fig 16-20.** Localized, gingival hyperplasia. (Courtesy F. Howell, San Diego.)

***Localized hyperplasia***

Gingival hyperplasia may occur as a localized overgrowth, limited to a certain area (Fig. 16-20). The etiology of such localized fibromas is unknown. Local irritation associated with a constitutional factor may be responsible for their development. Microscopically such overgrowths may be characterized by an increase in the fibrous as well as the cellular elements. Calcification and ossification may take place.*[18]

*Another noninflammatory localized gingival enlargement, rare in the dentate patient, is the carcinoma of the gingiva.

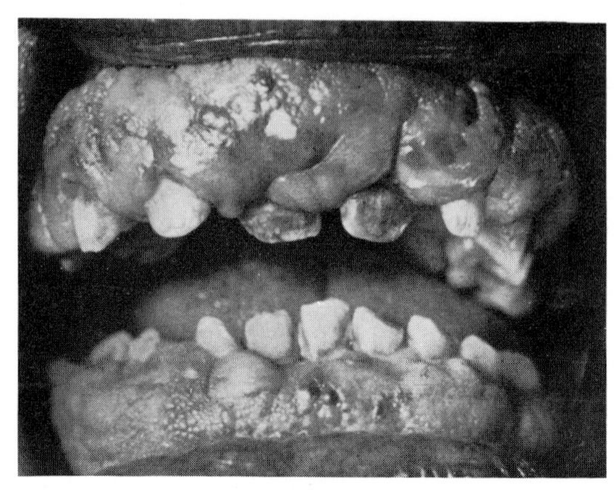

**Fig. 16-21.** Idiopathic gingival hyperplasia (fibromatosis). (Courtesy O. J. Shaffer, El Paso.)

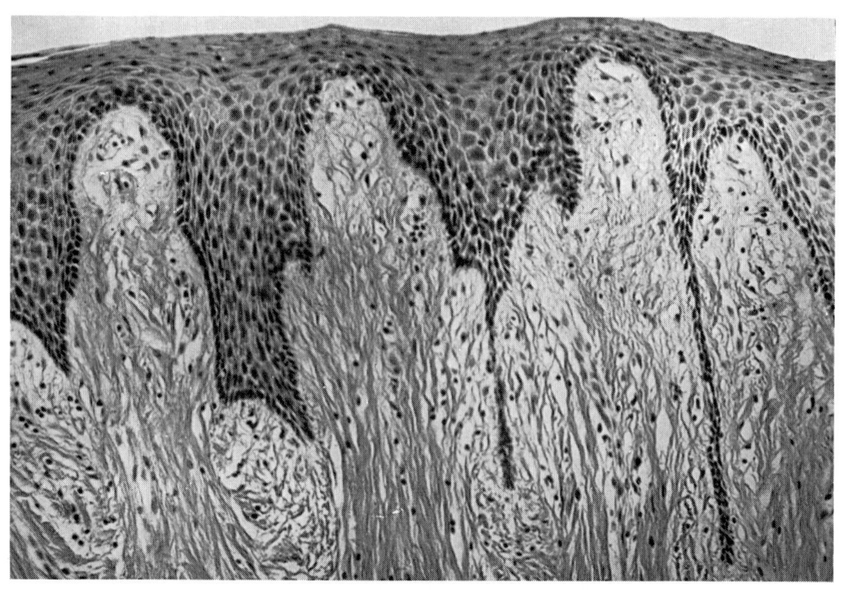

**Fig. 16-22.** Microscopic specimen of gingival hyperplasia showing extensive overgrowth of the fiber bundles with little inflammatory reaction.

Indicated therapy is the surgical removal and elimination of the particular local irritating factor. The prognosis is favorable, although these lesions sometimes recur. Complete removal and elimination of the local exciting factor (cavities, open contacts) is probably the only way to avoid this recurrence.

***Idiopathic generalized hyperplasia (fibromatosis)***

Generalized fibrous hyperplasia is a rare disease. It affects young persons and may be quite extensive.[19] A typical case is shown in Fig. 16-21, that of a 24-year-old man. The gingival tissues were removed surgically, all teeth were extracted, and an alveolectomy was performed. The microscopic examination revealed an increase in fibrous tissue elements (Fig. 16-22) with accompanying atrophic changes in the surface epithelium.[20] No etiologic factor could be established.

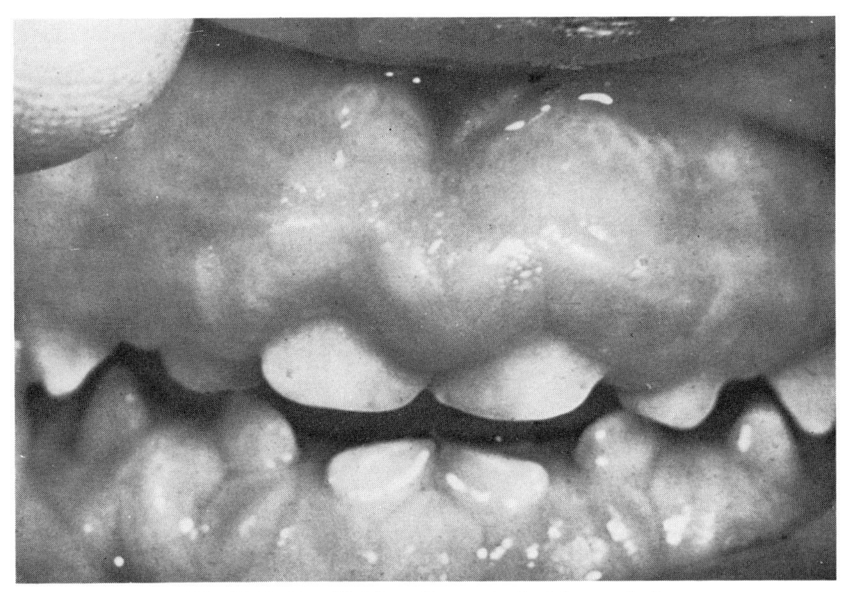

**Fig. 16-23.** Familial hereditary gingival hyperplasia.

A congenital constitutional factor frequently plays a major role, as shown in many reports of multiple occurrences in children of one family.[21-23] Such a case is reported in a family of eight children six of whom had fibrous hyperplasia. Fig. 16-23 shows the gingival condition of one of the children, who still had some of his primary teeth. The father had had a similar condition in childhood. He had had a gingivectomy at the age of 15, but the overgrowth had recurred. Finally, all his teeth were extracted, and dentures made. No systemic disease could be found in any member of this family.

Therapeutic judgment will govern the treatment for each specific case. The gingival enlargement has a tendency to recur after excision (gingivectomy) but not after extraction. Gingival fibromatosis thus has some semblance to keloid formation. However, these patients do not suffer from generalized keloids. A few are afflicted with idiopathic generalized gingival hyperplasia and show hirsutism and mental underdevelopment.[24]

Somewhere in between localized and generalized hyperplasia are cases of enormously enlarged tuberosities that extend orally, sometimes to the palatal midline, and mesially to the premolar area[25] (Fig. 16-24). The histologic makeup of these cases resembles that of gingival fibromatosis.

***Hyperplasia in diphenylhydantoin therapy***

Administration of diphenylhydantoin sodium (Dilantin, Epinutin) in the treatment of epilepsy is frequently followed by a hyperplastic and inflammatory overgrowth of the gingiva.[25-33] Such overgrowth has a tendency to disappear when the drug is discontinued. Not all patients taking diphenylhydantoin develop gingival hyperplasia.[31] Different investigators have reported widely differing incidences of hyperplasia in epileptic patients treated with diphenylhydantoin. The morbidity figure averaged from all published studies is about 40%.[30] The tendency toward hyperplasia varies considerably in amount and location. The hyperplasia is more pronounced about the anterior teeth and is more extensive on the vestibular than on the oral surfaces; it is also greater in the

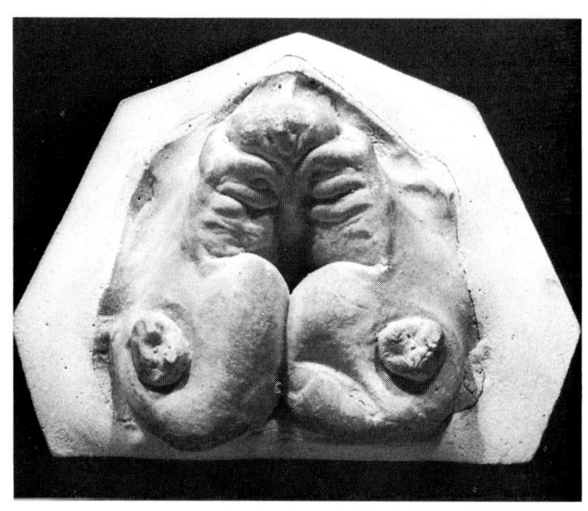

**Fig. 16-24.** Enormously enlarged tuberosities. (Courtesy H. Mathis, West Berlin.)

upper than the lower jaw. The overgrowth is probably more pronounced the greater the dosage.[29] Local etiologic factors may influence the amount and location of the enlargement.[32,33] About 1 to 1½ months are necessary for a patient on this medication to show typical signs of hyperplasia (latency period).[30]

The clinical picture of diphenylhydantoin-induced hyperplasia is somewhat different from that of idiopathic fibrous hyperplasia. The administration of diphenylhydantoin often leads to overgrowth of the papillae, leaving the margin unaffected or less affected (Fig. 16-25, *A*). Signs of inflammation are almost always present.

***Microscopic pathology***

The microscopic picture of diphenylhydantoin-induced hyperplasia also differs somewhat from that of idiopathic fibrous hyperplasia. In addition to an increase in the fibrous tissue elements,[32] there is a proliferative tendency in the epithelium (Fig. 16-25, *B*) and an increased accumulation of inflammatory cells.

The biologic mechanism for the gingival overgrowth in diphenylhydantoin therapy is not fully known. Local tissue chemistry is altered by this drug. Increased strength of scars in experimental animals on diphenylhydantoin has been demonstrated.[33] Diphenylhydantoin may be a fibroblastic stimulant[34] or cause interference with collagenolysis during turnover, leading to a piling up of collagen. There is increased diphenylhydantoin content in the saliva of patients on this therapy.[35] The fact that overgrowth can be prevented or minimized in some cases by good oral hygiene may indicate that as in other systemic conditions (pregnancy, diabetes, etc.), two elements must interact to produce periodontal disease—a systemic factor and a local triggering stimulus.

***Supplemental therapy***

If diphenylhydantoin therapy is instituted, some gingival hyperplasia is likely to occur; but with excellent oral hygiene the extent of the overgrowth can be kept to a minimum or avoided.[36] At the time of surgery and immediately thereafter, substitution for diphenylhydantoin may be made to avoid the recurrence of gingival enlargement during healing. Unfortunately many persons needing diphenylhydantoin therapy are not capable of following instructions for rigorous home physiotherapy. Some have a physical disability and a few are mentally retarded. At times the physician may be able to substitute other drugs (Mesantoin, Mysoline) that can control convulsions and do not induce hyper-

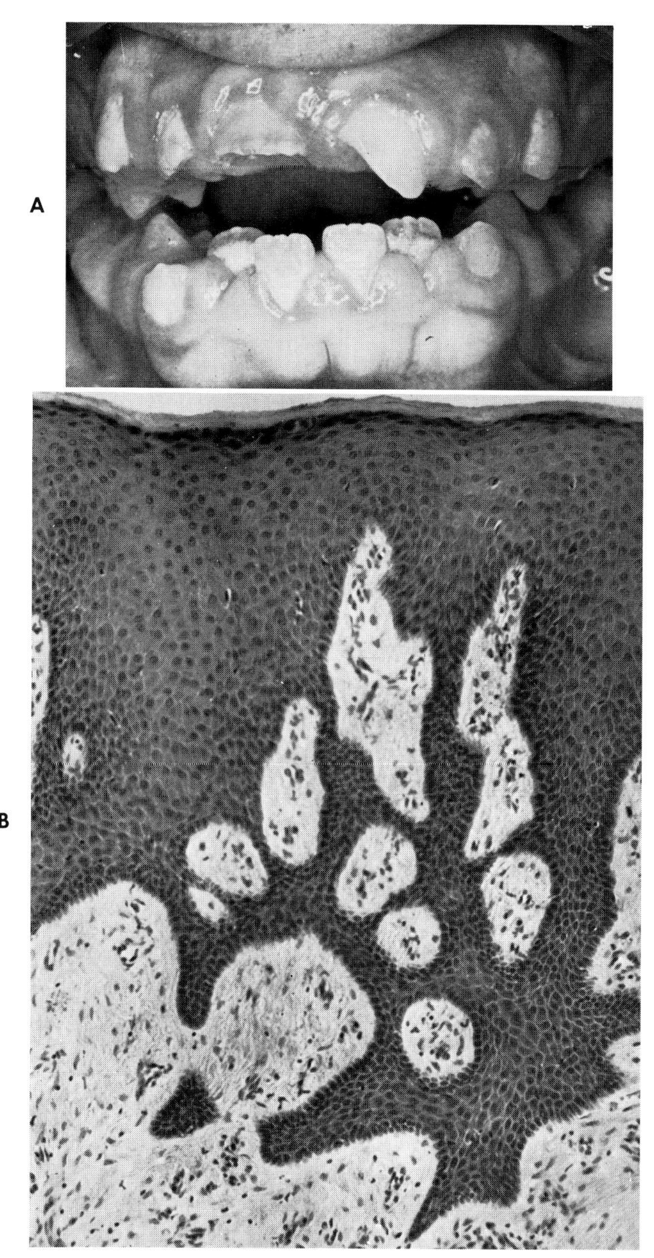


**Fig. 16-25. A,** Diphenylhydantoin-induced hyperplasia in a child. Note the migration of teeth resulting from the proliferation of dense connective tissue. The gingiva has become so enlarged that the greater portion of the crowns has become submerged. **B,** Gingival biopsy of diphenylhydantoin-induced hyperplasia. The section is characterized by overgrowth of the epithelium with accompanying inflammatory reaction and fibrous overgrowth. (**A** courtesy J. M. Nabers, Wichita Falls.)

plasia. At other times the dosage of diphenylhydantoin can be reduced by combinations with other drugs.[32,37,38] Since such substitution is sometimes impossible, however, it should be done only at the discretion of the attending neurologist. Despite the occurrence of gingival hyperplasia, diphenylhydantoin still remains the treatment of choice for grand mal; and although there is no effective drug therapy for the treatment of the gingival enlargement in diphenylhydantoin therapy, a program of diligent oral hygiene should be instituted to prevent or minimize the development of hyperplasia. Where overgrowth is already present, the following measures may be taken:

1. Institution of rigid oral hygiene practices
2. Application of pressure devices[39]
3. Gingivectomy-gingivoplasty when overgrowth is extensive

Gingival enlargement may be viewed as a spectrum extending from idiopathic gingival hyperplasia (fibromatosis), in which inflammatory elements are absent, to diphenylhydantoin hyperplasia, with its characteristic preponderance of hyperplastic over inflammatory elements, to hyperplastic inflammation, seen mainly in juvenile mouth breathers, to gingivitis in pregnancy, in which there is an almost complete lack of fibrous elements and an overwhelming predominance of inflammatory elements. These last two conditions are discussed in Chapter 14. The student may have difficulty understanding the difference between gingival hyperplasia and hyperplastic gingivitis. *Gingival hyperplasia,* which has been discussed in this chapter, is caused mainly by an increase in the number of local cellular elements and intercellular fibers. The enlargement in *hyperplastic gingivitis* is mainly the result of inflammation. The lesions can frequently be differentiated by their clinical appearance. When we deal with a lesion that is primarily hyperplastic, the enlarged gingiva will be pale and hard because the basis for the enlargement is the increase in fibrous connective tissue. When the gingival enlargement is primarily inflammatory, the gingiva will be red or bluish red and cyanotic. The consistency will be soft because the enlargement is due primarily to the presence of inflammatory elements and blood vessels. This latter condition has been discussed in Chapter 4.

### Cemental hypertrophy

Hypercementosis is most often seen in molars and premolars and is characterized by a bulbous or knoblike root form in roentgenograms. Such teeth gain in strength through the increase of root surface area. Presumably the overgrowth is initiated by functional stimuli and would be considered a hypertrophy. The increase in cementum due to regular apposition (Chapter 4) is a normal concomitant of ageing. The fusion of calcospherites or calcified epithelial rests with cementum, resulting in irregular protrusions, is also a characteristic of ageing.

## Periodontosis

Periodontosis is an infrequently seen disease of the periodontium characterized by a pattern of rapid, vertical loss of alveolar bone around the permanent first molars and incisors. Its etiology and pathology are not known. The rapidity and severity of its destruction seem out of proportion to local (extrinsic) factors.[1] The disease affects adolescents who are healthy otherwise, and it may be discovered in early adulthood. Since its etiology and pathology are unknown, for practical purposes the consistency of its clinical characteristics and incidence is diagnostic. Although the consistent finding of molar-incisor bone loss is pathognomonic in affected juveniles, other teeth may be affected.

*History*

The concept and understanding of periodontosis have undergone some changes in the 50 years since Gottlieb described the picture of "diffuse atrophy."[2,3] He envisioned a disease localized initially in the deeper periodontium and only secondarily involving the marginal periodontium. The name periodontosis was given to this condition in 1952 by Orban and Weinmann,[4] but the description of the disease had changed in the intervening period so as to involve primary changes in the marginal periodontium. Another basic concept of the present meaning of periodontosis was proposed by Wannenmacher in 1938.[5] He first described the molar-incisor type of juvenile periodontal disease, later reported in the United States by Miller.[6] The fusion of these two views has yielded today's concept of juvenile essential periodontosis.[7]

## Clinical features

Periodontosis is rarely diagnosed in its incipiency because at that time there are few subjective and objective symptoms. Early diagnosis is sometimes made fortuitously on examination of routine oral roentgenograms. In these cases the gingiva is largely free of gross clinical signs of inflammation. Late clinical features of the disease are migration of teeth, with the formation of diastemas, and elongation of teeth. By the time the patient seeks help, there usually are deep pockets present.

Several distinctive features of this disease justify its classification as a discrete clinical entity separate from periodontitis[8]:

1. Age of onset
2. Sex ratio
3. Familial tendencies
4. Lack of commensurate relationship between local (extrinsic) etiologic factors and severity of response (deep periodontal destruction)
5. Distinctive roentgenographic pattern of alveolar bone loss (Figs. 16-26 and 16-27)
6. Rate of progression

*Age of onset*

The onset of periodontosis is insidious and occurs sometime during the circumpubertal period, between the ages 11 and 13 years. Alveolar bone appears to develop normally, with the normal eruption of the teeth, and only subsequently undergoes resorptive changes. Thus the alveolar bone loss does not seem in most cases to be due to a developmental or congenital defect of the bone.

*Sex ratio*

Periodontosis affects more women than men[4]; a ratio of 3:1 (females to males) has been reported.[8,17]

*Familial tendencies*

There are familial tendencies in periodontosis.[8,17,18] It occurs in identical twins, parents and offspring, siblings, first cousins, and uncles and nephews. It tends to follow the maternal side of the line.

Another piece of evidence in favor of familial tendencies is the mirrorlike loss of attachment (Fig. 16-28) seen in some cases in which molars have been extracted.[19] Still another piece of evidence is the association with the prevalence of blood group B when compared with the known distribution of blood types in the population.[20] Such mirrorlike loss is likely due to some developmental defect and may be indicative of genetic involvement or predisposition.

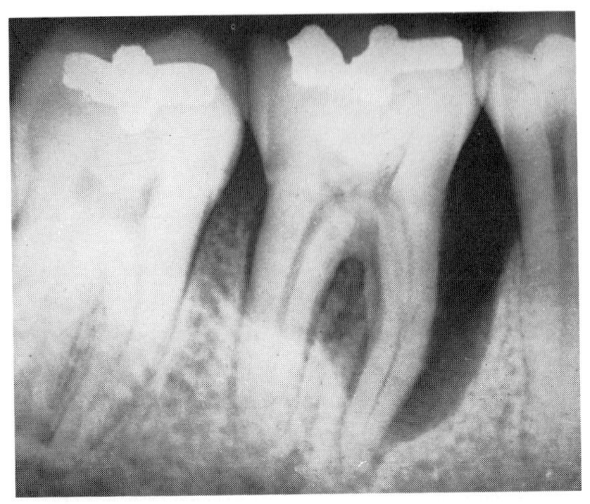

**Fig. 16-26.** Vertical type of bone resorption in periodontosis.

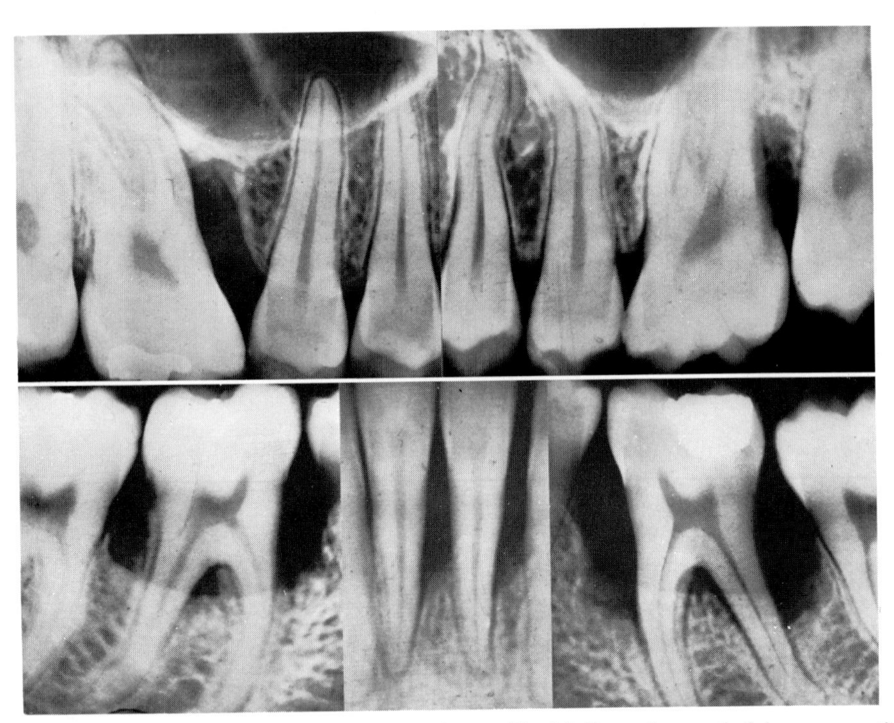

**Fig. 16-27.** Roentgenograms of the teeth of a 15-year-old girl. Extensive vertical bone resorption has occurred in the region of the mandibular first molars and incisors. (Courtesy C. L. Foss, San Diego.)

***Severity of response***

As stated at the beginning of the discussion of periodontosis, the rapidity and severity of the disease process seem out of proportion to local (extrinsic) factors.

***Distinctive roentgenographic pattern***

Contrary to certain oral manifestations in intrinsic diseases (e.g., Down's syndrome, cyclic neutropenia, hypophosphatasia, Papillon-Lefevre syndrome), the primary teeth in periodontosis are not affected and are not prematurely exfoliated. This disease seems to be entirely of the permanent dentition.

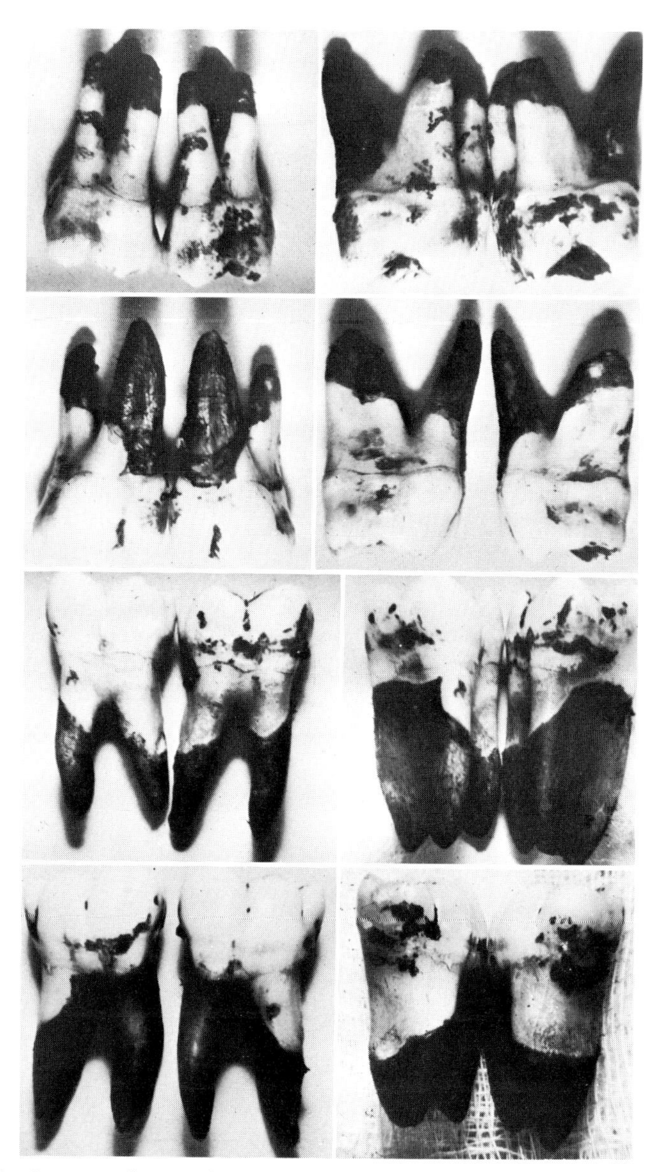

**Fig. 16-28.** Stained extracted teeth from two cases of periodontosis exhibiting a mirror-image pathologic condition. (From Kaslick, R. S., and Chasens, A. I.: Oral Surg. **25**:327, 1968.)

*Rate of progression*

Unlike periodontitis, which progresses at a slow rate, periodontosis progresses rapidly. The present available roentgenographic evidence, which admittedly is scanty, indicates that an affected tooth can lose approximately three fourths of its alveolar bone about one or more of its involved root surfaces in a period of 5 years or less from the time that the disease is first noted roentgenographically. This would be at least three to four times the rate of progression for periodontitis.

## Case reports

A typical first case is of a 17-year-old Negro girl (Fig. 16-29, *A*). Wide diastemas had appeared between the incisors, which were close together a few

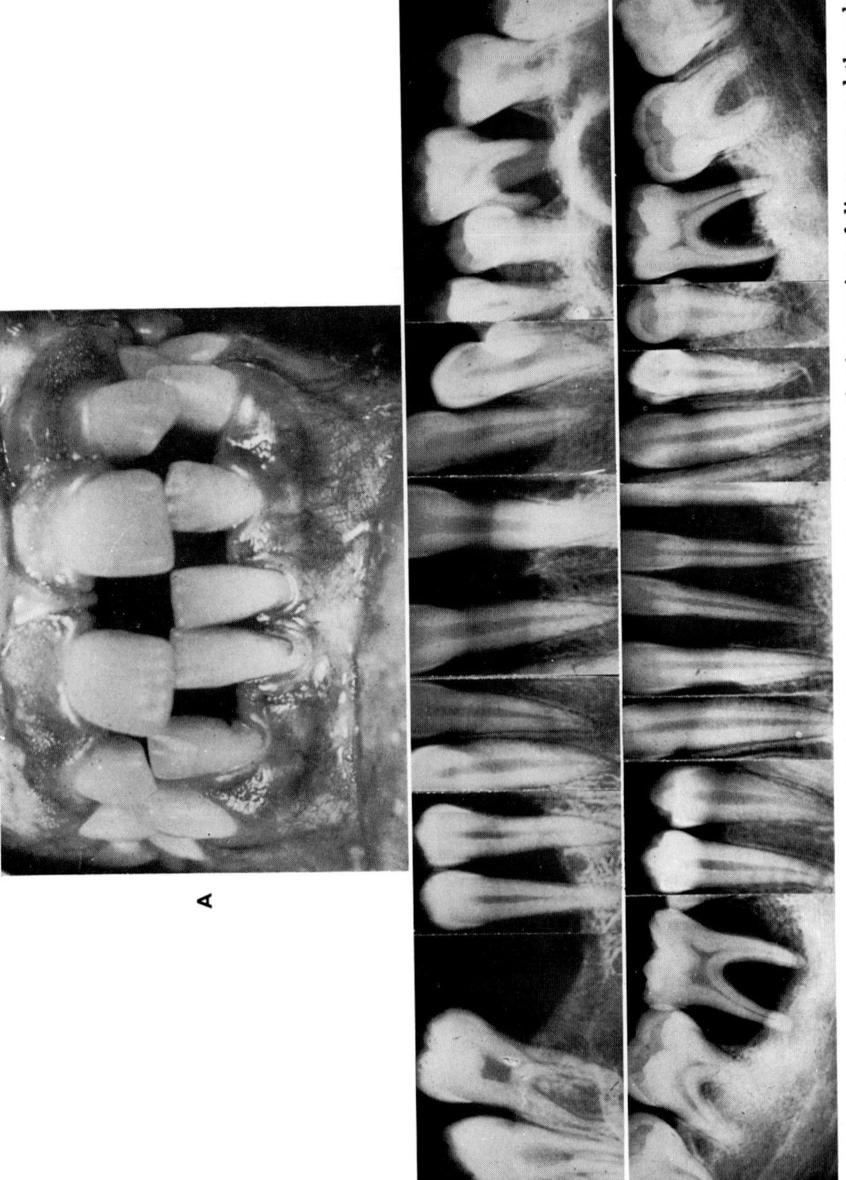


**Fig. 16-29. A,** Periodontitis in a 17-year-old girl. Note the migration of the teeth, the opening of diastemas, and the relative lack of inflammation. **B,** Roentgenograms of the same patient showing extensive bone destruction characteristic of periodontosis, which affects mainly the first molars and incisors.

years before. The gingiva was rather pale and without sign of inflammation. The roentgenograms (Fig. 16-29, *B*) revealed extremely severe bone loss, especially in the region of the incisors and first molars. One first molar had been lost a week prior to the consultation. Medical history was noncontributory. The patient was sent to a research hospital, and extensive examination failed to reveal any pertinent systemic factors.

A similar but not so extensive case is shown in the roentgenograms in Fig. 16-27. This case is of a 15-year-old white girl. Resorption of bone was limited to the four first mandibular molars and to two mandibular incisors. Medical history was also noncontributory.

### Prevalence

Some periodontists deny the existence of periodontosis[12]; and therefore a prevalence of zero is reported.[9] However, those who contend that periodontosis is a definable disease report a wide variation in its incidence.[8,13,14] These differences in prevalence may be due to the following circumstances: (1) inclusion in some studies of primary teeth and (2) inclusion in other studies of older age groups. Some differences are due to the fact that the studies were conducted in different parts of the world and with different populations or with varying standards for recognition and hence different populations and different diagnostic yardsticks. In yet other studies and in the previous editions of this text, cases of oral manifestations of systemic diseases were included but are not now considered in this category.

In the context of a definition of periodontosis that has become narrower than heretofore, the incidence in the United States among white people seems to be somewhat in excess of 0.1%.[8] Among American Indians the prevalence is higher,[8,17] and there may be differences in the incidence in other populations.[11,16]

### Etiology

The gingiva most frequently is almost normal in appearance, with a physiologic color and contour (at least in the early stages). In such very early stages therefore the diagnosis is often made fortuitously as a result of routine dental examination in which dental roentgenograms are used. When bone loss is evident roentgenographically, examination with the aid of a periodontal probe will reveal the presence of a periodontal pocket in such an area, even though the gingiva may have a near normal appearance. Gross deposits of subgingival calculus are uncommon in these patients, even when pockets extend almost to the apices. Plaque, however, is present whether the teeth are examined in the mouth with the aid of an explorer or visually after the affected teeth have been extracted because they were hopelessly involved. After extraction, when such teeth are decalcified, plaque will be seen under the microscope adhering to the root surfaces. In patients whose oral hygiene is poor and who have clinically obvious plaque and supragingival calculus, clinical gingival inflammation is more evident. Some signs of inflammation are also commonly seen in advanced cases. In the initial stages, however, this is not the rule, which is not to say that local etiologic factors are either absent or unimportant. The contrary is true. For example, there are cases with poor proximal contacts, permitting food impaction; and occlusal problems such as malalignment of the posterior teeth or some obvious premature contacts or interferences are occasionally seen.

In the vast majority of cases of periodontosis, however, the clinical impression remains that the extent of periodontal destruction is vastly out of proportion to the amount of demonstrable irritation. Hypothesizing on the etiology of this disease, Gottlieb considered continuous cementum formation to be the most important biologic feature of the periodontium and called periodontosis "deep cementopathia."[21] The senescence of certain areas of cementum may deny further attachment to the principal fibers and permit the apical progression of attachment epithelium. Studies have also shown that the cementum mantle is thinner in periodontally diseased teeth[22,23] and that the downward growth of the junctional epithelium is stopped at least temporarily if a barrier of hypercementosis or cementoid is present. Gottlieb's second contention—that periodontosis is a disease of eruption—also deserves consideration. Sometimes the symptoms of this disease are pathologic migration, sometimes rotation and elongation. The involved tooth or teeth, however, are prevented by their neighbors and chiefly by their antagonists from moving rapidly. An area of senescent cementum that the body wishes to exfoliate must be placed outside the epithelial covering, sometimes without the active movement of the tooth. In some cases the formation of infrabony defects is possibly the result of a frustration of exfoliation.

## Roentgenographic findings

Vertical bone destruction about the first molars and one or more incisor teeth in an otherwise healthy adolescent is a diagnostic sign of periodontosis. The pattern of bone loss in the well-established case (Fig. 16-26) is usually described as an arc-shaped loss of alveolar bone extending from the distal surface of the second premolar to the mesial surface of the second molar. The bone loss in the posterior regions occurs bilaterally, and the right and left sides are generally mirror images of each other. Whereas this is the so-called classical description, actually the patterns of bone loss are much more protean in nature. For example, in some instances the incisors are not involved but only the first molars are. At the onset the mesial surface of the first molar is most often affected. There are cases, however, in which the distal surface is involved. The degree and morphology of the bone loss are generally dependent on whether the disease is diagnosed in an early or an advanced stage. Only one proximal surface of the first molar in each arch may be initially involved. As the disease progresses, the other proximal surfaces usually become affected until all four first molars assume their classical mirror-image appearance. Since the vestibular and oral plates of alveolar bone are the last to resorb, the bifurcation areas of the molar teeth generally show radiolucencies only as a late manifestation of the disease.

As the disease progresses, the first molar and incisors tend to develop open proximal contacts. In late stages formation of diastemas, rotation, and elongation of individual teeth are seen. Migration always occurs away from the side of the pocket. Occasionally the disease involves teeth other than the first molars and incisors. This is particularly true in the advanced stages. On the other hand, single tooth involvement should not be classed as periodontosis because of the multiplicity of factors that may cause breakdown about a single tooth.[24]

In rare instances alveolar bone does not seem to be present on the coronal part of the root of the first molar but seems to resorb immediately after having formed (Fig. 16-30, *A* and *B*). Note the progression of bone destruction as illustrated in Fig. 16-30, *C*, which has occurred over a 2-year period.[13]

***Dental anatomy***

In some cases short or slender roots have been noted with periodontosis. These roots, disproportionate to the crown size, show a crown-to-root ratio of about 1:1 instead of the more usual 1:1½.

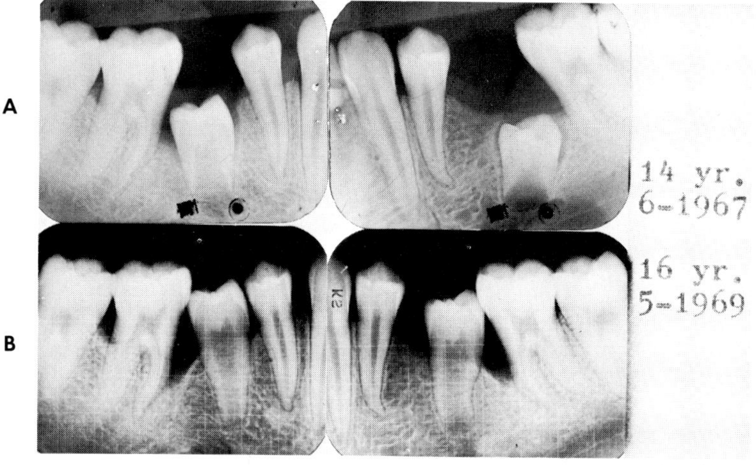


*Continued.*

**Fig. 16-30. A,** Roentgenograms (June 1967) of a 14-year-old girl with periodontosis. (Black marks are artifacts.) Note the bone loss in the upper and lower incisor areas and particularly the low level of alveolar bone at the mesial side of the first molar bilaterally prior to eruption of the second premolar. **B,** Same patient, May 1969. The defects in the incisor areas have progressed. In the molar areas the defects now appear as typical vertical alveolar resorptions. No bone has been lost in the area during the time between the two roentgenograms. Rather new bone has been added through the eruption of the second premolar.

Another associated but rarer finding is the presence of concurrent enamel hypoplasia.

*Remissions*

In some cases there are periods of remission. Roentgenograms show loss of alveolar bone progressing only to a certain point and then remaining stationary for many years.

*Microbiology*

No data exist to explain the special characteristics of periodontosis on the basis of microbial populations or immunology.

*Histopathology*

Insufficient microscopic evidence exists to allow conclusive analysis.[4,7,15,18]

## Therapy

The measures to be taken in the therapy of periodontosis with extensive vertical alveolar bone loss resemble those taken in the treatment of advanced periodontitis, with certain minor additions, modifications, and changes of emphasis:

1. When there are very deep vertical bone defects in a loose tooth next to firm teeth with excellent bone support, it is sometimes wise to extract the diseased tooth at an early date to give the sound neighbor a chance for survival.
2. Osseous surgery should be used judiciously. The sound neighbor should not be damaged for the sake of a questionable tooth. With newer methods of bone or bone marrow implant from a distant donor site, some such teeth can possibly be saved.[28]
3. Root amputation and hemisection in applicable cases of partly involved molars may be indicated.
4. Fixed splinting is beneficial and important for the aesthetic appearance of the patient.[25]
5. Orthodontic measures on the involved migrated teeth may improve the

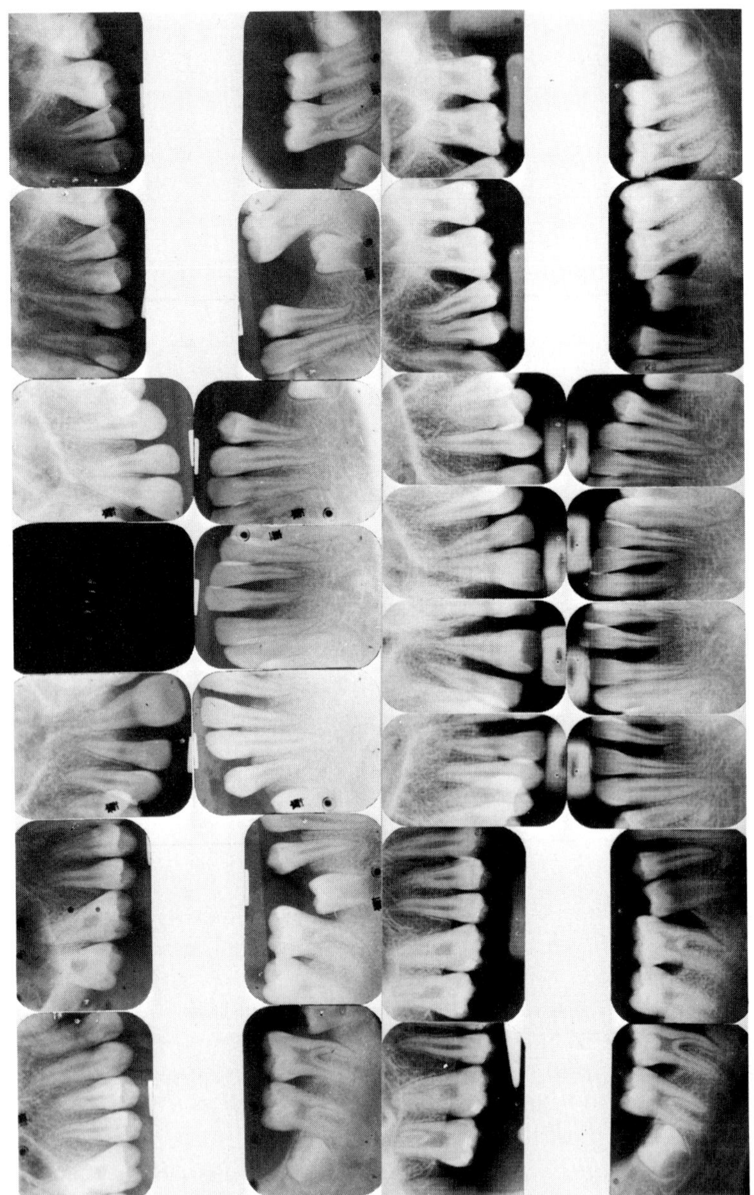


**Fig. 16-30, cont'd. C,** Compare the full-mouth roentgenograms of the patient in **A** and **B**, p. 279, taken in June 1967 (above) and May 1969 (below).

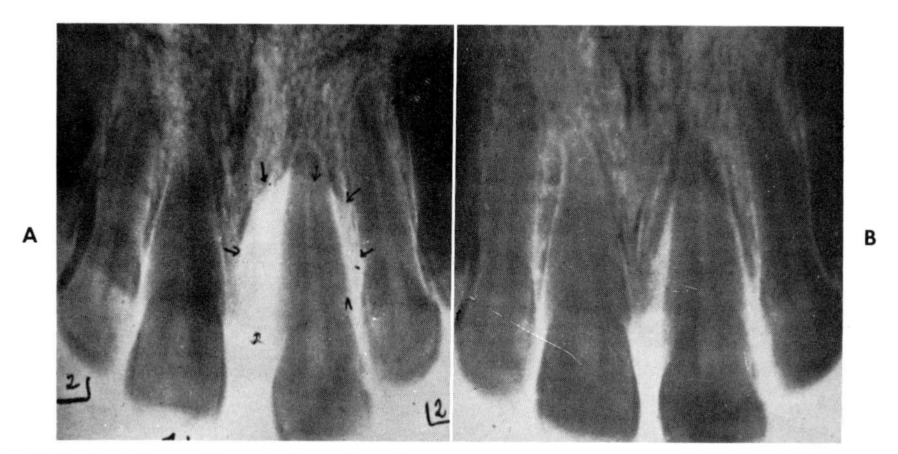


**Fig. 16-31. A,** Left maxillary incisor affected by periodontosis in a 28-year-old woman. Note the extent of bone resorption. **B,** Four years after periodontal orthodontic treatment.

clinical course of the disease. Fig. 16-31, *A,* shows the incisor area of a healthy 28-year-old white woman with periodontosis. The maxillary left central incisor was elongated and had shifted distally and vestibularly. This created a diastema between the central incisors and an unsightly appearance in the anterior region of the mouth. There was a deep pocket present on the oromesial aspect of the tooth. This pocket was eradicated surgically. A removable orthodontic appliance (Hawley) was used to move the tooth back to its original position. The tooth then was shortened by grinding of the incisal edge. Fig. 16-31, *B,* shows the same patient 4 years later. She was observed for another 4 years, and the tooth remained in good condition.

6. When occlusal traumatism is present, adjustment by selective grinding should be performed. (See the discussion on occlusal adjustment.)
7. Systematic and repeated grinding of the morsal surfaces to permit the involved tooth to erupt* is sometimes beneficial[26] (Figs. 16-32 and 16-33). In eruption of the tooth, cementum is deposited apically[29] and new bone is deposited at the crest.

In practice the last procedure follows these steps. The involved tooth is taken completely out of occlusion. Molars are narrowed orovestibularly as they are shortened. Periodontal therapy is performed, consisting of a flap operation, excochleation of the soft tissue content of the bone defect, and root planning with the Cavitron and scalers. In suitable cases autogenous bone implants may be utilized. After surgery occlusal grinding must be repeated approximately every 3 months, that is, at every visit for root planing. Grinding may be followed by tooth sensitivity. To minimize this inconvenience, the exposed dentin should be treated with an electrophoretic desensitizer to stimulate secondary dentin formation. Unusual sensitivity may require endodontic treatment to permit continued shortening of the crown by grinding.

8. Another approach to the treatment of periodontosis in teen-agers has been demonstrated by Baer and Gamble[27] (Fig. 16-34). The involved first molar is extracted, the empty socket is prepared to receive the third

*Not all teeth with infrabony pockets have an increased tendency to erupt.

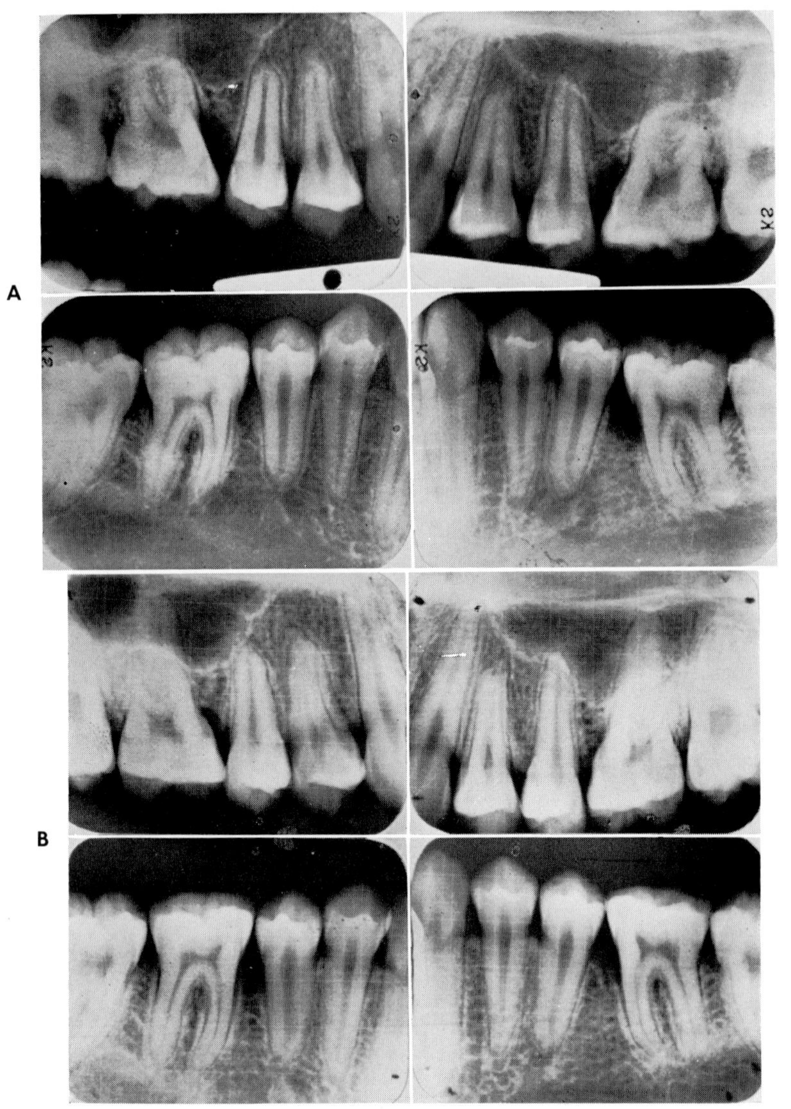


**Fig. 16-32.** **A,** Periodontosis in a 15-year-old girl. Roentgenograms show loss of bone on the mesial of the four first molars. **B,** Roentgenograms taken a year later show considerable improvement in all but the lower right first molar, where the bone defect has remained more or less stationary. Note the flattened masticatory contours of the treated molars.

molar germ, and the third molar is extracted and transplanted to the first molar alveolus. The right time for this operation is when the bifurcation of the third molar germ has just formed. In the operative procedure the bony septum separating the roots of the first molar should be removed and the transplanted tooth germ should be embedded in its new socket below the plane of occlusion; then the flap is sutured in place. The excellent success in these cases indicates that the lesion had been caused by the tooth since replacement of the lesion by the third molar permitted complete bone regeneration.

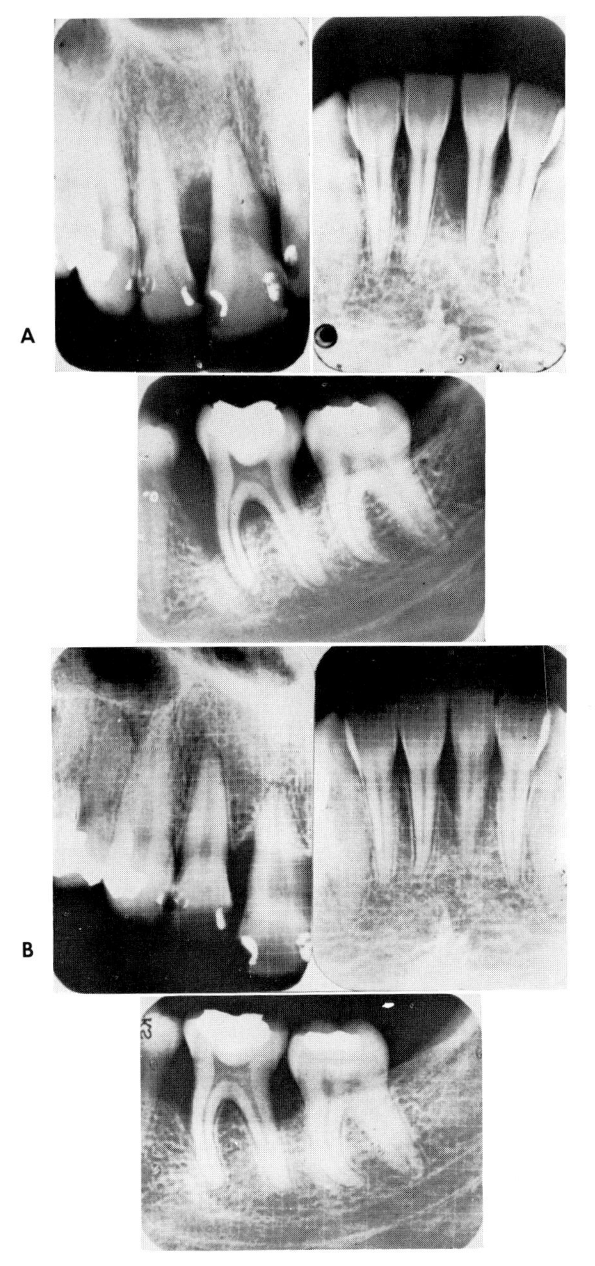


**Fig. 16-33. A,** Periodontosis in a 19-year-old girl. A diastema is present on the lower left between the second premolar and the first molar, and another between the lower two central incisors. **B,** Roentgenograms taken of the same areas 3 years later. Note the spontaneous closure of the diastemas and the greatly improved appearance of the alveolar bone. The masticatory contour in the treated molars is flattened. There has been not only bone apposition but also increased trabeculation.

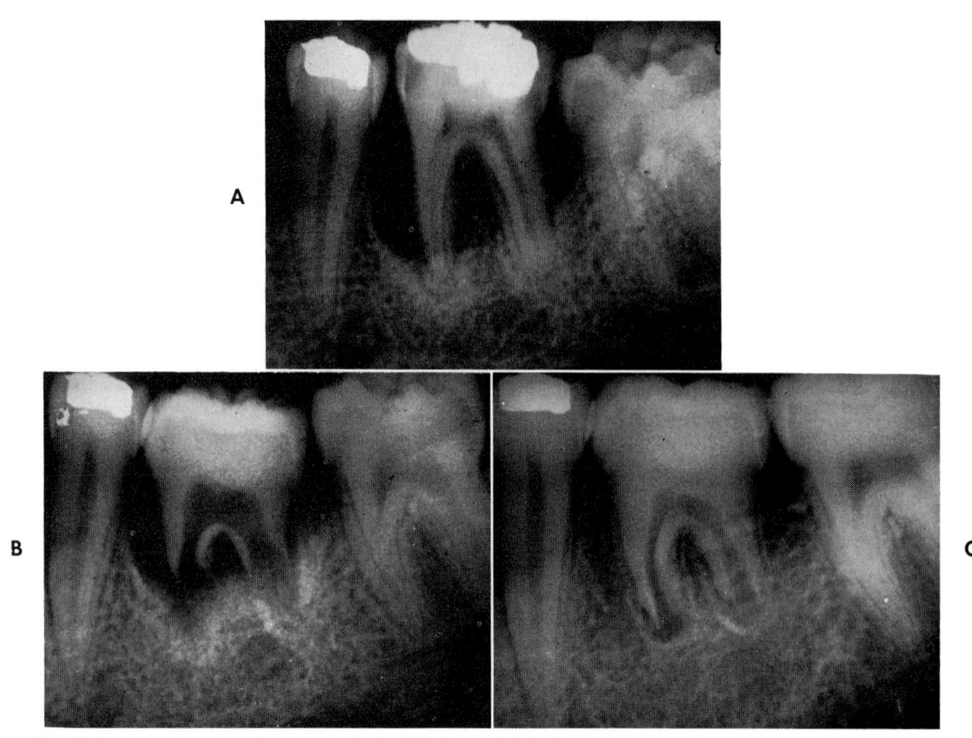


**Fig. 16-34. A,** Preoperative view (July 1964). **B,** Third molar autotransplanted into first molar site (August 1964). **C,** Eighteen months after transplant (February 1966). (Courtesy P. N. Baer, United States Public Health Service, and J. W. Gamble, Shreveport.)

The success of the grinding procedure and that of transplantation lends support to Gottlieb's contention that periodontosis is a disease of eruption and a cementopathia.

A few words of caution should be added about the rare occurrence of periodontosis during routine orthodontic therapy. Orthodontists who take a full mouth roentgenogram when they begin treatment would be well advised to continue such complete surveys at regular intervals to avoid the embarrassment of overlooking a developing periodontosis. It is next to impossible for the periodontist to convince parents that the destruction of periodontosis had occurred entirely independently of the orthodontic treatment.

## Prognosis

The prognosis of periodontosis should be viewed as guarded but not hopeless. We often do not know just when the bony changes seen in the roentgenograms have taken place; maybe the disease is in a state of complete remission and the changes have been present for years. To assess the acuteness of the disease, consult older roentgenograms when these are available. Periodontosis may occur cyclically, and it may show remissions lasting many years, during which time the disease does not progress. When the destruction is far advanced, the involved tooth may have to be sacrificed. In fact, some cases of periodontosis seem to go inexorably toward the loss of all the teeth. Fortunately the number of these hopeless cases is small by our present knowledge. The more we learn about this disease and the more refined our therapy becomes, the more teeth will be treated successfully. Only careful analysis and a great deal of clinical experience and technical know-how tells us how to proceed in a case of periodontosis. There always will be a factor of uncertainty as far as the prognosis for the health of the remaining teeth is concerned. If dentists and patients are aware of this, many difficulties can be avoided. The patient's confidence in the operator can be won by honesty and knowledge. No other problem in periodontics taxes this confidence as much as does that of periodontosis.

Much remains to be learned about the etiology and pathology of this disease. The clinical characteristics, however, of classical juvenile periodontosis are clearly defined. Since clinical inflammation is not a prominent feature (as a rule) and since the degree of periodontal destruction manifested seems far in excess of what could be provoked by the extrinsic irritants present, the preferred term for this clinical entity should be periodontosis.

**CHAPTER 16**

**References**

*Dystrophies*


1. Morris, M. L.: The position of the margin of the gingiva, Oral Surg. **11**:969, 1958.
2. Hirschfeld, L.: A study of skulls in the American Museum of Natural History in relation to periodontal disease, J. Dent. Res. **5**:241, 1923.
3. Everett, F. G.: The case of the disappearing clefts, J. Periodont. **39**:296, 1968.
4. Moskow, B. S., and Bressman, E.: Localized gingival recession, Dent. Radiogr. Photogr. **38**:3, 1965.
5. Hirschfeld, I.: The toothbrush: its use and abuse, Brooklyn, 1939, Dental Items of Interest Publishing Co.
6. Gorman, W. J.: Prevalence and etiology of gingival recession, J. Periodont. **38**:316, 1967.

6a. O'Leary, T. J., and others: The incidence of recession in young males; a further study, J. Periodont. **42**:264, 1971.

6b. Woofter, C.: The prevalence and etiology of gingival recession, Periodont. Abstr. **17**:45, 1969.

7. Gottlieb, B.: Der Epithelansatz am Zähne, Deutsch. Mschr. Zahnheilk. **39**:142, 1921.
8. Orban, B., and Köhler, J.: Die physiologische Zahnfleischtasche, Epithelansatz und Epitheltiefenwucherung, Z. Stomat. **22**:353, 1924.
9. Gargiulo, A. W., Wentz, F. M., and Orban, B.: Dimensions and relations of the dentogingival junction in humans, J. Periodont. **32**:261, 1961.
10. Merritt, A. H.: Periodontal diseases, ed. 3, New York, 1945, The Macmillan Co.
11. Ray, H., and Santos, H. A.: Consideration of tongue-thrusting as a factor in periodontal disease, J. Periodont. **25**:250, 1954.
12. Orban, G.: Clinical and histologic study of the surface characteristics of the gingiva, Oral Surg. **1**:827, 1948.
13. Wolff's law of transformation. Quoted in Weinmann, J. P., and Sicher, H.: Bone and bones, ed. 2, St. Louis, 1955, The C. V. Mosby Co.
14. Brescia, N.: Applied dental anatomy, St. Louis, 1961, The C. V. Mosby Co.
15. Kellner, E.: Histologische Befunde an antagonistenlosen Zähnen, Z. Stomat. **26**:271, 1928.
16. Weinmann, J. P., and Sicher, H., Bone and bones, ed. 2, St. Louis, 1955, The C. V. Mosby Co.
17. Kellner, E.: Das Verhältnis der Zement- und Periodontalbreiten zur funktionellen Beanspruchung der Zähne, Z. Stomat. **29**:44, 1931.
18. Bhaskar, S. N., and Jacoway, J. R.: Peripheral fibroma and peripheral fibroma with calcification, J. Amer. Dent. Ass. **73**:1312, 1966.
19. Ball, E. L.: Gingivoma, or elephantiasis of the gingiva, J. Periodont. **12**:96, 1941.
20. Orban, B.: Discussion of Ball, E. L.: Case of gingivoma, J. Periodont. **12**:100, 1941.
21. Savara, B. S., Suher, T., Everett, F. G., and Burns, A. G.: Hereditary gingival fibrosis; study of a family, J. Periodont. **25**:12, 1954.
22. Winstock, D.: Hereditary gingivofibromatosis, Brit. J. Oral Surg. **2**:59, 1964.
23. Zackin, S. J., and Weisberger, D.: Hereditary gingival fibromatosis, Oral Surg. **14**:828, 1961.

24. Willert, E.: Ein seltener Fall einer echten Fibromatosis Gingivae, Oest. Z. Stomat. **51**:663, 1954.
25. Mathis, H.: Zur Frage der Hyperplasie der Gingiva unter Dilantinbehandlung, Deutsch. Z. Zahnheilk. **9**:1280, 1954.
26. Kimball, O. P.: Treatment of epilepsy with sodium diphenyl hydantoinate, J.A.M.A., **112**:1244, 1939.
27. Staple, P. H.: Some tissue reactions associated with 5:5 diphenylhydantoin (Dilantin) sodium therapy, Brit. Dent. J. **95**:289, 1953.
28. Dummett, C. O.: Oral tissue reaction from Dilantin medication in the control of epileptic seizures, J. Periodont. **25**:112, 1954.
29. Aas, E.: Hyperplasia gingivae diphenylhydantoinea, Acta Odont. Scand., supp. 34, 1963. (Monograph contains an excellent and complete list of references.)
30. Triadan, H.: Ueber die parodontale Nebenwirkung der chronischen Hydantoinbehandlung, Heidelberg, 1968, Dr. Alfred Hüthig Verlag.
31. Babcock, J. R.: Incidence of gingival hyperplasia associated with Dilantin therapy in a hospital population, J. Amer. Dent. Ass. **71**:1447, 1965.
32. Panuska, H. J., Gorlin, R. J., Bearman, J. E., and Mitchell, D. F.: The effect of anticonvulsant drugs upon the gingiva. I, J. Periodont. **31**:336, 1960; II, J. Periodont. **32**:15, 1961.
33. Shafer, W. G., Beatty, R. E., and Davis, W. B.: Effect of Dilantin sodium on tensile strength of healing wounds, Proc. Soc. Exp. Biol. Med. **98**:348, 1958.
34. Shafer, W. G.: Response of radiated human fibroblast-like cells to Dilantin sodium in tissue culture, J. Dent. Res. **44**:671, 1965.
35. Babcock, J. R., and Nelson, G. H.: Gingival hyperplasia and Dilantin content of saliva, J. Amer. Dent. Ass. **68**:195, 1964.
36. Hall, W. B.: Dilantin hyperplasia; a preventable disease, J. Periodont. Res. supp. 4, p. 36, 1969.
37. Staple, P. H.: Regression of gingival hyperplasia following substitution of "Mysoline" for phenytoin sodium, Brit. Dent. J. **99**:432, 1955.
38. Trott, J. R., and Neuman, K.: Improved gingival and mental condition following reduction of diphenylhydantoin medication for epilepsy, J. Canad. Dent. Ass. **30**:518, 1964.
39. Babcock, J. R.: The successful use of a new therapy in Dilantin gingival hyperplasia, Periodontics **3**:196, 1965.

#### Additional suggested reading

Forscher, B. K., and Cecil, H. C.: Biochemical studies on acute inflammation. II, The effect of Dilantin, J. Dent. Res. **36**:927, 1957.

Mathur, R. M., and others: Study of gingival recession as it relates to oral cleaning habits, J. Indian Dent. Ass. **41**:159, 1969.

O'Leary, T. J.: The incidence of recession in young males, Periodontics **6**:109, 1968.

*Periodontosis*

1. Russell, A. L.: Epidemiology of periodontal disease, Int. Dent. J. **17**:1, 1967.
2. Gottlieb, B.: Zur Aetiologie und Therapie der Alveolarpyorrhoe, Z. Stomat. **18**:59, 1920.
3. Gottlieb, B.: Die diffuse Atrophie des Alveolarknochens, Z. Stomat **21**:195, 1923.
4. Orban, B., and Weinmann, J. P.: Diffuse atrophy of the alveolar bone (periodontosis), J. Periodont. **13**:31, 1952.
5. Wannenmacher, E.: Umschau auf dem Gebiete der Paradentose, Deutsch. Zahn- Mund-Kieferheilk. **3**:81, 1938.
6. Miller, S. C.: Precocious advanced alveolar atrophy, J. Periodont. **19**:146, 1948.
7. Petit, H.: Parodontite juvenile, Paris, 1970, Prelat.
8. Baer, P. N.: The case for periodontosis as a clinical entity, J. Periodont. **42**:516, 1971.
9. Waerhaug, J.: Preliminary report on WHO periodontal survey in Ceylon, October-December, 1960, Bull. WHO **175**:62, 1961.
10. Russell, A. L.: Some epidemiologic characteristics of periodontal disease in a series of urban populations, J. Periodont. **28**:286, 1957.
11. Emslie, R. D.: Periodontal diseases in tropical Africa, Parodontopathies **18**:26, 1966.
12. Häupl, K., and Lang, F. J.: Entgegnung auf die Randbemerkungen B. Orban's, Z. Stomat. **25**:1110, 1927.
13. Butler, H. J.: A familial pattern of juvenile periodontitis (periodontosis), J. Periodont. **40**:51, 1960.

14. Kaslick, R. S., and Chasens, A. I.: Periodontosis with periodontitis: A study involving young adult males. I, Oral Surg. 25:25, 305, 1968.
15. Baer, P. N., Stanley, H. R., Brown, K., and others: Advanced periodontal disease in the adolescent (periodontosis), J. Periodont. 34:533, 1963.
16. Rao, S. S., and Tewani, S. V.: Prevalence of periodontosis, J. Periodont. 39:27, 1968.
17. Benjamin, S. D., and Baer, P. N.: Familial patterns of advanced alveolar bone loss in adolescence (periodontosis), Periodontics 5:82, 1967.
18. Stambolieva, E., and Bourkova, T.: Comparative enzymatic histochemical investigation of gingival papillae in early parodontosis (periodontosis) and parodontitis (periodontitis) traumatica, J. Periodont. 42:532, 1970.
19. Kaslick, R. S., and Chasens, A. I.: Periodontosis with periodontitis: a study involving young adult males. II, Clinical, medical and histopatholic studies, Oral Surg. 25:327, 1968.
20. Kaslick, R. S., Chasens, A. I., Tuckman, M. A., and Kaufman, B.: Investigation of periodontosis with periodontitis; literature survey and findings based on ABO blood groups, J. Periodont. 42:420, 1971.
21. Gottlieb, B.: The new concept of periodontoclasia, J. Periodont. 17:7, 1946.
22. Harvey, B. L. C., and Zander, H. A.: Root surface resorption in periodontally diseased teeth, Oral Surg. 12:1439, 1959.
23. Müller, G., and Zander, H. A.: Cementum of periodontally involved teeth from India, J. Dent. Res. 39:385, 1960.
24. Gottlieb, B.: Parodontalpyorrhoe und Alveolaratrophie, Fortschr. Zahnheilk. 4:398, 1928.
25. Tenenbaum, B., Nahoum, H. I., Karshan, M., Beube, F. E., and Wiener, R.: Results of several types of treatment of periodontosis, J. Amer. Dent. Ass. 55:651, 1957.
26. Everett, F. G., and Baer, P. N.: A preliminary report on the treatment of the osseous defect in periodontosis, J. Periodont. 35:429, 1964.
27. Baer, P. N., and Gamble, J. W.: Autogenous dental transplants as a method of treating the osseous defect in periodontosis, Oral Surg. 22:405, 1966.
28. DeMarco, T. J., and Scaletta, L. J.: The use of autogenous bone marrow in the treatment of juvenile periodontosis, J. Periodont. 41:683, 1970.
29. Stallard, R. E.: The utilization of $H^3$ proline by the connective tissue elements of the periodontium, Periodontics 1:185, 1963.

**Additional suggested reading**

Baer, P. N., and Everett, F. G.: The maxillary sinus as a problem in the therapy of periodontosis, J. Periodont. 41:476, 1970.
Cohen, D. W., and Goldman, H. M.: Periodontal disease in children, P.D.M., July 1962.
Glickman, I.: Periodontal disease, New Eng. J. Med. 284:1071, 1971.
Kaslick, R. S., Chasens, A. I., Bressman, E., and others: Investigation of periodontosis with periodontitis: ultramicroanalysis of gingival fluid, gross examination of the periodontal ligament and approach to treatment, J. Periodont. 42:428, 1971.
Kluczka, J.: Infantile und juvenile Parodontopathien, Parodontopathies, p. 58, 1966.
Marks, M. H., and Corn, H.: The role of tooth movement in periodontal therapy, Dental Clinics of North America, Philadelphia, 1969, W. B. Saunders Co., vol. 13.
Nomenclature and Classification Committee report, J. Periodont. 21:40, 1970.
Ramfjord, S. P., Kerr, D. A., and Ash, M. M., Jr., editors: World workshop in periodontics, Ann Arbor, 1966, University of Michigan Press.
Spirgi, M., and Held, J. A.: Parodontolyses juveniles degeneratives, Parodontopathies, p. 41, 1966.
Weski, O.: Parodontopathien und Parodontosis, Berichte des 9ten internationalen Zahnärztekongresses der F.D.I., Vienna, 1936, Urban & Schwarzenberg.

PART VI

# Elements of therapeutic judgment

CHAPTER SEVENTEEN

# Doctor-patient relationship—psychologic aspects of periodontics



Although it is apparent that a degree of psychologic insight is required for the proper management of a dental practice, other relationships between psychology and dentistry are far less obvious but no less important. Psychoanalytic theory places great importance on the relationship of the oral cavity to the psyche. Other data also support the hypothesis that psychologic and social factors are involved in diseases of the oral cavity.

## PSYCHOSOMATIC FACTORS

Can periodontal disease be related to psychogenic causes? A study of hospitalized, emotionally ill population showed that the acutely disturbed patients had a higher incidence of periodontal disease than did the apathetic patients. Other reports have indicated a high degree of correlation between periodontal disease and neurotic tendency, measured anxiety (a symptom of neurosis), and factors such as strained family relationships, hysteria, and hypochondriasis.[1,2]

These studies support the existence of an association between periodontal disease and psychologic factors; that is, certain measurable factors of periodontal disease and psychologic status vary proportionately.[3,4] Causality is not involved in these measurements, yet such a presumption is tempting to make. Bruxism, NUG, poor oral hygiene, and poor diet may in fact be manifestations of psychologic states. To the extent that this is so, periodontal disease may be psychosomatic. Although a case can be made for this argument, it is not yet proved. On the other hand, case histories indicate that psychoanalysis sometimes permits the elimination of neurosis-induced periodontal symptoms.[3]

***Bruxism and clenching***

The extended muscular force produced during bruxism and clenching may result in occlusal traumatism. (See discussions on bruxism and occlusal traumatism in Chapter 36.) Therefore, a fuller understanding of how these muscle actions may have a psychologic origin could prove valuable.

The psychologic explanation for bruxism is a construction.* All persons have

*A construction in geometry is an assumption that leads to the derivation of a proof. In psychiatry and in periodontics, there are many constructions (working hypotheses) that facilitate treatment. These constructions need not be true for treatment based on them to work. It is possible for both treatment and construction to be related to other true but as yet unknown foundations.

drives that are associated with life goals. When these drives are blocked, the resultant frustration produces rage. Rage must have an outlet; for instance, an enraged child will not hesitate to bite. When the child learns that such biting behavior is socially unacceptable, the biting is repressed. Since the rage cannot be suppressed, new outlets for its dissipation must be found. Substitute satisfactions (sublimation) may be employed. When substitution is inadequate, one may still resort to biting to gain satisfaction. This satisfaction may be gained surrepticiously and symbolically on an unconscious level by bruxing or clenching. These activities may occur during the waking hours; but they are especially prevalent during sleep, when the unconscious is most emergent (night grinding). The patient may be completely unaware of these repeated and sustained forced contacts of the teeth that seem to have no functional significance in man (parafunction). There is evidence that bruxism in some primates is a tooth-honing mechanism.[4a]

The following evidence tends to support the psychologic correlation between bruxism and anxiety: In a word-association test given to a student with electrodes placed on the temporal muscles, spikes (muscle contractions) appeared with the emotional words and disappeared with the neutral words. Electromyographic recordings were made of the temporal and masseter muscles of eight dental students. During the recording, stress was provided by having the dean "unexpectedly" arrive on the scene and engage the student in a conversation that somehow turned to the subject of forthcoming examinations and the student's prospects. Action potentials increased with the stress.[6]

The electrical activity of the masseter and temporal muscles increases when a human experimental subject performs a task.[7] There are increases in amplitude of electromyograms when the subject makes a mistake in the performance of the task.[8] In a study of 103 patients with bruxism who were compared with a control group, the bruxing patients had a significantly higher degree of depression and anxiety symptoms. They also had symptoms of muscular tension and latent or manifest aggressiveness.[9] A striking enlargement of the masseter muscles has been observed in some mental patients, which could be a form of work hypertrophy related to clenching and oral-aggressive energy.[10,11]

Bruxism and circulatory phenomena may be interrelated in a psychophysiologic manner. Tooth contacts lasting up to 17 seconds have been reported concomitant with alterations in pulse rate and stroke. These periods of bruxing contact were directly related to periods of emotional reaction (stress and/or anxiety).[12] Although there may be an emotional basis for bruxism, the assumption that bruxism is diagnostic of emotional disturbance or psychopathology is not warranted.

***Saliva***

Just as "gnashing the teeth" and "shutting up like a clam" demonstrate emotional overtones, phrases like "spitting mad," "frothing at the mouth," and "drooling in anticipation" show that salivation has psychiatric implications. Although the relationship of emotionally controlled salivation to periodontal disease may not be so obvious as in the case of bruxism, it may be equally or more important. Psychologic factors are known to influence the rate of secretion and composition of saliva. Saliva, in turn, relates to plaque formation, calculus deposition, and antibacterial and proteolytic activities, all of which may have a bearing on periodontal disease.

A transient reduction of salivary flow and changes in salivary enzyme content of saliva can be produced by mental activity, stress, muscular effort, or emotional disturbance.[13-15] pH has also been observed to go up as salivation increases.[16]

These relationships between salivary physiology and psychologic status do not necessarily demonstrate causation of periodontal disease, but they may very well show that periodontal health is influenced by salivary changes.

***Circulation***

The tonus of the smooth muscle of blood vessels may be altered by the emotions via the autonomic nervous system. For example, dilatation and contraction may be related to blushing and blanching. Prolonged contraction could alter the supply of oxygen and nutrients to the tissues. There is very little evidence to support such a relationship with periodontal disease, however. Metabolic studies do indicate that the oxygen consumption of gingival tissues varies in health and disease, but this may relate to altered tissue activity.[16-20]

Rats caged in crowded conditions, in which movement is inhibited, demonstrate a lowered oxygen utilization by their oral tissues. This observation is related to the social stress provoked by the crowding.[20] Mice similarly treated have been observed to develop systolic hypertension.[21] Physical and psychologic stimuli (e.g., mental arithmetic) reduce the amplitude of the volume pulse of the gingiva as well as that of the finger. The gingival and cutaneous vascular responses occur simultaneously with other variables and are relatable to both the anticipation of stress and the actual cold pressor stimulation.[22,23]

***Diet and appetite***

Psychologic factors affect the choice of foods, the physical consistency of the diet, and the quantities of food eaten. These factors may have a direct or indirect influence on the periodontium.

***Habits***

Neurotic needs find oral expression. The mouth may be used to obtain satisfaction, to express dependency, to express hostility, and to inflict or receive pain. Sucking, biting, sensing, and feeling may become habitual as in thumb sucking, tongue thrusting, infantile swallowing, and biting of tongue, lip, cheek, or fingernail. These actions also figure in bruxing, clenching, tooth doodling, and smoking. Such habits may lead to tooth migration, occlusal traumatism, and occlusal wear.

***Oral hygiene***

It is obvious that proper oral hygiene is partially dependent on the mental health status of the patient. Some patients may be so disturbed or distracted psychologically that personal hygiene is neglected. Other patients may intentionally ignore oral hygiene to fulfill deep neurotic needs. Moulton and associates suggest that oral hygiene may be neglected during depression, deep anxiety, and rebellion against authority.[25] Dependent individuals may exhibit chronic neglect as if they were expecting such care to be the responsibility of others. The dentist's instructions concerning oral hygiene may be ignored as a form of "parental defiance."[25]

There are techniques available to the dentist for developing desired patient behavior with regard to oral hygiene. These techniques depend on psychologic approaches to reinforce desirable behavior and to extinguish undesirable behavior.

***Necrotizing ulcerative gingivitis***

Necrotizing ulcerative gingivitis (NUG) is a disease of special interest because it may have an emotional basis (Chapter 18). There is some evidence to indicate that the suggested relationship between emotional stress and NUG is more than conjecture. Of the hospitalized patients examined by Mellars and Herms, the acutely mentally ill were more prone to NUG than were the chronically mentally ill.[28] The disease among military personnel may be related to fatigue, nervousness, and unusual dependence.[29] A group of patients with this disease examined by

Moulton and co-workers exhibited a pattern of oral dependence as a central life problem.[24] The attacks of NUG among this group were brought on by acute anxiety. Case histories indicate that attacks of acute anxiety are often the precipitating factor.[30-31a]

Patients with NUG have a tendency to cutaneous vasodilatation in response to irritation and, in addition, show a longer latency period for flare reaction.[32]

*Smoking*

Other potentially harmful habits may act by affecting tissue moisture or temperature. Perhaps the most insidious of these is smoking, which according to some studies is related to NUG and probably to other oral diseases as well.[33,33a] Smoking is also inversely related to many psychosocial variables associated with mental health.[34] What is not known, however, is whether the smoking is in itself of direct etiologic significance or merely a symptom of some underlying psychologic disturbance that has a more important role in the pathogenesis of these diseases. This qualification would not minimize the direct local irritating effect of nicotine and tars on the tissue, nor would it probably influence the role of these irritants in the formation of calculus.[23]

*Coffee drinking*

Coffee drinking is another habit that may act extrinsically (through thermal or chemical properties) and intrinsically (through caffeine content). Coffee drinking is more frequent among smokers[34] and has also been shown to be greater among patients with NUG than among those with normal gingivae.[23]

## PSYCHOLOGIC FACTORS

An awareness of the patient's emotional structure can be significant, since the patient relates with emotional overtones to his disease and its treatment and to the dentist and since periodontal disease may have psychosomatic facets. It is possible for the dentist to have such an awareness without specific training. Although a capacity for warmth and feeling for people may occur naturally, it can also be developed if one learns to relax and to listen to what the patient is really saying. Qualities of sensitivity, perception, and insight can be nurtured by devoting adequate time to the interview. (See the discussion of patient interview in Chapter 18.) Some knowledge of this is as important to the dentist as it is to the physician.

Without being aware of it, patients exhibit clues to their emotional makeup and to what they are really thinking. The dentist who detects and interprets these clues correctly is in a position to help the patient so that a minimum of stress and a maximum of benefit are received from treatment.[35-39] Such an insight into the patient's behavior requires patience and diagnostic acumen. Everything the patient says or does usually has a reason. No reaction or response, not even a jest, is meaningless. Responses are clues to the unconscious. The unconscious is generally well hidden, and the patient is unaware of its influence on his behavior; but the observer can detect the behavior and through it interpret the unconscious.

The dentist, in a sense, symbolizes a parent; and a parent-child relationship may develop with many patients. With it, childhood attitudes of (among others) dependence, rebelliousness, and affection may be reenacted during the course of treatment. Since dentistry may be threatening or painful, ingrained attitudes toward sickness, pain, and death may be displayed. The patient may come to the dentist with many preconceived notions. These tend to set the stage for the actual relationship and color the technical aspects of treatment.

The mouth provides satisfactions and is used in eating, talking, fighting, sensing, and loving. Many neurotic conflicts are centered about the mouth. The dentist must deal with the patient's psychologic structure and the mouth as a center for emotional manifestations. Unfortunately the dentist is not a neuter in treatment, and his psyche enters into treatment via the patient-dentist relationship in a manner that is reflected in his treatment of the patient.

## Psychiatric manifestations

There are several relatively common situations that occur during treatment that are heavily laden with emotional significance. For example, some patients with mental distress may complain of an imbalance of occlusion, unconsciously hoping that a balancing of the occlusion will result in a "balancing" of the mind. Other patients, detesting some phase of their emotional structure and unconsciously wishing to have it removed, may repeatedly seek surgery of other structures (polysurgical addiction), including periodontal and dental. Naturally the dental treatment cannot eliminate the mental symptoms.

Some situations involve the patient, who, because of deep anxiety and rigidity, attempts to ensure the success of treatment by choosing a therapist who will serve in an omnipotent, godlike capacity. This distortion of the role of the therapist lends itself to the equally neurotic dentist who feels himself endowed with godlike abilities. Such an interaction results in an unhealthy dentist-patient relationship. Treatment is not regarded as a joint venture. The patient cannot tolerate untoward or unexpected developments. The situations can be traumatic to both neurotic personalities.

The degree to which behavior is logical, purposeful, and free of anxiety is a measure of mental health in both dentist and patient; and the reverse is a measure of neurosis. All people have neuroses. Neuroses should not bear disgrace or stigma since they are matters only of personal health. The neurosis represents some carefully self-selected adjustment to inner conflict. Although people are not consciously aware of the roots of their neuroses, they nurture and hold these neuroses dear on an unconscious level. Essentially we approve of our own neuroses, but we are critical of the neuroses of other people.

The dentist should treat his patient with friendliness and respect, not with criticism or condemnation. He should not develop "holier than thou" feelings, make snide remarks, or render value judgments. The patient should be treated with tact and courtesy. The dentist must be sincerely concerned with the welfare of his patients, for dentistry as a business is not his primary concern. He should try to understand the patient as well as the patients dental illness. In every instance he must be able to handle the patient and himself with proper psychologic controls. The dentist's training does not prepare him sufficiently to meet the psychologic demands made on him or to recognize the patient as he really is; nor does it prepare him to guide the development of new attitudes in patients concerning treatment and health, yet all facets of treatment, and in particular those require reeducation of the patient, require such training. On the other hand, although the dentist should conduct his practice in a psychologically oriented manner and although his dental treatment may be psychotherapeutic, he should not attempt psychotherapy per se.

Some dentists state that they have patients in their practice whom they regard as "a pain in the neck." After a particularly bad session with such a patient, the dentist may feel ready to give up dentistry. These feelings are indicative of the fact that not every dentist can treat every patient; nor can he truly understand what role the patient is acting out during the dental visit. If the dentist perceives his levels of nervousness increasing or his anger rising, he would be best advised to try to determine what he or the patient may be doing to produce this state of events and if possible alter the situation by handling its basic cause. When the situation appears to be unmanageable, the patient should be referred to another dentist or physician. On the other hand, the dentist may attempt to rectify the situation by minimizing his hostility toward the patient. The dentist feels less angry if he is under no compulsion to comply with impossible demands. This can be done by setting limits for the patient's behavior. In addition, he should not view the patient as a threat to himself or his competence.

The patient should be reassured, not threatened. He must not be manipulated, whether the dentist wishes to rehabilitate him mentally or dentally. The sympathetic, understanding, psychologically oriented dentist has an extended range of diagnostic ability. Moreover, by developing a therapeutically appropriate relationship with the patient, he is capable of providing the utmost of comfort and benefit to the patient.

## Summary

Psychologic factors may alter tissue physiology and contribute to periodontal disease. Knowledge concerning the definitive mechanisms of such alteration is lacking or incomplete. Nevertheless, understanding of periodontal disease and its treatment requires some awareness of the patient and his particular psychologic makeup. Although specific steps in treatment may be performed on a symptomatic basis, it is well to keep in mind that symptoms occur in people. Some dentists prefer to think of teeth, jaws, and mouth in an isolated sense. What in a living organism is really isolated? The patient of today readily accepts that psychologic stress affects other body organs, so why not the oral structures? Even in the most technical manipulation, the dentist is required to treat the whole patient, and only by so doing does he fulfill his professional responsibility.


**CHAPTER 17**

**References**

1. Ewen, S. J.: The dental interview, New York J. Dent. **21**:392, 1951.
2. Witkin, G. J.: Management of the patient with periodontal disease, J. Amer. Dent. Ass. **55**:625, 1957.
3. Saul, L. J.: A note on the psychogenesis of organic symptoms, Psychoanal. Quart. **4**:476, 1935.
4. Belting, C. M., and Gupta, O. P.: Incidence of periodontal diseases among persons with neuropsychiatric disorders, J. Dent. Res. **39**:744, 1960.

4a. Zingeser, M. R.: Canine tooth honing mechanism, Amer. J. Phys. Anthrop. **31**:205, 1969.

5. Manhold, J. H.: Report of a study on the relationship of personality variables to periodontal conditions, J. Periodont. **24**:248, 1953.
6. Perry, H. T., Lammie, G. A., Main, J., and Teuscher, G. W.: Occlusion in a stress situation, J. Amer. Dent. Ass. **60**:626, 1960.
7. Yemm, R.: Variations in the electrical activity of the human masseter muscle occurring in association with emotional stress, Arch. Oral Biol. **14**:873, 1969.
8. Yemm, R.: A comparison of the electrical activity of masseter and temporal muscles of human subjects during experimental stress, Arch. Oral Biol. **16**:269, 1971.
9. Molin, C., and Levi, L.: A psycho-odontologic investigation of patients with bruxism, Acta Odont. Scand. **24**:373, 1966.
10. Guggenheim, P., and Cohen, L. B.: The histopathology of masseteric hypertrophy, Arch. Otolaryng. **71**:906, 1960.
11. Guggenheim, P., and Cohen, L. B.: External hyperostosis of the mandible angle associated with masseteric hypertrophy, Arch. Otolaryng. **70**:674, 1959.

12. Butler, J. H., and Stallard, R. E.: Physiologic stress and tooth contact, J. Periodont. Res. **4**:152, 1969.
13. Winsor, A. L.: Effects of mental effort on parotid secretion, Amer. J. Psychol. **43**:434, 1931.
14. Brothers, J. D., and Warden, C. J.: Analysis of the enzyme activity of the conditioned salivary response in human subjects, Science **112**:751, 1950.
15. Bates, J. F., and Adams, D.: The influence of mental stress on the flow of saliva in man, Arch. Oral Biol. **13**:593, 1968.
16. Starr, H. E.: Hydrogen-ion concentration of mixed saliva considered as index of fatigue and emotional excitation, Amer. J. Psychol. **33**:394, 1922.
17. Glickman, I., Turesky, S., and Hill, R.: Determinations of oxygen consumption in normal and inflamed gingival tissue using the Warburg Manometric Technique, J. Dent. Res. **28**:83, 1949.
18. Glickman, I., Turesky, S., and Manhold, J. H.: The oxygen consumption of healing gingiva, J. Dent. Res. **29**:429, 1950.
19. Manhold, J. H.: Introductory psychosomatic dentistry, New York, 1956, Appleton-Century-Crofts.
20. Manhold, J. H., Doyle, J. L., and Weisinger, E. H.: Effects of social stress on oral and other bodily tissues. II, Results offering substance to a hypothesis for the mechanism of formation of periodontal pathology, J. Periodont. **42**:109, 1971.
21. Henry, J. P., Meehan, J. P., and Stephens, P. M.: The use of psychosocial stimuli to induce prolonged systolic hypertension in mice, Psychosom. Med. **29**:408, 1967.
22. Giddon, D. B., Cline, C. J., and Gustafson, L. A.: Studies of in vivo vascular reactions of normal human gingiva to cold pressor stimulation, J. Dent. Res. **43**:908, 1964.
23. Giddon, D. B.: Psychophysiology of the oral cavity, J. Dent. Res., vol. 45, supp., p. 1627, 1966.
24. Moulton, R., Ewen, S., and Thieman, W.: Emotional factors in periodontal disease, Oral Surg. **5**:833, 1952.
25. Sword, R. O.: Oral neglect—why, J. Amer. Dent. Ass. **80**:1327, 1970.
26. Winslow, E. K., and Ferris, R. T.: Developing desired patient behaviour, Dental Clinics of North America, Philadelphia, 1970, W. B. Saunders Co., vol. 14.
27. Ferris, R. T., and Winslow, E. K.: Reinforcing desired behaviour with periodontal patients, Dental Clinics of North America, Philadelphia, 1970, W. B. Saunders Co., vol. 14.
28. Mellars, N. W., and Herms, F. W.: Investigation of neuropathologic manifestations of oral tissues, Amer. J. Orthodont. **32**:30, 1946; **33**:812, 1947.
29. Carter, W. J., and Ball, D. M.: Results of a three year study of Vincent's infection at the Great Lakes Naval Dental Dept., J. Periodont. **24**:187, 1953.
30. Baker, E. G., Crook, G. H., and Schwabacher, E. D.: Personality correlates of periodontal disease, J. Dent. Res. **40**:396, 1961.
31. Davis, R. F.: Necrotizing ulcerative gingivitis in drug addict patients being withdrawn from drugs.
31a. Formicola, A. J., Witte, E. T., and Curran, P. M.: A study of the personality traits and acute, necrotizing, ulcerative gingivitis, J. Periodont. **41**:36, 1970.
32. Sekine, M., and Kakuda, Y.: Cited in Giddon, D. B.: J. Dent. Res., vol. 45, supp., p. 1627, 1966.
33. Goldhaber, P., and Giddon, D. B.: Present concepts concerning the etiology and treatment of acute necrotizing ulcerative gingivitis, Int. Dent. J. **14**:468, 1964.
33a. Everett, F. G.: Necrotizing ulcerative gingivitis. II, Treatment plan, Oregon Dent. J. **26**:2, 1957.
34. Matarazzo, J. D., and Saslow, G.: Psychological and related characteristics of smokers and nonsmokers, Psychol. Bull. **57**:493, 1960.
35. Raper, H. R.: The art of consultation with the dental patient, New York J. Dent. **33**:176, 1963.
36. Beldoch, M.: Sensitivity to the communication of feelings, Trans. N. Y. Acad. Sci. **24**:317, 1962.
37. Cinotti, U. R., and Grieder, A.: Applied psychology in dentistry, St. Louis, 1964, The C. V. Mosby Co.
38. Weckstein, M. S.: Practical applications of basic psychiatry to dentistry, Dental Clinics of North America, Philadelphia, 1970, W. B. Saunders Co., vol. 14.
39. Cowen, J., and Friedman, W. F.: Psychologic considerations in long-term dental care, Dent. Surveys, p. 34, 1971.

**Additional suggested reading**

Borland, L. R., and others: Psychology in dentistry: selected reference and abstract, Public Health Service Publication no. 929, Washington, D. C., 1962, U. S. Government Printing Office.

Boyens, P. J.: Value of autosuggestion in the therapy of "bruxism" and other biting habits, J. Amer. Dent. Ass. **27**:1773, 1940.

Cleary, M. F.: Postoperative psychiatric disturbance, Penn. Dent. J. **33**:269, 1966.

Dworkin, S. F.: Psychosomatic concepts and dentistry: some perspectives, J. Periodont. **40**: 647, 1969.

Golden, L. M.: Denial of dental problems by patients, Ann. Dent. **23**:103, 1964.

Land, M.: Management of emotional illness in dental practice, J. Amer. Dent. Ass. **73**:631, 1966.

Manhold, J.: Introductory psychosomatic dentistry, New York, 1956, Appleton-Century-Crofts.

Miller, A. A.: Psychologic considerations in dentistry, J. Amer. Dent. Ass. **81**:941, 1970.

Miller, S. C., Thaller, J. L., and Soberman, A.: Use of the Minnesota Multiphasic Personality Inventory as a diagnostic aid in periodontal disease—a preliminary report, J. Periodont. **27**:44, 1956.

Redman, R. S., Gorlin, R. J., Peagler, F. D., Vance, F., and Meskin, L.: A psychological component in the etiology of geographic tongue, Amer. J. Psychiat. **121**:805, 1965.

Ross, M. G.: The contributions of social and behavioral sciences to the health sciences, J. Dent. Res., vol. 44, supp., p. 1104, 1965.

Walsh, J.: Psychologic defense mechanisms in dentistry, Aust. Dent. J. **9**:455, 1964.

Winer, R. A., Cohen, M., Feller, R. P., and others: Composition of human saliva, parotid gland secretory rate, and electrolyte concentration in mentally subnormal persons, J. Dent. Res., vol. 44, supp., p. 632, 1965.

CHAPTER EIGHTEEN

# Examination and diagnosis



The natural teeth should be retained as long as they and their surrounding tissues are healthy and contribute to the patient's well-being. Dentistry helps people to go through life with an intact dentition. Periodontal disease is one threat to the realization of this goal. In the presence of periodontal disease, the preservation of the natural dentition is possible only when the dentist is capable of recognizing and successfully treating the disease.

Although the nature of periodontal disease is not completely known and only partially understood, most of the clinical signs can be easily recognized by the trained therapist. Moreover, therapeutic measures of demonstrated effectiveness have been developed. In essence, treatment consists of measures to control the etiologic factors presumed responsible for the disease and to remedy any damage that has occurred. The dentist notes the clinical signs of the disease and deduces their causes, and from the causes and clinical signs he arrives at the appropriate treatment.

The appropriate treatment will be performed only if the dentist can correlate the clinical signs and symptoms of the disease with a knowledge of the histology, histopathology, and physiology of the affected tissues. The sum of this knowledge permits him to exercise therapeutic judgment, to select proper treatment measures, and to treat the disease with predictable results.

To determine which periodontal disease is present and the precise clinical characteristics of the disease process in a given patient, the dentist must conduct a comprehensive examination. The signs of periodontal disease are often as varied and complex as are the possible causes. They occur in conjunction with other dental diseases and are superimposed on the specific intrinsic and emotional structure of the patient. Each person and each mouth is therefore an individual variant. In performing the examination and developing the treatment plan, the dentist must consider the patient as well as the oral cavity. He cannot categorize a patient as a type of case and then proceed with treatment according to set routines. Treatment must be regarded as individual as the patient. Moreover, most cases of periodontitis present a similar type of clinical and histologic picture, but each patient who has the disease is different. Thus his case of periodontitis is different. A disease entity has common characteristics. The manifestations are different in each patient who has the disease.

Since the approach to the patient is individualistic, effective therapy requires that a plan outlining treatment be developed. Such a plan should be based on the findings of the examination and also on the aims and specific objectives of treatment. Without preplanning, the dentist tends to proceed indecisively and the course of treatment meanders. Without an overall view, only limited treatment and a limited contribution to the patient's dental health are likely.

## EXAMINATION

A thorough examination is necessary to develop a plan for complete treatment. Such an examination contains the following elements: an interview, a roentgenographic examination, and an oral examination. All the information obtained should be charted, which is a simple means of documentation. Charting helps in the development of a considered diagnosis and treatment plan. Judgments may be made with greater objectivity. The findings of the examination, the diagnosis, the prognosis, and the treatment plan, all of which relate directly to each other, may be determined with a greater degree of accuracy on the basis of measured observations.

In addition to the disease process another threat to longevity of the natural dentition is lack of awareness on the part of the patient. He may not know about periodontal disease, or he may not be motivated toward treatment. It then falls on the dentist to educate the patient and to orient his motivation. This is possible when an appropriate dentist-patient relationship has been developed.

### Interview

The first step in an examination is the patient interview. It should be used with all new patients. However, it may be dispensed with for older patients if the objectives of the interview have been reached previously. The interview gives the dentist an opportunity to establish rapport,[1] to introduce patient education, and to acquaint the patient with the way in which the practice is conducted. During the interview the chief complaint, the medical history, and the dental history are obtained. Simultaneously the patient is observed for the purpose of making a preliminary evaluation of the individual. The successful observer combines the skills of a clinician with those of the lawyer, the psychiatrist, and the detective.[2]

***Dentist-patient relationship***

In the earlier days of medicine and dentistry, observation was all that the clinician had to go by. Today observation is still utilized to evaluate the type of individual who has come for treatment. Moreover, it enables one to know whether there is any relationship between the patient's general health and mental health and his dental disease. Such information can be gleaned by astute questioning, examining, recording, and observing.

A good share of observation consists of being attentive to the patient's manner of response. Much is revealed by the patient's choice of words, tone of voice, facial expression, and movements during the time he is answering your questions. These reactions tend to be heightened in the dental office since dentistry represents a stress situation to many patients.[3]

While the dentist is observing the patient, chances are that the patient will be appraising the dentist. Therefore the interview should be conducted in a relaxed, self-assured manner. A professional bearing is called for; but be attentive and sympathetic rather than aloof and cool. Let the patient do the talking. Should the patient ask questions, limit answers to the shortest and simplest possible. Above all, do not lecture the patient on the subject of dentistry.

Sometimes, when the patient asks questions concerning dentistry, he may be expressing anxiety rather than an interest in dentistry. The more experienced practitioner will sense this anxiety and reassure the patient, thus dealing with what is at the root of the question. In addition to words, the dentist's manner of approach will convey a sense of competence to the patient that will be reassuring to him. The less experienced practitioner will often deliver a long discourse that does not satisfy the patient's need, leaving the patient with a feeling of frustration.

On occasion the patient will ask a question that in reality reflects a doubt not expressed in his words. If this is sensed, attempt to make him verbalize the doubt so that it can be brought into the open and then dealt with. A question should be regarded as a clue. Unresolved doubts on the part of the patient may interfere with the course of treatment at a later time.

Preliminary information pertaining to the interview may be obtained through printed forms. These are not intended to supplant the interview but to supplement and expedite this step in the examination.

During the interview the following information should be elicited[4]: (1) vital statistics, (2) chief complaint, (3) medical history, and (4) dental history.

***Vital statistics***

The vital statistics include the patient's name, home and business addresses and phone numbers, age, sex, marital and family status, and occupation. These are all significant. They give information about the patient and his possible background. By the mode of response, the dentist may be able to gauge the patient's intelligence. He may also assay the degree of patient cooperation. The source of referral is important too. If the patient was referred by another patient who had periodontal treatment, chances are that he is partly informed about periodontal disease and less time for patient education will be required. The patient can be tested with a comment such as, "I guess that Mrs. ______ has told you all about periodontal disease." If the answer is negative, proceed as usual. If the answer is positive, the patient is rewarded with some remark about how unusual it is to have such a well-informed patient.

***Chief complaint***

What is the reason for the patient's visit? Does he have pain, discomfort, or any other complaint? Often he will present for a routine checkup. However, there will be times when he presents in an emergency, with pain, bleeding, or swelling. In these instances, attend to the emergency as soon as its location and cause have been determined. When there are no medical contraindications or precautions to be taken, the remainder of the interview may then be postponed. In any event the dentist may want to know when the condition started and whether it had ever occurred previously.

***Medical history***

To assist in assessing the medical status of a new patient, a questionnaire may be filled out by the patient prior to the actual interview. A typical questionnaire follows. This is only to provide a guide in obtaining a complete medical history. Some practitioners prefer a questionnaire; others work without such printed guides.

The patient should be asked, "How is your health?" Some patients will give a detailed answer. Most patients, however, will answer, "Fine." Test this answer by asking some of the following questions: "Have you ever been seriously ill?" "When were you last examined by a physician?" "Who is your physician?" "What was the reason for your last visit to him?" "What were the findings?" Are you under treatment now?" "Have you taken out insurance in the last few years?" "Did you have any difficulty with the insurance examination?" "Did you serve in

Name ______________________ Home address ______________________

Physician's name ______________________ Address ______________________

How old are you? Circle if you are: single, married, widowed, separated, divorced

Circle the highest year you reached in school: 1 2 3 4 5 6 7 8 (Elementary) 1 2 3 4 (High)

1 2 3 4 5 6 7 8 (College)

What is your occupation? ______________________

**Directions:** If your answer is yes to the question asked, put a circle around YES. If your answer is no, put a circle around NO. Answer all the questions. Answers to the following questions are for our records only, and they will be considered confidential.

1. Are you being treated for any condition by a physician now? .......... NO YES
2. Are you taking any medicines now? .......... NO YES
3. Have you been examined by your physician within the last year? .......... NO YES
4. Has there been any change in your general health in the last year? .......... NO YES
5. Have you ever been seriously ill? .......... NO YES
6. Have you ever been hospitalized? .......... NO YES
7. Have you ever had a major operation? .......... NO YES
8. Have you ever had a blood transfusion? .......... NO YES
9. Have you ever had any of the following diseases?
   - Rheumatic fever .......... NO YES
   - Inflammatory rheumatism .......... NO YES
   - Jaundice (yellow skin and eyes) .......... NO YES
   - Tuberculosis .......... NO YES
   - Venereal disease .......... NO YES
   - Heart attack .......... NO YES
   - Stroke .......... NO YES
10. Have you ever been told by a physician that you have a heart murmur? .......... NO YES
11. Do you ever have asthma or hay fever? .......... NO YES
12. Do you ever have hives or skin rash? .......... NO YES
13. Have you ever experienced an unusual reaction to any of the following drugs?
    - Aspirin .......... NO YES
    - Penicillin .......... NO YES
    - Iodine .......... NO YES
    - Sulfonamides (sulfa) .......... NO YES
    - Barbiturates (sleeping pills) .......... NO YES
    - Other medicines? .......... NO YES
14. Have you ever experienced an unusual reaction to a dental anesthetic? .......... NO YES
15. Do you have diabetes (sugar disease)? .......... NO YES
16. Do you have high blod pressure? .......... NO YES
17. Do you bleed for a long time when you cut yourself? .......... NO YES
18. Have you ever had an injury to your face or jaws? .......... NO YES
19. Have you ever had surgery or x-ray treatment for a tumor, growth, or other condition in your mouth or on your lips? .......... NO YES

**Systems review**

20. Do you have frequent severe headaches? .......... NO YES
21. Do you have any complaints regarding your eyes? .......... NO YES

22. Do you have any ear trouble? ........ NO YES
23. Do you have frequent colds? ........ NO YES
24. Do you have sinus trouble? ........ NO YES
25. Do you have nosebleeds? ........ NO YES
26. Do you have frequent sore throats? ........ NO YES
27. Do you have any sensitive teeth? ........ NO YES
28. Have you ever had a toothache? ........ NO YES
29. Do you have bleeding gums? ........ NO YES
30. Do you have frequent canker sores or cold sores? ........ NO YES
31. Have you ever had a severely sore mouth? ........ NO YES
32. Is it difficult for you to open your mouth as wide as you would like? .. NO YES
33. Does your jaw click when you chew? ........ NO YES

**Cardiorespiratory**

34. Do you have any chest pain on exertion? ........ NO YES
35. Are you ever short of breath on mild exertion? ........ NO YES
36. Do your ankles swell? ........ NO YES
37. Do you have a persistent cough? ........ NO YES
38. Do you ever cough blood? ........ NO YES

**Gastrointestinal**

39. Has your appetite changed recently? ........ NO YES
40. Are there any foods you cannot eat? ........ NO YES
41. Do you have any difficulty swallowing? ........ NO YES
42. Do you have frequent indigestion? ........ NO YES
43. Do you vomit frequently? ........ NO YES

**Genitourinary**

44. Do you have kidney trouble? ........ NO YES
45. Do you urinate more than six times a day? ........ NO YES
46. Are you thirsty much of the time? ........ NO YES

**Bones and joints**

47. Have you ever had painful and swollen joints? ........ NO YES

**Neuromuscular**

48. Do you have and numb or prickling areas on your skin? ........ NO YES
49. Do you ever have fits or convulsions? ........ NO YES
50. Do you have a tendency to faint? ........ NO YES

**Hematology**

51. Do you bruise easily? ........ NO YES
52. Do you have any blood disorder such as anemia (thin blood) ........ NO YES

**Endocrines and metabolism**

53. Does hot weather bother you more than it does other people you know? .. NO YES
54. Are you excessively nervous? ........ NO YES
55. Do you get tired easily? ........ NO YES

**Women**

56. Are you pregnant at the present time? ........ NO YES
57. Have you passed the menopause (change of life) ........ NO YES
58. Are your menstrual periods irregular? ........ NO YES

Courtesy A. E. Fry, University of Oregon Dental School

the Armed Forces?" "Were you discharged for any medical reason?" Have you ever been hospitalized?" "When and for what reason?" "Have you ever had any operations?" "Do you take any medication or drug regularly?" "Do you have any drug allergies?"

When questions concerning diseases of the various organ systems are answered in the negative, the negative answers need not be recorded.[5] Generally, specific inquiries should be made concerning the heart and circulatory system, respiratory system, genitourinary system, allergies, endocrinopathies, and blood dyscrasias. If all the answers are negative, the notation should read, "Medical history noncontributory." Certain negative answers, however, must be recorded. These are the answers to questions such as the following: "Have you ever had rheumatic fever?" "Have you had serum hepatitis?" "Have you ever had antibiotics?" "Are you allergic to any antibiotics?" "Are you sensitive to aspirin, or have you ever experienced any unusual reactions from local anesthetics or codeine?" All information of medical significance should be recorded. List briefly the essential factors in the patient's medical history that might be of significance to his periodontal disease (e. g., pregnancy, diabetes, dysfunction of ovaries, thyroid, or other endocrine gland) or that might affect the course of the treatment or require certain precautions (history of rheumatic or valvular heart disease, high blood pressure, use of anticoagulants, blood dyscrasia, hepatitis, syphilis, kidney disease). If the patient is taking anticoagulants, the dentist must confer with the patient's physician as to the feasibility of any proposed surgery; the use of aspirin, or drugs containing aspirin, is then contraindicated. Inquiry should be made regarding the adequacy of the patient's diet, disturbances of the digestive tract, diseases of the lungs, and allergic reactions.* Note should be made of the date and type of any general surgery that has been performed. Whether or not the patient has ever been uprated or rejected by an insurance company as an impaired risk should also be noted.

During this portion of the examination, the dentist-patient relationship tends to crystallize. Rapport is established, and this can be significant in all future relationships. Throughout the questioning period the examiner should be cancer-conscious and alert to any leads such as weight loss, swellings, ulcers. Most patients are cancer-conscious too, so the examiner must be careful never by word or action to arouse a patient's curiosity and then leave his fears unanswered. Even a chance remark such as "hhmm" will frighten some people. Observations of nervous habits and any abnormal condition of the skin, hair, and fingernails should be noted. Also any tic, ptosis, unusual expression, or unusual posture or gait should be recorded.

There are separate questions to ask women related to childbearing, menarche, and menopause. If the patient is married, ask her whether she has any children and how many. "Did you have any unusual trouble at the time of their birth?"

---

*Colored tags may be affixed to the patient's chart to alert the dentist to some systemic or local condition that must be considered. A red tag indicates the presence of a systemic condition such as cardiovascular disease, history of rheumatic fever, diabetes, ulcers, allergies, or that the patient is taking medication such as cortisone or anticoagulants. A yellow tag may be used to indicate that the patient is apprehensive and that some premedication such as a tranquilizer should be given or prescribed. A green tag may indicate tooth sensitivity to probing or to other instrumentation such as root planing. The condition may be entered in a prominent place on the chart entitled "Alert."

"Did you have trouble with your gums or teeth during pregnancy?" "Is your menstrual cycle regular?" If the patient is middle-aged, ask her whether she has reached menopause as yet.

An attempt should also be made to determine the patient's nervous state. "Do you get up tired?" may elicit a laugh and the answer "I'm always tired." Then the examiner must determine whether this is a joke or the patient is indeed serious. "Do you sleep well at night?" "Is your heartbeat regular?" "How is your appetite?" While asking these questions, reach out and gently take the patient's hand to examine the palm. Is it wet? Does the patient consider himself nervous? Any affirmative answers may be suggestive of neurosis. Develop the habit of watching the patient's upper lip and brow for perspiration, which may be a sign of nervous tension. The patient who yawns during the interview may be tense, not bored.

***Dental history***

When the chief complaint is of a nonemergency nature, obtain in the patient's own words the history of the present oral illness from its inception until the present time. "Have you ever had any treatment for this condition?" "What was it as you recall?" "Did you complete your treatment?" "Did you carry out your part of the treatment?" On occasion, the fact that the patient is stoic and has minimized an emergency situation will become evident. Conversely, an occasional anxious patient may present as an emergency what is actually a minor complaint. Whatever information the patient volunteers should be followed by questions in logical order so that as much as possible can be learned. Some particularly astute examiners pose the same question in two different ways to check the accuracy of the answers.

The dental history should include all dental treatments rendered in the past (orthodontics, prosthetic appliances, removal of impacted teeth). Additionally the history should include such items as the following: approximate dates of previous periodontal treatment (root planing, curettage, gingival surgery, osseous surgery, occlusal adjustment, splinting, home dental care instruction). Note the history of previous complaints (gingival bleeding, periodontal abscesses, pain, burning, bad taste, bad breath, pathologic tooth migration). Question the patient with regard to rapidity of new formation of stain and calcified deposits. The patient's periodontal complaint should be recorded in his own words. Entries such as the following should be made: "gums bleed on brushing," "gums hurt," "certain teeth loose," "some teeth moved," "teeth extremely sensitive to cold," "bad breath or bad taste" (subjective symptoms).

Many patients will present a preconceived idea of dentistry that does not include periodontics. Such patients will have to be educated as to why the examination is conducted as it is. They will have to be made aware of the existence of periodontal disease. Their education is best accomplished with casual sentences during the interview and the examination.

If the interview has progressed smoothly, a 1-minute introduction to periodontics (such as the following) may be in order, which will lead directly to the examination.

"At one time patients came to the dentist only when they had a toothache or wanted an extraction. Of course, each diseased tooth once had a very small cavity or beginning periodontal disease that could have been treated simply. It is now seldom necessary to extract a tooth unless caries or periodontal disease are far advanced. I am now going to make a careful examination to detect decay and periodontal disease. Do you approve?"

Most patients will consent to this examination. Some may ask what periodontal disease is. An explanation that this condition was once called "pyorrhea" should be sufficient. Then, give a brief, simple description of periodontal disease and mention that the word "pyorrhea" was used when the disease was considered hopeless. The disease can now be successfully treated so the word is no longer used.

Some patients will ask more detailed questions at this point, and these represent clues to the deeper-lying doubts. The examiner's objective is then to unmask the basic reason for the question and to properly educate the patient. Do not become hostile and argumentative. Responses should consist of a repetition of the preceding explanation and of gaining the patient's acceptance of the principle that it is important to find dental defects when they are just beginning. Elicit why the patient questions the need for the examinations. Once the patient has indicated the source from which his doubts stem, the examiner may effectively deal with the doubt in a way that reassures the patient.

***Medical consultation***

At times, after the interview, the dentist may believe that laboratory tests should be performed or that medical consultation might be desirable. Blood smears, biopsies, blood tests, and urine tests may be indicated. When medical consultation is called for, the dentist should contact the patient's physician. The clinical examination should follow the interview.

***Intraoral examination***

The intraoral examination consists of an inspection of the soft tissues (including the gingiva), the teeth, the occlusion, and the temporomandibular joint. Full-mouth roentgenograms should be taken. In addition, study models and Kodachrome photographs of the dentition may be helpful. It may be necessary to test the vitality of the teeth. The date of the examination should be noted. All data should be carefully charted, for these become a part of the patient's record and should be filed and stored in a systematic fashion so that they can be referred to with ease and not be lost.

## Roentgenographic examination

Roentgenograms are of greatest diagnostic value in periodontics when the angulation of projection and the density control are correct to show trabecular patterns and discrete changes in bone density. Roentgenograms can give some of the following information:

1. Interdental bone height and presence of a lamina dura
2. Trabecular patterns
3. Suggestive radiolucent areas of bone destruction that can be confirmed by probing
4. Bone loss in furcations
5. Width of periodontal ligament space
6. Crown-to-root ratio
7. Root shape and length
8. Caries, general quality of restorations, heavy calculus deposits
9. Location of antrum relative to alveolar crest
10. Missing teeth, supernumerary teeth, impactions

Roentgenograms give a two-dimensional representation of three-dimensional structures. They are most useful as a diagnostic tool when they are correlated with visual oral examination, clinical probing, and pocket charting.[14]

Surveys utilizing the long cone–paralleling technique of projection are desirable. A minimum of sixteen films should be used, the results in each area being

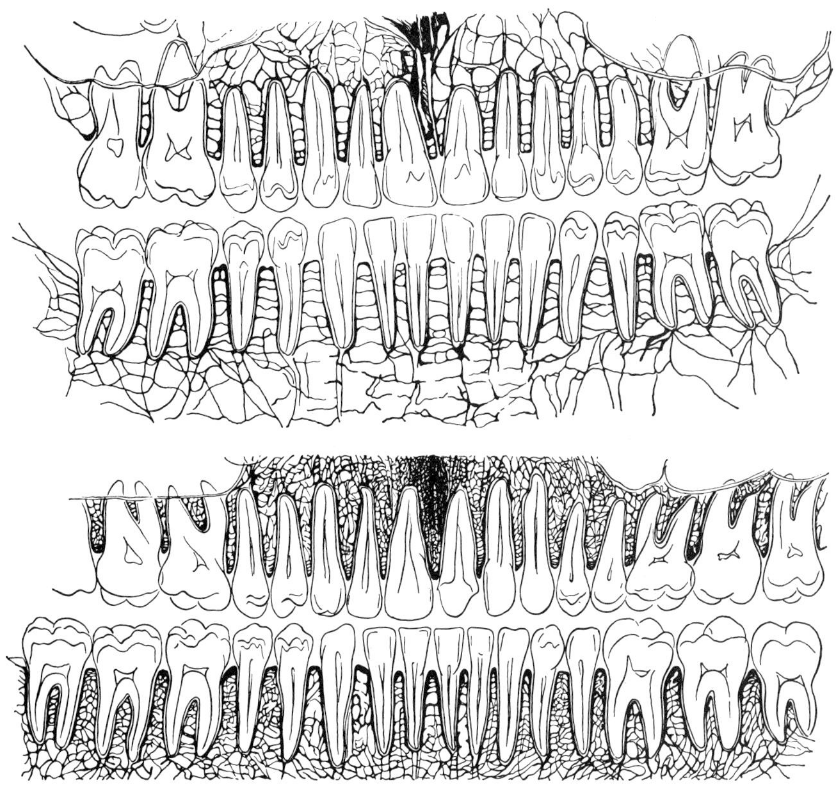

**Fig. 18-1.** Two types of normal trabecular arrangement. (From Brescia, N.: Applied dental anatomy, St. Louis, 1961, The C. V. Mosby Co.)

exposed from more than one angulation to produce a stereoscopic effect. Technical errors that produce elongation, foreshortening, and/or overlapping severely impair the diagnostic usefulness of the roentgenograms. Panoramic roentgenographic surveys may have limited use.

The place of the roentgenogram in periodontal diagnosis is important, on the one hand, and much misunderstood, on the other. Too often the diagnosis of periodontal disease is made from inspection of roentgenograms, at which time the disease is usually long established.

***Inspection before probing***

Before making a systematic oral examination, the clinician should study the roentgenograms in a sequential manner for gross oral pathology (cysts, granulomas, cementomas, foreign bodies, impactions, unerupted or supernumerary teeth, neoplasms). Next he should view the patterns of alveolar bone trabeculation. Several types of trabecular patterns have been described and are illustrated in Figs. 18-1 and 18-2.[15] Deviations from normal trabeculation, such as disuse atrophy, and rare general involvements, such as hyperparathyroidism and Paget's disease, should be noted. The loss of trabeculation caused by disuse atrophy will be readily apparent around teeth long out of occlusion and around extraction sites.

***Etiologic factors***

Roentgenograms should be inspected for the following: calculus, caries in the crown or root surfaces, and overhanging or defective restorations. Are there open contact points? Are these defects related to areas of bone loss? Is any immediate treatment necessary to prevent or cope with pulpal involvement? The

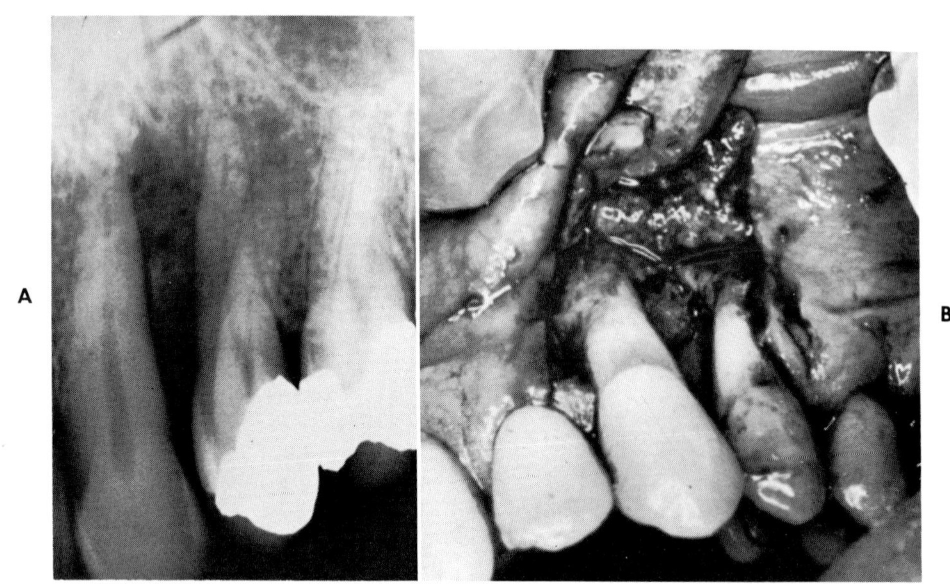


**Fig. 18-2.** Degree of density in a roentgenogram can mask obvious pathology. The bone loss shown in **B** is greater than the roentgenogram, **A**, would indicate.

roentgenograms should further be examined for height of septal bone, continuity of lamina dura, and width of periodontal ligament.

***Periodontal bone loss***

Osseous defects may become evident on the roentgenograms. The bone loss may be localized or generalized. The patterns of loss may be horizontal or vertical. Bony craters or troughs may be distinguishable. There may be roentgenographic furcation involvements. The maxillary antrum may come near the alveolar crest in the areas of bone loss.

After studying the roentgenograms, the therapist should make his clinical examination. When this is completed, he should peruse the roentgenograms once more to determine whether the findings agree or disagree with his impression of the patient's condition as far as prior findings are concerned. If there are any obvious differences, they should be accounted for. Reprobing may be necessary. Roentgenograms taken at predetermined angles may be needed to visualize bony defects. The use of calibrated silver points or grids may be helpful.[16,17]

***Occlusion***

The roentgenograms may reveal information about the occlusion. There may be evidence of occlusal traumatism. Roots may be long or they may be short and tapering. There may be root resorption, and the crown-to-root ratio may be low. There may be thickening of the periodontal ligament, and part of the root may actually be covered by bone. Teeth may be malaligned, tilted, overerupted, or depressed. There may be sclerotic areas related to overfunction.

***Limitations***

The value of roentgenograms is readily appreciated. However, their limitations should also be understood. Roentgenograms cannot give an accurate picture of pocket depth[14,17]; this can be judged only by probing. Roentgenograms do not show the earliest disease changes. They are rarely indisputable indicators of successful treatment. They may not depict bony deformities accurately or show bone changes on oral (lingual) and vestibular (buccal) aspects of teeth (Fig. 18-3). They show few soft tissue–to–hard tissue relationships. Despite these limitations, no accurate examination can be made without good roentgeno-

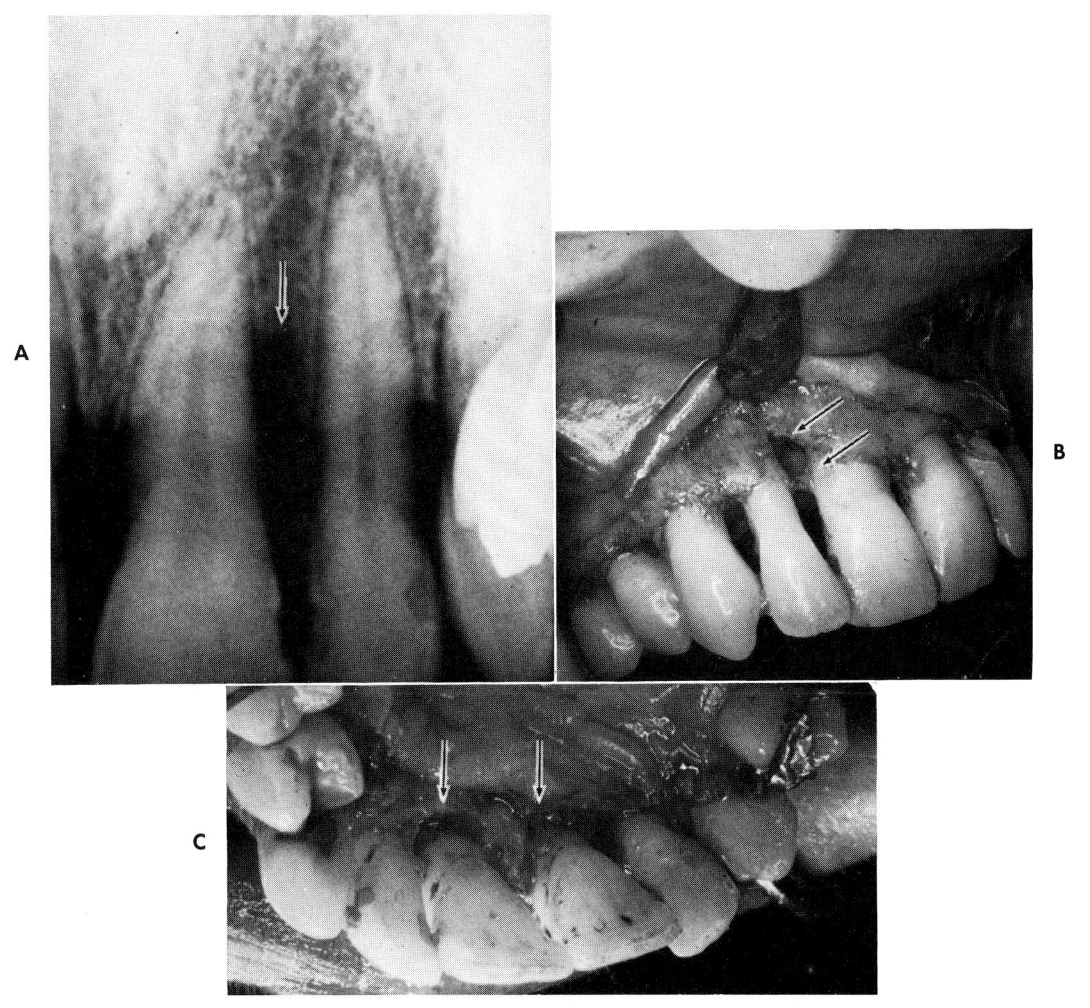

**Fig. 18-3. A,** Roentgenogram of the maxillary right central and lateral incisors shows an area of radiolucency interproximally bordering the central incisor. The bizarre bone configuration caused by the destruction was seen when a flap was retracted, **B.** An isthmus of bone is all that remains of the alveolar crest. A large area of bone destruction is apical to this and extends palatally. **C,** Troughlike, infrabony destruction can be seen on the palatal surface around the central incisor. The defect communicates with the bony defect on the interproximal and labial.

grams.[12] To summarize: good roentgenograms, viewed under good diffused light with a magnifying lens or loupes, and careful examination can reveal most bone lesions in periodontal disease. They are an essential part of the examination.

## Oral examination

The following description of the oral examination sequence will deal primarily with the periodontal status of the patient.

***Halitosis***

Halitosis (fetor ex ore) is important to the patient[7-11] and many times is the symptom that brings him to the dentist. It may originate in areas in which retention of food particles occurs. Decomposing soft deposits may cause it. Another frequent cause is acute necrotizing gingivitis. Deep carious lesions may also cause it. Halitosis is often seen in patients suffering from febrile diseases and

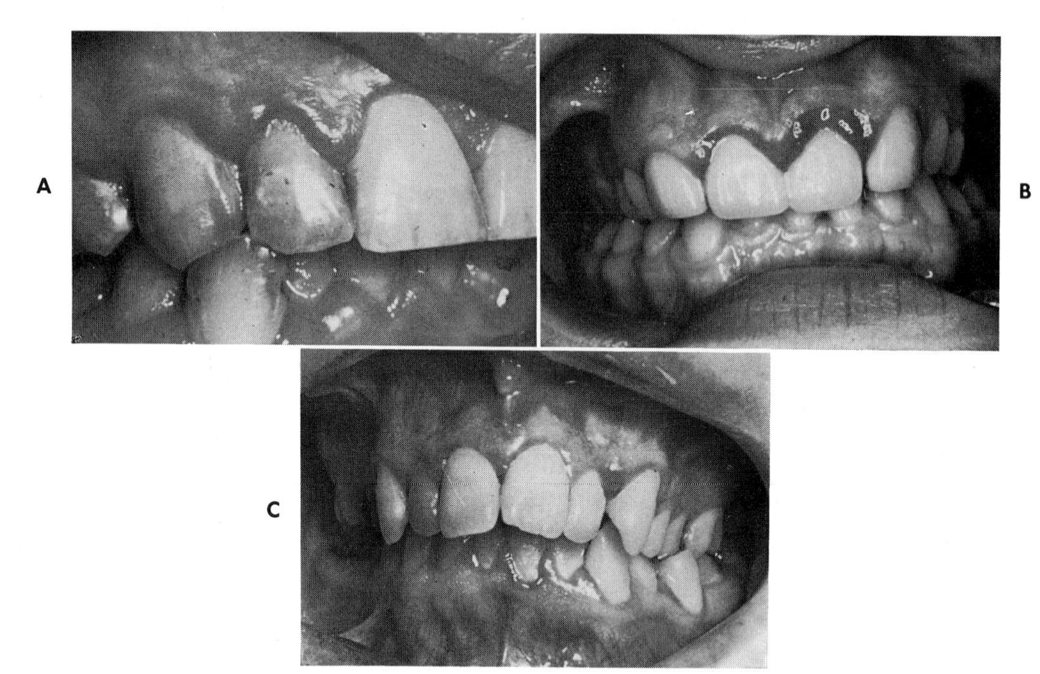

**Fig. 18-4.** Note the variations in form, color, firmness, and response of the gingiva to irritation. **A,** Fibrotic response to chronic irritation resulting in hyperplastic enlargement of the interdental papilla. **B,** Edematous response to irritation, localized around the central incisors. Gingival margins are enlarged because of the edema. There are no apparent changes elsewhere. **C,** Fibrotic and inflammatory response to irritation. The facial gingival margins are receded with a slight edematous border.

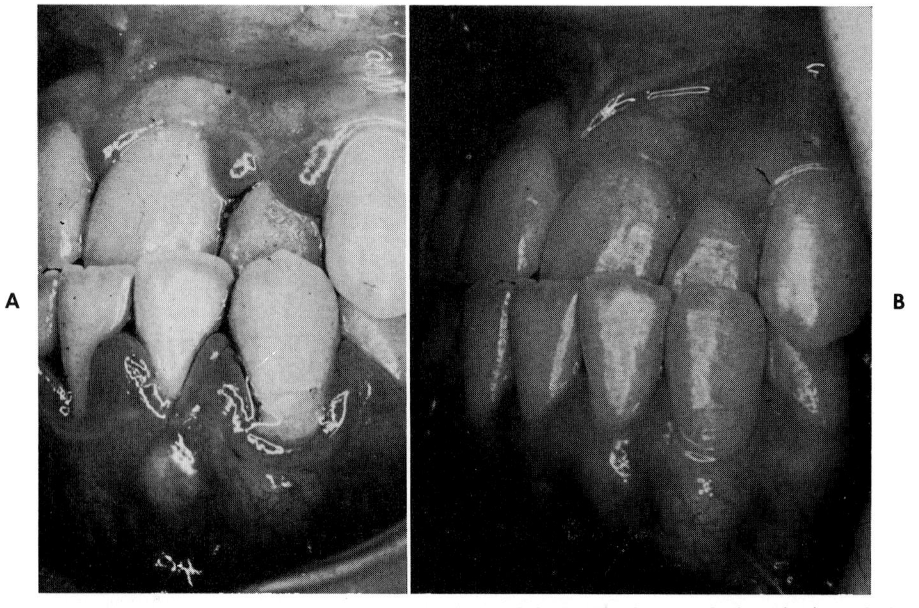

**Fig. 18-5.** Compare the nonphysiologic, **A,** and physiologic, **B,** forms of the gingiva (before and after treatment).

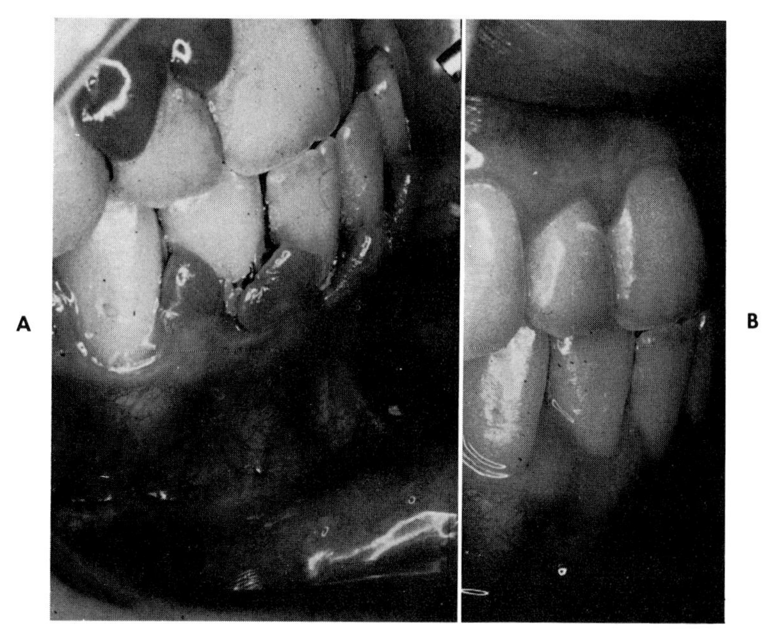


**Fig. 18-6.** Compare the retractable, **A,** and firm nonretractable, **B,** gingivae when subjected to a blast of air (before and after treatment).

from psychiatric depression. If after the elimination of dental and periodontal causes and the exclusion of offensive foods and drink bad breath persists, competent medical specialists should examine the nose, nasopharynx, tonsils, and lungs, because diseases of these organs may on occasion cause halitosis (Chapter 25).

***Soft tissues***

In the soft tissue area the dentist should concern himself particularly with abnormalities, and he should always note the location of such findings. The condition of the following should be observed: tongue, buccal mucosa, floor of the mouth, palate, frena, throat, and oral mucosa. Do the amount and consistency of saliva appear normal? Are there variations in the color, contour, or firmness of the gingiva (Fig. 18-4)? Is the form of the gingiva physiologic (Fig. 18-5)? Is the gingiva firm, or is it retractable and does it bleed easily (Figs. 18-6 and 18-7)? Is the vestibule shallow or deep? Is the zone of attached gingiva narrow or broad (Fig. 18-8)? Does the patient have pain? Are there areas of food impaction present? Are any other possible local causes evident? Did the patient relate a history of trench mouth or pyorrhea, recurrent cold sores, cankers or mouth blisters, dental abscesses, sinus trouble, swellings, or pain? Is there any evidence of these in the mouth?

The clinical gingival findings can be classified according to the following:

1. *Extent of lesions.* Localized or generalized
2. *Distribution of lesions.* Papillary, marginal, or attached gingival
3. *State of inflammation.* Acute or chronic
4. *Clinical features.* Hyperplasia, ulceration, necrosis, formation of pseudomembranes, depth of pockets, purulent exudation, serous exudation, hemorrhage, abnormal muscle attachments or frena, width of attached gingiva, relation of pockets to mucogingival junction

In examining the gingiva, the clinician must keep in mind a picture of the "normal" gingiva. With this as a guide, he can more readily observe the extent and state of inflammation and the distribution of the lesions.

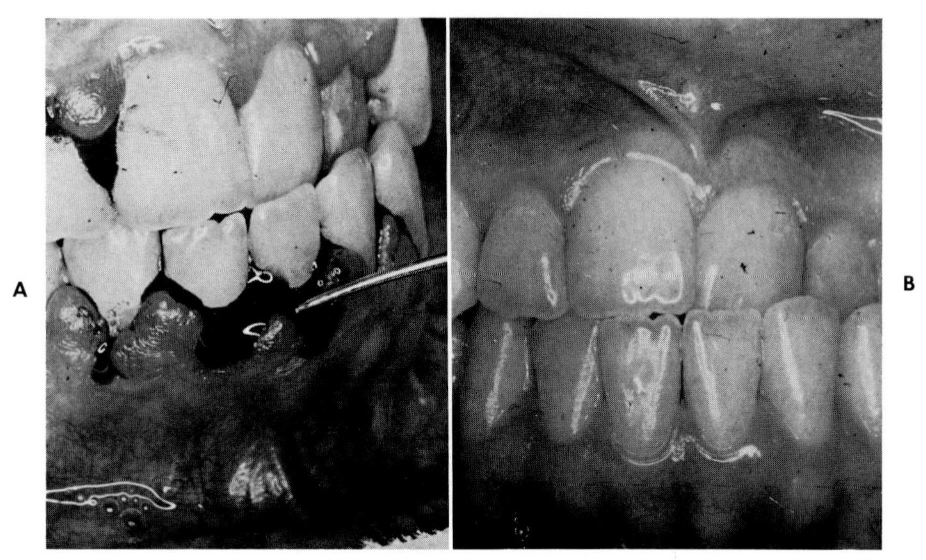

**Fig. 18-7.** Compare the edematous bleeding, **A,** and firm normal, **B,** gingivae (before and after treatment).

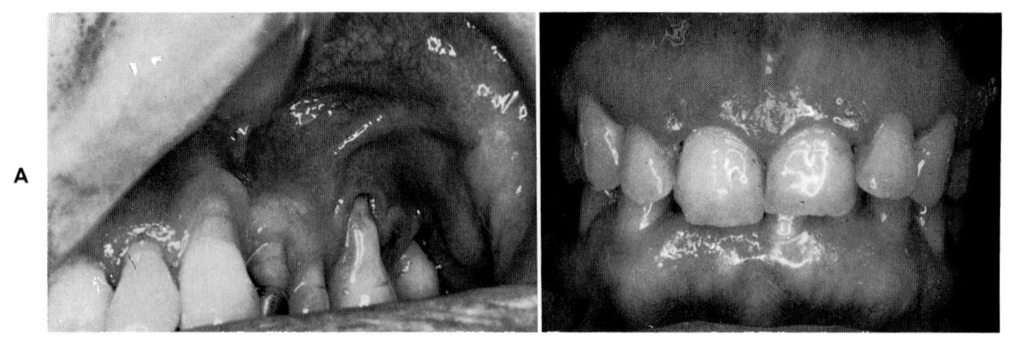

**Fig. 18-8. A,** Note the narrow zone of attached gingiva associated with pocket formation and recession. Pockets extend beyond the mucogingival junction. Note also the variation in level of the vestibular fornix. **B,** Wide zone of gingiva. Pockets are present but do not extend beyond the mucogingival junction.

***Teeth***

The size of the teeth should be noted, and the degree of caries susceptibility should be gauged by the presence of restorations. The type and quality of restorations should be evaluated. In addition, new carious lesions and erosions should be observed. The biting surfaces should be examined for excessive occlusal wear. When this is evident, the patient should be questioned as to whether he grinds his teeth or chews on one side only. Does he chew tobacco? Is he unhappy with the appearance of his mouth? Diastemas should be noted and proximal contacts tested with dental floss. Conditions such as toothbrush abrasion, tooth mobility, tooth malpositions, hypoplastic enamel, supernumerary teeth, nonvital teeth, and tooth sensitivity should be recorded. For tooth sensitivity, questions may be asked concerning the effects of temperature extremes and sweets. The teeth may be percussed and the tooth surfaces examined for caries.

*Oral hygiene*

The general status of oral hygiene should be ascertained. Note the presence of plaque, stain, and calculus. A disclosing solution may be used to graphically show the general status of oral hygiene. In addition, the patient may be questioned concerning the date of his last prophylaxis, his method and frequency of toothbrushing, and cleaning aids he uses, in an attempt to gauge the rate of calculus deposition.[6] (See also Chapter 12.)

Coronal findings may be recorded as follows:

1. Plaque
2. Subgingival deposits
3. Supragingival deposits
4. Materia alba
5. Location of dental caries
6. Erosion
7. Abrasion
8. Inadequate restorations

*Temporomandibular joint*

The patient should be questioned as to temporomandibular joint symptoms (e.g., pain, subluxation, clicking, popping).[13] The joint should be palpated in both protrusive and lateral excursions. In addition, the pathway of the chin point should be observed during mandibular movements. Deviation from a natural, smooth opening pattern may be indicative of joint or muscular dysfunction. In the majority of cases, however, the joints will be found to be functioning normally.

*Occlusion*

The dentition should be rated as complete or mutilated by extractions. When there are missing teeth, whether or not they have been replaced should be noted. Has the dentition then maintained itself or is the arch collapsing and are the teeth drifting? When the dentition is complete (or if the status can otherwise be ascertained), what is the orthodontic classification? Has the patient ever had orthodontic treatment? Has malocclusion or tooth malposition contributed to the patient's present disease status? Has perfect occlusion, when present, preserved good oral health? These factors are not always correlated. Does the patient have centric prematurities? Note their location. Does the patient have interferences in excursions (lateral and protrusive)? Are the teeth mobile to testing? Do they exhibit fremitus in function? Does the patient complain that his fillings squeak when he chews? Do the restorations contribute to pathologic changes, or do they promote oral health? Does the patient swallow with his mouth open or closed? Does he thrust his tongue between his teeth during swallowing? Does he have oral compulsions such as lip or tongue or cheek biting? Does he bite or chew on objects such as eyeglasses, pencils, fingernails? Does he lick his lips? Is he a mouth breather? Does he clench his masseters? The patient should be questioned concerning whether or not he grinds or clenches his teeth or sets his jaw in determination. The teeth should be checked for corroborative wear facets or mobility.

*Charting*

As one proceeds with the examination, the findings should be recorded on a suitable chart (Figs. 18-9 and 18-10). Missing teeth, impactions, anomalies, periapical pathology, caries, pain on percussion, poor contacts, food impactions, premature contacts, recessions, and rotations all have been entered by this time. If some notations have been overlooked, go back and enter them. Notations require more time in the beginning when one is unaccustomed to using them. Ultimately, when skill and accuracy are attained, they take only a short time. Standardized symbols should be used so that notations are universally understood and the charts may be readable in the future by others (Fig. 18-10). Auxiliary personnel may be used in recording the data.

At this point the all-important charting of mobility and pocket depth still remains. The patient should be told that some discomfort may be experienced

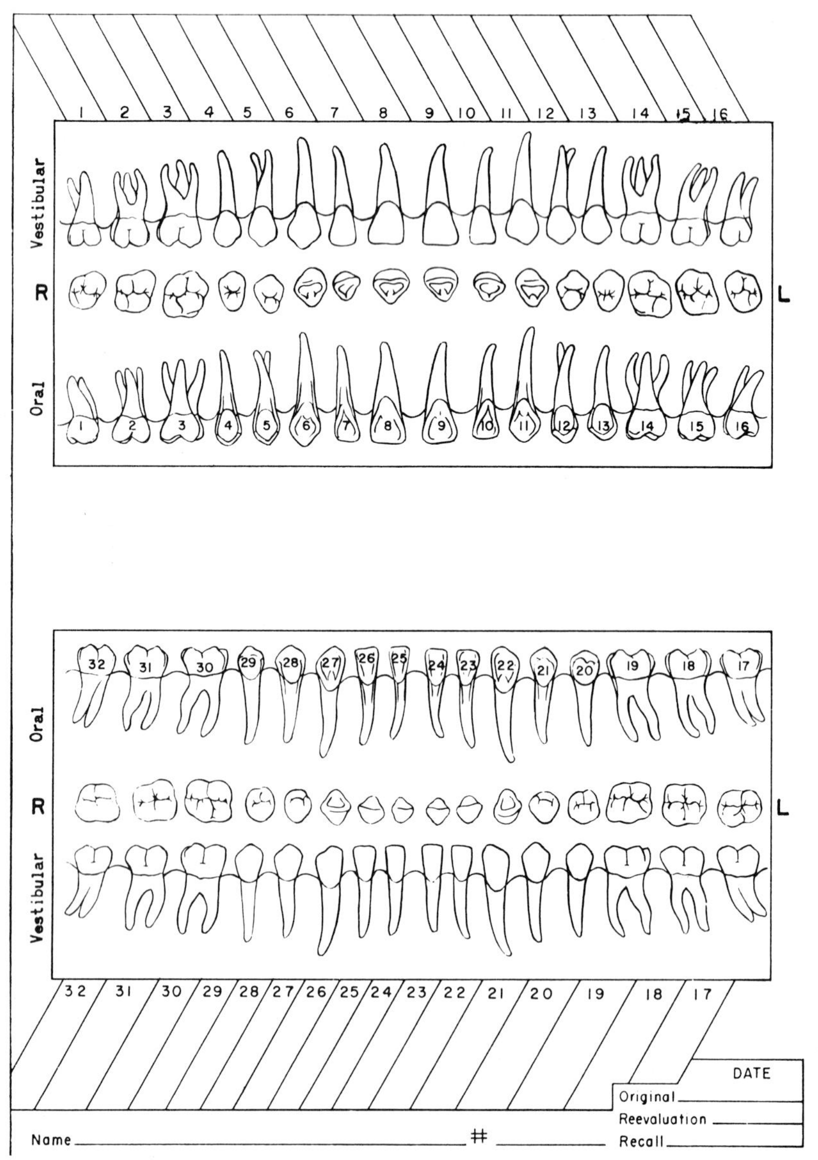


**Fig. 18-9.** Typical chart used for periodontal examination. Pocket depths and other findings may be indicated as shown in Fig. 18-14, *B*.

during the measurement of the pockets, particularly when inflammation is present. A topical anesthetic can usually minimize any pain. If the patient has reported a history of rheumatic fever with valvular involvement, he must be given an adequate dose of antibiotic prior to probing. When the case is to be documented with photographs or when study models are to be taken, it is best to obtain these prior to probing since the gingiva may bleed. Bleeding tends to mar the photographs and the models. The armamentarium used in the examination is shown in Figs. 18-11 and 18-12.

***Probing***

In determining pocket depth one may use either a pocket explorer or a peri-

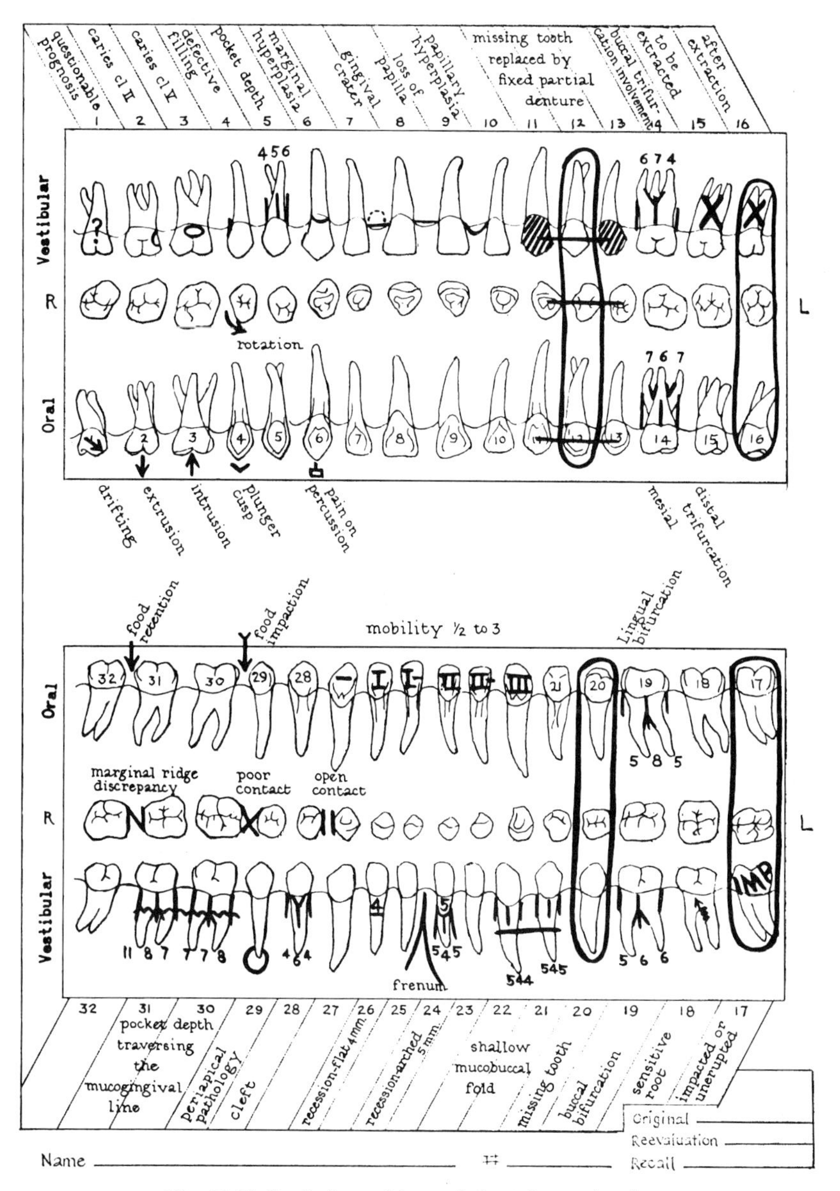


**Fig. 18-10.** Symbols used in periodontal examination.

odontal probe (Fig. 18-12, *A*). The periodontal probe is useful because it is calibrated. The explorer, on the other hand, is a finer instrument and can provide a better tactile assessment of the condition of the root surface. In general, the probe should be passed under the gingiva along the circumference of the tooth. Three measurements should be made on the buccal aspect and three on the lingual aspect of each tooth. The probe should be manipulated so that it is not blocked by the gingival calculus. In addition, the entire circumference of the pocket should be inspected in a sweeping traverse so as not to miss a narrow pocket entrance.

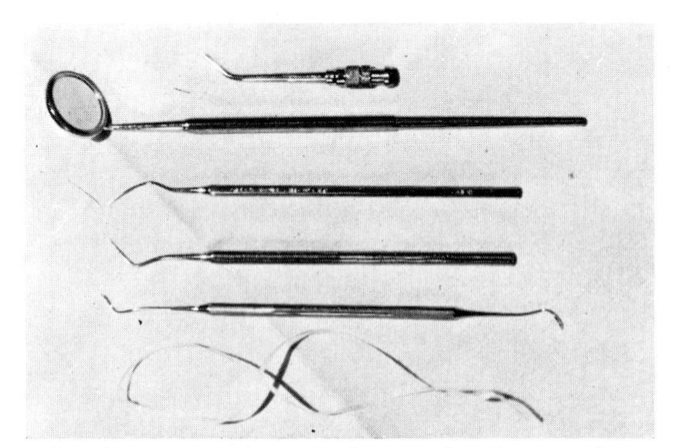

**Fig. 18-11.** Armamentarium for examination: air tip, mouth mirror, pocket explorer, periodontal probe, no. 2 explorer, dental floss.

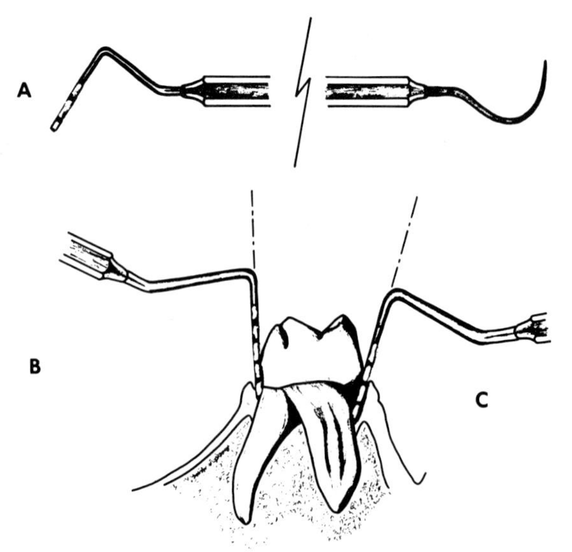


**Fig. 18-12.** Diagrammatic representation of, **A,** probe-explorer instrument that would be desirable in examination procedures; **B,** point or spot technique of probing in assessing the presence of pockets (three points on buccal and three on lingual aspect of each tooth recorded: mesial buccal, middle buccal, distal buccal, mesial lingual, middle lingual, distal lingual); and **C,** circumferential probing method, depicting schematically the drawing of the probe along the base of the pocket from proximal contact to proximal contact. (**B** and **C** courtesy J. Tussing, Lincoln, Neb.)

The probe may not reach to the bottom of the pocket.[21] How far it reaches will depend on the size of the probe, the force exerted, the dimensions of the pocket, the access, and the presence of deposits.

Calculus deposits often cause errors in probing by either preventing the probe from entering the sulcus at the proper angulation or impeding insertion to the depth of the pocket. In these instances the probe should be manipulated in several directions so as not to be blocked by the calculus deposits. It may be held horizontally when the shape of the interdental pocket is being explored; but, in general, it is held with a slight inclination to the long axis of the tooth (Fig. 18-13). In tortuous pockets, when the probe is held absolutely parallel to the

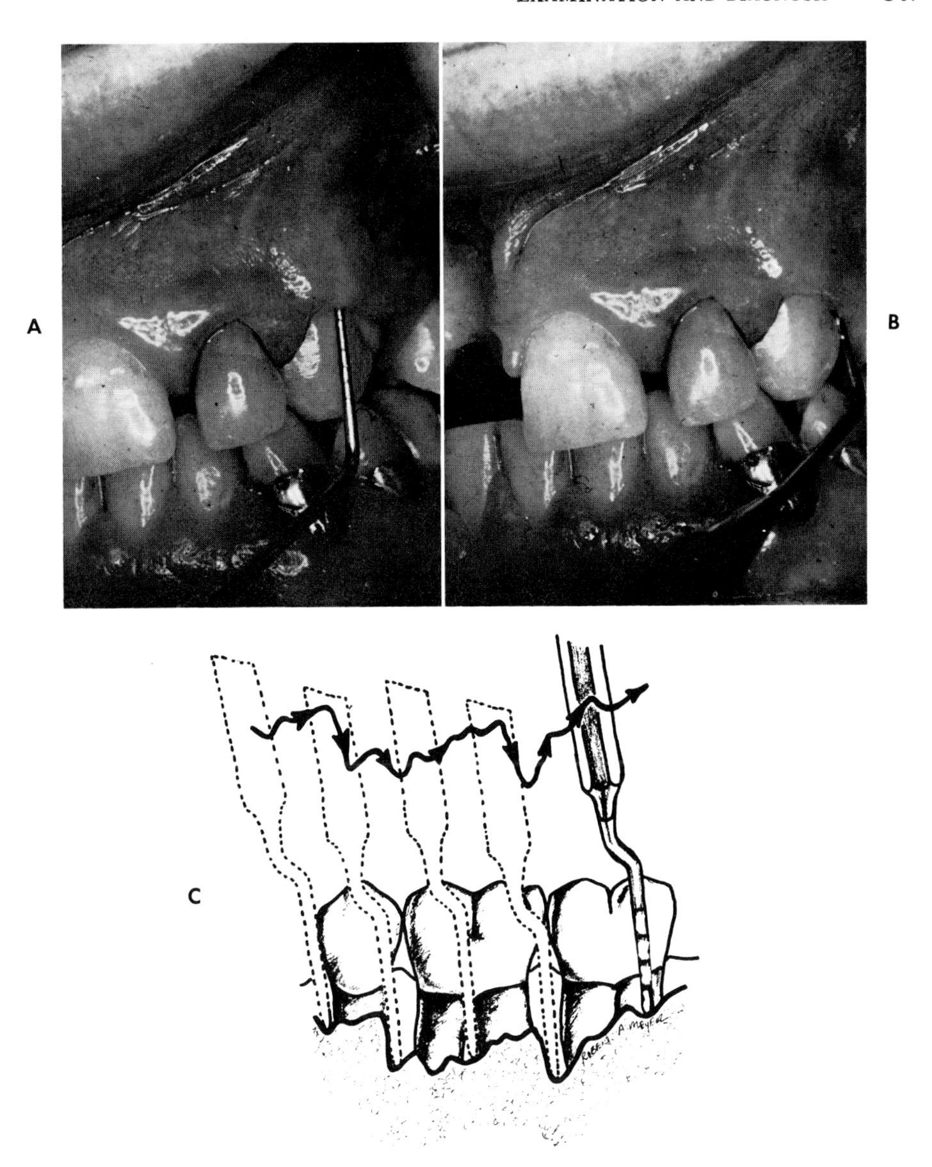


**Fig. 18-13.** Positioning of the probe for pocket measurement. **A,** The sulcular depth is 2 mm. on the labial surface of the canine (no pocket). **B,** On the distal surface of the same tooth, an 8 mm. pocket is present. Probe the sulci and pockets carefully since readings on different surfaces of the same tooth may vary extensively. **C,** Circumferential probing reveals the irregular character of bone loss in periodontitis. In this illustration the bone loss is shown along the vestibular tooth surfaces.

long axis of the tooth and is used for measuring and not exploring, the deepest portions of the pocket may be completely missed (Fig. 18-13).

Probing is particularly important because roentgenograms do not offer an accurate picture of pocket depth. Bone levels may be high and yet pockets may be deep. Extensive bone loss may exist and yet be unaccompanied by pockets if the gingiva has receded. A prime objective of periodontal therapy is the elimination of pocket depth. This cannot be achieved unless one realizes to what extent pockets are present. Patients may often be prejudged on the basis of the excellent

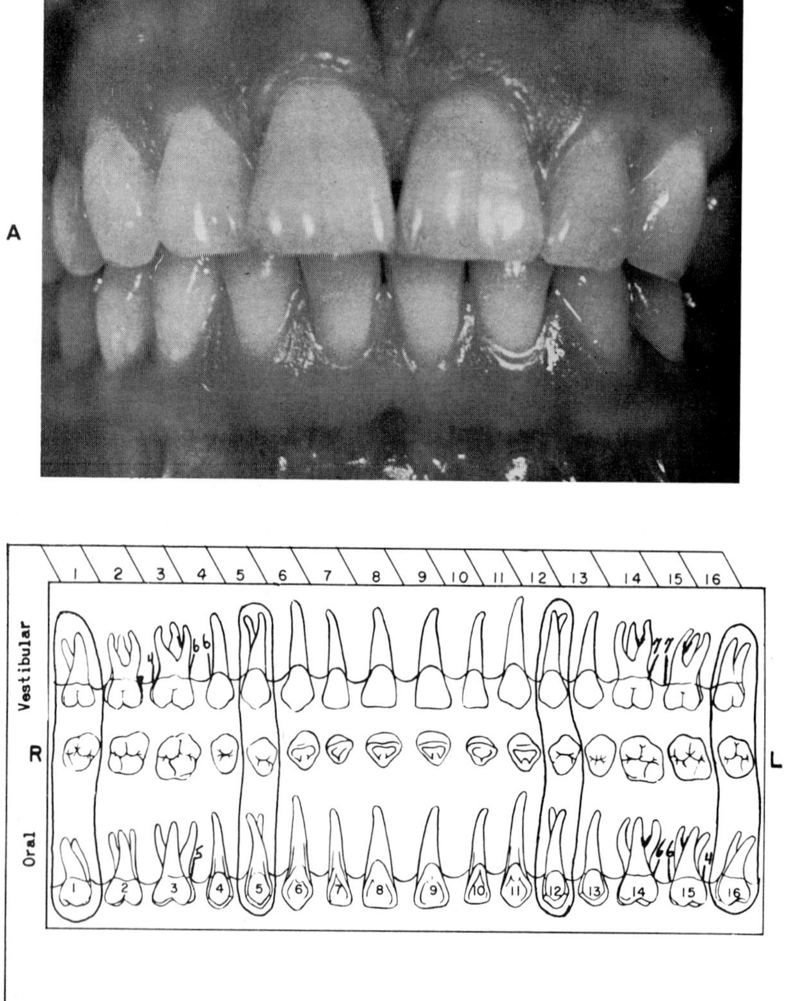


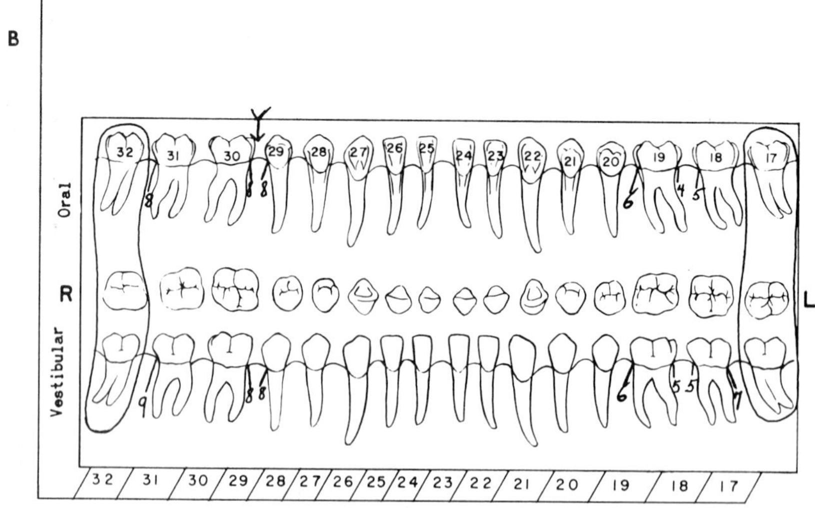


**Fig. 18-14. A,** Periodontitis in a case that appears fairly normal clinically. **B,** Recorded findings of the patient. Despite the excellent appearance, extensive periodontal disease is present. Note the pockets.

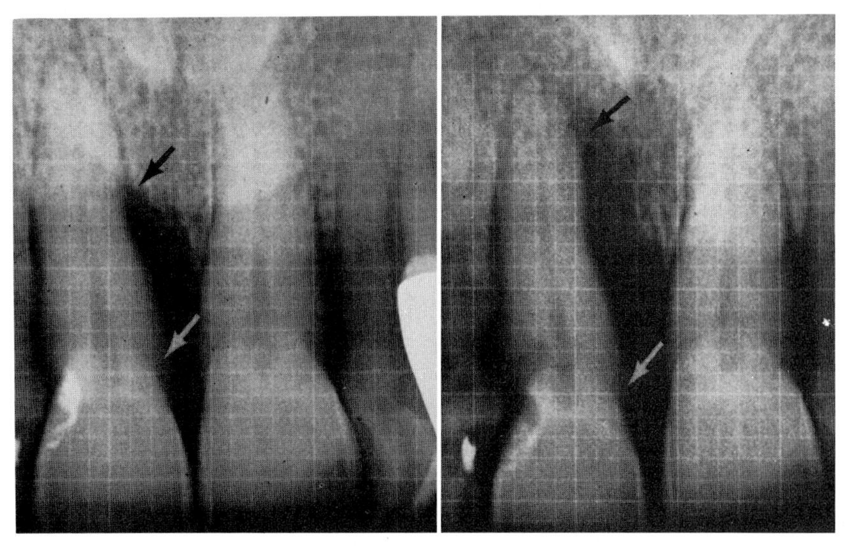

**Fig. 18-15.** A grid incorporated on the roentgenogram can be used to document and compare bone levels. The sequence is of an untreated case of periodontosis. Roentgenograms were taken a year apart and show rapid alveolar bone loss.

clinical appearance of the gingiva. The dentist may then decide that the patient is not a "periodontal case." These patients frequently have pockets that go undetected at a time when the condition could be rectified with greater ease (Fig. 18-14).

Once a surgical flap has been retracted, measurement of pocket depth can no longer be made. Defects of alveolar bone are often referred to as pockets. This is inaccurate. Although pockets are related to bony lesions, the terms are not synonymous. When one desires to document relationships for purposes of research, roentgenograms may be taken with calibrated silver points[16] or gutta-percha inserted in the pocket.[14] A grid incorporated on the roentgenogram has proved valuable in documenting alveolar crest and tooth relationships[17] (Fig. 18-15). It is also useful to obtain measurements from some fixed point on the tooth or to notch the tooth.

***Tooth mobility***

The prognosis of periodontally involved teeth depends, in part, on the initial mobility and whether it can be altered by treatment. Splinting and occlusal adjustment are therapeutic measures specifically concerned with the reduction of mobility. The measurement of mobility is essential in determining the therapy required and in evaluating the results of such treatment.

***Clinical measurement***

Mobility can be determined by luxating a tooth and observing its movement. The tooth may be moved between the handles of two instruments (Fig. 18-16) or between the fingers. The degree of movement is ascertained by comparison with adjacent teeth that are not being moved. Further information may be gained by having the patient move through lateral and protrusive glides with the teeth in contact and also by asking the patient to clench and rock his teeth. The occlusal contacts will cause the mobile teeth to move, and this can be perceived visually by observing highlights of reflected light on the tooth surface or by holding the fingertips partly on the teeth and partly on the gingivae. Visual perception may be enhanced by placing a piece of blue articulating paper be-

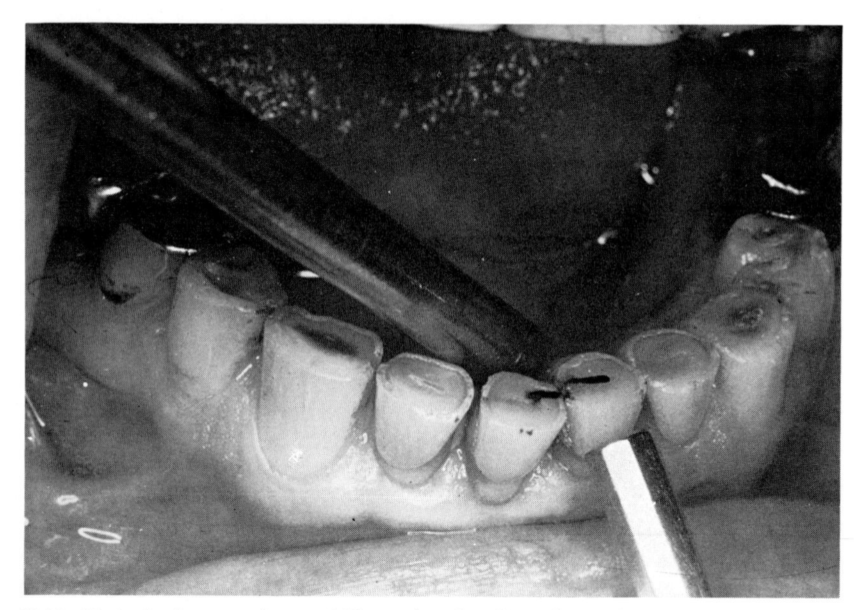

**Fig. 18-16.** Method of measuring mobility using handles of two instruments. Fix the jaw in place by hand and forearm. In this instance a line was drawn with indelible pencil to indicate the proximal relationship of the central incisors before movement. The lingual displacement of the mandibular left central incisor indicates a mobility of 2½.

tween the teeth during the glide movements. The movement of the teeth is more obvious against this dark background.

***Degree of movement***

The degree of movement is indicated on an arbitrary scale of 0 to 3. A reading of 0 indicates no perceptible movement; ½ refers to the barely perceptible movement of a healthy lower incisor; 1-1½ to 2-2½ are increasing degrees that end at 3, a degree of mobility indicating a hopeless prognosis. Teeth that can be depressed have a mobility of 3. The readings of trained observers correspond closely. Although these numbers are not precisely equated in millimeters, such measurements are possible in experiments that make use of mobility-measuring devices.

***Causes of mobility***

Normal teeth may have a range of mobility that is barely perceptible. Beyond this range, mobility is a symptom that occurs early in periodontal traumatism but late in periodontitis. The causes of mobility may be intrinsic, involving morphology or condition of the tissues, or extrinsic, involving the loading of these tissues. Thus the length and shape of the clinical root and crown, the height of the alveolar bone, and the width of the periodontal ligament may determine the firmness of a tooth. Firmness also depends on the biologic status of the supporting tissues. Teeth tend to loosen during acute inflammation, as may occur in infection or after surgery. Teeth may also loosen during pregnancy and in diabetes and severe nutritional deficiency. The alteration of tooth mobility in these instances may be mediated on a biochemical level.

***Primary and secondary traumatism***

Physical forces are exerted on the periodontium, superimposing their influence on whatever local and intrinsic factors are present. Habits, dental appliances, dental procedures, and traumatic impact may produce such forces. Stresses are also applied during mastication, swallowing, bruxism, and clenching. Primary traumatism is the production of mobility in a tooth with normal support subjected to a force in excess of physiologic limits. Secondary traumatism is the production of mobility by normal forces in a tooth with weakend support. When local and intrinsic factors such as inflammation and metabolic disturbance are present, normal forces may produce mobility in a tooth with a full osseous support (Chapter 39).

*Mobility-measuring devices*

Much knowledge concerning tooth mobility rests on subjective clinical observation. It would be desirable if laboratory techniques could be applied to the study of mobility. Mechanical and electronic devices for the quantitative measurement of tooth mobility have been developed for this reason.[18,20] Generally these may be either mechanical devices or electrical conductivity-sensing devices (transducer or strain gauge), through which tooth movement can be measured and recorded. A known load is applied to the tooth surface, and a measurement is obtained. The findings in these instances are experimental, but they may have clinical significance.

*Experimental findings in tooth mobility*

Experimental findings after the use of mobility-measuring devices on healthy teeth indicate that the application of small loads to the tooth will produce a considerable initial displacement. When increasing loads are applied, further displacement occurs but of lesser magnitude. The range of movement varies up to 0.2 mm. horizontally and 0.02 mm. vertically. In pathologic states this movement may be increased tenfold or more.

Mobility has been found to vary between individuals of the same age and between teeth in the same person. It is greater in children, young adults, and in some women. It decreases after completion of active tooth eruption. Anterior teeth are looser than posterior teeth. There are fluctuations during the day; a tooth is twice as mobile in the morning as it is in the evening. Lying down for a few moments will increase mobility. After a tooth is traumatically loosened, it slowly recovers in a matter of weeks. In some instances mobility may be increased during pregnancy or menstruation. Drugs that alter blood pressure may also alter mobility. The range of these experimental mobility measurements is enormmously increased in the presence of periodontal pathology.[19,20]

The opportunity to make objective measurements of tooth mobility and of force applied to the tooth will ultimately permit a better clinical evaluation of the factors that affect mobility.[20] This is important since mobility is a basic symptom of periodontal disease.

## DIAGNOSIS

The documented observations made in charting enable the clinician to make a diagnosis. Although the diagnostic statement is brief, it represents the information gathered from detailed, systematic observations. Treatment is planned from the observation and the diagnosis and a prognosis is projected.

The diagnosis of the patient's condition should be stated. For example, the dentist might indicate necrotizing ulcerative gingivitis (NUG), hyperplastic gingivitis, periodontitis (beginning, moderate, advanced), etc. In addition, the specific clinical characteristics of the gingiva should be stated. The salient findings that lead to this diagnosis should be enumerated. Further, the most likely primary and contributory etiologic factors should be summarized. As pointed out earlier, we reason from the findings to their causes and from the causes to the required treatment, all on a biologic basis. When the etiology is unknown, we must treat on a symptomatic basis. A differential diagnostic chart is presented in Table 18-1.

**Table 18-1.** Differential diagnostic chart—clinical symptoms and histologic findings of periodontal disease

| Disease | Clinical symptoms | Histopathologic findings |
|---|---|---|
| Gingivitis | A. 1. Inflammation localized to papillary or marginal gingiva; stippling of attached gingiva not appreciably affected<br>2. Pockets shallow<br>3. Plaque and calculus<br>4. Hemorrhage | A. Acute and chronic inflammation localized to gingiva (histopathologic picture will vary according to type of gingivitis—hyperplastic, pregnancy, NUG) |
| | B. Roentgenographic: no bone changes | B. No bone resorption |
| | C. No loosening of teeth | |
| Periodontis | A. 1. Change of gingival color to red or magenta | A. 1. Acute and chronic inflammation |
| | 2. Glossy surface, loss of stippling<br>3. Deep pockets with suppuration<br>4. Loss of firmness of gingiva<br>5. Subgingival deposits | 2. Apical proliferation of attachment epithelium; ulceration of pocket epithelium; progress of inflammation along blood vessels to alveolar bone |
| | B. Roentgenographic: resorption of bone at alveolar crest | B. Resorption of bone of alveolar crest |
| | C. Loosening and migration of teeth a late symptom | C. Late phase: extensive loss of alveolar bone; replacement of periodontal ligament by inflammatory tissue |
| Periodontosis | A. Formation of diastemas; migration of teeth; no inflammation<br>B. Roentgenographic: vertical type of bone resorption; irregular; not following anatomic landmarks<br>C. Development of isolated deep pockets with secondary inflammation in young patients | Insufficient data |
| Traumatism | A. Sensitivity to percussion | A. Side of pressure: necrosis of periodontal ligament; undermining resorption of bone |
| | B. Roentgenographic: widening of periodontal space at apex followed by widening of rest of periodontal space | B. Side of tension: damage to periodontal ligament by overstress; cemental tears; thrombosis; widening of periodontal ligament; new bone formation |
| | C. Loosening of teeth: depending on direction of overstress—if in one direction, tooth moves out of occlusal stress; if jiggling, tooth becomes loose | C. In constant jiggling, widening of periodontal space |

**CHAPTER 18**

**References**

1. Cinotti, W. R., and Grieder, A.: Applied psychology in dentistry, St. Louis, 1964, The C. V. Mosby Co.
2. Stern, I. B.: Case history and examination, University of Washington periodontics syllabus, Seattle, 1959, University of Washington Press.
3. Dember, W. N.: The psychology of perception, New York, 1960, Holt, Rinehart & Winston, Inc.

4. Cohen, H.: The nature, methods and purpose of diagnosis, Lancet **1**:23, 1943.
5. O'Leary, T. J., Shannon, I. L., and Prigmore, J. R.: Clinical and systemic findings in periodontal disease, J. Periodont. **33**:243, 1962.
6. Massler, M., Emslie, R. D., and Bolden, T. E.: Fetor ex ore, Oral Surg. **4**:110, 1951.
7. Hine, M. K.: Halitosis, J. Amer. Dent. Ass. **55**:37, 1957.
8. Burnette, E. W.: Limitations of roentgenograms in periodontal diagnosis, J. Periodont. **42**: 293, 1971.
9. Convery, L.: Halitosis, Irish Dent. Rev. **9**:44, 1963.
10. Spouge, J. D.: Halitosis, Dent. Pract. **14**:307, 1964.
11. Wright, W. H.: Local factors in periodontal disease, J. Periodont. **1**:163, 1963.
12. Everett, F. G.: Halitosis, Oregon Dent. J. **41**:13, 1971.
13. Prichard, J.: The role of the roentgenogram in the diagnosis and prognosis of periodontal disease, Oral Surg. **14**:182, 1961.
14. Brescia, N.: Applied dental anatomy, St. Louis, 1961, The C. V. Mosby Co.
15. Hirschfeld, L.: A calibrated silver point for periodontal diagnosis and recording, J. Periodont. **24**:94, 1953.
16. Everett, F. G., and Fixott, H. C.: Use of an incorporated grid in the interpretation of dental roentgenograms, Oral Surg. **16**:1061, 1963.
17. O'Leary, T. J., Rudd, K. D., and Nabers, C. L.: Factors influencing horizontal tooth mobility, Periodontics **4**:308, 1966.
18. Picton, D. C. A.: A study of normal tooth mobility and the changes with periodontal disease, Dent. Pract. **12**:167, 1962.
19. Mühlemann, H. R.: Tooth mobility; a review of clinical aspects and research findings, J. Periodont. **38**:686, 1967.
20. Everett, F. G.: Foreword. In Schroeder, H. E., and Listgarten, M. A., editors: Fine structure of the developing epithelial attachment of human teeth, Basel, 1971, S. Karger, AG.
21. Everett, F. G.: Grenzen der Behandlung parodontotischer Zähne, Deutsch. Zahnaerztekalender 1972. (In press.)

#### Additional suggested reading

Fröhlich, E.: Grenzen und Täuschungen bei der roentgenologischen Darstellung marginaler Zahnbetterkrankungen, Deutsch. Zahnaerztl. Z. **1**:225, 1956.

Green, E., Clayton, J. A., and Schork, M. A.: Longitudinal periodontometry, J. Periodont. Res. **6**:301, 1971.

Orban, B. J., and Orban, T. R.: Three-dimensional roentgenographic interpretation in periodontal diagnosis, J. Periodont. **31**:275, 1960.

Theilade, J.: An evaluation of the reliability of the radiographs in the measurement of bone loss in periodontal disease, J. Peridont. **31**:143, 1960.

CHAPTER NINETEEN

# Prognosis



*Definition*

Prognosis represents a considered judgment on the course of the disease and a prediction of the response to treatment. The accuracy of the prognosis therefore depends on the accuracy and completeness of the information gathered at the examination.

## CRITERIA FOR SUCCESSFUL PROGNOSIS

In general the prognosis depends on the dentist's ability to recognize and eliminate or control the factors causing the disease, on his ability to correct any damage that may have been caused by the disease, and on the patient's ability and determination in maintaining the health of the periodontium and teeth.

### Considerations

*Preserving the dentition*

The prime consideration is the preservation of the dentition as a functioning unit. This means that the loss of individual components can be tolerated provided the remaining dentition can be retained and restored properly. Therefore the strategic importance of individual teeth and of arch segments and the number of remaining teeth and their distribution cannot be overemphasized.

*Objectives of treatment*

Several treatment considerations should be evaluated. Can treatment objectives of a firm nonretractable gingiva that does not bleed be reached? Can the pocket be eliminated?[1] Can the tooth be stabilized? Can the teeth be restored? Can the patient tolerate the treatment? If not, alternative treatment, compromise or extraction, may be advisable.

*Prostheses*

The complexity and extent of any necessary associated prosthesis should be carefully evaluated. If extensive restoration of the dentition is necessary, if fixed splinting is necessary, if orthodontic movement and other procedures are necessary, the patient's ability to have all associated procedures performed must be considered.

### Factors

The prognosis should be stated as good, guarded, or hopeless. Often some teeth have one prognosis, and other teeth have another. In such cases the prognosis must be made tooth by tooth. The following factors will affect the prognosis:

1. *Pocket formation—extent, location, depth, and complexity*. Shallower pockets have a better prognosis. Deep pockets can have a more favorable prognosis when bone levels are high (pseudopockets). Pockets around single-rooted teeth

are usually easier to eliminate; pockets around multirooted teeth present special problems when furcations are involved. In general, the more accessible the pocket, the better will be the prognosis.

2. *Bone loss—extent, location, and complexity.* Greater and more irregular bone loss has a poorer prognosis. When the pattern of bone loss is horizontal, pocket elimination is usually easier. When irregular, vertical, or troughlike bone defects are present, the feasibility of osteoplasty, reattachment attempts, or bone grafts and transplants must be evaluated. As a rule, the more complex the treatment required, the more guarded will be the prognosis. The situation is more serious when furcations are involved.

3. *Tooth mobility and its cause.* Teeth with pocket depth and bone loss have a more favorable prognosis when the teeth are firm rather than loose. With further involvement, including extensive bone loss, tooth mobility becomes increasingly important. Teeth with only 4 or 5 mm. of remaining bone or with a mobility of class 2 to class 3 have a doubtful, if not hopeless, prognosis. When the cause of tooth mobility can be eliminated and when the mobility can be controlled or eliminated, the prognosis is better.[2]

The term *firm* is an oversimplification since all teeth, unless they are ankylosed, have a range of mobility. In general, however, a direct association exists between increasing mobility and worsening prognosis. Prognosis is poor in the presence of advanced bone loss and uncorrected systemic factors. A tooth that can be rotated or depressed is more seriously involved than a tooth that can be luxated buccolingually or mesiodistally. Mobility that relates to a widened periodontal ligament rather than to loss of alveolar support has a more favorable prognosis. Occlusal adjustment and stabilization through splinting are procedures intended to reduce tooth mobility. Successful application of these procedures will also alter prognosis.

Mobility must be correlated with other clinical and roentgenographic findings in determining prognosis. Unfortunately mobility is not always reflected in roentgenograms. Unless its etiology is understood, mobility cannot be properly evaluated in the assessment of prognosis. Tooth mobility directly reflects disturbance, and its measurement is useful in planning treatment and evaluating results. Mobility need not be progressive; some mobile teeth remain equally mobile for years.

4. *Etiology.* When the signs of periodontal disease can be attributed to inflammation, the situation is less grave than when inflammation does not appear to be the cause. When the causative factors of the disease are easily recognized, such as poor oral hygiene or the presence of deposits, the correction can be more easily accomplished. When teeth have tilted, drifted, or rotated, hygiene may be more difficult and elimination of pockets may be impaired; then the prognosis is poorer. In general, the more obvious the etiology, the easier will be the treatment.[3]

5. *Duration of the disease, extent and nature of the involvement.* Prognosis is also related to the extent, nature, and duration of the involvement. When extensive involvement occurs in an older patient, there is more likelihood of stretching the serviceability of the dentition to match the patient's life expectancy than there is when a young patient presents with an advanced condition. A patient with a systemic involvement presents more of a problem than does a patient who is in excellent health. A patient's health and associated capacity for repair are important. Some information concerning prognosis can be obtained if past records permit evaluation of the rate of breakdown. The quicker the breakdown,

the poorer will be the prognosis. The patient who presents a severe response to minimal irritation has a poorer prognosis than does the patient who presents a resistant response in the presence of considerable irritants.[4]

6. *Tooth morphology—crown form, root form, crown-to-root ratio.* The more favorable the crown-to-root ratio, the better will be the prognosis. Teeth with short slender or tapering roots have a poorer prognosis than do those with long broad roots. Multirooted teeth usually resist traumatic forces better than do single-rooted teeth. Broad occlusal tables can contribute to mobility. Teeth with deflecting contours, favoring proper food deflection patterns, have a better prognosis.

***Furcation involvement***

Involvement of furcations in pocket formation presents problems that require special consideration.[5-7] Pocket formation and bone destruction may involve the trifurcations of maxillary molars and the bifurcations of maxillary first premolars and mandibular molars. The involvement may be partial when the lesion extends into the buccal or lingual aspects of the furcation, or it may be total with the exposure extending from the buccal to the lingual aspect. Hemisection and root amputation are often the treatment of choice when the bifurcations and trifurcations of strategically important teeth are involved. Mandibular molars may be hemisected to retain one or both parts, functioning as splinted premolars. This will open the furcation area for care and permit restoration of exposed root surfaces. Maxillary molar teeth may have one or two roots removed, and the remaining portion may then be restored with a properly constructed crown. Pockets may be eliminated and a physiologic gingival form created by such measures.

In partial furcation involvements of mandibular molars, osseous surgery or bone grafts should be considered. These procedures are less successful on trifurcated maxillary molars. Bifurcated maxillary premolars are difficult to treat, except when hemisection is possible.

The following factors should be considered in projecting a prognosis for teeth with furcation involvements[6,7]:

a. *Extent of involvement.* Is the furcation partially or totally involved? Examine by clinical probing; and correlate with roentgenograms.
b. *Status of adjoining interproximal, oral, and vestibular areas.* If these areas are relatively sound or treatable, the effort to save the tooth is justified even when extensive clinical furcation involvement is present.
c. *Mobility.* Class 2 or class 3 mobility makes for an unfavorable prognosis unless this mobility can be eliminated.[8] The root length and crown-to-root ratio must be considered.
d. *Angulation of root spread.* Teeth with widely spread roots are more easily treated.
e. *Health of neighboring teeth.* When good abutment teeth are present mesial as well as distal to the involved tooth, extraction should be considered if the furcation involvement is difficult to treat and the outcome of treatment is doubtful.
f. *Position of tooth in the arch.* Isolated teeth or those most distal in the arch may be retained and treated when access for oral hygiene is good and retention of the tooth is desirable for prosthetic reasons.
g. *Age and health of the patient.* Retention of teeth with furcation involvements in older patients may be desirable. The life expectancy of the patient and of the tooth should be considered.

h. *Oral hygiene and caries index.* Treatment is indicated only when oral hygiene performance is acceptable and caries incidence is not high.

7. *Can treatment objectives be reached and maintained?* The dentist must be able to realize treatment objectives of creating a healthy gingiva, of eliminating pockets, and of establishing conditions whereby the patient can maintain the health of his mouth. If these objectives can be reached, the prognosis is good.

8. *Complexity and extent of any associated prosthesis.* When complex and extensive prostheses are involved, the prognosis tends to be more guarded than when the integrity of the dentition can be maintained with less involved prostheses.

9. *Attitude and desires of the patient, ability and resolution in home dental care procedures.* The patient must be interested in retaining his teeth. If he is not, chances are that the therapy will be less effective.[9,10]

## EVALUATION OF RESULTS

Unfortunately dental treatment is often conceived of in terms of absolutes. Good and poor prognoses or success and failure are viewed as black and white. In addition, a minimal time period of 15 to 20 years is often made a qualifying measure of success or a favorable prognosis. In actuality, a wide zone of gray exists between black and white in periodontal prognosis. Some confusion exists because of our inability to perceive all the criteria for prognosis in advance. The inexperienced diagnostician will often recognize and treat only the most overt periodontal conditions. These become more obvious with the severity of the situation. Moreover, such conditions are often treated inadequately. Naturally, then, the rate of failure is high. Disillusionment with the effectiveness of periodontal treatment may follow. The pendulum may swing to the other extreme, and further attempts at periodontal therapy may be abandoned in a retreat to the forceps. Neither approach is rational. There are times when extractions are indicated; and there are other times when periodontal treatment is indicated. It is important to be able to differentiate between the two.

Judgments should be made on a tooth-to-tooth basis with the entire dentition in mind. In some instances the extraction of a single tooth will make the whole situation untenable. In other situations isolated extractions will simplify the problem.

**CHAPTER 19**

**References**

1. Williams, C. H. M.: Rationalization of periodontal pocket therapy, J. Periodont. **14**:67, 1943.
2. Everett, F. G., and Stern, I. B.: When is tooth mobility an indication for extraction? Dental Clinics of North America, Philadelphia, 1969, W. B. Saunders Co., vol. 13.
3. Wade, A. B.: Causes in failure of treatment of localized pocketing, Dent. Health **4**:9, 1965.
4. Homan, B. T.: A prescription for periodontal therapy; curettage, Aust. Dent. J. **9**:515, 1964.
5. Everett, F. G., Jump, E. B., Holder, T. D., and Williams, G. C.: The intermediate bifurcational ridge; a study of the morphology of the bifurcation of the lower first molar, J. Dent. Res. **37**:162, 1958.
6. Staffileno, H. J.: Surgical management of the furca invasion, Dental Clinics of North America, Philadelphia, 1969, W. B. Saunders Co., vol. 13.
7. Everett, F. G.: Bifurcation involvement, Oregon Dent. J. **28**:2, 1959.
8. Forsberg, A., and Hägglund, G.: Mobility of teeth as a check of periodontal therapy, Acta Odont. Scand. **15**:305, 1957.
9. Awwa, I., and Stallard, R. E.: Periodontal prognosis. Educational and psychological implications, J. Periodont. **41**:183, 1970.
10. Derbyshire, J. C.: Patient motivation in periodontics, J. Periodont. **41**:630, 1970.

CHAPTER TWENTY

# Treatment plan



*Definition*

The treatment plan is an organized schedule of measures to eliminate the signs and symptoms of disease and to restore health. A treatment plan based on the findings of the examination, the diagnosis, the presumptive etiology of the condition, and the prognosis should be developed. A planned, cooperative effort between patient and doctor is required; and, except in early and uncomplicated cases of periodontal disease, a treatment period of months is necessary.[1]

## RATIONALE

The rationale for periodontal treatment is to arrest the process of breakdown, which may otherwise lead to ultimate loss of teeth, and to establish oral conditions conducive to periodontal health.[2] Within limits one should be able to use therapeutic measures on a predictable basis. In general, treatment should be on an ordered schedule and limited to the direct measures necessary to achieve the result.[3] The treatment plan should also project a tentative schedule to maintain the treated state without further significant encroachments of periodontal disease for a reasonable length of time. This, of course, depends on the presenting condition of the patient and the objectives of treatment. The treatment plan is developed on the basis of the patient's needs and the findings of the initial examination.

## ORDER OF TREATMENT

### Preliminary therapy

Treatment consists of a number of steps. The initial effort should be directed toward the elimination of inflammation and the institution of a program of oral hygiene. This may require a number of visits to remove all deposits and to establish effective plaque control. The patient's level of oral hygiene performance should be evaluated at each visit (with the aid of a plaque index) and further coaching in home dental care given as necessary.

### Reevaluation

At the end of this phase of treatment, an all-important reevaluation should be made on the basis of the degree of improvement obtained. The results of initial treatment should be checked against the charting. Residual inflammation and its presumptive causes should be noted, and changes in pocket depth and tooth mobility should be recorded. The treatment plan should be reevaluated and any appropriate changes made.

### Restorations

Usually periodontal therapy should precede restorative interventions. At times, however, caries may be so deep as to require immediate attention. Depending on the patient's needs, these restorations should be temporary since the completion of periodontal treatment may be followed by reconstruction. Provisional splinting during the treatment period may be necessary, and the necessity for this measure should be evaluated.

### Extractions

Teeth with hopeless prognosis should be extracted early in treatment unless they are being retained temporarily for aesthetics or for space maintenance.[2,3] The failure to remove such teeth at this time can lead to complications. Hopeless teeth can interfere with treatment and make it more complex. The patient may forget that a hopeless prognosis had been made for this tooth in the beginning and later feel that treatment is unsuccessful when extraction is ordered.

### Orthodontics

Orthodontic tooth movement may precede or follow any surgical interventions. When orthodontic tooth movement is done to eliminate inflammation resulting from tooth position or bony deformities resulting from tooth malalignment, tilting, or drifting, this measure should precede surgery. When orthodontic tooth movement is done for purposes of reconstruction or aesthetics, it may follow any surgery. A schedule should be made for frequent, regular scaling during orthodontic interventions and for appraisal of plaque control.

### Occlusal adjustment

Occlusal adjustments may be made after scaling and root planing, when inflammation has been eliminated. When teeth show significant mobility, some gross occlusal adjustments may be done as a first step to reduce mobility. After surgery and orthodontic therapy, further occlusal adjustment may be necessary.

## SUMMARY

In summation, the procedures to be followed in examination, diagnosis, prognosis, and treatment planning are outlined below:

*1. Examination
   a. Interview
      (1) Vital statistics
      (2) Chief complaint
      (3) Medical history

*Obligatory steps in all patients.

b. Intraoral examination
c. Roentgenographic examination
*2. Diagnosis
*3. Prognosis
*4. Treatment plan
*a. Initial scaling and root planing
*b. Plaque control instruction (repeated at subsequent visits)
c. Initial occlusal adjustment
*d. Root planing
†e. Elimination of other extrinsic factors (e.g., overhanging margins), extractions, temporary fillings
*f. Reevaluation
†g. Temporary splinting
†h. Surgery
†i. Minor tooth movement
†j. Definitive occlusal adjustment
*k. Root planing and plaque control instruction
*l. Posttreatment examination
†m. Reconstructive treatment plan
†n. Establishment of a maintenance schedule (after treatment) for preventive periodontal care

*Records*

The treatment performed should be recorded carefully at each visit. An exact record of every step that has been taken is essential. Note the drugs that have been prescribed, the type of toothbrush recommended, and the method of toothbrushing and other oral hygiene procedures demonstrated. Step by step, as treatment is executed, the items should be checked off against the treatment plan; and an orderly and complete record should be kept at each visit. Appointments for reevaluation should be included at appropriate times.

## CASE PRESENTATION

When the treatment plan has been made, the findings, the diagnosis, and the prognosis should be presented to the patient and explained. These items are the result of the examination and must be understood by the patient before a treatment plan is presented. The treatment plan is presented only to patients who understand their condition and who are properly motivated. This is basic to obtaining an informed consent. Such patients frequently ask what can be done for them. At this point, the case presentation should be made. Attempt to be objective with the patient. Never do an "off the cuff" presentation. All the needed facts should be known, fully digested, and a written plan prepared before a presentation is made. Do not make rash promises, great pronouncements, or profound judgments. The expectations of the patient stem, in part from the case presentation. Do your best to ensure that the expectations are realistic and that the patient understands them.

---

*Obligatory steps in all patients.
†To be used as needed.

**CHAPTER 20**

**References**

1. Despeignes, J.: Synthesis of current periodontal therapy; on the need for a system in treatment planning, Bull. Acad. Dent. **10**:9, 1966.
2. Everett, F. G., and Stern, I.: When is tooth mobility an indication for extraction? Dental Clinics of North America, Philadelphia, 1969, W. B. Saunders Co., vol. 13.
3. Corn, H., and Marks, M. H.: Strategic extractions in periodontal therapy, Dental Clinics of North America, Philadelphia, 1969, W. B. Saunders Co., vol. 13.

**Additional suggested reading**

Grieder, A., and Cinotti, W. R.: Periodontal prosthesis, St. Louis, 1968, The C. V. Mosby Co.

PART VII

# Conditions requiring immediate treatment

CHAPTER TWENTY-ONE

# Necrotizing ulcerative gingivitis



Necrotizing ulcerative gingivitis (NUG) is an acute infection of the gingiva. It is also known as *Vincent's gingivitis,* because of the description by Vincent of the organisms associated with the disease, and *trench mouth,* because of the heavy incidence among soldiers in trenches during World War I. Actually the disease has been known since ancient times under a variety of names.[1] The current name is derived from the key symptoms—necrosis, ulceration, and inflammation of the gingiva.[2]

## DIAGNOSTIC FEATURES

The classical signs and symptoms from which diagnosis may be made include the following[2,3]:

1. Ulceration of the tips of the interdental papillae
2. Bleeding
3. An apparent sudden onset
4. Pain
5. Foul odor (fetor oris)

The disease may present, however, in an early mild stage in which only two clinical signs are present[3,4]:

1. Necrosis of the tips of the interdental papillae (Fig. 21-1).
2. Tendency toward easy gingival bleeding

Although during this early stage pain may be absent, when the area is probed, the patient complains of pain. Local irritational factors may be minimal.

The disease has been classified into acute, subacute, and chronic forms. This

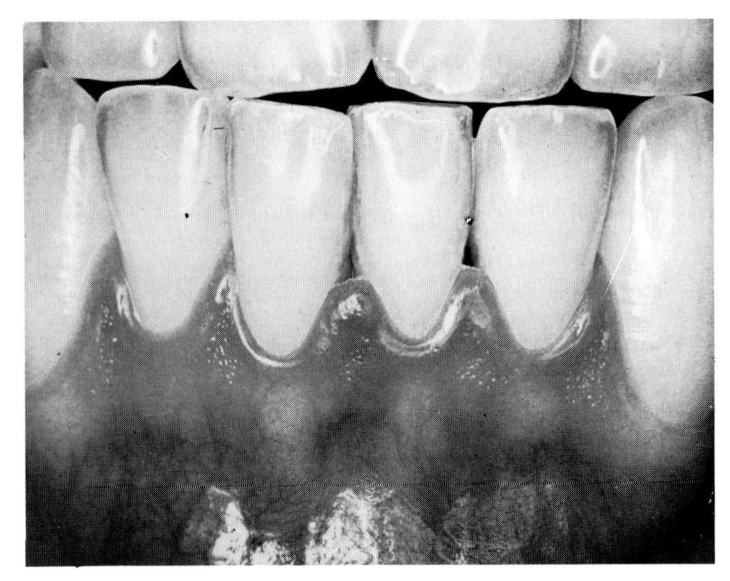

**Fig. 21-1.** Early necrotizing ulcerative gingivitis. The initial signs are ulcerations at the tips of the papillae. Pain may be absent. (From the collection of H. E. Grupe, Sr.)

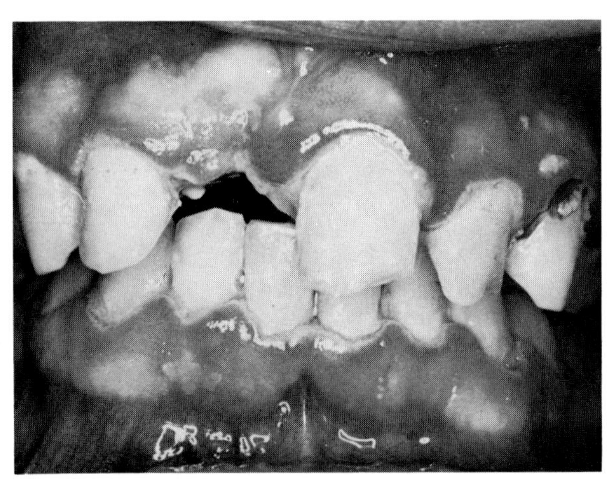

**Fig. 21-2.** The marginal and papillary gingivae are extensively involved, most severely in the anterior region.

clinical differentiation is based on the severity, duration, and onset of the infection and not on the type of inflammation. Some disagreement exists concerning the subacute and chronic forms. Most authorities believe that these terms refer to the recurring acute form of the disease. Classification of the disease into these categories is primarily of academic importance. Recognition and treatment are the most significant aspects to the dentist and his patient.

Diagnosis rests on the clinical appearance of the lesions.[5] The interdental papillae may appear eroded, punched out, or clipped off because of the ulcerative destruction. The ulcerations may progress to include the marginal and,

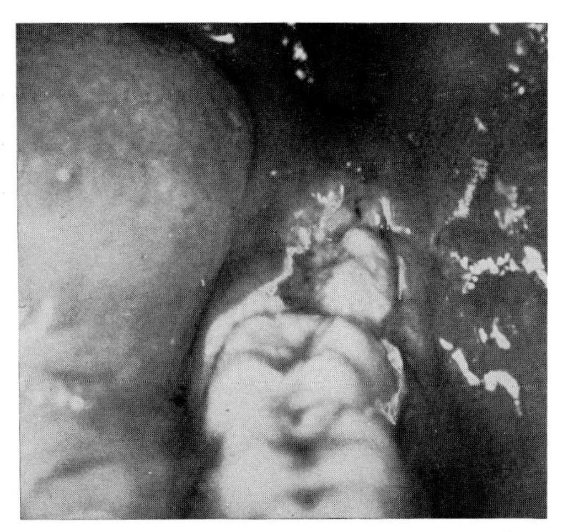

**Fig. 21-3.** Necrotizing ulcerative gingivitis. Note the ulceration of the third molar flap.

rarely, the attached gingivae. The lesions may be covered with a whitish, yellowish, or gray pseudomembrane. The gingiva around the ulcerations is an angry red color. Bleeding occurs when it is touched. The regional lymph glands may be swollen and painful.

### Site and extent of involvement

The tips of the interdental papillae (Fig. 21-1) are characteristically involved first, although the disease may progressively involve the gingival margins (Fig. 21-2). The gingivae of any area of the mouth may be affected. However, the entire mouth need not be involved. The distribution of the disease does not follow any consistent pattern and may differ from mouth to mouth. Initially involvement of the incisor regions and third molar flaps seems to occur most frequently (Fig. 21-3). (See Chapter 19.) The infection may spread to other parts of the mucosa, although this rarely occurs. Direct contact may cause lip and tongue ulcers. Pharyngeal involvement (Vincent's angina) may also accompany the gingival infection (Fig. 21-4). Pain is usually the patient's main complaint. It may be so severe as to interfere with mastication and toothbrushing. The patient may state that his teeth feel as if they were separating or were wooden.

### Alterations in tissue form with repeated attacks

With more extensive involvement the interdental tissue may become cratered (Fig. 21-5). At the same time slight proliferation of the tissue adjacent to the necrotic area may take place (Fig. 21-6). This combination of necrosis and proliferation can produce various outlines in the marginal and papillary gingivae (e.g., punched-out tips, flaplike and papilla-less types) (Figs. 21-5 and 21-6). These forms are usually indicative of repeated attacks.

When the papillae are deeply cratered, the ulceration may occur at the base of a crater or in a col; at the same time the tips of the papillae may proliferate. In such instances the buccal and lingual portions of the papillae may form movable flaps. Such ulcerations remain hidden unless the flap is depressed and the cratered area is inspected. When roots are closely approximated, the septum may be lost, resulting in the formation of a deep cleft. Even when the disease

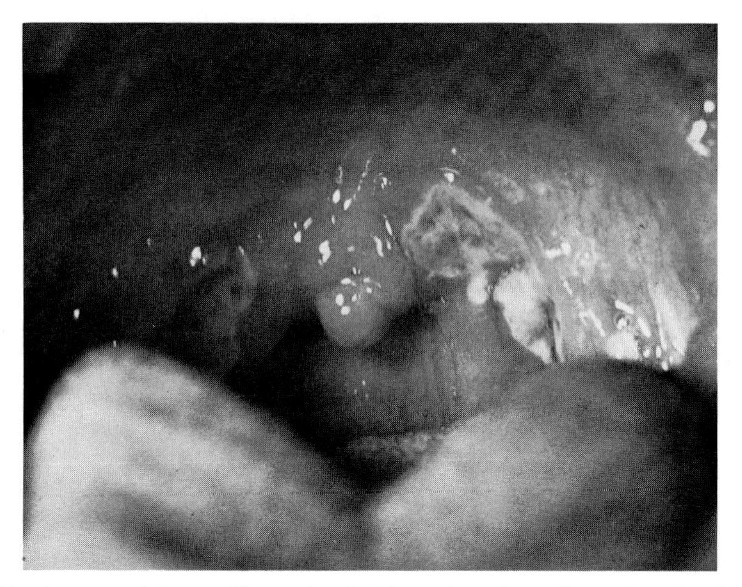

**Fig. 21-4.** Involvement of the tonsillar region in Vincent's angina. (From the collection of H. E. Grupe, Sr.)

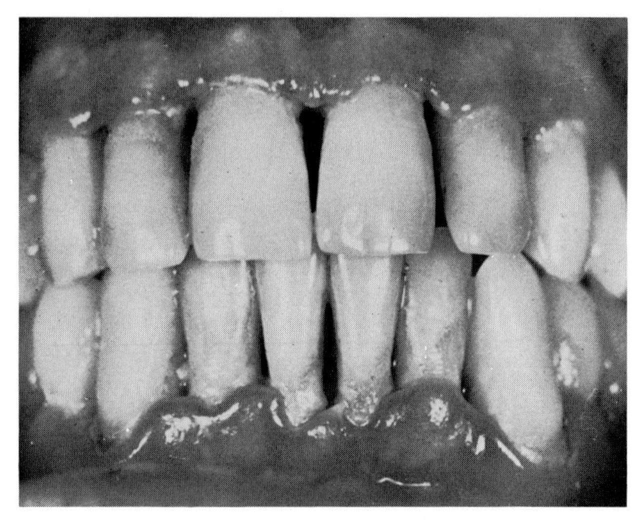

**Fig. 21-5.** Recurrent necrotizing ulcerative gingivitis. The repeated acute attacks have caused the loss of the interproximal gingiva. Interdental craters and troughs mark this destruction.

process is arrested, the deformity of reverse architecture may remain. Needless to say, gingival and osseous deformities are produced that may have a bearing on the production of periodontitis and therefore require surgical correction.

## Recurrent NUG

The reasons for the recurrence of NUG are as incompletely known as are the reasons for the primary appearance of the disease. Apparently the acute phase can be brought under control by a variety of techniques and medications. Unfortunately, as soon as the symptoms abate, many patients tend to discontinue

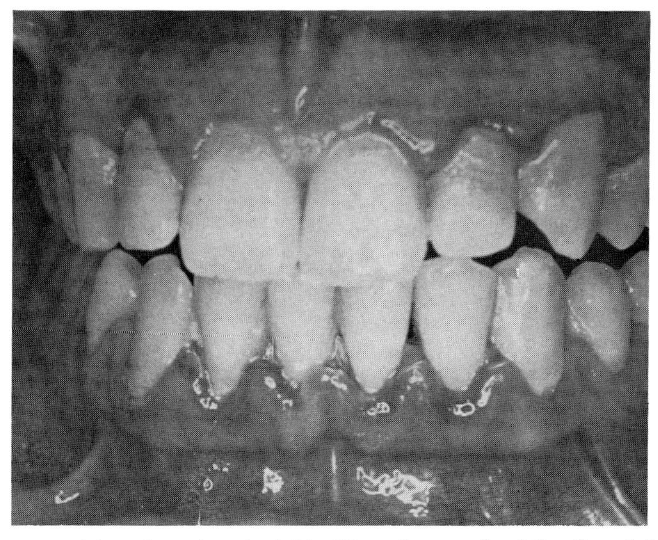

**Fig. 21-6.** Acute necrotizing ulcerative gingivitis. There is necrosis of the tips of the gingival papillae and edema of the area.

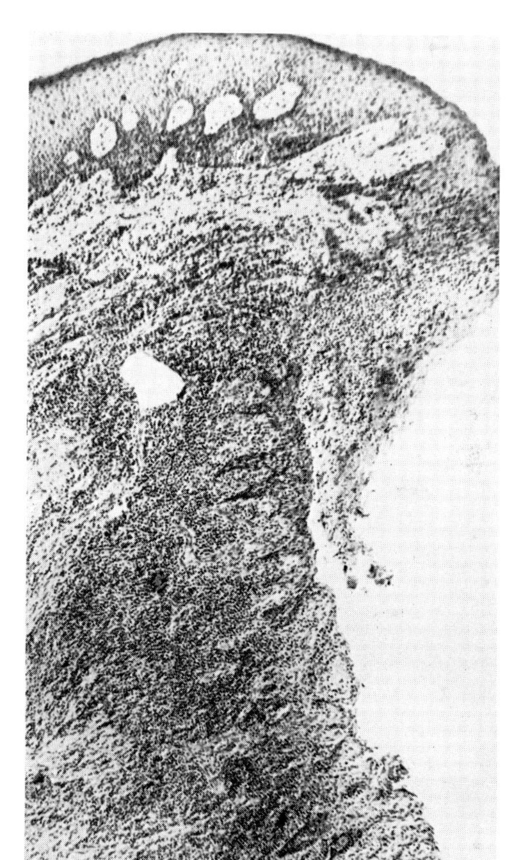

**Fig. 21-7.** Biopsy of the gingiva of a patient with necrotizing ulcerative gingivitis. The surface shows a pseudomembranous ulceration.

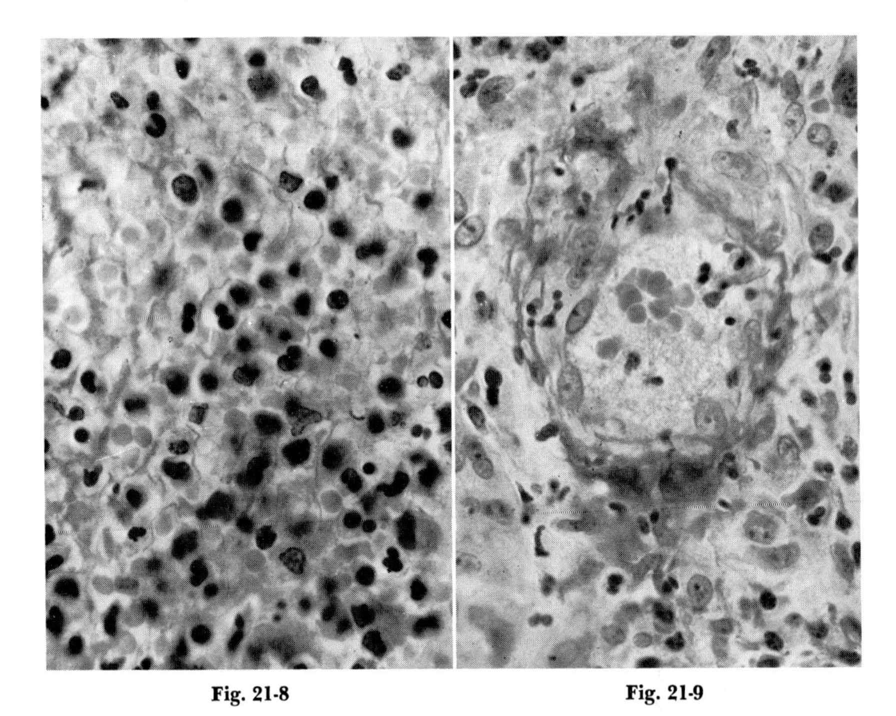

Fig. 21-8 Fig. 21-9

**Fig. 21-8.** High magnification of a pseudomembrane of a patient with necrotizing ulcerative gingivitis. The fibrinous network enmeshes erythrocytes, leukocytes, and macrophages.
**Fig. 21-9.** Fibrinous exudate surrounding a capillary with migrating leukocytes in a case of necrotizing ulcerative gingivitis.

treatment and proper oral hygiene. The underlying extrinsic, intrinsic, and psychogenic causative factors may then continue or reappear and may contribute to a relapse. Incomplete or insufficient treatment plays an important role in such recurrence. However, the tendency for the disease to recur is great no matter what basic treatment has been used.

The patient and therapist must clearly understand that this tendency for recurrence exists. The patient should be made aware that easy bleeding is an early and significant sign of recurrence and that, on noticing this symptom, he must return for treatment regardless of when his next appointment may be. The practitioner should continue to observe the patient at regular intervals for at least a year after "cure." Otherwise, treatment may have been terminated prematurely.

Recurrent NUG may become a chronic condition in some patients. Acute exacerbations of the disease occur superimposed on a basic periodontitis. The chronic inflammation of the patient's periodontitis often leads to hyperplastic changes in the gingivae. The necrotizing phase leads to a severe loss of tissue, especially in the interproximal areas. The result is often a combination of the two phenomena (Fig. 21-5).

## Histopathology of NUG

The microscopic picture of NUG reveals an acute inflammatory process with ulceration and the formation of a pseudomembrane on the surface (Fig. 21-7). In subacute cases leukocytes may be seen in the pseudomembrane (Fig. 21-8) and

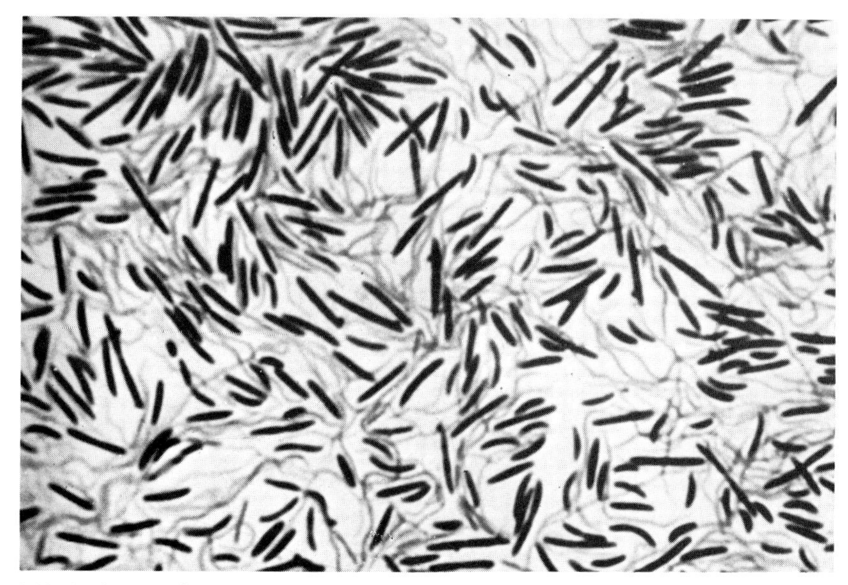

**Fig. 21-10.** Oral smear from a patient with necrotizing ulcerative gingivitis demonstrating spirochetes and fusiform microorganisms. (From the collection of E. D. Coolidge.)

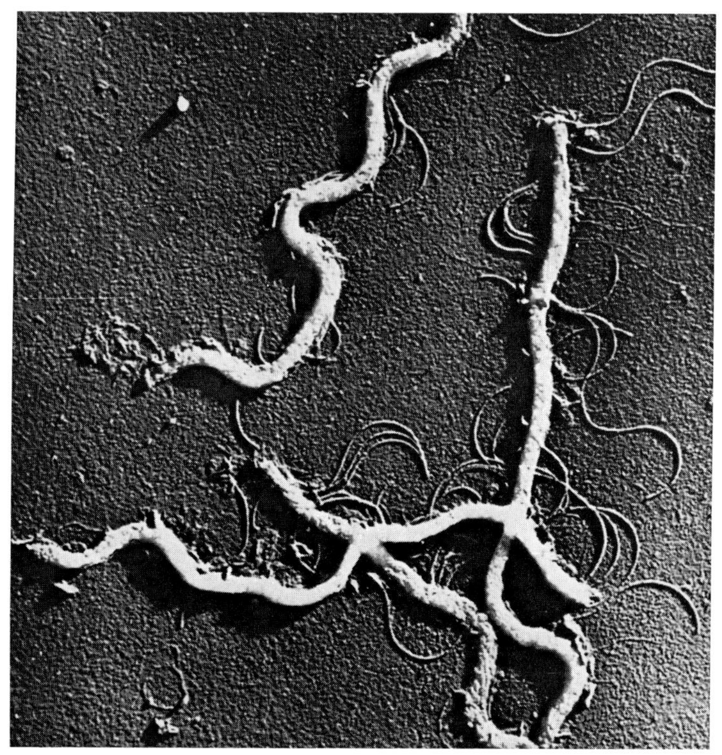

**Fig. 21-11.** Electron micrograph of *Borrelia vincentii.* (Shadowed preparation; ×11,000.) (Courtesy E. G. Hampp, Bethesda.)

in the tissue (Fig. 21-9). In the deeper layer large masses of plasma cells may accumulate in such recurrent cases, and tissue necrosis may become a prominent feature. Spirochetes can be seen invading the tissue (Fig. 21-12).

### Differential diagnosis and concurrent conditions

More rarely NUG may have to be differentiated from herpetic gingivostomatitis, streptococcal stomatitis,[6] erythema multiforme, and infectious mononucleosis. The possibility that NUG may be superimposed on an underlying agranulocytosis[7] (malignant neutropenia), acute leukemia,[8] or heavy metal poisoning should not be ignored. These conditions may be accompanied by mild gingival swelling and ulceration and may become complicated by NUG. Whenever severe NUG does not improve in the first few days of treatment, a differential blood count is indicated. The possibility of missing the underlying disease is real. Any unusual complication warrants medical consultation and/or hospitalization.

## PREVALENCE

In the United States and in Europe, acute NUG occurs mostly among adolescents and young adults. Reports of epidemics of NUG in the United States probably represent misdiagnoses.[9] Reports from other continents stress that, under conditions prevailing in those areas, NUG occurs frequently among children. Noma may follow in conditions of famine[10-13] (Fig. 11-2).

The diagnosis of NUG must be made primarily on clinical criteria and sometimes on the patient's response to treatment. Conditions such as herpetic gingivostomatitis, agranulocytosis, and streptococcal gingivitis have been confused with this disease. They will be discussed later in this chapter.

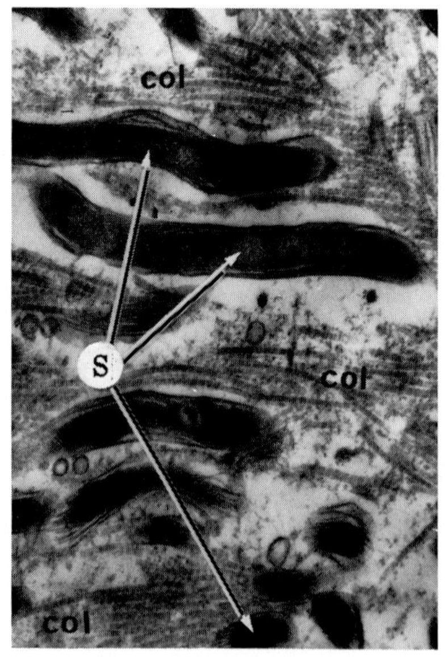


**Fig. 21-12.** Zone of spirochetal infiltration. *S,* Spirochetes infiltrating the connective tissue beneath the ulcerated lesion; *col,* collagen fibers. (From Listgarten, M. A.: J. Periodont. **36**:328, 1965.)

## ETIOLOGY

The etiology of NUG is not fully understood. Bacteria and other extrinsic factors as well as intrinsic and psychogenic factors have all been incriminated.

### Bacteria

The disease is accompanied by an increase in the numbers of spirochetes and fusiform bacilli and is an infection. However, since spirochetes and fusiform bacilli are present in a majority of mouths, positive smears and dark fields are inconclusive in the absence of clinical symptoms. The presence of overwhelming numbers of these organisms can serve as corroborative evidence. Plaut in 1894 and Vincent in 1896 first noted these organisms. *Fusobacterium fusiforme* is a gram-negative or weakly gram-positive anaerobic bacillus 8 to 16 $\mu$ in length, occurring in straight or curved paired rods whose blunt ends are together and whose pointed outer ends give the characteristic cigar-shaped appearance to this bacterium (Fig. 21-10). *Borrelia vincentii* is a loosely wound spirochete 8 to 12 $\mu$ in length, with three to eight irregular shallow spirals[14,15] (Fig. 21-11). It is gram negative. (See Chapter 5.)

Attempts to transmit the disease in humans have failed almost without exception.[16] There are reports of severe, foul-smelling infections associated with human bite wounds. These do not represent the same disease. The conclusion has been drawn that the disease is not communicable.[17] However, evidence is, as yet, incomplete.[9]

***Microbiologic experimentation***

Experimentation, on the other hand, has yielded some interesting results. When mixed cultures obtained from acute cases are injected subcutaneously into the groin of guinea pigs, abscess formation and necrosis result.[17] *Borrelia vincentii* and *Fusobacterium fusiforme* can be recovered from such lesions. This infection can be passed through several transfers. In experimental transmission into guinea pigs, MacDonald and his associates found the presence of *Bacteroides melaninogenicus* essential.[18] Hampp and Mergenhagen insisted that spirochetes cannot be dismissed as causative agents because abscesses can be produced in the guinea pig by injection of *Borrelia vincentii* and *Borrelia buccalis*.[19] More recently these same investigators produced intracutaneous abscesses by injection of oral fusobacteria separately or in combination with a strain of oral spirochetes.[20] Listgarten and Socransky stressed that the major spirochete in NUG is distinctly different from *Borrelia vincentii*.[21] Spirochetes can be seen invading the tissues immediately beneath the epithelium[22] (Fig. 21-12). An immunofluorescent study failed to show a significant rise in antibody titers against *Borrelia vincentii, Fusobacterium fusiforms,* and *Bacteroides melaninogenicus* in patients suffering from acute NUG.[23] This study tends to place a rather secondary function on these organisms. (For further study of bacterial activities, refer to Chapter 5.)

Although these experiments are important, the relationship to the clinical disease entity remains tenuous. None of the experiments has produced oral lesions typical of NUG. The weight of evidence, however, indicates that the organisms are in some way implicated. The administration of antibiotics is effective in treatment. Koch's first and second postulates (Chapter 6) are satisfied because the organisms are always present in the lesions and can be isolated in pure culture. However, his third postulate is not satisfied because the disease cannot be reproduced in humans or animals in its typical clinical form. No single organism or combination has yet been proved to be the causative agent in NUG.

### Extrinsic predisposing factors

In addition to the microbiologic factors, other coincident or predisposing findings such as unfilled cavities, food impaction, defective dentistry, poor oral hygiene, calculus, pericoronal flaps and crypts, periodontal pockets, and excessive smoking are common.[24-26] The onset of the disease may be promoted by the lowering of tissue resistance because of the tissue insult. The disease may occur, however, in the absence of any or all of these factors. NUG may occur in nonsmokers and in mouths that are scrupulously clean.[4] Since brushing is painful for these patients, poor hygiene may be an effect rather than a cause.

### Intrinsic predisposing factors

Oral fusospirochetal infection occasionally follows acute febrile or debilitating diseases such as nutritional deficiency, leukemia, agranulocytosis, pernicious anemia, infectious mononucleosis, and erythema multiforme. Intrinsic factors may modify the ability to resist and repair. In these instances NUG is superimposed on the basic condition, and the clinical appearance of the disease is unchanged. Should the patient fail to respond to local treatment of the oral disease, the possible presence of a systemic disease should be investigated.

### Psychogenic causes

A psychogenic origin has been suggested for NUG.[27-29] (See discussion on psychologic aspects of periodontal disease in Chapter 17.) Psychogenic factors probably predispose to the disease. The microorganisms may act secondarily as facultative pathogens. Pseudoepidemics can be attributed to the fact that populations may be simultaneously subjected to similar noxious and disturbing circumstances.

## TREATMENT

The objectives of treatment of NUG are (1) the reduction of acute symptoms (elimination of the necrotizing process), (2) the elimination of predisposing factors (restoration of the tissues to health), and (3) the correction of tissue deformities by surgery. Initial treatment may be varied and/or supplemented according to the needs of the patient.

### Reduction of acute symptoms

The acute symptoms must be reduced. Medication, debridement, and the institution of oral hygiene procedures may all be used for reduction of the acute symptoms. Some 100 different medications have been advocated. Such remedies may afford a spurious cure by causing a temporary remission of symptoms.[26] (See discussion of recurrent NUG earlier in this chapter.) The apparent amelioration of symptoms leads to the increased usage of medications whereas, in essence, medication is only one step in treatment.[30,31]

### Elimination of predisposing factors

The extrinsic and intrinsic predisposing factors must be eliminated when possible. Otherwise, they may continue to operate and influence the course of the disease. The patient should be placed in a generally healthful situation. Factors that could possibly lower tissue resistance, such as fatigue, alcoholism, and excessive smoking, should be reduced or eliminated. Bed rest may be advisable in very severe cases, especially when fever is present. The possible role of psychogenic stress should be mentioned and gently investigated.

***First appointment***

The mouth is examined and a diagnosis made. The mouth is sprayed to remove slough. Preliminary debridement is performed. A topical anesthetic may be used if necessary. Ultrasonic debridement has a special place in the treatment of NUG.[32] The lavage is an asset in the bacterial and necrotic tissue debridement. Wound healing appears to be facilitated.

The patient is instructed in the use of hot-water rinses as a home treatment. A mouthful of water, as warm as the patient can endure, is forcefully swished back and forth between the teeth for several minutes. Rinsing should be performed several times a day. The necrotic pseudomembranes will be loosened, and anaerobic organisms diminished in number. In 24 hours subjective and objective improvement should be noted.

Dilute hydrogen peroxide solution (1 part in 4 parts of warm water) may be used instead of hot water. This solution appears to be beneficial, but whether the therapeutic effect is a result of the oxygenating or the bubbling effervescence of the mouthwash is not known. The topical application of Proxygel (an oral antiseptic and cleanser) or Gly-Oxide (a hydrogen peroxide–urea preparation in glycerin) seems also to be beneficial. Oxygenating drugs were originally introduced in the treatment of NUG on the rationale that the causative organisms were anaerobic. The dentist should carefully supervise the use of oxygenating drugs and should discontinue their prescription after 2 weeks. Longer use may lead to the formation of black (hairy) tongue and the decalcification of tooth substances.

Antibiotics, either locally or systemically,* may be utilized in treatment. Local administration should be limited to those antibiotics† that are not frequently used systemically or that are known to have little sensitizing effect. Most patients with NUG can be treated successfully without the use of antibiotics.[30] The advantage of using antibiotics lies in the quick abortion of the ulcerative necrotizing process, thus minimizing permanent tissue damage. The disadvantage of using antibiotics lies in the possibility of sensitization of the patient to the drug. Topical penicillin constitutes a distinct danger to the patient, and its use is ill advised. Antibiotics may also cause changes in the ecology of the oral cavity, with the promotion of candidiasis (thrush). However, this reaction has been observed to be only temporary.

Dietary recommendations should include fruit juices when needed. The diet may be soft and bland for the first few days after an acute attack.

Vitamin supplementation is suggested when indicated. A preparation containing at least 150 mg. of ascorbic acid, 50 mg. of riboflavin, and double the minimal amounts of the other components of the B complex group may be prescribed twice daily.

***Second appointment (1 or 2 days later)***

The patient should now show considerable clinical improvement. Pain should be greatly reduced or absent. Further root planing is carried out under topical anesthesia. Instruction in oral hygiene procedures with a soft, multitufted toothbrush are given.

---

*All antibiotics administered systemically should be given in adequate dosage.

†Grupe and Wilder have suggested the use of a 250 mg. capsule of chlortetracycline (Aureomycin) powder mixed in equal parts with gum tragacanth (denture powder).[4] The resulting mixture is blown on the diseased mucosa by means of an insufflator until a yellow, leathery coating protects the ulcerated surface. The danger of sensitization and side reactions is minimal.[33]

*Subsequent appointments*

The patient should now be seen at least once a week. During these visits scaling and polishing of the teeth should be completed. Oral hygiene can be evaluated and altered according to the needs of the patient.

### Correction of tissue deformities

Surgery, extractions, and general anesthesia are usually deferred until the infection has been cured. During the height of the disease, septicemia or bacteremia may follow surgery. Third molar flaps (Fig. 21-3) and other nidi of infection should be eliminated. The disease may be superimposed on or lead to the development of periodontitis. In either event, gingival and osseous deformities may remain after the acute phase has been resolved. When the cratering is mild, rigorous application of oral hygiene principles may lead to complete recovery of normal papillary form. When deformities persist, gingival and osseous surgery may be necessary; otherwise these deformities may predispose to recurrent NUG or periodontitis.

## HERPETIC GINGIVOSTOMATITIS

A primary infection with one of the oral herpesviruses may lead to a disease known as acute primary herpetic gingivostomatitis. This disease is frequently misdiagnosed as NUG. Acute primary herpetic gingivostomatitis is found in children from 6 months to 10 years of age, and less frequently in adolescents and young adults. NUG, by contrast, is not found in children under 12 years of age in the United States.

The lesion in herpetic gingivostomatitis is the single or multiple bulla (blister). Oral bullae break readily and leave shallow, yellowish ulcerations. The ulcers in herpetic gingivostomatitis are *not* confined to the gingiva but may be seen anyplace in the oral cavity, including the lips, cheeks, palate, tongue, and pharynx. In fact, bullae or groups of bullae may be seen at the time of the oral eruption also on the face; or they may be reported by the patient on other parts of his body.

Herpetic gingivostomatitis has a sudden onset. It runs its course in 10 to 16 days. The patient is febrile and debilitated. Temperatures may rise to 104°. The patient has malaise and his mouth becomes so painful that the intake of solid food is difficult or impossible. In adults weight loss of 10 pounds in 1 week is not uncommon. In young children dehydration becomes a specific problem.

In the case history the patient may report contact with a relative or friend who had an active herpes labialis lesion present. After he has recovered from the primary attack, subsequent symptoms may occur as herpes labialis or localized oral attacks characterized by one or two isolated clusters of bullae.

Since there is more than one oral herpes strain, the patient may have a second primary infection. Moreover, immunity to subsequent attacks has not been unequivocally proved to follow a primary attack.

*Differential diagnosis*

Herpetic gingivostomatitis is a self-limiting disease that usually lasts about 2 weeks.[34-37] Treatment includes the use of antibiotics to combat secondary invaders and supportive intravenous fluids in very severe cases. Penicillin is ineffective and has been reported to be detrimental, protracting the duration and aggravating the course of the disease. Therefore its use is contraindicated. Topical application of chlortetracycline, however, may be beneficial. Gamma globulin has been tried, but the results are inconclusive. Hydrogen peroxide mouthwashes are ineffective and serve to irritate the mouth further. Mild, soothing mouthwashes* or mucosal ointments (Orabase) are helpful. Eating can be painful for these patients. Bland foods and supplements (Metrecal, Sego, Nutrament) are recommended.

**CHAPTER 21**

**References**

1. Hirschfeld, I., Beube, F., and Siegel, E. H.: The history of Vincent's infection, J. Periodont. **11**:89, 1940.
2. Schaffer, E. M.: Necrotizing ulcerative gingivitis, Northwest Dent. **33**:267, 1954.
3. Goldhaber, P., and Giddon, D. B.: Present concepts concerning the etiology and treatment of acute necrotizing ulcerative gingivitis, Int. Dent. J. **14**:468, 1964.
4. Grupe, H. E., and Wilder, L. S.: Observations of necrotizing gingivitis in 870 military trainees, J. Periodont. **27**:255, 1956.
5. Grant, D. A.: Necrotizing ulcerative gingivitis, J. S. Calif. Dent. Ass. **23**:21, 1955.

5a. Knolle, G., and Strassburg, M.: Die ulzeröse stomatitis und differentialdiagnostisch wichtige Krankheitbilder. In Hardt, E., editor: Deutscher Zahnärtzekalender 1972, Munich, 1971, Carl Hanser Verlag.

6. Blake, G. C., and Trott, J. R.: Acute streptococcal gingivitis, Dent. Pract. **10**:43, 1959.
7. Anday, G., and Orban, B.: Acute agranulocytosis, Arch. Path. **39**:369, 1945.
8. Lynch, M. A., and Ship, I.: Initial oral manifestations of leukemia, J. Amer. Dent. Ass. **75**: 932, 1967.
9. Everett, F. G.: Necrotizing ulcerative gingivitis, a reportable disease? J. Periodont. **27**:198, 1956.
10. Sheiham, A.: An epidemiological survey of acute ulcerative gingivitis in Nigerians, Arch. Oral Biol. **11**:937, 1966.
11. Emslie, R. D.: Periodontal disease in tropical Africa, Parodontopathies **18**:26, 1966.
12. Pindborg, J. J., Bhat, M., Devanath, K. R., and others: Occurrence of acute necrotizing ulcerative gingivitis in South Indian children, J. Periodont. **37**:14, 1966.
13. Zinserling, W. D.: Ueber die spirochetöse Gangrän und einige verwandte Prozesses vorzugsweise bei Kindern, Jena, 1928, Gustav Fischer.
14. Appleton, J. L. T.: Bacterial infection, ed. 4, Philadelphia, 1950, Lea & Febiger.
15. Hampp, E. G., Scott, D. B., and Wyckoff, R. W.: Morphological characteristics of certain cultured strains of oral spirochetes and Treponema pallidum as revealed by the electron microscope, J. Bact. **56**:755, 1948.
16. King, J. D.: Nutritional and other factors in trench mouth with special reference to the nicotinic acid component of vitamin B complex, Brit. Dent. J. **74**:113, 1943.
17. Rosebury, T.: The role of infection in periodontal disease, Oral Surg. **5**:363, 1952.
18. MacDonald, J. B., Socransky, S. S., and Gibbons, R. J.: Aspects of mixed anaerobic infections of mucous membranes, J. Dent. Res. **42**:529, 1963.
19. Hampp, E. G., and Mergenhagen, S. E.: Experimental infections with oral spirochetes, J. Infect. Dis. **109**:43, 1961.
20. Hampp, E. G., and Mergenhagen, S. E.: Experimental intracutaneous fusobacterial and fusospirochetal infections, J. Infect. Dis. **112**:84, 1963.
21. Listgarten, M. A., and Socransky, S. S.: Ultrastructural characteristics of a spirochete in the lesion of acute necrotizing ulcerative gingivostomatitis (Vincent's infection), Arch. Oral Biol. **9**:95, 1964.
22. Listgarten, M. A.: Electron microscopic observations on the bacterial flora of acute necrotizing ulcerative gingivitis, J. Periodont. **36**:328, 1965.
23. Lehner, T., and Clarry, E. D.: Acute ulcerative gingivitis, Brit. Dent. J. **121**:366, 1966.
24. Lado, R. A., and Carranza, F. A.: Estudio sobre incidencia de la gingivitis ulceronecrotizante, Rev. Asoc. Odont. Argent. **49**:87, 1961.
25. Pindborg, J. J.: The epidemiology of ulceromembranous gingivitis showing the influence of service in the Armed Forces, Parodontologie **10**:114, 1956.
26. Everett, F. G.: Necrotizing ulcerative gingivitis. Parts I and II, Oregon Dent. J. **26**:2 (April), 2 (May), 1957.

---

*Warm water (⅔ tumbler)
White Karo syrup (⅓ tumbler)
Xylocaine viscous (1 tablespoon)
Sig: Rinse 5 times a day before meals.

27. Moulton, R., Ewen, S., and Thieman, W.: Emotional factors in periodontal disease, Oral Surg. **5**:833, 1952.
28. Formicola, A. J., Witte, E. T., and Curran, P. M.: A study of personality traits and acute necrotizing ulcerative gingivitis, J. Periodont. **41**:36, 1970.
29. Giddon, D. B., Zackin, S. J., and Goldhaber, P.: Acute necrotizing ulcerative gingivitis in college students, J. Amer. Dent. Ass. **68**:381, 1964.
30. Schaffer, E. M.: The effects of drugs in the treatment of necrotizing ulcerative gingivitis, J. Amer. Dent. Ass. **48**:279, 1954.
31. Stern, I. B.: Necrotizing ulcerative gingivitis. In Kutscher, A. H., Zegarelli, E. V., and Hyman, G. A., editors: Pharmacotherapeutics of oral disease, New York, 1964, McGraw-Hill Book Co.
32. Fitch, H. B., Bethart, H., Alling, C. C., and Munns, C. R.: Acute necrotizing ulcerative gingivitis, J. Periodont. **34**:422, 1963.
33. Goodman, L. S., and Gilman, A.: The pharmacological basis of therapeutics, ed. 4, New York, 1970, The Macmillan Co.
34. Dodd, K., Johnson, L. M., and Buddingh, G. J.: Herptic stomatitis, J. Pediat. **12**:95, 1938.
35. Scott, T. F. M., Steigman, A. J., and Convey, J. H.: Acute infectious gingivostomatitis, J.A.M.A. **117**:999, 1941.
36. Chilton, N. W.: Herpetic stomatitis, Amer. J. Orthodont. (Oral Surg. section) **30**:335, 1944.
37. Ziskin, D. E., and Holden, M.: Acute herpetic gingivostomatitis, J. Amer. Dent. Ass. **30**:1697, 1943.

**Additional suggested reading**

Emslie, R. D.: Treatment of acute gingivtis, Brit. Dent. J. **122**:307, 1967.

Fröhlich, E.: Die Pathologie der postulzerösen Zahnfleischnische und ihre Therapie, Deutsch. Zahnaerztl. Z. **27**:284, 1972.

Holroyd, S. V.: Antibiotics in the practice of periodontics, J. Periodont. **42**:584, 1971.

Malberger, E.: Acute infectious oral necrosis among young children in the Gambia, J. Periodont. Res. **2**:154, 1967.

CHAPTER TWENTY-TWO

# Pericoronitis



*Definition*

Pericoronitis is defined as the inflammation of gingival and contiguous soft tissues about the crown of an incompletely erupted tooth.[1-3] The mandibular third molars are the most frequently involved. However, the mandibular second molars may become involved when they are the most distal teeth in the arch. Less often the most distal maxillary teeth are involved.

## ANATOMIC RELATIONSHIPS

The occlusal surface of an involved tooth may be partly covered by a flap of tissue, the operculum, which exists during the eruption of the tooth and may persist afterward (Fig. 22-1). Various degrees of eruption, malposition, or impaction may further complicate the soft tissue architecture. In addition, pocket formation and body deformities are not uncommon.

### Signs and symptoms

The operculum is particularly vulnerable to irritation and is often directly traumatized when it is caught between the crown that it covers and the antagonist tooth during closure. The cryptlike form of the pericoronal tissues favors the retention and stagnation of food and the proliferation of microorganisms; the performance of adequate oral hygiene in this area is difficult. These factors predipose to streptococcal and staphylococcal infection, and the flaps may occasionally be involved in NUG.[1]

## TREATMENT

In the treatment of pericoronitis, the following factors should be considered[4]:

1. Severity of the inflammatory process
2. Systemic complications
3. Advisability of retaining the involved tooth

Before undertaking treatment, the dentist should review the medical history to determine whether the patient is a health risk because of valvular heart disease or uveitis or because he has a cardiovascular prosthesis. In these cases immediate coverage with ample doses of antibiotics is indicated.

Steps in the treatment of pericoronitis are as follows:

1. Cleanse the area by lavage and gentle curettage to remove debris from

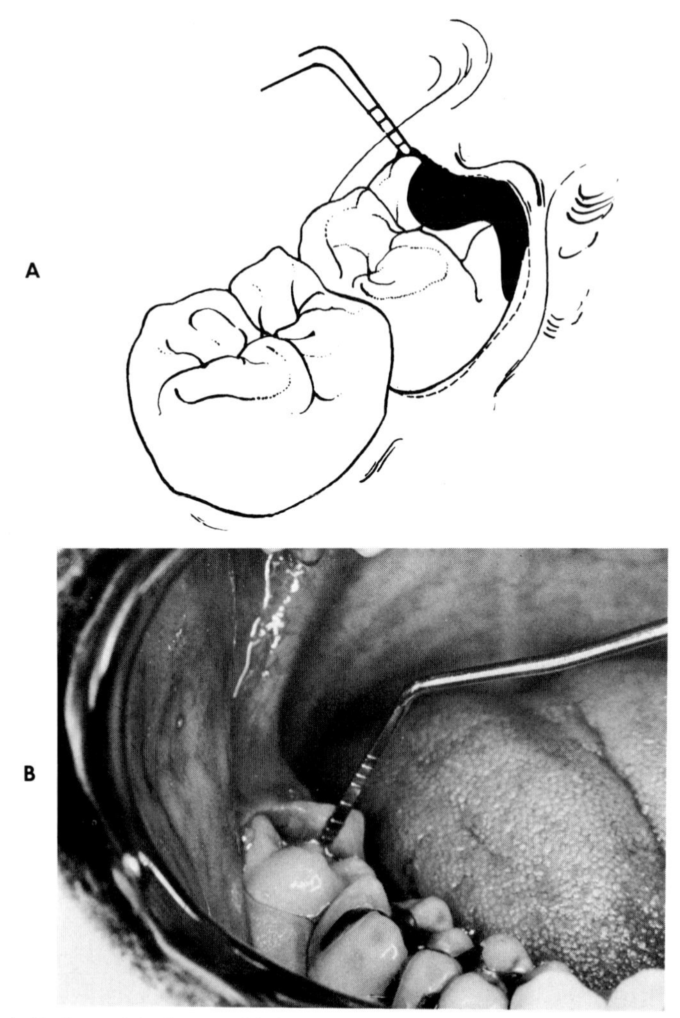


**Fig. 22-1. A,** Pericoronitis about a third molar. The tooth is partially enveloped by tissue, and the operculum covers the distal portion of the occlusal surface. In addition, a pocket has developed. **B,** Operculum retracted by a probe.

below the operculum. Establish drainage. Possibly obtain culture for an antibiotic sensitivity test.

2. Insert a single thickness of ¼-inch iodoform gauze below the operculum.
3. If adequate drainage cannot be established and palpation reveals fluctuation, you may have to incise and drain through the incision.
4. If fever and lymphadenopathy are present, systemic antibiotic therapy should be considered.
5. Instruct the patient to rinse frequently with warm solutions of saline (1 teaspoonful of salt to a pint of warm water).
6. At the second appointment (24 hours later), remove the drain. Insert a new drain for another 24 hours. The patient should feel improvement.
7. Decide either to extract or retain the offending tooth and remove the operculum. If NUG was an etiologic factor in the pericoronitis, appropriate treatment should be given. (See Chapter 21.)

The muscular floor of the oral cavity proper terminates mesially at the mandibular third molar. An infection in the lingual aspect of the mandibular third molar may therefore descend in the lymph spaces of the neck and mediastinum.

## PREVENTION

Elimination of third molar flaps (opercula) about the most distal, incompletely erupted teeth can prevent pericoronitis. When this condition exists, it should be corrected. Semi-impacted teeth should be removed carefully at an early time. This not only corrects pericoronitis but may enhance the potential for osseous repair on the distal surface of the adjacent tooth.

A pericoronal flap may be asymptomatic, but it is a potential site for gingival enlargement with concomitant deepening of the pocket. It thus provides for additional retention of bacteria and exudate. Acute exacerbation may ensue. Further enlargement of the tissue then acts to inhibit drainage from the sulcus, inducing deeper spreading of the process beyond the gingival tissues. Often the enlarged tissues become traumatized during mastication, adding to the discomfort of the patient. Pus may issue from under the operculum. As the condition becomes more severe, swelling increases, mandibular movement is limited (trismus), and temperature is elevated. In addition, there may be leukocytosis, lymphadenopathy, foul breath (fetor oris), and referred pain to the ear. Pus may accumulate in the tissues subjacent to the buccal (vestibular) fornix.

## COMPLICATIONS

If the initial infection is not contained or is carried more deeply during surgical procedures, it may spread along fascial planes into the surgical spaces of the head and neck. Retropharyngeal, peritonsillar, masseter space, and temporal space abscesses, Ludwig's angina, laryngeal edema, cavernous sinus thrombosis, and acute meningitis are relatively rare but serious consequences of pericoronitis.

**CHAPTER 22**

**References**

1. Kay, H. L. W.: Investigation into the nature of pericoronitis, Brit. J. Oral Surg. **4**:52, 1966.
2. Andrews, A. G.: Pericoronitis, Appl. Ther. **8**:688, 1966.
3. Wallace, J. R.: Pericoronitis and military dentistry, Oral Surg. **22**:543, 1966.
4. Kay, H. L. W.: The management of pericoronitis, Dent. Pract. **11**:80, 1960.
5. Bean, L. R., and King, D. P.: Pericoronitis; its nature and etiology, J. Amer. Dent. Ass. **83**: 1074, 1971.

CHAPTER TWENTY-THREE

# Abscesses and cysts



## ABSCESSES

A dental abscess is a circumscribed, acute, purulent inflammation of the soft tissues in or about the teeth. It is caused by a mixed infection of oral organisms.[1] The area involved may be swollen and painful. It may be accompanied by malaise, elevation of temperature, and lymphadenopathy. Pus may distend the gingiva and extend into the tissues subjacent to the vestibular fornix.

Bacteria are not normally present in the tissues. When they gain entrance, a rapid migration of leukocytes occurs to contain the infection. The area is walled off by thrombosis of the vessels and by a fibrinous blockade. The numbers of leukocytes and microorganisms continue to increase. This is followed by necrosis and liquefaction of the central area, with formation of pus.

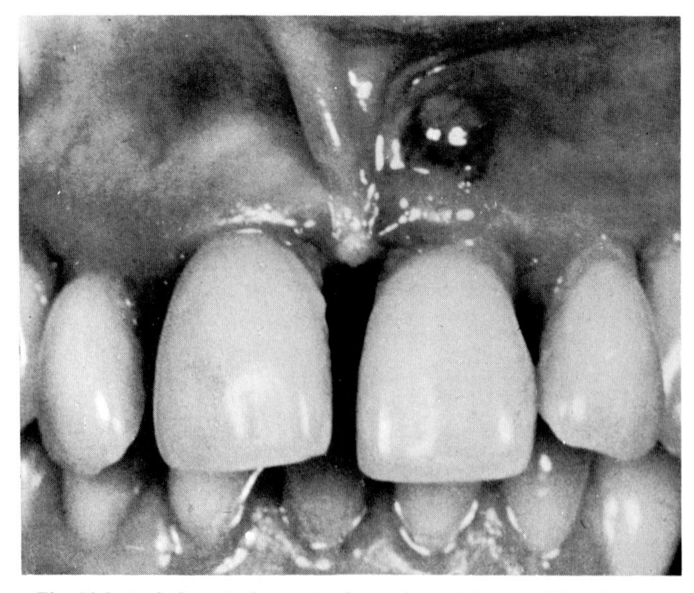

**Fig. 23-1.** Periodontal abscess in the region of the maxillary incisor.

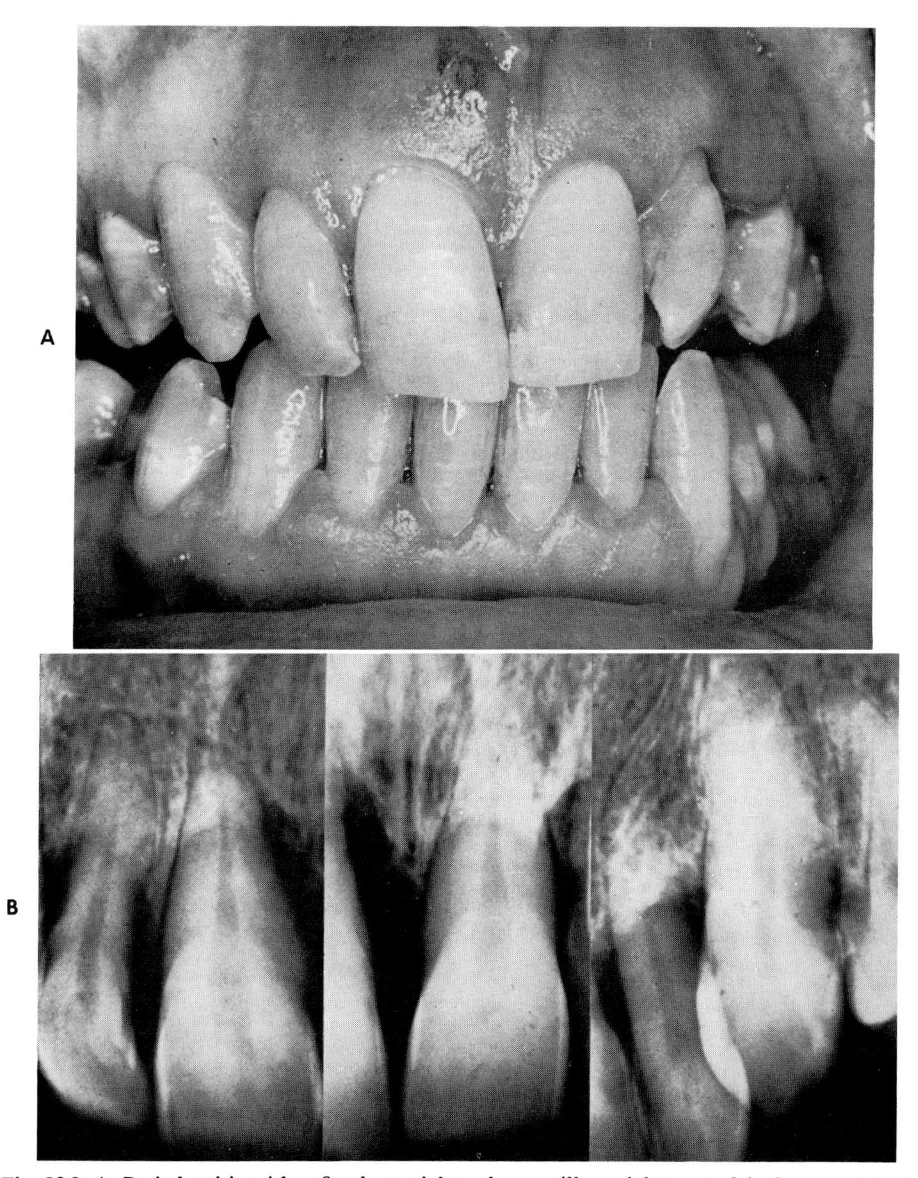


**Fig. 23-2. A,** Periodontitis with a fistula mesial to the maxillary right central incisor, next to the frenum. **B,** Roentgenograms of the same patient showing considerable bone destruction in the maxillary anterior region.

## Periodontal abscess

The periodontal abscess can be an acute exacerbation of chronic periodontal disease. It may occur when the infection passes into the tissues through the pocket epithelium. Such abscesses are frequently the result of the occlusion of the narrow mouths of tortuous or deep intra-alveolar pockets (Figs. 23-1 and 23-2). Since the virulence of the organisms is an important factor, even shallow pockets may become involved. Occasionally, lateral periodontal cysts (Fig. 23-10) may abscess.[2,3]

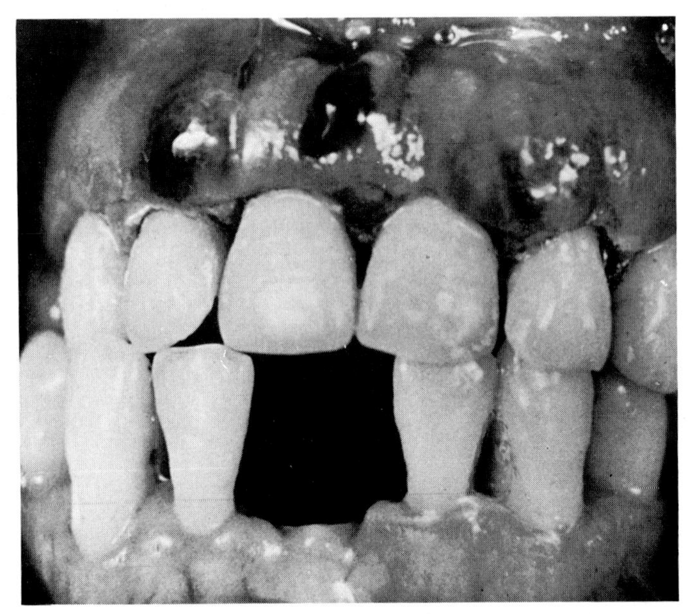

**Fig. 23-3.** Acute abscesses (gingival abscesses) produced by mechanical injury to the gingival tissues.

## Gingival abscess

The gingival abscess is a relative rarity that occurs when the bacteria invade through some break in the gingival surface. Such abrasions may be the result of mastication, oral hygiene procedures, or dental treatment (Fig. 23-3). Although the gingival sulcus is not involved at the onset, the abscess may extend deep into the connective tissue, involving the alveolar bone and communicating with the sulcus. The resistance of the patient is an important factor. The patient with an uncontrolled diabetes, for example, may be more susceptible to abscesses.

## Periapical abscess

The periapical (dentoalveolar) abscess is the result of pulpal infection that extends through the apical foramen to the periapical tissues. Such abscesses may develop fistulous tracts that communicate with the oral cavity. They may also develop a communication with the periodontal pocket or the gingival sulcus. It is possible for the pulpal infection to reach these periodontal tissues through an aberrant canal, a root fracture, or a perforation. Of all the dental abscesses, the periapical is the most common type.

## Differential diagnosis

The differential diagnosis of an abscess may involve periapical, periodontal, and gingival abscesses. Periodontal treatment, however, is concerned primarily with periodontal and gingival abscesses. Dental abscesses may resemble each other clinically yet differ in their origin. The periapical abscess is from pulpal infection, the periodontal abscess develops via the pocket, and the gingival abscess is an infection that occurs through a break in the gingival surface (Fig. 23-4). Although an abscess may originate in any one place, it may extend to involve

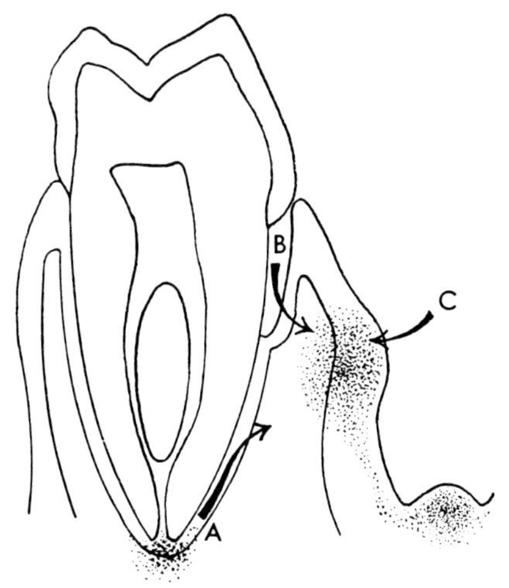


**Fig. 23-4.** Portals of entry in abscess formation: *A,* Periapical abscess; *B,* periodontal abscess; *C,* gingival abscess. A primary infection in any one area may travel to the other areas and involve them secondarily. In addition, extension to the vestibular fornix may occur.

other areas. For example, the periodontal abscess may cause pulpal necrosis and periapical abscesses and may ultimately lead to pocket formation.

The infective process and clinical symptoms of the various dental abscesses tend to resemble each other. The abscesses differ only in origin and avenue of infection. Many periodontal abscesses are misdiagnosed as periapical abscesses and the teeth extracted because the dentist is reluctant to treat this condition. Proper diagnosis, on the other hand, could lead to proper treatment and retention of many abscessed teeth. Diagnosis depends on clinical findings, roentgenographic examination, and pulp testing. Caries, pulpal involvement, and periapical pathosis are suggestive of periapical abscess, whereas pocket formation, alveolar bone loss, and periodontal pathology are suggestive of periodontal abscess. When neither set of circumstances is obvious, a gingival abscess should be suspected. Periodontal abscesses can occur about nonvital teeth; and, conversely, periapical abscesses can occur in periodontally involved teeth. Moreover, the infection can spread from periodontium to pulp and vice versa so that an abscess may be both periodontal and periapical. (See Chapter 35.) Fortunately complications such as these are infrequent. Abscesses tend to have periods of exacerbation and remission. Repeated exacerbations are responsible for bizarre and extensive loss of bone.

## Prognosis

The purpose of the diagnosis is to establish which type of abscess is present, the prognosis, and the choice of treatment. The prognosis of an abscessed tooth depends on the amenability of the infection to treatment. The gingival abscess is completely treatable and its prognosis favorable. The prognosis of the periapically abscessed tooth depends on whether root canal therapy is possible. The prognosis of the periodontally abscessed tooth depends on the amount and nature of the bone loss and the strategic position of the tooth. During the height of the abscess, mobility is increased and is an inconclusive symptom. The prognosis

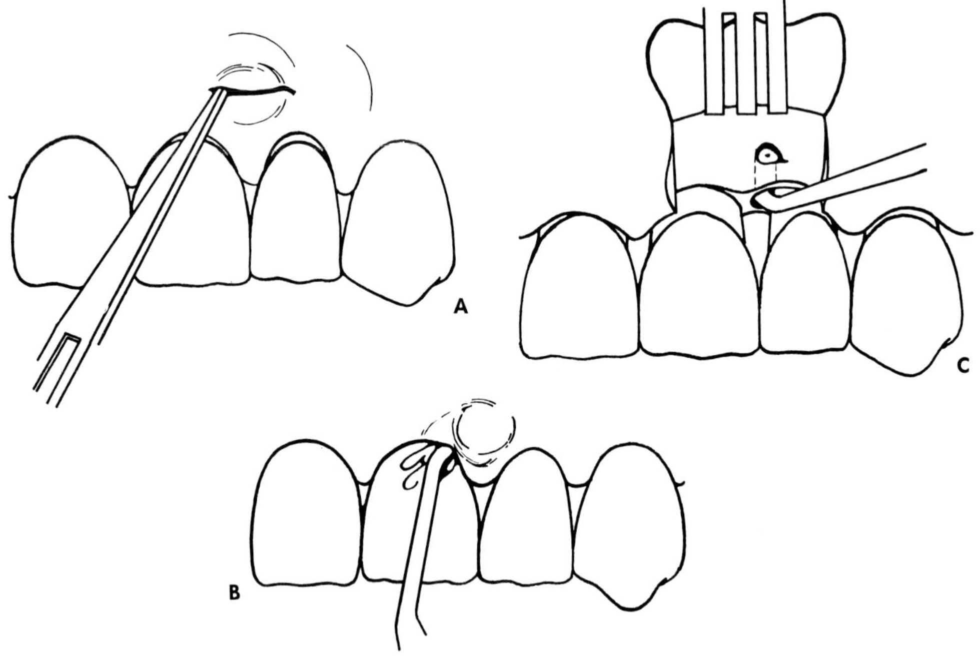


**Fig. 23-5.** Means of establishing drainage. **A,** Horizontal incision. **B,** Curettage through the gingival sulcus. **C,** Raising a small flap.

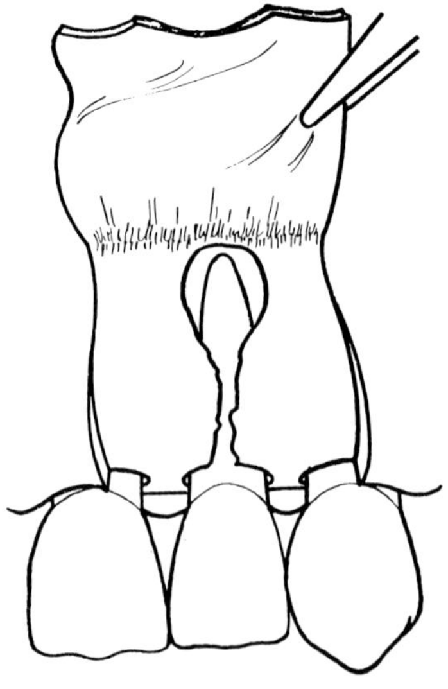

**Fig. 23-6.** Flap raised to give access to periapical and periodontal tissues. Apical resection and root curettage can be performed in instances requiring simultaneous endodontic and periodontal treatment. (Adapted from Trott, J. R.: J. Canad. Dent. Ass. **25:**601, 1959.)

of a tooth with a periodontal abscess is generally promising, except in rare cases when a localized osteomyelitis follows.[4]

## Treatment

Treatment of the abscessed tooth varies with the decision to retain or to extract the tooth and with the type of abscess present. Treatment therefore has exodontic, periodontal, and endodontic aspects. The details of periodontal treatment are dealt with more fully in Chapters 24, 26, and 29. The first step in treatment is the reduction of the abscess. The administration of antibiotics is indicated in the presence of fever and malaise. Drainage should be established if it is not already present. This may involve curetting the pocket or incising the abscess (Fig. 23-5). When necessary, the extraction of the tooth will serve to establish drainage. Reduction of the abscess should be followed by the appropriate treatment.

In some instances rinsing the mouth with hot water every 2 hours will help the abscess to point. If an incision is needed, a horizontal cut over the center of the abscess is favored. Iodoform gauze may be inserted. Vertical incisions involving the gingival margin may lead to unsightly recessions and should be avoided. On occasion a flap may be reflected (Figs. 23-5 and 23-6).

During the acute stages of the abscess, portions of the alveolar bone may become necrotic. Small sequestra may form. When a sequestrum forms, the abscess will not resolve in the usual manner and the sequestrum may have to be removed (preferably by a flap approach unless it is exfoliated). Observations of the presence of pus and necrotic bone associated with periodontal abscesses may have influenced the development of the early mistaken concept of periodontal abscesses as a flow of pus from the bone (pyorrhea alveolaris) and the mistaken concept for surgical procedures to remove necrotic bone.

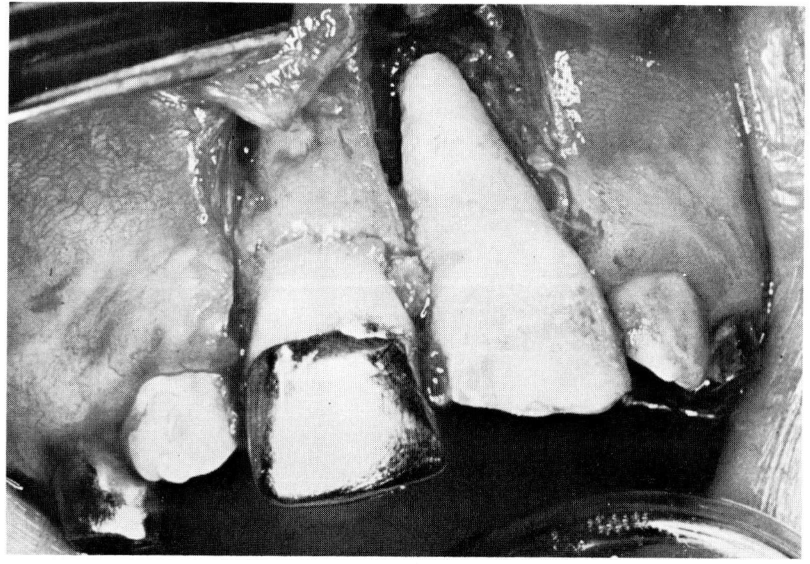

**Fig. 23-7.** A flap has been elevated to show the bone destruction caused by an abscess. The vestibular bone is completely destroyed, the apex of the tooth is involved, and the bone destruction extends orally to the palatal surface of the apical half of the tooth.

After the abscess is reduced, further treatment is determined by diagnosis and prognosis. If a tooth is hopelessly involved, it should be extracted. The gingival abscess will usually resolve completely after drainage. Periapical lesions are treated by endodontic procedures, and the involved sulcus may subsequently heal.

Since the bone loss associated with periodontal abscesses may be extensive, osseous surgical procedures that might require further sacrifice of bone may be contraindicated. Reattachment or bone graft procedures are more conserving of bone and are therefore preferable. Moreover, after periodontal abscesses the potential for reattachment is enhanced.[5-7] Successful treatment is often followed by regeneration of bone. Reattachment attempts depend on the location of the abscess and access to the area. In addition, adequate stabilization and minimization of occlusal traumatism may be called for. These can be achieved by splinting and occlusal adjustment. (See Chapters 29 and 30.)

If an abscess has involved both periapical and periodontal tissues, combined treatment may be necessary (Chapter 33). This can be accomplished by exposing the area with a broad flap to gain access to the root surface and the apex (Figs. 23-6 to 23-8). In this way both curettage and apicoectomy can be performed in one operation.[6,8]

## CYSTS

### Gingival cyst

The gingival cyst occurs as a painless, bluish gray nodule in the gingiva (Fig. 23-9) and has the appearance and consistency of a mucocele.[2] Because such a cyst is located superficially, it is not apparent on the roentgenogram.

### Periodontal cyst

A periodontal cyst (sometimes called a lateral periodontal cyst) may be seen on roentgenograms (Fig. 23-10) as a well-defined radiolucent lesion adjacent to

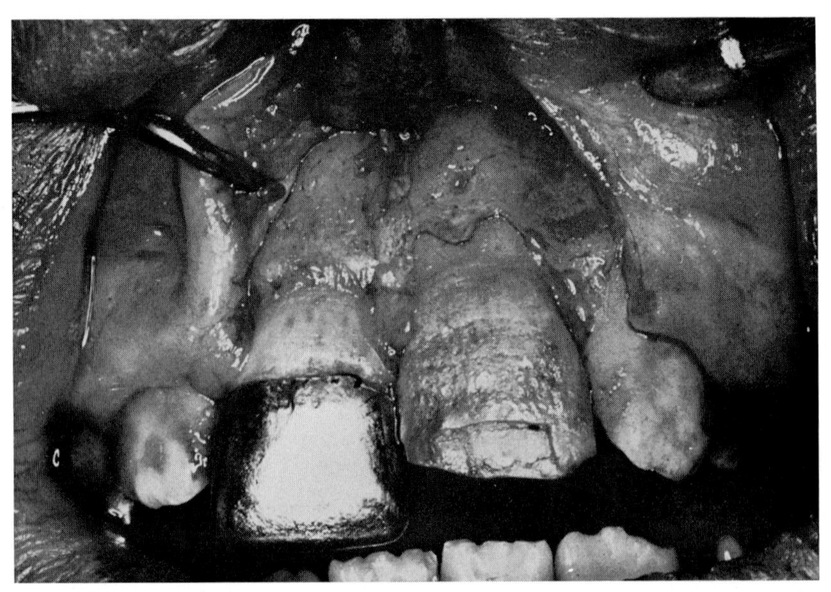

**Fig. 23-8.** Reoperation showing remarkable regeneration of vestibular bone after successful endodontic treatment. (Courtesy W. H. Hiatt, Denver.)

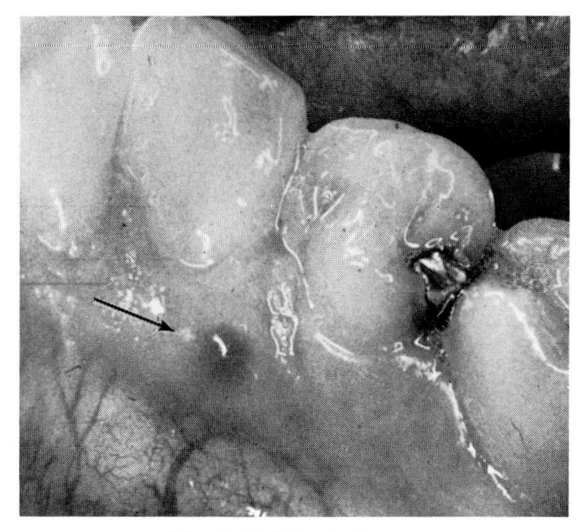

**Fig. 23-9.** Gingival cyst.

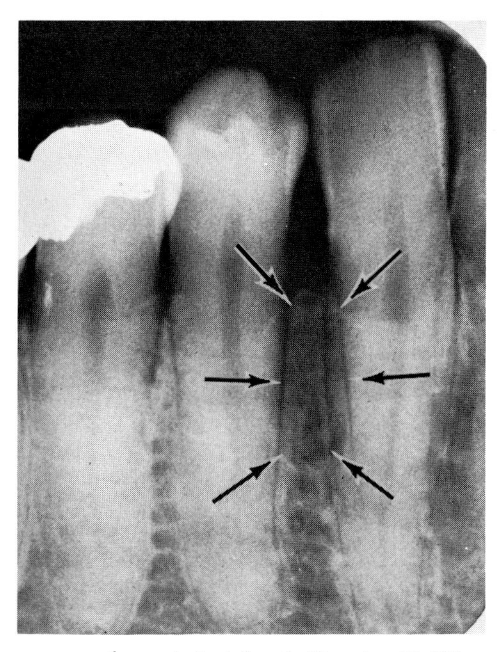

**Fig. 23-10.** Roentgenogram of a periodontal cyst. (Courtesy T. Gilmore, Portland, Ore.)

a root.[2,3] It lies mainly in the bone, sometimes breaking through the cortical plate, resulting in a swelling of the gingiva.

## Incidence and origin

Gingival and periodontal cysts are rather rare. They most frequently arise from remnants of odontogenic epithelium in the periodontal ligament or the gingiva. Other mechanisms leading to the formation of such cysts undoubtedly operate occasionally. These include traumatic implantation of surface epithelium that later undergoes cystic degeneration, development from heterotopic glandular epithelium, or cystic development within a lateral periodontal abscess. It is interesting that most gingival and periodontal cysts occur in the region of the mandibular cuspid. Such a cyst may on occasion become infected and then form a puzzling abscess in a vital tooth with no demonstrable pocket.

In general, insufficient importance is attached to tooth vitality in periodontal treatment. Extensive and precipitous bone loss may have pulp pathology as an associated cause. Proper diagnosis of such cases will continue to further success in treatment.

**CHAPTER 23**

**References**

1. Ludwig, T. G.: An investigation of the oral flora of suppurative oral swelling, Aust. Dent. J. **2**:259, 1957.
2. Rickles, N. H., and Everett, F. G.: Gingival and lateral periodontal cysts, Parodontologie **14**:41, 1960.
3. Moskow, B. S., Siegel, K., Zegarelli, E. V., and others: Gingival and lateral periodontal cysts, J. Periodont. **41**:249, 1970.
4. Moskow, B. S., Wasserman, B. H., Hirschfeld, L. S., and Morris, M. L.: Repair of periodontal tissues following acute localized osteomyelitis, Periodontics **5**:29, 1967.
5. Prichard, J. F.: Management of the periodontal abscess, Oral Surg. **6**:474, 1953.
6. Trott, J. R.: The acute periodontal abscess, J. Canad. Dent. Ass. **25**:601, 1959.
7. Knewitz, K. W., Devine, K. D., and Waite, D. E.: Differential diagnosis of cervicofacial swellings, Oral Surg. **25**:43, 1968.
8. Hiatt, W. H.: Regeneration of the periodontium after endodontic therapy and flap operation, Oral Surg. **12**:1471, 1959.

**Additional suggested reading**

Knolle, G.: Der Paradontalabscess, Deutsch. Zahnaerztl. Z. **27**:290, 1972.

Nabers, J. M., Meador, H. L., Nabers, C. L., and O'Leary, T. J.: Chronology, an important factor in the repair of osseous defects, Periodontics **2**:304, 1964.

Ritchey, B., and Orban, B.: Cysts of the gingiva, Oral Surg. **6**:765, 1953.

PART VIII

# Therapy

CHAPTER TWENTY-FOUR

# Root planing



*Definition*

Root planing is the instrumentation applied to the root surface to divest the surface of deposits and softened or roughened cementum. When it is thoroughly performed, it can produce a smooth, clean, hard, polished root surface. Root planing is the primary treatment for periodontal inflammation. In simple cases it may be the only treatment necessary (by the dentist); in severe, advanced cases in which other treatment is not possible, root planing may be the only treatment that is feasible. In all other cases the patient is maintained after treatment by regular root planing and a program of plaque control. Since the removal of irritants is the definitive treatment for periodontal inflammations, root planing is used more than any other type of periodontal therapy.

Inflammation, pockets, tooth mobility, and tooth migration are the classical signs of periodontal disease against which most therapy is directed. Such therapy may include root planing, occlusal adjustment, periodontal surgery, orthodontic tooth movement, splinting, and other operative and prosthetic interventions as well as a program of meticulous plaque control at home. The sequence in which any or all of these measures are performed will vary according to the needs of the patient. Except in emergencies, a thorough diagnosis and the projection of a treatment plan should precede any therapeutic effort. We shall first consider root planing, which is used in the treatment of almost all patients with periodontal disease. Together with plaque control, root planing is vital in the prevention of inflammatory periodontal disease. In an epidemiologic study Russell has noted: "The conclusion seems inescapable that much of the current high tooth mortality from periodontal disease could have been prevented by early and adequate scaling."*

## RATIONALE

The fact that the periodontal pocket must be eliminated is obvious, for the pocket is a haven for bacterial activity. It contains concealed spicules of calculus

*From Russell, A. L.: Epidemiologic research 1960-1963, J. Amer. Dent. Ass. 68:820, 1964.

covered by plaque, which are a source of irritation and serve as a focal spot of the inflammatory process; the spicules may also promote the further deepening of the pocket. Obviously therefore the elimination of deposits is basic to therapy. Root planing is a prerequisite for the cure of periodontal disease and with plaque control is an integral part of the effort to prevent the disease.

When calcified and uncalcified deposits are removed, the diseased dento-gingival junction can heal. The chronic inflammatory tissue in the lamina propria can be replaced by a young connective tissue consisting of reserve cells, other fibrous elements, and blood cells. The greater portion of this tissue organizes to form a healthy lamina propria. The ulcerated sulcular epithelium heals and forms an intact barrier to exogenous substances, and the pocket thus is converted into a healthy sulcus.

## INDICATIONS

Root planing is a part of every treatment of gingivitis and periodontitis. It may bring about the eradication of some of the shallower pockets through the resolution of the inflammation. It should precede most surgical procedures since it creates a cleaner environment, reduces hyperemia and edema, and improves the healing tendencies of the tissues. It is also repeated during some surgical procedures and after healing to ensure the complete debridement and thorough polishing of the teeth so that the patient can maintain gingival health by proper oral hygiene.

When pocket depth is accompanied by edematous gingivae, it may be reduced or eliminated entirely by root planing. When the gingivae are largely fibrotic, chances for pocket elimination by shrinkage of the gingiva are much less. Although some reduction in pocket depth of highly fibrotic gingivae may take place, this can be a long drawn-out process. Attempts to reduce the depth of fibrotic pockets by root planing and oral hygiene will fail in many instances. Pocket depth may also be reduced by reattachment, although the root planing approach to reattachment does not yield predictable results.

## INSTRUMENTATION

Successful root planing requires the skillful use of instruments carefully adapted to the needs of the operation. The extent and direction of the application of this well-designed armamentarium will be guided by the operator's intimate knowledge of the tissues involved as gained from the examination.

All instruments used in root planing are generally called scalers. The objectives of root instrumentation go beyond scaling for the removal of deposits, however. The results of scaling should include a root surface that is not only divested of deposits[2,2a] but also glass-hard and smooth to touch; and the removal of the deposits should cause the least amount of injury to the soft and hard tissues forming the pocket.[3-9]

***Designs for specific needs***

The purpose of an instrument should be well understood. Some instruments are more efficient in removing bulky, calcified deposits but are not made to reach to the bottom of the pocket. Others are made so that their blades can be carried below the apical end of the calculus at the bottom of the pocket without causing undue damage to the attachment tissues.

The names given to the instruments usually describe the shape and design of the blades or the mode of action of the instruments. There are five groups: chisels, hoes, sickles, files, and curettes. Each of the five types is designed for a

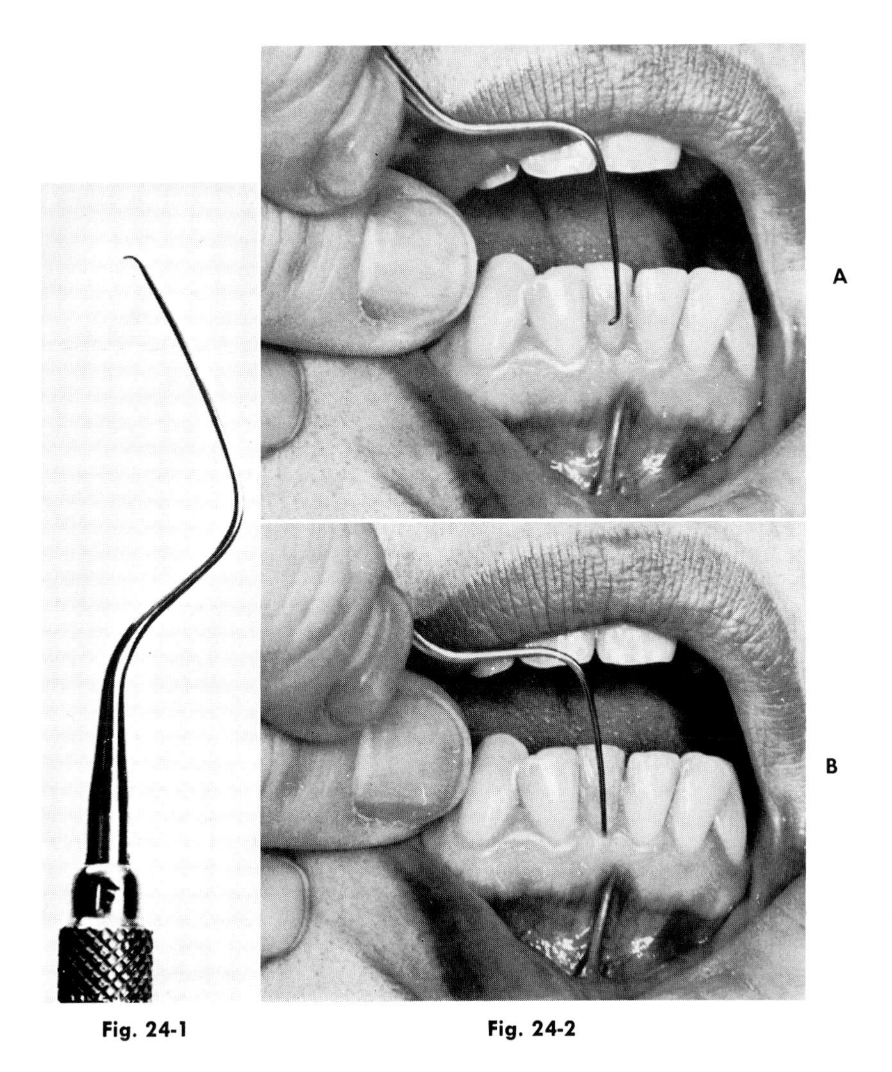


Fig. 24-1 Fig. 24-2

**Fig. 24-1.** Pocket explorer, an indispensable instrument in periodontal diagnosis.
**Fig. 24-2. A,** Place the pocket explorer with the side of the tip toward the surface of the tooth. **B,** Guide the tip of the explorer easily to the bottom of the sulcus or pocket. Surface irregularities will be transmitted to the fingers.

specific use and sometimes for access to a specific tooth surface. The chisel, hoe, and sickle are designed for the removal of heavy calculus, whereas curettes and files are intended for the finer and final planing of the root surface to the bottom of the pocket.

## Pocket explorer

The explorer (Fig. 24-1) is used to determine the depth of the pocket and the amount of calculus and its configuration in the pocket before debridement is started. This instrument is indispensable for determining the texture and character of the root surface. When the small, bent tip of the instrument is placed with its side to the surface of the tooth and guided into the pocket (Fig. 24-2), it transmits to the operator's fingers a feeling of the character of the root surface.

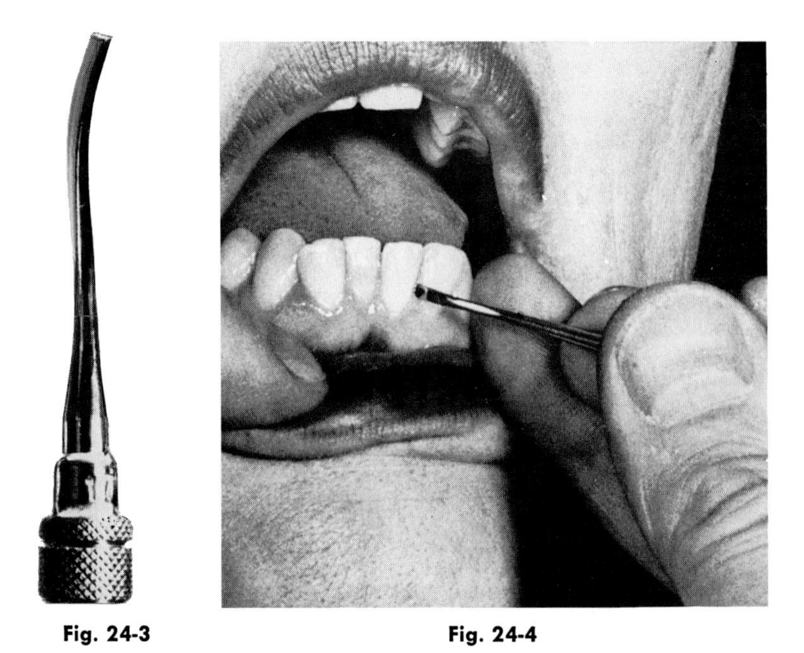

Fig. 24-3 Fig. 24-4

**Fig. 24-3.** Periodontal chisel.
**Fig. 24-4.** Proper application of the periodontal chisel used as a push instrument.

Accretions, indentations, furcation, or ledges can be determined more easily than they can with a straight explorer. The bottom of the pocket can be probed without injury to the soft tissues. The explorer will indicate the proper extent and direction for the application of instruments in the pocket.

## Chisel

The chisel (Fig. 24-3) is designed for removal of extensive supragingival calcified deposits, especially those located in the mandibular anterior region. When calculus occupies the interproximal and lingual area, the chisel is used in a labiolingual direction with a push stroke to dislodge the gross mass.

Some chisels have very sharp corners that may nick the tooth surface and traumatize the tissues. These corners may be rounded without affecting the efficacy of the instrument.[6] Fig. 24-4 shows the proper use of the chisel.

## Hoe

Hoe-shaped instruments (Fig. 24-5, *A*) are intended for the removal of easily accessible calculus. These pull instruments should be used subgingivally only when the gingivae are easily displaced.

## Sickle

The blades of some sickles (Fig. 24-5, *B*) are rectangular and extremely thin, sometimes as fine as 0.2 to 0.4 mm. They may be used in a push or a pull stroke. The blades of other sickles are triangular in cross section and may be used only in pull strokes. A large, hooked sickle is helpful when used on the lingual surface

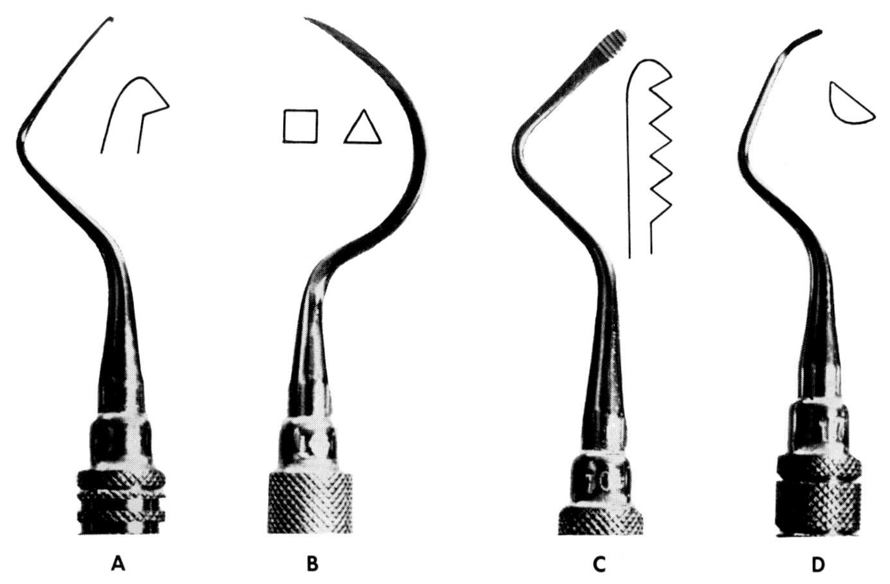


**Fig. 24-5. A,** Hoe-shaped periodontal instrument. The diagram shows the working blade. **B,** Sickle-shaped periodontal instrument. The blade has four cutting edges (90-degree angle). Triangular blades also are used (diagram). **C,** Periodontal file. The blades simulate the cutting edges of three to five hoe-shaped instruments. **D,** Periodontal curette. The cutting blade is spoon shaped.

of mandibular incisors, an area difficult to reach with shorter instruments. Double contra-angled sickles such as the Jaquette scalers are well adapted for interproximal use in the premolar and molar areas.

### File

Files (Fig. 24-5, *C*) may be considered as having an action similar to that of three to five hoes in gang. These instruments are designed for use in deep, narrow-mouthed pockets and in tortuous pockets inaccessible to other instruments. However, they are difficult to sharpen, which limits their usefulness.

### Curette

Curettes (Fig. 24-5, *D*) are spoon shaped, similar to spoon excavators used in operative dentistry. The curette has two cutting edges and therefore performs two functions: it removes the soft tissue wall of the pocket and it serves as a root planer. Frequently both functions are performed simultaneously. The term *curettage,* however, should be reserved for the intentional removal of soft tissues. Curettes are designed as pull or push instruments. The tool angles of pull curettes are approximately 80 degrees, and those of push curettes approximately 40 degrees. One can distinguish the two types of instruments by examining their faces. Each instrument should be used in the manner for which it was designed. The pull curette (e.g., McCall) is applied to the tooth so that its face makes an 80- to 85-degree angle (negative rake). The push curette is applied to the tooth to make a 15- to 25-degree angle. The rake angle is defined as the angle that the cutting blade makes with a line perpendicular to the surface of the tooth (Fig. 24-6). The push curette may sometimes be used as a pull instrument, and

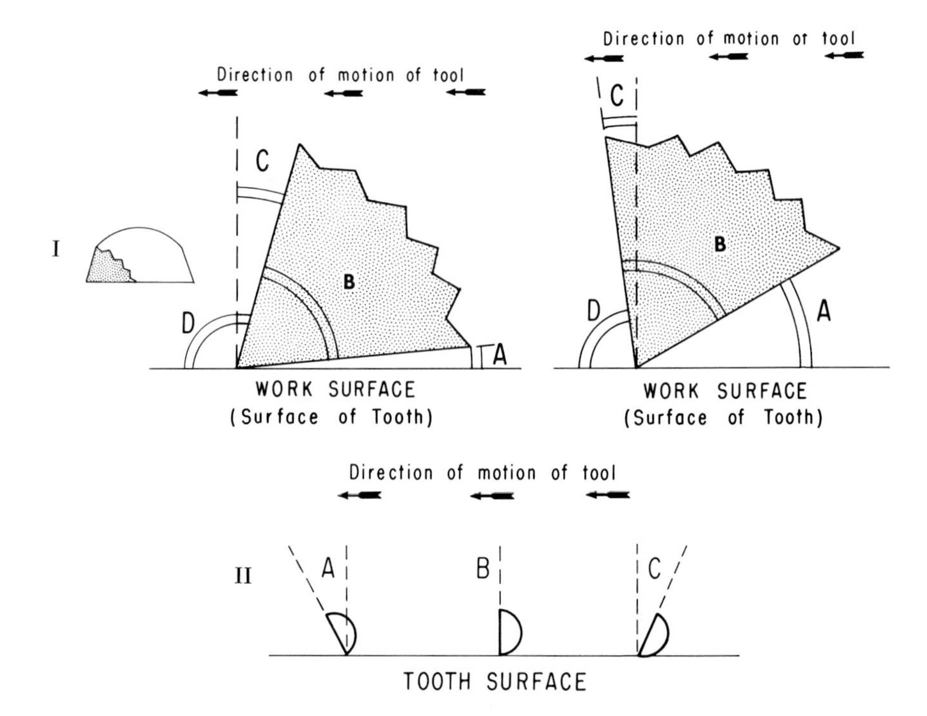


**Fig. 24-6. I,** The dotted areas are magnifications of the cutting part of the small curette at the left. *A,* Clearance angle; *B,* tool angle; *C,* rake angle; *D,* angle of application. The rake angle *(C)* is positive in the left illustration because the inclination of the tool is more acute than when the rake angle is zero (90 degrees to the working surface). The rake angle is negative in the illustration to the right. **II,** A curette is used with varying rake angles: *A,* negative; *B,* zero; *C,* positive.

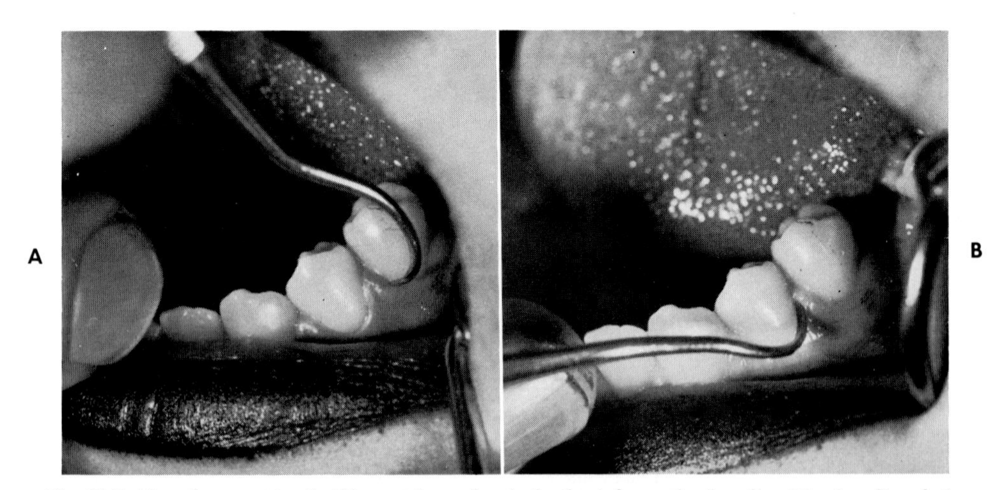


**Fig. 24-7.** Use of a curette. **A,** The cutting edge is farthest from the handle. The handle of the instrument is in the long axis of the tooth. **B,** If the cutting edge nearest the handle is applied, the instrument is lowered to make the handle more perpendicular to the long axis of the tooth. (Courtesy H. A. Zander, Rochester, N. Y., and E. M. Schaffer, Minneapolis.)

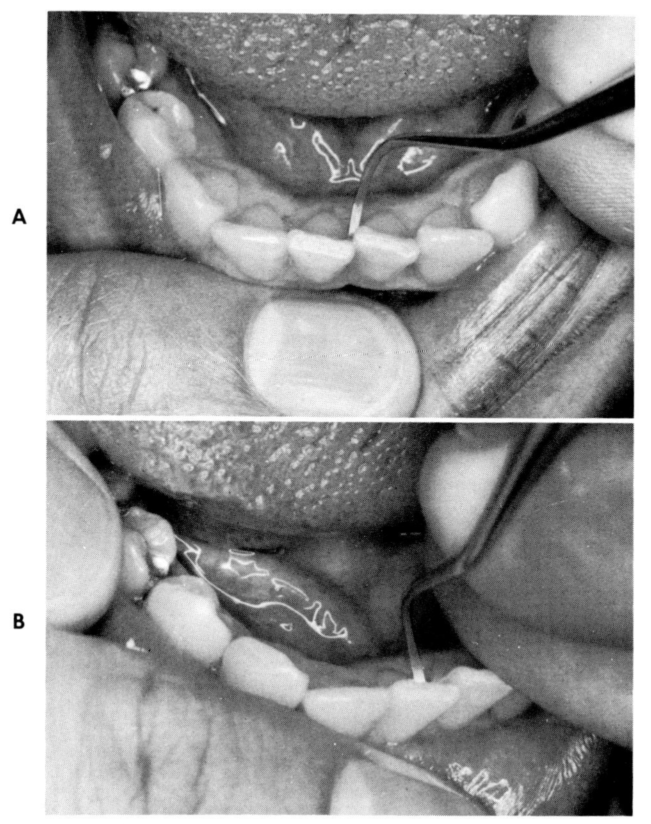


**Fig. 24-8.** Proper angulation for curettes when used on lingual and interproximal surfaces, **A**, and on mesial and distal surfaces, **B**. (Courtesy C. Amen, Denver.)

the pull curette as a push instrument, by a mere turn of the wrist to obtain a changed rake angle. If the angle of application is too acute, the tooth surface may be nicked. If, on the other hand, it is too obtuse, the deposits may be burnished rather than removed.

The curette is the most commonly used instrument for root planing and curettage. Its design permits easy entrance into pockets for the removal of deposits, and it is easily sharpened.[3-9]

Some of the more commonly used curettes are the Gracey and McCall types, which are applied with the curvature of the curette corresponding to the convex surface of the tooth. The McCall instrument is primarily a *pull* curette; the Gracey is a *push* instrument. The edge farthest from the handle is employed most frequently. When this edge is used, the handle of the instrument is held parallel to the long axis of the tooth (Figs. 24-7 and 24-8). To use the cutting edge nearest the handle for root planing, hold the instrument at an angle to the tooth and turn it to be more perpendicular to the long axis of the tooth (Fig. 24-8, *A*). When this edge is used, there is a greater chattering effect and an increased possibility of nicking the root surface. The edge farthest from the handle can also be used for root planing, by either of two means: (1) turning the wrist so that the blade contacts the tooth at 85 degrees or (2) holding the instrument at right angles to its usual position (Fig. 24-8, *B*) to use the instrument like a sickle scaler.

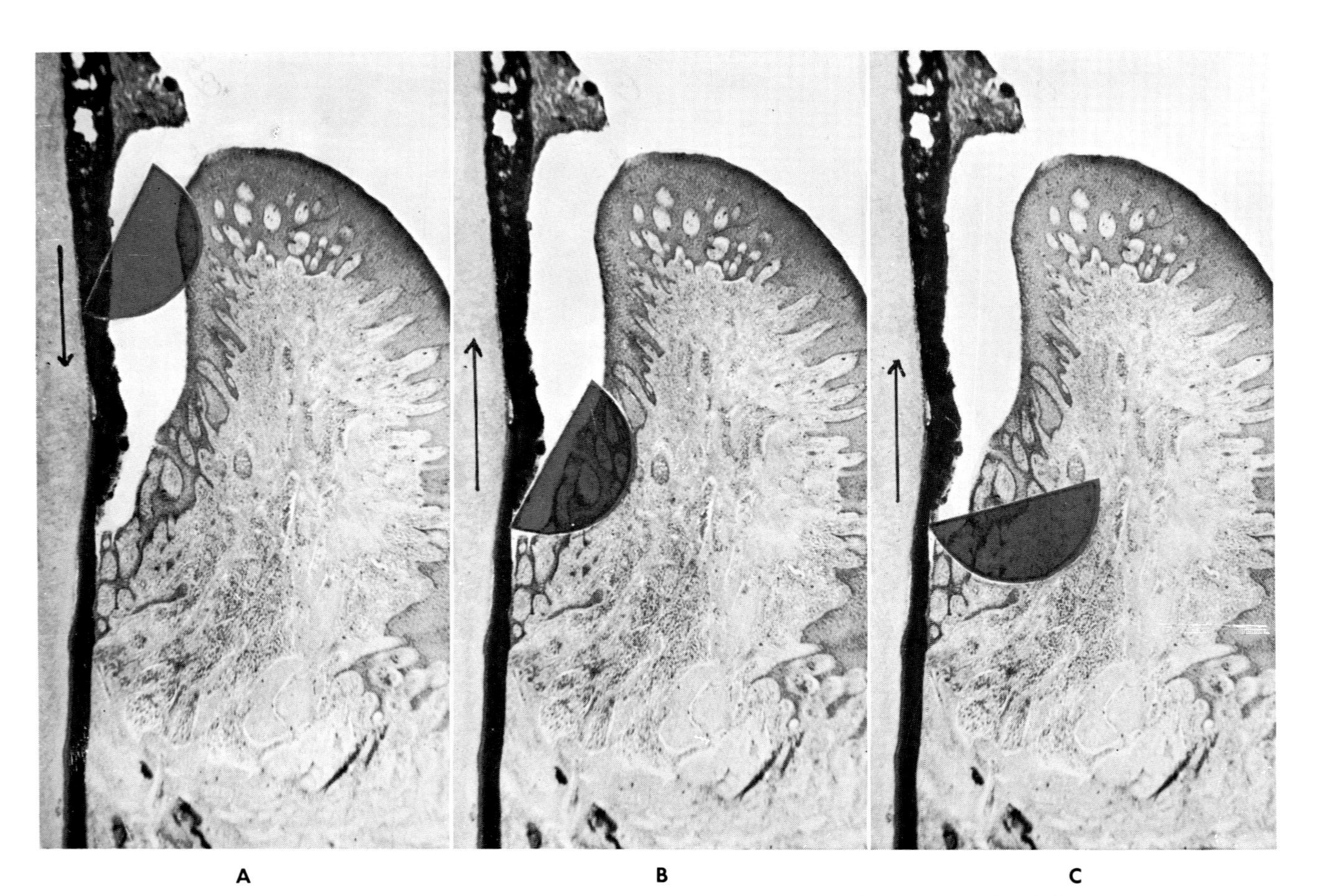


**Fig. 24-9.** Curette in a pocket. **A,** With a 25-degree clearance angle used as a push instrument (effective). **B,** With a 25-degree angle of application used with a pull stroke (ineffective). **C,** With an 85-degree angle of application used with a pull stroke (will also curette tissue).

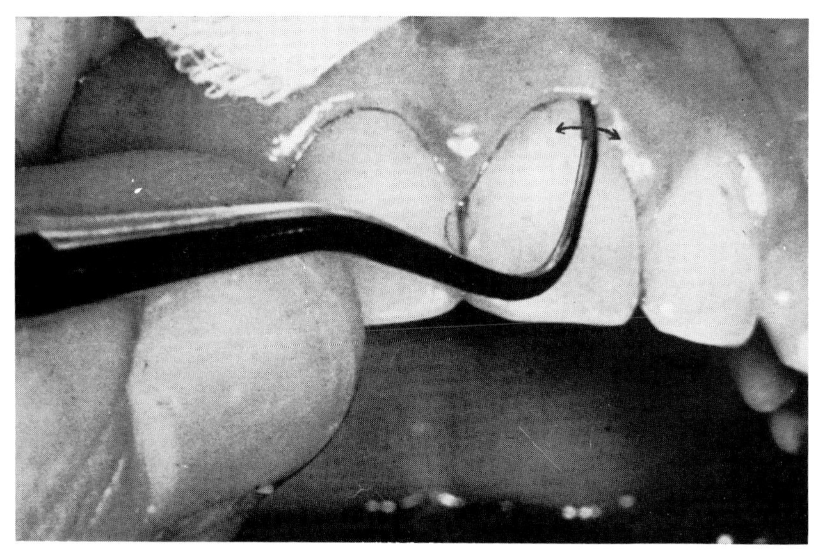

**Fig. 24-10.** The modified Younger-Goode curette is used with an alternating, lateral horizontal stroke. (Courtesy E. Robinson, San Francisco.)

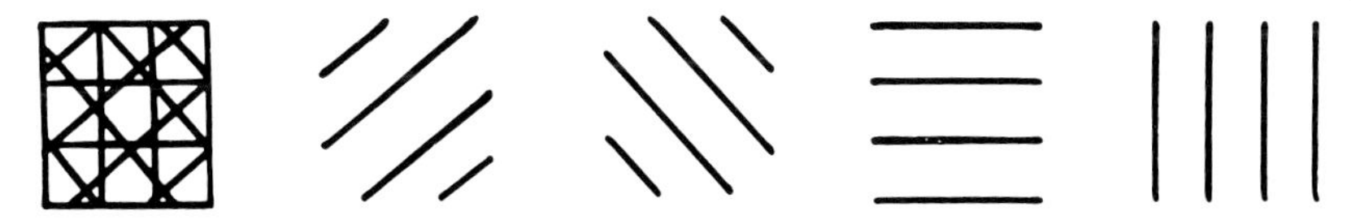

**Fig. 24-11.** Effective root planing requires that the instrument be manipulated in several directions so that calcified deposits can be removed and a smooth hard cemental surface produced. The diagrams illustrate the directions of manipulation of the instrument that are required to accomplish this objective. (Courtesy E. M. Schaffer, Minneapolis.)

Fig. 24-9 shows cross sections of the tip of a curette in a pocket. When the curette is used with a push stroke (*A*), deposits at the root surface are removed, root planing is accomplished, and the soft sulcular tissue is not affected. If the instrument were used at this angle with a pull stroke (*B*), instrumentation would be ineffective for the removal of hard deposits. At this angle the instrument would not engage the calculus effectively. If the removal of large, hard deposits is attempted with a pull curette (*C*), an angle of application of 85 degrees (negative rake) should be used.[8]

The modified Younger-Goode curette (Fig. 24-10) is used as a pull curette, but it can also be used differently in planing root surfaces. It may be introduced into a pocket with the handle perpendicular to the long axis of the tooth and the blade parallel. The stroke of the instrument is then at a right angle to the tooth in an alternating, lateral horizontal motion.

Curettes are usually preferred for final root planing because they tend to leave smoother root surfaces.[9]

In final root planing, strokes of different directions should be used (up and down, crosswise, back and forth) so that the entire root surface is covered (Fig. 24-11).

## DESIGN OF INSTRUMENTS

In a consideration of the biologic requirements of successful root planing, no substitution should be made for an instrument of choice. A hoe should not be used for fine planing at the bottom of the pocket, nor should a curette be used for the removal of heavy calculus when a hoe can be employed to greater advantage with more efficiency and speed. An instrument whose size and design are equal to the task should be selected. Heavy instruments should be used for heavy deposits, progressively more delicate instruments for finer deposits and root planing.

To obtain good results in an operation that involves root planing, the operator must divest the root surface completely of all calcareous deposits and make the surface perfectly smooth.[4,9] Since the operation is painstaking and laborious and requires skill,[5] the operator should consider thoughtfully the design of the instruments to be used for the job[6]:

1. The instruments should be well balanced.
2. The working edges of the instruments should function efficiently.[7]
3. The working edges should cause as little damage to the gingival tissues and tooth structure as possible.
4. The instruments should be made of steel alloy to retain a cutting edge capable of repeated sharpening and autoclaving.
5. The dimensions should be fine to minimize damage to soft tissues.[6,6a]

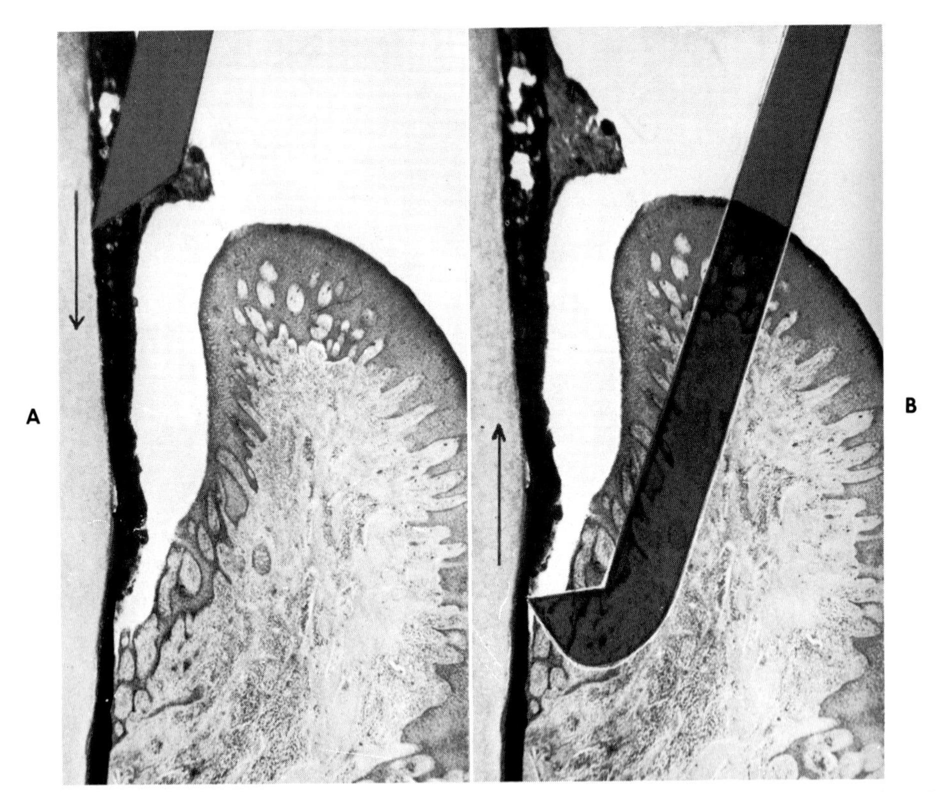


**Fig. 24-12.** Four conventional instrument types in the periodontal pocket to show the size of these instruments relative to their site of operation rather than their use. Superimposed instruments are in a magnification equivalent to that of the photomicrograph. **A,** Chisel. **B,** Hoe. **C,** Sickle. **D,** File.

Enlargements of instruments superimposed on photomicrographs of the same magnification make possible correct visualization of the relation of the instrument to both soft and hard tissues. Four of the five conventional types of instruments are shown in a pocket in this manner (Fig. 24-12).

***Chisel in pocket***

Fig. 24-12, *A*, shows the relative dimensions of a chisel and a pocket. The instrument is usually applied horizontally from labial to lingual (Fig. 24-4), mainly on anterior teeth.

***Hoe in pocket***

Fig. 24-12, *B*, shows a cross section of a hoe in a pocket. This instrument would obviously displace the tissue greatly and, if thrust to the very bottom of the pocket, would injure the attachment. Therefore it is used for the larger, superficial pieces of calculus only.

***Sickle in pocket***

Fig. 24-12, *C*, shows a cross section of the tip of a sickle in a pocket. From the illustrations, the sickle would appear to be most suitable for reaching the bottom of the pocket. However, there is a problem in placing a sickle in a pocket without injuring the buccal or lingual gingiva. Nevertheless, this instrument is efficient for removing hard and bulky pieces of calculus found in interproximal areas.

The four-edged sickle may be used in either a push or a pull stroke, provided the rules of angulation are observed. Extreme care should be exercised in the push stroke so that neither the instrument nor a mobilized piece of calculus is forced into the soft tissues. Very short strokes should be used, and the instrument should be held in a firm and balanced grip with good finger rest to prevent slipping.

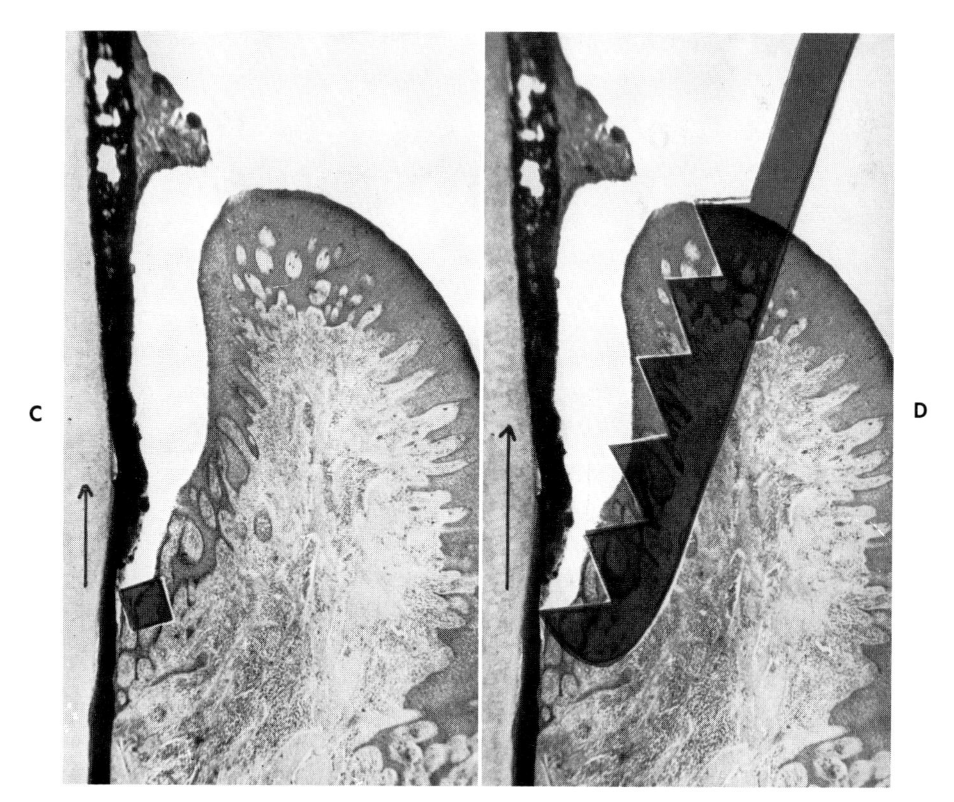


**Fig. 24-12, cont'd.** For legend see opposite page.

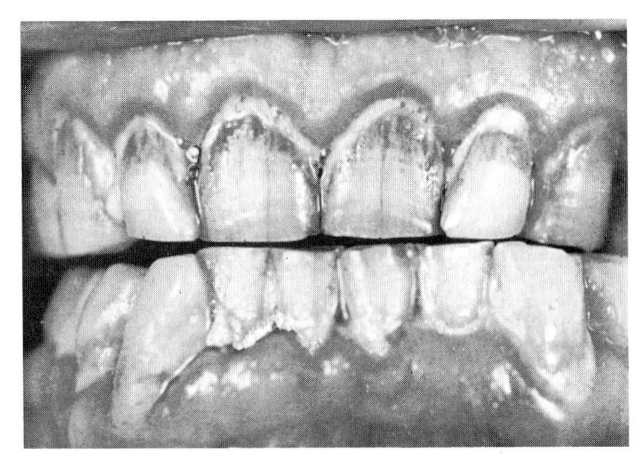

**Fig. 24-13.** Extensive amount of plaque and materia alba on teeth.

*File in pocket*

The file (Fig. 24-12, *D*) is a finer instrument than the hoe and can reach the bottom of the pocket with little tissue displacement.[12] The angle of each blade of the file resembles that of the cutting blade of the hoe. The file should not be used with its cutting edge angled to the tooth more than 90 degrees; 85 degrees is considered ideal.

## PRINCIPLES OF ROOT PLANING

### Cleansing field of operation

The field of operation should be cleansed as thoroughly as possible. If, as shown in Fig. 24-13, the exposed surfaces are covered with large masses of plaque and materia alba, start by using fine pumice, Silex, or zirconium silicate[10,11] in a motor-driven rubber cup to remove these soft deposits. This will make the field cleaner for operation and give a clearer view.

### Anesthetic

It is unnecessary to use an anesthetic unless gingival or tooth sensitivity is present. If the root surfaces are not too sensitive, use a topical anesthetic, applying it on cotton pellets and carrying it into the pockets with instruments. If considerable root sensitivity is present, use block or infiltration anesthesia. Analgesia has also been successfully employed. Patients with a history of rheumatic fever, valvular disease, or uveitis should be appropriately protected with antibiotics before treatment because instrumentation may cause a transient bacteremia.

### Finger rest

The correct finger rest is the first requirement for careful instrumentation. It is important in preventing injury to the patient's teeth and periodontal tissues and also for the patient's comfort. The operator who maintains an insecure grip or applies excessive pressure during instrumentation may be stigmatized as having a "heavy hand." A sharp instrument is the second requirement for correct instrumentation because less force is necessary when using such a tool. Various finger rests are shown in Figs. 24-14 and 24-15. The former shows the rest with the fourth finger on the teeth. Many operators feel that this position permits greater dexterity since the finger rest is farther from the instrument, which

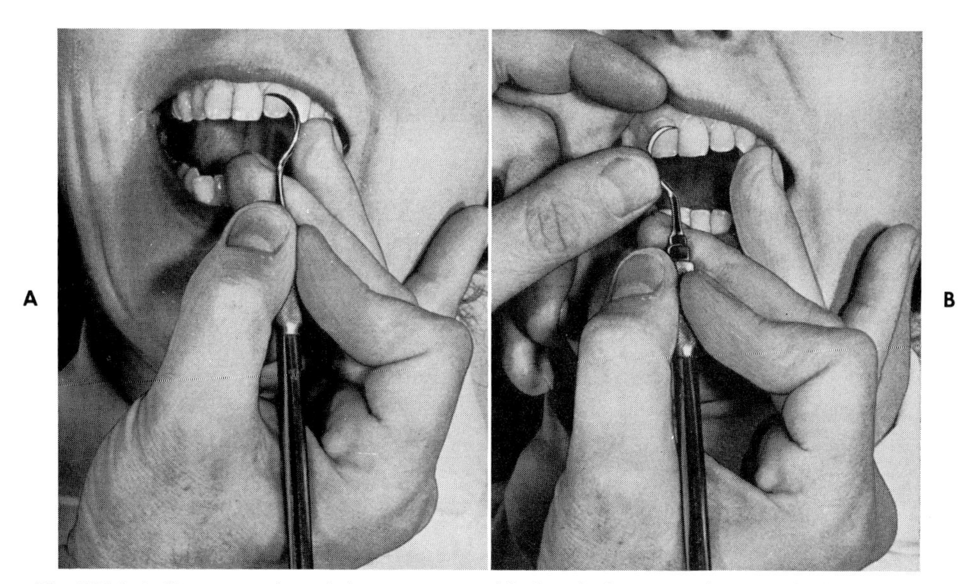


**Fig. 24-14. A,** Demonstration of the pen grasp with fourth finger rest in root planing. **B,** Fourth finger rest with assistance of the thumb of the other hand in root planing.

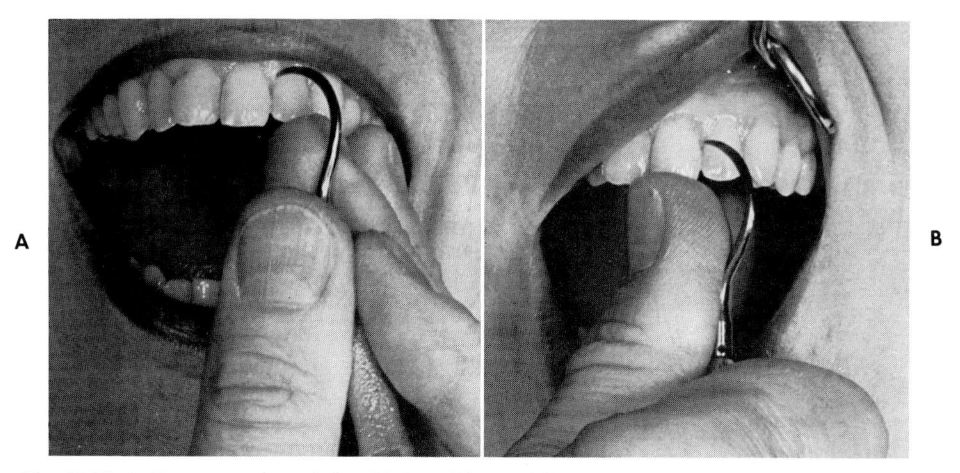


**Fig. 24-15. A,** Demonstration of the third or third and fourth finger rest in root planing. **B,** Palm and thumb grasp in root planing.

enhances digital tactile perception. In addition, the third finger is free to secure a better instrument grasp. The latter (Fig. 24-15) shows the third finger rest (*A*). Practitioners who use this rest like it because it brings the rest finger in contact with the instrument. It is believed, by virtue of this fact, to provide greater control. Fig. 24-15, *B,* shows the thumb rest of instrument to tooth. This position is advantageous when extremely adherent pieces of calculus are being removed and great pressure must be exerted. It brings a great controlled force on the instrument. However, the firmer the grasp, the less will be the digital perception; and the lighter the grasp, the greater the digital perception.

## Systematic sequence

Teeth should be planed in a systematic order and sequence. Two approaches are possible: one is to plane each tooth as thoroughly as possible before starting on the next, making a complete circuit of the mouth (this may be repeated at subsequent visits); the other is to select a specific quadrant and use one instrument on all applicable tooth surfaces (one instrument on the mesial and another on the distal surfaces and then change the instruments and repeat the pattern until all quadrants are completely and thoroughly planed). The second method of scaling requires several visits, that is, one quadrant per visit. Nevertheless, it is an efficient method of operation. Haphazard or spot scaling is time consuming and inefficient, and it fails to remove all deposits.

The extent of planing should depend on the condition of the tissues, the amount of calculus, and the time reserved for the patient. In very severe cases it may not be possible to plane more than a few teeth or a quadrant. Whatever is done should be done thoroughly before proceeding to another area. If two quadrants are scaled in one visit, it is advisable to instrument *both* quadrants on *one* side of the mouth. This will permit the patient to chew comfortably on the uninstrumented side. Except in severe cases, the patient should not experience more than mild discomfort.

The deliberate removal of extensive amounts of tooth structure cannot be justified. The attachment of calculus in spaces formerly occupied by Sharpey's fibers and in cemental irregularities, however, makes the removal of cementum necessary.[2,16] Clinical and histologic investigations have shown that over half the cementum is removed during subgingival root planing. Dentin is exposed, and any remaining cementum is very thin when the root surface feels clinically hard and smooth. Clinicians have not been able to determine by touch whether cementum or dentin is being instrumented.[7] Overinstrumentation should be avoided. It can lead to root sensitivity and unnecessary removal of root structure.

## Dressings

A preoperational displacement pack may be used to reduce edema and to facilitate visualization of deposits (Fig. 24-16). The pack is placed 1 to 3 days before instrumentation. Gingival tissues are retracted, deposits may be visualized, hemorrhage is reduced, and instrumentation is facilitated. A displacement pack is removed one tooth at a time.

Postoperative dressings may be used in selected cases after root planing. This tends to reduce bleeding and postoperative pain and makes the patient more comfortable.

## Ultrasonics

*How the instrument works*

Ultrasonic instruments are commonly used for root planing and removal of calculus. These instruments function according to the principle of magnetostriction.[13,14] When the metal stack, which is part of the ultrasonic handpiece, is placed in an electromagnetic field, its length is reduced slightly and the working tip is withdrawn by this amount. When the alternating current changes direction, the tip is thrust forward and then back to its original position. This alternating sequence drives the tip back and forth in line with the stack at a frequency of approximately 25,000 cycles per second.[14] The length of travel is approximately 0.001 inch.

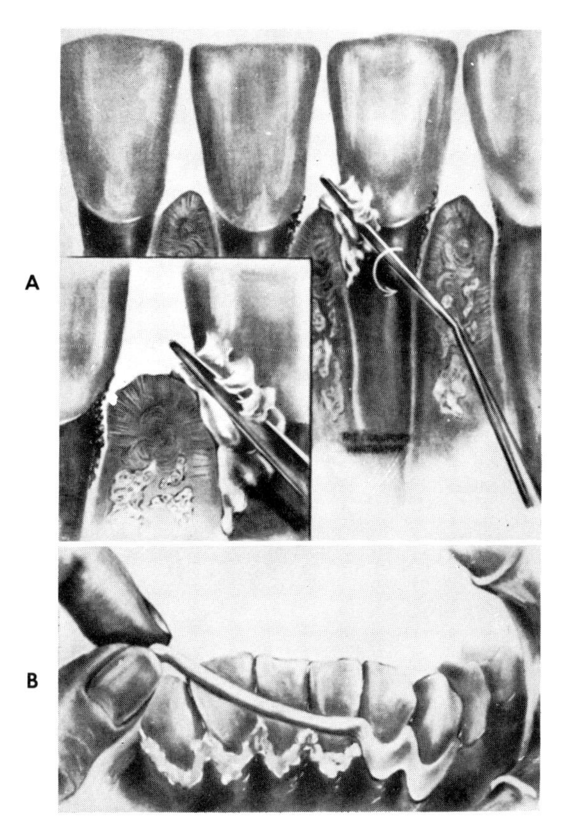


**Fig. 24-16.** Application of a sedative displacement pack. **A,** The pack is teased into the pocket with a thin plastic instrument. **B,** The thin, rolled section of the pack is then placed over the previously applied displacement pack. After 1 to 3 days, it is removed tooth by tooth, and the pocket is left open with the deposits visible. (Courtesy J. W. Gallagher, Seattle.)

***Influence on hard and soft tissues***

The effect of ultrasonic energy on the teeth and gingivae may range from little or no change to a characteristic, fine, stippled or granular[15] pattern of varying depth[17] (Fig. 24-17). The main effect on the soft tissue is a fragmenting and washing away of the sulcular lining and adjacent tissue[18,19] (gingival curettage). Coagulation has also been reported.[14] The depth and degree of these tissue effects are governed by the quantity of ultrasonic energy applied,[14] and this quantity is determined by the following factors[20]: (1) power setting (amplitude of tip motion), (2) applied pressure, (3) relative sharpness of the tip, (4) angle of application, and (5) time of exposure per unit area. The healing of wounds produced by ultrasonic instrumentation appears to be similar to that of wounds produced by hand instrumentation. Both the time required for epithelization and the reappearance of an inflammatory infiltrate in the adjacent connective tissue during healing have been studied.[21-23] These instruments are mainly employed for the removal of calculus.

***Clinical application***

Ultrasonic instruments are mainly employed for the removal of calculus. In general, the lowest power setting consistent with effectiveness should be used. After the instrument has been prepared for use, the tip should be run between the fingers to guard against excessive vibration and heat production.[17] The handpiece and tip should be applied with very light pressure—a feather

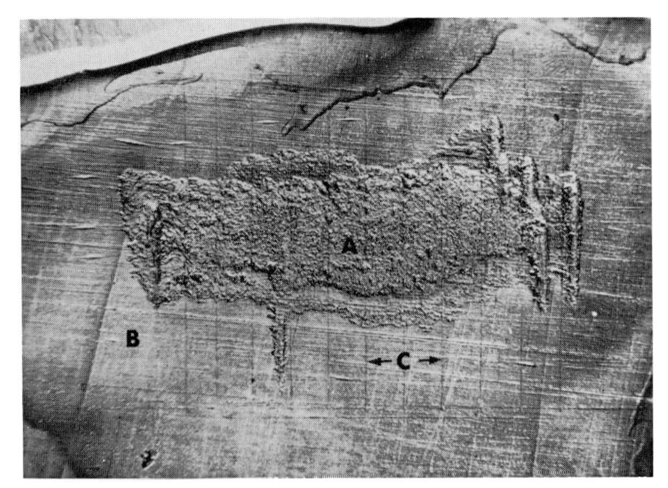


**Fig. 24-17.** Metal-shadowed replica of a specimen tooth showing, *A,* the defect produced by ultrasonic instrumentation in, *B,* the center of the prepared surface, and, *C,* lines produced by a diamond stylus during profile tracing. The force of application was very light (75 gm.), and the setting of the power knob was medium. (Courtesy S. M. Clark, Portland, Ore.)

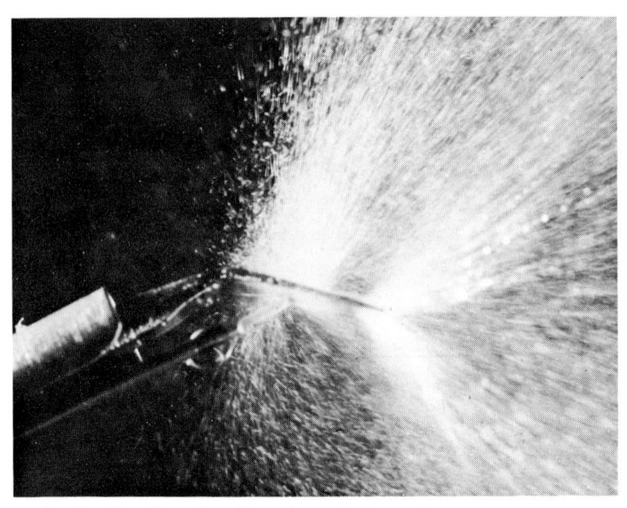

**Fig. 24-18.** Ultrasonic tip showing the direction of the reflected water spray (cavitation). The water spray is used primarily as a cooling device for the tip, which would otherwise become too warm. The water, however, is also useful for lavage and the removal of debris.

touch or brush stroke.[20] The time of application should be kept as short as practical. A reasonable guide for a given area of tooth surface is a maximum of six back-and-forth strokes. As the instrument is being used, the tip should be kept in motion at all times when the machine is on. A periodontal feeling instrument should always be used during ultrasonic instrumentation in pockets. An ample amount of water spray should be used (Fig. 24-18), particularly in areas where the flow at the tip may be impaired (subgingivally). It is important not to use tips that have rough surfaces or spurs, which would scratch the tooth surface.

*Indications and contraindications*

Ultrasonic curettage is particularly useful in the early phase of treatment and when tissues are hemorrhagic. The washed field also makes the instruments convenient for calculus removal during periodontal surgery. In addition, the instrumentation with lavage is helpful in the treatment of acute necrotizing ulcerative gingivitis; and it enhances resolution of the acute phase of this disease. The instrumentation is further useful in patients with heavy supragingival calculus deposits. Contraindications for the use of ultrasonics have not been clearly defined. Some patients have experienced pain; others have reported tooth sensitivity after repeated use. Caution is called for in the presence of baked porcelain inlays or jacket crowns. Root surfaces treated with an ultrasonic scaler should be finally finished with curettes.[24] For tooth surfaces coronal to the epithelial attachment, it seems reasonable that the smoothest surface possible would be most satisfactory to minimize the recurrence of deposits, to present a smooth surface against which the free gingiva could rest, and to facilitate plaque removal by the patient.

## Reexamination

Areas once scaled should be carefully reexamined on subsequent visits. Probably with even the most meticulous instrumentation some fragments of calculus remain and cause persistent inflammation. The reddish or bluish color of the gingiva in such instances may contrast with the pink color of areas where the root has been completely divested of calcified deposits, making such areas obvious. With the resolution of inflammation, remaining fragments of subgingival deposits may become supragingival.

## Polishing

After root planing has been completed, the teeth should be polished thoroughly with fine polishing agents.[10,11] Polishing can be done adequately with the motor-driven rubber cup (Fig. 24-19, *A*) on accessible areas of the tooth. The use of the rubber cup rather than the brush for the buccal and lingual areas allows surfaces below the gingival margins to be polished simultaneously. Interproximal areas should be polished with shaped balsa wood sticks or a porte polisher and wide waxed dental tape or with fine linen strips. In polishing with a porte polisher, use soft orangewood points *(B)*. These can be shaped with a knife to fit any area. The fine polishing agent should be carried to the area to be polished and the tape applied in a shoeshine fashion *(C)*. Fine cuttlefish disks may be used on tooth surfaces that need more than pumice polishing *(D)*. A special contra-angle handpiece for cleansing and polishing interproximal surfaces is also available (Eva handpiece, Dentatus, Sweden).

The most widely used polishing agent is a paste consisting of flour of pumice and glycerine with flavoring and color correctives added. Sodium fluoride or stannous fluoride may be added to this mixture for a desensitizing effect. Other polishing agents such as zirconium oxide or kaolinite pastes have been suggested.

## Disclosing solution

It is advisable to use a disclosing solution (0.2% basic fuchsin, erythrosin, Skinner's or Churchill's iodine) after the polishing has been completed to be sure that all deposits are removed. The solution is applied and the mouth rinsed with water. The red or brown spots that remain are material that has not been removed. Drying the tooth may also help to visualize deposits. These areas should be planed and polished until the deposit is removed.

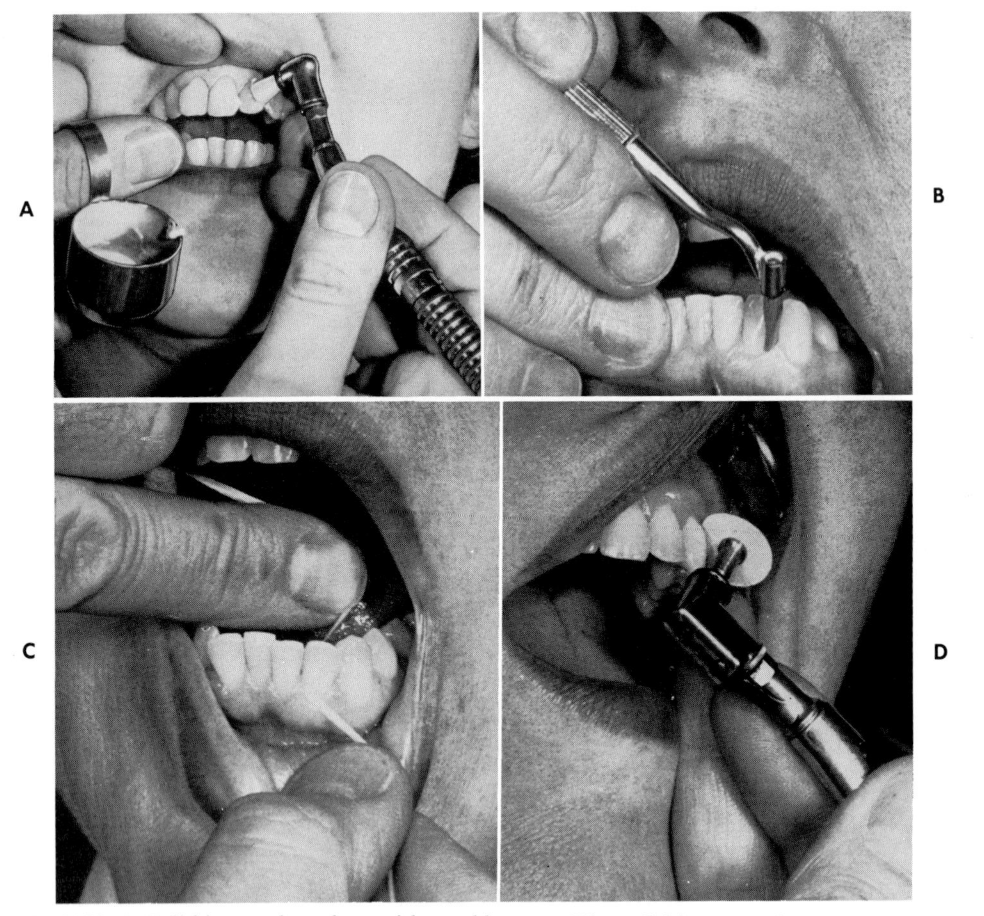


**Fig. 24-19. A,** Polishing tooth surfaces with a rubber cup. The polishing agent is retained in the thumb cup. **B,** Use of porte polisher as an aid in root polishing. **C,** Use of waxed dental tape for interproximal polishing of tooth surfaces. **D,** Use of cuttlefish polishing disks for polishing the teeth.

The treatment of simple gingivitis entails more than excellent root planing. All extrinsic etiologic factors discussed earlier must be eliminated, and the patient trained to keep his teeth clean by correct home care (home physiotherapy). The latter feature cannot be overemphasized. It is best to practice toothbrushing with the patient at every session until he is competent. Methods of home dental care (plaque control) will be discussed in Chapter 25.

Cases of chronic and acute gingivitis caused primarily by extrinsic factors (the overwhelming majority) can be treated successfully by local measures and carry a favorable prognosis.

## Sharpening instruments

All instruments used in root planing, currettage, and surgical procedures must be absolutely sharp.[6,25] A sharp instrument will do less injury to the hard and soft tissues than a dull one. A sharp instrument does not have to be grasped or pressed as firmly. Consequently, since less force is used, there is less danger of slipping off the tooth or grossly nicking the tooth surface.

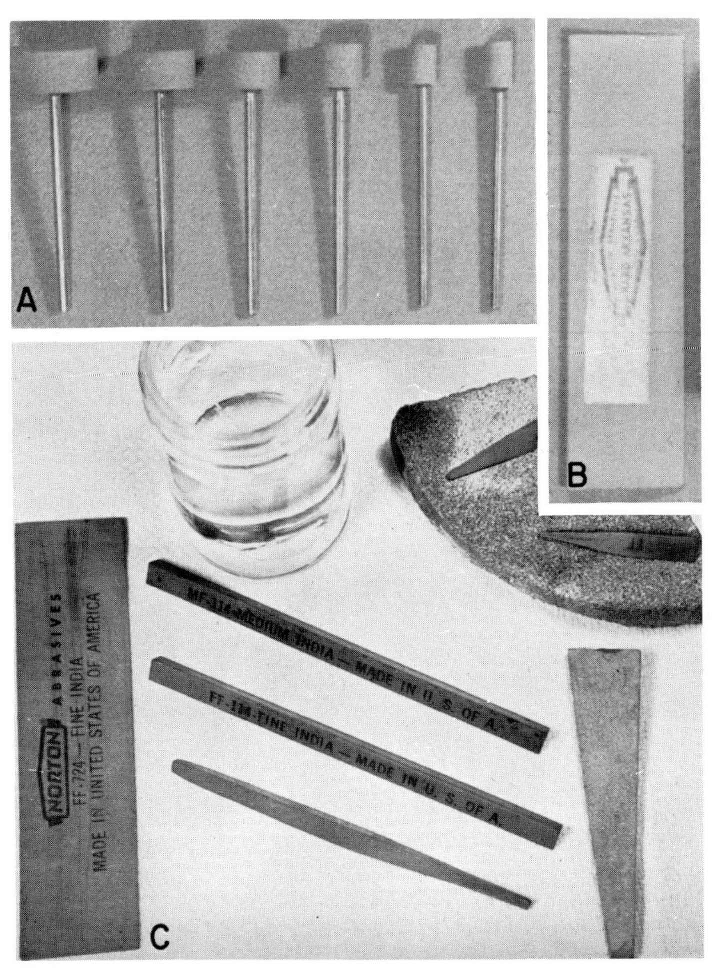


**Fig. 24-20.** Armamentarium for sharpening periodontal instruments. **A,** Mounted Arkansas stones, used mainly to sharpen sickles. **B,** Arkansas slip stone for sharpening hoes and files. **C,** Fine India stone for sharpening hoes and curettes. (Courtesy C. L. Foss, San Diego, and T. R. Orban, Denver.)

Sharpening instruments must be learned, just as any other mechanical technique must be mastered. It is advisable to have a special corner in the laboratory fixed for sharpening. A mounted magnifying glass or dissecting microscope should be used in performing some sharpening operations, especially in sharpening files and hoes. To sharpen these instruments, use either fine Arkansas slip stones (Fig. 24-20, *B*) or India stones (Fig. 24-20, *C*).[25] The edges of these stones must be ground according to the inclinations of the blades of the instruments.

To sharpen sickle-shaped instruments, use mounted Arkansas or ruby stones (Fig. 24-20, *A*) as shown in Fig. 24-21. Care should be exercised not to overheat the instrument, for this ruins the temper of the steel.

Sharpen curettes on a conically shaped India or Arkansas stone (Fig. 24-22), pushing and pulling the instrument along the stone, following the curvature of the instrument. A flat stone may be used instead of a curved one. Some Arkansas and diamond hones also are now made for sharpening instruments.

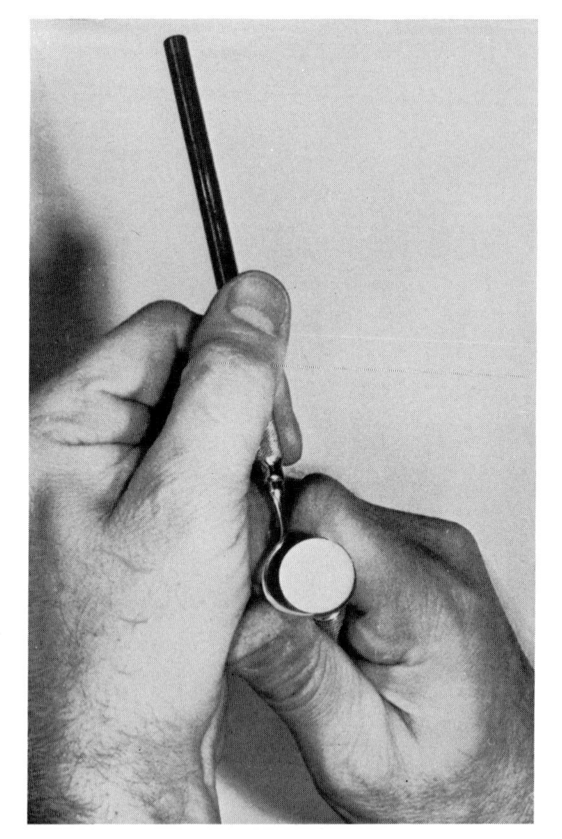

**Fig. 24-21.** Use of a mounted stone in sharpening a sickle.

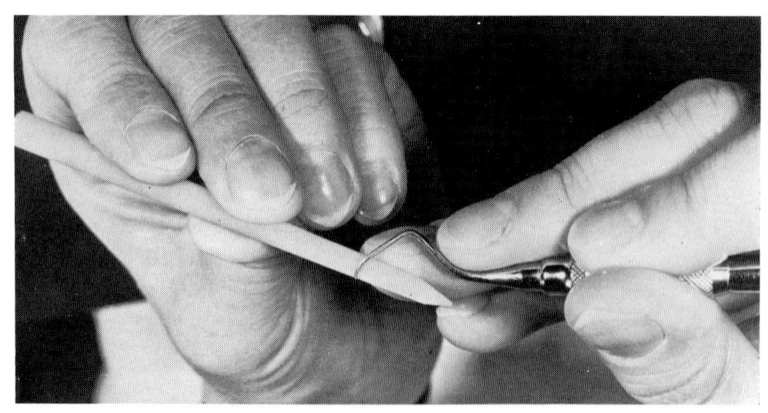

**Fig. 24-22.** Sharpening a curette on a conical Arkansas stone.

## SUMMARY

The removal of calculus and soft deposits will aid in the reduction of inflammation and pocket depth and is the first step in the care of periodontal disease. Supragingival plaque may be removed by oral hygiene measures. Supragingival calculus is removable only by instrumentation. Rough subgingival calculus may be a mechanical irritant, providing entry for toxins. Subgingival calculus itself serves as a reservoir for toxins.[21b] The exact removal of calculus is therefore necessary.

Elimination of the periodontal pocket can be achieved in several ways, depending on the extent of the pocket and the relation of the pocket to the rest of the periodontium. The operator with a knowledge of the basic principles of periodontics will treat a pocket with regard to its unique situation. Not every pocket can be eliminated by root planing, any more than every pocket can be eradicated by surgery. In many cases it is necessary to use several different techniques for various situations in the mouth, including special surgical procedures, which will be discussed later.

**CHAPTER 24**

**References**

1. Russell, A. L.: Epidemiologic research 1960-1963, J. Amer. Dent. Ass. **68**:820, 1964.
2. Zander, H. A.: The attachment of calculus to root surfaces, J. Periodont. **24**:16, 1953.
3. Schaffer, E. M.: Histological results of root curettage of human teeth, J. Periodont. **27**:296, 1956.
4. Björn, H., and Lindhe, J.: The influence of periodontal instruments on the tooth surface. Odont. Rev. **13**:355, 1962.
5. Frumker, S. C., and Gardner, W. M.: The relation of the topography of the root surface to the removal of calculus, J. Periodont. **27**:292, 1956.
6. Orban, B., and Manella, V. B.: A macroscopic and microscopic study of instruments designed for root planing, J. Periodont. **27**:120, 1956.

6a. Waerhaug, J., Arno, A., and Lovdal, A.: The dimensions of instruments for removal of subgingival calculus, J. Periodont. **25**:261, 1954.

7. Everett, F. G., Foss, C. L., and Orban, B.: Study of instruments for scaling (root planing), Parodontologie **16**:61, 1962.
8. Hirschfeld, I.: Subgingival curettage in periodontal treatment, J. Amer. Dent. Ass. **44**:301, 1952.
9. Green, E., and Ramfjord, S. P.: Tooth roughness after subgingival root planing, J. Periodont. **37**:396, 1966.
10. Muhler, J. C., Dudding, N. J., and Stookey, G. K.: Clinical effectiveness of a particular particle size distribution of zirconium silicate for use as a cleaning and polishing agent for oral hard tissues, J. Periodont. **35**:481, 1964.
11. Stoll, F. A., and Werner, A. R.: New polishing agent for dental prophylaxis, J. Amer. Dent. Hygienists Ass. **37**:79, 1963.
12. Burke, S. W., and Green, E.: Effectiveness of periodontal files, J. Periodont. **41**:39, 1970.
13. Sweeney, W. T.: Characteristics of ultrasonic vibrations, J. Amer. Dent. Ass. **55**:819, 1957.
14. Ewen, S., and Glickstein, C.: Ultrasonic therapy in periodontics, Springfield, Ill., 1968, Charles C Thomas, Publisher.
15. Belting, C. M., and Spjut, P. J.: Effects of high-speed periodontal instruments on the root surface during subgingival calculus removal, J. Amer. Dent. Ass. **69**:578, 1964.
16. Kopczyk, R. A., and Conroy, C. W.: Attachment of calculus to root planed surfaces, Periodontics **6**:78, 1968.
17. Clark, S. M., Grupe, H. E., and Mahler, D. B.: Effect of ultrasonic instrumentation on root surfaces, J. Periodont. **39**:135, 1968.
18. Goldman, H.: Curettage by ultrasonic instrument, Oral Surg. **13**:43, 1960.
19. Frisch, J., Bhaskar, S. N., and Shell, D.: Effect of ultrasonic instrumentation on human gingival connective tissue, Periodontics **5**:123, 1967.
20. Clark, S. M.: The ultrasonic dental unit: a guide for the clinical application of ultrasonics in dentistry and in dental hygiene, J. Periodont. **40**:621, 1969.

21. Sanderson, A. D.: Gingival curettage by hand and ultrasonic instruments: a histologic comparison, J. Periodont. 37:279, 1966.
21a. Jones, S. J., Lozdan, J., and Boyde, A.: Tooth surfaces treated in situ with periodontal instruments, Brit. Dent. J. 132:57, 1972.
21b. Baumhammers, A., and Rohrbaugh, E. A.: Permeability of human and rat dental calculus, J. Periodont. 41:279, 1970.
22. Schaffer, E. M., Stende, G., and King, D.: Healing of periodontal pocket tissues following ultrasonic scaling and hand planing, J. Periodont. 35:140, 1964.
23. Goldman, H. M.: Histologic assay of healing following ultrasonic curettage versus hand-instrument curettage, Oral Surg. 14:925, 1961.
24. Stende, G., and Schaffer, E. M.: A comparison of ultrasonic and hand scaling, J. Periodont. 32:312, 1961.
25. Foss, C. L., and Orban, T. R.: Sharpening periodontal instruments, J. Periodont. 27:135, 1956.

**Additional selected reading**

Stewart, J. L., Drisko, R. R., and Herlach, A. D.: Comparison of ultrasonic and hand instruments for the removal of calculus, J. Amer. Dent. Ass. 75:153, 1967.

Stone, S., Ramfjord, S. P., and Waldron, J.: Scaling and gingival curettage; a radioautographic study, J. Periodont. 37:415, 1966.

CHAPTER TWENTY-FIVE

# Oral hygiene (plaque control) and gingival massage, root sensitivity, and halitosis



## Oral hygiene (plaque control) and gingival massage

*Definition*

Oral hygiene and gingival massage are procedures performed by the patient to remove plaque, soft deposits, and debris from the teeth, to make the gingiva firm, and to increase cornification of the epithelium.

Adequate oral hygiene is necessary to help cure inflammatory periodontal disease and to maintain the cure.[1] This is mainly done by the regular removal of plaque, which is regarded as a primary cause of gingival inflammation. Oral hygiene therefore can be both therapeutic and prophylactic. In addition, effective care is important in managing problems of gingival recession (atrophy) and gingival enlargement (hyperplasia).

### OBJECTIVES

The immediate objectives of oral hygiene at home are as follows:

1. To reduce the number of microorganisms on the teeth[2]

   All accessible dental plaque and debris should be removed from the gingival margin, proximal tooth surfaces, and (where possible) gingival sulcus. In doing this, the dentist can eliminate the causative factors that produce irritation and inflammation.[3] One of the causes of halitosis is also removed by these measures.

2. To promote circulation
3. To promote cornification of the epithelium and to render the gingival tissues more resistant to mechanical irritation[4]

The role of the patient as an active participant in the treatment of disease and in the maintenance of oral health must be emphasized. The success or failure of treatment may hinge on the patient's ability to understand and cooperate in carrying out oral hygiene procedures.

Definitive, purposeful techniques of patient education must be used to emphasize the importance of oral hygiene.

## REQUIREMENTS

Requirements for care will vary from patient to patient and even in different areas of the same mouth.

### Clinical examination

*Anatomic considerations and patient interview*

Clinical examination will enable the dentist to evaluate the needs of each patient. This evaluation should include an appraisal of the anatomy and alignment of the teeth, the relationship of the teeth to the gingiva, and the type and amount of deposits present. The patient should be questioned as to his current oral hygiene practices. During the discussion the dentist should note the responses of the patient to both oral hygiene questions and suggestions regarding the home dental care program. (See Chapter 17.) Some patients may be free of gingival disease or resistant to it. These people will pose few problems in oral hygiene.

*Diet*

Apparently diet plays little part in cleansing the teeth of plaque.[5-8] Recent reports tell of little effect of the so-called detergent foods in eliminating plaque from tooth surfaces. However, in some patients portions of teeth seem to be free of plaque even in the absence of brushing. It may be that the function of lips, cheeks, and tongue on tooth surfaces eliminates some plaque.[8] The passage of food over the teeth may have some cleansing effect, for astronauts on tube-fed diets formed more plaque than did their comrades who masticated their food, despite prescribed oral hygiene measures.[5]

### Patient evaluation and education

Evaluate the patient. Note the quality of his oral hygiene and try to determine his attitude toward home dental care. Discuss his daily schedule. Does he work in an office or does he travel? Construction workers may have different facilities available for oral hygiene from those that lawyers or traveling salesmen have, and they may have differing social attitudes toward oral hygiene. This does not mean that such attitudes cannot be altered; what it does mean is that the dentist may perceive a basis from which to proceed in his educational efforts.

*Disclosing solutions and plaque index*

Show the patient the plaque in his mouth. It may not be readily visible. Use an explorer or other instrument to collect a small amount of this material. When a phase microscope is available, take a smear from the interdental tooth surfaces, place it on a slide, add a drop of water and a cover slip, and demonstrate to the patient the motile bacteria.[10] This can be dramatic. Now ask the patient to rinse with a disclosing solution (0.2% basic fuchsin, Chayes Beta-Rose, Butler Two-

Tone) or to chew a disclosing tablet (X-Pose, Red-Cote).[9] Using a hand mirror and good light, show the patient the stained areas on his teeth.[11] Tell him that this stain represents plaque and that he must remove all plaque from all tooth surfaces at least once every 12 hours. Take a plaque index (Fig. 12-1). At subsequent visits the plaque index may be repeated to show the patient the improvement (hopefully) or lack thereof.

In brushed mouths most plaque will be found primarily on the interdental tooth surfaces and secondarily at the gingival margins. Show the patient how to remove plaque. Because interdental areas are rarely cleansed as well as other areas and tend to have the deepest pockets, start here.

*Flossing*

Instruction in flossing techniques are as follows:

1. Give the patient a hand mirror and have him observe.[11]
2. Start with unwaxed floss.
3. Demonstrate the use of the floss in the patient's mouth. Floss all proximal tooth surfaces, starting at the most posterior tooth in the maxillary right quadrant, completing all maxillary teeth, and progressing from the mandibular left quadrant to end on the mandibular right.
4. When using the unwaxed dental floss, discuss the composition of plaque, the role plaque plays in producing inflammation, the relative invisibility of plaque, and therefore the need for the daily use of disclosing tablets or solution to make plaque readily visible. Emphasize that daily plaque removal can eliminate most inflammation and that after cure this care can prevent or minimize future periodontal disease.
5. Emphasize that the floss can remove plaque in areas where the toothbrush cannot or where the toothbrush is inefficient.[12-14] Tell the patient that plaque is gluelike and that firm pressure is necessary to remove it.
6. Avoid value judgments concerning the patient's oral hygiene. Establish a visual objective that he can reach, such as removal of all the red stain on the visible tooth surfaces. Where tooth stains such as those from tobacco are found or where calculus is present, explain that you will remove these.

A procedure for the use of floss is as follows:

1. Draw an 18- to 24-inch length of unwaxed dental floss from the container, using the small sharp device on the container for cutting the desired length.
2. Twist the floss three times around the middle finger of the right hand and three times around the middle finger of the left hand, leaving a space of 1 to 4 inches between the hands. The thumbs and forefingers should be left free. Use them to guide the floss (Fig. 25-1, *A*).
3. Work the floss gently through the contact points to avoid damaging the gingiva[10] (Fig. 25-1, *B* and *C*).
4. Make the floss firm by stretching it. Press the floss against the tooth and carry it carefully under the free gingival margin of the papilla (Fig. 25-1, *D*).
5. Once the floss is in the sulcus, wrap it firmly against the mesial tooth surface by applying pressure with both hands (toward the distal). Carry the floss apically until resistance is met (Fig. 25-1, *E*). Then, engaging any plaque, move it incisally or occlusally toward the contact point. You do not have to pass through the contact point at this time. Repeat the procedure for the adjacent (distal) proximal tooth surface.

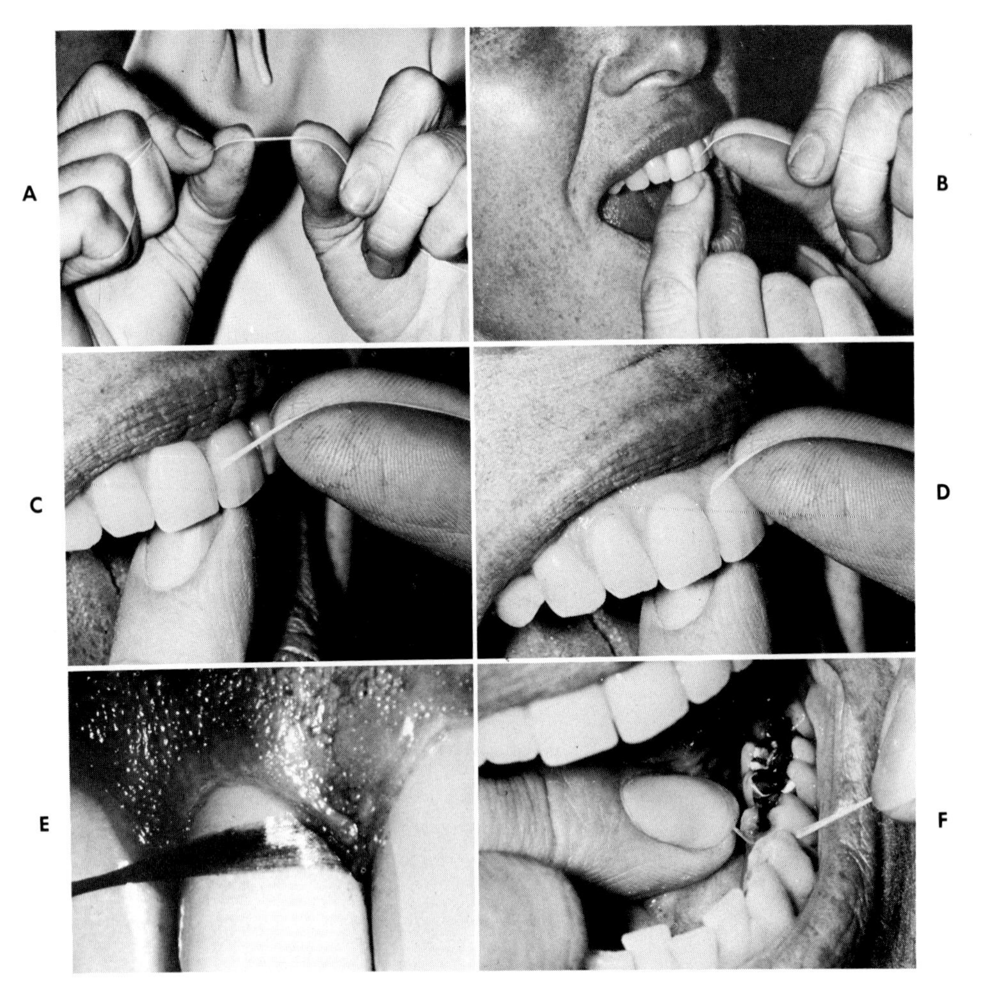


**Fig. 25-1. A,** Wrap most of the floss on the middle finger of the right hand and the rest around the middle finger of the left hand. As you are flossing, take up the floss on the other finger like a scroll to provide fresh floss. Use index fingers and thumbs as guides for flossing the upper teeth, and index fingers for the lower teeth. **B,** Hold the floss tightly and work it gently between the teeth. Be very careful not to snap the floss between teeth and under gums, for this can harm the delicate tissue. **C,** Curve the floss around the tooth and carefully work it apically. **D,** Work the floss into the sulcus. **E,** Holding the floss tightly against the tooth, scrape toward the point where the tooth touches its neighbor. Repeat this step on the adjacent tooth. **F,** Set a pattern for flossing and follow the same pattern every time so that all the teeth are flossed.

Thumbs and forefingers are appropriate for all teeth (Fig. 25-1, *F*). For additional cleansing efficiency, apply a dentifrice or stain remover to the tooth before using the floss.

Although unwaxed floss is efficient for plaque removal, some people lack the dexterity to use it. For these patients a floss carrier should be recommended (Fig. 25-2).

## TRAINING ROUTINE

In order to establish an educational procedure that will train the patient, advise him to embark on a program of regular, closely spaced visits. Programs

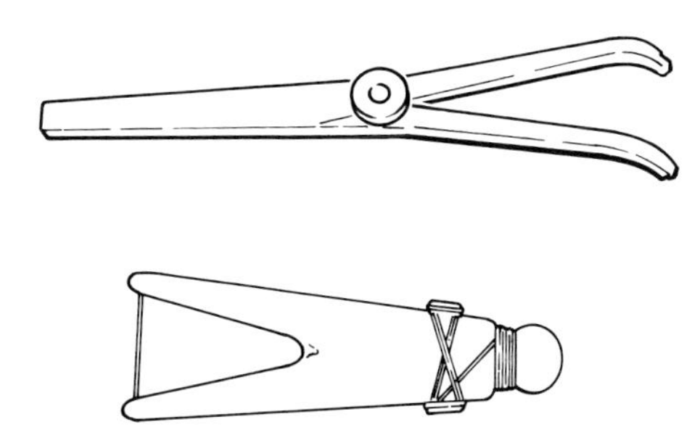

**Fig. 25-2.** Two types of floss carriers. These are particularly useful for patients with poor digital dexterity.

of daily visits (or visits every other day) encourage learning retention and permit patient feedback. They also permit the dentist to reinforce learning and to help in the establishment of new habit patterns by the patient.[15,16]

Such repeated instruction is valuable, for the patient is actively involved in the treatment procedure. He is shown what to do and then allowed to do it himself. The daily visits or visits every other day should be followed by several weekly visits to further establish habit patterns.[17]

At one visit, have the patient rinse with a disclosing solution or use a disclosing tablet and take another plaque index. Point out areas of successful accomplishment and areas of deficiency.

Then have the patient demonstrate flossing. If he is found to injure himself with floss, the use of flat dental tape may be indicated in place of the floss.[18] Praise his accomplishments and correct his errors in its use.

When larger interproximal spaces are present or near posterior pontics, 4-ply cotton yarn may be helpful. When necessary, the yarn can be reduced in width by unraveling. Attach the yarn to the floss by knotting and introduce it into the interproximal areas by drawing the floss through the contact followed by the yarn through the embrasure (Fig. 25-19). The yarn can remove plaque in such areas. Its size and surface are effective where floss is sometimes inefficient because of tooth anatomy (e.g., fluting of the root) or embrasure form.

The patient would be overwhelmed if instruction in the use of all the oral hygiene aids that he might need were given to him at once. Therefore one technique should be presented at a time, in this case flossing.

When the patient shows reasonable progress in mastering the use of floss, begin the education in the use of toothbrush and other aids.

## Brushing

*Perio-Aid*

A device that is useful in reducing dental plaque at gingival margins and interproximally is called the Perio-Aid (Fig. 25-3). This instrument consists of a plastic handle that will receive round polished toothpicks and permit the patient to cleanse the teeth at gingival margins where accessible and in areas of difficult access. The tip can be dipped into the sulcus.

*Interproximal brushes*

Interproximal brushes (Fig. 25-4) are useful in cleansing interdental areas. Some patients prefer these brushes to floss since less dexterity is required.

*Home dental care aids*

Home dental care aids fall into one of two categories—those for cleansing and those for massage. They are listed under the category of their greater effectiveness. However, most of the aids are effective, primarily or secondarily, in *both*

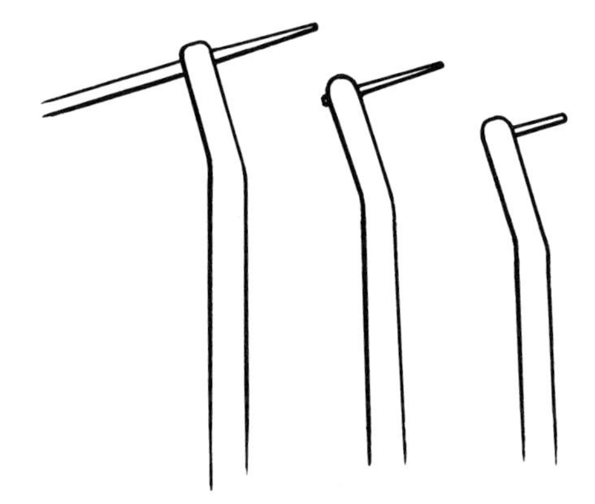

**Fig. 25-3.** Toothpick holder (Perio-Aid) useful for cleansing at the gingival margin and interdentally. A tapered, round toothpick is inserted into the hole in the carrier and is then broken off; the tip is left and is used in a tracing motion along the gingival margins.

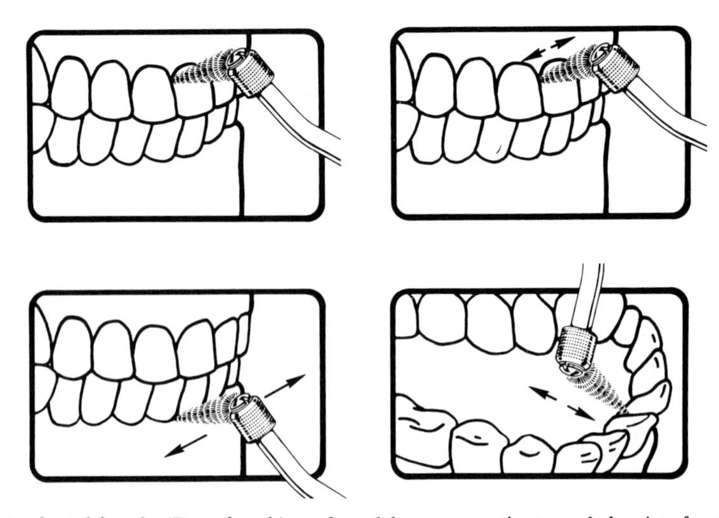

**Fig. 25-4.** Interdental brush (Proxabrush) preferred by some patients and dentists for interdental cleansing. The brushes are replaceable.

categories. Brushing, for example, is almost as important for massage as it is for cleansing. An armamentarium for oral hygiene instruction is shown in (Fig. 25-5).

*Primarily important as cleansing aids:*

1. Toothbrush (manual or electric)
2. Dental floss (waxed or unwaxed)
3. Disclosing solutions or tablets
4. Cotton 4-ply yarn
5. Toothpicks
6. Single-tufted brush (manual or electric)
7. Gauze strips
8. Water irrigation device

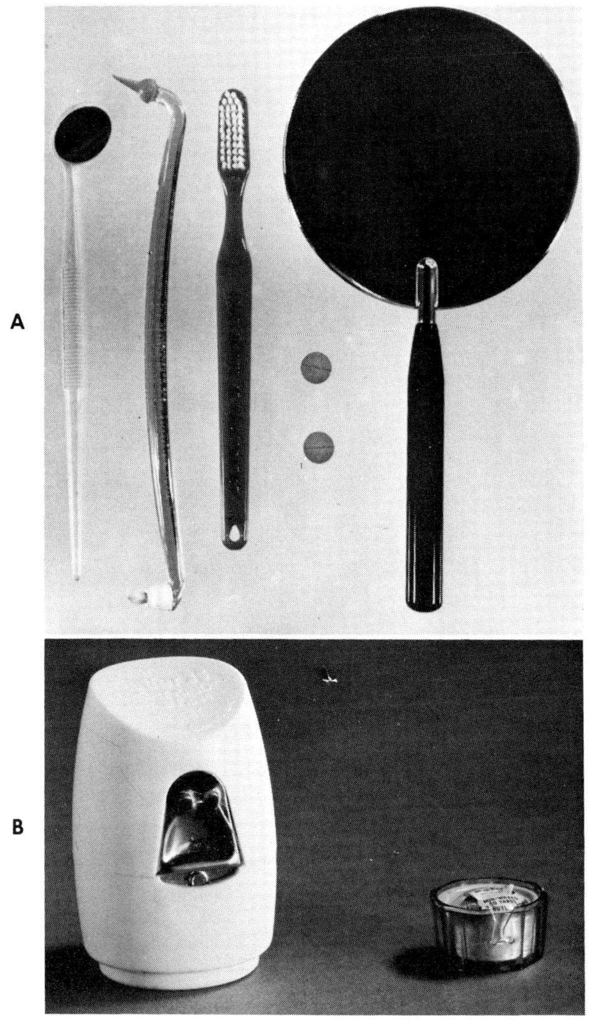


**Fig. 25-5. A,** Basic armamentarium for oral hygiene. Hand mirror, disclosing tablets, toothbrush, interdental stimulator, and mouth mirror. **B,** Unwaxed dental floss. (Courtesy E. Moser, San Francisco.)

9. Dentifrice
10. Mouthwash
11. Interdental brushes

*Primarily important as massaging aids:*

1. Balsa wood wedges (Stim-U-Dents) or other toothpicks
2. Interdental stimulator (plastic, rubber)
3. Rubber cup gingival stimulator
4. Digital massage

Before any instruction in brushing begins, make the patient aware of several concepts:

1. *Frequency of brushing.* The necessity of brushing once or twice daily to remove all plaque and debris and to stimulate the surrounding tissue should be impressed on the patient.

2. *Nature and composition of debris.* The location of debris and the consequences of the presence of debris to the gingiva and supporting structure should be explained. The use of diagrams is most helpful, if not indispensable, as a teaching aid.
3. *Relationship of plaque and debris to periodontal disease.* The patient should be made aware of what you are attempting to accomplish and what favorable results can be obtained. Although this may be repetitive, it helps to reinforce motivation.
4. *Type of toothbrush to be used.* Toothbrush recommendations should be based on the patient's individual needs, with emphasis on the fact that two brushes are to be used daily at alternate sessions. They should be rinsed thoroughly and air dried.

***Frequency of brushing***

The frequency of toothbrushing and cleansing should be timed with the aim of preventing gingival disease and caries. Based on interpretations of recent studies, only daily cleansing or cleansing every other day may be necessary to prevent gingivitis.[19] However, the requirements for caries control or the control of breath odors are more demanding. Acidogenic microorganisms can, in the presence of a proper substrate, lower the pH on the tooth surface in an incredibly short time. Breath odors are found directly after ingestion of foods. Moreover, the feeling of personal comfort that clean teeth can give requires frequent brushing. On the basis of these factors, consider twice daily brushing to be empirically necessary.

Once the patient is aware of the reasons for brushing, begin the technical instruction. Visual aids will help to convey the message to him. The recommended sequence for instruction is as follows:

1. Tell him which brush or brushes to use.[21,22,29]
2. Demonstrate the technique of brushing on a model.
3. Demonstrate the maxillary and mandibular anterior areas in his mouth. He should observe with a mirror.
4. Have him brush his own teeth, using a moistened brush.
5. Point out any errors in his technique, including placement of the brush and position of his hand and arm.
6. Correct his efforts in subsequent demonstrations until the desired technique is perfected in the anterior area.
7. Repeat the sequence of instruction for other areas of the mouth.

***Disclosing solutions and tablets***

Disclosing solutions and tablets will provide an objective criterion for adequate oral hygiene that the patient can see. Their use at home will encourage greater brushing effort since plaques are visualized and the stain must be removed. Disclosing solutions also stain the mucosa of lips, tongue, cheeks, and gingiva, however. Most of the tissue discoloration can be removed by rinsing with a mouthwash. Reassure the patient that the coloration of the soft tissues can be removed by rinsing and brushing. The residual mucosal coloration disappears in a few hours (Fig. 25-6). Have the patient use a disclosing tablet at each subsequent appointment before treatment begins. Show him the areas missed. Then take corrective educational measures.

***Toothbrushes***

The following should be taken into consideration when recommending a toothbrush:

1. *Type.* Decide which type or types of toothbrush should be used.[20] There are manual and mechanical brushes. In the majority of cases, the manual

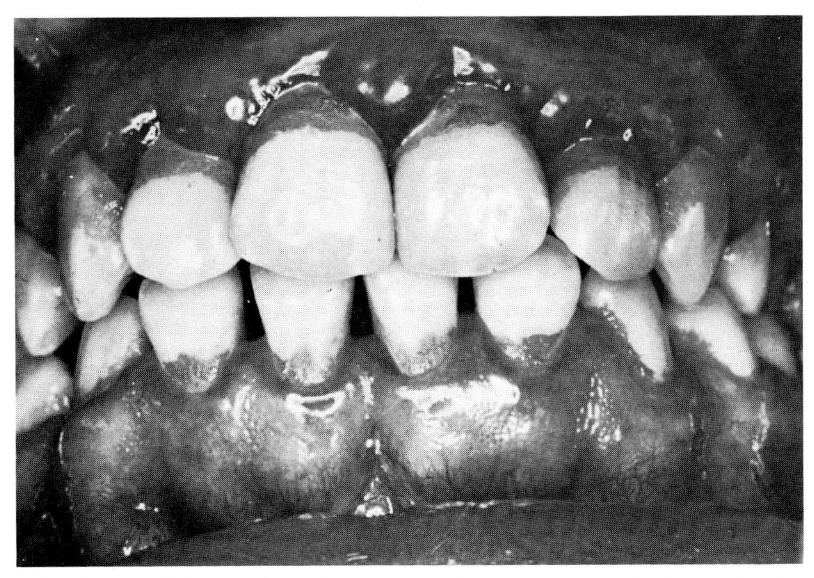

**Fig. 25-6.** Disclosing solution used to visually emphasize the presence of plaques, deposits, stains, and materia alba.

brush is the instrument of choice. There are instances, however, in which the mechanically operated brush should be recommended.[23]

2. *Size.* The handle of the hand-operated brush should be shaped for a firm, comfortable grip. The head of the brush should be small enough for easy insertion into all areas of the mouth yet large enough to cover several teeth at once.
3. *Bristles.* The bristles should be of equal length. If they are soft, they should be arranged closely in two or more rows. If they are hard, they should be arranged in two or three rows and be more widely spaced (Fig. 25-7). They may be of either synthetic or natural boar fibers. The synthetic variety has been improved in resiliency. The ends are rounded, with a diameter of 0.007 to 0.011 inch, so that the bristles can be used to advantage in either the soft[21a] (Fig. 25-8) or the hard type of brush.[22] Synthetic bristles are more easily cleansed and are more durable, and their stiffness is not so easily affected by water.[20] Brushes are available with supersoft synthetic bristles arranged in two or three rows. These types are generally employed for only a short time, usually during the healing period after periodontal surgery following the removal of the dressing.

***Sequence of brushing***

Instruct the patient to brush systematically, starting posteriorly and moving progressively toward the anterior region and then returning to the posterior region on the opposite side of the same arch.

The length of time required for mouth cleansing will vary for each patient, depending in part on the frequency of brushing. Suggest a prescribed time, emphasizing the fact that initially more time (10 to 20 minutes) will be required until the patient becomes adept in the use of the several home dental care aids. (Later, 3 to 5 minutes may suffice.)

Brushing should be performed before a mirror with a good light so that the patient can check the placement of the brush and bristles. Some patients who

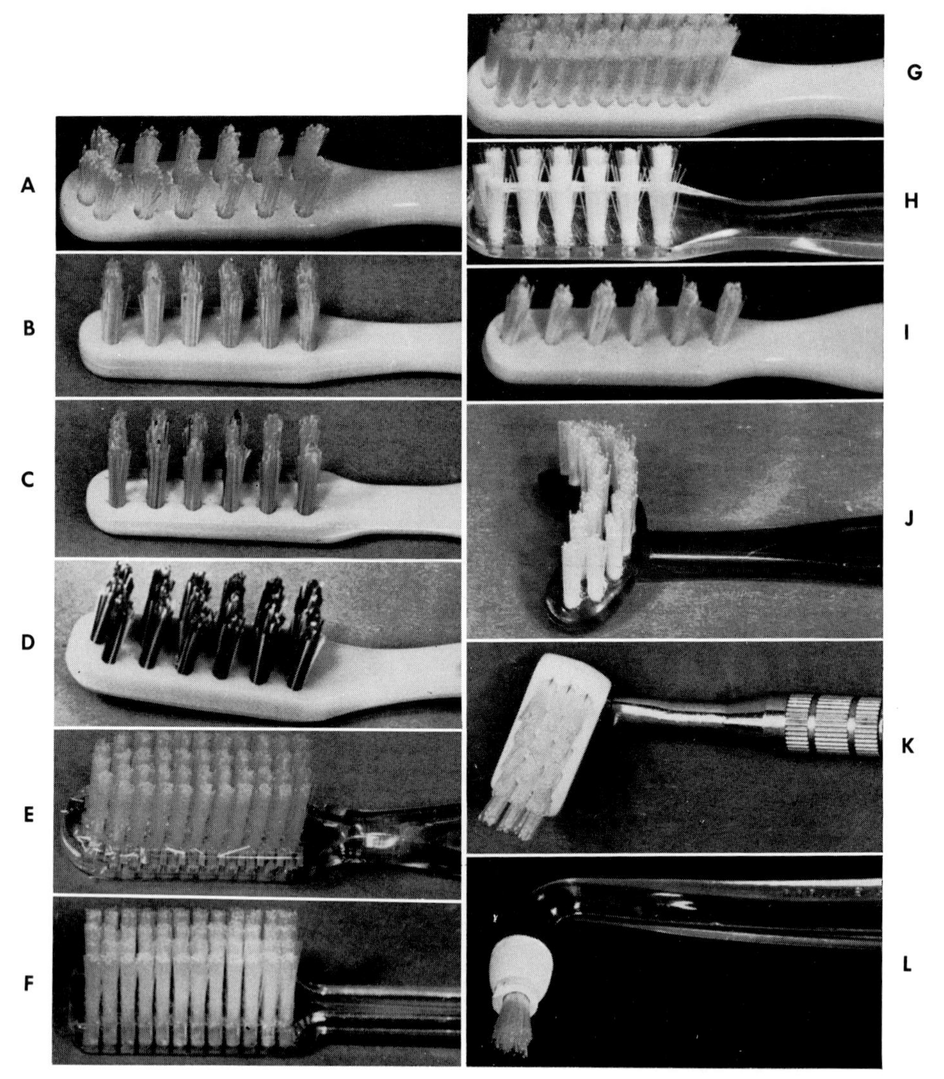


**Fig. 25-7.** Different types of brushes. All may be used to advantage if used correctly. **A** and **B,** Two-row, hard, nylon-bristled brushes. **C,** Two-row, hard, boar-bristled (bleached) brush. **D,** Three-row, hard, boar-bristled (unbleached) brush. **E** and **F,** Multitufted, four-row, soft, nylon-bristled brush. **G,** Three-row, multitufted, soft, nylon-bristled brush. **H,** Three-row, soft, nylon-bristled brush with space sufts. **I,** Single-row, hard, boar-bristled (bleached) brush. **J,** Curved-head, two-row nylon-bristled brush. **K,** Three-row, nylon-bristled brush with adjustable head. **L,** Single-tufted brush tip.

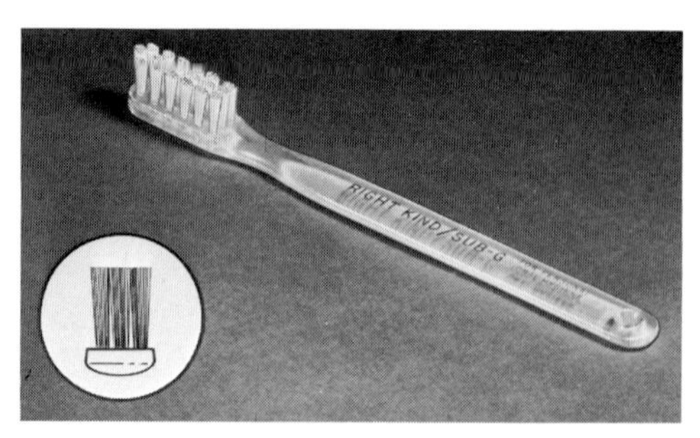


**Fig. 25-8.** Soft-bristled brush with rounded ends for sulcular brushing.

claim to brush often may not accomplish as thorough a debridement as others who may brush conscientiously once a day.[15] The patient should brush at night before going to bed. Thus during the hours of sleep, the mouth will be as clean as possible and plaque will not be left in situ for 12 or more hours.

At successive appointments, examine the patient's mouth to evaluate the oral hygiene program. If there are areas in which plaque remains, examine his technique and correct any errors. In many cases several months may elapse before the patient is able to carry out his home dental care regimen successfully. Monitor the efficacy of his oral hygiene throughout treatment and suggest changes as necessary in home dental care methods or in the treatment plan based on this evaluation.

***Intersulcular method***

No single method of toothbrushing has been demonstrated to be totally adequate for all patients.[17] The intersulcular method advocated by Talbot in 1899[24] and by Bass in 1944[21] is currently popular since it includes an attempt to cleanse the sulcus. This method is efficient in removing dental plaque from the exposed gingival margin of the tooth and approximately a half millimeter or so into the sulcus. The interdental sulci are better cleansed with floss. The occlusal surface must be cleansed by a vibrating motion of the bristle ends over the occlusal surfaces. In mouths where periodontal disease has created large interproximal spaces, the Charters method of toothbrushing may be used after the intersulcular method to be followed by dental floss or cotton yarn.

***Modified intersulcular method***

In the modified intersulcular method a brush with soft multitufted synthetic bristles is used. The bristles have rounded polished ends 0.007 inch in diameter. Place the brush so that the sides of the bristles are flat against the facial, palatal, or lingual surfaces of the teeth, the inside bristles are next to the teeth, and the ends of the bristles are at the gingival margin of these teeth (Fig. 25-9, *A*). Rotate the handle of the brush slightly so that the outer two or three rows of bristles overlap both the gingival margin and the attached gingiva adjacent to that margin *(B)*. Impart a vibrating (reciprocating) motion to the brush in an anteroposterior direction, allowing the fine bristles next to the tooth to be introduced into the gingival sulcus. At the same time the vibrating motion by the outer two or three rows of bristles will cleanse the plaque from that part of the attached gingiva under the bristle ends and stimulate the gingiva. This vibrating motion should be applied for about 10 seconds. The sides of the bristles next to the tooth impart the friction, which helps to loosen the plaque. After the vibrating motion, roll the brush toward the occlusal surface. Begin the sequence of brushing in the posterior part of the mouth on the maxillary arch and at the facial surfaces *(C)*. Place the brush as described to complete the cycle. Then move it to the next segment toward the mesial *(D)*, overlapping the segments slightly *(E)*. Repeat the cycle until the last tooth of the opposite side of the arch is cleansed. Brush the distal surface of the last tooth in the arch by placing the ends of the bristles against this surface and vibrating the brush. Repeat the procedure, this time moving back to the palatal surface on the opposite side of the arch *(F* to *H)*. Next, place the bristle ends on the occlusal surface at one end of the maxillary arch and vibrate them into the occlusal fissures, moving around to the opposite side *(I)*.

When the maxillary arch has been completed, brush the mandibular teeth, starting at the posterior segment on the facial surface and moving around the arch on the facial and lingual surfaces in the same manner as described for the maxillary arch. Place the bristle ends at the gingival margins with the sides of the

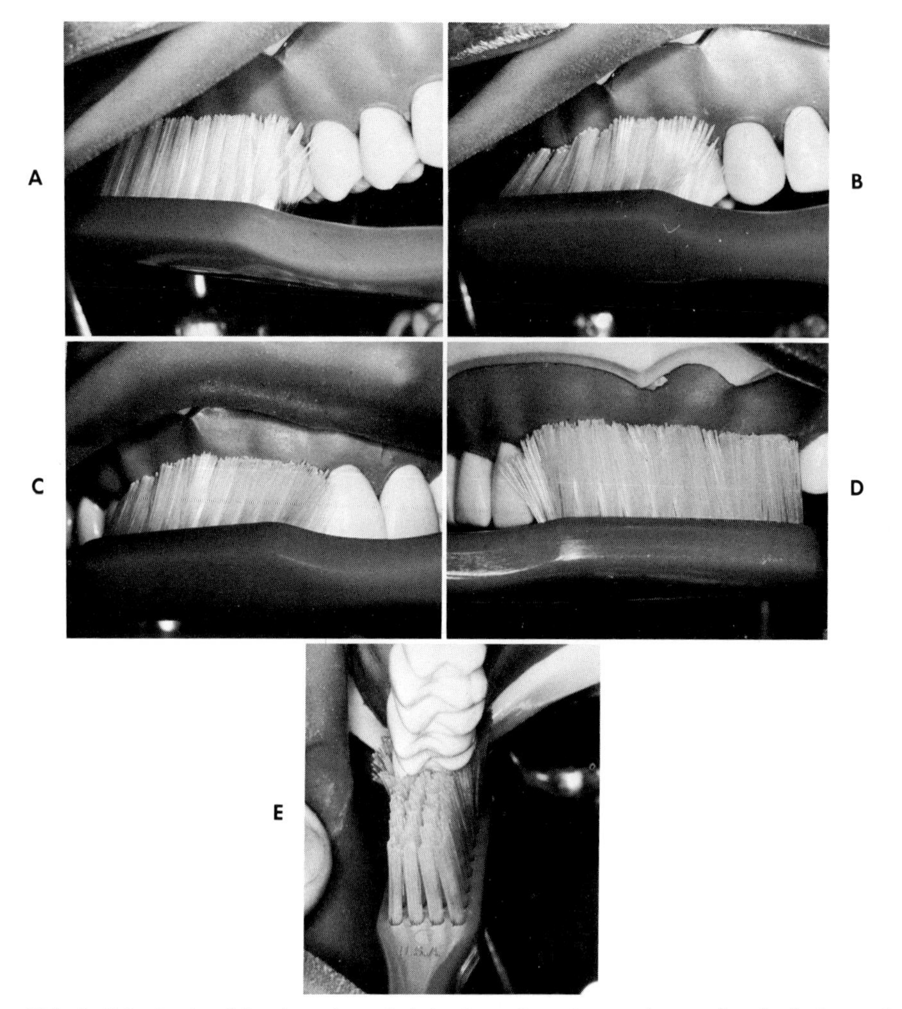


**Fig. 25-9. A,** Sulcular brushing introduces bristles into the sulcus and over the gingival margin. **B,** The bristles are shimmied in place. **C,** Brush each segment in turn, overlapping the segments. Start on the upper right. **D,** Even pressure should be applied. **E,** Brush the distal surface of the last tooth (upper left).

bristles against the tooth surface. Turn the brush handle so that the outer two or three rows of bristle ends are in contact with the attached gingiva and then vibrate the brush in a slightly anteroposterior direction, permitting the bristle ends of the inside row to be introduced into the sulcus. After approximately 10 seconds (eight or ten vibrations), rotate the wrist to carry the bristle ends toward the occlusal surfaces. Do this in segments around the arch on the facial surfaces of the teeth and repeat it on the lingual surfaces as described for the maxillary arch. Brush the posterior surfaces of the last teeth in the arch and the occlusal surfaces.

Brush the anterior lingual segment as any other segment. Be sure to choose a brush with a small head that will fit the curved segments.

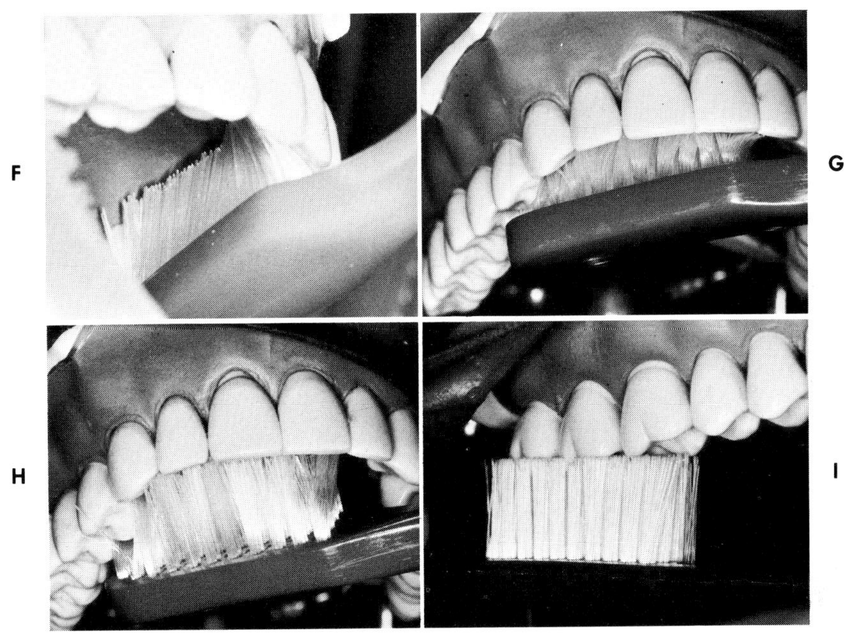


**Fig. 25-9, cont'd. F,** Palatal brushing is difficult for some persons. Bristles should be placed carefully against the margin and in the sulcus. **G,** Overlapping and even pressure are used. **H,** Work the brush downward after the sulcus and gingiva are brushed. **I,** Finish on the upper right. The occlusal surfaces are now brushed, and you can repeat the procedure for the mandibular area. (Courtesy E. Moser, San Francisco.)

***Modified Stillman's method***

The modified Stillman brushing method[25] has enjoyed widespread popularity, for it permits good cleansing and excellent massage. Because of the stimulation that it provides, it is sometimes recommended in managing problems of gingival hyperplasia.

In this technique, place the bristles first on the attached gingiva just coronal to the mucogingival junction (Fig. 25-10, *A*). Direct the tips of the bristles apically at a 45-degree angle. With the sides of the bristles pressed firmly against the gingiva, introduce a slight mesiodistal vibratory motion simultaneously with the gradual movement of the brush toward the occlusal plane. This slight yet firm mesiodistal massage is believed to clean the teeth effectively, especially since the vibratory movement forces the bristles into interproximal spaces and adjoining tooth areas (the so-called unclean area of the tooth). The gingiva is also massaged simultaneously. The ill effects of improper placement of bristles should be shown so that injury to the soft tissues is avoided (Fig. 25-11, *A*). Be sure that the patient knows how easy it is to miss the gingiva *(B)* and the cervical areas of the teeth, thus leaving materia alba (*C*). Instruct him to apply sufficient pressure to produce a blanching of the tissues (*D*). In brushing the vestibular areas of the maxillary molars, show him how cheek clearance for the brush can be obtained by moving the mandibular toward the side being brushed (*F*). Show him how to brush the distal surfaces of the last molars, working the bristles up and around these areas.

Demonstrate the placement of brush to teeth and gingiva on the palatal and lingual surfaces. The technique can be shown first in the mandibular anterior

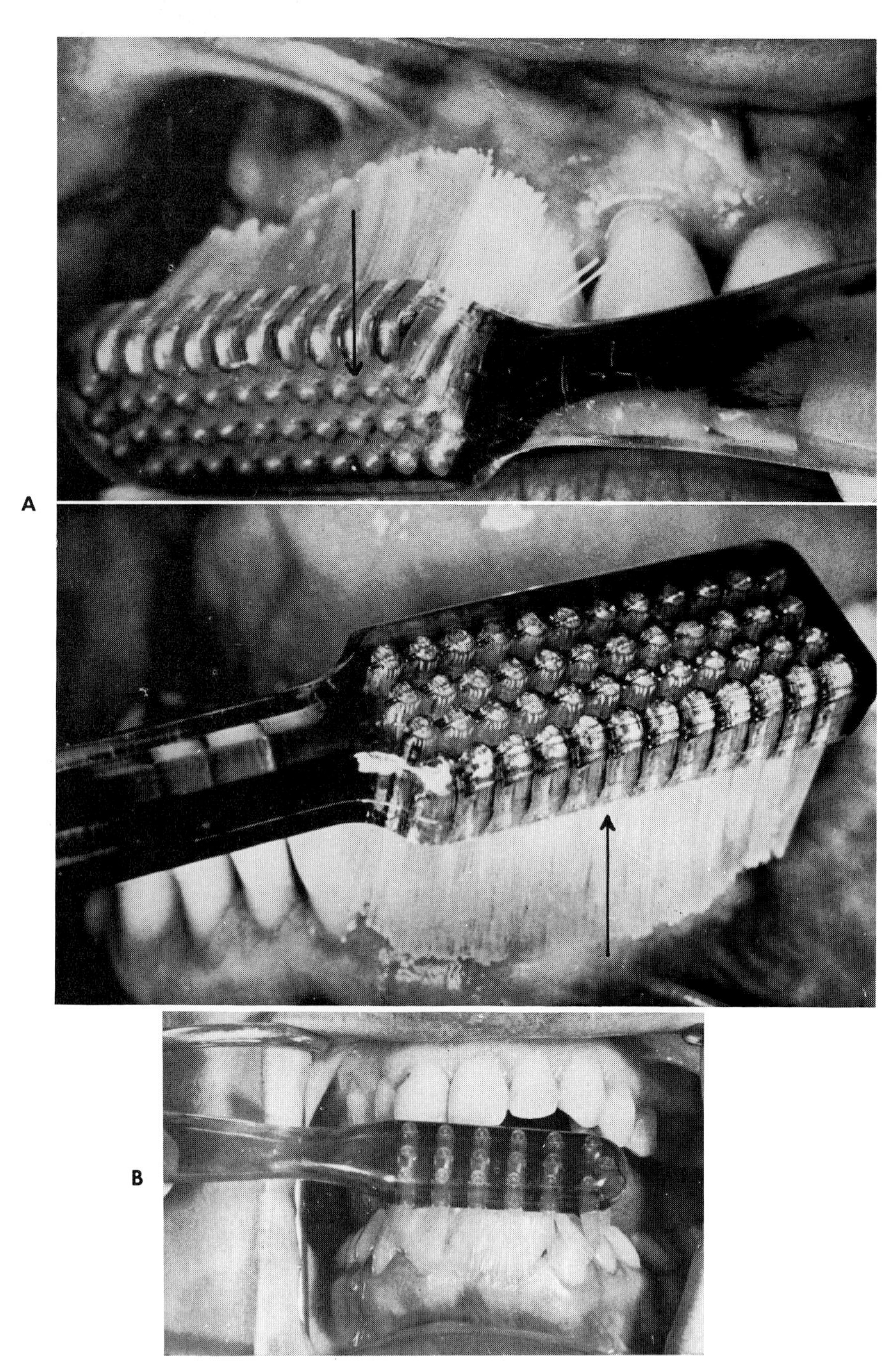


**Fig. 25-10. A,** Placement of the toothbrush at a 45-degree angle on the attached gingiva. Press the brush against the tissues until blanching is achieved. Then shimmy or pump the brush with a reciprocal motion of the handle and carry the brush coronally without turning or twisting the brush head in the direction of the arrows (modified Stillman's technique). **B,** Brush with the bristle tips toward the gingiva and into the sulci to cleanse the interdental spaces and the sulci. This is the modified Stillman technique. The massaging action is shown in the blanching of the gingiva.

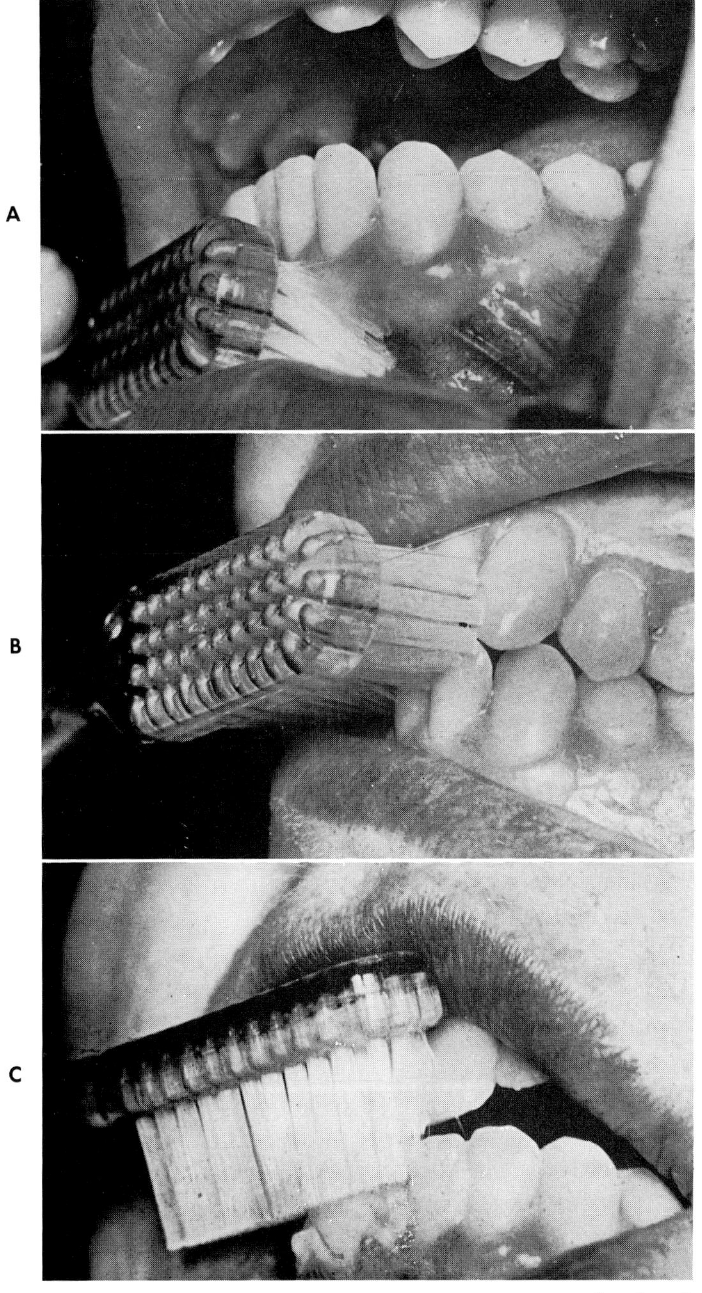


*Continued.*

**Fig. 25-11.** Modified Stillman's technique. **A,** Do not place the brush on the alveolar mucosa. **B,** If the brush is placed on the teeth, the gingiva may be missed completely. **C,** If the cervical areas of the teeth are missed in brushing, materia alba will remain on the teeth and gingiva.

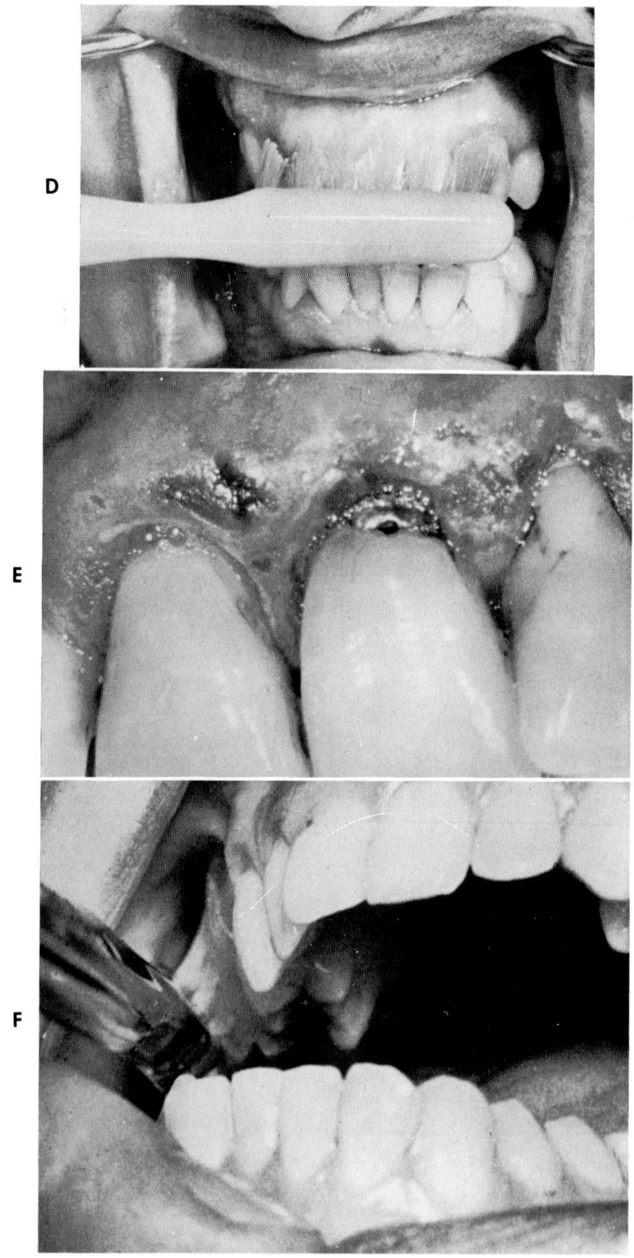


**Fig. 25-11, cont'd. D,** Press the brush against the gingiva with sufficient pressure to produce blanching. **E,** Improper brushing may cause tissue injury. **F,** To brush the vestibular surfaces of maxillary molars, do not open the mouth too wide. Shift the mandible laterally to the side that is to be brushed. This will create more free working area.

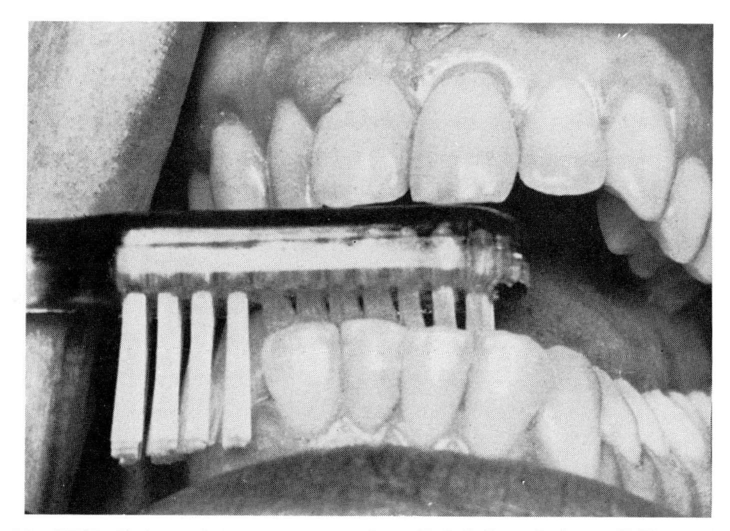

**Fig. 25-12.** If the arch is narrow, use the split-bristle technique (Stillman's).

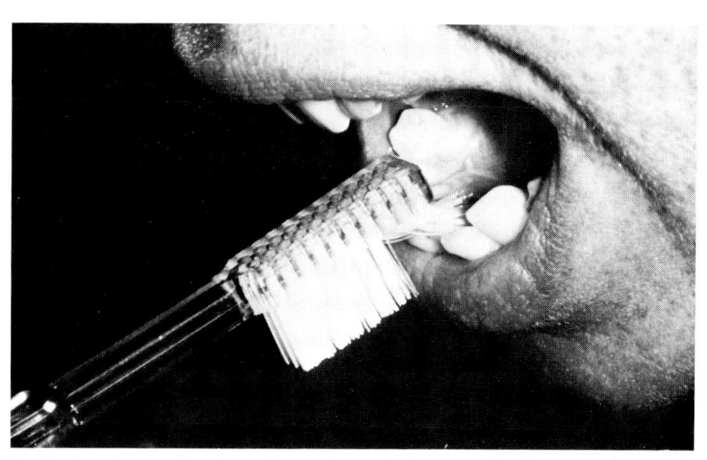

**Fig. 25-13.** Effectively cleanse the lingual surfaces of the mandibular anterior teeth by chewing on the brush to push bristles into the interproximal areas.

region. Those patients with a narrow arch should use only part of the bristles (split-brush technique) (Fig. 25-12). In some cases the patient can effectively cleanse the mandibular incisors by biting on a finely textured brush, as shown in Fig. 25-13. Another effective way to brush the lingual surfaces of mandibular incisors is as follows: hold the brush at the end and, bending over the basin, bring the full force of the arm to bear in the stroke. Since the lingual surfaces of the mandibular incisor teeth often are difficult areas to clean, many types of brushes can be employed (stiff, one-row bristled brushes for cases of crowding or buckling or during orthodontic treatment, lingual brushes with bristles inserted on a curved head, brushes with a small head that can be turned on an adjustable swivel to various positions) (Fig. 25-7).

Emphasize to the patient that the entire lingual surface of mandibular molars must be reached (Fig. 25-14, *A*). Show him how the last molar may be missed

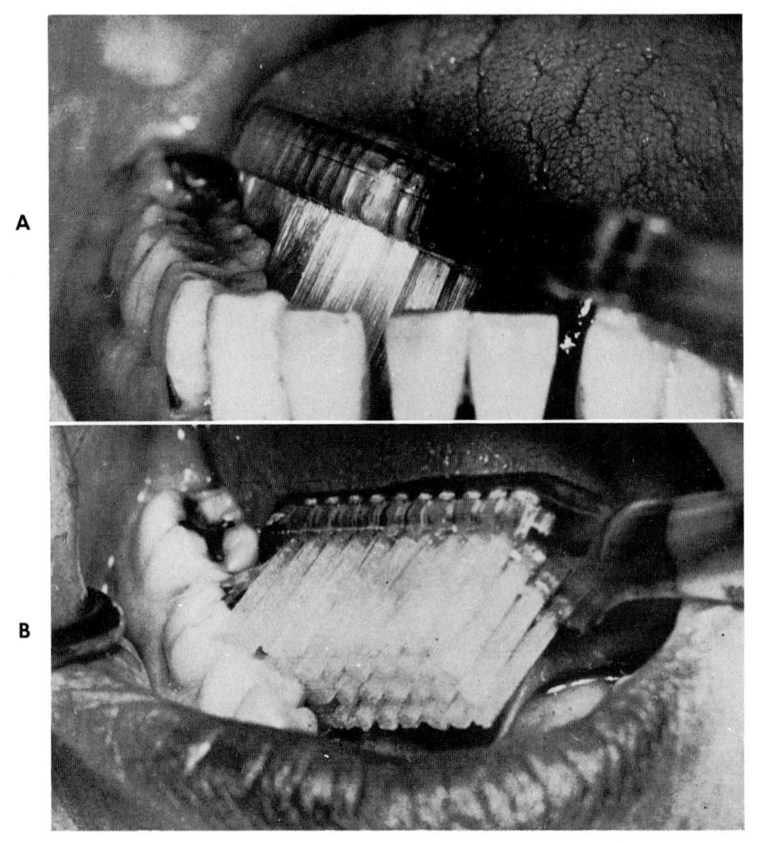


**Fig. 25-14. A,** Proper placement of the brush for lingual surfaces of molars and premolars. **B,** Improper placement of the brush on the lingual area of molars (modified Stillman's technique).

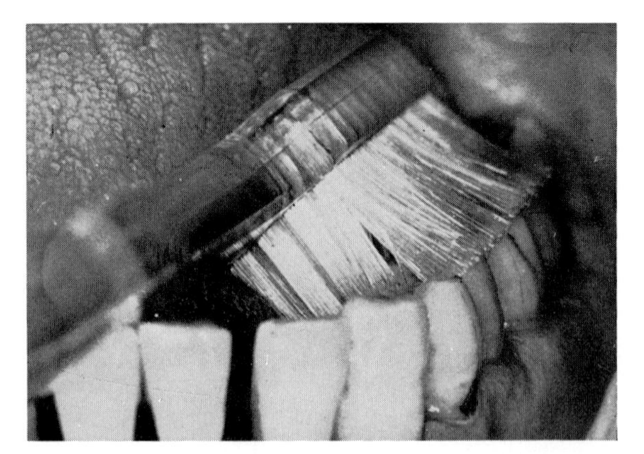

**Fig. 25-15.** Lingual surfaces of the mandibular molar and premolar areas are difficult to keep clean. Instruct patients to place half the bristles on the occlusal surface of the teeth and to carry half to the gingiva, using a slight back-and-forth movement (modified Stillman's technique).

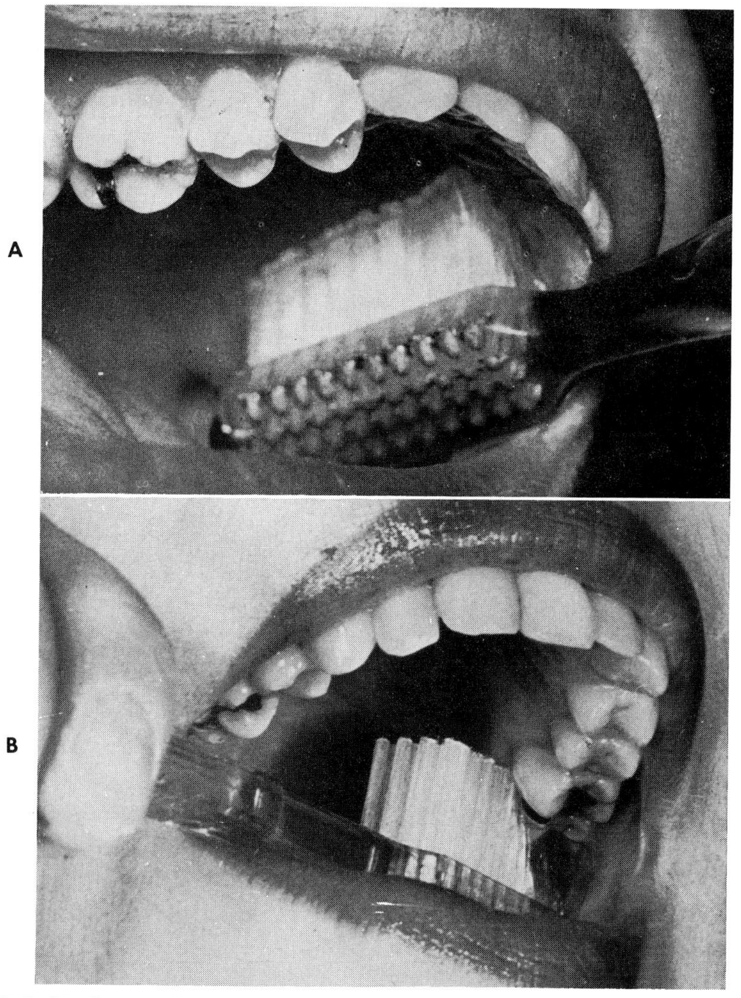


**Fig. 25-16. A,** In the maxillary molar and premolar area, hold the brush parallel to the arch. The handle should touch the central incisors. **B,** If the handle is held to the side, brushing becomes ineffective (modified Stillman's technique).

completely if the brush is not carried down on the gingiva and far enough back (Fig. 25-14, *B*).

When a patient is troubled by gagging or difficulty of access, instruct him to place the bristles on the occlusal surfaces, retaining half the bristles in this position and carrying the remaining bristles toward the gingiva (Fig. 25-15).

On the oral surfaces of the maxillary premolars and molars, hold the brush so that it is parallel to the median line of the maxilla (Fig. 25-16, *A*). In this manner the bristles reach all areas evenly. If the handle is held to one side (Fig. 25-16, *B*), all bristles may not touch the teeth and cleansing and massage will be ineffective.

The benefits of the modified Stillman method are as follows:

1. The attached gingiva is mechanically stimulated.
2. The gingival third of the tooth is contacted with a short vibratory motion

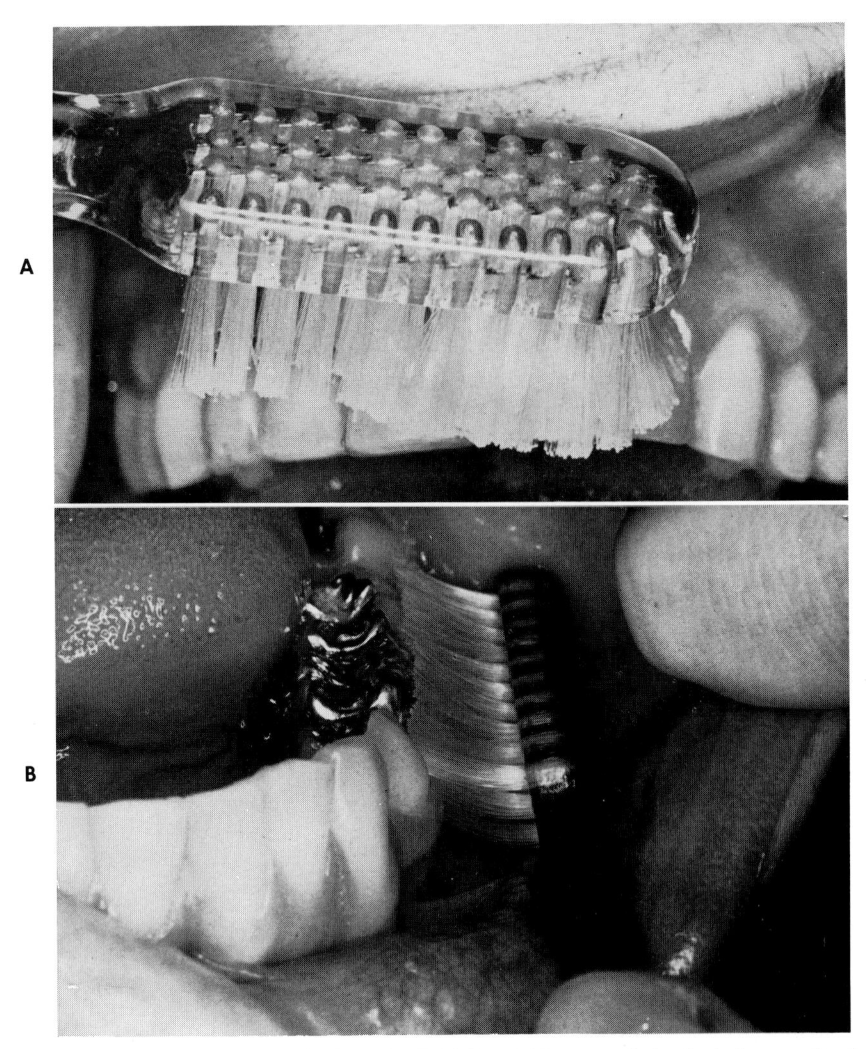


**Fig. 25-17. A,** Place the bristles firmly at a 45-degree angle toward the incisal or occlusal edges of the teeth. Brush the interdental spaces by a gentle shimmying motion. **B,** Position the brush for interdental brushing as shown on the mandible (Charters' technique).

over the surface, and plaque is removed between the gingival margin and the height of contour.

3. The tips of the bristles tend to reach the interproximal areas and to clean and stimulate the interdental papillae without injury.

The preceding is a description of the *modified* Stillman method. In the original method there is no brush movement toward the occlusal plane.[25] The bristles are placed on the gingival margin and the cervical portion of the tooth, and the mesiodistal vibratory pressure is applied without any movement of the bristle tips from their original placement.

For the management of gingival hyperplasia, a hard brush may be prescribed for the modified Stillman method.

***Charters' technique (interdental brushing)***

When the interdental papillae are receded, leaving interdental areas open, the method of oral hygiene and physiotherapy should be adapted to this dento-gingival terrain. Work the bristles between the teeth and point them incisally or occlusally at a 45-degree angle. After the bristles are engaged interproximally, use a firm but gentle shimmying motion for 10 to 15 seconds in each area.[26] The proper placement of the brush for the labial area of the maxillary anterior teeth is shown in Fig. 25-17, *A*, and that for the buccal area of the mandibular teeth in Fig. 25-17, *B*. For lingual brushing the same procedure is employed, except that only the tip of the brush may be used effectively (Fig. 25-18). On the lingual and palatal areas of the maxillary posterior teeth, advise the patient to place the brush head against the palate to permit the bristles to work between the teeth. If the proper angle is not maintained, some bristles may impinge on the gingiva and prevent the patient from working the rest of the bristles interdentally. The Charters, Stillman, and intrasulcular methods are difficult for many patients to master. Just as important, no method is particularly efficient in removing debris once it has been loosened. Therefore a thorough and vigorous rinsing should follow each brushing procedure.

***Roll technique***

The roll technique is probably the most universally taught method of brushing and is most easily performed by the patient. It is most appropriate when there is only a minimal change in the normal dentogingival relationship.

In this technique the bristles are placed well up on the attached gingiva at a 45-degree angle. Press the sides of the bristles against the tissue and simultaneously move them incisally or occlusally against the gingiva and teeth in a rolling motion, similar to the turning of a latch key.

***Electric toothbrush***

More than a passing glance should be given the electric toothbrush, for this implement can no longer be considered just a lazy man's way of brushing. Experience has shown that it is both efficient and surprisingly appealing to patients. Because of these reasons, it has a definite place in the oral hygiene program.[23,27]

The electric toothbrush is especially indicated for the handicapped and for patients who do not have the digital dexterity to manipulate an ordinary toothbrush properly. The use of an electric brush is also valuable in patients with complicated fixed bridgework and in those who were fixed orthodontic appliances that tend to entangle food debris. Currently there are three types of actions or movements of electric toothbrushes. All three brushes have small removable heads of synthetic fibers. The bristles are of a soft texture, and damage to the tissues is rare since the brush action stops immediately on the application of excessive pressure. Also, in any of the three types of brushes, the action can be modified by a mere turning of the handle.

In the first type of brush action (arc oscillating), the bristles rotate vigorously in an arc of approximately 60 degrees. In using this instrument, hold the brush lightly against the teeth so that the bristles move in a gently sweeping arc from the incisal edge to the attached gingiva and back again.

The second type provides a reciprocating horizontal movement. The action of this brush is somewhat comparable to that used in the Charters, intrasulcular, and Stillman methods. When a reciprocating-type brush is used in a Bass-like stroke, the bristles are believed to enter into the sulci better and to cleanse them better.

A third type (elliptic) combines the oscillating with the reciprocating.

## Cleansing agents

***Dentifrices and mouthwashes***

The rationale for using a dentifrice is that the dentifrice contains very fine abrasives and detergents mixed with some flavoring agents.[27a] The detergents are an aid in polishing the teeth since they foam and help in the mobilization of the debris. The flavoring agents make toothbrushing more pleasant and leave

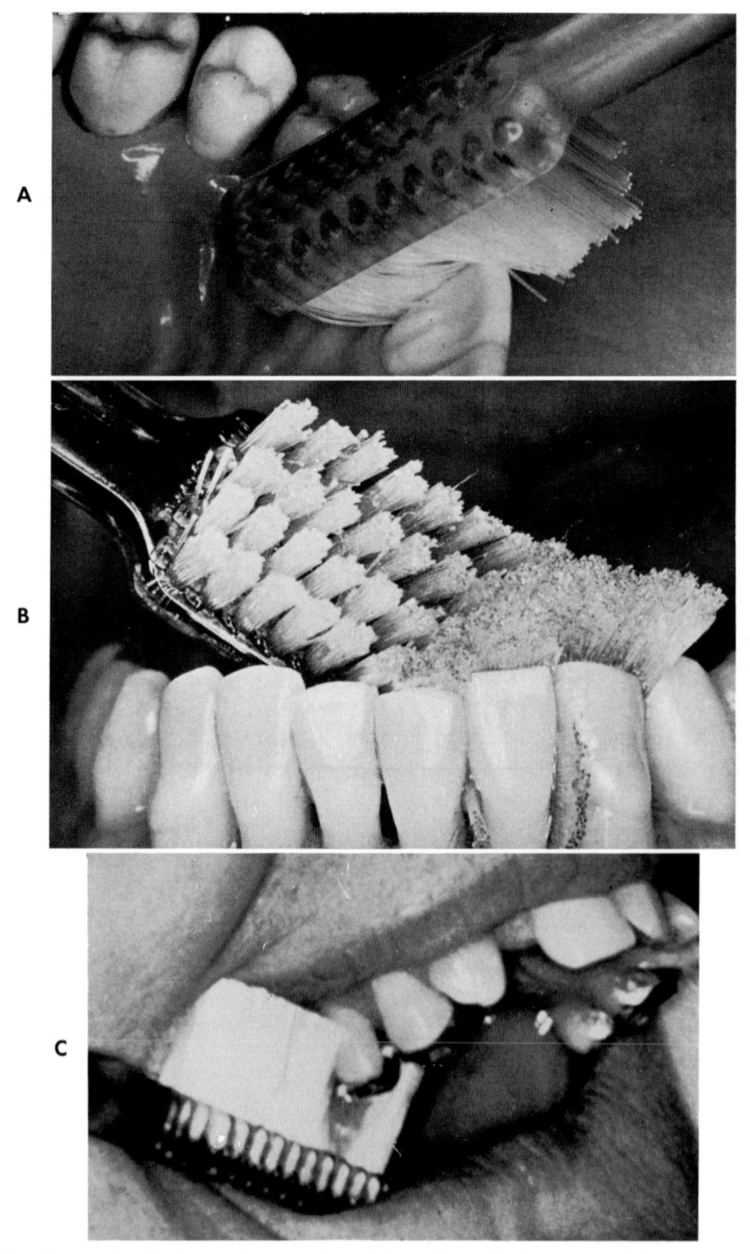


**Fig. 25-18.** Charters' technique. **A,** Interdental brushing of the oral surfaces of the maxillary teeth. **B,** Interdental brushing of the oral surfaces of the mandibular teeth. **C,** Teeth adjacent to edentulous areas must be brushed by a right-angle application of the brush to the tooth.

the mouth feeling refreshed; however, the actual job of cleansing is done by the patient with the brush.

Should a patient ask for the recommendation of a dentifrice, inquire of him what dentifrice he is now using. If it is a reputable one, recommend that he continue to use it. This avoids giving an erroneous impression of endorsement by the dentist of some particular commercial dentifrice or that a brush or dentifrice has therapeutic properties that will do the work for the patient.

Various therapeutic agents may indeed be incorporated in the dentifrice, such as cariostatic agents (fluorides), desensitizing agents (Thermodent, Sensodyne), proteolytic enzymes (Caroid), chelating agents, (X-Tar) and, possibly in the future, plaque-control agents.

The commercially available mouthwashes are of little help in preventing or treating periodontal diseases. Most of them rely on a strong aromatic and flavoring agent to suppress halitosis temporarily. A fleeting antiseptic effect is also obtained, but the salivary bacterial population returns to full strength not long after the patient uses the mouthwash. However, inasmuch as the mouthwash may make the performance of oral hygiene more pleasant, it may have a minor place in the home care program.

***Gauze strips***

Teeth bordering edentulous areas (Fig. 25-18, *C*) may be cleansed with a brush rotated so that the bristles strike the proximal surfaces. Four-ply cotton yarn or gauze strips may be used when the tooth surfaces are not readily accessible to a brush (Fig. 25-19). The gauze material for this technique may be 1-inch gauze bandage cut into strips 6 inches in length and folded down the center. Place the fold gingivally on the tooth and carry the gauze as far to the gingiva as possible, even under the margin. Move the gauze, in a shoeshine motion, several times across the area.[13]

Floss or tape can be threaded through the embrasures and pontics and abutment teeth can be cleansed (Fig. 25-20).

***Pipe cleaners***

Pipe cleaners are sometimes effective in cleansing inaccessible interproximal areas and exposed bifurcations and trifurcations. The cleaners are carefully teased between the exposed roots of the furcations and pulled through (Fig. 25-21).

## Massage

***Balsa wood toothpicks***

The proper use of balsa wood toothpicks (Stim-U-Dents) as a daily regimen in oral hygiene should be emphasized for those in whom interdental topography indicates such use. These picks (triangular in cross section) are small enough to fit into most interdental spaces. As a supplement to brushing, they are useful for dislodging interproximally trapped debris often missed by the most meticulous brushing and for massaging the underlying interproximal gingiva. First, teach the patient to use his hand as a fulcrum by placing it on the chin, cheek, or gingiva, depending on the area to be cleansed. Then, have him moisten the balsa wood toothpick to make it less brittle and then place it interdentally with the base of the triangle toward the tissue. It is inserted in a slightly coronal direction so as not to injure the gingiva. Wedge the toothpick into the interproximal space and partially withdraw it. Repeat this in-and-out motion several times without completely disengaging the toothpick from the area (Fig. 25-22). Balsa wood toothpicks may also be used to cleanse plaque on proximal tooth surfaces facing edentulous areas.

***Interdental stimulator***

The interdental stimulator consists of a rubber tip of smooth or ribbed conical shape attached to a plastic handle or to the end of a toothbrush handle.

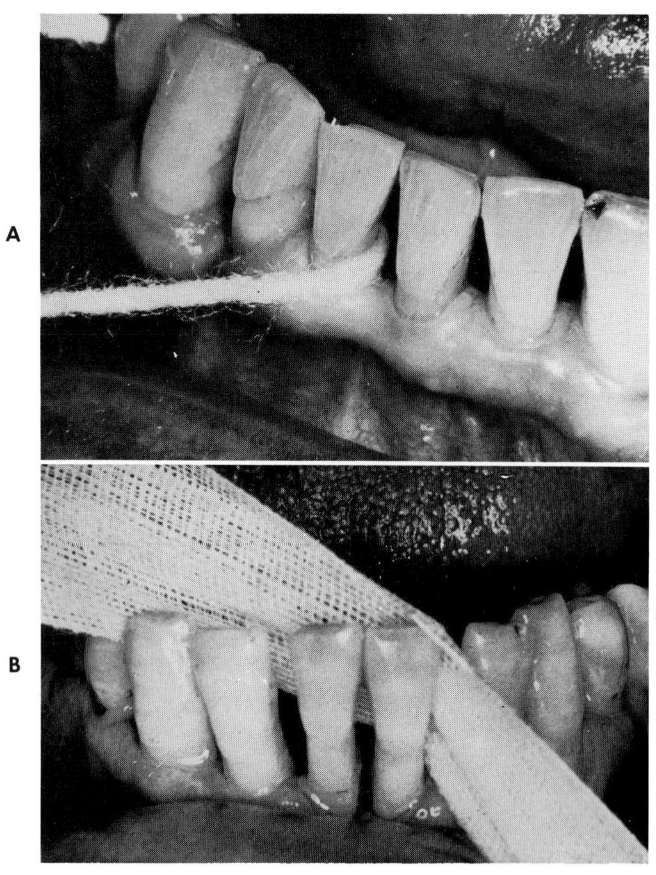


**Fig. 25-19. A,** Use yarn for interdental cleansing and stimulation. **B,** Use gauze strips to cleanse proximal areas of widely spaced teeth. (**A** courtesy D. Keene, Daytona Beach.)

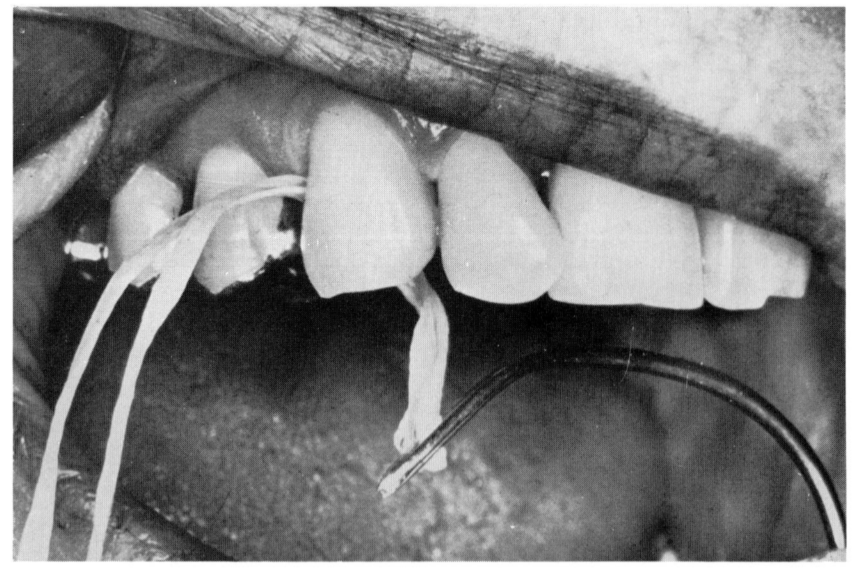

**Fig. 25-20.** Threading dental tape or floss between abutment teeth or pontics with the help of a large, curved needle. Plastic needles (Zon, Explac, Butler) are also available for this purpose.

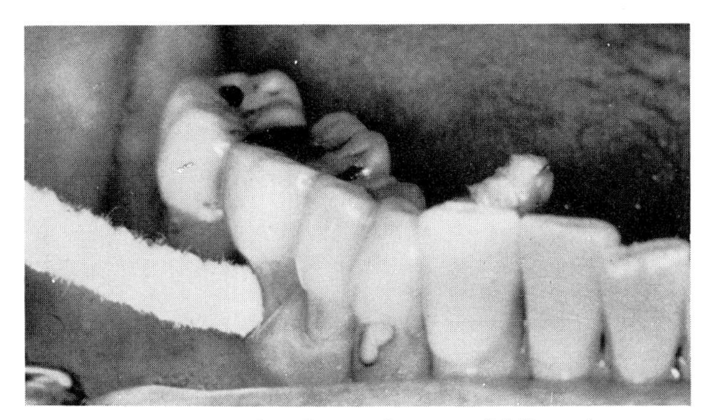

**Fig. 25-21.** Use pipe cleaners in exposed bifurcations.

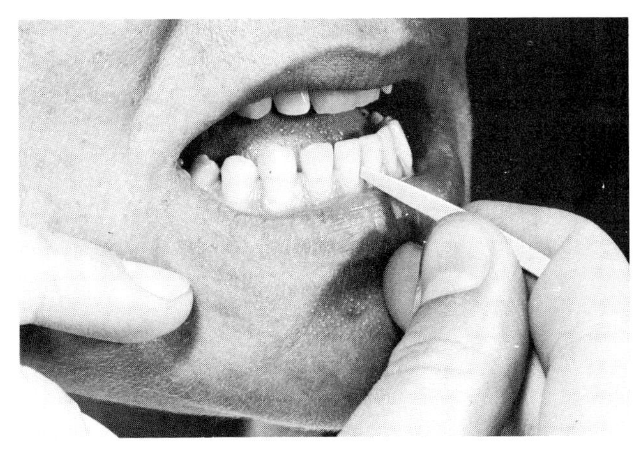

**Fig. 25-22.** Use Stim-U-Dents for interproximal cleansing and gingival stimulation. A to-and-fro motion works best.

Plastic tips are also available. Its action massages and stimulates circulation of the interdental gingiva and may increase the tone of the tissue. It can also aid in cleansing debris from interproximal areas where papillary height is reduced and embrasures are open. It is not recommended for areas in which the papillae are normal and fill the interproximal spaces, for the patient may try to force the tip interproximally by applying excessive pressure and thus cause injury to the gingival tissue.

Interdental stimulation is needed in nearly all areas in which gingivectomy or other surgical procedures have been performed. This physiotherapy is also useful in areas in which the interdental tissue has been destroyed by disease, such as necrotizing ulcerative gingivitis. Instruct the patient who needs interdental stimulation to use the interdental stimulator at least once a day. Have him place the tip of the stimulator interdentally and slightly coronally. Pressure is exerted on the gingiva in a horizontal motion, and interdental stimulation is applied from both the buccal and the lingual aspects (Fig. 25-23).

## Special situations

In the presence of gingival recession (atrophy), only a soft, multitufted hand brush with rounded bristle tips should be recommended and a nontraumatizing

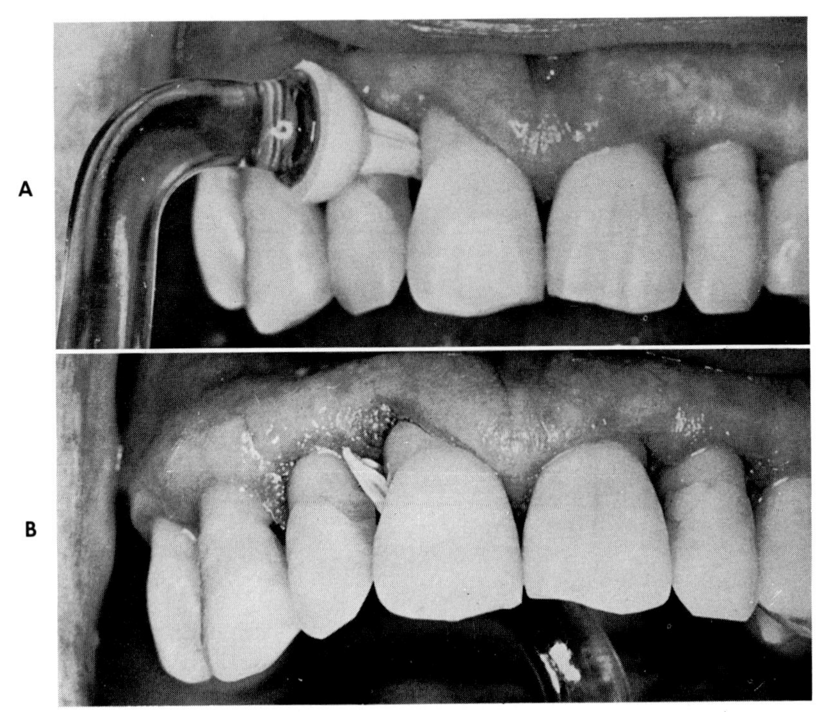


**Fig. 25-23. A,** Use the rubber-tipped stimulator in a rotary motion, exerting pressure on the gingiva—vestibular (labial) application. **B,** Rubber-tipped stimulator—oral (palatal) application.

method of toothbrushing used, such as Stillman's (modified). In addition, a dentifrice with extremely fine polishing agents should be prescribed. Similar instructions are given for patients suffering from chronic desquamative gingivitis and for patients in the early postsurgical stages. In the presence of gingival hyperplasia, such as in patients on diphenylhydantoin (Dilantin), vigorous brushing and massaging with a somewhat stiffer brush may be recommended. Massage of the hyperplastic gum with the tip of the index finger is also beneficial in such cases.

Supplemental massaging devices may occasionally be useful, however, such as the soft rubber cup made by Denticator. In addition, a gingival area that refuses to assume good color and tonus after meticulous debridement and despite good oral hygiene will sometimes respond to massage with the forefinger.

Correct cleansing and massage are of inestimable value in the treatment of periodontal disease and in the maintenance of a treated case (Fig. 25-24). Strict attention should be given to the needs of each patient. The topography of the teeth and tissues, digital dexterity, and patient idiosyncrasies will create problems in individual cases.

***Rinsing***

After brushing and interdental stimulation, mouth rinsing is essential.[28] Lukewarm water should be flushed vigorously through all interdental spaces. The brush, toothpicks, and tape often will loosen but may not remove the materia alba and other debris.

***Water irrigation devices***

Water irrigation devices may be used. There are several types. One uses faucet water to irrigate between and around the teeth. The water pressure is steady and is controlled by turning the faucet handle (Fig. 25-25). Another is

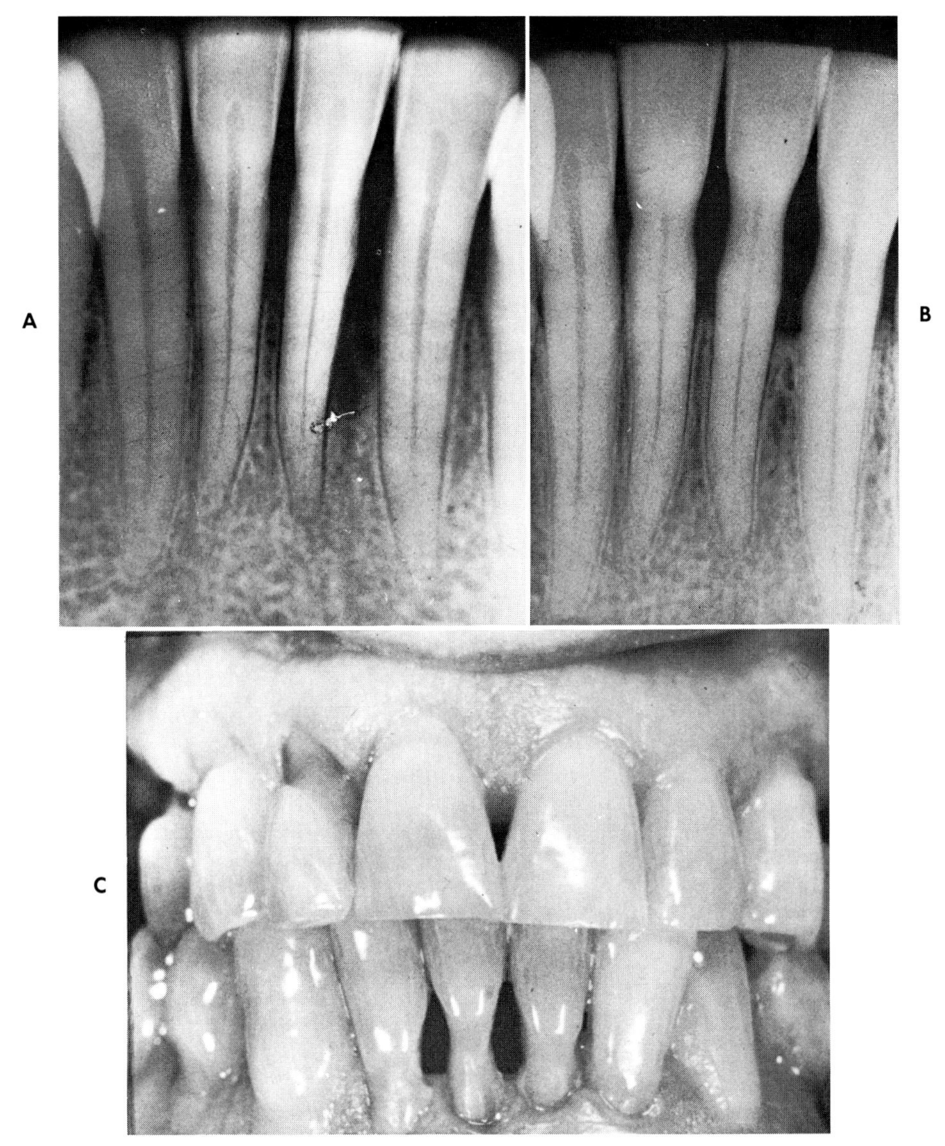


**Fig. 25-24. A,** Lower anterior teeth of a patient 1 year after the start of treatment consisting of root planing and home dental care. **B,** Roentgenogram of the same patient 27 years later. Note the improved appearance of the alveolar bone. The shape of the cervical areas of the teeth has been altered as a result of the regular instrumentation. This is commonly seen in patients on a regular program of periodontal maintenance. **C,** Clinical appearance of the patient's teeth and gingiva at the time of a regular maintenance visit and before any instrumentation. (Courtesy G. Ivancie, Denver.)

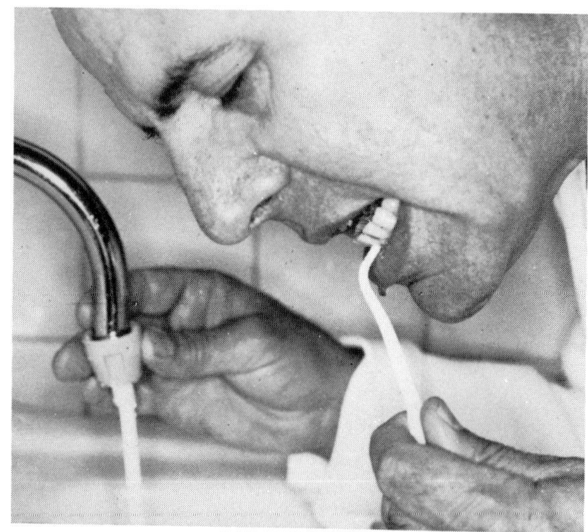

**Fig. 25-25.** Water irrigation device (faucet-controlled) for interdental cleansing. (Courtesy E. Moser, San Francisco.)

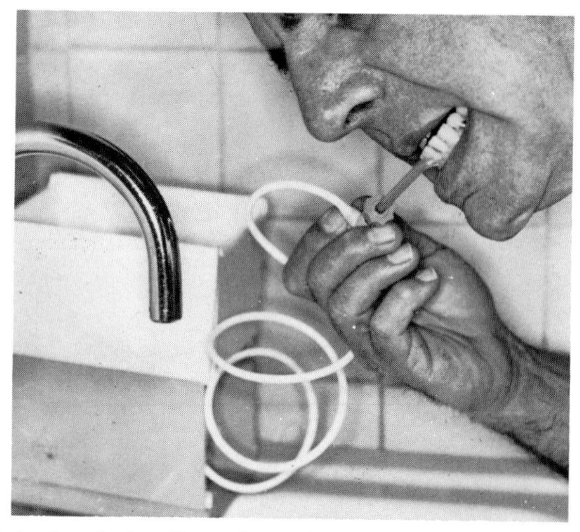

**Fig. 25-26.** Water irrigation device (intermittent jet type). (Courtesy E. Moser, San Francisco.)

the intermittent water jet.[29,30] Water is placed in a receptacle and is propelled by a jumper; controlled intermittent pressure can be delivered to the teeth and gingiva (Fig. 25-26).

When complicated bridgework and fixed orthodontic appliances are present in the mouth, they tend to accumulate debris. The rinsing device helps to keep the mouth clean and to prevent irritation in such cases. For some patients it is useful to add an irrigation device to the oral hygiene regimen for more effective removal of debris. The impression prevails that water pressure helps to remove food debris and even some materia alba but does not remove all the tough film of dental plaque.

There have been reports of injury and abscess formation caused by water pressure devices, but no evidence of a cause-effect relationship has been presented. Above all, remember that rinsing, necessary as it may be, only readily removes loose material; it complements but does not replace the use of the toothbrush and interdental stimulation. Water irrigation techniques have long been employed in Europe in the treatment of periodontal disease. There they are referred to as balneotherapy.

## CHEMICAL PLAQUE CONTROL

The chemical control of bacterial plaque is being investigated intensively. Given the well-known inability or lack of desire of many individuals to remove plaque daily from the tooth surfaces, research has been directed toward drugs administered in mouthwashes, dentifrices, chewing gums, and other vehicles, in an effort to control dental plaque. Theoretically it is possible to interfere with dental plaque by the following means:

1. Making the tooth surface unfavorable to microbial colonization *(tensioactive agents, antiseptics)*
2. Reducing the numbers of those organisms that are capable of colonizing on the tooth surface *(antibiotics, antiseptics)*
3. Degrading the cementing intermicrobial matrix *(enzymes)*
4. Interfering with the metabolism of plaque bacteria, thereby reducing their pathogenicity *(antiseptics, dietary substances, fluorides)*

### Tensioactive agents

Dental deposits have been described as less common in people living in areas with a high fluoride content in the drinking water.[57] In vitro experimentation has shown that fluoride reduces the ability of hydroxyapatite powders to adsorb protein and diminishes the surface energy[58,59] of enamel surfaces and the formation of plaque on them. Although laboratory and animal investigations have shown fluorides to inhibit bacterial multiplication[60] and, topically applied, to reduce plaque formation,[61] clinical trials in humans have failed to demonstrate a plaque-reducing effect in fluoride-containing mouthwashes.[62,63]

Application of silicones seemed to reduce calculus formation in vitro,[64] but further studies have indicated that the application of various kinds of films involves technical difficulties, must be frequently repeated, and has only a limited effect on plaque formation. Such methods have proved of little practical value to date.[65,66]

### Antibiotics

Several antibiotics can depress oral microorganisms (penicillin,[67,68,85] tetracyclines,[69] vancomycin,[67,68] actinobolin,[72] cc 10232[73-75]) and thereby plaque formation in vivo and in vitro. Results of animal experiments with drugs directed against gram-positive microorganisms have proved promising, but clinical trials in humans have generally been unsuccessful.[76,77] Although several antibiotics (especially the broad-spectrum ones), when applied topically, have a marked plaque-reducing effect, the use of such drugs in long-term trials in humans involves the potential risks of sensitization, candidiasis, and the development of resistant strains of microorganisms. Thus serious objections can be raised against local antibiotic prophylaxis.

### Enzymes

Enzymes are theoretically capable of degrading the intermicrobial cementing matrix of plaque and thereby the framework for bacterial colonization.

It has been shown in vitro that established plaque is dissolved by dextranases[78] and that the addition of dextranase to animal diets containing sucrose inhibits plaque formation.[79,80] Dextranase preparations tested in humans, however, have had little[61,81,82] or no[83,84] effect on the microbial plaque. Apart from dextranase, enzyme preparations such as trypsin, chymotrypsin, pancreatin, amylase, lipase, and elasterase have been tested for their ability to degrade dental plaque. At this time, it seems justified to state that clinical trials with enzymes have not been encouraging.

### Antiseptics

In recent years plaque inhibition in vivo has been demonstrated with sodium ricinoleate,[85] mercurials (e.g., sodium parahydroxymercuribenzoate[86]), and substances such as chloramin T, cetylpyridinium chloride, benzalkonium chloride,[73,87-89] and chlorhexidene salts.[90-92,96,97] These substances have attracted great attention. The assumption is that the chlorhexidene effect is the result of a local antibacterial action of the antiseptic since the antiseptic is bound to organic or inorganic components of the tooth surface.[93,94]

Some undesirable side effects are present. Discoloration of the teeth, silicate fillings, and the tongue is clearly seen in chlorhexidene rinsers. Some persons have complained of a bitter taste and an interference with their sense of taste for a long time.[89,90,95]

Laboratories all over the world are working on problems related to chemical plaque control, and the day is doubtlessly approaching when topical application of antibacterial substances will facilitate achievement of a dentition free of microbial plaque.

## Root sensitivity

### Sensitivity of exposed root surfaces

Sensitivity of an exposed root surface is a vexing problem for the patient and is a not infrequent and distressing sequel to instrumentation and surgical procedures in the treatment of periodontal disease. Basically such sensitivity is the result of irritation of organic matter in exposed dentinal tubules. This excludes from the discussion sensitivity from occlusal trauma and other pulpal changes caused by such factors as caries and restorative procedures.

Even though they may not have been especially sensitive originally, surgically exposed root surfaces often become hypersensitive. Routine, thorough brushing and use of adjunctive aids in oral hygiene, such as toothpicks, stimulators, and dental tape, help to desensitize root surfaces. Plaque and food debris, if allowed to remain on exposed root surfaces, often lead to increasing sensitivity. A vicious cycle[31] may be created. Exposed root surfaces are not kept clean and become hypersensitive. Because of the discomfort involved in brushing them, the patient tends to avoid these areas, and the hypersensitivity is aggravated. In such cases root surfaces must be desensitized and an adequate oral physiotherapy regime must be instituted. Without effective home care, however, even the improvement that follows desensitization is likely to be short lived.

The stimuli responsible for hypersensitivity reactions to mechanical, chemical, or thermal stimuli include the following:

**Mechanical stimuli**

1. Periodontal instrumentation (especially postsurgically and after extensive root planing)
2. Toothbrushing

**Chemical stimuli**

1. Sweet or sour foods and drink
2. Plaque allowed to remain on the tooth surface (It has been noted by many clinicians that the tooth sensitivity is often proportionate to the unhygienic conditions around the denuded cemental surface. A vicious cycle ensues in which the patient does not or cannot cleanse the area adequately, deposits collect, and sensitivity increases.)

**Thermal stimuli**

1. Hot and cold liquids or foods
2. Dental procedures (use of hot or cold fluids, compounds, hydrocolloid)

The rationale of desensitization procedures is not fully understood. Some techniques may depend on denaturation of the superficial ends of Tomes' fibers or of nerve endings in dentin. Other procedures are designed to deposit an insoluble substance on the ends of the fibers or nerves to act as a barrier to stimuli. Still others are designed to stimulate secondary dentin formation, thus insulating the pulp from external stimuli. The anti-inflammatory and antihyperemic properties of corticoids may prevent or relieve hypersensitivity by reducing hyperemia in the pulp. Evidence for each of these rationales is incomplete at present.

Grossman has suggested the following requirements for a satisfactory method of treating hypersensitivity[32]: the method should be nonirritating to the pulp, painless on application, easily applied, and rapid acting; it should be consistently effective for long periods of time; and it must not discolor the teeth. None of the methods described next meets all these requirements.

Some procedures for treatment may be carried out in the office. Others may be done by the patient at home. A combination of both is sometimes indicated.

## Desensitization

*Office treatment*

In all patients in whom office treatment is used, the root surfaces must be clean, dry, and carefully isolated.

Silver nitrate has been a traditional "nostrum" in dental offices. This treatment is obsolete since it produces unsightly discoloration. In its stead Gottlieb's impregnation has been used successfully.[33] Cleanse and dry the tooth with a solution of benzene (U.S.P.). Apply a 40% aqueous solution of zinc chloride for 1 minute. (Care should be taken to protect adjacent soft tissues.) Follow this by the application of a 20% aqueous solution of potassium ferrocyanide to the root surface still moist from the zinc chloride. Rub the potassium ferrocyanide into the root surface with a cotton pellet or porte polisher for 1 minute. A whitish, curdy, insoluble precipitate forms, which reduces hypersensitivity.

Sodium fluoride* may be used for office treatment of hypersensitive root surfaces.[34] It is in the form of a paste, consisting of equal parts of sodium fluoride, kaolin, and glycerin.[35] After cleansing the hypersensitive areas, rub the paste into the exposed root surfaces with a porte polisher and orangewood stick or a rubber cup for 1 to 5 minutes. Satisfactory results are usually obtained. No caustic effects on gingiva or mucosa result from contact with the paste; however, it is toxic if accidentally ingested.

*Fluoride solutions should be stored in plastic bottles to avoid reactions with the glass, which would cause deterioration of the solutions.

A modification of the fluoride treatment for hypersensitive teeth is the use of sodium silicofluoride.[36] A saturated watery solution (0.7% to 0.9%*) is applied for 5 minutes to the cervical areas and rubbed into the surface for 5 minutes. The patient may also use the solution at home. Results are said to be better than are those with the sodium fluoride paste.

For use in the dental office, stannous fluoride prophylactic paste containing 8.9% stannous fluoride in the mixture has been introduced and seems to have desensitizing properties when used in prophylaxis.[37] Such preparations are available commercially.

Iontophoresis has also been used in the obtunding of hypersensitive exposed root surfaces.[38-41] Watery sodium fluoride solutions (1% to 2%) are the electrolytes used. Low-voltage batteries creating a galvanic current of fractions of 1 ma. are employed. The appliances are so used that a sable brush serves as the cathode, which is wetted with the fluoride solution and brought into contact with the sensitive root surface. The desensitization achieved by iontophoresis is the result of stimulation of secondary dentin formation by the current.[37] Acidulated phosphofluoride solutions have also been employed.

Corticoids have been used in periodontal practice with some success for the desensitization of exposed root surfaces.[42]

***Home care procedures***

Home care procedures may include the use of a paraformaldehyde tooth powder (2%) of the following formula:

| | (%) |
|---|---|
| Trioxmethylene (paraformaldehyde) | 2.0 |
| Calcium carbonate precipitate | 73.9 |
| Magnesium carbonate, light (U.S.P.) | 5.0 |
| Sodium bicarbonate (U.S.P.) | 10.0 |
| Castile soap powder (U.S.P.) | 5.0 |
| Saccharin soluble | 0.1 |
| Oil of peppermint | 3.0 |
| Methyl salicylate | 0.5 |
| Oil of cloves | 0.5 |

A toothpaste containing paraformaldehyde, the active ingredient of this powder, may give good results with prolonged use.[43] Another desensitizing toothpaste containing strontium chloride has also been used.[44] Reports of good results with sodium monofluorphosphate have been published.

Office treatments and home treatment often must be combined for best results. Office treatment may have to be repeated. Home treatment alone may produce desensitization after several weeks, but usually several methods must be tried before satisfactory results are obtained. Oftentimes diligent oral hygiene alone solves the problem.

# Halitosis

Fear of offending by bad breath is a powerful motivating force driving people to seek dental attention, perhaps third in importance after cosmetic considerations and pain. If a person has any doubts, he need only watch television to see a substantial number of commercials recommending mouthwashes that purport to prevent or cure this condition.

---

*Sodium silicofluoride is soluble in cold water up to 0.7%, in boiling water up to 0.9%.

Two terms appear in the literature—halitosis and fetor ex ore (fetor oris). Some authors make a distinction between the two: bad mouth odor not arising in the mouth is halitosis, and those odors that are caused orally are fetor ex ore.[45] This distinction does not seem to be important, and the term halitosis is used in this book for any kind of bad breath.

An important clinical feature of halitosis is that the offending person may be unaware of his condition. Howe stated in 1874 that "few of the afflicted persons detect the cause of their isolation."[46]

Attempts have been made to measure the intensity of bad breath by means of an instrument called an osmoscope,[47,48] and lately by spectrometer analysis and a titrilog,[49] which is an instrument capable of measuring volatile oxidizable sulfur components (hydrogen sulfide, methyl mercaptan, methyl disulfide), thought to be responsible for oral bad breath. A number of other instruments have also been employed for objective measurement of halitosis.

Breath comes from the lungs and is exhaled through bronchi, trachea, larynx, and nose or mouth. Therefore bad breath may arise in any of these areas, the lungs, the breathing passages, the nose, or the mouth. Among breath odors originating in the lungs are the smell of garlic and of alcohol. These odors are caused by the excretion into the lungs of the volatile oils flavoring these foods. Similarly there may be acetone on the breath of uncontrolled diabetics. In addition, bronchiectasis, advanced malignancy, and some other diseases in the respiratory tract may impart bad odor to the breath. There are furthermore a certain number of cases of bad breath due to conditions of the nose and the nasopharynx, for instance, chronic atrophic rhinitis (ozena), purulent sinusitis, and adenoids.

In the older writings diseases of the stomach and the gastrointestinal tract were also mentioned as possible causes.[46] However, such conditions are no longer considered to be etiologic factors for halitosis.

In the majority of cases, bad breath originates in the oral cavity; there it may be due to one of the following forms of tissue destruction: acute necrotizing ulcerative gingivitis, bad oral hygiene, advanced chronic periodontal disease, Plaut-Vincent's angina, open gangrenous pulps, and large unfilled cavities containing decomposing food remnants. Smoking imparts a characteristic odor offensive to many. Bad mouth odors are also found in the leukemias and the terminal stages of cirrhosis of the liver; these are due to the decomposition of blood oozing from the hemorrhagic gingiva.[50]

A rather common cause for halitosis is mouth breathing[51]; this habit prevents the mucosa and teeth from being washed and flushed with saliva and thereby interferes with the removal of squames, bacteria,[52] and their products. A specific microorganism responsible for bad breath has not been determined, however. A coated tongue may sometimes be the source of halitosis; and reduction of salivary flow in febrile diseases and old age often contributes heavily to bad breath. Other situations in which bad breath is often observed include morning breath and hunger breath. The latter condition is more strongly manifested the longer the time passed since the last meal. Some women have a characteristic bad breath during menstruation.[50]

A promising new drug, dimethyl sulfoxide (DMSO),[53] which seems to be quite effective in the treatment of rheumatic fever and a number of other diseases, gives the breath a characteristic unpleasant odor of not quite fresh oysters. DMSO can as yet be used only by qualified scientists in the United States although it is freely dispensed in Europe.

## Treatment

In view of the many etiologic factors causing or contributing to bad breath, the taking of good medical and dental history is essential. As stated before, keep in mind the possible systemic ramifications of this problem; however, the majority of cases will be seen to be caused by local oral factors.

Early extraction of broken down root stumps is recommended as well as the restoration of carious teeth. Strive for sufficiently wide embrasure spaces, well-contoured and well-polished restorations, removal of overhangs, and well-placed contact points. These measures will prevent food retention and the attending bad odors and irritation of the underlying gingiva. Furthermore, be sure to institute a regimen of good oral hygiene using a toothpaste. Brushing of teeth, gingivae, and tongue produces a sizable reduction of bad odor for 2 hours.[54] Several years ago claims were made touting chlorophyll toothpastes for use in halitosis; these claims have not been fully proved.

The use of mouthwashes may have a temporary effect in reducing halitosis. The Food and Drug Administration, however, citing a study of the National Academy of Sciences–National Research Council Drug Efficacy Group,[55] has advised manufacturers of nine brands of mouthwashes to stop using such advertising claims as "effectively destroys bacteria that cause bad breath in the mouth." The study had concluded that there was a lack of substantial evidence for such claims. These mouthwashes may be advertised as "aromatic mouth fresheners," "an aid to the daily care of the mouth," and "causing the mouth to feel clean."[56]

Antiseptic mouthwashes may help to reduce halitosis for as long as 2 to 3 hours.[48] However, the effect of proper personal periodontal care is in only small part the result of a masking effect. To a much greater degree it is the result of the friction of brushing, the removing of squames and their bacterial colonies, and the increased salivary flow due to flavoring agents. Prolonged use of so-called deodorants, such as sodium perborate or hydrogen peroxide, is discouraged because of the attending undesirable side effects, which include the possible production of a black hairy tongue. Mouth breathing and lack of lip seal should be stopped whenever possible. To do this, first establish whether an obstacle to normal respiration exists (e.g., deviated nasal septum or large adenoids). To combat the accompanying halitosis, suggest that the patient brush his teeth, gums, and tongue vigorously three times a day using a mild dentifrice and a mildly aromatic mouthwash. In older patients sometimes the use of sour lozenges not containing sugar may be suggested in the interval between brushing to increase salivary flow.

In conclusion, halitosis for objective as well as subjective reasons is most important to the patient. It may interfere with married life, dating, and business and social contacts. The dentist himself may offend his patients.[55,56] More important yet, bad breath may indicate the presence of an underlying systemic condition. Therefore, whenever local measures prove ineffective, the consultation of a competent internist is indicated.

**CHAPTER 25**

**References**

1. Hirschfeld, I.: The toothbrush; its use and abuse, Brooklyn, 1939, Dental Items of Interest Publishing Co.

2. Arnim, S. S.: Microcosms of the human mouth, J. Tenn. Dent. Ass. **39**:3, 1959.
3. Schultz-Haudt, S. D., Bruce, M. A., and Bibby, B. G.: Tissue-destructive products of gingival bacteria from non-specific gingivitis, J. Dent. Res. **33**:624, 1954.
4. Stahl, S. S., Wachtel, N., DeCastro, C., and Pelletier, G.: The effect of toothbrushing on the keratinization of the gingiva, J. Periodont. **24**:20, 1953.
5. Wilcox, C. E., and Everett, F. G.: Friction on the teeth and gingiva during mastication, J. Amer. Dent. Ass. **66**:513, 1963.
6. Egelberg, J.: Local effect of diet on plaque formation and development of gingivitis in dogs, Odont. Rev. **16**:50, 1965.
7. Lindhe, J., and Wicen, P. O.: The effect on the gingivae of chewing fibrous food, J. Periodont. Res. **4**:193, 1969.
8. Wade, A. B.: Effect on dental plaque of chewing apples, Dent. Pract. **21**:194, 1971.
9. Hartley, J. L.: Aspects of oral hygiene and emergency dental care for long-term space flight stomatologic evaluation, USAF-NASA nutrition study, 1966.
10. Arnim, S. S.: The use of disclosing agents for measuring tooth cleanliness, J. Periodont. **34**:227, 1963.
11. Everett, F. G., and Passmore, D. J.: Mirror as an aid to toothbrushing and oral physiotherapy, J. West. Soc. Periodont. **6**:104, 1958.
12. Parfitt, G. J.: Cleansing the subgingival space, J. Periodont. **34**:133, 1963.
13. Smith, J. H., O'Connor, T. W., and Radentz, W.: Oral hygiene of the interdental area, Periodontics **1**:204, 1963.
14. Bass, C. C.: Optimum characteristics of dental floss for personal oral hygiene, Dent. Items Interest **70**:921, 1948.
15. Goldman, H. M.: Effect of single and multiple toothbrushing in the cleansing of the normal and periodontally involved dentition, Oral Surg. **9**:203, 1956.
16. Stanmeyer, W. R.: Measure of tissue response to frequency of toothbrushing, J. Periodont. **28**:17, 1957.
17. Kimmelman, B. J.: Teaching two toothbrushing techniques: observations and comparisons, J. Periodont. **39**:36, 1968.
18. Everett, F. G., and Kunkel, P. W., Sr.: Abrasion through the abuse of dental floss, J. Periodont. **24**:186, 1953.
19. Löe, H., Greene, J. C., Arnim, S. S., and Ariado, A.: How frequently must patients carry out effective oral hygiene procedures in order to maintain gingival health? J. Periodont. **42**:309, 1971.
20. Hine, M. K., Jr., Wachtl, C., and Fosdick, L. S.: Some observations on the cleansing effect of nylon and bristle toothbrushes, J. Periodont. **25**:183, 1954.
21. Bass, C. C.: The optimum characteristics of toothbrushes for personal oral hygiene, Dent. Items Interest **70**:696, 1948.
21a. Gilson, C. M., Charbeneau, G. T., and Hill, H. C.: A comparison of physical properties of several soft toothbrushes, J. Mich. Dent. Ass. **51**:347, 1969.
22. Puckett, J. B.: Bristles in hand-manipulated toothbrushes, J. Periodont. **41**:398, 1970.
23. Bechlem, D. N., Saxe, S. R., and Stern, I. B.: A histologic study of the effect upon the gingivae of using an electric toothbrush in the presence of marginal periodontitis, Periodontics **3**:90, 1965.
24. Talbot, E. S.: Interstitial gingivitis, Philadelphia, 1899, S.S. White Dental Mfg. Co.
25. Stillman, P. R., and McCall, J. O.: A textbook of clinical periodontia, ed. 2, New York, 1937, The Macmillan Co.
26. Charters, W. J.: Proper home care of the mouth, J. Periodont. **19**:136, 1948.
27. Aronovitz, R., and Conroy, C. W.: Effectiveness of the automatic toothbrush for handicapped persons, Amer. J. Phys. Med. **48**:193, 1969.
27a. Jefopoulos, T.: Dentifrices, Park Ridge, N. J., 1970, Noyes Data Corp.
28. Everett, F. G., and Bettman, M. M.: Mouth rinsing, J. Periodont. **23**:213, 1952.
29. Crumley, P. J., and Sumner, C. F.: Effectiveness of a water pressure cleansing device, Periodontics **3**:193, 1965.
30. Krajewski, J. J., Robach, W. C., and Higgenbotham, T. L.: Current status of water pressure cleansing in oral hygiene, J. Calif. Dent. Ass. **42**:433, 1966.
31. Everett, F. G., Hall, W. B., and Phatak, N. M.: Treatment of hypersensitive dentin, J. Oral Ther. **2**:300, 1966.
32. Grossman, L. E.: The treatment of hypersensitive dentin, J. Amer. Dent. Ass. **22**:592, 1935.

33. Gottlieb, B.: Technique of impregnation for caries prophylaxis, J. Missouri Dent. Ass. **28**:366, 1948.
34. Lukomsky, E. H.: Fluorine therapy for exposed dentin and alveolar atrophy, J. Dent. Res. **20**:649, 1941.
35. Hoyt, W. H., and Bibby, B. G.: Use of sodium fluoride for desensitizing dentin, J. Amer. Dent. Ass. **30**:1372, 1943.
36. Bhatia, H. L.: Use of sodium silicofluoride as a desensitizing agent for exposed sensitive cementum and cervical dentin, Bur **54**:4, 1953.
37. Bixler, D., and Muhler, J. C.: Effect of dental caries in children in a nonfluoride area: combined use of three agents containing stannous fluoride: a prophylactic paste, a solution, and a dentifrice, J. Amer. Dent. Ass. **68**:792, 1964.
38. Siemon, W. H.: A new approach in solving the problem of hypersensitivity and postoperative distress in dentin and cementum, J. Conn. Dent. Ass. **34**:5, 1960.
39. Schlegel, P. L., Stowell, E. C., and Emmerson, C. C.: The influence of an electrical potential on topically applied fluorides, J. S. Calif. Dent. Ass. **30**:321, 1962.
40. Jensen, A. L.: Hypersensitivity controlled by iontophoresis, J. Amer. Dent. Ass. **68**:216, 1964.
41. Lefkowitz, W., Burdick, H. C., and Moore, D. L.: Desensitization of dentin by bioelectric induction of secondary dentin, J. Prosth. Dent. **13**:940, 1963.
42. Bowers, G. M., and Elliott, J. R.: Topical use of prednisolone in periodontics, J. Periodont. **35**:486, 1964.
43. Toto, P. D., Staffileno, H., and Gargiulo, A. W.: A clinical evaluation of a desensitizing toothpaste, J. Periodont. **29**:192, 1958.
44. Ross, M. R.: Hypersensitive teeth: effect of strontium chloride in a compatible dentifrice, J. Periodont. **32**:49, 1961.
45. Crohn, B. B., and Drosd, R.: Halitosis, J.A.M.A. **117**:2242, 1941.
46. Howe, J. W.: The breath and diseases which give it a fetid odor, New York, 1874, Appleton-Century.
47. Brening, R. H., Sulser, G. F., and Fosdick, J. S.: Determination of halitosis by use of osmoscope and cryoscopic methods, J. Dent. Res. **18**:127, 1939.
48. Morris, P. P., and Read, R. R.: Halitosis, J. Dent. Res. **28**:324, 1949.
49. Richter, V. J., and Tonzetich, J.: The application of instrumental technique for the evaluation of odoriferous volatiles from saliva and breath, Arch. Oral Biol. **9**:47, 1964.
50. Massler, M., Emslie, R. D., and Bolden, T. E.: Fetor ex ore, Oral Surg. **4**:110, 1951.
51. Fox, N., and Kesel, R. G.: Hyperplastic sino-pharyngitis, Arch. Otolaryng. **42**:368, 1945.
52. Berg, M., and Fosdick, L. S.: Studies in periodontal disease. II. Putrefactive organisms in the mouth, J. Dent. Res. **25**:73, 1946.
53. Kutscher, A. H., Zegarelli, E. V., and Everett, F. G.: DMSO in stomatologic research, Ann. N. Y. Acad. Sci. **141**:465, 1967.
54. Sulser, R. H., Lesney, T. A., and Fosdick, L. S.: Reduction of breath and mouth odors by means of brushing teeth, J. Dent. Res. **19**:193, 1940.
55. Everett, F. G.: Halitosis, Oregon Dent. J. **41**:13, 1971.
56. Morgenroth, J.: Ueber den Foetor ex ore, Deutsch. Zahnaerztl. Z. **20**:67, 1966.
57. Möller, I. J.: Dental fluorose og caries, Copenhagen, 1965, Rhodos, International Science & Art Publishers.
58. Ericsson, T. and Ericsson, Y.: Effect of partial fluorine substitution on the phosphate exchange and protein absorption of hydroxyapatite, Helv. Odont. Acta **11**:10, 1967.
59. Glantz, P.-O.: On wettability and adhesiveness, Odont. Rev., vol. 20, supp. 17, 1969.
60. Bibby, B. G., and Van Kestern, M.: The effect of fluorine on mouth bacteria, J. Dent. Res. **19**:391, 1940.
61. Keyes, P. H., Rowberry, S. A., Englander, H. R., and Fitzgerald, R. J.: Bio-assays of medicaments for the control of dentobacterial plaque, dental caries and periodontal lesions in Syrian hamsters, J. Oral Ther. **3**:157, 1966.
62. Koch, G., and Lindhe, J.: The effect of supervised oral hygiene on the gingiva of children, J. Periodont. Res. **2**:64, 1967.
63. Theilade, J., and Fitzgerald, R. J.: Dental calculus in the rat: effect of diet and erythromycin, Acta Odont. Scand. **21**:571, 1963.
64. Draus, F. J., Leung, S. W., and Miklos, F.: Towards a chemical inhibition of calculus, Dent. Progr. **3**:79, 1963.
65. Schaffer, E. W., Schindler, C. H., and McHugh, R. B.: The effects of two ion exchange resins on the inhibition of calculus-like deposits in vitro, J. Periodont. **35**:296, 1964.

66. Bowen, W. H.: The prevention or control of dental plaque. In McHugh, W. D., editor: Dental plaque, Edinburgh, 1970, E & S Livingstone, Ltd.
67. Littleton, N. W., and White, C. L.: Dental findings from a preliminary study of children receiving extended antibiotic therapy, J. Amer. Dent. Ass. **68**:520, 1964.
68. Mühlemann, H. R., Meyer, R. W., König, K. G., and Marthaler, T. M.: The cariostatic effect of some antibacterial compounds in animal experimentation, Helv. Odont. Acta **5**:18, 1961.
69. Löe, H., Theilade, E., Jensen, S. B., and Rindom Schiött, C.: Experimental gingivitis in man, J. Periodont. Res. **2**:282, 1967.
70. McCormick, M. H., Stark, W. M., Pittenger, G. E., Pittenger, R. C., and McGuire, J. M.: Vancomycin, a new antibiotic. I. Chemical and biologic properties, Antibiot. Ann., p. 606, 1956.
71. Jordan, D. C., and Mallory, H. D. C.: Site of action of vancomycin and Staphylococcus aureus, Antimicrob. Agents Chemother. **4**:489, 1964.
72. Armstrong, P. J., and Hunt, D. E.: In vitro evaluation of actinobolin as an antibiotic for the treatment of periodontal disease, I.A.D.R. abstract no. 142, 1971.
73. Volpe, A. R., Schulman, S. M., Goldman, H. M., King, W. J., and Kupczak, L. J.: The long term effect of an antimicrobial formulation on dental calculus formation, J. Periodont. **41**:463, 1970.
74. Stallard, R. E., Volpe, A. R., Orban, J. E., and King, W. J.: The effect of an antimicrobial mouthrinse on dental plaque, calculus and gingivitis, J. Periodont. **40**:683, 1969.
75. Hazen, S. P., Rokita, J., and Volpe, A. R.: Histologic study of a potential plaque inhibiting agent, I.A.D.R. abstract no. 285, 1971.
76. McFall, W. T., Shoulars, H. W., and Carnevale, R. A.: Effect of vancomycin in the inhibition of bacterial plaque formation, I.A.D.R. abstract no. 46, 1968.
77. Jensen, S. B., Löe, H., Rindom Schiött, C., and Theilade, E.: Experimental gingivitis in man. IV. Vancomycin induced changes in bacterial plaque, J. Periodont. Res. **3**:284, 1968.
78. Fitzgerald, R. J., Spinell, D. M., and Stoudt, T. H.: Enzymatic removal of artificial plaques, Arch. Oral Biol. **13**:125, 1968.
79. Fitzgerald, R. J., Keyes, P. H., Standt, T. H., and Spinell, D. M.: The effects of a dextranase preparation on plaque and caries in hamsters. A preliminary report, J. Amer. Dent. Ass. **76**: 301, 1968.
80. König, K. G., and Guggenheim, B.: In vivo effects of dextranase on plaque and caries, Helv. Odont. Acta **12**:48, 1968.
81. Jensen, S. B., and Löe, H.: The effect of dextranase on plaque and gingivitis in man. In The prevention of periodontal disease, proceedings of a European symposium, London, 1971, Henry Kimpton.
82. Lobene, R. R.: A clinical study on the effect of dextranase on human dental plaque, J. Amer. Dent. Ass. **82**:132, 1971.
83. Caldwell, R. C., Sandham, H. J., Mann, W. V., Jr., Finn, S. B., and Formicola, A. J.: The effect of a dextranase mouthwash on dental plaque in young adults and children, J. Amer. Dent. Ass. **82**:124, 1971.
84. Nyman, S., Lindhe, J., and Jansson, J.-C.: The effect of a bacterial dextranase on human dental plaque formation and gingivitis development, Odont. Rev. In press.
85. Dossenbach, W. F., and Mühlemann, H. R.: Effect of penicillin and ricinoleate on early calculus formation, Helv. Odont. Acta **5**:25, 1961.
86. Hanke, M. T.: Studies on the local factor in dental caries. I. Destruction of plaques and retardation of bacterial growth in the oral cavity, J. Amer. Dent. Ass. **27**:1379, 1940.
87. Strålfors, A.: Disinfection of dental plaques in man. In Mühlemann, H. R., and König, H. G., editors: Caries symposium, proceedings of an international symposium (Zurich), Berne, 1961, Hans Huber Medical Publisher.
88. Renggli, H.: Zahnbeläge und gingivale Entzündung unter dem Einfluss eines Antibakteriellen Mundspülmittels, Zurich, 1966, K. Schippert.
89. Schroeder, H. E.: Formation and inhibition of dental calculus, Berne, 1969, Hans Huber Medical Publisher.
90. Löe, H., and Rindom Schiött, C.: The effect of mouthrinses and topical application of chlorhexidine on the development of dental plaque and gingivitis in man, J. Periodont. Res. **5**:79, 1970.
91. Rindom Schiött, C., Löe, H., Jensen, S. B., Kilian, M., Davies, R. M., and Glavind, K.: The effect of chlorhexidine mouthrinses on the human oral flora, J. Periodont. Res. **5**:84, 1970.

92. Gjermo, P., Baastad, K. L., and Rölla, G.: The plaque-inhibiting capacity of eleven anti- and salivary mucins, J. Periodont. Res. 5:90, 1970.
bacterial compounds, J. Periodont. Res. 5:102, 1970.
93. Rölla, G., Löe, H., and Rindom Schiött, C.: The affinity of chlorhexidine for hydroxyapatite
94. Lindhe, J., Hamp, S.-E., Löe, H., and Rindom Schiött, C.: Influence of topical application of chlorhexidine on chronic gingivitis and gingival wound healing in the dog, Scand. J. Dent. Res. 78:471, 1970.
95. Löe, H., and Rindom Schiött, C.: In International conference on periodontal research, J. Periodont. Res., supp. 4, p. 38, 1969.
96. Turesky, S., Glickman, I., and Sandberg, R.: Chemical inhibition of in vitro plaque formation, I.A.D.R. abstract no. 143, 1971.
97. Davies, R. M., Jensen, S. B., Rindom Schiött, C., and Löe, H.: The effect of topical application of chlorhexidine on the bacterial colonization of the teeth and gingiva, J. Periodont. Res. 5:69, 1970.

**Additional suggested reading**

Arnim, S. S.: Effect of thorough mouth cleansing on oral health, Periodontics 6:41, 1968.
Ash, M. M., Jr.: A review of the problems and results of studies on manual and power tooth brushes, J. Periodont. 35:202, 1964.
Baer, C., and Baer, P. N.: Story of the toothpick, J. Periodont. 37:158, 1966.
Ball, D. M., and Ball, E. L., Jr.: Comparative effectiveness of two mouthwashes used after gingivectomy, J. Periodont. 38:395, 1967.
Chace, R., Robinson, R. E., and Gottsegen, R.: What are the most effective methods of controlling hypersensitivity of teeth following periodontal therapy? Peridont. Abs. 13:10, 1965.
Chasens, A. I., and Marcus, R. W.: Evaluation of the comparative effectiveness of manual and automatic toothbrushes in maintaining the periodontal patient, J. Periodont. 39:156, 1968.
Dabelsteen, I.: Om elektriske tandborster, Tandlaegebladet 68:257, 1964.
Derbyshire, J. C., and Mankodi, S. M.: Gingival keratinization with hand and electric toothbrushes; a cytological comparison, J. Amer. Dent. Ass. 68:255, 1964.
Editorial: Manual toothbrushes are not obsolete, J. Amer. Dent. Ass. 68:279, 1964.
Fanning, E. A., and Henning, F. R.: Toothbrush design and its relation to oral health, Aust. Dent. J. 12:464, 1967.
Geist, H.: Halitosis in ancient literature, Dent. Abstr. 2:417, 1957.
Graham, C. J.: Home care effectiveness upon planed teeth and scaled teeth following surgery, J. Periodont. 37:43, 1966.
Harrington, J. H., and Terry, I. A.: Automatic and hand tooth brushing abrasion studies, J. Amer. Dent. Ass. 68:343, 1964.
Iwersen, A. E., and Werking, D. H.: Hand and automatic tooth brushes, J. Amer. Dent. Ass. 68:178, 1964.
Lobene, R. R.: Effect of an automatic toothbrush on gingival health, J. Periodont. 35:137, 1964.
Lobene, R. R.: Evaluation of altered gingival health from permissive powered toothbrushing, J. Amer. Dent. Ass. 69:585, 1964.
Rainey, B. L.: A clinical study of short stroke reciprocating action electric toothbrush, J. Periodont. 35:455, 1964.
Reilly, E. B.: Halitosis, New Zeal. Dent. J. 59:129, 1963.
Rost, A.: Histologische Pulpauntersuchungen bei Zahnhals Hypersensibiltät, Deutsch. Zahnaerztl. Z. 22:680, 1967.
Smith, B. A., and Ash, M. M., Jr.: Evaluation of a desensitizing dentifrice, J. Amer. Dent. Ass. 68:639, 1964.
Smith, B. A., and Ash, M. M., Jr.: A study of a desensitizing dentifrice and gingival hypersensitivity, J. Periodont. 35:222, 1964.
Soparkar, P. M., and Quigley, G. A.: Power versus handbrushing; effect on gingivitis, J. Amer. Dent. Ass. 68:182, 1964.
Spouge, J. D.: Halitosis: a review of its causes and treatment, Dent. Pract. 14:307, 1964.
Stookey, G. K., Hudson, J. R., and Muhler, J. C.: Polishing properties of zirconium silicate on enamel, J. Periodont. 37:200, 1966.

CHAPTER TWENTY-SIX

# Preparations for periodontal surgery



## PREOPERATIVE EVALUATION

Sometime before undertaking surgery (approximately a week), the dentist should reexamine the medical and dental history of the patient. The initial charting should be reviewed and a new evaluation made to determine any changes in pocket depth as a result of prior root planing, curettage, and oral hygiene instruction. The patient's ability to care for his mouth should be carefully evaluated. Tooth sensitivity should be noted, and measures should be taken to control it.

### Examination

Presurgical examination includes recharting to evaluate changes in pocket depth and to note the form, contour, color, and texture of the gingiva.

*General indications for surgery*

The general indications for surgery are the presence of pockets and unphysiologic gingival form. Specific indications are discussed in appropriate chapters on surgical procedures.

*General contra-indications*

Surgery may be contraindicated in patients with certain organic or metabolic diseases (Addison's disease, poorly controlled diabetes, severe cardiac disease, hemorrhagic problems) and in those patients who have responded poorly to previous surgery. In addition, patients with a high caries index may be poor risks when cemental areas are exposed after surgery. When systemic or bleeding problems are present or anticoagulant therapy is being administered, consultation with a physician and appropriate laboratory tests are mandatory.

*Emotional status of the patient*

In selecting the best treatment for the patient, the dentist should also consider the patient's emotional status. When the patient feels threatened by proposed surgery, alternative treatment may be indicated.

*Aesthetics*

Any surgery should be approached cautiously when the patient is wary of aesthetic deformity that may be caused by the apical displacement of the gingival margins.

*Poor home dental care*

Finally, the patient who is unwilling or unable to perform properly the measures for oral hygiene is a poor candidate for surgical procedures. The seeds for future recurrence of the disease are present in this situation.

## Planning

If surgery is indicated, presurgical evaluation should be made. The area to be operated on, the type and extent of surgery, and the steps common for the procedure should be carefully planned. All this should be noted in the patient's treatment record. The patient should be advised of the plans for the forthcoming surgery so that he may fit them in with his social or business schedule and so that the dentist can deal with any anxiety.

*Premedication*

Premedication should be given when indicated. It may include the administration of antibiotics to patients with valvular heart disease or other conditions requiring antibiotics. In such cases the medication should be started 24 hours before surgery to provide adequate levels. Antibiotic medication should be adequate in amount and should be continued for several days after surgery.

*Apprehension*

Anxiety or apprehension is present in most patients who are facing surgery. At times verbal reassurance is all that is needed to allay anxiety. At other times premedication with a tranquilizer or barbiturate may be indicated. Premedication may be given at the time of surgery. Currently, intramuscular or intravenous administration or scopolamine or meperidine-antihistamine combinations are widely used. If oral or intramuscular premedication is used in the office, it should be administered 30 to 45 minutes before local anesthetic injections. If the premedication, anesthesia, or postmedication given may affect the patient's ability to drive or to care for himself properly, preparations should be made for the patient to have adequate transportation and care.

At the time of surgery, the surgeon should resurvey the operative site for the purpose of familiarization.

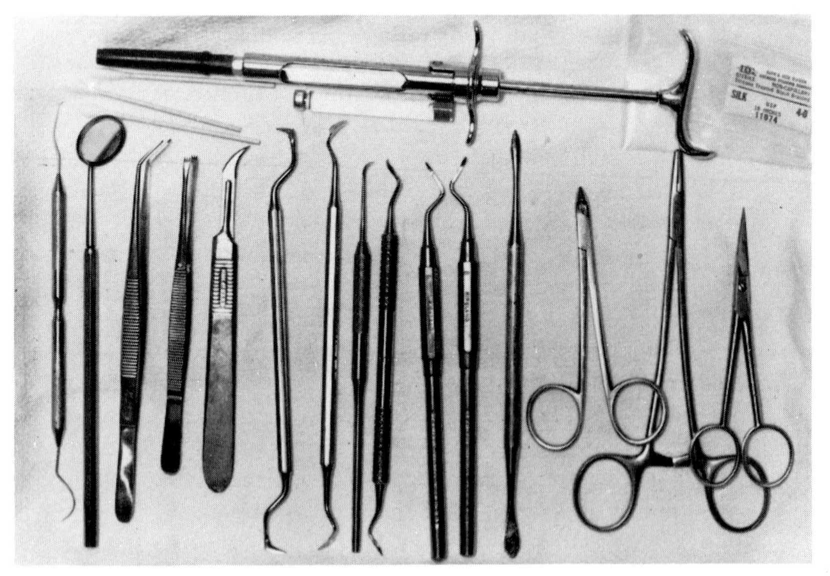

**Fig. 26-1.** Surgical tray containing instruments most commonly used in flap and gingivectomy procedures. From left to right, the tray holds explorer, mirror, cotton forceps, tissue forceps, scalpel with no. 12 removable blade, interdental knife and kidney-shaped knife, hawk-beaked anterior curette, double-ended posterior curette, Kirkland nos. 8 and 9 soft tissue curettes, periosteal elevator, soft tissue rongeurs, needle holder, serrated tissue scissors, suture, anesthetic syringe, sponges, and applicators.

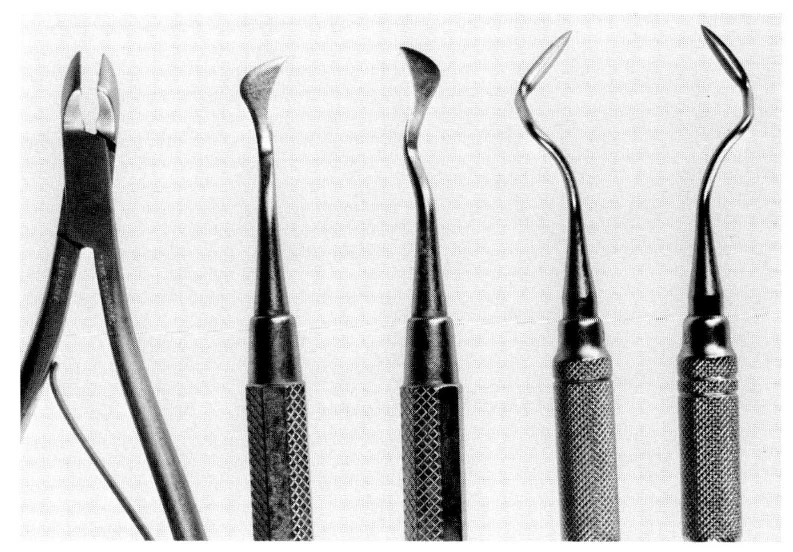

**Fig. 26-2.** Periodontal scalpels (knives) and soft tissue rongeurs.

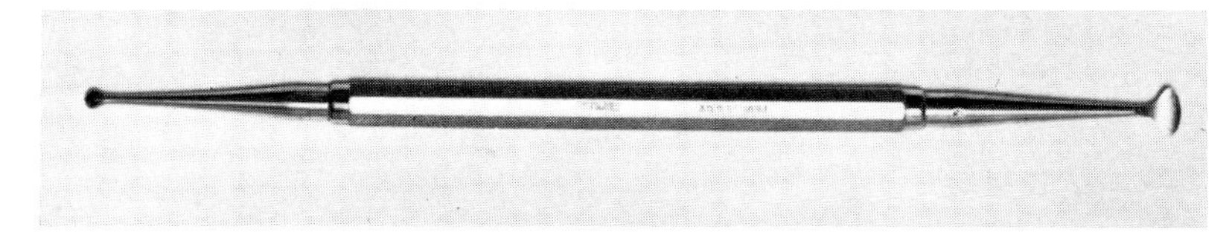

**Fig. 26-3.** Double-ended Molt curette for obtaining cortical bone for grafts and transplants.

Before the anesthetic is given, the surgeon and assistant must scrub. The patient's partial dentures, eyeglasses, earrings, or other items that may interfere with surgery should be removed to a safe and convenient place. The patient should be suitably draped. Sterile technique, including rubber gloves, is recommended.

***Instruments***

Surgical trays (Figs. 26-1 and 26-2) containing those instruments for an indicated procedure are recommended. The tray should be placed in a position that is readily accessible to the dentist and his assistant. The tray may be placed above and in front of the patient, out of the patient's view, or behind the patient so that no instruments are visible. In addition to the surgical instruments, a good supply of suction tips, mirrors, retractors, and gauze sponges should be at hand. Other instruments for special procedures should be kept in sterile packs, readily accessible for use (Figs. 26-3 and 26-4).

***Local anesthetic***

An anesthetic may then be given. Local infiltration and block anesthesia are the methods of choice. Standard techniques of dosage and administration should be used. After the initial administration it may be desirable to inject a drop of anesthetic directly into the interdental papilla. This is particularly useful in gingivectomy. It makes the gingiva firmer and easier to incise and has a hemostatic effect because of the vasoconstrictor in the anesthetic solution.

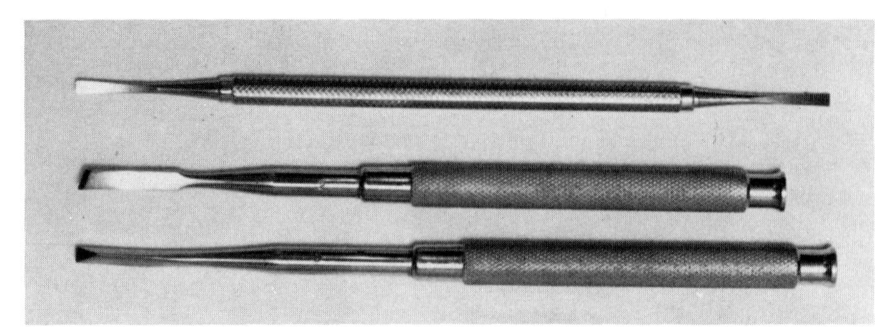

**Fig. 26-4. Bone chisels used in osseous surgery for bone grafts.**

*Pocket marking*

When gingivectomy is to be performed, pocket depth should be marked to permit precise planning of the incisions. This may be done with a pocket-marking forceps or with a millimeter probe and an explorer, which will create a bleeding point that can be seen by the clinician. Bleeding points should be placed on the facial and interdental areas on both the buccal and lingual surfaces. Pocket marking is not necessary in flaps or mucogingival procedures.

Once premedication and a local anesthetic have been given, the patient should not be left alone. The assistant or the dentist should be present.

*Communications*

During the operation verbal instructions to the assistant should be worded to avoid creating anxiety. Requests for instruments and other materials should be made in a professional manner or by signals to maintain a calm atmosphere. Careless orders, remarks, angry glances, or unnecessarily rapid movements are alarming to the patient and may result in a tense and unsatisfactory atmosphere. The patient may interpret such events to mean the operation is progressing poorly.

## SURGICAL ASSISTANT

The assistant is an active participant in all surgical procedures.[1] He serves as a second pair of hands for the dentist. It is his duty to aspirate, to retract, to pass and retrieve instruments, and to cleanse the surgical surface with water spray. The assistant should explain to the patient in brief, simple, and nonalarming terms the use of the aspirator so that the patient will not be apprehensive when the machine is used. The assistant should also inform the patient that, if his muscles tire from holding his mouth open, he will be given the opportunity to close his mouth and rest. Adroit explanation will properly prepare the patient for surgery and permit the operation to progress smoothly.

### Lighting of surgical field

It should be the function of the assistant to control the lighting so that the operative field is adequately illuminated at all times. The dental spotlight may be posititoned to provide proper illumination. In certain cases a small intraoral spotlight or headlamp may be necessary to provide additional lighting.

### Retraction for surgery

It should also be the duty of the assistant to retract the lips, cheeks, and tongue to permit adequate access for the therapist and to facilitate the surgical procedures. Retraction may be accomplished with a no. 4 mouth mirror, which can be used to hold the tongue away (Fig. 26-5) and to distend the cheek (Fig.

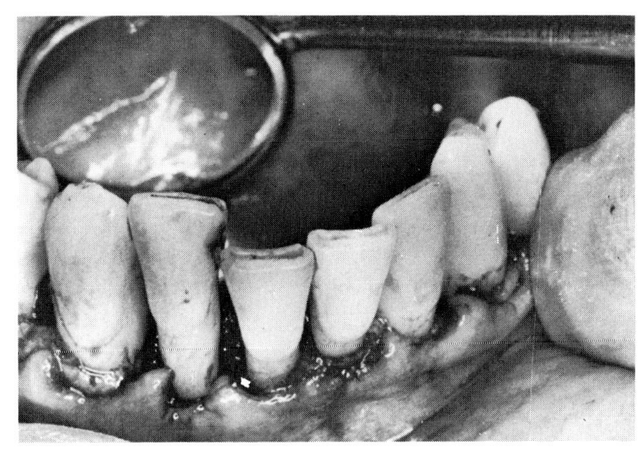

**Fig. 26-5.** Use the no. 4 mouth mirror to retract the tongue.

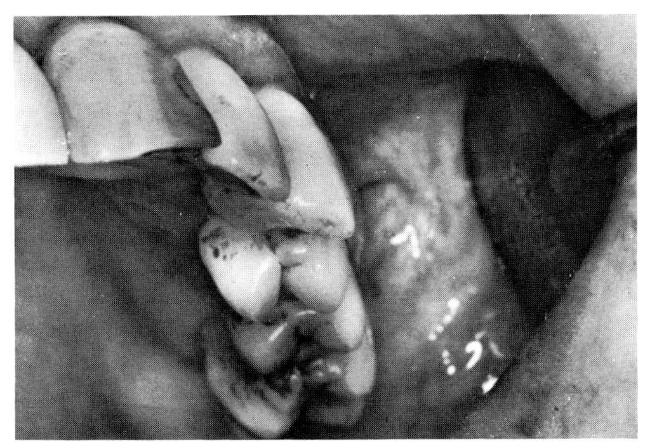

**Fig. 26-6.** Use the no. 4 mouth mirror to retract the cheek.

26-6). Also the assistant may use a finger placed in the vestibule to retract the cheek. The aspirator tip, in addition to keeping the field clear of blood and saliva, may occasionally be used to keep the tongue from the field of surgery (Fig. 26-7). The assistant may sometimes be responsible for retracting flaps while osseous surgery is being performed. Various instruments are used to retract flaps, including the periostome and tissue retractors (Figs. 26-8 to 26-10).

## Protection of cheek, lips, and tongue

Protection of cheek, lips, and tongue is especially important when surgical burs, stones, or chisels are used (Fig. 26-11). A mirror, a periostome, cheek retractors, or a surgical aspirator tip should be kept between the cheek or tongue and the revolving bur or other surgical instrument.

## Removing fluids and debris

The assistant will use an aspirator to remove blood, oral secretions, and water or saline solution spray. The size and shape of the aspirator tip used will de-

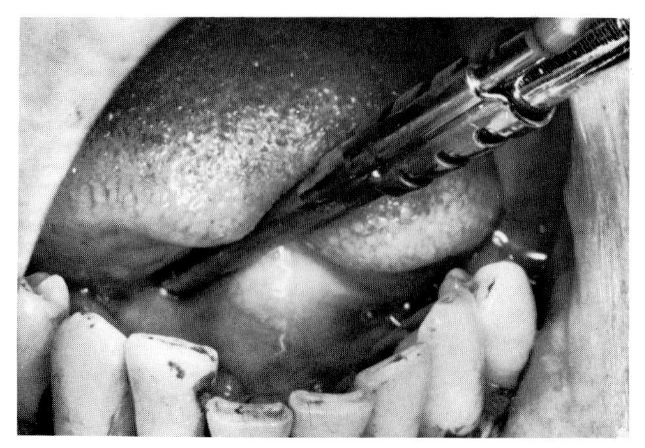

Fig. 26-7. Use the aspirator tip to keep the tongue away from the surgical field.

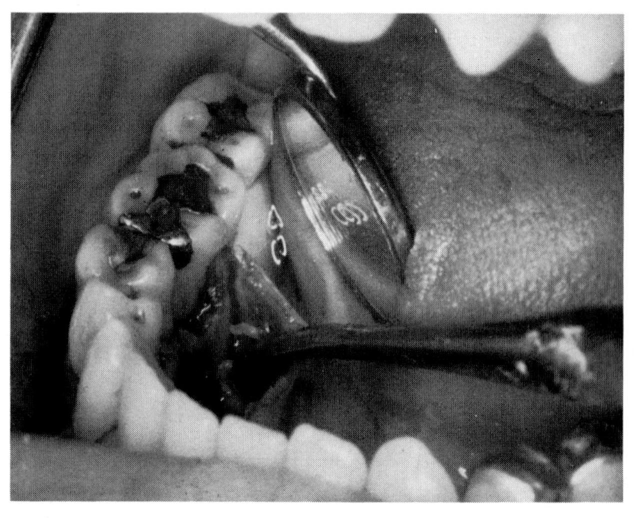

Fig. 26-8. Use the mirror to retract the tongue and reflect light. With the aspirator tip, aspirate, retract the flap, and protect the tongue and sublingual tissues during instrumentation.

pend on the type of instrument and on the specific requirements of the surgical intervention. In general, it is desirable to have both a small and a larger tip available. A device that incorporates the spray on the tip of the aspirator is desirable (Fig. 26-12). The assistant may control the device by a foot pedal. The spray cleanses the surgical field of blood and removes small pieces of tissue loosened by the curette or scalpel. Flakes of calculus are also removed. Small bits of excised tissue, blood, and debris may be lifted from the end of surgical instruments by a touching motion with the aspirator tip (Fig. 26-13). A saliva ejector is not desirable since it occupies space, is inconvenient, and is not under direct control of the assistant or the dentist. Proper surgical aspiration can adequately remove fluids and debris from the mouth.

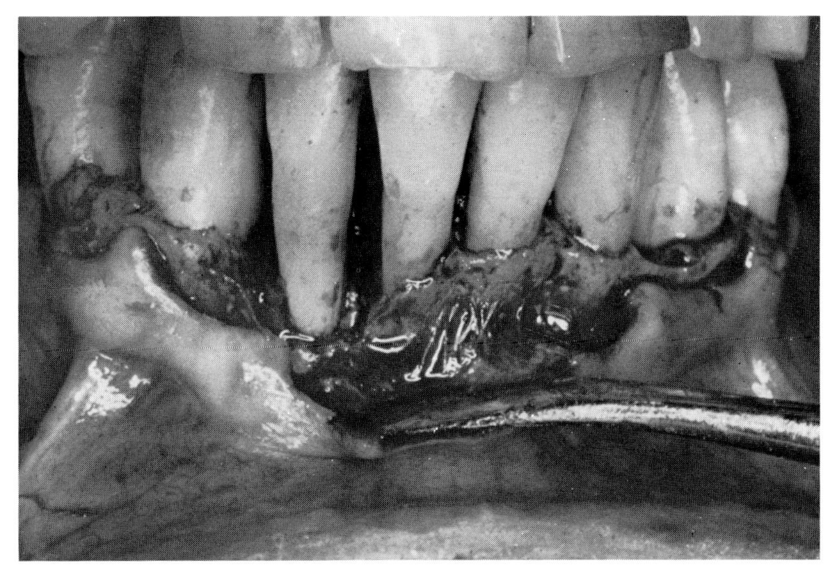

**Fig. 26-9.** The assistant retracts a full-thickness modified flap with a periosteal elevator.

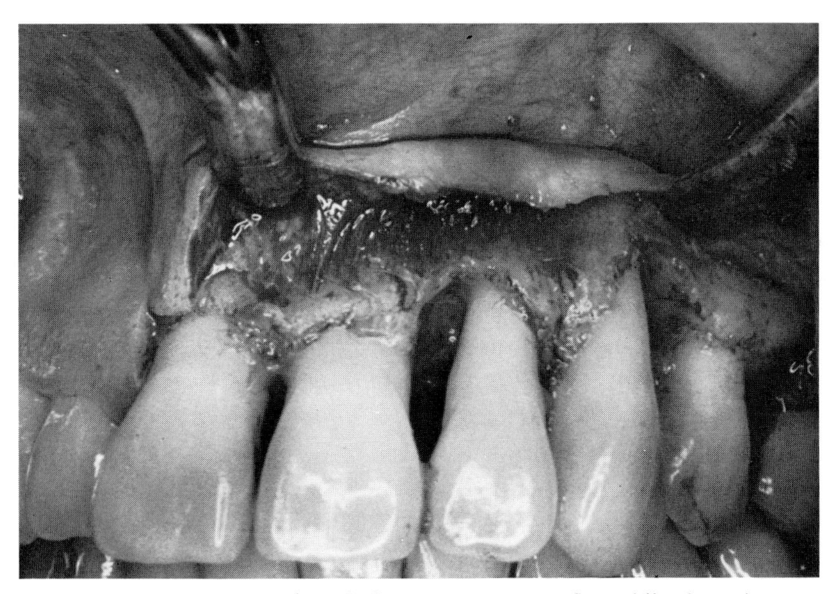

**Fig. 26-10.** The surgeon uses a periosteal elevator to retract a flap while the assistant uses the tip of the aspirator to retract and aspirate.

## Control of bleeding

On completion of the surgery, before suturing or applying the dressing, the assistant may carry out measures to control bleeding (when indicated) and to permit conclusion of the operating procedure. Bleeding may be controlled by sponges (Fig. 26-14). Capillary bleeding can be controlled by pressure; arterial bleeding requires suturing. Bleeding on incision may be more profuse and may diminish as the operation progresses. The dentist may at times apply local

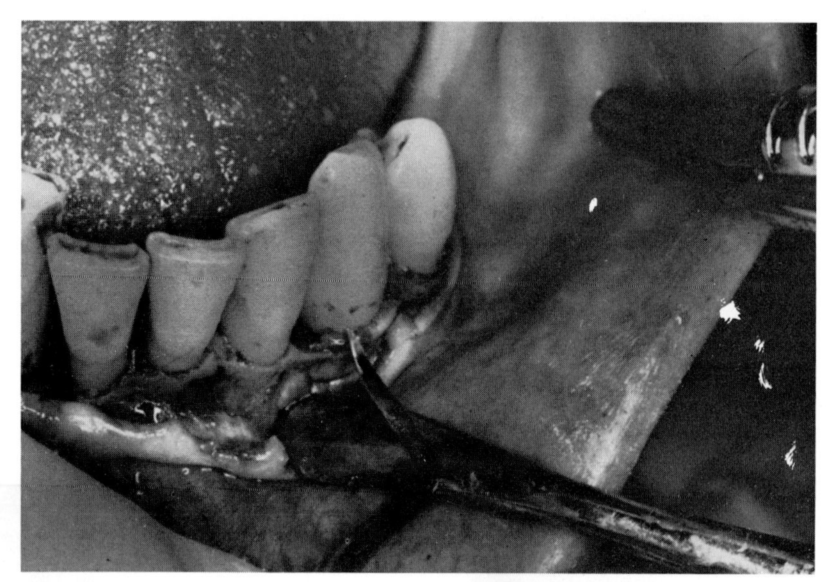

**Fig. 26-11.** Use the aspirator tip to distend the cheek to provide better access for instrumentation during surgery.

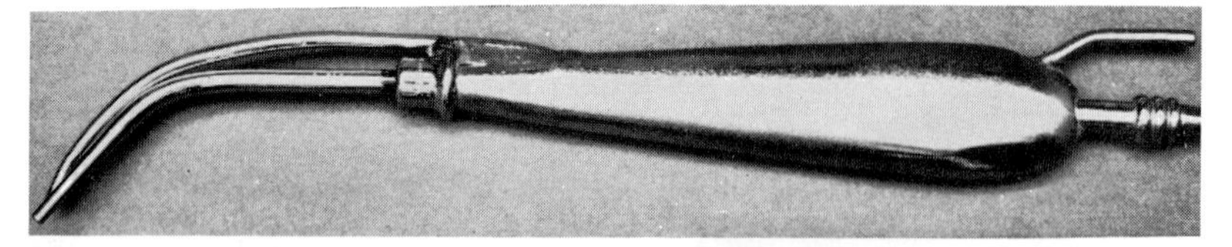

**Fig. 26-12.** Suction-spray equipment. (Courtesy C. L. Foss, San Diego.)

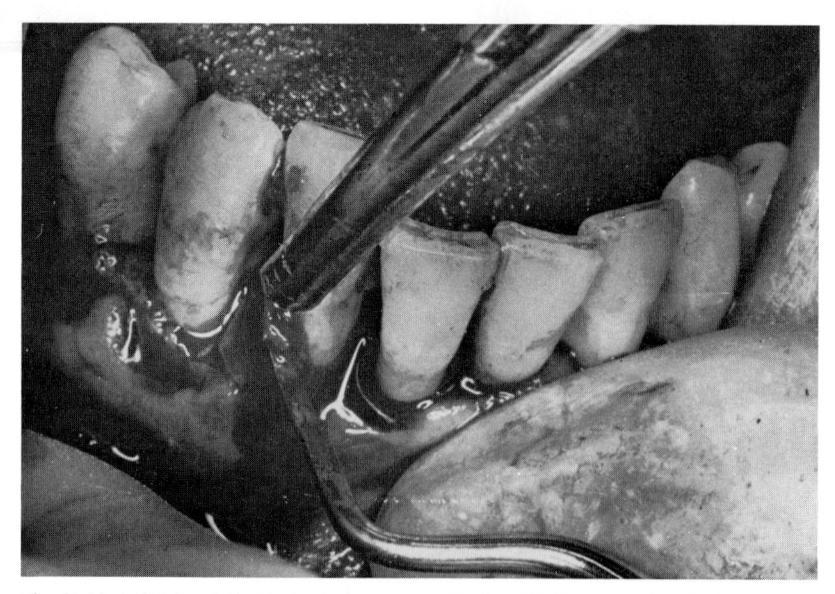

**Fig. 26-13.** Lift bits of tissue from the curette blade with the aspirator during surgery.

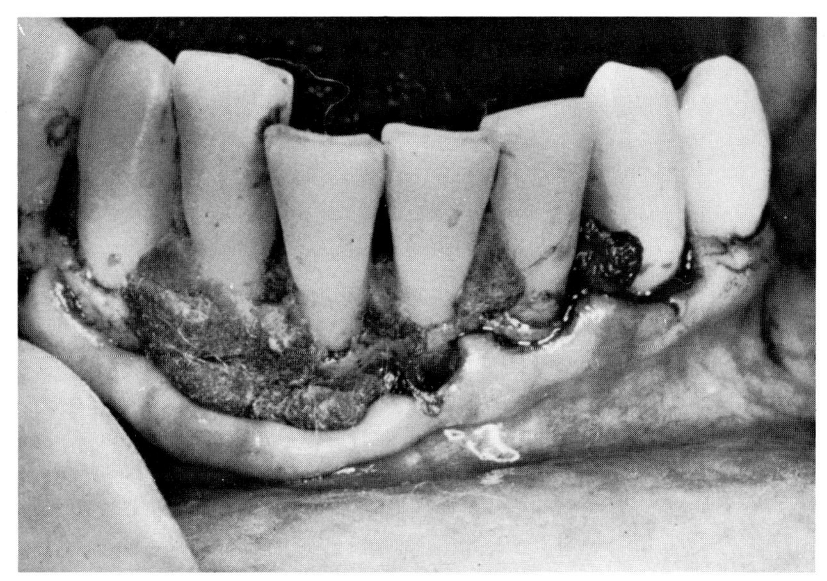

**Fig. 26-14.** Use sponges and cotton pellets to control bleeding prior to osseous corrections.

hemostatic pellets (1:1000 Adrenalin chloride solution) under pressure to control hemorrhage (Fig. 26-14). Usually a wait of 3 to 5 minutes will then permit the surgery to proceed without excessive bleeding.

### Suturing

Flaps may now be sutured. This procedure alone may achieve hemostasis. A dressing may be applied. When needed, a dressing is placed to cover the wound surface. During suturing the efforts of the assistant are extremely important. Assisting with the placement of sutures is a highly developed art. The assistant usually holds the loose end of the suture to prevent it from being drawn out of the tissue. In addition, he uses the other hand to retract the cheek or lip. He may also support the flaps with a tissue forceps so that the needle can be more easily passed through. After the tie is made, the surgeon retracts the lips, cheek, or tongue and extends the suture while the assistant cuts the ends. (See discussion on suturing in Chapter 29.)

### Postoperative appointment

After the operation the assistant takes the patient to the desk and gives instructions to the secretary for the date and time of the postoperative appointment.

## PERIODONTAL DRESSINGS

Periodontal dressings are used to cover and protect wound surfaces after surgery. They are cementlike in character and shield the incised tissues from irritation by foods, air, tongue or cheek movements, etc.

Several types of dressings are available:

1. Zinc oxide–eugenol base dressings
2. Ready-mix dressings (Peripak [De Trey])
   (These do not contain eugenol. The ingredients are calcium sulfate, zinc oxide, acrylate, and corrigents for taste and color.)

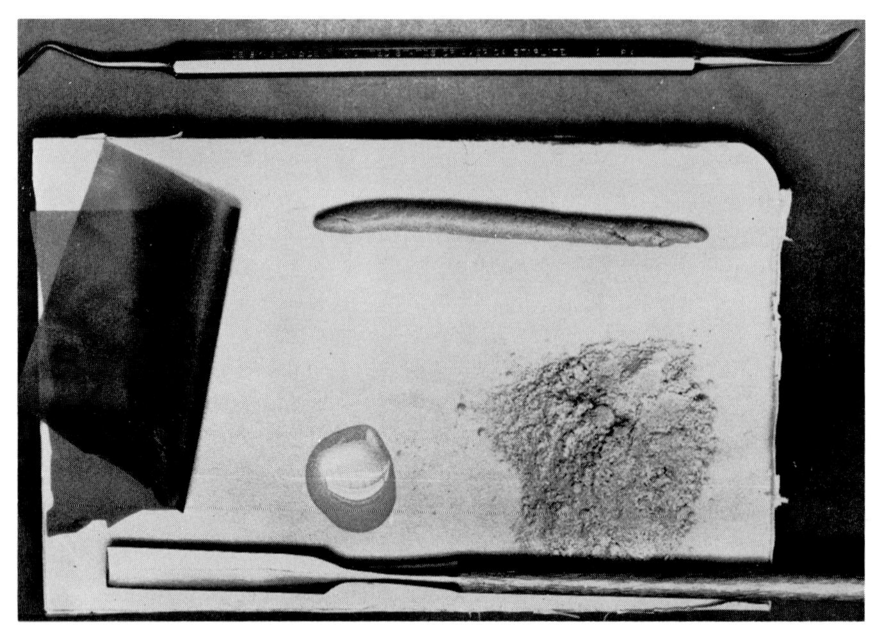

**Fig. 26-15.** Waxed-paper pad and instruments for mixing and applying surgical dressing.

3. Rosins
4. Combinations of water-soluble metallic oxides and nonionizing carboxylic acids (Coe Pak)
   (These do not contain eugenol.)
5. Fat-base dressings.

The zinc oxide–eugenol base dressings are most commonly used and are marketed commercially. A widely used formula follows:

| *Powder* | *(%)* |
|---|---|
| Zinc oxide | 43.5 |
| Rosin | 45.0 |
| Kaolin | 3.0 |
| Fine asbestos fibers | 4.0 |
| Tannic acid (powdered) | 3.0 |
| Zinc acetate (powdered) | 1.5 |
| *Liquid* | *(%)* |
| Eugenol | 85.0 |
| Cottonseed oil | 14.0 |
| Thymol | 1.0 |

The powder and liquid are mixed to a semidry, firm, puttylike consistency. The dressing may be applied directly (Fig. 26-15) or stored by refrigeration for future use. In applying the dressing, divide the mass into small wedges for interproximal placement and into strips for application to buccal and lingual wound surfaces. If sutures are present, cover the cut ends with Gelfoam to prevent their incorporation into the pack. Apply the strips to the wound surface and gently knead them into interproximal spaces to connect the buccal and lingual segments. A moistened cotton swab may be used to shape the mass after application. The dressing should cover the wound but should not interfere with full jaw closure and tooth articulation. Impingement on motile tissues may cause painful ulcerations. (In other words, the dressing should be muscle trimmed.)

*Other types*

Considerable work has been done on the compounding and testing of periodontal dressings. One type (Coe Pak) is easily applied and leaves a smooth nonirritating surface. It cannot be prepared in advance for storage. Noneugenol formulas[2,3] are believed to be less irritating to bone, although this belief has been challenged.[4] Another noneugenol formula (Baer et al.[5]) follows:

| | |
|---|---|
| *Powder* | |
| Rosin | 0.52 gm. |
| Zinc oxide | 0.41 gm. |
| Bacitracin | 3000 units |
| *Liquid* | *(%)* |
| Zinc oxide | 5 |
| Hydrogenated fat | 95 |

Thermoplastic materials and oral adhesives are also marketed.[6] A liquid application dressing is reported to be advantageous in healing,[7] but it is not yet available commercially.

The possible advantages of bacteriocidal and bacteriostatic drugs in dressings have not been fully investigated. Sensitization, allergy, and candidiasis should be considered when they are used.[8]

Some periodontists use no dressing when flaps are coapted and sutured. When reattachment operations and bone grafts are attempted, tinfoil, Telfa, or Adaptic may be placed over the suture wound before placement of the pack.

## POSTOPERATIVE PERIOD

### Instructions

After the completion of suturing and the placing of any dressings, the assistant should give the patient postoperative instructions and any prescriptions that the doctor may have written. It is wise to prepare the postoperative instructions on a printed sheet since the patient may forget it only verbal instructions are given. An example of such a printed sheet is shown in the box. After surgery has been completed, the patient's face should be washed and the patient conducted from the operating room by the assistant.

**POSTOPERATIVE INSTRUCTIONS TO PATIENT AFTER PERIODONTAL SURGERY**

1. Do not eat or drink for 2 hours after surgery.
2. Do not investigate the dressing with tongue or fingers. This dressing serves as a bandage to protect the wound.
3. Avoid tart or spicy foods.
4. Drink fruit juices with a straw.
5. If the dressing breaks or falls off, call the doctor. As an emergency measure the wound may be covered with Orabase or paraffin.
6. For postoperative comfort, take pills per instructions in the prescription given you.
7. Brush unoperated parts of mouth. Brush only the biting surfaces of the teeth where surgery was performed. Be sure to brush!
8. Rinse the mouth carefully after eating. Clean the outside of the dressing with a moistened cotton swab.

In emergency, call the doctor!

Dr. ________________, D.D.S.
Telephone: ________________

*Diet*

The patient should be instructed to avoid tart or spicy foods since these may cause pain. Fruit juices should be taken by straw for the same reason. As a rule, a normal diet may be adequate; but, when dietary supplements such as vitamins are indicated, these should be prescribed.

## Medication

Postoperative medication for pain, sedation, hemorrhage, swelling, or infection may be needed. Analgesics and narcotics are used for relief of pain. Depending on the degree of pain, aspirin, Darvon compound-65 or codeine may be prescribed. Dosage of aspirin is usually two 5-grain tablets every 3 hours, with smaller doses for children. Darvon compound-65 is given, one or two Pulvules every 4 hours as needed. Empirin compound no. 3 (with ¾ grain of codeine) is usually prescribed, one tablet every 4 hours as needed. Patients on anticoagulant therapy should not be given aspirin. Tylenol may be prescribed.

*Pain*

In cases of severe pain, meperidine hydrochloride (Demerol) may be administered intramuscularly (50 or 100 mg.) or orally in 50 mg. tablets every 4 hours.

*Sedation*

Sedation after surgery may be prescribed for those patients who are anxious or apprehensive, or when postsurgical pain warrants. Tranquilizers or barbiturates are most frequently prescribed. Meprobamate, 200 or 400 mg., one or two tablets q.i.d., may be used or librium, 5 or 10 mg., one capsule t.i.d. Phenobarbital, 0.016 Gm. b.i.d., may be prescribed when tranquilizers are contraindicated.

*Bleeding*

Postsurgical bleeding at home can usually be controlled by local measures, unless it is arterial. Lavage, pressure packs, or a wet tea bag (tannic acid) as a rule are adequate. When the patient cannot control the bleeding, he should be seen promptly by the doctor. Steps to be taken at this time follow:

1. Cleanse the wound.
2. Find the area of bleeding.
3. Ligate, apply pressure, or use electrocautery as appropriate.
4. Apply oxidized cellulose (Oxycel) on the wound with pressure.

*Swelling*

Swelling after surgery is best prevented by the use of ice packs. After swelling develops, hot moist packs and frequent lavage with warm saline solution are preferred. Digestive and bacterial enzymes such as trypsin (Tryptar), papain (Papase, Ananase), streptokinase-streptodornase (Varidase) are often helpful in reducing edema. When these enzymes are used, it is advisable to protect the patient with antibiotics to reduce the possibility of spread of infection. Not all postoperative swelling is caused by inflammation alone; some swelling may be caused by bleeding into tissues. This may occur after flap operations and be accompanied by discoloration under the cheek or eye.

*Antibiotics*

Antibiotics may be prescribed after surgery to treat or to prevent infections. They are used regularly when bone grafts or reattachments operations are performed. Their routine use after all periodontal surgery has been advised.[9-11] Broad-spectrum antibotics are recommended, and sound pharmacologic principles should be followed in all prescriptions.

## Cleaning and sterilizing

After the patient is dismissed, the operating room must be carefully cleaned and inspected. Surgical instruments are taken to a sterilizing area where all instruments may be washed, sharpened, and autoclaved. The equipment in the operating room is washed and disinfected, particularly the handle of the dental spotlight, the chair controls, and handles of the handpiece, Cavitron, aspirator tubing, and water spray controls.

## Records

A full report of the operation (including number of sutures) and medications should be made in the patient's chart.


**CHAPTER 26**

**References**

1. Prichard, J. F.: Advanced periodontal disease; surgical and prosthetic management, ed. 2, Philadelphia, 1972, W. B. Saunders Co.
2. Eberle, P., and Mühlemann, H. R.: Ein neuer Parodontal-Verband, Schweiz. Mschr. Zahnheilk. **69**:1095, 1959.
3. Rateitschak, K. H., Graf, H., and Guldener, P.: Periodontal pack without eugenol, J. Periodont. **35**:290, 1964.
4. Frisch, J., and Bhaskar, S. N.: Tissue response to eugenol-containing dressings, J. Periodont. **38**:402, 1967.
5. Baer, P. N., Sumner, C. F., III, and Scigliano, J.: Studies on a hydrogenated fat-zinc bacitracin periodontal dressing, Oral Surg. **13**:494, 1960.
6. Ewen, S. J.: Periodontal uses of a tissue adhesive, J. Periodont. **38**:138, 1967.
7. Bhaskar, S. N., and Frisch, J.: Use of cyanoacrylate adhesives in dentistry, J. Amer. Dent. Ass. **77**:831, 1969.
8. Fraleigh, C. M.: An evaluation of topical Terramycin in postgingivectomy pack, J. Periodont. **27**:201, 1956.
9. Collings, C. K., and Redden, D. R.: Further studies on the experimental production of periodontitis in dogs, J. Periodont. **30**:284, 1959.
10. Vargas, B., Collings, C. K., Polter, L., and Haberman, S.: Effects of certain factors on bacteremias resulting from gingival resection, J. Periodont. **30**:196, 1959.
11. Schafer, T. J., Collings, C. K., Bishop, J. G., and Dorman, H. L.: Antibiotics on healing following osseous contouring in dogs, Periodontics **2**:243, 1964.

**Additional suggested reading**

Prichard, J. F.: The advantages of periodontal surgery with local anesthetic agents: report of 100 cases, J. Periodont. **41**:502, 1970.

CHAPTER TWENTY-SEVEN

# Gingival curettage—curettage of the pocket wall



Gingival curettage is a planned and systematic operation to remove some or all of the ulcerated, chronically inflamed gingival lining of a pocket.

## OBJECTIVES

To be successful, gingival curettage must be based on well-understood indications, deliberate objectives, and a disciplined procedure. The objectives are ultimately those of all periodontal treatment: to eliminate inflammation, to eradicate pockets, and to restore gingival health. More specifically, gingival curettage is frequently used to reduce clinical edema, hyperemia, or cyanosis and to cause a shrinkage of the free gingiva. The elimination of inflammation and the eradication of some or all of the gingival pocket may thereby be accomplished. Frequently this leaves a physiologic gingival contour so that further surgery is unnecessary.

The procedure (called by some soft tissue curettage) should be differentiated from root planing, which is the instrumentation applied to the tooth surface to divest the surface of calcareous deposits and to smooth it. The procedure also should be differentiated from subgingival curettage and from surgical curettage by flap, which are procedures used in reattachment operations and intentionally extend to alveolar bone. The term *curettage,* as used herein, will refer only to the treatment afforded the soft tissue side of gingival or periodontal pockets. Pioneers in the field used it more frequently and more extensively than any other procedure, with the exception of root planing.[1,2]

## INDICATIONS AND CONTRAINDICATIONS

In some instances gingival curettage may be done simultaneously with root planing. In others, when a gingival inflammation persists after careful and thorough root planing, the operator may attempt to curette the diseased lining of the pocket to reduce inflammation and to encourage a shrinkage of the margin of the gingiva. In general, patients with edematous and granulomatous inflammations respond better to curettage than do those with conditions characterized primarily by fibrous hyperplasia. This treatment may also be valuable in patients in whom more extensive surgery is contraindicated because of emotional resistance or systemic impairment.

The presence of long-standing fibrosis is a contraindication to curettage when shrinkage of the marginal gingiva is the aim. Wide or tortuous intra-alveolar pockets are not amenable to gingival curettage. Bony craters are treated by osseous procedures or bone grafts.

## METHOD

Gingival curettage attempts to cut or strip the lining of the pocket and to remove subjacent inflammatory tissue. Since this is a surgical procedure, local anesthesia (topical, conduction, or infiltration) should be administered. The surgeon should plan to operate around a single tooth or a segment of the arch at one sitting. Whether he can do this will depend on the accessibility and topography of the pockets and the character of the tissue. He should not attempt to curette thin, friable gingiva. The danger of perforating or tearing such tissue would be too great. He should hold the instrument in a modified pen grasp, using the third or fourth finger as a rest. He should cut rather than tear or mutilate the soft tissue pocket wall. Placement of the thumb and index finger against the buccolabial or lingual surface of the gingiva during instrumentation will support the tissue and aid in performing the curettage. Using a definite pattern and short strokes, he should bring the diseased tissue to the surface and each time wipe the blade of the curette clean with sterile gauze. After curettage he should wash the pockets with sterile normal saline solution, using a Luer-Lok syringe with a blunt (25-gauge) needle, and should inspect the surgical area to be sure that complete debridement of the root surfaces has been achieved. Tissues should be approximated carefully to the tooth surface and, where necessary, a surgical dressing applied. Within 2 weeks he may be able to evaluate results and to determine the possible need for further treatment.

*Armamentarium*

Many periodontists have sets of curettes to be used only on soft tissue. These instruments are kept exquisitely sharp. They are delicate in construction, with thin blades to enter narrow, deep, and circuitous pockets. This armamentarium frequently is obtained by altering standard curettes to the operator's desires. The use of a curette in gingival curettage is illustrated in Fig. 27-1.

In Fig. 27-2, *A*, an interproximal area can be seen. Calculus extends to the bottom of the pocket on both teeth. The soft tissue side of the pocket is lined with epithelium of varying thickness, ulcerated in some areas. Epithelial strands project into the lamina propria, where plasma cells, some lymphocytes, macrophages, and a few polymorphonuclear leukocytes can be seen close to the bottom of the pocket. Chronically inflamed gingival connective tissue consists mainly of plasma cells, proliferating epithelial strands, and some fibrous connective tissue elements and ground substance.

To eliminate such a pocket by gingival curettage, the surgeon should first remove all calculus by root planing (Fig. 27-2, *B*). When the root surface is thoroughly planed and smooth, he should remove the pocket lining and some of the inflammatory tissue by curettage *(C)*. The result of tissue shrinkage after curettage is illustrated diagrammatically in *D*.

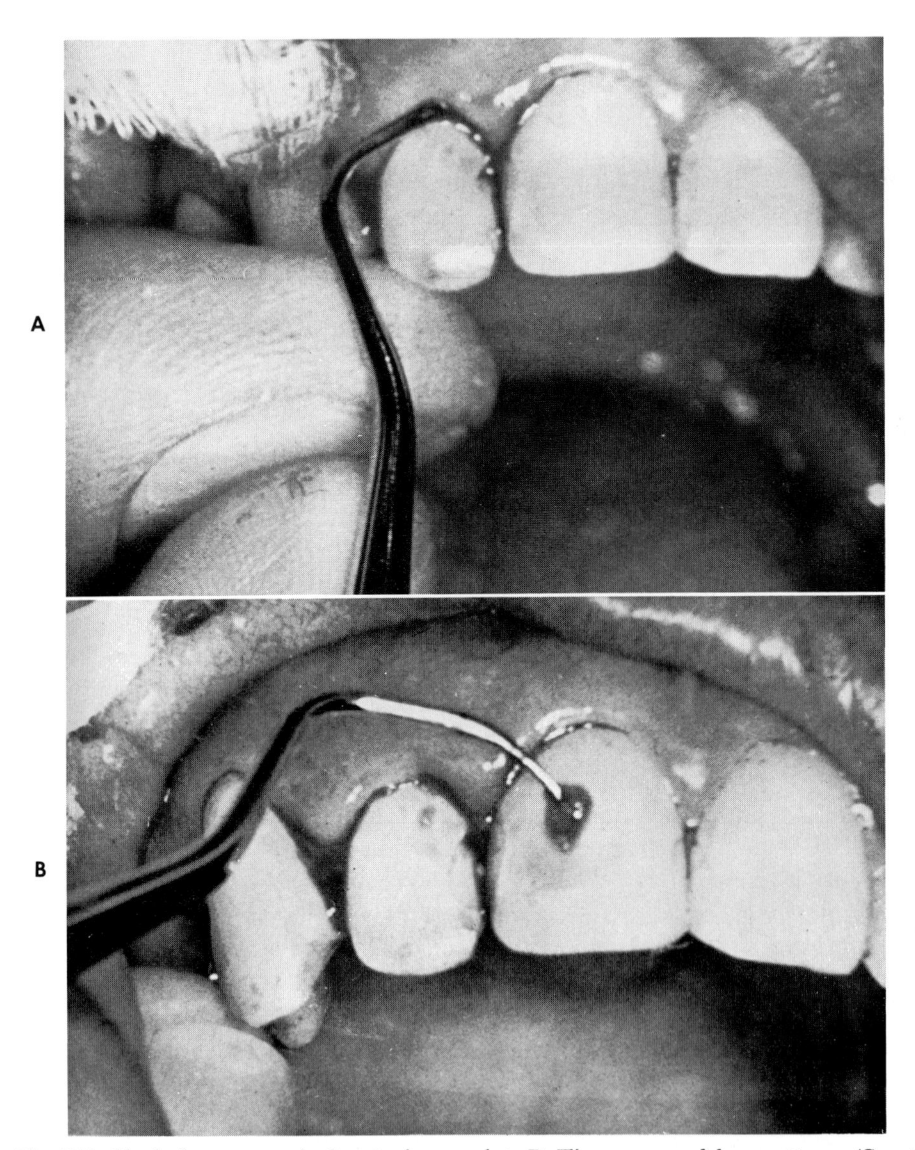


**Fig. 27-1.** Gingival curettage. **A,** Curette in a pocket. **B,** Tissue removed by curettage. (Courtesy E. Robinson, San Francisco.)

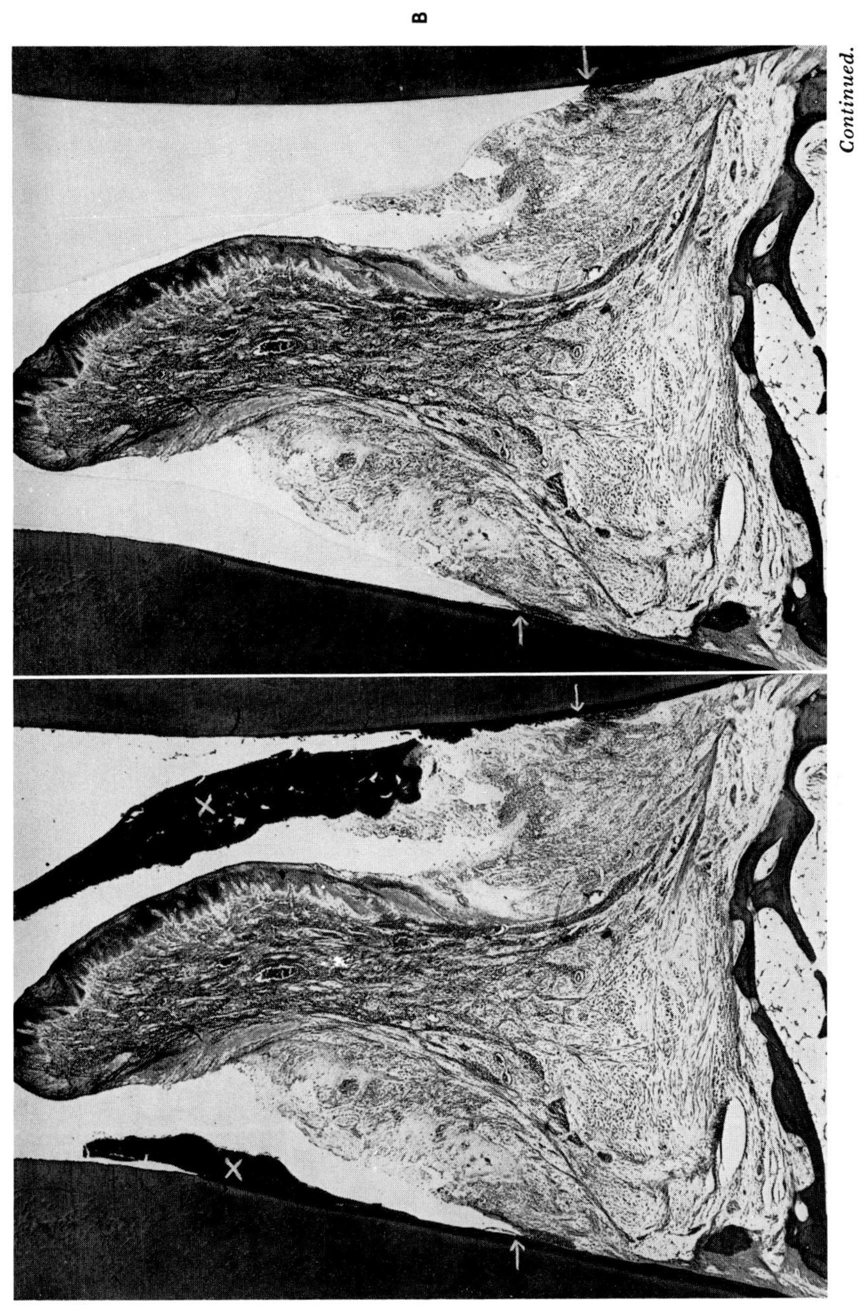


**Fig. 27-2.** **A,** Severe periodontitis in an interproximal area. *x,* Calculus. Arrows designate bottom of the pockets. **B,** After calculus removed by root planing. *Continued.*

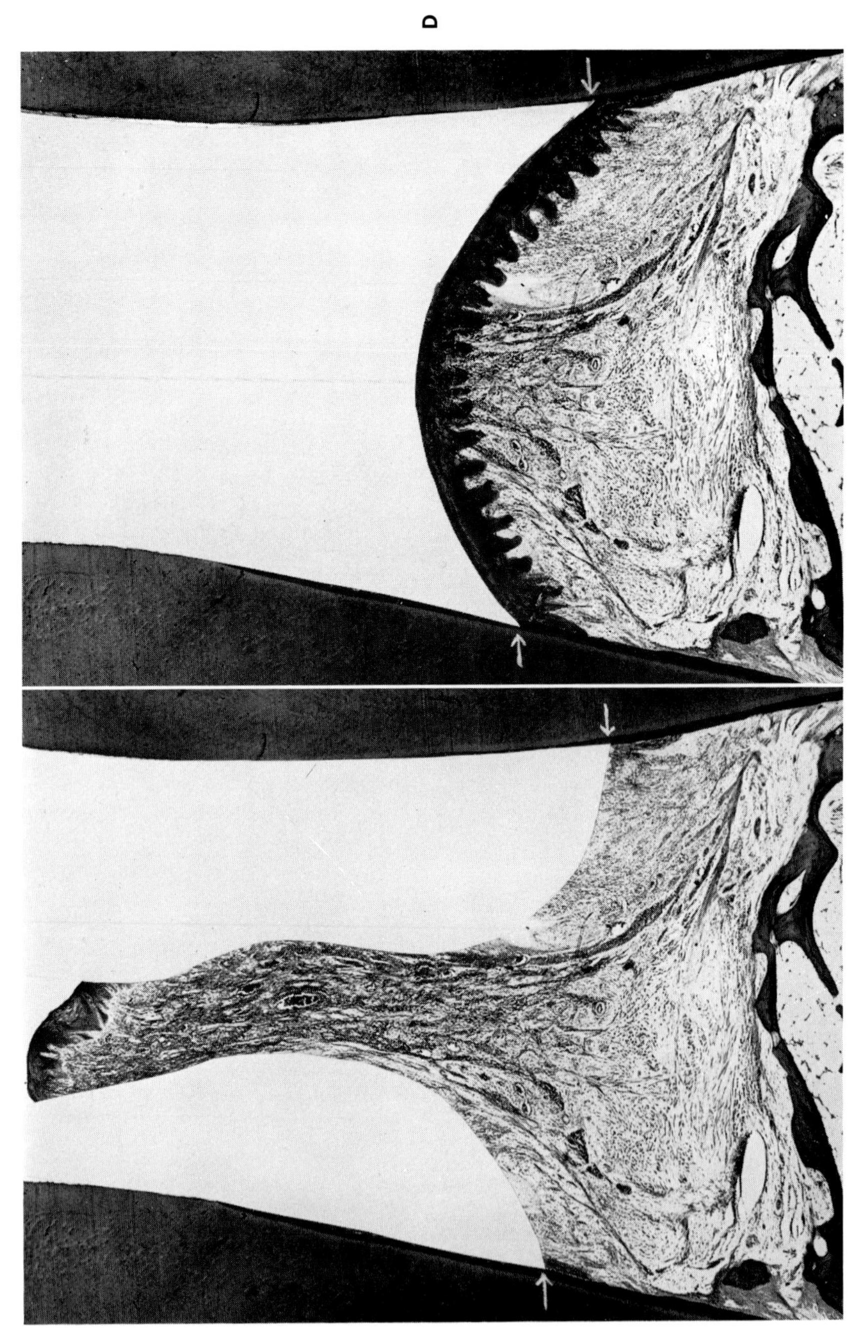


**Fig. 27-2, cont'd. C,** Pocket lining removed by curettage. **D,** Tissue shrinkage and healing as expected after gingival curettage. (Retouched.)

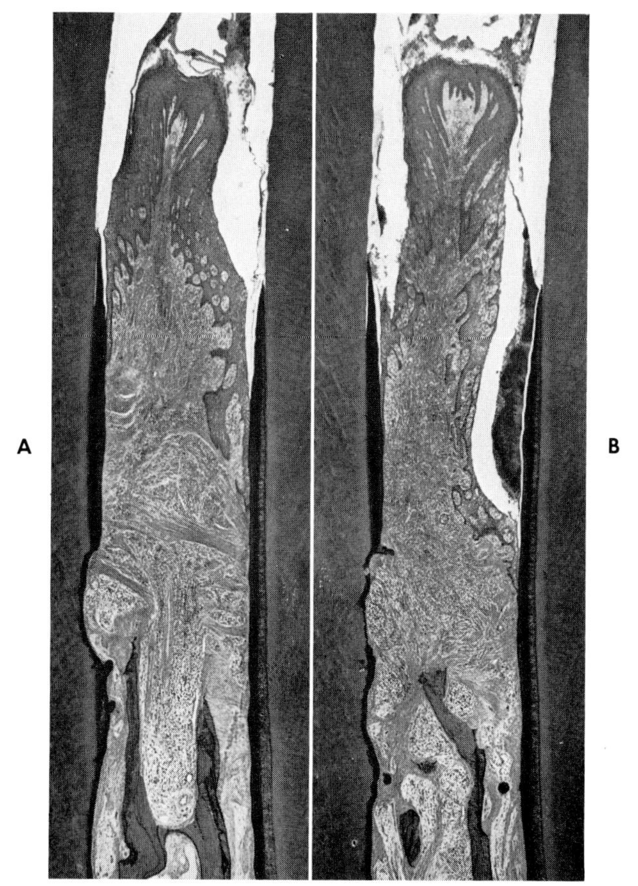


**Fig. 27-3.** Two histologic sections of the same interproximal area in a patient with periodontitis. **A,** Labially located section. **B,** More centrally located section. The inflammatory process extends into the bone marrow spaces.

## Granulation tissue

The connective tissue alongside and directly beneath the periodontal pocket is usually chronically inflamed (Figs. 27-3 and 27-4). This chronically inflamed connective tissue has been called granulation tissue. It was thought to be infected,[3-7] and its removal in treatment was recommended. However, the term granulation tissue is a misnomer in this case. Granulation tissue is found in healing wounds and is composed of fibroblasts and proliferating capillaries, which also give it a granular appearance. With healing, granulation tissue reforms into a normal fibrous connective tissue.

## Chronic inflammatory tissue

On the other hand, the chronically inflamed tissue near the pocket cannot proceed to complete healing. It is unable to isolate and remove the irritants, which lie outside the tissue, in the pocket. The chronic inflammatory tissue is not infected, however.[7] If the irritants are removed, it will reform into a fibrous connective tissue. Many clinicians prefer to remove the chronic inflammatory tissue during gingival curettage in the belief that more rapid healing will ensue.

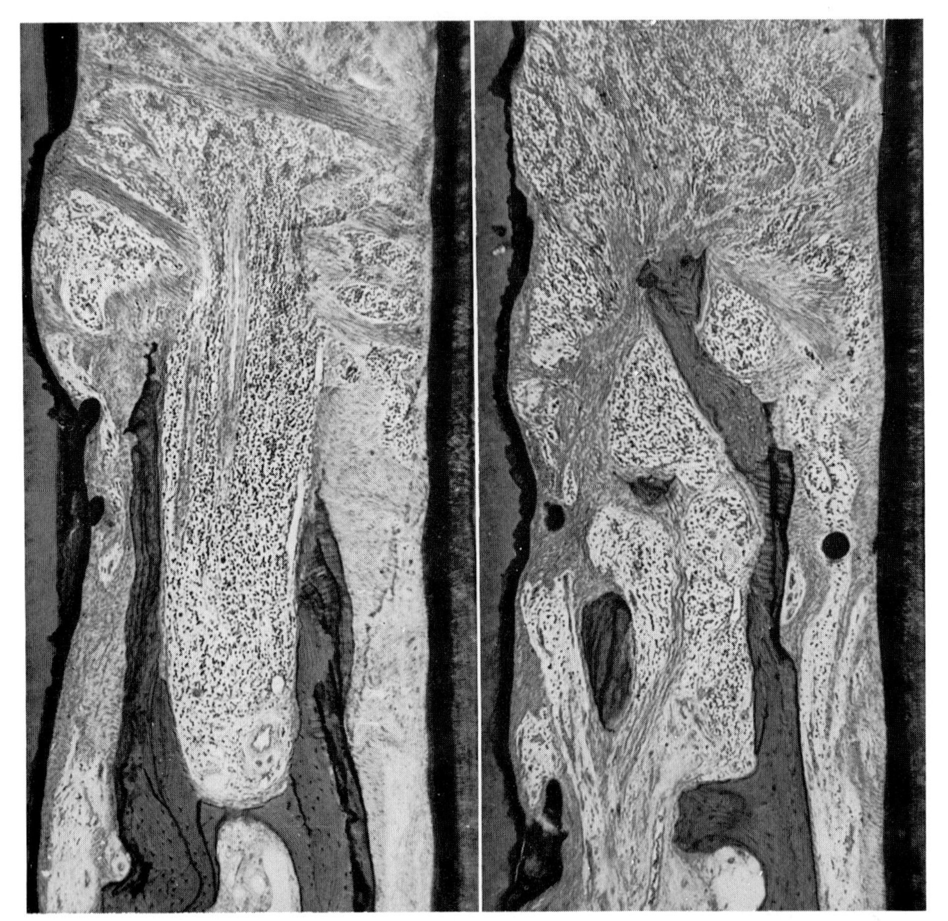

**Fig. 27-4.** High magnification of the alveolar crestal areas shown in Fig. 27-3. Note the extension of the chronic inflammatory process into the bone marrow spaces.

## ULTRASONIC INSTRUMENTATION

The ultrasonic instrument may be used for curettage of the soft tissue wall of a periodontal pocket (Fig. 27-5). Histologic studies have shown ultrasonics to be effective in the removal of ulcerated pocket epithelium. The separation of the epithelium and the connective tissue portion of the gingiva seems to be at the basement membrane. Sound energy absorbed at tissue junctions may take the form of heat, resulting in coagulation.[8] The coagulated epithelium is probably removed by the mechanical action of the vibrating tool and/or the steady stream of water. Epithelization occurs within 3 days after ultrasonic curettage, and fewer inflammatory cells are found in the lamina propria than are seen after hand instrumentation.[9,10]

## OTHER TYPES OF INSTRUMENTATION

Other instruments and chemicals have been used for gingival curettage. Some operators have obtained excellent results using bipolar electrocautery (Fig. 27-6). Gingival curettage will remove the sulcular epithelium and some underlying connective tissue. A clot forms and becomes organized, and re-epithelization usually occurs within a week (Fig. 27-7).

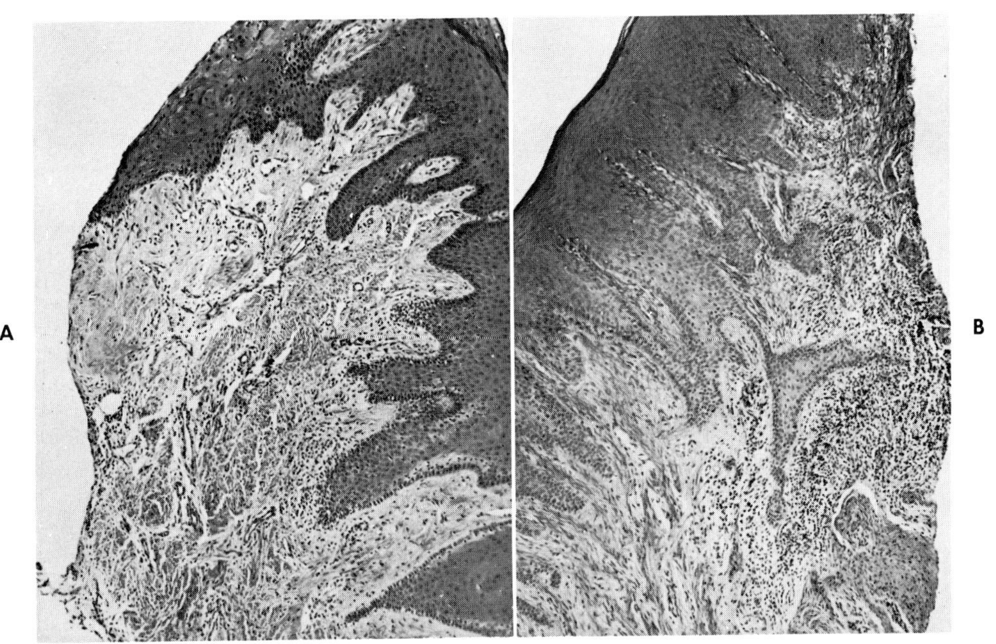


**Fig. 27-5. A,** Photomicrograph of the sulcular epithelium and underlying connective tissue 7 days after ultrasonic curettage. Note that the sulcular epithelium is intact and that there are few inflammatory cells in the lamina propria. **B,** Seven days after hand instrumentation, epithelial continuity is interrupted and a mild inflammatory infiltrate is present in the lamina propria. (Courtesy J. R. Wilson, Columbus, Ohio.)

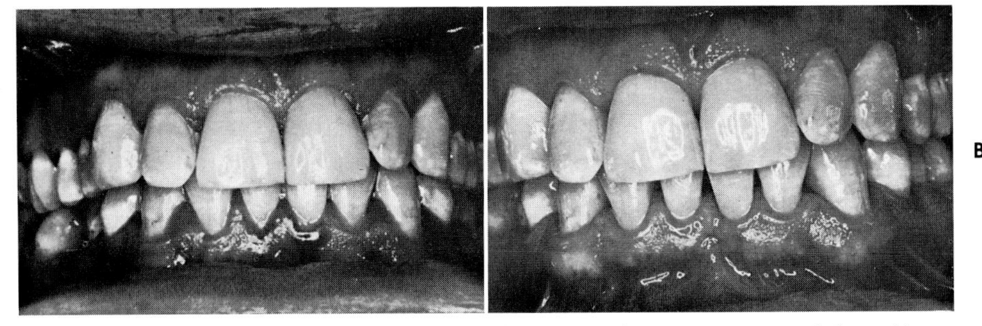


**Fig. 27-6. A,** Chronic, marginal, papillary gingivitis. **B,** After treatment consisting of root planing and gingival curettage with bipolar electrocautery. Tissue repair and resolution of inflammation are evident. (Courtesy W. Hiatt, Denver.)

Postoperative instrumentation in the area should be delayed for at least 2 weeks because, although regeneration of an epithelial lining and attachment takes less than 1 week, a longer period is necessary for connective tissue maturation.[11-13a] With good plaque control, however, gingival health will ensue and can be maintained.

## CASE REPORT

A localized, acute, marginal, papillary gingivitis in a 34-year-old woman is shown in Fig. 27-8, *A*. Calcified deposits covered the cervical third of the

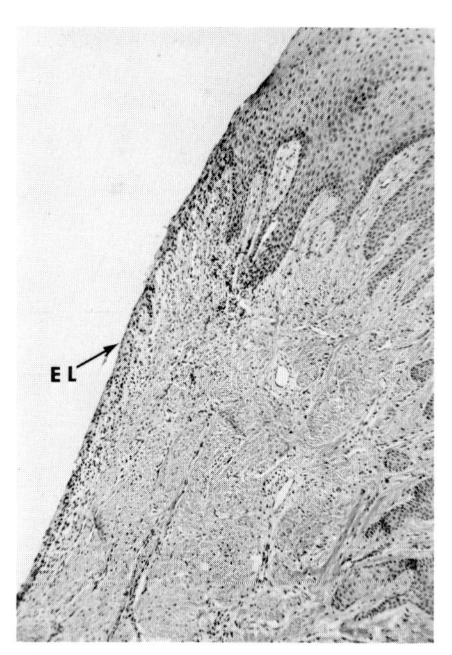


**Fig. 27-7.** Intact epithelial lining, *EL,* 8 days after gingival curettage. (Courtesy B. S. Moskow, Columbia, University, New York.)

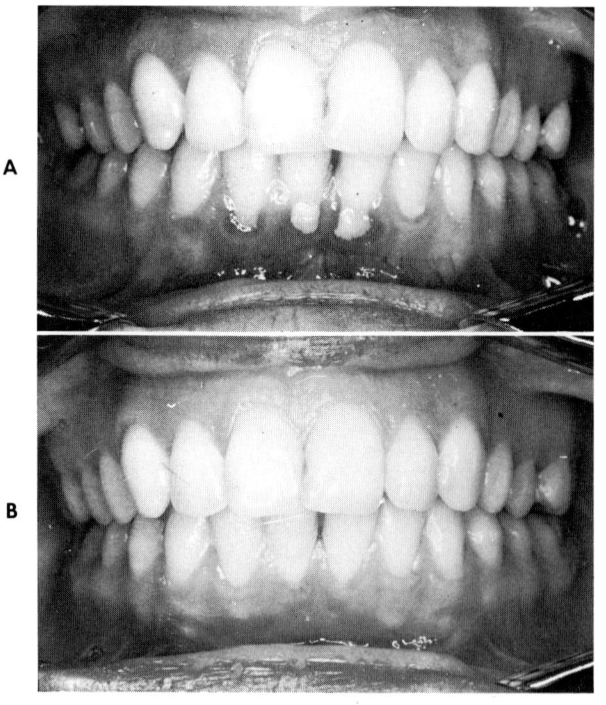


**Fig. 27-8. A,** Large calcified deposits are present on the cervical third of the crowns of the mandibular central incisors. The gingival margins have receded and adjoin the mucogingival junction. A pocket probe inserted into the pockets extended beyond the mucogingival junction. Elsewhere in the mouth, a marginal gingivitis is present and some alteration in tissue form is apparent. **B,** Three months later, after root planing, gingival curettage, and improved oral hygiene, a physiologic gingiva is present. No mucogingival surgery was performed.

crowns of the mandibular central incisors. Some marginal gingiva had been destroyed and the receded gingival margins now approximated the mucogingival junction. A therapeutic problem involving the mucogingival junction and the alveolar mucosa seemed to be present. A periodontal probe inserted into pockets extended 1 mm. beyond the mucogingival junction. The vestibular gingiva around the incisors was deep red in color and bled easily on touch. The papillae were enlarged and blunted.

Treatment consisted of root planing and gingival curettage to remove the edematous tissue, as well as coaching in home dental care. Three months later a remarkable regeneration of tissue had taken place (Fig. 27-8, *B*). The gingiva throughout the mouth had the clinical characteristics of health, including shallow sulcus, physiologic form, and a functionally adequate zone of gingiva. Despite the seeming presence of a mucogingival problem, cure was effected without mucogingival surgery. Too often a hasty resort to more extensive surgery aborts the regenerative potential of periodontal tissues. The experienced therapist will select the most conservative measures that are indicated to reach his therapeutic goals without compromise of results.

**CHAPTER 27**

**References**

1. Bell, D. G.: Clinical procedures in periodontal therapy, J. Periodont. **27**:301, 1956.
2. Younger, W. J.: Pyorrhea alveolaris; remarks on the treatment, Int. Dent. J. **20**:413, 1899.
2a. Sachs, H.: Die Behandlung lockerer Zähne, Berlin, 1929, Berlinische Verlagsanstalt.
2b. Halek, F. J.: The role of subgingival curettage in periodontal therapy, Dental Clinics of North America, Philadelphia, 1969, W. B. Saunders Co., vol. 13.
3. Zentler, A.: Suppurative gingivitis with alveolar involvement. A new surgical procedure, J.A.M.A. **71**:1530, 1918.
4. Crane, A. B., and Kaplan, H.: The Crane-Kaplan operation for the prompt elimination of pyorrhea alveolaris, Dent. Cosmos **73**:643, 1931.
5. Ward, A.: Consideration of periodontal pocket elimination, Acad. Rev. **4**:64, 1956.
6. Raust, G. T., Hall, W. B., Moskow, B. S., Kenney, E. B., and Ramfjord, S. P.: What is the value of gingival curettage in periodontal therapy? Periodont. Abstr. **17**:142, 1969.
7. Orban, B.: To what extent should the tissues be excised in gingivectomy? J. Periodont. **12**:83, 1941.
8. Ewen, S. J.: The ultrasonic wound. Some microscopic observations, J. Periodont. **32**:315, 1961.
9. Goldman, H. M.: Histologic assay of healing following ultrasonic curettage versus hand instrument curettage, Oral Surg. **14**:925, 1961.
10. Frisch, J., Bhaskar, S. N., and Shell, D. D.: Effect of ultrasonic instrumentation on human gingival connective tissue, Periodontics **5**:123, 1967.
11. Morris, M. L.: The removal of pocket and attachment epithelium in humans: a histological study, J. Periodont. **25**:7, 1954.
12. Moskow, B. S.: The response of the gingival sulcus to instrumentation: a histological investigation. II. Gingival curettage, J. Periodont. **35**:112, 1964.
13. Kon, S., Novaes, A. B., Ruben, M. P., and Goldman, H. M.: Visualization of microvascularization of the healing periodontal wound. II. Curettage, J. Periodont. **40**:96, 1969.
13a. Stahl, S. S., Weiner, J. M., Benjamin, S., and Yamada, L.: Soft tissue healing following curettage and root planing, J. Periodont. **42**:678, 1971.

**Additional suggested reading**

Bhaskar, S. N., Grower, M. F., and Cutright, D. E.: Gingival healing after hand and ultrasonic scaling, J. Periodont. **43**:31, 1972.
Held, A. J., and Chaput, A.: Les parodontolyses, Paris, 1959, Prelat.

CHAPTER TWENTY-EIGHT

# Gingivectomy and gingivoplasty



***Definition***

Gingivectomy may be defined as the excision of the soft tissue wall of a pocket (Fig. 28-1, *A*). Its objective is the elimination of pockets. Gingivoplasty is the recontouring of gingiva that has lost its physiologic outer form (Fig. 28-1, *B*). Its objective is the creation of physiologic gingival form rather than the elimination of pockets. Gingivectomy and gingivoplasty are most often performed together, although they may be considered separately for teaching purposes. The two names reflect only the two different objectives of the same procedure.[1-4]

In the elimination of the signs and symptoms of gingival disease, nonsurgical therapy (root planing, proper oral hygiene) or minor surgical intervention (curettage) will often suffice. In some cases inflammation and consequent periodontal disease may recur or remain unresolved. Often such failures are the result of inadequate scaling or poor performance of oral hygiene procedures. Frequently, however, recurrence is the result of a preexisting pocket depth that was not reduced or eliminated.[5] The pocket remains as a locus minoris resistentiae and predisposes to further extension of the disease. In such cases only the removal of the pocket can permit cure (Fig. 28-2) and proper long-term maintenance by the dentist, with good home dental care by the patient.

## PREREQUISITES

The gingivectomy-gingivoplasty surgical technique is used in the treatment of a variety of situations. However, before gingivectomy-gingivoplasty is performed, the basic prerequisites for gingivectomy must exist. These are as follows:

1. The zone of attached gingiva must be wide enough that excision of part of it will still leave a functionally adequate zone.

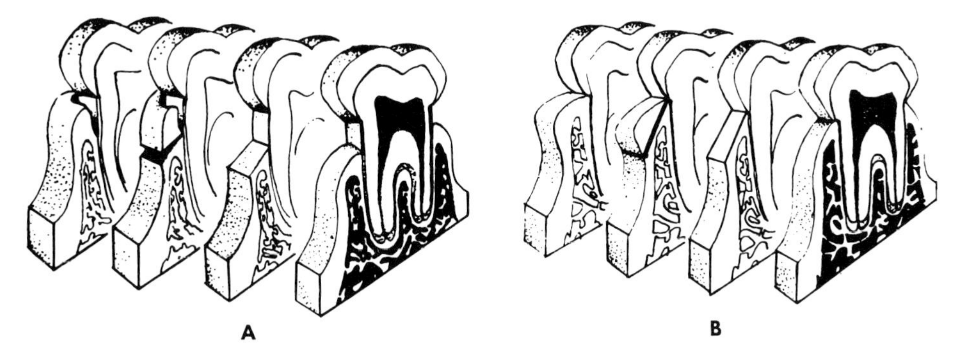


**Fig. 28-1. A,** Sequence in the performance of gingivectomy. **B,** Sequence in the performance of gingivoplasty. (After Fröhlich, E.: Die chirurgische Behandlung der marginalen Parodontitis; from Häupl, K., Meyer, W., and Schuchardt, K.: Die Zahn-, Mund-, und Kieferheilkunde, Munich, 1957, Urban & Schwarzenberg, vol. 3, pt. 1.)

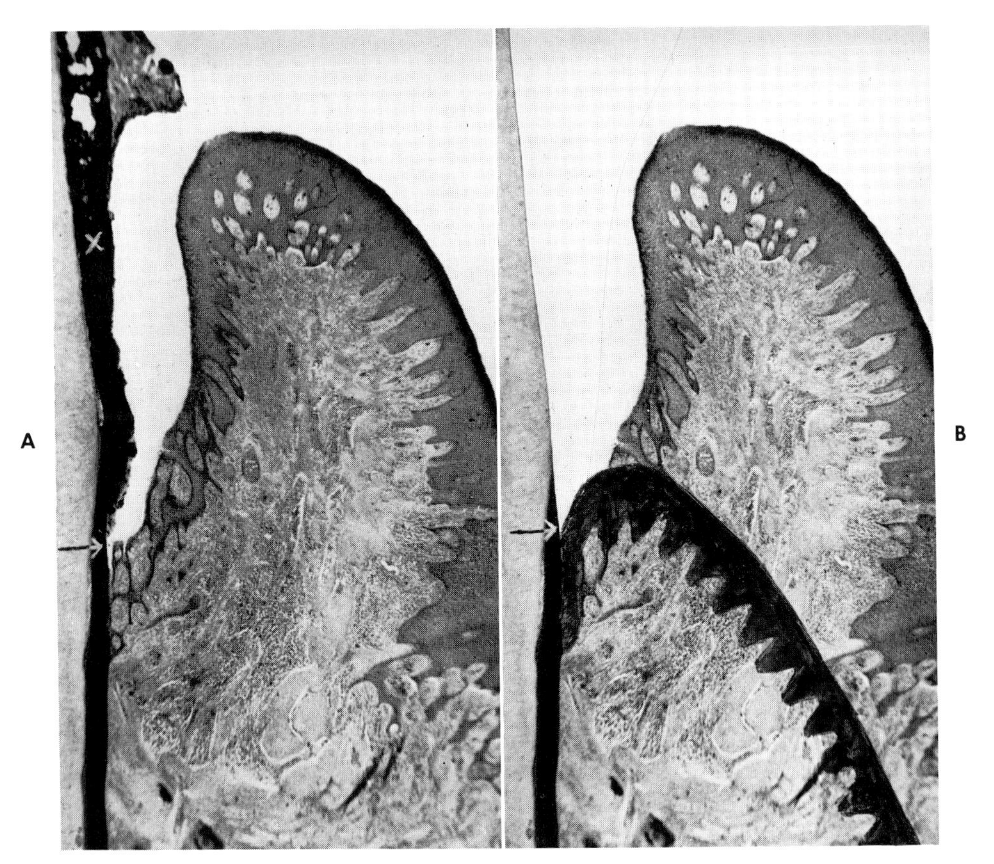


**Fig. 28-2.** Illustration to show the objective in gingivectomy. In **A,** calculus is indicated by *x;* arrow indicates the bottom of the pocket. **B,** Calculus removed by root planing and excision of gingiva, with resultant healing indicated by reduced gingival contour. (Simulated)

2. The underlying alveolar crest must be normal in form. If bone loss has occurred, the loss must be horizontal in nature, leaving a relatively regular crestal bone form at the new lower level.[6]
3. There should be no infrabony (intra-alveolar) defects or pockets.

## INDICATIONS AND CONTRAINDICATIONS

If these prerequisites are met, gingivectomy-gingivoplasty may be used to do the following:

1. Eliminate supra-alveolar pockets and pseudopockets (see classification of pockets, Chapter 29)
2. Remove fibrous or edematous enlargements of the gingiva
3. Transform rolled or blunted margins to ideal (knife-edge) form
4. Create more aesthetic form in cases in which exposure of the anatomic crown has not fully occurred
5. Create bilateral symmetery where the gingival margin of one incisor has receded somewhat more than that of its adjacent incisor
6. Expose additional clinical crown to gain added retention for restorative purposes, to provide access to subgingival caries, or to permit a clamp to be seated in endodontic treatment
7. Correct gingival craters

In addition, gingivectomy-gingivoplasty may be used as a compromise when other procedures are ordinarily indicated but are not feasible. For example, a maxillary molar (Fig. 28-3) may have an intra-alveolar defect on the mesial aspect that can ordinarily be corrected by osseous surgery. However, in this instance the proximity of the antrum can limit the extent of the osseous surgery. Still retaining the molar to serve as an abutment tooth might be advantageous. Therefore in this situation possibly gingivectomy can be used as a compromise procedure. Pocket depth will be reduced but not eliminted. The effectiveness of such a course will depend on the dentist's and the patient's ability to maintain the tooth. Sometimes long-term success will be obtained. However, it is only fair to say that compromise surgery may result in recurrence and extension of pocket depth.

Gingivectomy-gingivoplasty is not indicated in the following situations:

1. In the presence of thick oral and vestibular alveolar ledges, interdental craters, or bizarre crestal bone form

   The position of the gingival margin and the contour of the gingiva relate to the thickness of the gingiva as well as the form of the underlying bone. Tooth position and form also play a role in gingival morphology. Perhaps the most important of these factors to the success or failure of the gingivectomy-gingivoplasty is bone form. In such situations one would expect a coronal regrowth of the interdental papillae and to a lesser extent of the oral and vestibular gingivae.

2. If intra-alveolar (infrabony) pockets are present

   If the pocket dips below the alveolar crest, its base cannot be eliminated by gingivectomy alone. The remnant pocket will cause pocket depth to reform.

3. If excision of the gingiva would leave an inadequate zone of attached gingiva

   If the pocket dips below the mucogingival junction, surgery will excise most or all of the attached gingiva. Alveolar mucosa is not an adequate

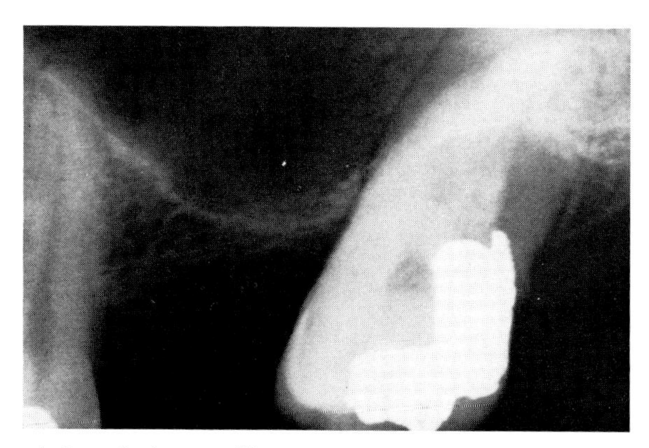

**Fig. 28-3.** The proximity of the maxillary antrum may contraindicate the performance of osseous surgery.

substitute for attached gingiva. Further breakdown often follows in such situations.

4. If oral hygiene performance is poor

   If the patient cannot or will not perform his oral hygiene adequately, surgical therapy will fail.

5. If adequate patient-dentist rapport is lacking or if patient management is a problem

   In treating the patient the dentist should consider the patient's emotional status. When the patient's emotional security is threatened by proposed surgery, the dentist may elect to discontinue treatment. Such patients can be handled with empathy and with careful guidance. Consultation with the patient's physician may be necessary. If the patient is rigid and inflexible, caution is advisable and alternative treatment may be necessary. A particular concern to the management of the patient's psyche is the influence of surgically induced gingival recession (particularly around the maxillary anterior teeth, where some patients may show a great deal of gingiva). When aesthetic deformity is anticipated or unavoidable, the patient must be prepared for it in advance.

6. When certain diseases and conditions exist

   For example, surgery should not be performed in Addison's disease and uncontrolled diabetes and in patients who are anticoagulated, weak, or debilitated or who generally respond poorly to surgery. (See Chapter 26.)

7. When the patient complains of tooth sensitivity before any surgery

   The cause of any complaint should be investigated and surgery considered carefully if the sensitivity cannot be controlled.

A good therapist knows the advantages and disadvantages of his treatment.[21,22] He recognizes his own limitations and knows his patient and how the patient will respond.

## METHOD[7-10]

### Gingivectomy-gingivoplasty, surgical steps

Careful examination of the tissue form and measurement of pocket depth will give the operator a three-dimensional picture that will permit more precise

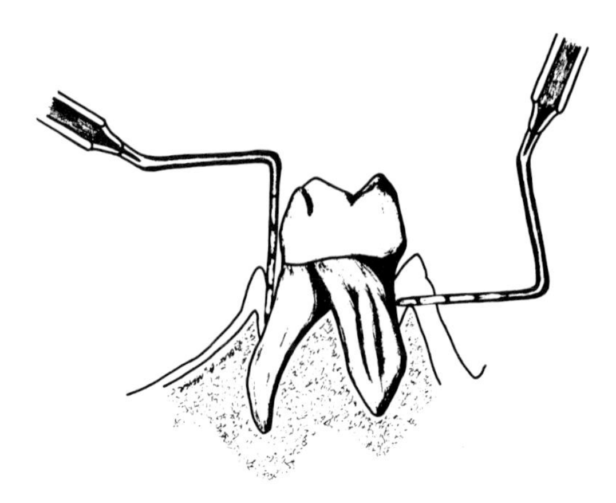

**Fig. 28-4.** Diagrammatic representation of the sounding approach to analyze alveolar bone topography by piercing the soft tissues until the bone is contacted. A systematic stepping procedure is utilized until the bony architecture is ascertained. Delineate the pocket depth by marking bleeding points with a pocket probe. This will guide you in positioning the blade for the initial incision. (Courtesy J. Tussing, Lincoln, Neb.)

execution of the surgery. Mark the pockets with a periodontal probe or with pocket-marking forceps. When the millimeter probe is used, measure and mark on the outer surface of the gingiva (Fig. 28-4) by puncturing the gingiva with a probe or an explorer. When the pocket-marking forceps are used, insert the probing (straight) beak to the bottom of the pocket and mark the depth with the puncturing beak. Make bleeding points in all areas with pocket depth, including the interdental papilla.

***Incision***

Make the incision apical to the bleeding point and extend it through the gingiva to end at the tooth at the level of the bottom of the pocket, that is, at the level of the bleeding point (Fig. 28-2). Exactly how far apical to this marked point the incision should start will depend on the thickness of the gingiva and the axial inclination of the teeth. Where the gingiva is thick, the bevel may be long. Conversely, in the presence of a thin, finely textured gingiva, a short bevel will produce the desired sloping form. Undulate the incision mesiodistally in imitation of ideal scalloped form (similar to the festooning of dentures). The periodontal knife should be keenly sharp so that the incisions are made with ease and the tissues are not torn or lacerated.

You should feel the blade contacting the tooth surface at the depth of the cut. Interdentally the incision should extend deeper into the tissue. When heavy, fibrotic gingiva is present, the stroke may have to be retraced within the initial incision to sever the gingiva completely.

Blend the incision with the tissues lateral to the site of operation so that good form prevails throughout the operated and adjacent areas. In order to do this, you may have to sacrifice a strip of normal gingiva to obtain proper tissue form.

When the surgery involves the gingiva around the last tooth in the arch, start the incision distal to this tooth. Appropriately angled knives (Fig. 28-5) are sometimes used to incise this area and to provide proper bevel. Make the initial incision with a broad-bladed, kidney-shaped knife (using the heel of the instrument) or with similar instruments (Figs. 26-2 and 28-9).

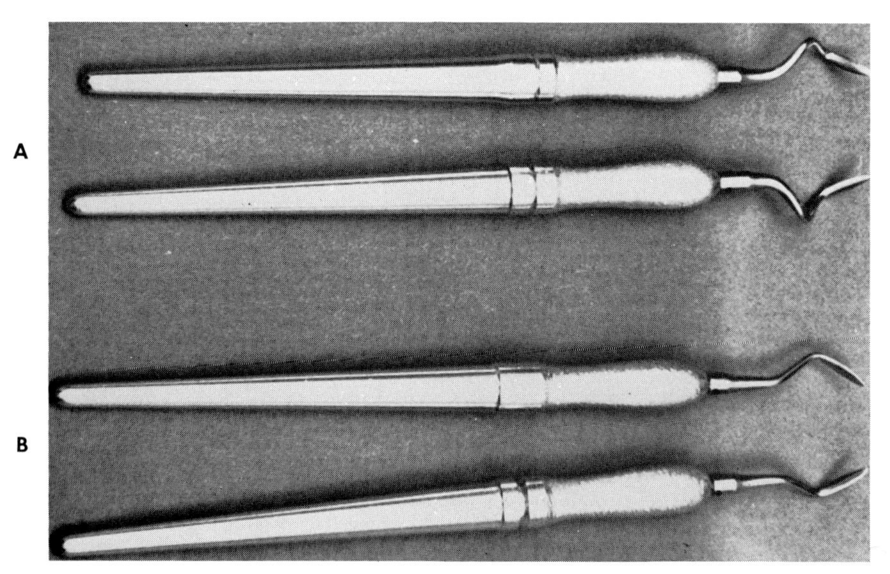


**Fig. 28-5. A,** Gingivectomy knives. **B,** Special knives for distal surfaces of the posterior teeth.

Use a thin-bladed gingivectomy knife such as the Orban knife to sever the interdental gingiva and to connect the incisions between the teeth (Fig. 28-10). The incised gingival tissue can then be removed by holding one end of the partially detached tissue with a tissue forceps and then severing its remaining connection with a scalpel or knife.

*Beveling and festooning*

If the incisions are well planned and performed, (1) pockets will be eliminated, (2) the incision will produce a surface that slopes coronally (called a bevel), (3) the bevel will end in a knife-edge margin, and (4) the remaining tissue will be scalloped about each tooth (festooned) (Fig. 28-14).

It is sometimes necessary to accentuate the festooning to ensure that the physiologic form and a shallow sulcus both persist after healing.[10] Such correction can be made with the Orban knife, although some operators prefer to use surgical shears, tissue rongeurs, or electrocautery. Interdental spillways can be created with the same instruments.

The proper angulation of the initial incision in gingivectomy will create coronally sloping gingival contours and thin gingival margins. Should corrections be necessary, use kidney-shaped or interdental knives in a scraping motion to correct bevels. Scrape the edge lightly but with a firm, even pressure over the resistant fibrous tissue (Fig. 28-12). Be careful to avoid jagged incisions. When done properly, such scraping can be used to make minor corrections, to lengthen, deepen, or blend bevels, or to help in the creation of a more prominent festooning. Diamond stones may be used in a similar fashion to festoon or bevel gingival surfaces when the tissue is firm[11] (Fig. 28-21, *C*). Rotate the wheel-shaped stones in a direction away from the tooth at moderate or high speeds. This will prevent damage to the tooth surface and avoid catching the loose areolar tissue of the fornix. A stream of water or saline should be directed on the stone and tissue to serve as a coolant and to prevent clogging of the stone. Small round stones or spear-shaped stones are available for tissue contouring in interdental or furcation areas.

*Electro-cautery*

Electrocautery can also be used to correct gingival contours or to bevel the cut surface after the initial incision.[12,13a] A number of differently shaped electrodes are available that offer access to specific areas and are designed to facilitate particular corrections of form. The electrodes can remove flat or concave tissue slices, and thin sections of tissue can be excised with ease. In addition, the cautery can be used to eliminate tissue tags and to correct ragged incisions. Be careful, however, not to touch metal restorations, bone, or periosteum because of the danger of injury to bone and pulp. Use a wooden tongue blade to retract the cheeks or to depress the tongue; and to eliminate the offensive odor of burning, quickly blow air over the surgical area.

Soft tissue rongeurs (nippers) and sharp scissors are particularly useful for the creation of interdental grooves and for the removal of tissue tags.

When used correctly, within its indications, gingivectomy-gingivoplasty should not create aesthetic deformity. Scraping knives, diamond stones, electrocautery, nippers, or scissors may improve gingival form, and their use constitutes the gingivoplasty part of the procedure.

## Gingivoplasty alone

Gingivoplasty can be performed without gingivectomy as a procedure in its own right when the gingival margins are blunted and fibrotic and when pocket depth is minimal. Although preliminary root planing, curettage, and proper oral hygiene will usually eliminate or reduce some of the deformity caused by the edema and cellular infiltrate of inflammation, fibrotic (hyperplastic) deformities may resist these measures and these are best eliminated by surgery.

The relation of dentogingival form to function (i.e., the relation of tooth contour and gingival topography to the effectiveness of food deflection) is an important concept.[10] Generally the proper interrelationship of these two factors can make the maintenance of periodontal health much easier. When gingiva-protecting tooth surfaces are absent, food deflection during mastication cannot occur. Food retention and impaction during mastication may become more pronounced. The gingiva loses its thin margin and becomes blunted. This vicious cycle can be corrected by proper restorations and gingivoplasty.

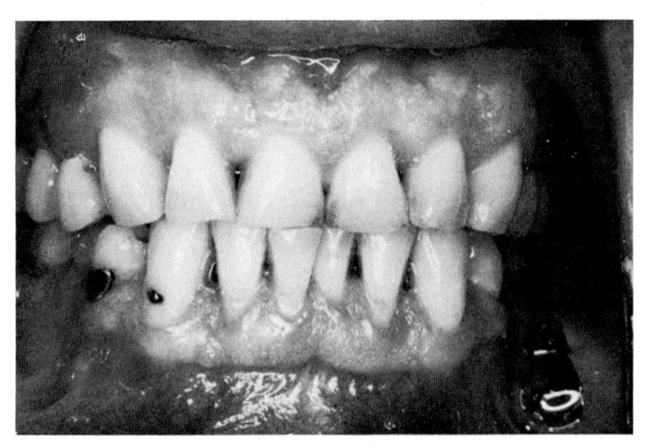

**Fig. 28-6.** Fibrotic inflamed mandibular gingival margins are evident in a 38-year-old man. Note the tissue form in the lower anterior region.

## Illustrative cases

At this point let us review some actual gingivectomy-gingivoplasty procedures. In the first case the procedure was done in the mandible (Figs. 28-6 to 28-16). Although the maxillary gingiva was clinically fibrotic and lacked ideal contour, particularly between the right lateral and central incisors, the clinical health of the area and the lack of pocket depth indicated that no surgery was necessary in the upper jaw. Clinical success in maintaining health confirmed this judgment (Fig. 28-16).

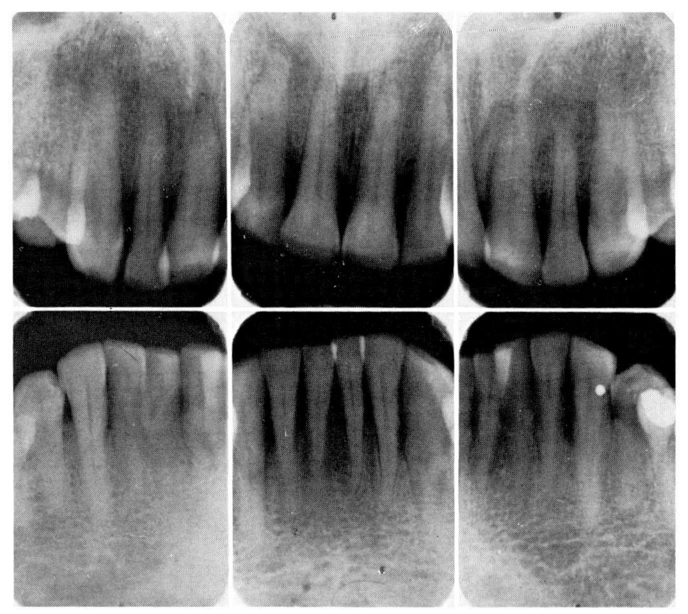

**Fig. 28-7.** Roentgenogram showing some horizontal bone loss but a regular crestal outline.

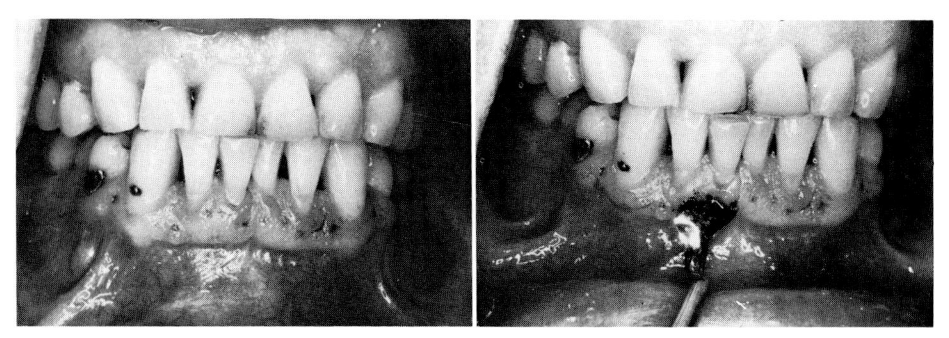

**Fig. 28-8** **Fig. 28-9**

**Fig. 28-8.** Root planing and home dental care have reduced the clinical inflammation but have failed to eliminate pocket depth or to change the fibrotic gingival contours. A broad zone of gingiva is present. Pockets ranging in depth 3 to 5 mm. were present around the mandibular incisors and canines. Bleeding points illustrate the distribution of pocket depth.

**Fig. 28-9.** A kidney-shaped knife is used to make the initial incision. Start the incision apical to the bleeding points and angulate it to eliminate pockets and to provide a coronally sloping bevel. A mesiodistal scalloped form will thus be maintained.

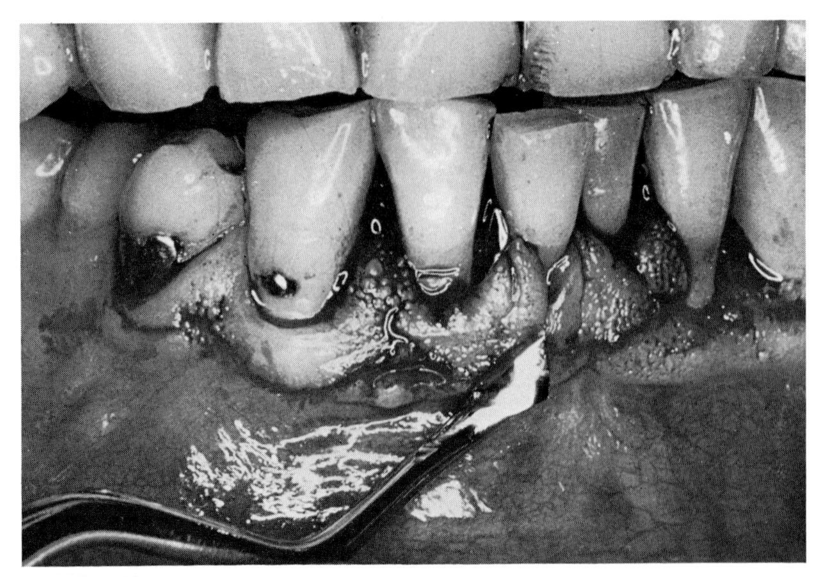

**Fig. 28-10.** Sever the interdental papillae with a thin interproximal knife and join the oral (lingual) and vestibular (buccal) incisions. Then remove the detached gingiva with a curette or sickle scaler.

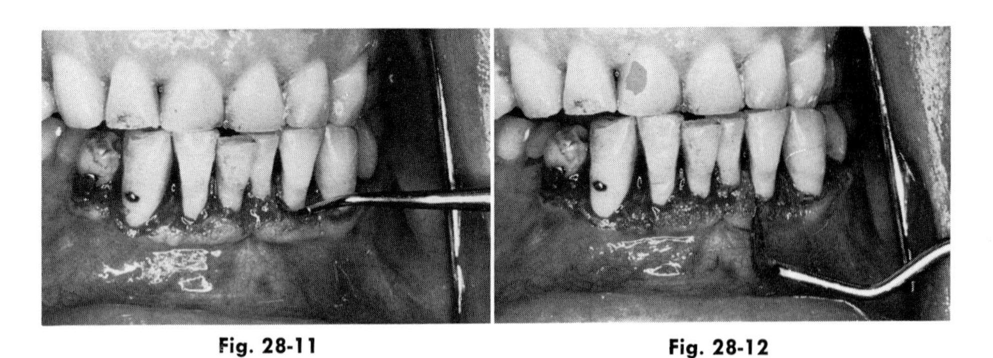

**Fig. 28-11** **Fig. 28-12**

**Fig. 28-11.** A curette removes tissue tags and any remaining deposits.

**Fig. 28-12.** A scalpel, used in a scraping motion, provides proper bevel and scalloped mesiodistal form. Interdental grooves are accentuated.

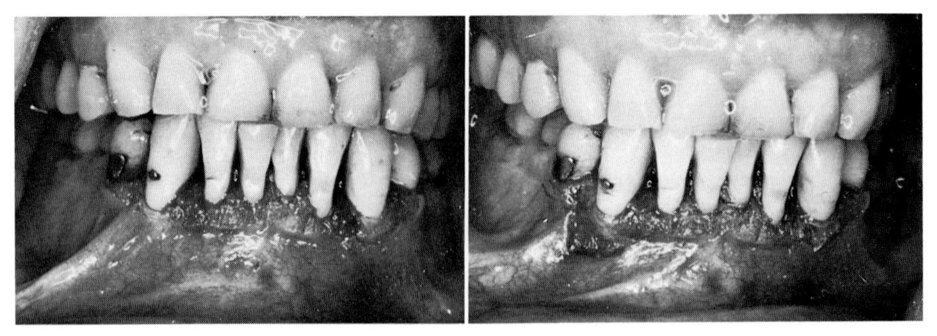

**Fig. 28-13** **Fig. 28-14**

**Fig. 28-13.** Contoured wound. Note that a mucogingival problem (lack of gingiva and pull of the frenum) exists on the vestibular surface of the right canine.

**Fig. 28-14.** An incision is made at the mucogingival junction around the right canine, and the alveolar mucosa is permitted to sag apically. The alveolar surface remains covered only by periosteum.

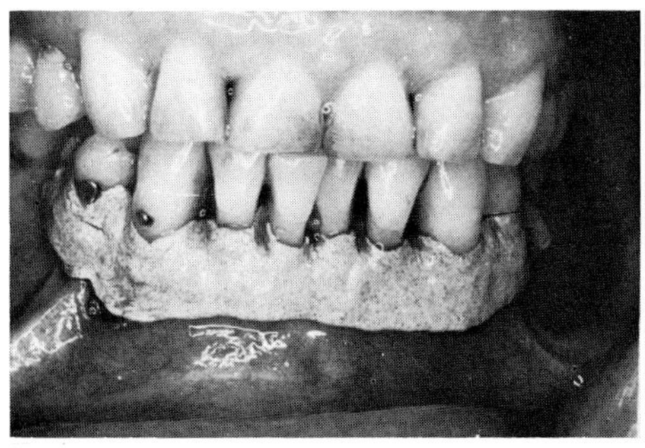

Fig. 28-15

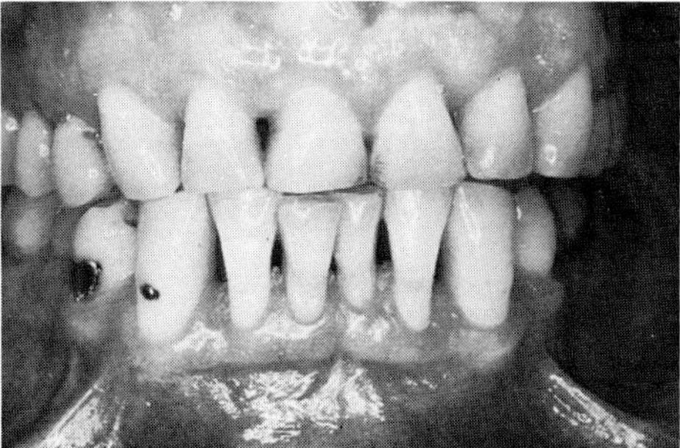

Fig. 28-16

**Fig. 28-15.** After hemorrhage has been controlled, a dressing is carefully placed.
**Fig. 28-16.** Physiologic gingival form 1 year later. Maintenance procedures consisted of root planing and oral hygiene.

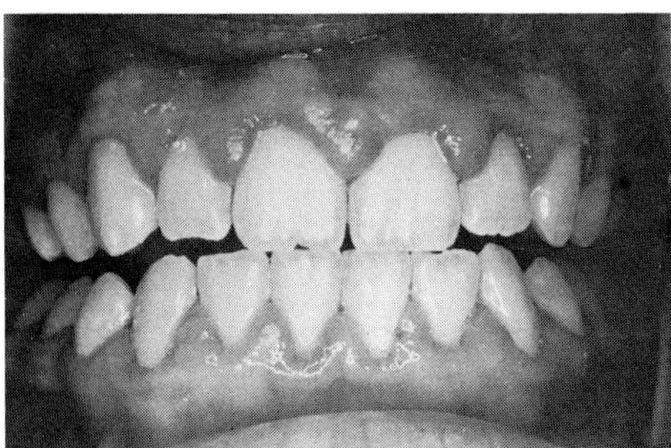

Fig. 28-17

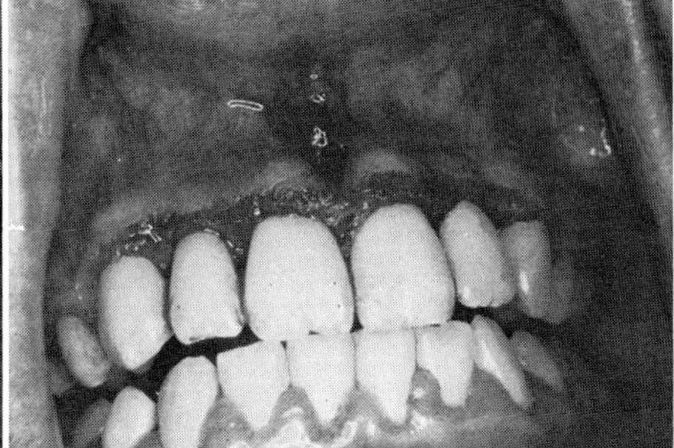

Fig. 28-18

**Fig. 28-17.** Generalized, marginal, hyperplastic gingivitis in a 15-year-old white girl. The gingival enlargement is mostly the result of hyperplasia.
**Fig. 28-18.** Gingivectomy was performed in the upper anterior segment. The frenum was excised since it infringed on the surgical field. Note that root planing had not corrected the gingival enlargement, still visible in the lower arch. Gingivectomy was performed later in the lower anterior region.

An important therapeutic principle is illustrated in this case. The selection of treatment procedures is based on the individual needs of the patient, not on presumptions of ideal gingival form or on rote prescriptions of surgery. Gingivectomy is not another means to help remove calculus.

Another illustrative case is that of a 15-year-old girl (Figs. 28-17 to 28-20). Enlarged gingival margins and hyperplastic papillae were evident. Initial treatment consisted of root planing and oral hygiene instruction. The remaining fibrotic tissue was then removed by gingivectomy and gingivoplasty.

In still another case, gingivectomy-gingivoplasty was performed. On one side of the mouth, the gingivoplasty portion was done by scraping with a knife and on the other side by using a coarse diamond stone (Fig. 28-21).

Gingivoplasty also is employed in the attempt to bring about resolution of a disease process in which improper gingival form persists. Such a case is seen in Fig. 28-22, showing the gingival condition of a 29-year-old white man who pre-

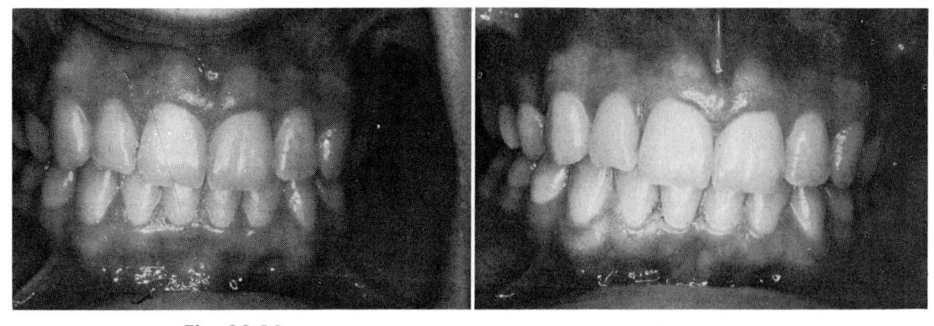


**Fig. 28-19.** Six months after therapy the inflammation is corrected and gingival form is acceptable. **Fig. 28-20.** Five years later the patient has maintained a physiologic gingival form.

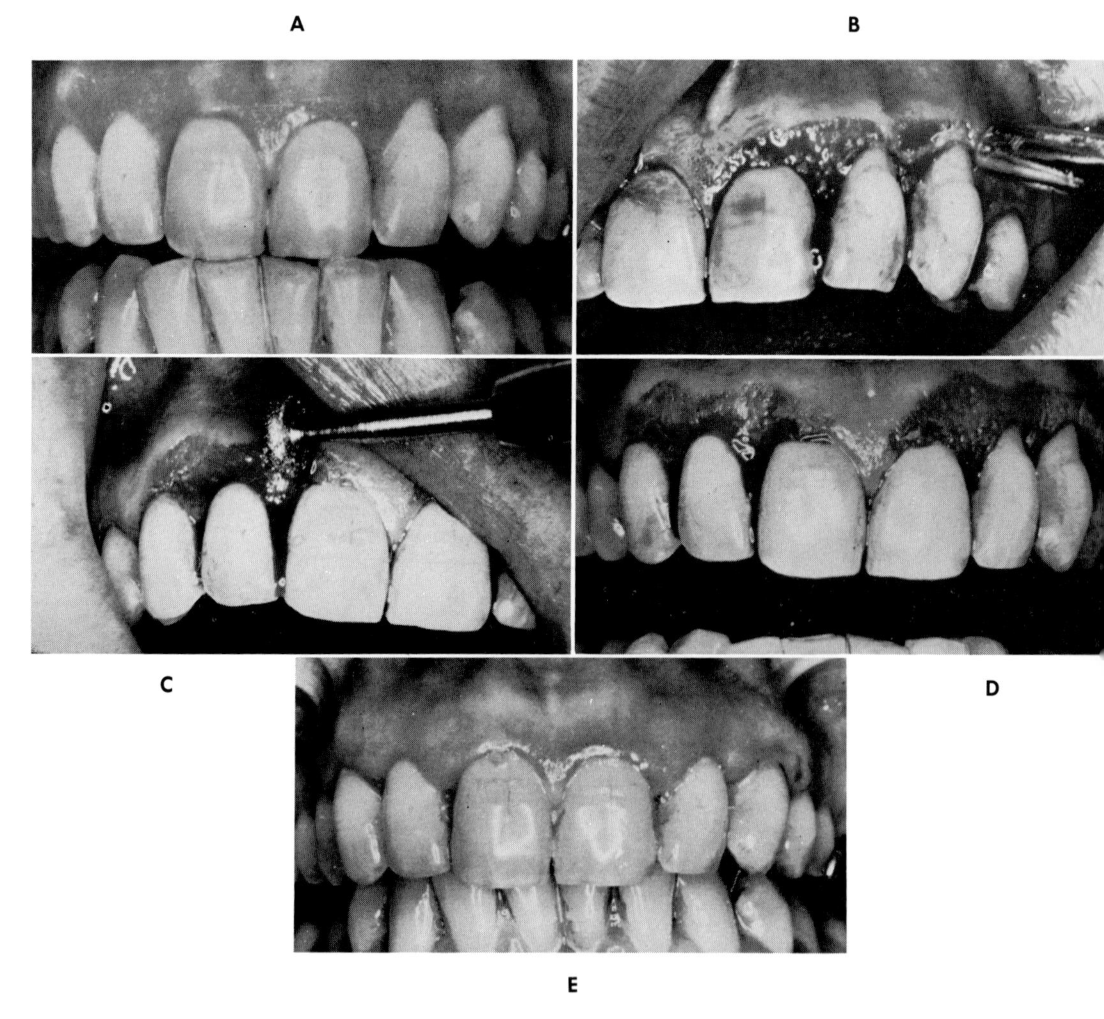


**Fig. 28-21.** Recontouring tissues by gingivoplasty. **A,** Preoperative condition. **B,** Gingivoplasty performed by scraping with a scalpel. **C,** Gingivoplasty performed by use of a coarse diamond stone. **D,** Immediately after surgery. **E,** View after complete healing. (Courtesy S. Schluger, Seattle.)

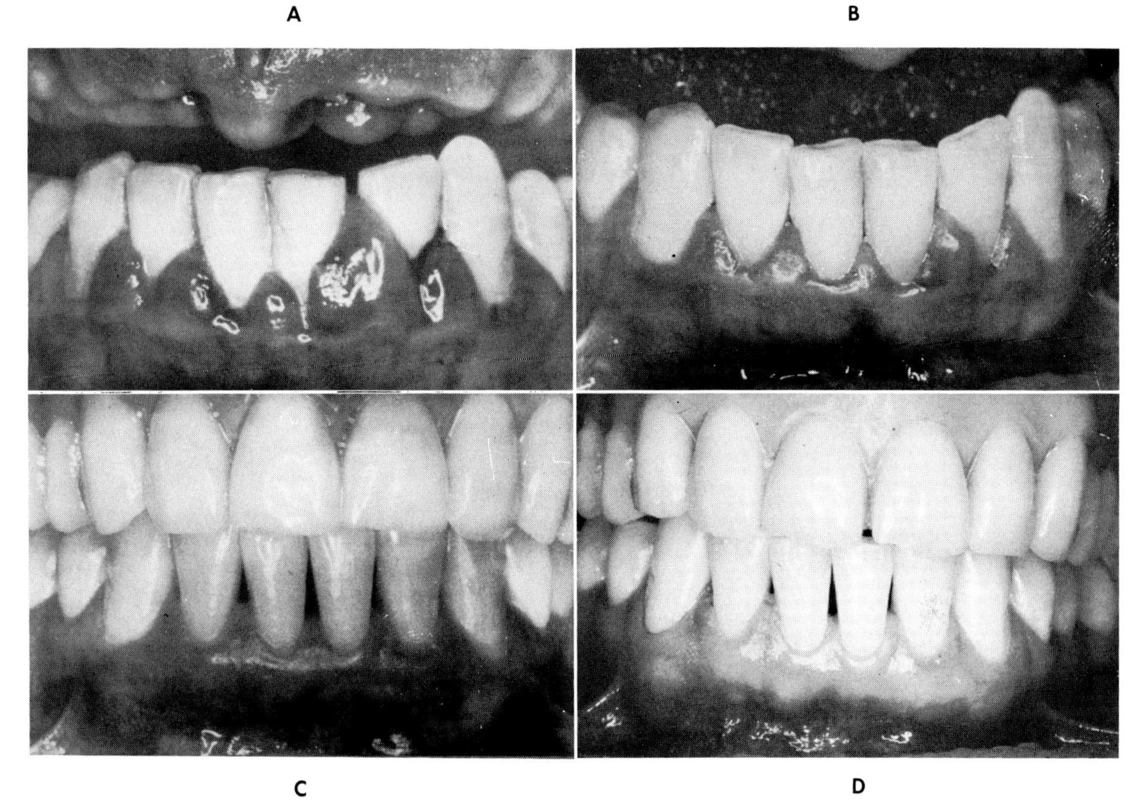


**Fig. 28-22. A,** Hyperplastic periodontitis in a 29-year-old white man. **B,** Two months later, after root planing and gingival curettage. Note the closed contact between the mandibular left central and lateral incisors where there previously was a diastema. **C,** Six months after gingivoplasty. **D,** Six years later.

sented a chronic, hyperplastic periodontitis. There was a diastema between the mandibular left central and lateral incisors. The maxillary teeth had all been extracted. Root planing, gingival curettage, and oral hygiene instruction were carried out over a period of 2 months, leading to considerable improvement of the condition and closure of the diastema. At that time the tissues appeared fibrous, and there was still papillary and marginal enlargement present. Gingivoplasty was performed.

Another case in which gingivoplasty was performed is that of a 40-year-old man. A gingivectomy had been performed a year previously but was done inadequately. The heavy gingival ledge on the labial side of the mandibular incisors had not been beveled or festooned at the time (Fig. 28-23, *A*). The gingiva was slightly red and edematous, and the patient had difficulty in maintaining good oral hygiene. Gingivoplasty was performed (Fig. 28-23, *B*), and healing took place within 2 weeks. The gingival contour was improved, maintenance of good oral hygiene was enhanced, and the tissues appeared healthy.

Gingivoplasty is a logical adjunct to gingivectomy. Properly performed gingivectomy includes contouring of the gingival margin. Cases such as the one shown in Fig. 28-23 would not have needed special care and added surgery if the gingivectomy had been done with attention to gingival architecture. On the other hand, some patients who appear to require gingivoplasty can be treated sucess-

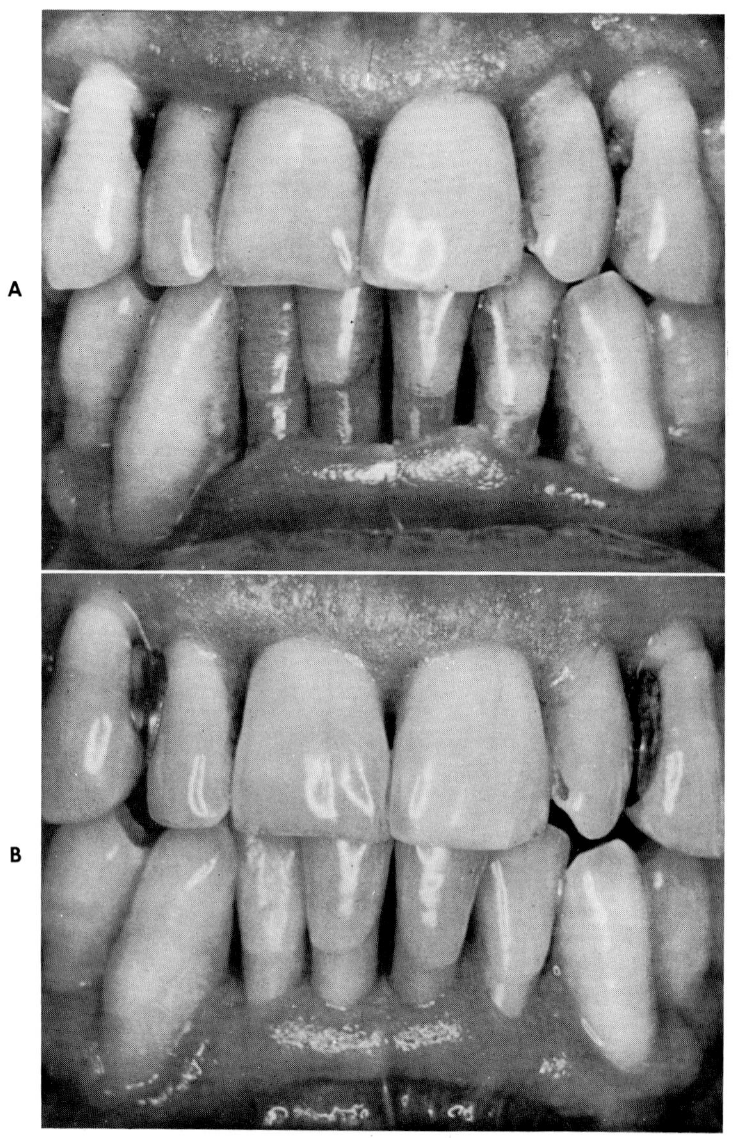


**Fig. 28-23. A,** Heavy, fibrous ledge of tissue apparent on mandibular teeth 1 year after gingivectomy. **B,** Gingivoplasty has produced a good gingival contour.

fully by proper root planing, gingival curettage, and good oral hygiene (Fig. 28-11, upper jaw). It remains the decision of the operator as to which method he will choose in treating a given patient.

## PERFORMING FIRST GINGIVECTOMY-GINGIVOPLASTY

Now that the steps of the gingivectomy-gingivoplasty have been reviewed, the student is ready to proceed with surgery. He needs only a few additional pointers before he does his first gingivectomy-gingivoplasty.

### Presurgical period

*Scaling*

The patient's tissues must be prepared for surgery by the removal of all calcified deposits and plaque. The patient must also be taught to be effective in his oral hygiene. If he cannot maintain proper oral hygiene prior to surgery, he will not be able to do any better after surgery. Surely, then, surgery will not result in a cure for the condition.

*Oral hygiene*

If the patient demonstrates his ability in oral hygiene, much of the inflammation will have been resolved by the time of surgery. During surgery there will be less bleeding, the tissues will have a firmer consistency, and ragged wound edges and tissues will be avoided.

*Premedication*

Premedication for apprehension has been discussed in Chapter 26. In addition, antibiotic coverage[13b] for systemic complications has been discussed. Prescriptions for premedication should be written at the final visit before the surgery, when the area to be operated on is reexamined and reevaluated and changes in pocket depth are noted.

*Mixing the dressing*

The periodontal pack may be mixed prior to surgery and stored in the refrigerator to prevent its premature setting. For gingivectomy-gingivoplasty, mix the pack to a stiff consistency similar to that of putty.

*Planning the surgery*

The charting and roentgenograms of the area to be operated on should be studied. Generally the student will do only a limited area. In practice a quadrant or half a mouth may be operated on and the other side of the mouth left uninvolved so that the patient is able to masticate comfortably.

Gingivectomy may be performed about a single tooth for access in operative procedures or to seat a clamp for endodontic procedures. Sometimes further treatment (endodontics or operative dentistry) may immediately follow the surgery. In such cases these steps should be planned in advance and the appropriate instruments be available so that the procedures may be done smoothly and without interruption.

## Surgery

*Anesthesia*

Local infiltration is the method of choice. Standard techniques of dosage and administration should be followed. After anesthesia is obtained, inject a drop into each interdental papilla involved. This increases the turgor of the gingiva and makes it easier to incise. In addition, the vasoconstrictor will reduce bleeding during surgery.

After confirming that the tissues are completely anesthesized, probe the pockets, mark the pocket depths, and perform the surgery as outlined in the preceding pages.

*Control of bleeding*

Carefully inspect the wound and tooth surfaces after the surgery. Remove any remaining deposits or tissue tags. At this point it will be necessary to obtain good hemostasis before a pack is placed. This may be accomplished by rinsing the wound surfaces with sterile saline solution or water and then packing gauze sponges over the area. If this does not produce hemostasis, pack the interproximal areas with pledgets containing dilute (no greater than 1/1000) epinephrine. Strong epinephrine solutions (8%) could produce undesirable systemic effects.

*Placing the dressing*

The purpose of the dressing is to keep the patient more comfortable postoperatively. The dressing serves to prevent formation of exuberant granulation tissue and thereby acts as a template. It should cover the wound and protect the wound from mechanical trauma during chewing and from irritation by highly seasoned foods. However, the dressing itself should not become irritating, and this can be assured only if it is placed firmly. The dressing should be placed along the necks of the teeth and should not cover the occlusal surfaces. If the dressing interferes with the occlusion, the patient may fracture the dressing after it has set. If not, the hardened dressing acts as an occlusal interference.

Place the dressing interdentally in cone-shaped pieces. Then adapt flat strips of dressing to the interproximal cones. Force the pack into place by instrument and finger pressure. Inspect the dressing to be sure that it does not impinge on muscle attachments or the orovestibular mucosa. If it does, muscle trim the pack in much the same way that full denture impressions are muscle trimmed. In some cases the dressing may be covered with adhesive Burlew tinfoil. The foil helps to hold the dressing in place.

*Stents*

It is sometimes difficult to apply the pack around posterior teeth when a shallow vestibule is present. Performed acrylic stents may be used to retain the dressing. When the surgery involves an isolated tooth, tie dental floss around the neck of the tooth, leaving dangling ends of the floss 3 to 4 mm. in length. The dressing will then adhere to the floss.

If aesthetics demands, a plastic gingival veneer may be made prior to the operation and placed over the dressing. Such a veneer will also stabilize the dressing.

### Postsurgical checklist and procedures

*Instructions to patient*

Instruct the patient to avoid eating or drinking after surgery for 1 hour or until the pack is set. Tart or spicy foods should be avoided. Brushing should be limited to occlusal and incisal tooth surfaces in the operated area. The dressing should be cleansed gently with a soft multitufted toothbrush. Frequent, gentle rinsing after meals is advisable. Any prescription for postmedication is made at this time. (See discussion of postmedication in Chapter 26.) Instructions for emergency situations should be presented in printed form together with the dentist's home phone number. Emergencies are rare, but the patient feels comforted to know that he can call the dentist should the need arise.

*Dressing changes*

Instruct the patient to return for postoperative dressing change in 3 to 5 days, or earlier if the dressing is dislodged. In minor cases the dressing may be removed at this time. Other cases may require one or two dressing changes. At each dressing change, inspect and clean the wound and root surfaces. If exuberant granulation tissue is present, it can be removed with a curette.

*Dressing removal*

On removal of the final dressing advise the patient that there must be no letup in oral hygiene. Some patients are fearful of bleeding and let up on brushing. In those cases exuberant granulation tissue may form, or the tissue may not mature properly. Gingivectomy may fail without proper postoperative oral hygiene. Special extrasoft brushes (Prophylactic) may be used immediately after dressing removal for 1 or 2 weeks (Chapter 26).

## WOUND HEALING

Wound healing[14-17,21,22] takes place by the development of an acute inflammatory process and the formation of granulation tissue. This process takes place both in the depth of the tissue and on the surface. In the deeper tissues an acute inflammatory reaction occurs soon after surgery, consisting of dilatation of blood vessels (Fig. 28-24, *A*) and migration of leukocytes into the tissue (*B*). This occurs during the first few days postoperatively. The connective tissue surrounding the blood vessels responds by proliferation characterized by mitotic activity in the fibroblasts (*C*), in the endothelial cells (*D*), and in the undifferentiated mesen-

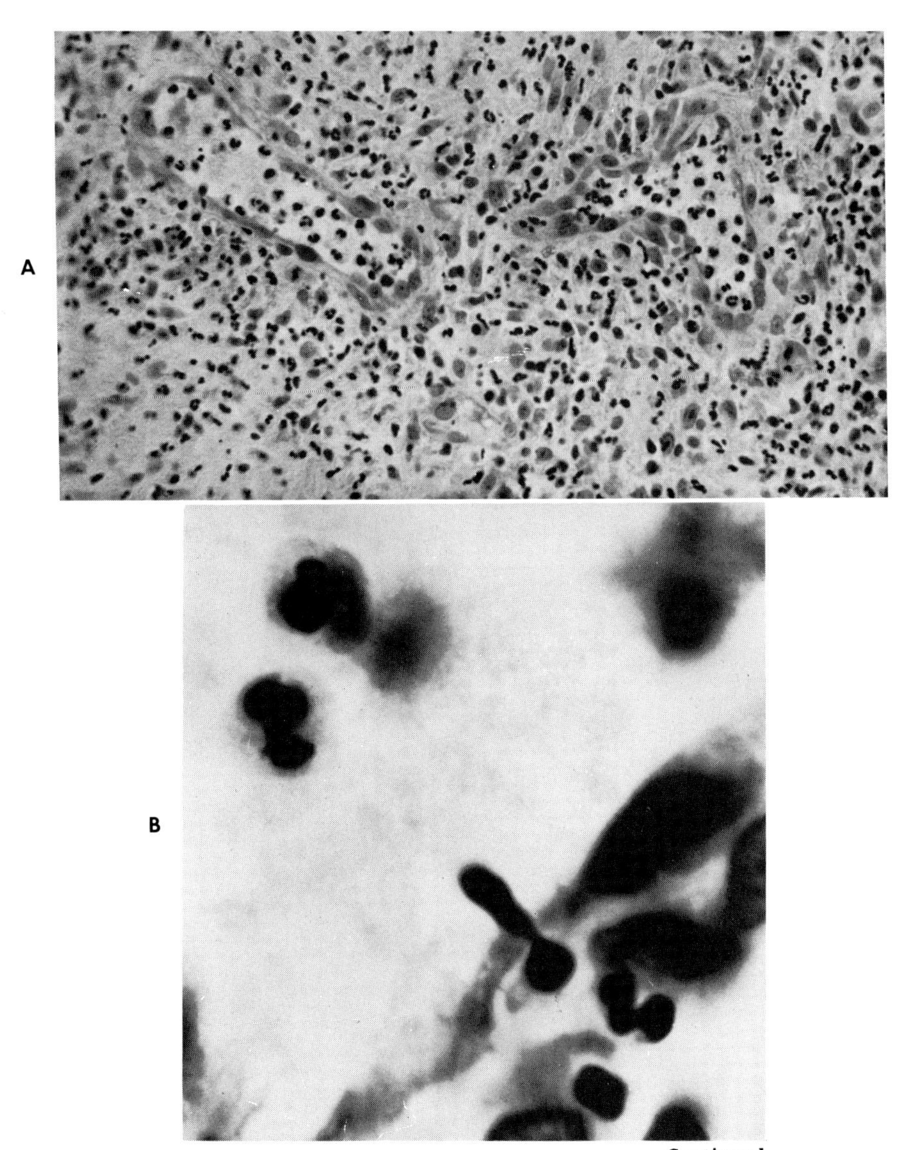


*Continued.*

**Fig. 28-24. A,** Acute inflammatory reaction 2 days after gingivectomy—dilated capillaries, filled with leukocytes migrating from the capillaries into surrounding tissue. **B,** High magnification of a capillary with a leukocyte migrating through the endothelial wall.

chymal cells (*E*). This is called fibroplasia and constitutes the development of true granulation tissue.

While this process is occurring in the deeper tissues, the surface is also undergoing changes. Immediately after surgery the blood clot covers the exposed connective tissue. Two days after surgery the blood clot consists of three distinct layers (Fig. 28-25, *A*). The surface of the blood clot becomes necrotic, and the innermost layer appears to be fibrinous; between these two layers is a stratum rich in leukocytes (leukocyte band), which separates the necrotic surface from the fibrinous layer. The epithelium grows under the blood clot. Four days after the surgery the necrotic surface of the blood clot is cast off (*B*), and the epithelium then proceeds to cover the surface at a rate of 0.5 mm./day. Eight days

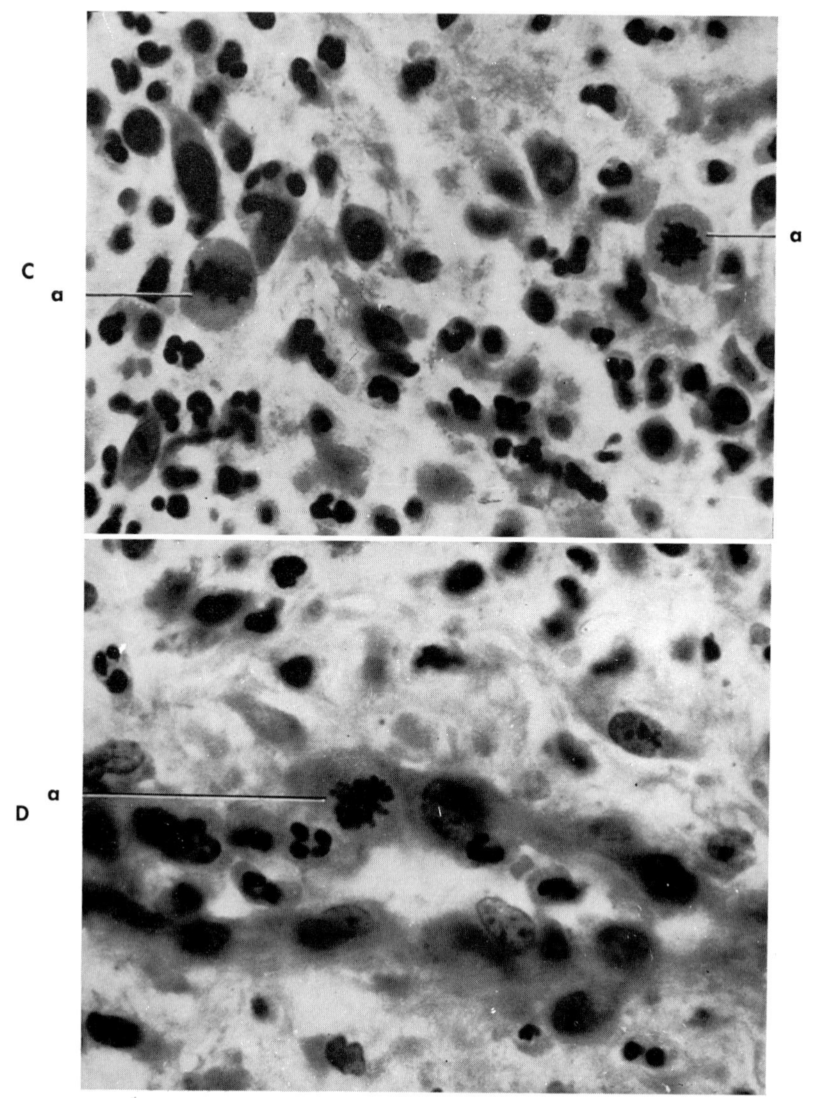


**Fig. 28-24, cont'd. C,** Histologic section from a healing gingivectomy wound showing mitosis, *a,* of fibroblasts. **D,** Histologic section from a healing gingivectomy wound showing mitosis, *a,* of an endothelial cell in the wall of a capillary.

after surgery, only a small part of the wound surface is not epithelized (*C*). The granulation tissue extends above the surface, and in 14 days the entire wound is covered by the epithelium (*D*).

Healing proceeds by proliferation of capillaries (Fig. 28-25, *E*) and fibroblasts (*F*) under the fibrinous inner layer of the blood clot. A large, massive blood clot has been found to delay healing because the bacterial activity is greater. The dressing should be closely adapted so that the extent of the blood clot can be minimized.

During this process of healing (by secondary intention), the problem of secondary infection of the granulation tissue may occur. The ever-present

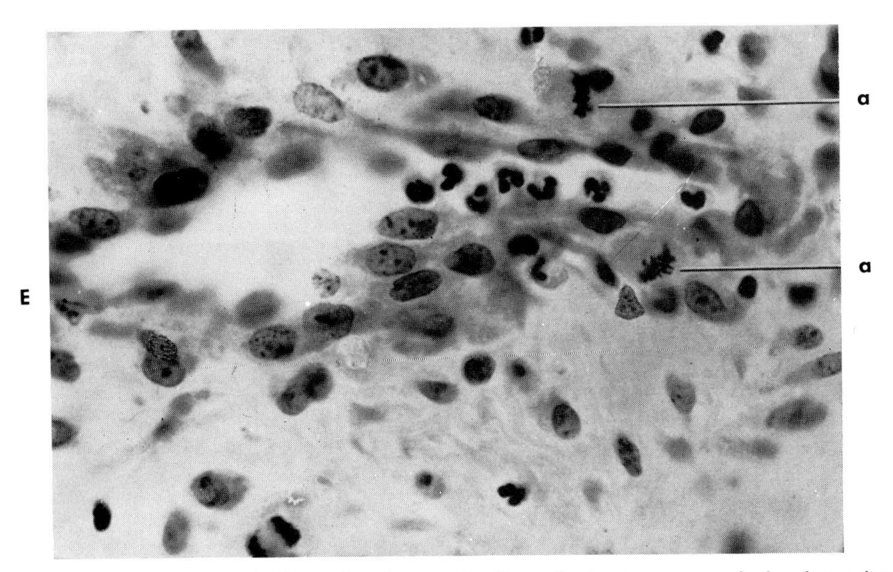


**Fig. 28-24, cont'd. E,** Histologic section from a healing gingivectomy wound showing mitosis, *a,* in undifferentiated mesenchymal cells.

bacterial flora, though not virulent, grows readily on the blood clot and surface of the young granulating connective tissue. These bacteria may produce toxins that are irritating to the healing wound surface. As a reaction to this irritant and ensuing inflammatory reaction, the granulation tissue may proliferate more rapidly and grow over the surface as proud flesh or infected granulation tissue. Careful root planing, refined surgical techniques, proper placement of the dressing, and proper postoperative wound care will keep surface infection to a minimum. The epithelium that must cover the exposed connective tissue can grow only if the granulation tissue is not infected and does not proliferate in an exuberant fashion.

## Aids in the healing process

Experiments have shown that frequent change of dressing is advantageous to wound healing[8] (Fig. 28-26). The tissue underneath a dressing that had been left on without change for 10 days showed an accumulation of exudate and necrotic material and severe inflammation in the underlying connective tissue with poor epithelization of the wound surface, whereas a postoperative wound of 10 days in which the dressing had been changed at 3-day intervals showed good healing tendency.

The following steps are helpful in aiding the healing process:

1. Use fastidious surgical technique to reduce tissue laceration and trauma.
2. Use scrupulous aseptic methods even though the oral cavity may be considered a contaminated site. Avoid the possible introduction of organisms not commonly found in the oral cavity.
3. Minimize the size of the clot.
4. Protect the wound surface with a well-placed surgical dressing.
5. Change the dressing every 3 to 5 days.
6. Remove all debris and any remaining calculus at each dressing change.

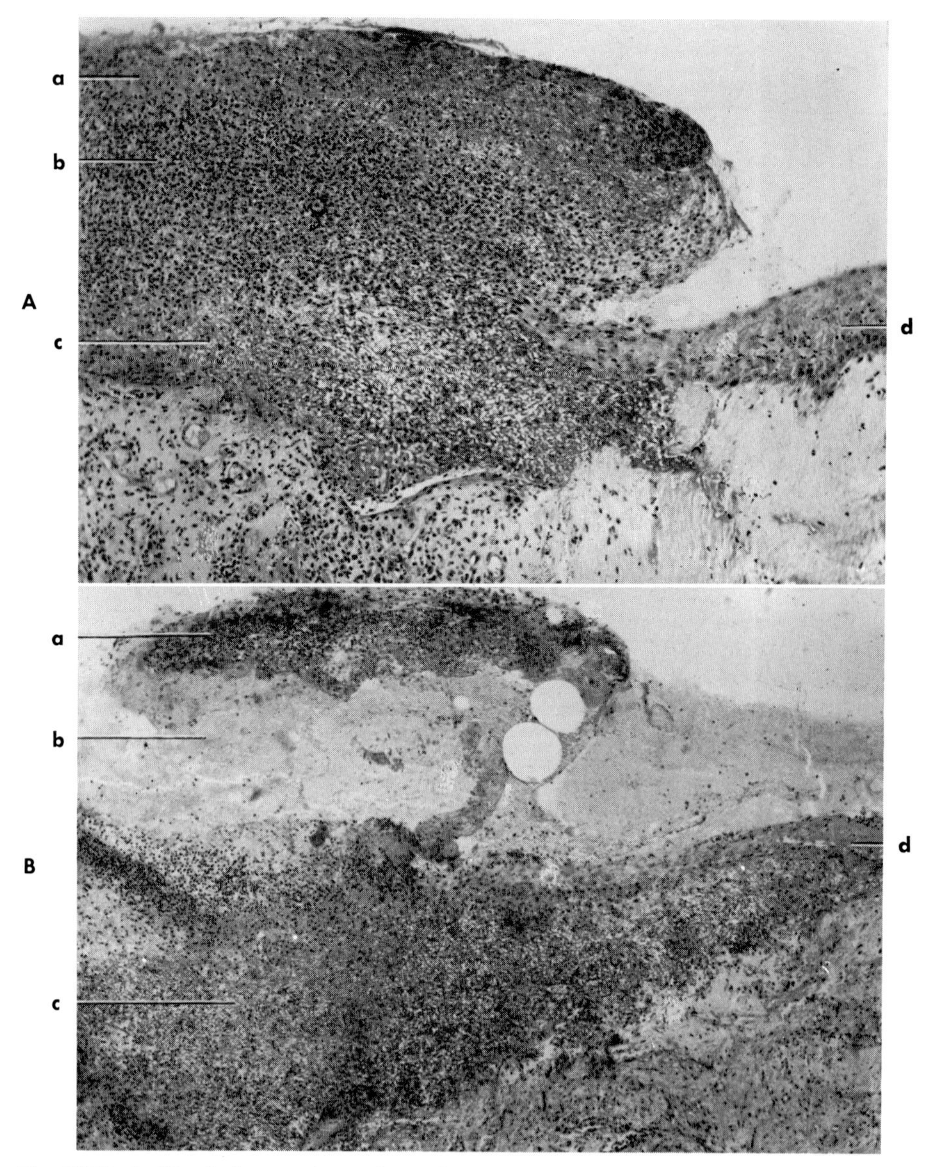


**Fig. 28-25. A,** Blood clot on the surface of a healing wound 2 days after gingivectomy. The blood clot is separated into three layers: the outermost, *a,* is necrotic; the innermost *c,* is fibrinous; and the middle, *b,* consists of a wall of leukocytes limiting the outer from the inner layer. The epithelium, *d,* then proceeds to cover the wound surface. **B,** Four days after gingivectomy the outer necrotic layer, *a,* of the clot is cast off. The migration of the epithelium, *d,* progresses.

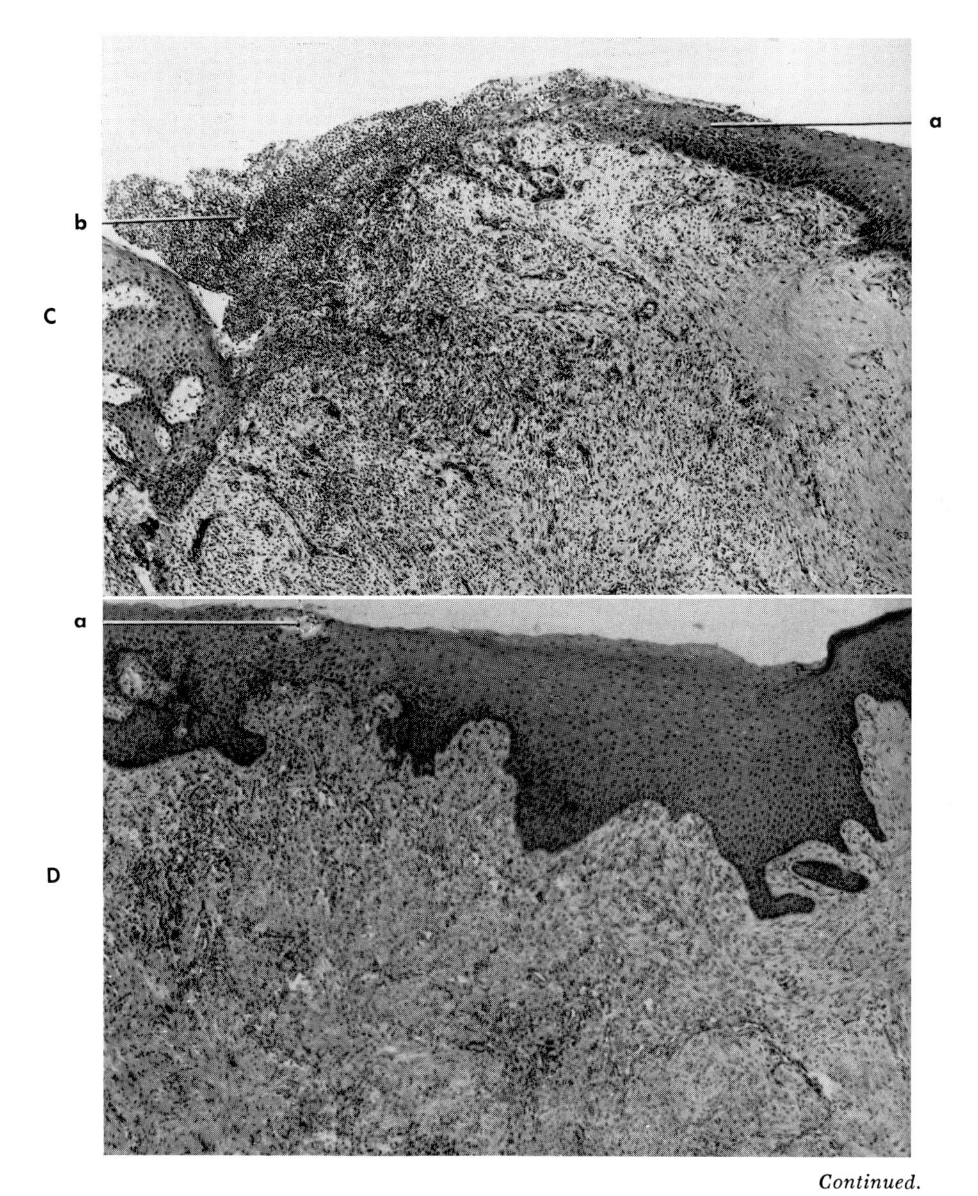


*Continued.*

**Fig. 28-25, cont'd. C,** Eight days after surgery, only a small area of the wound is not covered by epithelium, *a*. Granulation tissue, *b,* covers the surface. **D,** Fourteen days after surgery the wound surface is completely epithelized. However, there is a small area, *a,* that shows the migration of inflammatory cells to the surface.

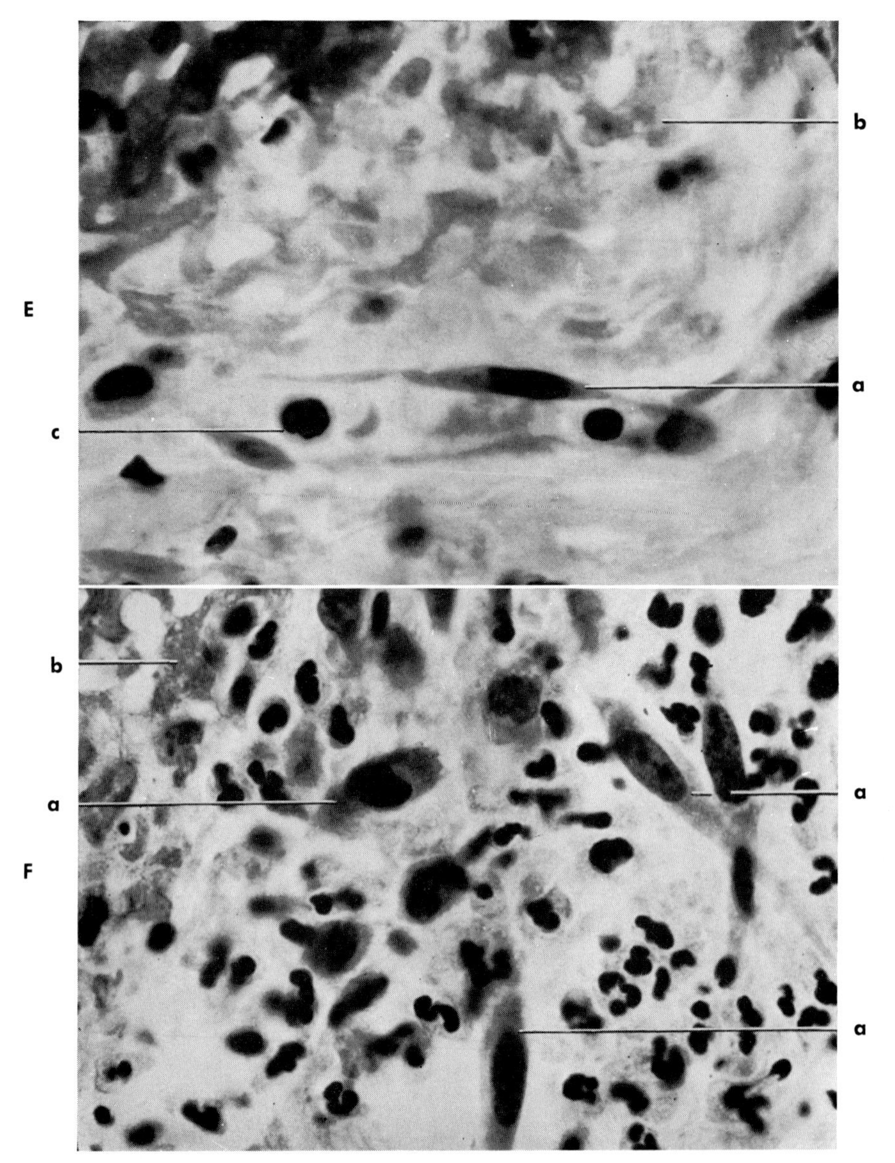


**Fig. 28-25, cont'd. E,** Histologic section of wound healing showing proliferation of endothelial cells, *a,* forming new capillaries. *b,* Fibrinous network; *c,* white blood cells in the new capillary. **F,** Proliferating fibroblasts, *a,* organizing remnants of the blood clot, *b.*

Remember, little, if anything, can be done to accelerate healing. However, infection, contamination, and debris may all retard healing.

## ELECTROSURGERY

Some surgeons prefer to use electrosurgery for gingivectomy-gingivoplasty.[12-13a] This method employs either bipolar electrocoagulation or single-pole electrodes. Both can be used as adjuncts to the knife, especially in areas where access is limited and difficult. Gingivoplasty often is difficult to perform in an isolated area and electrosurgery is useful in such cases (Fig. 28-27).

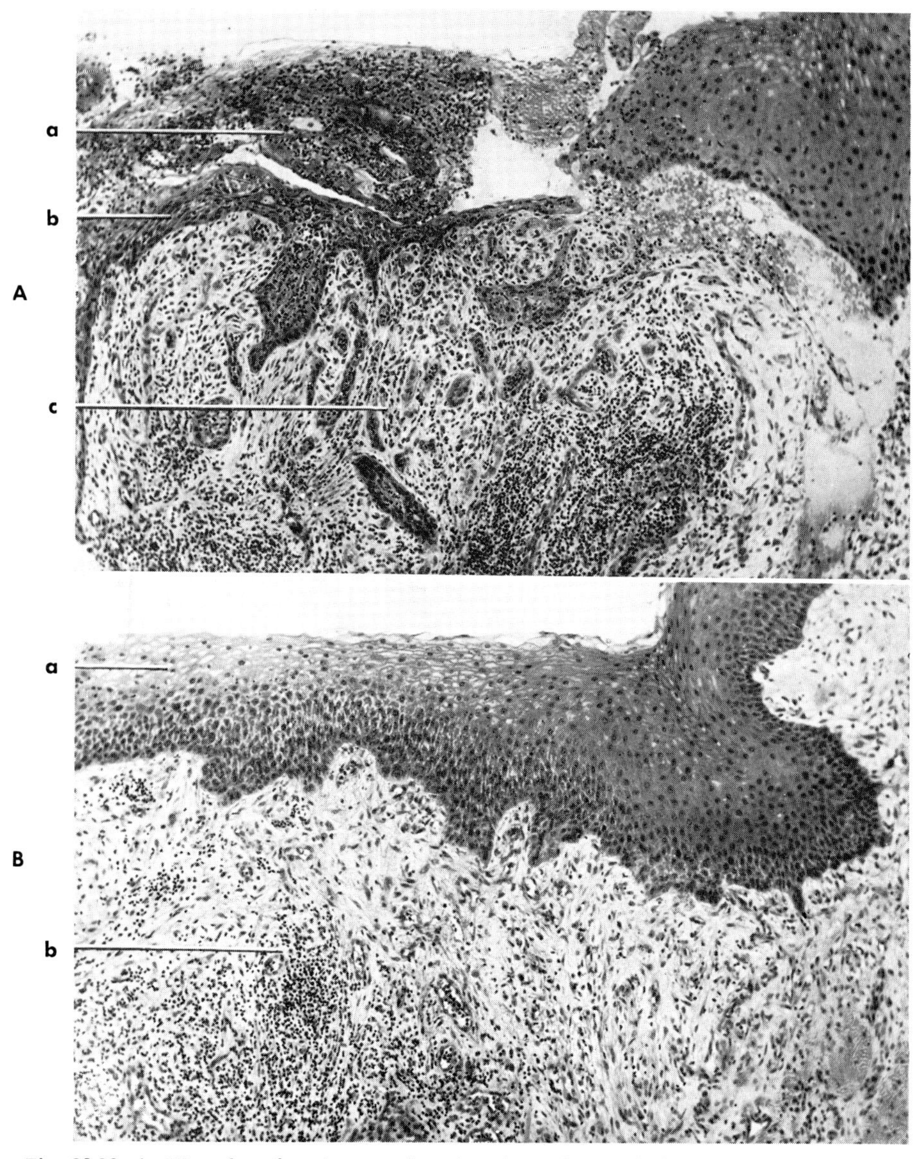


**Fig. 28-26. A,** Wound surface in a patient in whom the surgical dressing was unchanged for 10 days. There was an accumulation of exudate and necrotic material, *a;* the epithelium was thin and proliferative, *b;* and a severe inflammatory reaction could be seen below the surface, *c.* **B,** Wound surface in a patient in whom the dressing was changed three times in 10 days. The epithelization, *a,* of the wound surface is good. There is no necrotic blood clot on the surface. The subepithelial inflammatory reaction, *b,* is moderate.

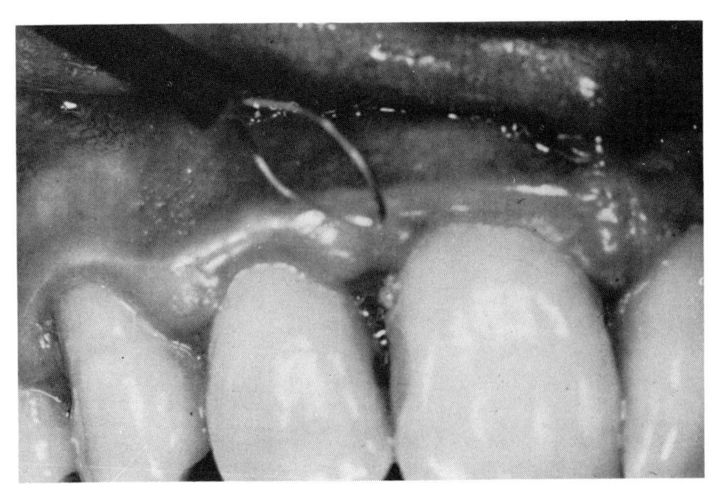

**Fig. 28-27.** Use of the unipolar electrode in the performance of gingivoplasty. (Courtesy G. P. Ivancie, Denver.)

Electrosurgery may be more painful postoperatively than surgery with a scalpel. One of the arguments in favor of electrosurgery is that a rather bloodless operation may be performed, which is in part true. However, there are other ways of controlling bleeding incident to surgery without resorting to cautery.

The histopathologic features of tissue healing after electrocoagulation[21] can be seen in Fig. 28-28. In *A* the immediate result of coagulation is seen. A blister was formed in the epithelium, and necrosis and hemorrhage could be seen in the adjacent areas. Two days later (*B*) the necrotic, coagulated tissue was separated from the underlying tissue by migration of leukocytes and demarcation of the living from the dead tissue. In 14 days epithelization and shrinkage of the wound surface took place (*C*). In one area, however, two small bone sequestra were found beneath the epithelium (*D*), which were eliminated by either sloughing or resorption. This sequestration process can delay healing considerably. It can occur whenever the current used is too strong or applied too long or when the instrument is used close to bone.

## EVALUATION OF RESULTS

*Success* If the prerequisites of gingivectomy-gingivoplasty are met and the procedure is carefully performed as described, the objectives will be achieved and permit long-term maintenance.

*Failure* On occasion the desired ends are not gained or the result cannot be maintained. Such developments are labeled failures. Most often failures are predictable. They occur if the basic prerequisites were not met, if the performance of the surgery was not adequate, or if the procedure was used when contraindicated.[19,20]

### Errors in surgical technique

Failures or partial failures can occur immediately after healing. They may be caused by careless or inexact performance of surgery. Early failure can occur because of any of the following situations:

1. Poor and inaccurate probing and pocket marking that leads to incomplete pocket elimination

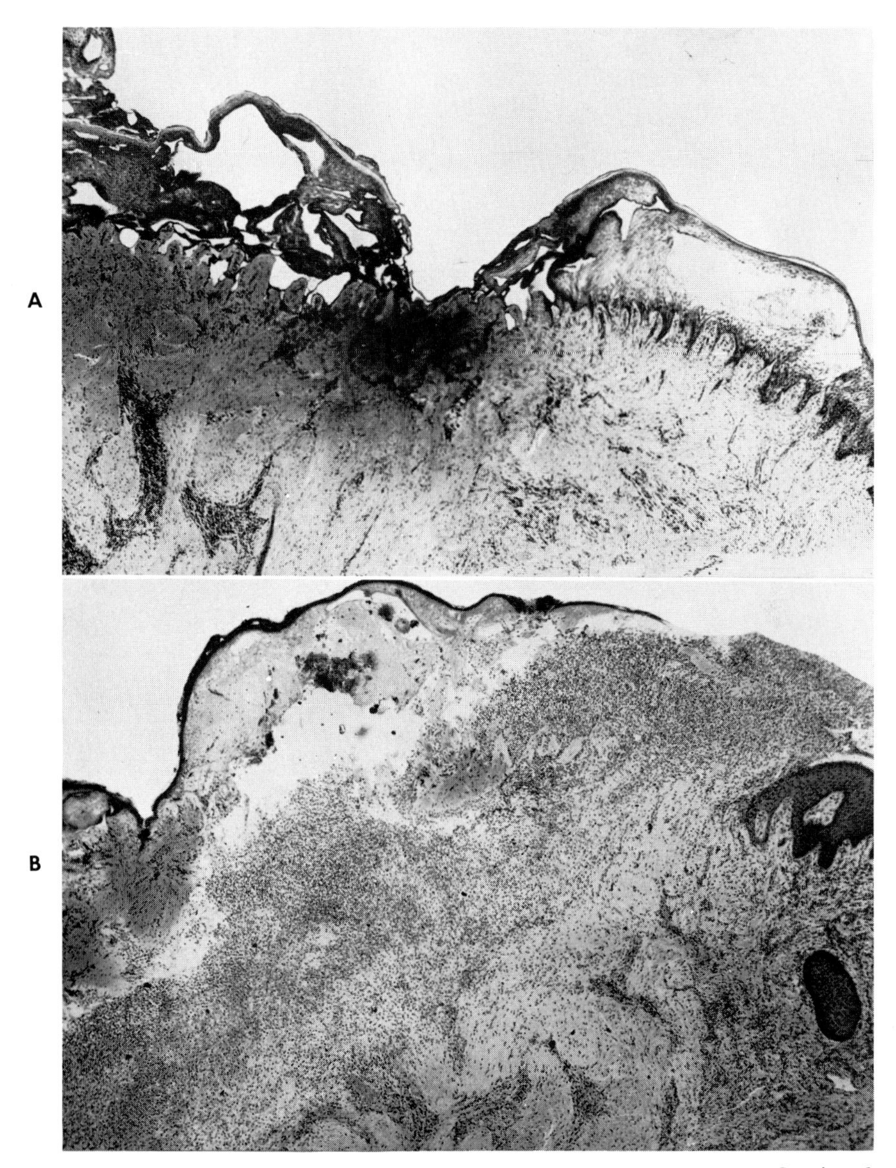


*Continued.*

**Fig. 28-28.** Histologic features of tissue healing after electrocoagulation. **A,** Blister formation and necrosis immediately after coagulation. **B,** Demarcation of the necrotic from the viable tissue.

2. Timidity in making the initial and subsequent incisions so that some pocket depth remains
3. Failure to examine after surgery for residual pocket depth

   If residual pockets are found, they should be eliminated.
4. Failure to create a proper bevel leaving blunt gingival margins
5. Failure to create adequate festooning

   If a mesiodistal scalloped form is not achieved, the gingival margin produced may be horizontal (without interdental papillae) or, even less desirable, may be one of reverse architecture. In reverse architecture the interdental tissues are lower than the oral and vestibular gingival margins.

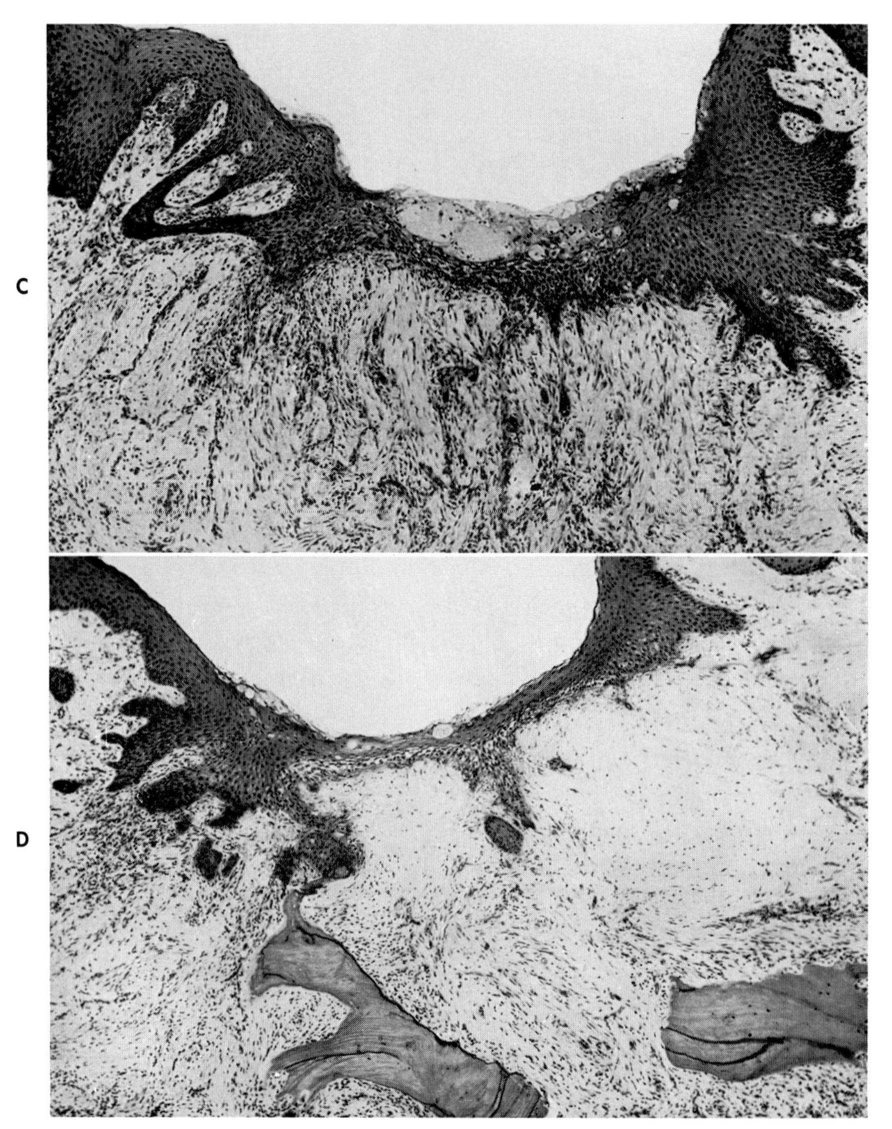


**Fig. 28-28, cont'd. C,** Complete epithelization and shrinkage of the wound surface. **D,** Formation of sequestra, delaying the healing.

If this is specially pronounced, interdental defects may be produced, making oral hygiene more difficult to perform.

6. Failure to be technically proficient

   If dull instruments are used, the tissue becomes lacerated and tissue tags result, which should be removed. If presurgical scaling was inadequate, calculus may remain. Any remnant of calculus must be removed at the time of operation. If the dressing is not properly mixed or placed, it may loosen and irritate the tissue. In some instances the dressing may not be placed firmly over the tissue and clots may form. Larger clots organize poorly. If the dressing is not changed in time, the tissue fluids, desquamated cells, saliva, and bacteria below the dressing may become putrescent.

Any of these situations can lead to a coronal and lateral proliferation of granulation tissue and the reestablishment of pocket depth.

If such a failure should result (caused by the foregoing factors), reoperation may become necessary.

**CHAPTER 28**

**References**

1. Pickerill H. P.: Stomatology in general practice, London, 1912, Henry Frowde, Hodder & Stoughton.
2. Fröhlich, E.: Die chirurgische Behandlung der marginalen Parodontitis. In Häupl, K., and Schuchardt, K., editors: Die Zahn-, Mund-, und Kieferheilkunde, Munich, 1957, Urban & Schwarzenberg, vol. 3, pt. 1.
3. Hiatt, W. H., Stallard, R. E., Grant, D. A., and Kramer, G. J.: Is the simple gingivectomy obsolete? Periodont. Abstr. **13**:62, 1965.
4. Ward, A. W.: Consideration of periodontal pocket elimination, Acad. Rev. **4**:64, 1956.
5. Orban, B.: To what extent should the tissues be excised in gingivectomy? J. Periodont. **12**:83, 1941.
6. Prichard, J.: Gingivoplasty, gingivectomy, and osseous surgery, J. Periodont. **32**:275, 1961.
7. Orban, B.: Surgical gingivectomy, J. Amer. Dent. Ass. **32**:701, 1945.
8. Orban, B.: Indications, technique and postoperative management of gingivectomy in treatment of the periodontal pocket, J. Periodont. **12**:89, 1941.
9. Goldman, H. M.: Gingivectomy, Oral Surg. **4**:1136, 1951.
10. Goldman, H. M.: The development of physiologic gingival contour by gingivoplasty, Oral Surg. **3**:879, 1950.
11. Fox, L.: Rotating abrasives in the management of periodontal soft and hard tissues, Oral Surg. **8**:1134, 1955.
12. Saghirian, L. M.: Electrosurgical gingivoplasty, Oral Surg. **2**:1549, 1949.
13. Sugarman, M. M.: Electrosurgical gingivoplasty—a technic, J. Periodont. **22**:156, 1951.

13a. Oringer, M. J.: Electrosurgery in dentistry, Philadelphia, 1962, W. B. Saunders Co.

13b. Spitzy, K. H.: Neue Aspekte in der antibakteriellen Chemotherapie, Oest. Z. Stomat. **68**: 445, 1971.

14. Archer, E. A., and Orban, B.: Dynamics of wound healing following elimination of gingival pockets, Amer. J. Orthodont. (Oral Surg. section) **31**:40, 1945.
15. Ramfjord, S. P., and Costich, E. R.: Healing after simple gingivectomy, J. Periodont. **34**:401, 1963.
16. Stahl, S. S., Witkin, G. J., Cantor, M., and Brown, R.: Gingival healing. II. Clinical and histologic repair sequences following gingivectomy, J. Periodont. **39**:109, 1968.
17. Orban, B.: Tissue healing following electrocoagulation of gingiva, J. Periodont. **15**:17, 1944.
18. Pope, J. W., Gargiulo, A. W., Staffileno, H., and Levy, S.: Effects of electrosurgery on wound healing, Periodontics **6**:30, 1968.
19. Swenson, H. M.: Success or failure in periodontal surgery, J. Amer. Dent. Ass. **67**:193, 1963.
20. Wade, A. B.: Where gingivectomy fails, J. Periodont. **25**:189, 1954.
21. Nakata, T. M.: Epithelial regeneration in wounds, Periodont. Abstr. **19**:105, 1971.
22. Parham, D.: Current concepts of wound healing and healing of the excisional type of gingival wound, Periodont. Abstr. **19**:112, 1971.

**Additional suggested reading**

Bloom, J.: The justification for surgical procedures employed in periodontal therapy, Oral Surg. **15**:531, 1962.

Burch, J. G., Conroy, C. W., and Ferris, R. T.: Tooth mobility following gingivectomy—a study of gingival support of the teeth, Periodontics **6**:90, 1968.

Donnenfeld, O. W., and Glickman, I.: A biometric study of the effects of gingivectomy, J. Periodont. **37**:447, 1966.

Glickman, I.: The results obtained with an unembellished gingivectomy technique in humans, J. Periodont. **27**:247, 1956.

Grant, D. A.: Experimental periodontal surgery: gingivectomy, excision to the alveolar crest, J. Dent. Res. **43**:790, 1964.

Hirschfeld, L., and others: Is surgical pocket elimination necessary for successful periodontal therapy? J. West. Soc. Periodont. **11**:88, 1963.

Hulin, C.: Les parodontoses pyorrhéiques ou pyorhées alvéolaires, Paris, 1941, Foulon.
Korn, N. A., Schaffer, E. M., and McHugh, R. B.: An experimental assessment of gingivectomy and soft tissue curettage in dogs, J. Periodont. 36:96, 1965.
Ramfjord, S. P., Engler, W. O., and Hiniker, J. J.: A radioautographic study of healing following simple gingivectomy. II. The connective tissue, J. Periodont. 37:179, 1966.

CHAPTER TWENTY-NINE

# Periodontal flap



*Definition*

In periodontics a flap is a unit (segment) of gingiva and (most often) adjoining alveolar mucosa that is partially detached by surgical means. The base of the flap remains attached to provide adequate vascular supply.

## CLASSIFICATION

Flaps may be classified into full-thickness and partial-thickness flaps. The full-thickness flap includes all the gingiva or alveolar mucosa covering the tooth and bone. Tooth and bone are left bared on reflection of this type of flap. The partial-thickness flap is elevated by sharp dissection so as to leave bone covered by soft connective tissue, including the periosteum.

## DESIGN

Flaps are designed to provide good access to underlying tissues and to retain adequate circulation to the partially detached tissues. The shape that the surgeon gives to the flap will depend on specific needs, such as to provide adequate surgical access or to reposition the gingiva.[1-3] Flap design is divided into two categories—the full flap[4,5] and the modified flap.[6]

*Full flap*

Full flaps (Fig. 29-1, *A*) are reflected by vertical or oblique releasing incisions at both its lateral ends. These ends are connected by a horizontal incision at the gingival margin or apical to it. When vertical incisions are used, they should extend far enough into the gingiva and, where necessary, into the alveolar mucosa to relieve tissue tension and permit good surgical access.

*Modified flap*

Modified flaps (Figs. 29-1, *B*, and 29-2) differ from full flaps in that they have either only one vertical or oblique incision or no vertical incision.

### Access and blood supply

Surgical judgment will govern the selection of the type of flap and the extent of the area to be involved. Adequate access must be obtained as well as a satisfactory blood supply to the flap. The base of the flap should be at least as broad as the detached tissue, but the unnecessary involvement of areas adjacent to the surgical field should be avoided. The design and management of a flap can be critical in determining the success of periodontal surgery.

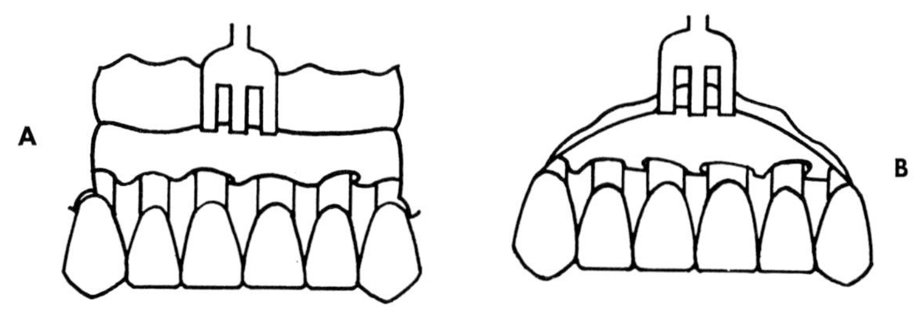


Fig. 29-1. **A,** Full flap. **B,** Modified flap with no vertical incisions.

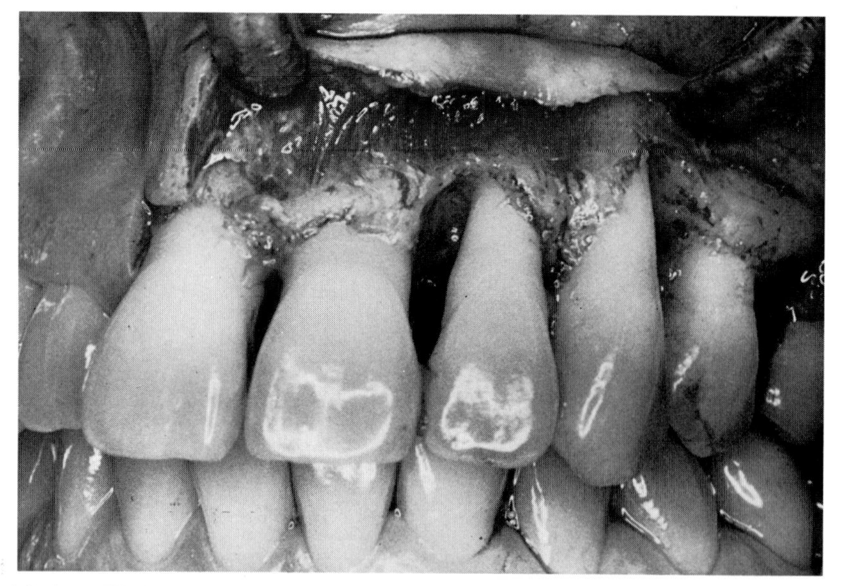

Fig. 29-2. A modified flap with one vertical incision (distal to the right central incisor) has been elevated, showing osseous defects.

## ELEVATING THE FLAP

Flaps may be reflected by blunt or sharp dissection. Blunt dissection is used when surgical remodeling of lateral alveolar surfaces is planned or when reattachment, bone graft, or bone transplant procedures are to be done. Blunt dissection can divest the bone of soft tissue and expose the alveolar surface for inspection and any extensive surgery.

### Blunt dissection

*Full-thickness flaps*

Blunt flap reflection is accomplished by insertion of a periosteal elevator between the gingiva and the tooth or bone. The instrument is worked mesially, distally, and apically to reflect the gingiva, alveolar mucosa, and periosteum. The initial incision, prior to the insertion of the elevator, may be made with a scalpel or periodontal knife. In this way a full-thickness flap may be elevated.

*Thick gingival margins*

When the gingiva is thick and bulbous, the flap margin may be trimmed and beveled. Do this by performing a partial gingivectomy before reflecting the flap, by trimming the flap after other surgery, or by reflecting the flap with an undermining horizontal incision (reverse bevel) (Fig. 29-3).

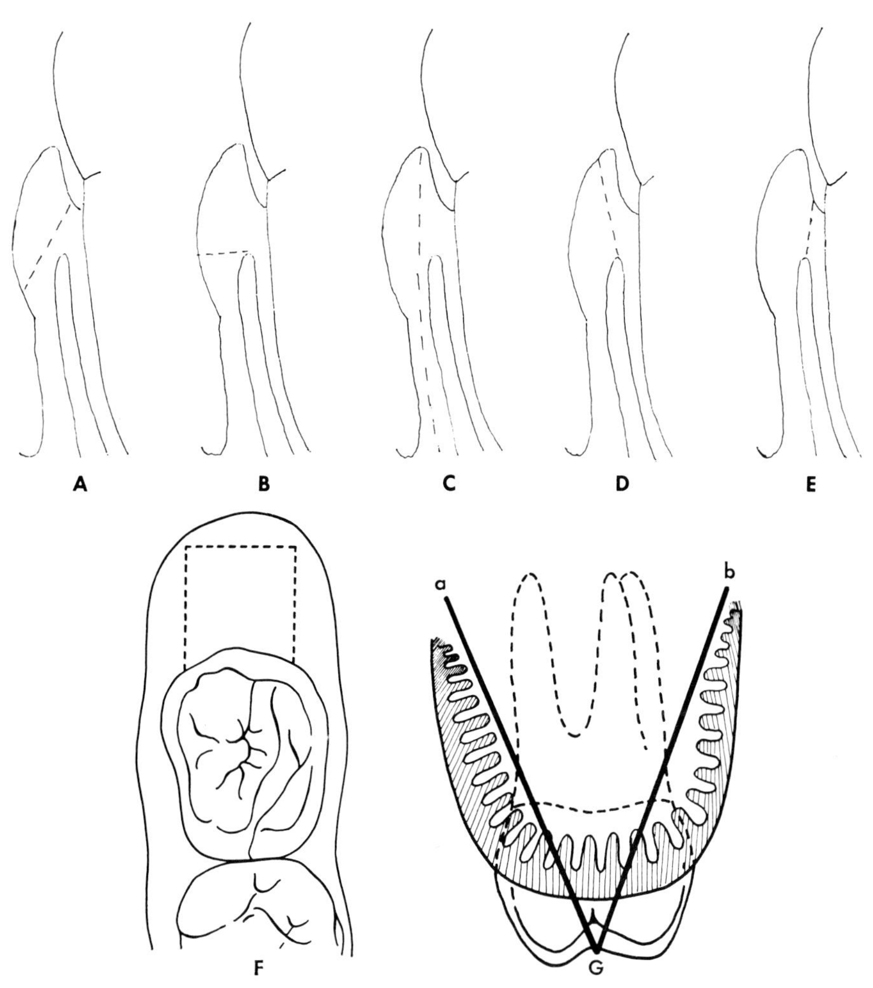


**Fig. 29-3.** Initial incisions prior to reflecting a flap. **A,** Beveled gingivectomy. **B,** Excision to the alveolar crest. **C,** Split-thickness flap. **D,** Internal (reverse) bevel. **E,** Incision via the pocket. **F,** Square cut distal wedge incision. **G,** Internal beveling by undermining incisions. (**E** and **F** courtesy R. E. Robinson, San Mateo, Calif.)

*Retromolar incisions*

When flap incisions involve retromolar tissues, special attention must be given to the thick, fibrous bulk. In addition, deep pockets and furcation involvements may be present. To reduce the bulk of this tissue, undermine and excise some of the tissue. This will permit both access to the bone and reduction of the tissue bulk for flap coaptation after surgery.

The tissue may be excised as triangular, rectangular, or trapezoidal wedges. Such tissue reduction (called distal wedge operation[7]) may be accomplished by initial undermining incisions as in Fig. 29-3, *F* and *G*. When the tissue is not bulky, two simple linear undermining incisions meeting at the surface will suffice.

## Sharp dissection

*Split-thickness flaps*

Sharp dissection may be done with a replaceable surgical blade or with a kidney-shaped scalpel. It is indicated when the surgeon wants to avoid exposure of bone. The scalpel may be inserted into the gingiva or the sulcus to dissect through the lamina propria without removing the soft tissue over the bone. This is desirable in the presence of thin bony plates or when the surgical correction of the bone involves only alveolar margins. Sharp dissection in the lamina propria will leave the bone protected by the covering connective tissue, including the periosteum. This may reduce the extent of any postsurgical bone resorption.[8,8a]

*Thin gingival margins*

When the gingiva is thin, sharp dissection from the sulcus is difficult. In this situation, insert the blade via the vertical releasing incision to sharply dissect and undermine; then work the blade coronally from the base of the flap. This method is difficult but can result in a split-thickness flap.[5,8]

## MANIPULATION

*Treatment of the gingival margin of the flap*

The gingival margin of a flap may be left intact if it is thin; or if it is thick, it may be excised, trimmed, or beveled. The excision, trimming, or beveling may be done before the flap is reflected by an undermining incision or by partial gingivectomy. The flap may also be trimmed or beveled after reflection by the use of tissue shears, scalpel, or electrocautery. The electrocautery is particularly valuable in thinning the flap margin after the flap has been reflected, when holding the flap for surgical manipulation is difficult. Care must be exercised to avoid postoperative tissue slough.

*Replacement of the flap*

After any surgical procedures have been performed, the flap may be replaced in its original position, or repositioned apically, coronally, or laterally. Wherever possible, bone should be covered to avoid the destruction that takes place when it is left exposed.[8-12]

## SUTURING

The extensive use of flap techniques has forced the dentist to be conversant with various suturing procedures. Suturing is used for the post-operative replacement and readaptation of the flap.[13,14] (See discussion on the role of the assistant in suturing, Chapter 26.)

Sutures and needles should be selected for the particular procedure: nos. 3-0, 4-0, 5-0, and 6-0 silk, synthetic, or gut sutures as required. Needles should be the swaged, atraumatic type: ⅜-circle reverse cutting, ⅜-circle conventional cutting, ½-circle layer, and ½-circle conventional cutting needles as appropriate.

*Suturing for the replacement of reflected tissues*

It is important to accurately replace or reappose the flap. This is necessary for hemostasis, for reducing the size of the wound to be repaired, to permit healing by first intention, and to prevent unnecessary bone destruction.[2,8-11] In addition, when flaps are repositioned apically or laterally, it is necessary to properly suture and fix them in place to maintain the desired position.[12]

*Interdental ligation*

Interdental ligation is the most frequently used form of suturing and has several modifications (Figs. 29-4 to 29-7). It produces the firmest adaptation of soft tissue to underlying tooth and bone and is of greatest value when both buccal and lingual flaps are to be coapted and tightly adapted to the bone and tooth surfaces. Silicone-treated silk no. 4-0 noncapillary type suture, which is swaged to a ⅜-circle reverse cutting needle, is commonly used. There are situations, particularly when the tissue is very thin and laterally repositioned flaps are attempted, in which a no. 5-0 or 6-0 suture may be necessary. In other cases, when a particularly heavy and fibrous tissue is present, a no. 3-0 suture may be used. Some dentists prefer dermal or synthetic suture material.

Grasp the needle firmly in the needle holder or hemostat and insert it into

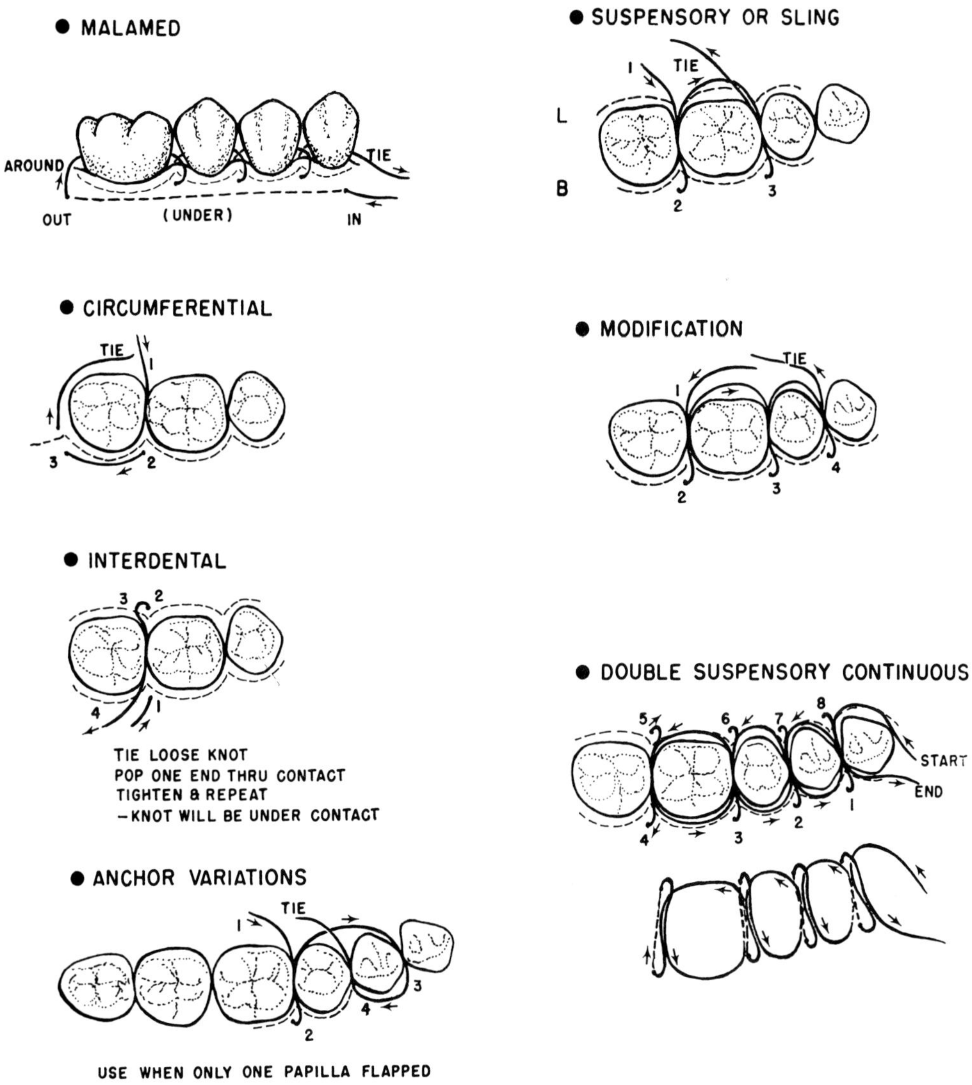

**Fig. 29-4.** Diagram of several popular suturing techniques. (Courtesy R. La Belle, Minneapolis.)

the more mobile flap, usually the buccal flap, from the buccal aspect. Pass it through the interdental space and pierce the lingual or palatal flap from the inner aspect. Then pass it back through the interdental space to the vestibule for tying. Double ties are made to prevent the suture from becoming loosened or displaced. When firmest adaptation to both tooth and bone is desired, snap one end of the suture back through the contact point or pass it beneath the contact. Tighten the knot by pulling one end of thread toward the oral surface and one end toward the vestibular surface. Passage between teeth is simple where wide embrasures exist. When the needle cannot be passed between teeth, passage of the suture through the contact is difficult. Care must be exercised to avoid tearing tissues or breaking the suture. Dental floss may be used to force the suture through the contact.

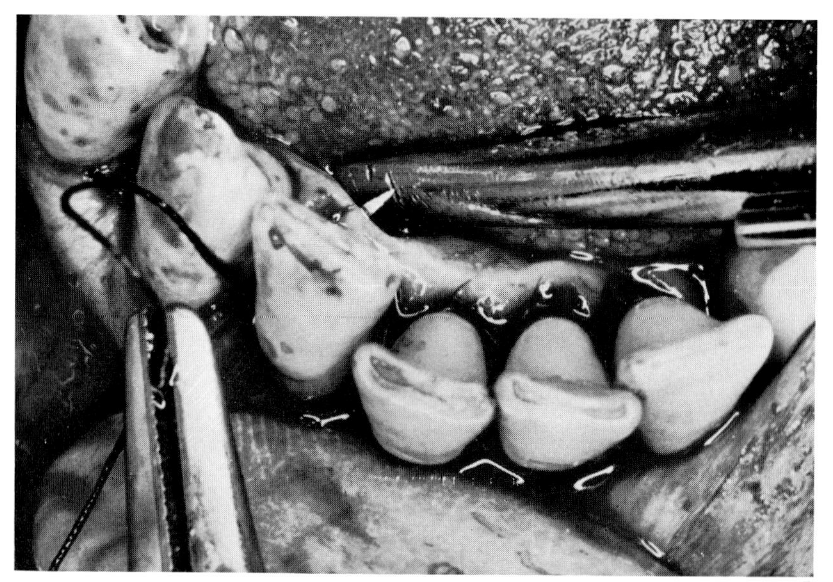

**Fig. 29-5.** The surgeon has passed the needle under the contact to pierce the lingual flap from its inner aspect. The assistant supports the flap with the aspirator tip to permit passage of the needle.

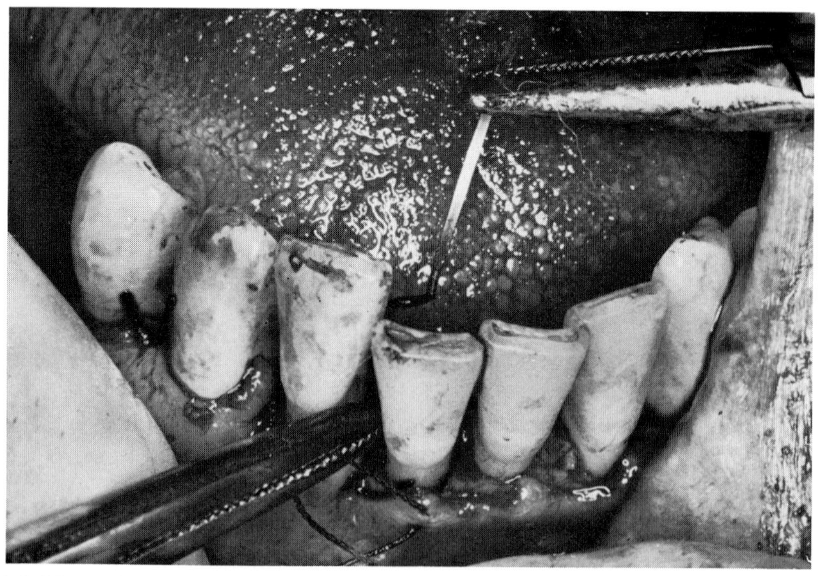

**Fig. 29-6.** The assistant grasps the end of the suture with a needle holder while the surgeon draws the suture through the flaps (interdental ligation).

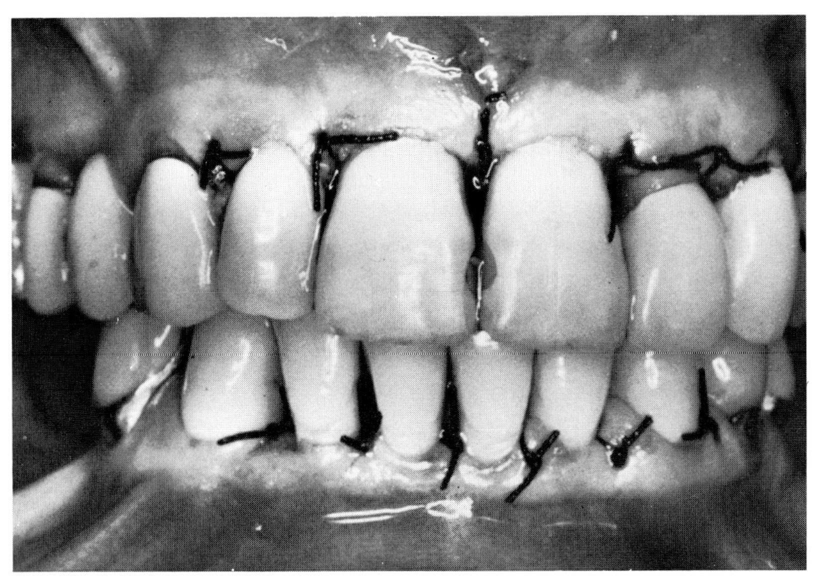

**Fig. 29-7.** Interdental ligation. Cut the suture ends short. A dressing may not be necessary when flap margins are coapted.

A modification of the procedure is used when the needle does not penetrate the inner aspect of the opposite flap. Reverse the needle after passing it through the interdental space; next, pierce the lingual flap from the lingual surface and pass the needle through the interdental space again for tying. This method will provide a firmer adaptation of tissue to tooth and bone. It is sometimes used for this purpose alone.

***Suspensory ligation***

Suspensory ligation encircles the tooth and is used mostly when a flap is reflected on only one surface, such as the buccal or the lingual, or when tying the buccal flap to the lingual flap is impossible or undesirable (Fig. 29-4). Such a situation may be present when one of the flaps is repositioned apically while the other is replaced in its original position. Another situation in which this suturing may be used is when inserting a curved needle through contact points is difficult or impossible, when the therapist finds inserting the needle into one of the flaps difficult, or when a flap is reflected on only one surface. In suspensory ligation, pass the needle through the outer surface of the flap, around the neck of the tooth, and through the embrasure and reinsert it through the flap from the outer or epithelial aspect. Make the knot on either the facial or the lingual surface of the tooth.

***Continuous ligation***

Continuous ligation (Fig. 29-8) is useful to suspend the flap at a predetermined level.[13] In this technique a continuous mattress-type suture is used for an entire quadrant or for an area involving several teeth. No. 4-0 or 3-0 suture with a medium-sized no. 2 curved needle is preferred. Each flap will be sutured and fixed to place individually. Pass the curved needle through the outer aspect of the flap at the most mesial border. Penetrate the flap about 2 mm. distal to the edge of the anterior releasing incision close to the mucogingival junction. The needle will enter from the outside and exit on the inside of the tissue flap. Lead the suture along the inner surface of the flap to the distal border. Then perforate the inner surface of the flap to exit on the outer surface. Circle the neck of the

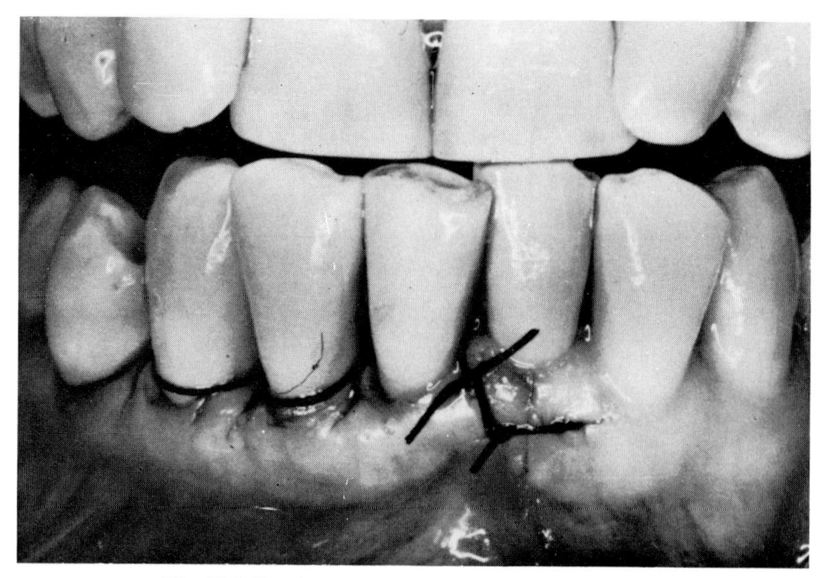

**Fig. 29-8.** Continuous suspensory ligation (modified).

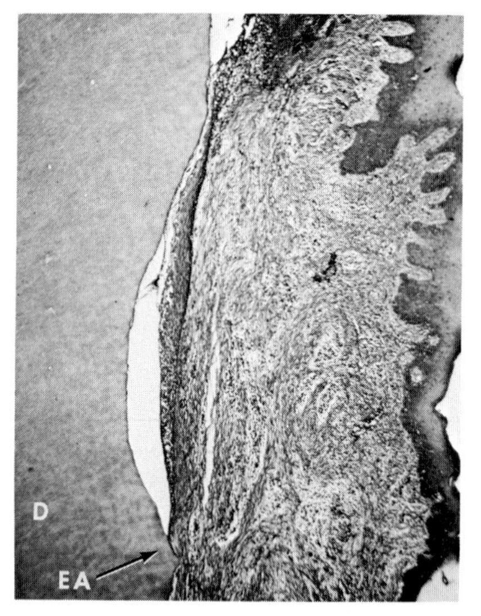


**Fig. 29-9.** Vertical section of a surgically created pocket showing an epithelial attachment, *EA*, on dentin, *D*.

tooth with the suture and pass the suture back at the next embrasure to enter the flap on the inner aspect. Then reverse the needle and repeat the procedure. Thus the entire flap is held in suspension while the suture runs along the inside of the flap slightly coronal to the level of the mucogingival junction and around the necks of the teeth. Make first a loose double tie at the mesial end of the flap where the tail end of the thread remains from the insertion of the needle. Press a gauze square against the flap to position the flap accurately to the desired level. Then, while an assistant holds the flap in place with a gauze square, tighten

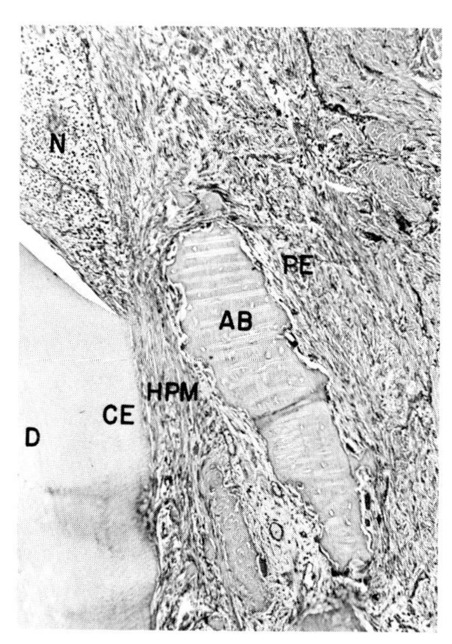


**Fig. 29-10.** Vertical section of a surgically created pocket. The healing periodontal ligament, *HPM,* consists of fibers aligned parallel to the long axis of the root between bone, *AB,* and cementum, *CE.* (Courtesy M. L. Morris, Columbia University, New York.)

the tie and make a double knot. If the opposite (lingual or buccal) area is similarly involved, use a continuous suture separately for this flap.

## SUMMARY

To summarize, precise flap design and suturing are necessary for accurate adaptation of the flap to tooth and bone and for accurate placement of the flap in its original position. These factors are also necessary to coapt flaps and to reposition flaps coronally, apically, or laterally. Close adaptation of the flap to bone may help to reduce postoperative pain and result in an improved tissue form after surgery. Perfect coaptation of flap margins is essential in bone grafting operations to enclose the grafted material and permit a take. Cooperation between the dentist and the assistant is necessary during the suturing procedure. Careful training and practice will permit these procedures to be performed with relative ease.

## WOUND HEALING

There are a number of histologic reports on the healing of flaps.[15-22] Close reapposition of the flap is necessary.[20] Any space due to loose fixation of the tissues will interfere with first intention healing. If an attachment epithelium can regenerate promptly, it acts as a seal and allows connective tissue healing to procede unhindered. However, the clot must be of minimal bulk. A thin clot is more easily replaced by collagen.

The new attachment epithelium may form on either cementum or dentin[20] (Fig. 29-9) by the elaboration of an extracellular material composed of a protein and mucopolysaccharide complex and of hemidesmosomes.[23-26]

The attachment epithelium is reestablished in 1 week. By the end of the second week, a collagenous reunion with the root has formed.[17]

Resorptions may occur on both cementum and dentin. They are more prominent in deep root concavities. However, at approximately 40 days new cementum appears in the concavities and nicks.[22]

An interlacing network of collagen fibers forms parallel to the root surface[8] (Fig. 29-10). Histologic observations up to 106 days and clinical records over 10 years attest to the integrity of the union. This attachment does not require a new cemental surface but may exist on dentin or old cementum.

In summary, the reunion of a periodontal flap and root may be successfully accomplished if firm apposition of tissues is realized. Although an epithelial attachment is formed by 1 week and a collagenous attachment by the second, this area is best left unprobed for at least 1 month.

**CHAPTER 29**

**References**


1. Johnson, W. N., Groat, J. E., and Romans, A. R.: The periodontal flap; literature review, Periodont. Abstr. **15**:11, 1967.
2. Nabers, C. L.: Repositioning the attached gingiva, J. Periodont. **25**:38, 1954.
3. Dahlberg, W. H.: Incisions and suturing, Dental Clinics of North America, Philadelphia, 1969, W. B. Saunders Co., vol. 13.
4. Neumann, R.: Atlas der radical-chirurgischen Behandlung der Paradentosen, Berlin, 1926, Hermann Meusser.
5. Everett, F. G., Waerhaug, J., and Widman, A.: Leonard Widman, surgical treatment of pyorrhea alveolaris, J. Periodont. **42**:571, 1971.
6. Kirkland, O.: Modified flap operation in surgical treatment of periodontoclasia, J. Amer. Dent. Ass. **19**:1918, 1932.
7. Robinson, R. E.: The distal wedge operation, Periodontics **4**:256, 1966.
8. Staffileno, H., Wentz, F. M., and Orban, B.: Histologic study of healing of split thickness flap surgery in dogs, J. Periodont. **33**:56, 1962.

8a. Hoag, P. M., Wood, D. L., Donnenfeld, O. W., and Rosenfeld, L. D.: Alveolar crest reduction following full and partial thickness flaps, J. Periodont. **43**:141, 1972.

9. Wilderman, M. N., Wentz, F. M., and Orban, B.: Histogenesis of repair after mucogingival surgery, J. Periodont, **31**:283, 1960.
10. Grant, D. A.: Experimental periodontal surgery: sequestration of alveolar bone, J. Periodont. **38**:409, 1967.
11. Pfeiffer, J. S.: The reaction of alveolar bone to flap procedure in man, Periodontics **3**:135, 1965.
12. Carranza, F. A., Jr., and Carraro, J. J.: Effect of removal of periosteum on postoperative result of mucogingival surgery, J. Periodont. **34**:223, 1963.
13. Morris, M. L.: Suturing techniques in periodontal surgery, Periodontics **3**:84, 1965.
14. Malamed, E. H.: A technique of suturing flaps in periodontal surgery, Periodontics **1**:207, 1963.
15. Linghorne, W. J., and O'Connell, D. C.: Studies in the regeneration and reattachment of supporting structures of the teeth, J. Dent. Res. **29**:419, 1950.
16. Persson, P.: The regeneration of the marginal periodontium after flap operation, Acta Odont. Scand. **20**:43, 1962.
17. Hiatt, W. H., Stallard, R. E., Butler, E. D., and Badgett, B.: Repair following mucoperiosteal flap surgery with full gingival retention, J. Periodont. **39**:11, 1968.
18. Morris, M. L.: The reattachment of human periodontal tissues following surgical detachment: a clinical and histological study, J. Periodont. **24**:220, 1953.
19. Morris, M. L.: Healing of human periodontal tissues following surgical detachment and extirpation of vital pulps, J. Periodont. **31**:23, 1960.
20. Morris, M. L.: Healing of human periodontal tissues following surgical detachment from vital teeth: the position of the epithelial attachment, J. Periodont. **32**:108, 1961.
21. Morris, M. L., and Thompson, R. H.: Healing of human periodontal tissues following surgical detachment: factors related to the deposition of new cementum on dentin, Periodontics **1**:189, 1963.

22. Morris, M. L.: Healing of human periodontal tissues following surgical detachment: the arrangement of the fibers of the periodontal space, Periodontics **1**:118, 1963.
23. Toto, P. D., and Sicher, H.: The epithelial attachment, Periodontics **2**:154, 1964.
24. Stallard, R. E., Diab, M. A., and Zander, H. A.: The attaching substance between enamel and epithelium—a product of the epithelial cells, J. Periodont. **36**:130, 1965.
25. Stern, I. B.: Electron microscopic observations of oral epithelium, Periodontics **3**:224, 1965.
26. Listgarten, M. A.: Periodontal tissue repair over surgically exposed dentin and cementum surfaces, I.A.D.R. abstract no. 474, 1971.

**Additional suggested reading**

Kirkland, O.: The suppurative periodontal pus pocket: its treatment by the modified flap operation, J. Amer. Dent. Ass. **18**:1462, 1931.

Levine, H. L.: Periodontal flap surgery with gingival fiber retention, J. Periodont. **43**:91, 1972.

Levine, H. L., and Stahl, S. S.: Repair following flap surgery with retention of gingival fibers, J. Periodont. **43**:99, 1972.

Manly, R. S.: Adhesions in biological systems, New York, 1970, Academic Press, Inc.

Östman, B.: Zur differentiellen Therapie der marginalen Paradentosen, Vjschr. Zahnheilk. **41**:49, 1925.

Rennefarth, I.: Biosuturen als Nahtmaterial in der chirurgischen Stomatologie, Deutsch. Stomat. **19**:455, 1969.

Tilly, G., Armstrong, J., Salem, J., and Cutcher, J.: Reaction of oral tissues to suture materials, Oral Surg. **26**:592, 1968.

Zemsky, J. L.: Surgical treatment of periodontal diseases with the author's open-view operation for advanced cases of dental periclasia, Dent. Cosmos **68**:465, 1926.

Zentler, A.: Suppurative gingivitis with alveolar involvement. A new surgical procedure, J.A.M.A. **71**:1530, 1918.

CHAPTER THIRTY

# Surgical curettage by flap



## OBJECTIVES

The purpose of surgical curettage by flap is to remove chronic inflammatory tissue (granulation tissue, Chapter 27) and any remaining calcified deposits. When this surgery is successful, it will result in (1) resolution of inflammation and (2) reduction of pocket depth or elimination of pockets by inducing recession of the gingival walls of the pockets. It may also result in some reattachment and some favorable remodeling of bone.

## INDICATIONS

Surgical curettage is generally used in the management of deep pockets with extensive bone loss when scaling and gingival curettage are not enough and when other procedures (gingivectomy, osseous surgery, retachment, or bone grafting) are not indicated (Fig. 30-1).

## METHOD

***Reflecting a full-thickness flap***

Make the initial incision with a no. 12b or 11 removable blade to bisect the papillae (Fig. 30-1, *C*). Then insert a periosteal elevator into the sulci and work it against tooth and bone to elevate a full-thickness flap by blunt dissection (Fig. 30-1, *D*).

***Curettage***

The excellent access and visibility obtained will permit the removal of adherent inflammatory tissue from tooth and bone and the planing of the exposed root surface (Fig. 30-1, *E*). Remove the inflammatory tissue from the inner surface of the reflected flaps by cutting with scissors or scraping with a kidney-shaped periodontal knife blade. Then replace the flap and fix it by interdental sutures (Fig. 30-1, *F*). The successful result 2 years later can be seen in Fig. 30-1, *G*.

## DISCUSSION

With the removal of chronic inflammatory tissue bordering pockets and from bony margins facing pockets, a number of events may follow. Some bone resorption undoubtedly occurs after the reflection of the flap and the instrumentation. Some reattachment may also take place. With the resorption of thin bony plates and spicules and with some bone regeneration, irregularities tend to be corrected and a more regular crestal alveolar form may be created.

Surgical curettage has a long history, and its current acceptance may indicate its usefulness.[1-6]

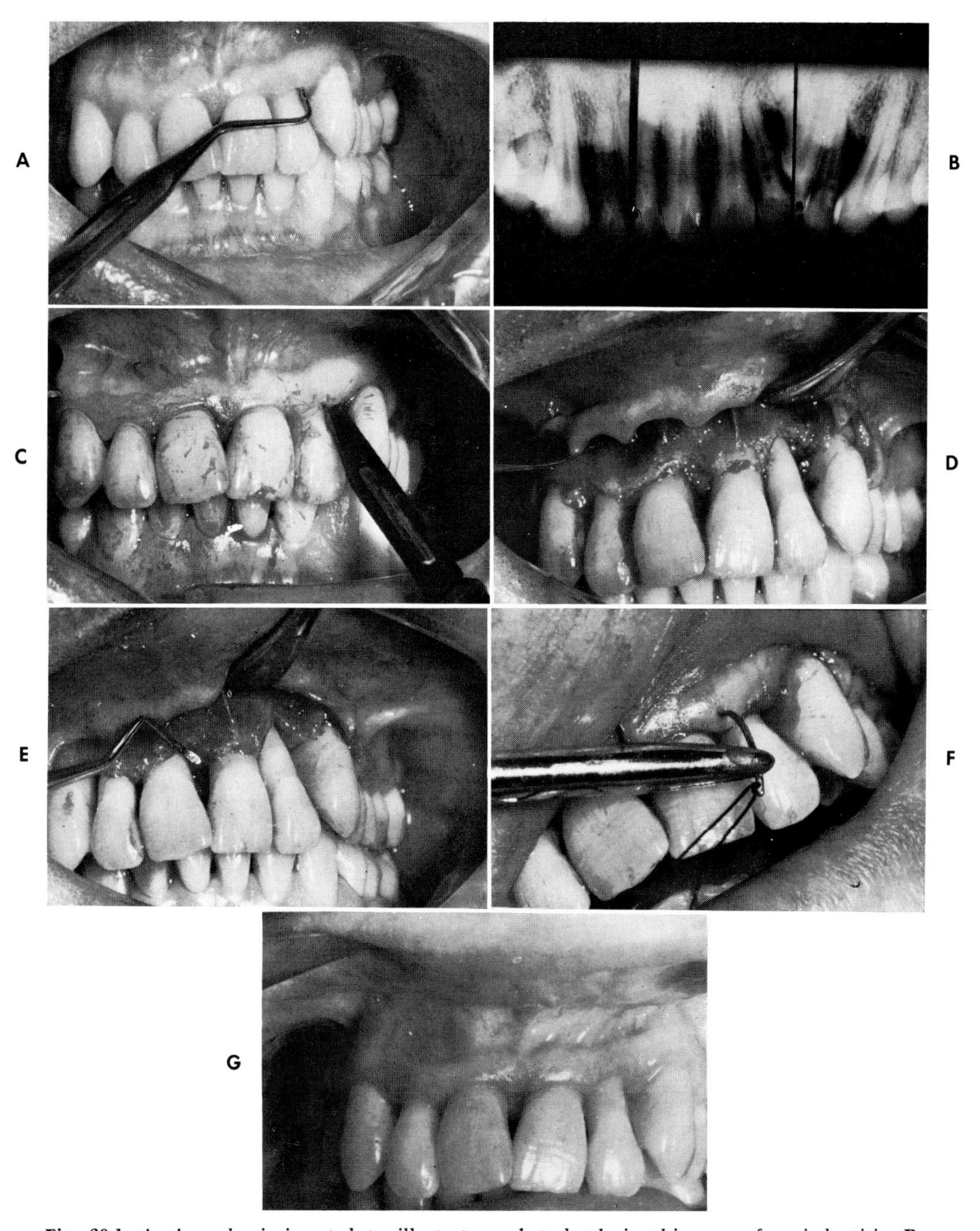


**Fig. 30-1. A,** A probe is inserted to illustrate pocket depth in this case of periodontitis. **B,** Roentgenograms reveal extensive alveolar resorption. **C,** A no. 11 removable surgical blade is used to incise the papillae and marginal gingiva. **D,** The flap with periosteum is reflected by blunt dissection. **E,** A curette is used to remove deposits, plane the root surface, and debride both tooth and bone of adherent inflammatory tissue. **F,** The flap is carefully sutured, and a dressing is then placed. **G,** Two years later an excellent result is evident. Gingival form is physiologic with only an insignificant gingival deformity visible between the maxillary incisors. (Courtesy J. Ingle, Los Angeles.)

**CHAPTER 30**

**References**

1. Patur, B., and Glickman, I.: Clinical and roentgenographic evaluation of the posttreatment healing of infrabony pockets, J. Periodont. **33**:164, 1962.
2. Gilson, C. M.: Surgical treatment of periodontal disease, J. Amer. Dent. Ass. **44**:733, 1952.
3. Kirkland, O.: The suppurative periodontal pus pocket: its treatment by the modified flap operation, J. Amer. Dent. Ass. **18**:1462, 1931.
4. Kirkland, O.: The surgical flap and semiflap technique in periodontal surgery, Dent. Dig. **42**:125, 1936.
5. Ingle, J. L.: Periodontal curettement in the premaxilla, J. Periodont. **23**:143, 1952.
6. Stern, I. B., Everett, F. G., and Robicsek, K.: S. Robicsek—a pioneer in the surgical treatment of periodontal disease, J. Periodont. **36**:265, 1965.

CHAPTER THIRTY-ONE

# Reattachment operations



The restoration of previously destroyed periodontal structures is the most attractive treatment result possible for both patient and dentist. The operations to create such tissue regeneration are generally called *reattachment operations.*[1]

## OBJECTIVES

When reattachment operations are successful, new attachment is created coronal to the preoperative level. New bone and new cementum are deposited and new periodontal ligament fibers are formed and become organized. The attachment epithelium reforms coronal to its presurgical level. The bottom of the sulcus (pocket) is shifted coronally, and pocket depth is reduced or eliminated (Fig. 31-1).

The term reattachment operation is applied to two distinct surgical procedures: (1) extension of subgingival curettage beyond the sulcular and attachment epithelium to bone and (2) surgical curettage by flap of three-walled (and sometimes two-walled) infrabony craters.

## INDICATIONS

The most favorable situation for reattachment is found in the three-walled infrabony (intra-alveolar) pocket.[2,3] Although reattachment may occur in any infrabony or suprabony pocket,[4,5] the pocket with three bony walls yields the greatest percentage of success (Fig. 31-2).

Infrabony defects may occur interdentally (Figs. 31-2 to 31-5) or on vestibular (labiobuccal) or oral (palatolingual) surfaces of teeth (Fig. 31-6). When infrabony defects are found interdentally, one tooth generally has a deep pocket whereas its neighboring tooth has a shallow pocket or no pocket (Fig. 31-4).

Since two different surgical procedures are known as a reattachment operation, they will be discussed individually.

## SUBGINGIVAL CURETTAGE

The classical reattachment operation is by subgingival curettage via the lumen of a pocket.[4,5] This technique requires that the area be anesthetized and

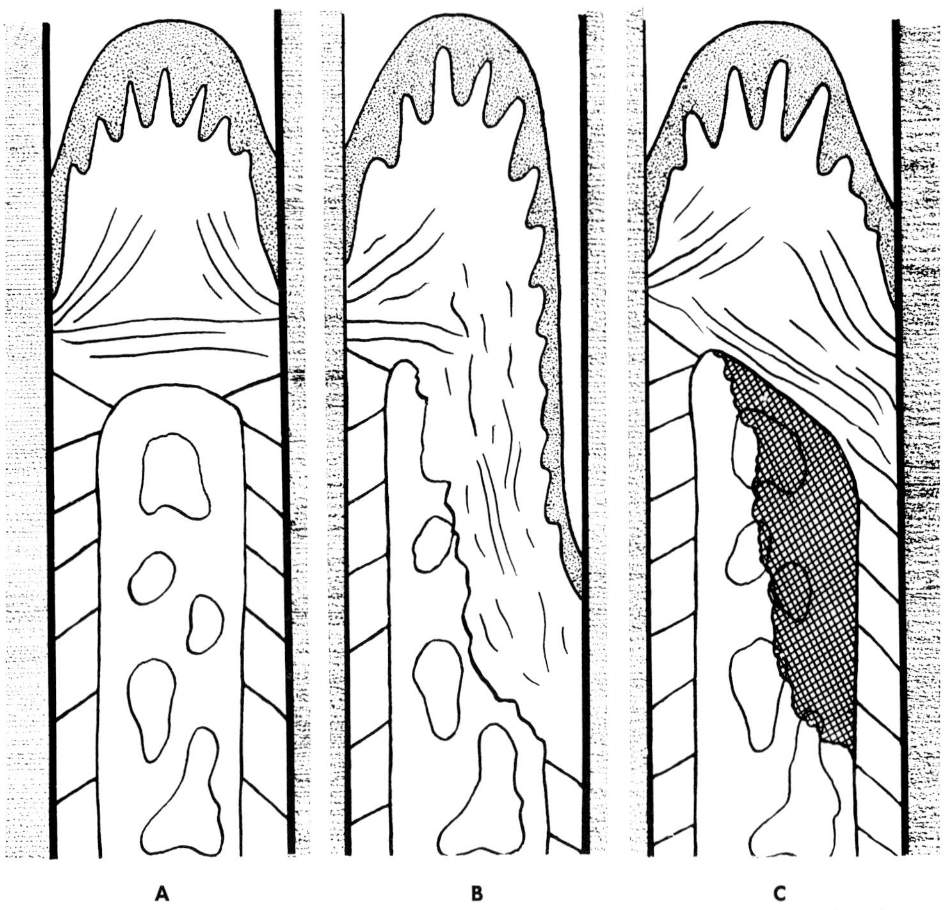


**Fig 31-1.** Diagrammatic illustration of, **A,** healthy interdental area, **B,** development of an intra-alveolar pocket, and, **C,** postoperative result after successful reattachment operations. New periodontal ligament and new alveolar bone have developed where the pocket was.

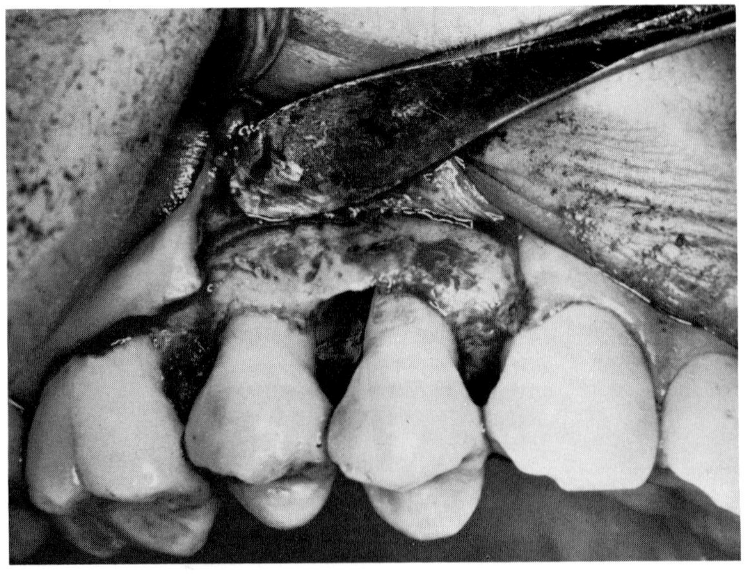

**Fig. 31-2.** Three-walled infrabony (intra-alveolar) crater between the premolars seen after the reflection of a modified full-thickness flap.

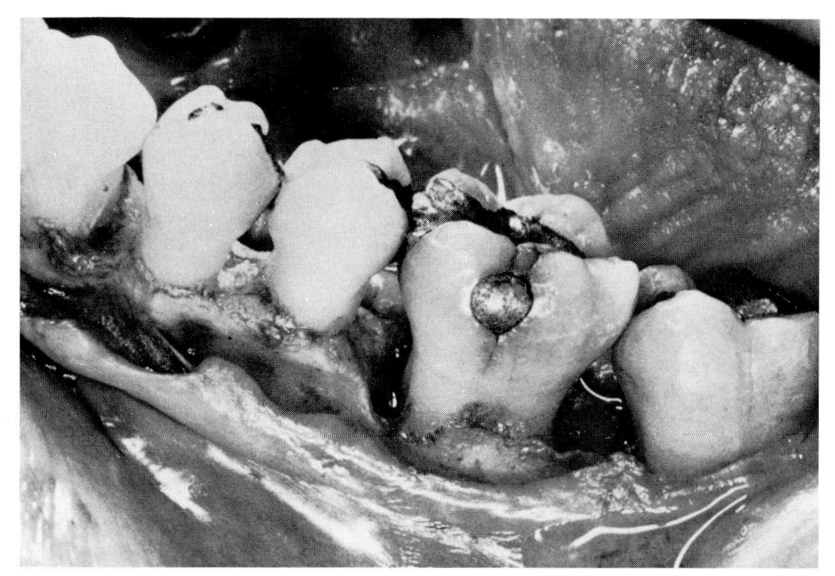

**Fig. 31-3.** Interdental osseous craters on a mandibular molar. The crater on the mesial has three walls at its greatest depth. Near the crest the buccal (vestibular) bony wall is lost and the defect becomes two walled. On the distal a two-walled crater is found. The interdental septum has been destroyed, leaving buccal and lingual bony walls to form a deep osseous defect.

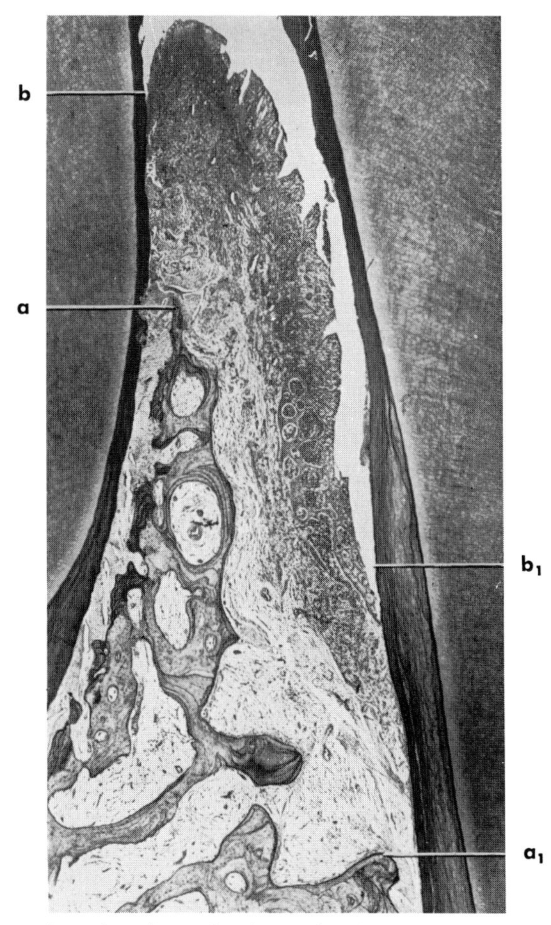


**Fig. 31-4.** Histologic section of an intra-alveolar pocket between two molars. The alveolar bone on one side is high, *a,* and the pocket on the side is shallow, *b*. Where the pocket is deep, $b_1$, the alveolar bone is resorbed, $a_1$.

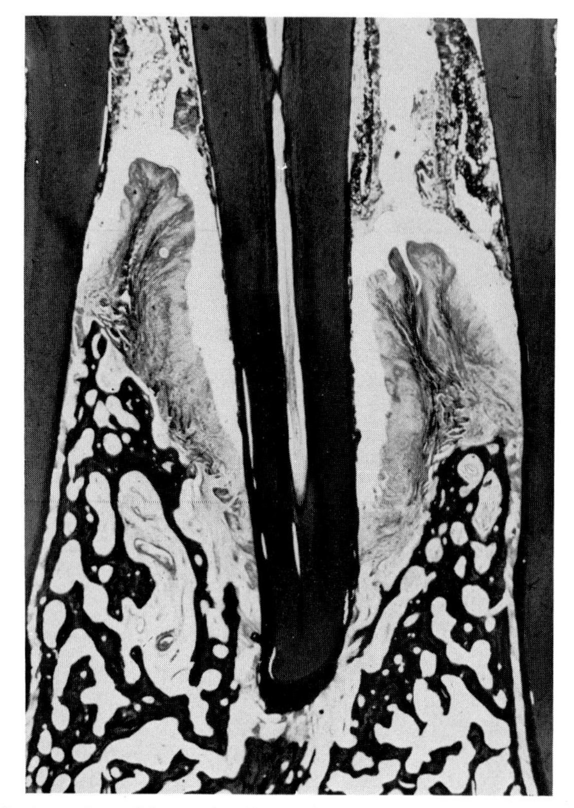

**Fig. 31-5.** Histologic section of intra-alveolar pockets on both sides of a mandibular incisor.

that general surgical preparations, including sterility, be followed (Chapter 26). The instrumentation with curettes is similar to that described in Chapter 27, on subgingival curettage. For reattachment, however, all attachment epithelium must be removed as well as some or all of the soft connective tissue adjacent and subjacent to the pocket. This is best accomplished by planing and curetting until the blade of the instrument contacts bone.

After subgingival curettage the gingiva should be pressed against the tooth to coapt the soft tissue to the tooth and to minimize the size of the blood clot. Protect the clot by placing adhesive foil or Telfa over the lumen of the pocket before placing a periodontal dressing. A well-placed dressing is necessary to avoid disturbing the clot and to shield it from mechanical insult and the entrance of foreign substances. Administer or prescribe antibiotics at the time of surgery and for 3 to 4 days thereafter.

When reattachment is attempted, it may be successful (Figs. 31-7 and 31-8), partly successful (Fig. 31-1, *C*), or unsuccessful. Proper case selection and careful technique tend to increase the percentage of success.

## Summary

The steps and objectives of the reattachment operation by subgingival curettage are summarized as follows:

1. Removal of the epithelium to permit connective tissue reattachment

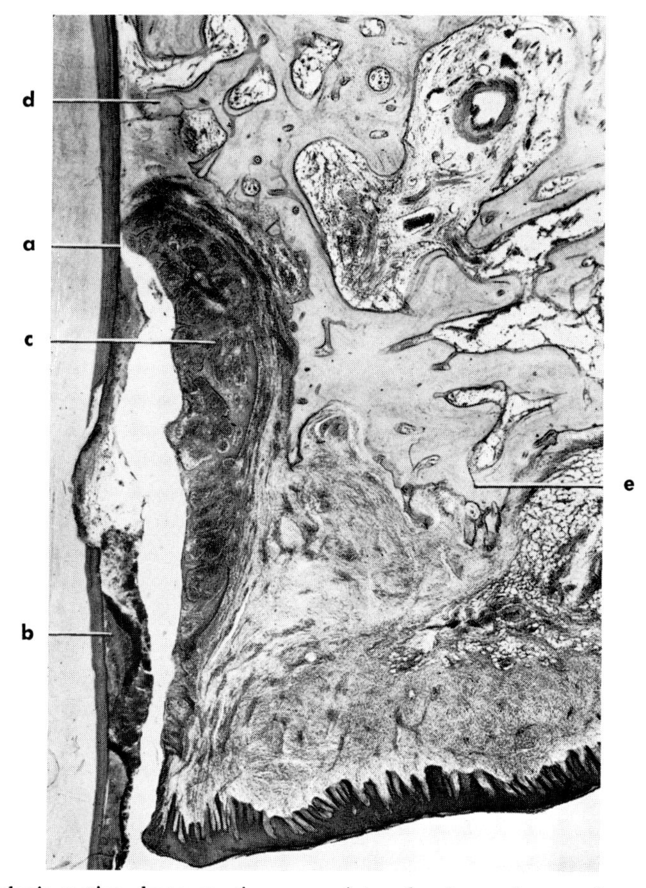


**Fig. 31-6.** Histologic section demonstrating, *a,* an intra-alveolar pocket on the palatal side of a maxillary central incisor, *b,* with much calculus on the root surface, and, *c,* severe inflammation in the wall of the pocket. *d,* Alveolar bone; *e,* crest of the palatal bone.

2. Removal of the underlying inflammatory tissue
3. Approximation of the gingiva close to the tooth to minimize the size of the blood clot and to maintain the clot so that wound healing will be enhanced
4. Encouragement of the formation of new cementum, new bone, and new periodontal ligament fibers (Fig. 31-1, *C*).

This new connective tissue attachment (reattachment) is a restoration of tooth support destroyed previously by disease.

## FLAP OPERATION

Reattachment by flap operation has been a standard procedure in recent years[3] and is discussed in Chapter 30. The method permits better access and visibility in the field of operation. The three-walled infrabony pocket offers the best opportunity for success (Fig. 31-9, *A* and *B*). Full-thickness flaps are reflected to expose the bony defect (*B*). The soft tissue contents of the bony crypt are enucleated by curettage and the root is planed. The flap is debrided of inflammatory tissue and epithelial strands. The flap margins are coapted and sutured to place.

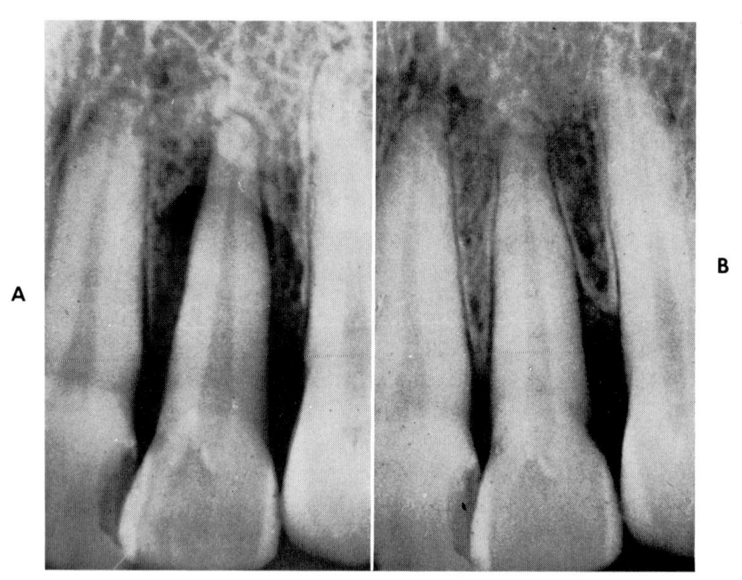


**Fig. 31-7. A,** Preoperative roentgenogram in a case of reattachment by subgingival curettage. Bone destruction appears in a semilunar pattern. **B,** Roentgenogram of the patient 1 year after the reattachment operation. Note the height and density of the alveolar processes.

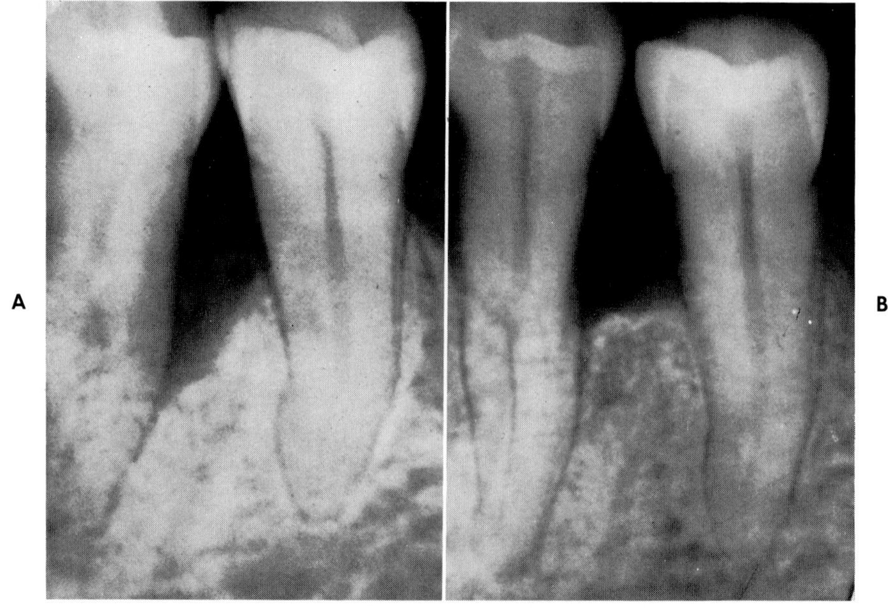


**Fig. 31-8. A,** Roentgenogram of a mandibular premolar with a distal pocket. A flap operation and subgingival curettage were performed. **B,** Roentgenogram of the patient 1 year postoperative. (Courtesy T. Messinger, Colorado Springs.)

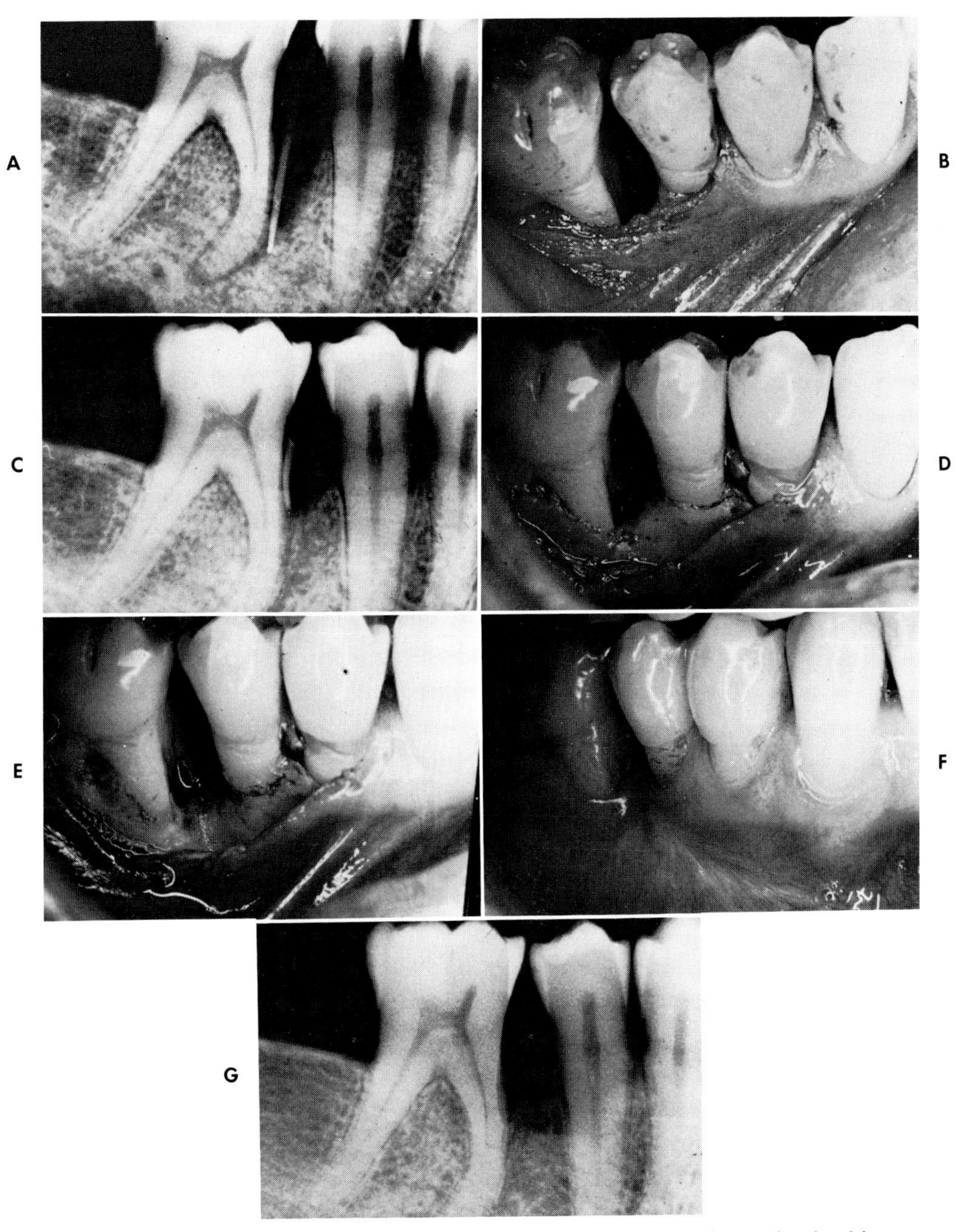


**Fig. 31-9. A,** A gutta-percha point has been inserted into an intra-alveolar pocket in this preoperative roentgenogram. **B,** A modified flap has been reflected in a reattachment operation to reveal the three-walled osseous defect on the mesial surface of a mandibular first molar. **C,** Roentgenogram taken 6 months later shows that considerable regeneration of bone has taken place. **D,** A modified flap is reflected to reveal the residual osseous defect, a two-walled hemiseptum. **E,** Osseous surgery was performed to eliminate the defect. **F,** Two years later the clinical appearance of the area is good. **G,** Roentgenogram confirms the clinical findings. No pocket remains, and a physiologic osseous and gingival form has been created. (Courtesy J. Prichard, Fort Worth.)

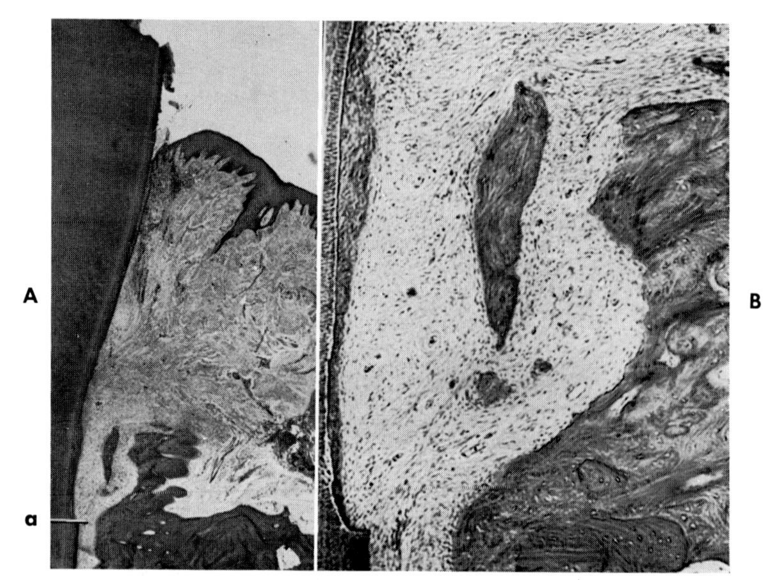


**Fig. 31-10. A,** Human biopsy specimen. The histologic section shows the result of an experimental reattachment operation. The notch on the surface of the cementum, *a,* and the corresponding bone defect show to what point curettage has been performed. **B,** Higher magnification of the apical end of the curettage showing new formation of cementum on the curetted cemental surface, with attachment of periodontal fibers and formation of new bone. The interpretation that reattachment occurred in the area of a previously existing pocket is suspect, and this specimen may indicate only healing after surgical wounding with a curette rather than reattachment.

Adhesive foil is placed over the wound site, and a protective periodontal dressing is placed over the foil. The succesful result can be seen in *E* to *G*.

For many years successful reattachment was believed to be rare or impossible to obtain.[6,7] However, whereas clinical evidence (Fig. 31-10) that reattachment can occur is strong, good experimental evidence is lacking.

Although the three-walled infrabony defect is believed to have the greatest chance of success in reattachment operations, sometimes one-walled or two-walled infrabony defects are successfully treated. In a 37-year-old woman who presented with advanced periodontal disease, vertical bone destruction was found around the mandibular right first premolar and first molar (Fig. 31-11, *A*). After repeated scaling and instruction in plaque control, the clinically visible inflammation was eliminated or sharply reduced (*B*). A flap was reflected to reveal the osseous deformities (*C*). Despite repeated scaling, some calcified deposits remained. Although the outer surface of the gingiva appeared healthy, granulomatous tissue was found in the pockets. A reattachment operation was done. One year later the healthy-appearing, physiologic gingiva could be seen (*D*). Minor pocket depth remained; but reflection of a flap showed a remarkable regeneration of bone (*E*).

## Summary

The clinician can evaluate the relative success of reattachment operations by careful clinical probing and roentgenograms. For investigative purposes, however, more critical criteria for evaluation are required. Reduction in pocket depth may be caused by gingival recession as well as by coronal displacement of the

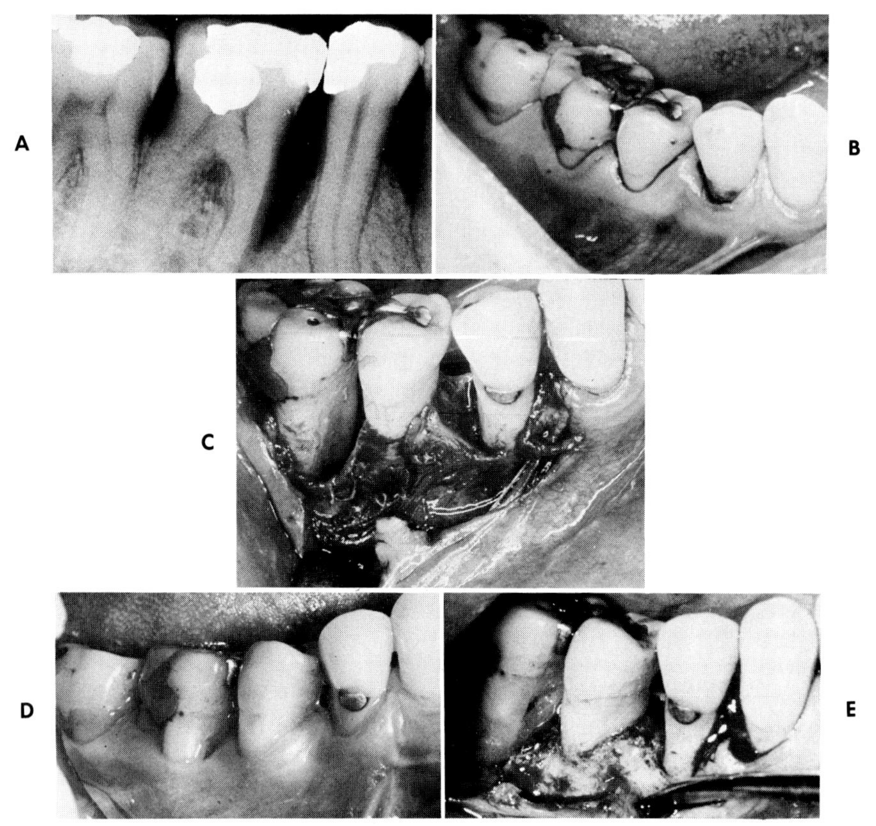

**Fig. 31-11. A,** Roentgenogram of the mandibular right molar and premolar area showing vertical bone destruction. **B,** After root planing and instruction in plaque control, clinical inflammation was reduced or eliminated. Pocket depth remained. **C,** A modified flap was reflected in an attempt to stimulate reattachment. One- and two-walled osseous defects are present. **D,** One year later a physiologic gingival form is present. **E,** A flap was reflected so that osteoplasty could be performed. A remarkable regeneration of bone had taken place.

attachment epithelium. Increased density of bone may be caused by an increase in trabeculation of existing bone after treatment rather than by the formation of new bone. Roentgenograms alone cannot provide indisputable evidence of success or failure.[8-10] Variables in roentgenography, such as angulation, density, voltage, and amperage, make the x-ray film less than fully reliable as an evaluative tool. However, when standardized methods of taking the roentgenogram are used together with parallel projection techniques and measuring devices such as grids[10] and calibrated silver points placed in the same plane,[11] the critically evaluated roentgenogram can be a useful clinical tool for measuring bony reattachment.

**CHAPTER 31**

**References**

1. Box, H. K.: Treatment of the periodontal pocket, Toronto, 1928, University of Toronto Press.
2. Black, G. V.: Special dental pathology, Chicago, 1915, Medico-Dental Publishing Co.
3. Prichard, J.: The infrabony technique as a predictable procedure, J. Periodont. 28:202, 1957.

4. Goldman, H. M.: A rationale for the treatment of the intrabony pocket; one method of treatment, subgingival curettage, J. Periodont. **20**:83, 1949.
5. Schaffer, E. M., and Zander, H. A.: Histological evidence of reattachment of periodontal pockets, Parodontologie **7**:101, 1953.
6. Skillen, W. G., and Lundquist, G. R.: An experimental study of peridental membrane reattachment in healthy and pathologic tissues, J. Amer. Dent. Ass. **24**:175, 1937.
7. Orban, B.: Pocket elimination or reattachment, New York J. Dent. **14**:227, 1948.
8. Orban, B., and Orban, T.: Three-dimensional roentgenographic interpretation in periodontal diagnosis, J. Periodont. **31**:275, 1960.
9. Friedman, N.: Reattachment and roentgenograms, J. Periodont. **29**:98, 1958.
10. Everett, F. G., and Fixott, H. C.: Use of an incorporated grid in the diagnosis of oral roentgenograms, Oral Surg. **16**:1061, 1963.
11. Hirschfeld, L.: Calibrated silver point for periodontal diagnosis and recording, J. Periodont. **24**:94, 1953.

**Additional suggested reading**

Beube, F. E.: The problem of reattachment, J. Periodont. **31**:310, 1960.

Beube, F. E.: A radiographic and histologic study on reattachment, J. Periodont. **23**:158, 1952.

Carranza, F. A.: A technique for reattachment, J. Periodont. **25**:272, 1954.

Kramer, G. M., and Kohn, J. D.: Postoperative care of the infrabony pocket, J. Periodont. **32**: 95, 1961.

Patur, B., and Glickman, I.: Clinical and roentgenographic evaluation of the post-treatment healing of infrabony pockets, J. Periodont. **33**:164, 1962.

Prichard, J.: The etiology, diagnosis and treatment of the intrabony defect, J. Periodont. **38**: 455, 1967.

Ramfjord, S.: Reattachment in periodontal therapy, J. Amer. Dent. Ass. **45**:513, 1952.

Smith, T. S.: The treatment of two periodontal cases, J. Periodont. **20**:129, 1949.

CHAPTER THIRTY-TWO

# Bone grafts and transplants



*Definition*

A graft is living tissue, which, after having been taken from a donor site, is implanted to form an organic union with the host tissue.[8] In the case of bone grafts into the periodontium, the living bone becomes incorporated in the healing process and survives afterward as a functioning part of the periodontium. A transplant may be living or nonliving tissue. An example of a living tissue transplant is a third molar transplanted into the socket of a first molar of the same person. This can also be called a graft. An example of a nonliving tissue transplant is despeciated bone placed in an osseous defect. An example of a foreign material used for this purpose is plaster of Paris. In this case we speak of an implant. When the transplant is bone, it does not survive indefinitely but is progressively resorbed and replaced by newly formed bone.[11] The transplant serves as a scaffold in the healing process.

## CLASSIFICATION

Bone grafts may be autogenous (from the same individual), isogenous (from an identical twin), homogenous (from an individual of the same species), or heterogenous (from another species).* Autogenous grafts obviously yield the best results; they do not provoke immune reactions, which cause graft rejection.

Grafts may consist of cancellous or cortical bone, or a combination of both. Cancellous grafts are considered preferable. The marrow spaces and the greater vascularity and cellularity are presumed to permit easier incorporation in the healing process. When cortical bone is used, thin scrapings are best.

Grafts may be structurally classified as free or pedicle grafts. An example of a free graft is a marrow graft; an example of a pedicle graft is the laterally repositioned flap.

## REQUIREMENTS

The requirements for periodontal bone grafts and transplants are bone from an acceptable site or donor, a prepared recipient bed, and enclosure of the implanted bone in the bed by coapted flap margins. When flap margins cannot be coapted because of technical difficulties, dry foil may be used to cover the wound.

*See references 1-7, 9, 10, 12-14, 18, 19, 21, 22, 24.

Postsurgical infection must be prevented, and antibiotic administration at the time of surgery and for 4 to 14 days thereafter has been suggested.

The bone for grafting (donor bone) is most often obtained from the patient (autograft) and may be cancellous or cortical bone from the alveolar processes; or it may be hematopoietic marrow from the iliac crest. Homografts of banked cancellous bone from which the organic stroma and cells have been removed are also used. Heterografts of despeciated bovine bone were used in the past, but these have been largely abandoned.

*Hematopoietic marrow in cancellous bone*

Autogenous hematopoietic marrow in cancellous bone has been reported to yield excellent results. Cellular and/or other factors in these tissues apparently enhance the chances of the graft's taking and seem to induce an osteogenic effect in the graft site. Autogenous hematopoietic marrow in cancellous bone has even been used succesfully in furcation defects, where other materials and methods invariably fail. Studies to support the clinical use of such grafts are inconclusive, however. Reports of root resorption and ankylosis after the implantation of fresh marrow (with viable cells) indicate the need for caution and further study.

*Swaging*

A procedure analogous to bone grafting is called swaging[12] or contiguous autogenous transplant.[13] The procedure involves a greenstick fracture of bone bordering an infrabony defect and the displacement of bone to eliminate the osseous defect. Successful results have been reported, but further evaluation is needed.

## INDICATIONS

The relative degree of success of periodontal bone grafting is reported to vary directly with the number of bony walls of the defect (vascularized, osseous surface area) and inversely with the surface area of the root against which the graft is implanted. Thus a narrow, three-walled infrabony defect usually yields the greatest success, a two-walled defect the next best, and a one-walled defect the least. There is even some take reported when the bone graft is piled on the crest of the interdental septum.

Clinically the chances for success are best in a three-walled infrabony (intraalveolar) pocket and least in a through-and-through furcation defect on a maxillary molar.

## METHOD

Thorough root planing must precede any attempts at grafting or transplantation to provide a clean recipient site and to permit the placement of the graft in as little time as possible. The cleanliness of the recipient site and the expeditious placement of the graft enhance the possibility of a take.

After inflammation has been reduced by prior root planing and home dental care, examine the receptor site by probing and roentgenograms (Fig. 32-1, *A* to *C*) to visualize the topography of the osseous defect. Donor bone should be at hand or an intraoral donor site should be selected before the operation.

### Homografts, nonoral autografts

When homografts or nonoral autografts are used, prepare them at the start of the operation. Homografts of freeze-dried,[19] banked,[20,20a] cancellous bone must be reconstituted in blood, normal saline, or lactated Ringer's solution.

*Obtaining, storing, and using marrow*

Hematopoietic marrow may be obtained by a physician from the posterior, superior iliac crest and spine using a Westerman-Jensen bone marrow biopsy needle or by direct access. The former method requires only local anesthesia and

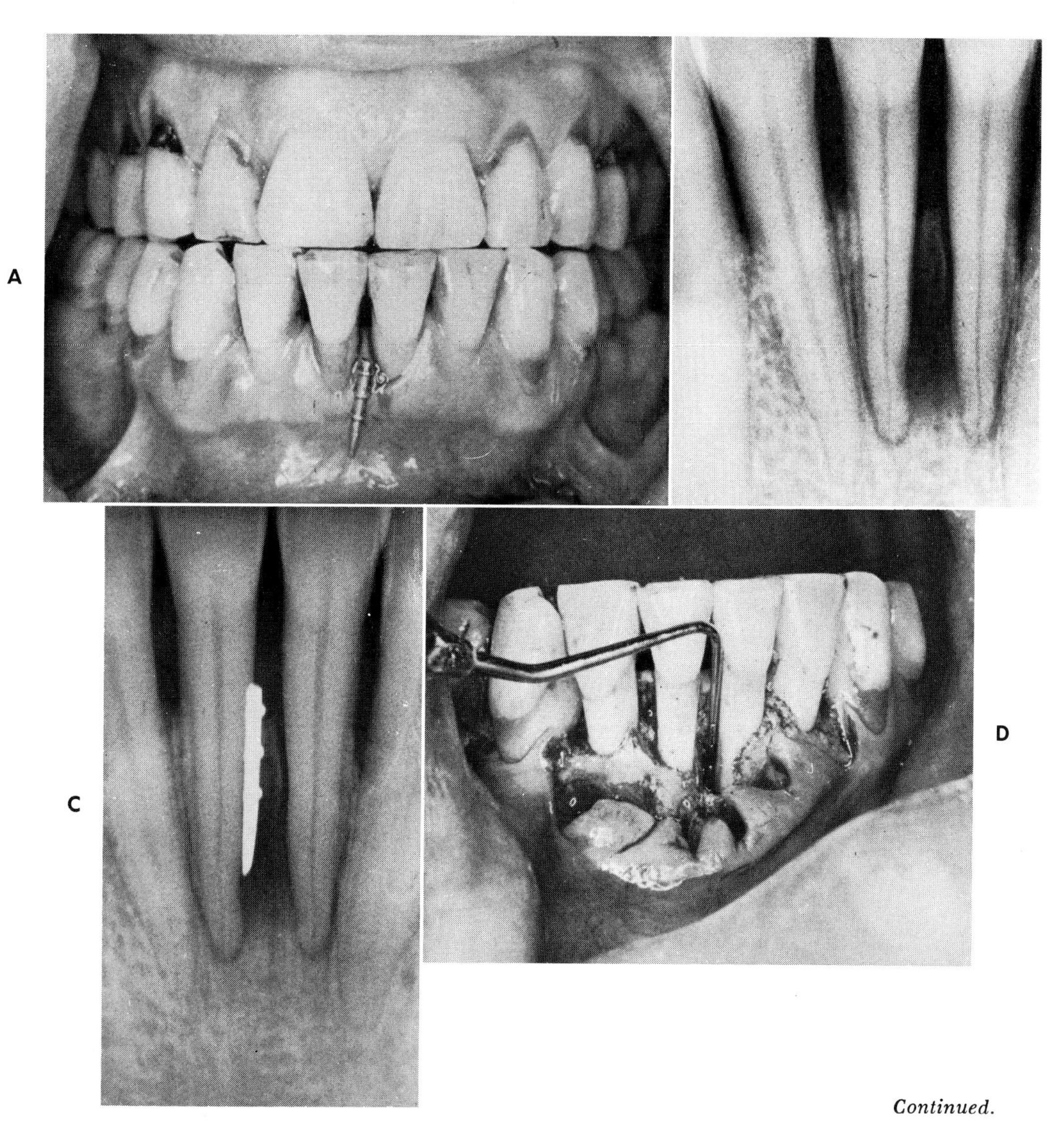


*Continued.*

**Fig. 32-1. A,** Clinical appearance of a mouth prior to bone grafting. A calibrated silver point indicates pocket depth on the mandibular incisor. **B,** Roentgenogram indicating bone loss. **C,** The calibrated silver point placed in the pocket shows a 9 mm. depth. **D,** A modified flap is reflected to reveal a two-walled osseous defect.

may be performed in the office whereas the latter requires hospitalization and general anesthesia. The one to eight cores obtainable with the biopsy needle are adequate for most periodontal procedures.[23,23a,23b,23d,25]

When the graft is to be used immediately, Schallhorn and co-workers suggest placing it in minimum essential tissue culture media, lactated Ringer's solution, or blood.[23] For short-term storage (3 hours to 1 week), these investigators employ minimum essential media with 5% to 15% glycerol as a cryoprotective agent. The graft is sealed and refrigerated at 4° C. (with a cooling curve of 1° to 2° C./min.). At the time of implantation, it is quickly warmed to 37° C. Deglycerolization is said to be unnecessary. For long-term storage (1 week to 6 months) these investigators place the graft in 25% glycerol in minimum essential

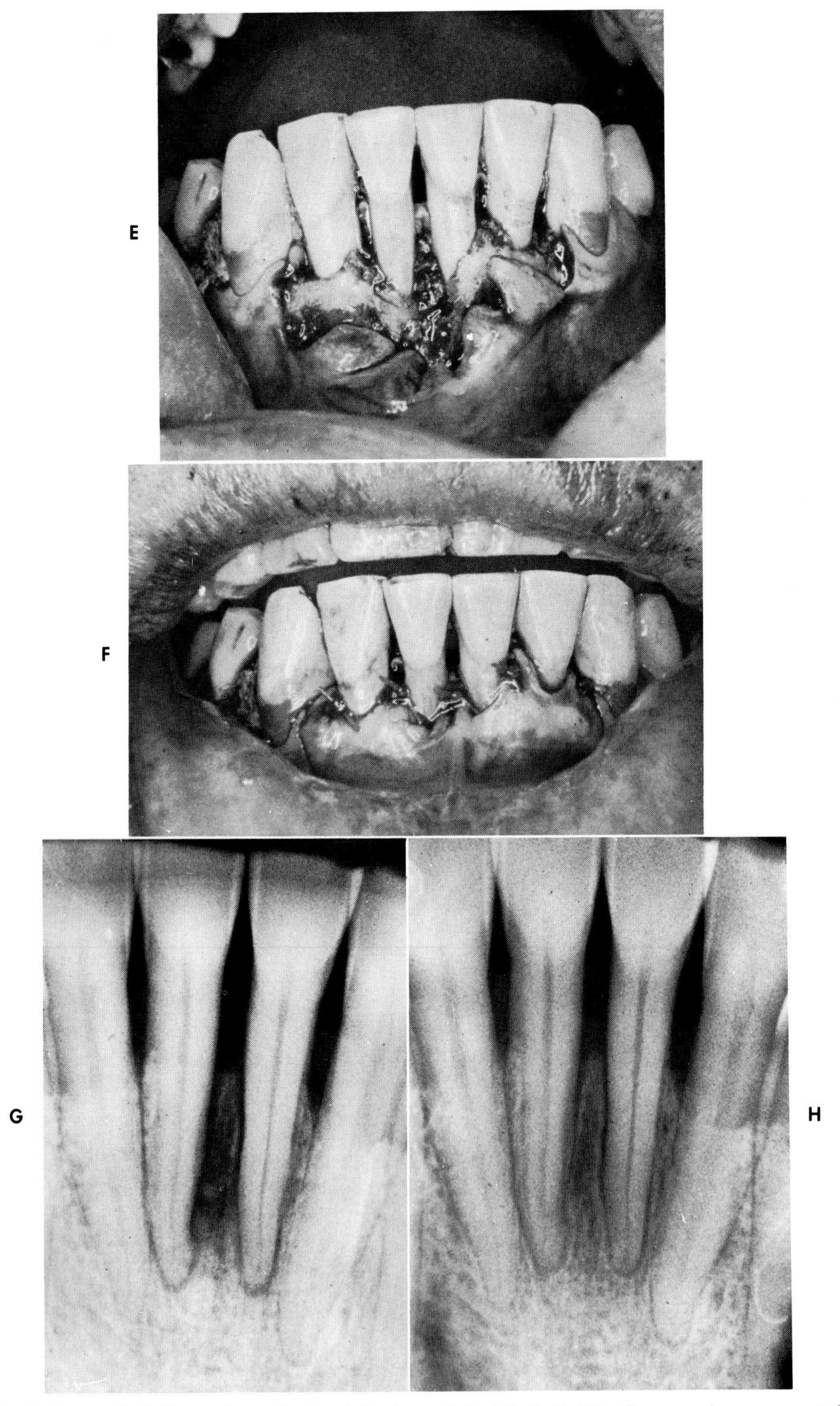


**Fig. 32-1, cont'd. E,** Donor bone is placed in the recipient bed. **F,** The flap margins are coapted and then sutured to place. **G,** Roentgenogram showing the graft in place 1 week after surgery. **H,** Seventh month postoperative roentgenogram. The graft has taken, and the pocket is eliminated. (Courtesy J. Nabers, Wichita Falls.)

media, permit it to reach equilibrium at room temperature, and then place it in a refrigerator for several hours; finally, they store it in a freezer at −79° C. For use they thaw the graft rapidly to 37° C. and modify it to reestablish a compatible osmotic gradient.

There has been some effort to maintain cell viability. However, viability may not be essential for the success of the graft. Better osteogenesis has been noted with frozen marrow implants, in which there is poor or no cell viability, than with fresh marrow implants.

*Recipient site*

The recipient site is prepared first. Reflect a full-thickness flap, retaining the interdental papillae (Fig. 32-1, *D*). Curette the osseous defect to remove all soft tissue and to expose marrow spaces. Plane the root, wash the osseous defect with sterile saline solution, and control bleeding to prepare the recipient bed for the graft. Any other osseous procedures to adjacent areas should be done before the graft is placed.

*Donor site*

At this time the intraoral donor site is operated. Obtain donor bone from edentulous sites such as ridges, the maxillary tuberosity, or extraction sockets. Reflect a flap in the donor site by making a mesiodistal incision on the ridge, with relieving incisions if needed. Remove bone with a rongeur, curette, trephine, or bur. Be careful not to mutilate or remove the lateral cortical plates. The maxillary tuberosity frequently provides an adequate amount of cancellous bone for implantation. When the tuberosity is used, the incision should extend into the mucosa beyond. The removal of a triangular wedge of gingiva will permit later coaptation of the flap margins. Remove the bone with a curved, end cutting rongeur with narrow beaks. Cut or shell the thin cortical plates of the graft material away prior to implantation. Be careful not to enter the maxillary sinus. Have good roentgenograms at hand.

## Oral osseous autografts

*Cancellous bone*

For cancellous bone autografts, take bone fragments from the oral donor site and place them loosely in the osseous defect* (Fig. 32-1, *E*). Coapt the flap margins of the receptor site and suture them to place (Fig. 32-1, *F*). Protect the wound by adhesive foil and place a dressing carefully so that the graft is not dislodged. Suture the donor site and dress the wound as neded. Give postoperative instructions and medication.

The dressing may be changed or removed 5 to 7 days postoperatively. Sutures are removed when the flaps are fixed in place, when wound closure is obtained, or when the operated surface is covered by granulation tissue.

The postoperative roentgenogram (Fig. 32-1, *G*) shows the graft in place. Seven months later the graft has taken and the pocket has been eliminated (Fig. 32-1, *H*).

*Cortical bone shavings*

Cortical bone may be used as a transplant when autogenous cancellous bone is not readily available.[15] Small scrapings of cortical bone yield better results than do larger fragments of bone. The tiny fragments offer a large surface area for incorporation in the healing process, and they facilitate the invasion of blood vessels into the transplanted bone mash. Used in this form, the fragments act as a scaffold; and when the operation is successful, they are progressively resorbed and replaced by newly deposited bone (Fig. 32-2). Pre- and postsurgical treatment is the same as for periodontal bone grafting.

---

*For the purpose of records, take roentgenograms after the donor site is prepared and after the graft is placed.

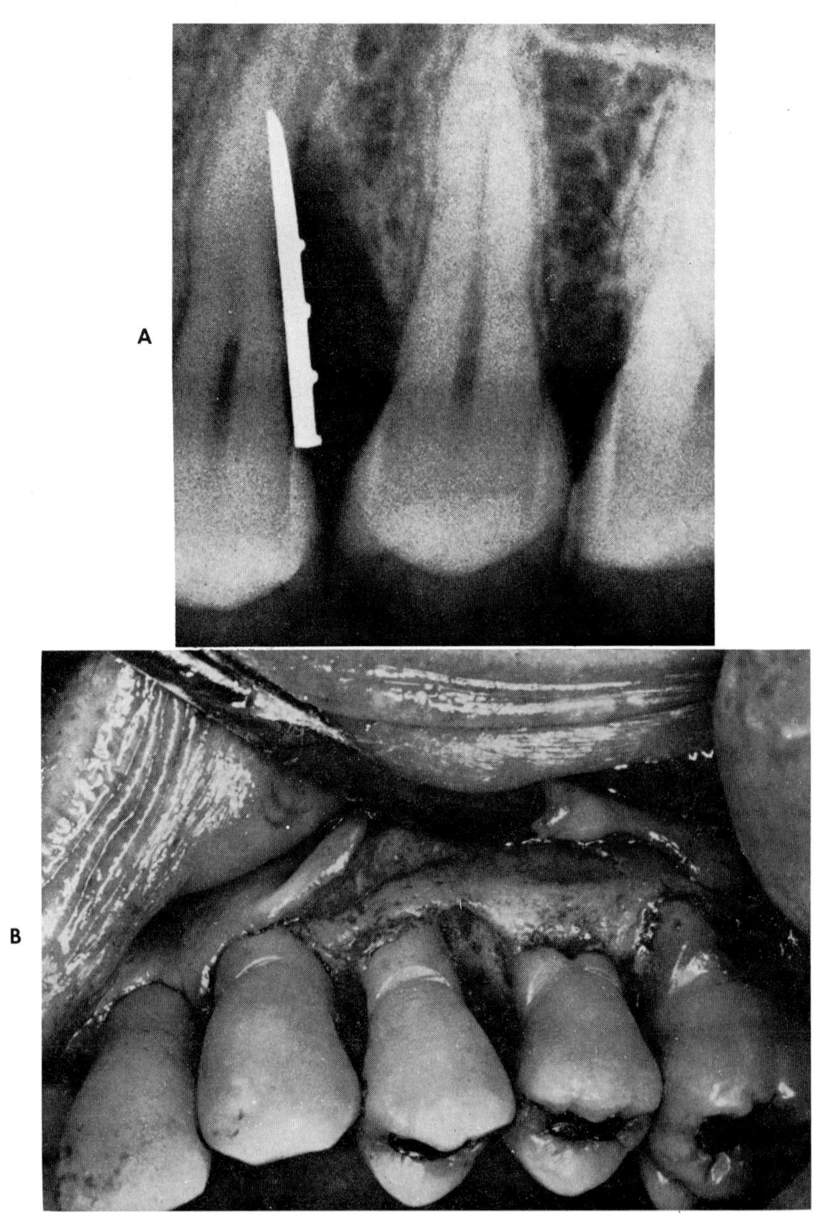


**Fig. 32-2. A,** Roentgenogram with a calibrated silver point illustrating the extent of the bony lesion. **B,** A modified flap has been reflected to expose a two-walled infrabony crater on the distal of the maxillary first premolar.

A troughlike, osseous defect in a 57-year-old man is seen in Fig. 32-3, *A*. The pockets before reflection of the flap measured 6 to 9 mm. in depth. The tooth had a grade 2 mobility. An osseous coagulum[14,15] was obtained with a Molt curette placed in the crater (*B*), and the flap margins were coapted and sutured to place (*C*). Six months later a successful result was obtained (*D*).

## WOUND HEALING

Bone, cementum, and dentin chips have been introduced into surgically created pockets in animals in attempts to stimulate osseous regeneration.[15-19,20a] Autogenous bone grafts in bifurcations in dogs with periodontitis have produced

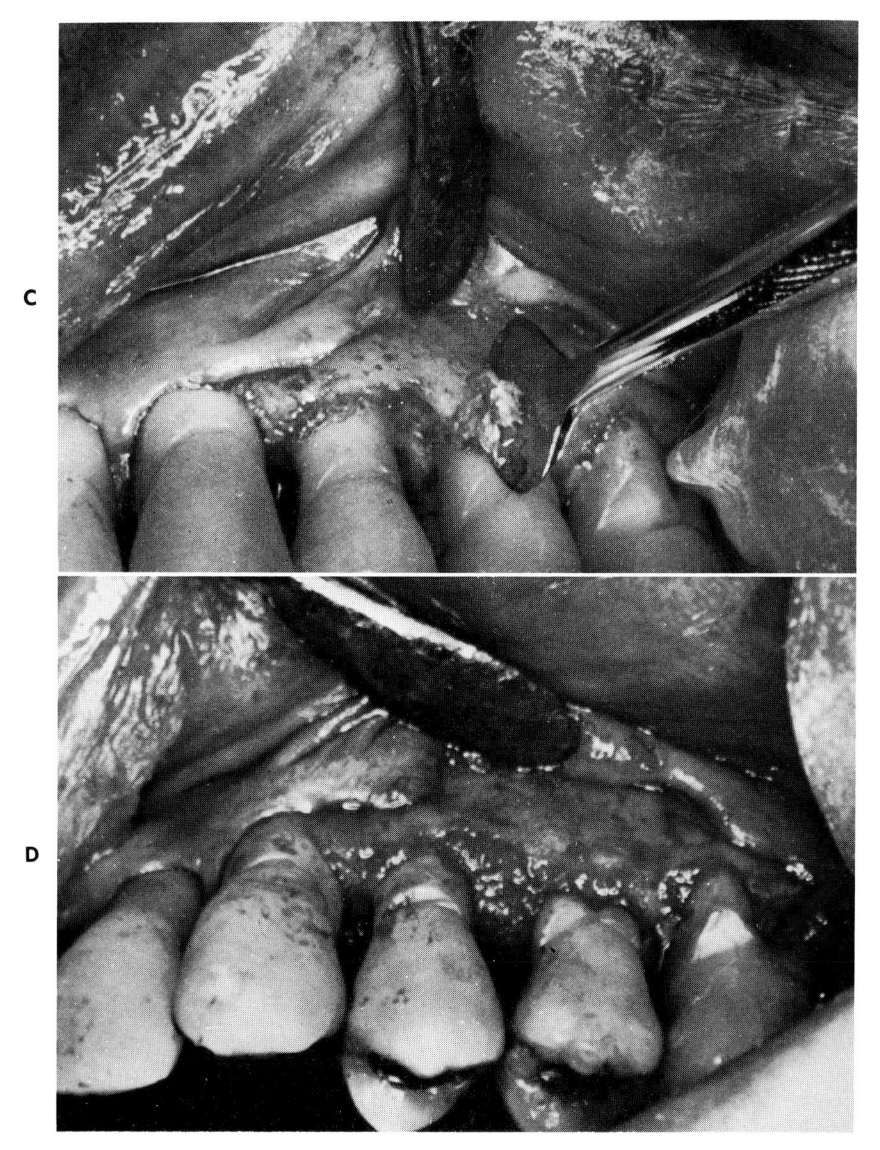


**Fig. 32-2, cont'd. C,** Cortical bone is obtained when the alveolar surface is scraped with a Molt curette. **D,** Cortical bone scrapings (donor bone) placed in the osseous defect. The finely scraped bone particles form a mash when moistened by blood.

bony and cemental growth; but there is no convincing proof of a new ligament coronal to the original pocket depth.[21]

Reports on clinical cases with bone and/or marrow implants have shown convincing photographic evidence of reentry bone growth, but the roentgenographic evidence is less convincing.[14,23-26] Human histologic material is scarce. New bone lacking osteocytes has been shown 8 months postoperatively, but there was no evidence of its attachment to new cementum by a periodontal fiber system.[22]

In successful bone grafts (e.g., fractures) the graft is progressively resorbed and replaced by new bone. Root resorption after bone and marrow implantation has been observed clinically,[23c] with the resorption often extending into dentin and the pulp chamber. However, the resorptive area may be filled in with new bone and ankylosis may ensue, which would be a pathologic manifestation of the progressive resorption and replacement just noted. Other postoperative prob-

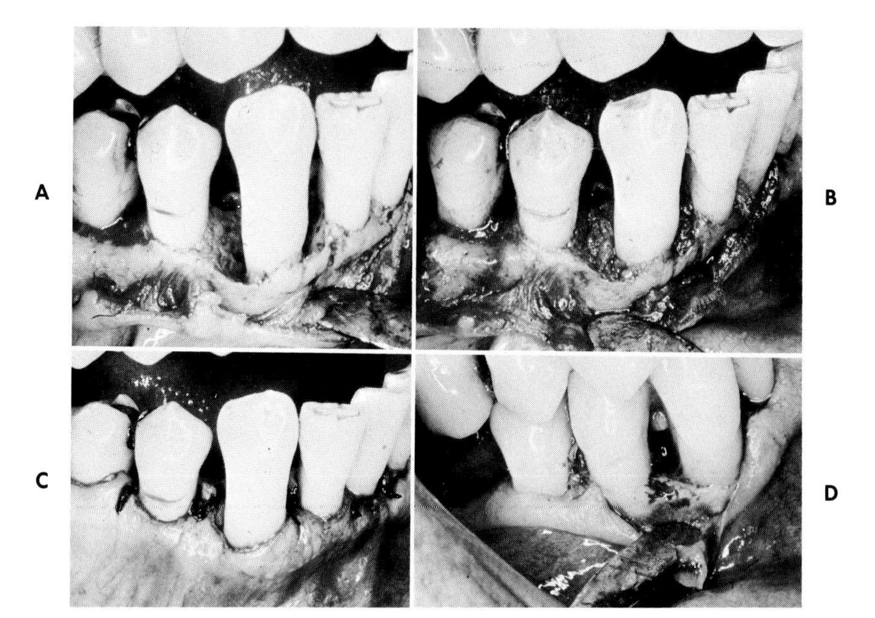


**Fig. 32-3. A,** Troughlike osseous crater around a tooth with grade 2 mobility. **B,** An osseous coagulum has been placed in the defect. **C,** Flap margins are coapted and sutured to place. **D,** Six months later, bone has regenerated to eliminate the defect.

lems occurring occasionally after osseous or marrow transplants are infection, exfoliation of the graft, various and sometimes prolonged rates of healing, and rapid recurrence of the defect.[23c]

## SUMMARY

The future realization of periodontal reconstruction may depend on the implantation of a substance with a high potential for osteoblastic, not hematopoietic, formation. Only controlled experiments will be able to determine the proper biologic additive that will not only grow bone but also stimulate the formation of the highly specialized periodontal apparatus and eliminate the possibility of root resorption.

The grafting of bone and cartilage for restoring periodontal support is a feasible operation. Autogenous cancellous bone offers the best opportunity for success. However, the procedure requires careful case selection, precise instrumentation, and proper postoperative care for best results.

**CHAPTER 32**

**References**

1. Cross, W.: Bone implants in periodontal disease—a further study. J. Periodont. **28**:184, 1957.
2. Krømer, H.: Bone homografts in surgical treatment of cysts of the jaws and periodontal pockets, Oslo, 1960, Oslo University Press.
3. Yuktanadana, I.: Bone graft in the treatment of intrabony periodontal pocket in dogs, J. Periodont. **30**:17, 1959.
4. Nabers, C. L., and O'Leary, J.: Autogenous bone transplants in the treatment of osseous defects, J. Periodont. **36**:5, 1965.
5. Nabers, C. L., and O'Leary, T. J.: Autogenous bone grafts, Periodontics **5**:251, 1967.
6. Schreiber, H. R., Harder, E. W., and Thompson, L. B.: Cartilage and bone grafts in suprabony pockets in dogs, J. Periodont. **30**:291, 1959.
7. Patterson, R. L., Collings, C. K., and Zimmerman, E. R.: Autogenous implants in the alveolar process of the dog with induced periodontitis, Periodontics **5**:19, 1967.

8. Billingham, R. E.: The immunobiology of tissue transplantation, Int. Dent. J. 21:478, 1971.
9. Mann, W. V.: Autogenous transplant in the treatment of an infrabony pocket, Periodontics 2:205, 1964.
10. Heiple, K. G., Chase, S. W., and Herndon, C. H.: A comparative study of the healing process following different types of bone transportation, J. Bone Joint Surg. 45:1593, 1963.
11. Ham, S. W., and Harris, W. R.: Repair and transplantation of bone. In Bourne, G. H., editor: The biochemistry and physiology of bone, New York, 1956, Academic Press, Inc.
12. Ewen, S. J.: Bone swaging, J. Periodont. 36:57, 1965.
13. Ross, S. E., Malamed, E. H., and Amsterdam, M.: The contiguous autogenous transplant—its rationale, indications and technique, Periodontics 4:246, 1966.
14. Rivault, A. F., Toto, P. D., Levy, S., and Gargiulo, A. W.: Autogenous bone grafts; osseous coagulum and osseous retrograde procedures in primates, J. Periodont. 42:787, 1971.
15. Robinson, R. E.: Osseous coagulum for bone induction, J. Periodont. 40:503, 1969.
16. Linghorne, W. J., and O'Connell, D. C.: Studies in the regeneration and reattachment of supporting structures of the teeth. II. Regeneration of alveolar process, J. Dent. Res. 30:604, 1951.
17. Linghorne, W. J.: Studies in the reattachment and regeneration of the supporting structures of the teeth. IV. Regeneration in epithelized pockets following organization of a blood clot, J. Dent. Res. 36:4, 1957.
18. Stallard, R. E., and Hiatt, W. H.: The induction of new bone and cementum formation. I. Retention of mineralized fragments within the flap, J. Periodont. 39:273, 1968.
19. Hurt, W. C.: Freeze dried bone homografts in periodontal lesions in dogs, J. Periodont. 38:89, 1968.
20. Hiatt, W. H., and Schallhorn, R. G.: Human allografts of iliac cancellous bone and marrow in periodontal osseous defects. I. Rationale and methodology, J. Periodont. 42:642, 1971.
20a. Schallhorn, R. G., and Hiatt, W. H.: Human allografts of iliac cancellous bone and marrow in periodontal osseous defects. II. Clinical observations, J. Periodont. 43:67, 1972.
21. Patterson, R. L., Collins, C. K., and Zimmermann, E. R.: Autogenous implants in the alveolar process of the dog with induced periodontitis, Periodontics 5:19, 1967.
22. Ross, S. E., and Cohen, D. W.: The fate of a free osseous tissue autograft; a clinical and histologic case report, Periodontics 6:145, 1968.
23. Schallhorn, R. G., Hiatt, W. H., and Boyce, W.: Iliac transplants in periodontal therapy, J. Periodont. 41:566, 1970.
23a. Haggerty, P. C., and Maeda, I.: Autogenous bone grafts: a revolution in the treatment of vertical bone defects, J. Periodont. 42:626, 1971.
23b. Dragoo, M. R., and Irwin, R. K.: A method of procuring iliac bone utilizing a trephine needle, J. Periodont. 43:82, 1972.
23c. Schallhorn, R. G.: Postoperative problems associated with iliac transplants, J. Periodont. 43:3, 1972.
23d. Rosenberg, M. M.: Free osseous tissue autografts as a predictable procedure, J. Periodont. 42:195, 1971.
24. Ross, S. E., Malamed, E. H., and Amsterdam, M.: The contiguous antogenous transplant—its rationale, indications and technique, Periodontics 4:246, 1966.
25. Seibert, J. S.: Reconstructive periodontal surgery: case report, J. Periodont. 41:113, 1970.
26. Mann, W. V.: Autogenous transplant in the treatment of an intrabony pocket: case report, Periodontics 2:205, 1964.

#### Additional suggested reading

Chaput, A., Marc, A., Barelle, J., and others: Greffes et parodontolyses; étude préliminaire, Rev. Franc. Odontostomat. 6:1191, 1959.

DeMarco, T., and Scaletta, L. J.: The use of autogenous hip marrow in the treatment of periodontosis, J. Periodont. 41:683, 1970.

Mühlemann, H. R., and Wolf, H. F.: Ein Beitrag zur Parodontalchirurgie, Schweiz. Mschr. Zahnheilk. 76:891, 1967.

Schallhorn, R. G.: Eradication of bifurcation defects utilizing frozen autogenous hip marrow implants, Periodont. Abstr. 15:101, 1967.

Schallhorn, R. G.: The use of autogenous hip marrow biopsy implants for bony crater defects, J. Periodont. 39:145, 1968.

Shaffer, C. D., and App, G. R.: The use of plaster of Paris in treating infrabony periodontal defects in humans, J. Periodont. 42:685, 1971.

CHAPTER THIRTY-THREE

# Periodontal osseous resection



Periodontal osseous resection is one of several tools in the dentist's repertoire. In most cases it is used with other procedures such as reattachment operations, curettage by flap, and bone grafts.

Periodontal osseous surgery consists of procedures that (1) remove alveolar bone so that pockets may be eliminated and physiologic bony contours may be created and (2) permit the gingiva to be maintained in health.[1-11,33]

## OSTECTOMY AND OSTEOPLASTY

Osseous resection may be classified into ostectomy and osteoplasty.[5] Ostectomy is the removal of bone that provides attachment for periodontal ligament fibers; osteoplasty is the reshaping of bone that does not provide attachment for periodontal ligament fibers. The procedures are usually performed together and are generally referred to as osseous surgery.

## INDICATIONS

Osseous resection is indicated when the alveolar bony profile must be changed to facilitate the elimination of pockets and to make physiologic gingival contours possible.

Bone destruction that occurs in periodontal disease may vary in form, extent, and distribution and frequently results in bizarre or sharp bone configurations differing from the conceptual ideal of alveolar form (Figs. 33-1 and 33-2). On the one hand, unlike the bone that is resorbed, the gingival margins may be unchanged in height (Fig. 33-1) or may become enlarged and blunted. On the

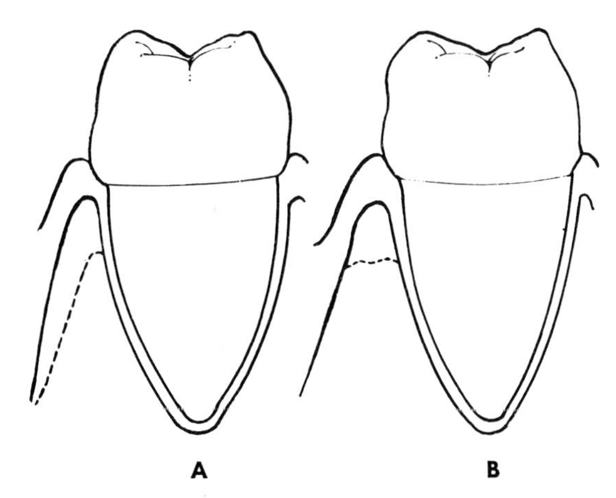


**Fig. 33-1. A,** If bone resorption were to occur as in this illustration, osseous surgery would be unnecessary. Thin margins and a coronally sloping profile would be present. **B,** More often, bone resorption is irregular. This produces deformities such as the broad, thick margin shown here. In this instance, pocket elimination by gingivectomy would fail. Osseous surgery would be necessary to provide for lasting pocket elimination and the creation of physiologic gingival form.

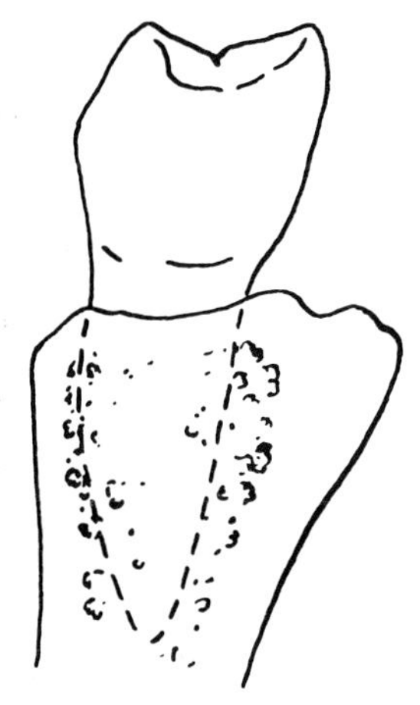

**Fig. 33-2.** Normal bone form seen in the human mandibular third molar area. (After Sicher, H., and DuBrul, E. L.: Oral anatomy, ed. 5, St. Louis, 1970, The C. V. Mosby Co.)

other hand, when a finely textured, thin gingiva (and thin underlying bone) is present, the gingiva may recede. Both enlargement and recession may be present in different areas of the same mouth or even at opposite surfaces of the same tooth. Furthermore, bone resorption without pocket formation is seen occasionally in human histologic specimens. This may be correlated with the clinical observation of alveolar deformities sometimes noted on surgical reflection of a flap in areas without pocket depth.

## CONTRAINDICATIONS

Local anatomic features that sometimes interfere with osseous surgery and thus constitute a contraindication to periodontal osseous surgery include the following[23]:

1. Maxillary antrum

2. Zygomatic process
3. Retromolar triangle and inner or outer oblique lines
4. Mental foramen and anterior palatine foramen
5. Thin bony plates
6. Alveolar dehiscences or fenestrations[13,24] (Figs. 3-26 and 3-27)
7. Enlarged marrow spaces
8. Hamulus and pterygoid plates

Other contraindications include impaired health of the patient.

Some bone resorption inevitably follows any surgical insult in proximity to bone.[25-32] This resorption may range from slight to extensive and may go undetected unless it is accompanied by a dramatic recession of the gingival margin by sequestration or by the appearance of a pocket. Bone may be lost because the oral and vestibular plates that invest the root are thin, particularly near the crest, at the canine eminence, and over the mesiobuccal root of the maxillary first molar. Alveolar dehiscences (Figs. 33-3, *D,* and 33-7, *C*) or fenestrations may also be present, and these characteristics make bone vulnerable to surgical insult. Careful manipulation of tissues may reduce the extent of resorption and the occurrence of sequestration in some instances, but it will not prevent these aftereffects in others.

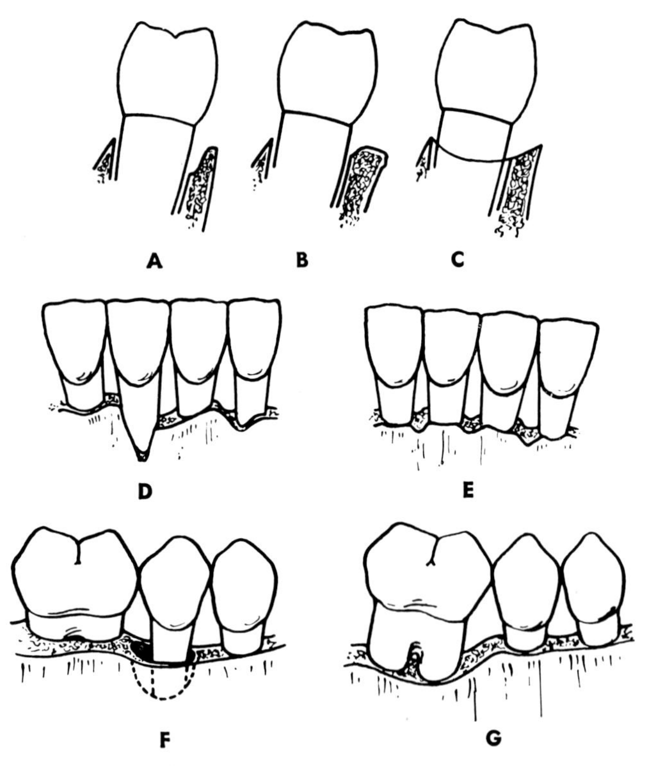


**Fig. 33-3.** Some common oral and vestibular bone defects as a result of periodontal disease. **A,** Vestibular intra-alveolar defect. **B,** Thick vestibular ledge. **C,** Thick ledge with spine. **D,** Vertical groove or notch (dehiscence), reverse architecture, and hemiseptum. **E,** Reverse architecture. **F,** Troughlike, circumferential intra-alveolar crater. **G,** Inclined septum associated with tilted tooth.

## CONCEPTUAL IDEAL OF BONE FORM AS GOAL IN THERAPY

A conceptual ideal of normal osseous architecture may be therapeutically useful.[1,6,7] When this osseous form is surgically created, it helps to prevent the reestablishment of pocket depth. It may also help to create gingival contours that favor better oral hygiene. This bone form serves as a therapeutic goal and resembles the festooned shape given to the gingiva of dentures. Such a conceptual ideal would have the alveolar bone sloping in a coronal direction (on oral and vestibular surfaces) and ending in a thin margin 1 to 2 mm. below the cementoenamel junction. The mesiodistal outline of bone would be scalloped and would parallel the oral and vestibular outlines of the cementoenamel junctions.

### Normal anatomic bony features

The marginal bone form would therefore depend on (1) root form, (2) outlines of the cementoenamel junctions, and (3) proximal relationships of the teeth to each other. The crests of the interdental septa would arc slightly or pyramidally from buccal to lingual, depending on (1) the shape and the proximal relationships of the cementoenamel junctions, (2) the shape of the crowns, and (3) the contact relationships of the teeth. Concave grooves, much like sluiceways would indent the outer surface of the septa.

### Rationale

Osseous resection is not new in periodontal treatment. Early procedures were based on the mistaken notion that the surface bone was infected or necrotic because of inflammation and suppuration of the gingiva.

The alveolar bone does not become infected in chronic periodontal disease despite any inflammation or suppuration from pockets. The inflammatory process in periodontitis extends into bone marrow spaces and causes fatty marrow to change to fibrous marrow. The tissue changes under such circumstances can be classified as osteitis, an extension of inflammation from the pocket area into the bone. However, there is no disease of the bone per se. If the irritation in the pocket is eliminated, the inflammation may be reduced or may disappear although pocket depth will probably remain. Periodontal osseous resection has evolved as a method that permits pocket elimination in such cases.

Some of the early concepts and techniques of bone surgery, however, contained much that is currently regarded as valid. Black, Carranza, Weski, Neumann, Widman, Zentler, Orban, Goldman, Emslie, Manson, Zemsky, Kirkland, and others recognized that changes might have to be made in bone form to eliminate pockets. Neumann proposed that the shape of the bone that had been changed by bone destruction be altered surgically to make it resemble the normal form.[2] Schluger postulated the principle of a harmonious, consistent relationship between gingival form and the underlying osseous contours.[3] He proposed that in health the form of the normal gingiva duplicates that of the underlying bone. He revived Widman's[33] and Neumann's thesis that bone altered by disease should be surgically changed to resemble the normal form.

### Justification

To conceive that normal gingival form always parallels underlying osseous form may be rational; and although the concept is not entirely true,[8,21] it may be a useful teaching tool. It enables us to construct a rationale and to estab-

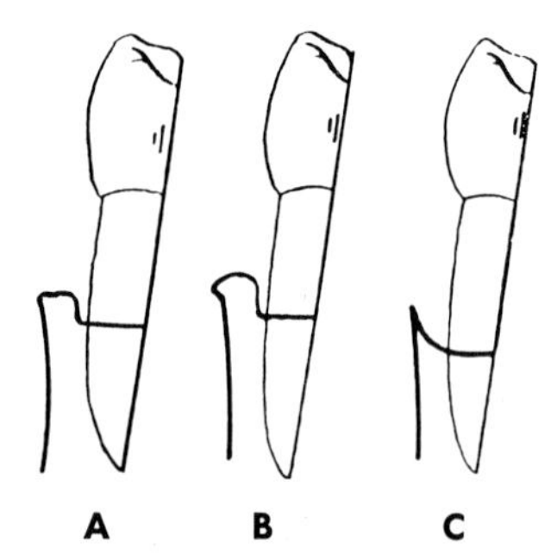


**Fig. 33-4.** Some frequently occurring oral and vestibular bone defects. **A,** Flattened, bulging crest. **B,** Beaded bone margin. **C,** Spine.

lish goals for the performance of osseous surgery.* For the sake of accuracy, however, we should note that although in some patients with normal gingiva there may be a similarity between gingival and osseous form in others a dissimilarity may exist and such disparity is normal. Beaded bone margins may be present and the overlying gingiva may still slope gently and end firmly in a knife-edge margin. Bony protuberances or exostoses may be present (Fig. 33-2) without deformities of the gingival margin or detachment of the coronal gingiva. The mesiodistal scalloping may be insignificant, and the interdental septa may be flat, particularly in the molar areas.

The types of bone deformities resulting from resorption that may need surgical alteration may be classified according to location and to form.

## CLASSIFICATION OF BONE DEFORMITIES ACCORDING TO LOCATION AND TYPE

The following deformities may be so severe that periodontal osseous surgery is called for:

1. Interdental bone defects[12] (Fig. 33-3)
   a. Shallow cupping or craters
   b. Hemisepta (one- or two-walled intra-alveolar defects)[9]
   c. Three-walled intra-alveolar (infrabony) defects
   d. Combinations of the foregoing
2. Oral and vestibular osseous defects or anatomic features (Figs. 33-5 and 33-6)
   a. Reverse architecture
   b. Thick bony ledges, beaded margins, spines, notches, and other irregular resorptions
   c. Exostoses and tori
   d. Thin bony plates and dehiscences
3. Root furcation involvements
   a. Bifurcation involvements that are partial or complete (through and through)
   b. Trifurcation involvements that are partial or complete

*We must recognize the distinction between the justification for the use of a therapeutic procedure and the rationale that is offered to explain it. The justification for the use of periodontal osseous surgery is its clinical success in reaching specific objectives. The rationale for the idealized bone form in osseous surgery is a construct of logic. Although the evidence for the rationale is persuasive, it is by no means conclusive according to scientific standards.

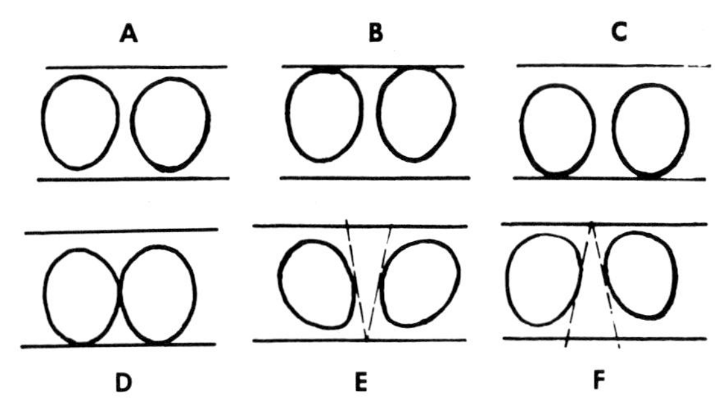


**Fig. 33-5.** Occlusal view of root location within the alveolar process. **A,** Normal or ideal location of roots in relation to oral, vestibular, and septal bone. **B,** Roots malaligned toward the oral surface, producing a thin bony plate on the oral surface and a thick bony plate on the vestibular. **C,** Teeth malposed toward the vestibular surface, producing thin labial bone plate and thick lingual plates. **D,** Roots too closely approximated or touching so that septal bone is very thin or absent. **E** and **F,** Rotated teeth. Tooth malpositions may predispose the patient to gingival pathology. The thickness of the bone will influence the pattern of any bone resorption that may occur. The location of remaining bone will influence the choice of surgical approach. When bone is thin on one surface (e.g., oral or vestibular) and thick on the opposing surface, a flap is usually reflected where the bone is thicker.

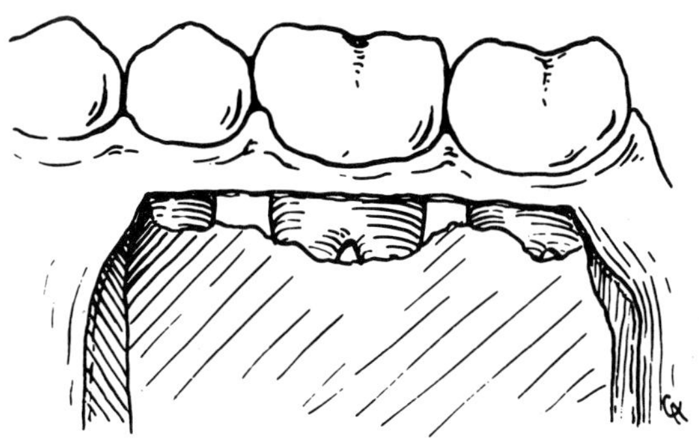

**Fig. 33-6.** A regular gingival margin may mask an irregular bony outline as a result of resorption in periodontal disease. (After Friedman, N.: J. Periodont. **26**:257, 1955.)

4. Bone resorption bordering on edentulous areas
   a. Shallow or deep intra-alveolar (infrabony) defects with one to three crater walls
   b. Angular or vertical mesiodistal bone inclines (defects) found proximal to tilted, drifted teeth

To deal with problems of osseous deformity successfully, dentists have employed a variety of surgical procedures.[1,6,7,9-11,33] These have changed constantly in past years. Currently the emphasis on plaque control and presurgical preparation, such as root planing and subgingival curettage, has minimized the need for and use of osseous resection when compared to the era 1950-1967. The dentist who examines properly and can read tissue will be able to anticipate the need for osseous surgery with a high degree of accuracy.

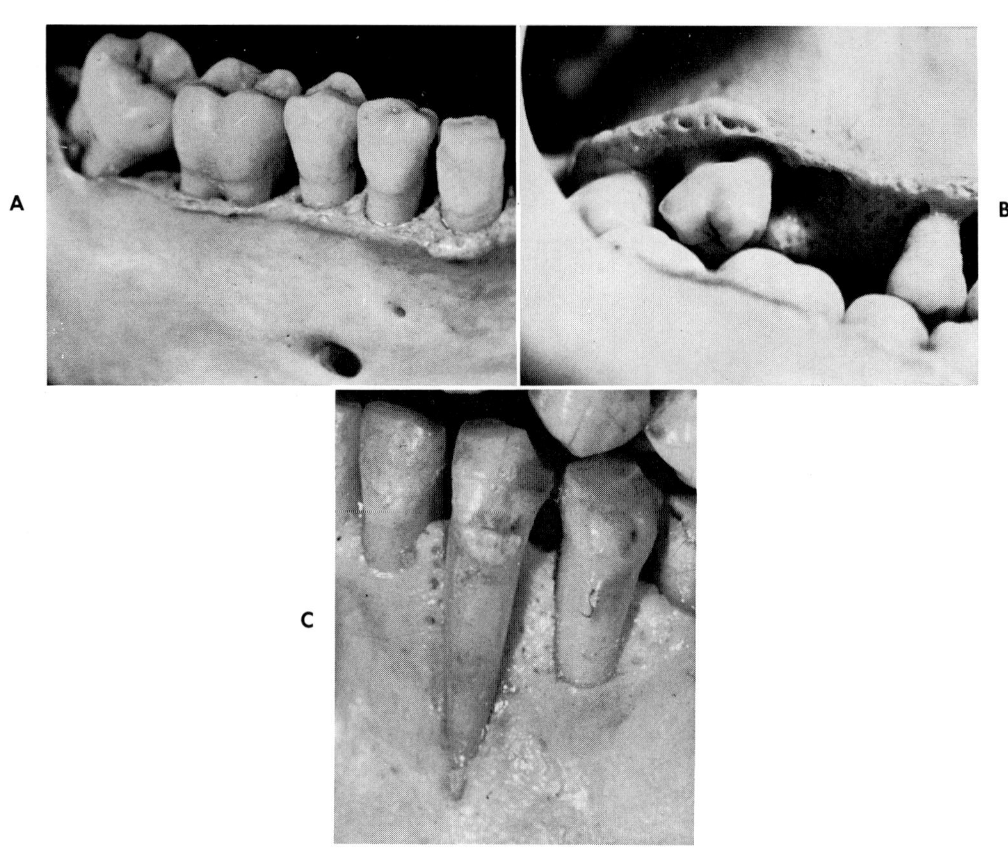


**Fig. 33-7. A, Irregular, troughlike bone destruction is apparent around the second mandibular** molar. Minimal interdental bone deformities are present in the premolar region. These marginal alveolar defects might not be discernible in roentgenograms. Careful examination and correlation with roentgenograms would be necessary for treatment planning before any osseous resection. **B,** Intra-alveolar (infrabony) osseous defects and beaded bone margins are present in the maxillary molar and premolar areas. The proximity of the maxillary antrum to the alveolar crest and osseous defects would be an important consideration in treatment planning. **C,** Complete absence of the buccal alveolar plate of this mandibular canine would not be apparent on roentgen study.

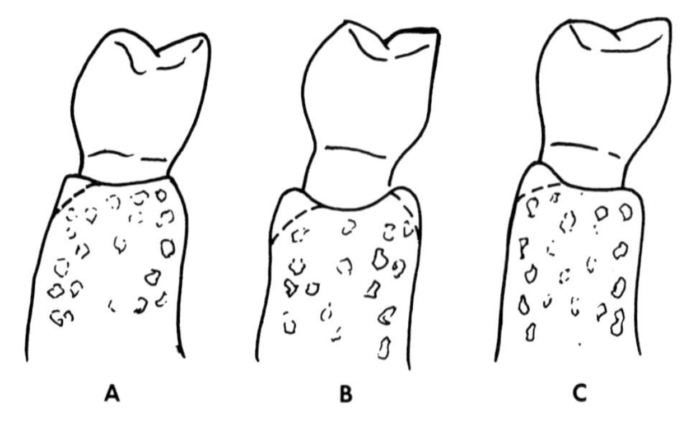


**Fig. 33-8.** Osseous corrections applied to interdental bone deformities. **A,** Blunted alveolar margin is beveled. **B,** Shallow interdental crater is eradicated, and a convex septal form created. **C,** Spinelike vestibular bone margin is removed in this deeper septal crater. The bone is ramped from vestibular to oral, and the septal crest is placed toward the oral alveolar bone surface.

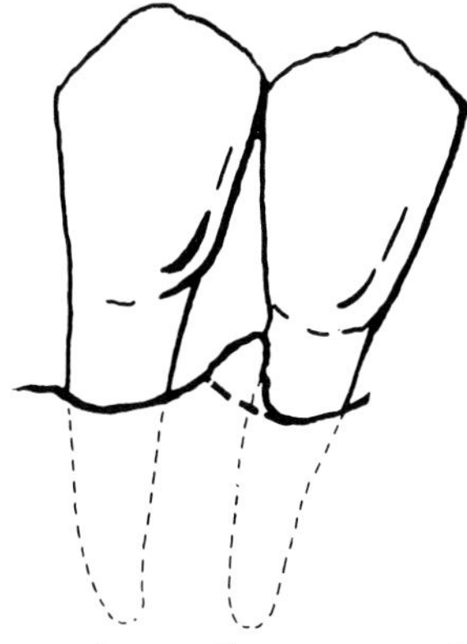

**Fig. 33-9.** A hemiseptum is removed to eradicate a two-walled intra-alveolar bone defect.

## Interdental bone defects

*Shallow cupping or craters*

Shallow cupping or craters are managed best by re-creation of a convex or flat septum. Do this by lowering the oral and vestibular bone margins to a level slightly below the base of the crater. It is sometimes necessary also to lower the oral or vestibular bone margins of the adjacent teeth for proper festooning. The oral and vestibular bone margins may be beveled as needed (Fig. 33-8).

*Hemisepta (one- or two-walled bony defects)*

Bone destruction may leave mesial or distal portions of the interdental septum standing alone. If such a defect is extensive, it can present a vexing problem since one-walled intra-alveolar defects are poor candidates for reattachment. When ostectomy is possible, use small round burs to reduce the hemiseptum, leaving on the root a thin layer of bone that is then removed by enamel chisels or curettes (Fig. 33-9). When possible, manage the defect by bone graft. Sometimes a tooth is so seriously involved that it must be extracted.

Two-walled intra-alveolar defects,* consisting of a hemiseptum with either the oral or the vestibular bone margins standing, may be treated by ostectomy if the resorption is shallow. If the resorption leaves deep precipitous inclines, employ a combination of bone graft and ramping.

*Three-walled intra-alveolar defects*

Shallow three-walled intra-alveolar (infrabony) defects (Fig. 33-3, *E*) are best managed by eradication of the deformity to reestablish a flat or convex buccolingual septal crest. Lower the adjacent buccal or lingual plate to the level of the septal crest or, if possible, slightly apical to it. The management of deep three-walled intra-alveolar defects is discussed under reattachment in Chapter 31 and under bone grafts, Chapter 32.

## Oral and vestibular osseous defects

*Reverse architecture, thick ledges, beaded margins, spines, notches*

Reverse architecture is a common defect of bone form. It is created when greater bone resorption occurs interdentally than on vestibular or oral surfaces. As a result the oral and vestibular bone margins over roots are left at a more coronal level than the interdental septa. The condition may be complicated by the presence of thick ledges, beading, exostoses, spines, notches, or other irregular resorptions.

---

*The number of walls in an intra-alveolar (osseous) defect refers to the bony walls. In every case the tooth surface forms an additional wall that is not included in the count.

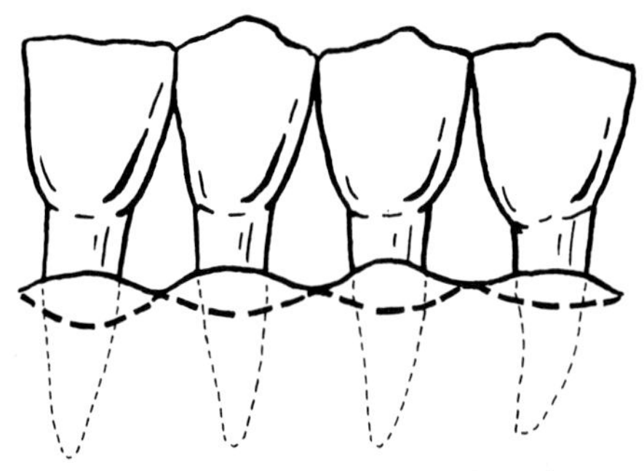

**Fig. 33-10.** Reverse architecture is corrected by the creation of a mesiodistal scalloped form so that interdental crests are at a more coronal level than the alveolar margins over the oral or vestibular root surfaces. Interrupted lines show bone form after surgery.

The ideal correction would create a mesiodistal scalloped bone form that sloped coronally and ended in a thin margin (Fig. 33-10). When such festooning and beveling procedures removed excessive amounts of bone, the mesiodistal outline might have to be made flat or straight rather than scalloped. In the case of precipitous irregularities, long slopes would permit pocket elimination and enable the gingiva to follow this form. In extremes, compromises would be inevitable. When retention of the tooth was important, the dentist might have to be content to leave residual bony deformities.

*Thick bony plates, exostoses, and tori*

Intra-alveolar (infrabony) craters and other bone deformities are frequently seen adjacent to thick bony plates, tori, and bony exostoses. When indicated, reattachment or bone graft should be attempted. When reattachment is not possible, such bony enlargements may be removed to eliminate pockets and to create a physiologic gingival form. Prophylactic removal of tori and exostoses, however, is not indicated.

## Root furcation involvements

The treatment of osseous problems involving furcated teeth[14-18] will depend on the tooth involved, the extent and pattern of bone loss, the anatomy of the involved and adjacent areas, and the accessibility of the area to treatment and oral hygiene. Prognosis wil depend on the extent and pattern of bone destruction in the furcation, the width of the space, the root length, and tooth mobility.

*Partial or complete bifurcation*

Bifurcated teeth, in general, are more amenable to treatment than are trifurcated teeth, with the exception of maxillary first premolars, in which root anatomy and poor accessibility for oral hygiene make for a guarded or poor prognosis. The mandibular first molar offers a better prognosis than the second molar because of better access and the absence of problems involving the ascending ramus, the retromolar triangle, external or internal oblique ridges, and muscle attachments or mucosal reflections (Fig. 33-11).

Treat incomplete bifurcation involvements of mandibular molars by grooving the bone between the roots and then festooning and beveling the bone over the roots.[16] When access for thorough debridement is present, attempt bone grafts.[17] Manage complete furcation involvements by opening the furcation and appropriately festooning the adjacent bone. Some success may be obtained by root canal therapy followed by hemisection (saving one or both halves)[22] or root

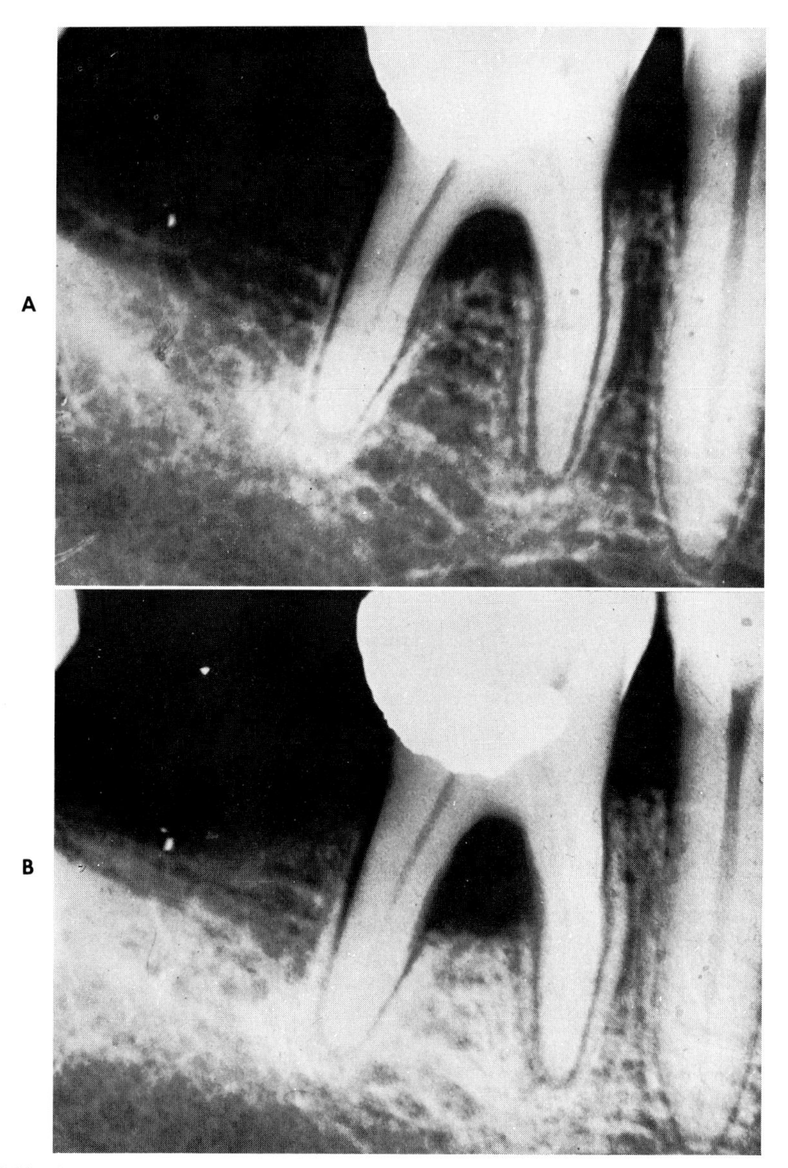


**Fig. 33-11. A,** Roentgenogram showing bifurcation involvement of a mandibular molar. The mesial and distal alveolar crests are not involved. **B,** Roentgenogram showing the enlargement of the space in the bifurcation after surgery to open the bifurcation. Maintaining the health of a tooth with an exposed bifurcation can be a problem because of the difficulty in oral hygiene and the danger of root caries incident to inadequate oral hygiene procedures.

amputation. Such procedures may produce acceptable results and solve vexing problems (Chapter 35).

***Partial or complete trifurcation***

The trifurcation of maxillary molars may be involved from the mesial, distal, or vestibular aspects. Such teeth are poor candidates for reattachment.[15,18] Consequently ramping and festooning should be applied to create as manageable a situation as possible. An effort should be made to provide access to the involved furcations for oral hygiene (Figs. 33-11, 33-12, and 33-17). In the case of extensive involvements, consider root amputation or extraction.

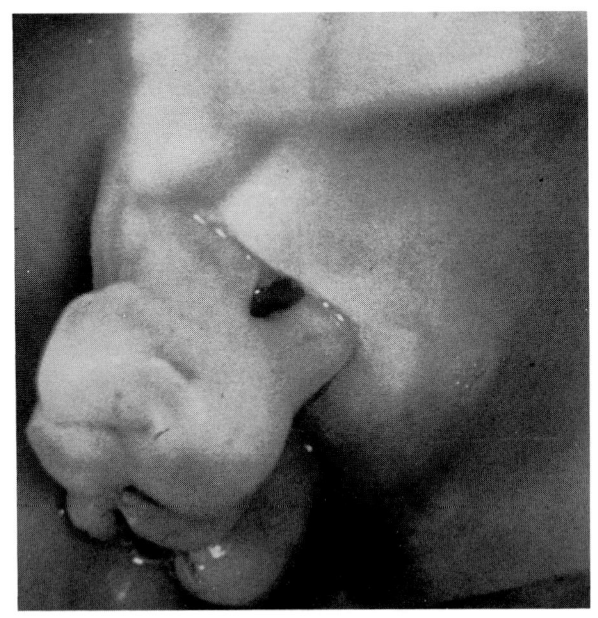

**Fig. 33-12.** Trifurcation involvement in a maxillary first molar exposed by surgery. The area was made accessible for home care maintenance.

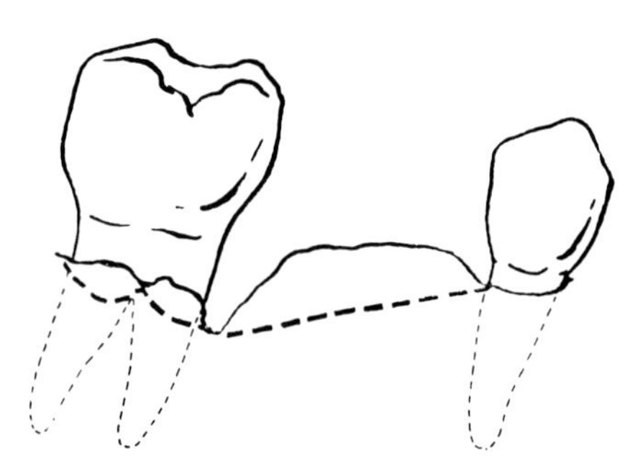

**Fig. 33-13.** The edentulous area proximal to a tilted mandibular molar is ramped to remove a one-walled intra-alveolar bone defect. A gradual ascending slope (ramping) from distal to mesial has been created to permit pocket elimination. An incipient furcation involvement has been treated by grooving the bone between the roots and festooning the adjacent alveolar bone margins. This will permit the formation of a papilla in the furcation area that will be protected by the deflecting cervical tooth convexity.

## Bone resorption bordering on edentulous areas

*Shallow (or deep) intra-alveolar defects with one to three walls*

Intra-alveolar (infrabony) defects adjacent to edentulous tooth surfaces may be corrected by osseous surgery, reattachment attempt, bone graft, or a combination of methods.[19,20] Orthodontic tooth movement can sometimes eliminate bone defects associated with tilted teeth without surgery (Chapter 38). When the defects are shallow, totally ediminate them by ramping and beveling. Deep effects may require bone graft or ramping and narrowing of the edentulous area, or a combination of these procedures (Fig. 33-13). Reshaping of the crown with stones or by crowns or inlays may correct the crown inclination and reestablish a more favorable tooth-to-tissue relationship.

After osseous surgery the flaps should readapted to the alveolar surface and retained by sutures. When necessary, the flap may be repositioned apically to obtain an adequate zone of attached gingiva. Problems involving the mucogingival junction may occur with osseous problems and are discussed separately for teaching purposes (Chapter 34).

***Angular or vertical mesiodistal bone inclines***

## THERAPEUTIC PROCEDURE

### Presurgical preparation

***Planning the surgery***

The preparations for periodontal osseous surgery are similar to those for other periodontal surgery, except for the need of preparing a special armamentarium and possible antibiotic premedication. Pocket depths should be rechecked directly before the actual performance of osseous surgery. Any changes resulting from presurgical preparation should be noted. An effort should be made to visualize the alveolar topography in a three-dimensional view to relate the form of the gingiva with pocket depth and the underlying osseous form[13] (Figs. 33-6 and 33-7). This may enable the therapist to plan surgical intervention more precisely. Sometimes the insertion of calibrated silver points or gutta-percha points into pockets for additional roentgenographic studies is helpful. Roentgenograms taken at varying angles may further assist in visualizing altered bony contours and intra-alveolar (infrabony) defects. After administration of the anesthetic, the alveolar surface may be probed with the injection needle or a fine explorer inserted through the gingiva to further reveal the bony configurations.

Osseous resection is time consuming. When extensive procedures are planned, limiting the surgery to sextant or quadrant operations may be judicious and may make the postsurgical period more comfortable for the patient.

***Armamentarium***

Osseous surgery requires special instrumentation. The armamentarium (Chapter 26) should include a kidney-shaped knife, an interdental knife, a scalpel with a no. 12b removable blade, hawk-beaked curettes and scaling instruments (Fig. 26-1), a periosteal elevator and retractor, round burs, a bone file, bone chisels, rongeurs, a needle holder, and suture. Large round burs (nos. 10 to 12 and 26 to 30) are used for making gross bony reductions. Smaller round burs (nos. 6 to 9) may be used to enter embrasures. High-speed dental apparatus may also be used, in which case smaller burs should be employed (nos. 6 to 8 round surgical). Rotary instruments should be used under saline spray. Rongeurs are sometimes necessary for gross reductions in edentulous areas and for exostoses. Bone chisels and files can be used for marginal bone corrections close to tooth surfaces, and the Molt bone curette (Fig. 29-11) can be used to collect bone shavings for transportation (grafting and transplanting procedures). The therapist should avoid nicking or gouging the root surface.

The surgical remodeling of alveolar bone requires access, which is best gained by the flap. Direct visualization of the bone surface is thus obtained, and the flap can be reapposed to cover the bone after the surgery. Other methods are used infrequently.

***Flaps for access***

Depending on the need for access, a full flap or a modified flap may be used. The flap may be full or partial (split) thickness. Surgical judgment will govern the type and length. The thickness of the bony plate will also influence the choice. When only marginal osseous corrections are to be attempted, a partial-thickness flap is most desirable. A partial-thickness flap should also be used when the bone is exceptionally thin. When extensive osseous corrections, reattachment, or bone grafts or transplants are anticipated, a full-thickness flap retaining all of the gingiva, including the papillae, is more suitable.

This should be elevated by blunt dissection. It will permit coaptation of the flap margins postsurgically and complete coverage of the bone. In order to obtain this coaptation interdentally, retain papillae on the flap. Neumann suggested lengthening the interdental gingival tongues (papillae) by accentuating festooning in preparing the flap.[2] After the flap is reflected, remove soft tissue from osseous defects by curettage. Inspect the roots and remove any remaining calculus. Then make any necessary osseous corrections. Do not discard any bone removed but place it in sterile dappen dishes for possible grafting.

## Management of osseous problems

The management of specific osseous lesions requires surgical judgment. Although the defects are classified separately, they may blend with or be superimposed on one another in any given surgical field. The techniques for their management may also be blended. These include festooning, ramping, and beveling. Procedures such as bone grafting and reattachment operations are also frequently combined with these steps.

***Reproducing bone form***

The ideal normal form of the alveolar bone should be used as a pattern when it can be applied. Beveling may be used to thin bone margins to create coronally inclined slopes. Festooning may be used to alter the mesiodistal bone form to create a scalloped marginal outline. Ramping may be used to create interdental sluiceways, concave grooves, or gradual slopes such as those made in edentulous areas next to tilted teeth.

For the most part, the ideal form can be created surgically. When this is not possible, a compromise may be indicated. Where precipitous or extensive bone resorption has occurred, further surgical removal of bone might weaken tooth support or threaten the survival of the teeth. To preserve bone in such cases, the dentist may alter the desired mesiodistal scalloped form to make gradual slopes and inclines. When there are interdental problems, the crests of the septa may be placed toward the oral or vestibular margins and ramped toward the opposite surface, to which the gingiva may adapt. The purpose of such a compromise is to create an acceptable although not perfect bone form. Similar techniques may be used for defects on the proximal surface of a last standing or isolated tooth.

Complete bone exposure should be minimized. Experimental evidence has indicated that bone exposure is followed by more bone loss.[21] Consequently, techniques (such as the split flap) that avoid complete exposure of bone should be employed when possible.[32-34] The only areas where bone exposure may be well tolerated are those where the bone is thick. An example is the interdental septum,[35-37,39,41-43] where repair will probably maintain the bone level.

***Covering bone***

Whenever possible, after osseous surgery the bone should be covered by gingiva (Figs. 33-14 and 33-15). Occasionally the surgeon may be faced with an area where the gingival margin is alveolar mucosa and no gingiva is present. Where there is no gingiva, he may elect to use a laterally transposed flap or a free gingival graft (Chapter 34) to cover bone and to create an adequate zone of gingiva. When some postsurgical exposure of bone is unavoidable, the bone should be covered with Gelfoam, Telfa, or Adaptic before the surgical pack is placed.

***Placing the dressing***

When good flap coaptation exists, no dressing may be necessary. Adequate hemostasis should be obtained when a dressing is used. The pack should be slightly softer in consistency than that used for gingivectomy. This will enable

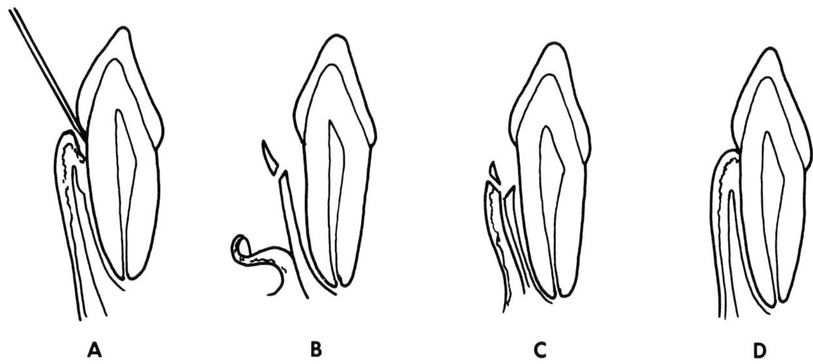


**Fig. 33-14. A,** A full-thickness flap is reflected by either sharp or blunt dissection. In sharp dissection, introduce a scalpel into the pocket to detach the gingiva from the level of the alveolar crest. Then work a periosteal elevator against the bone to elevate a flap. In blunt dissection, introduce a periosteal elevator directly into the pocket and work it between the gingiva and bone (retaining the periosteum) to reflect a flap. **B,** Ostectomy-osteoplasty is performed in an attempt to eliminate the bony deformity. **C,** When necessary for pocket elimination, trim the gingiva and suture the flap to place to cover the bone. **D,** Resultant physiologic gingival and osseous form without pocket depth.

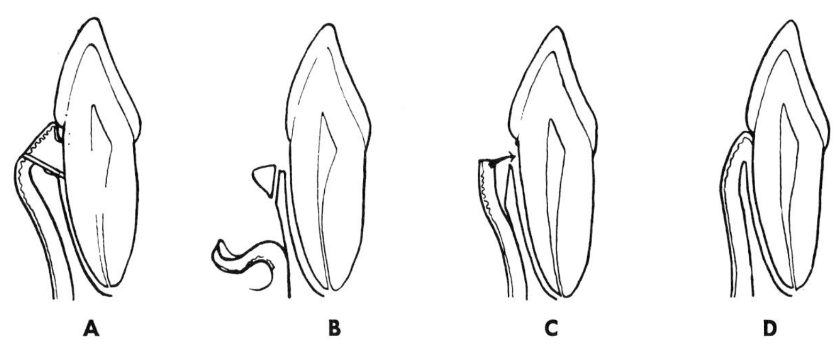


**Fig. 33-15. A,** Excise the gingiva to the level of the bulbous alveolar crest prior to reflecting a flap. **B,** Perform osteoplasty to provide a more ideal form. **C,** Reappose the flap. **D,** The blunted, beaded osseous margin has been corrected and pockets have been eliminated.

the surgeon to place the dressing without displacing the flap margins. The use of a too soft pack, however, might permit the material to become interposed between the flap and bone.

***Postsurgical medication***

Postsurgical medication to reduce pain and swelling should be prescribed as necessary. The patient should be given postoperative instructions (Chapter 26).

***Dressing changes***

The dressing should be changed after 5 days. The wound should be cleansed, sutures removed, and a new dressing placed when necessary. A week later the dressing may be removed and the healing wound inspected and usually left uncovered. After removal of the dressing, oral hygiene procedures should be reviewed. The patient should be cautioned to expect tenderness on brushing. Any root sensitivity should be treated at this time (Chapter 25).

The successful use of osseous surgical procedures results in pocket elimination and the establishment of a physiologic gingival form with the gingival margin usually at a more apical position.

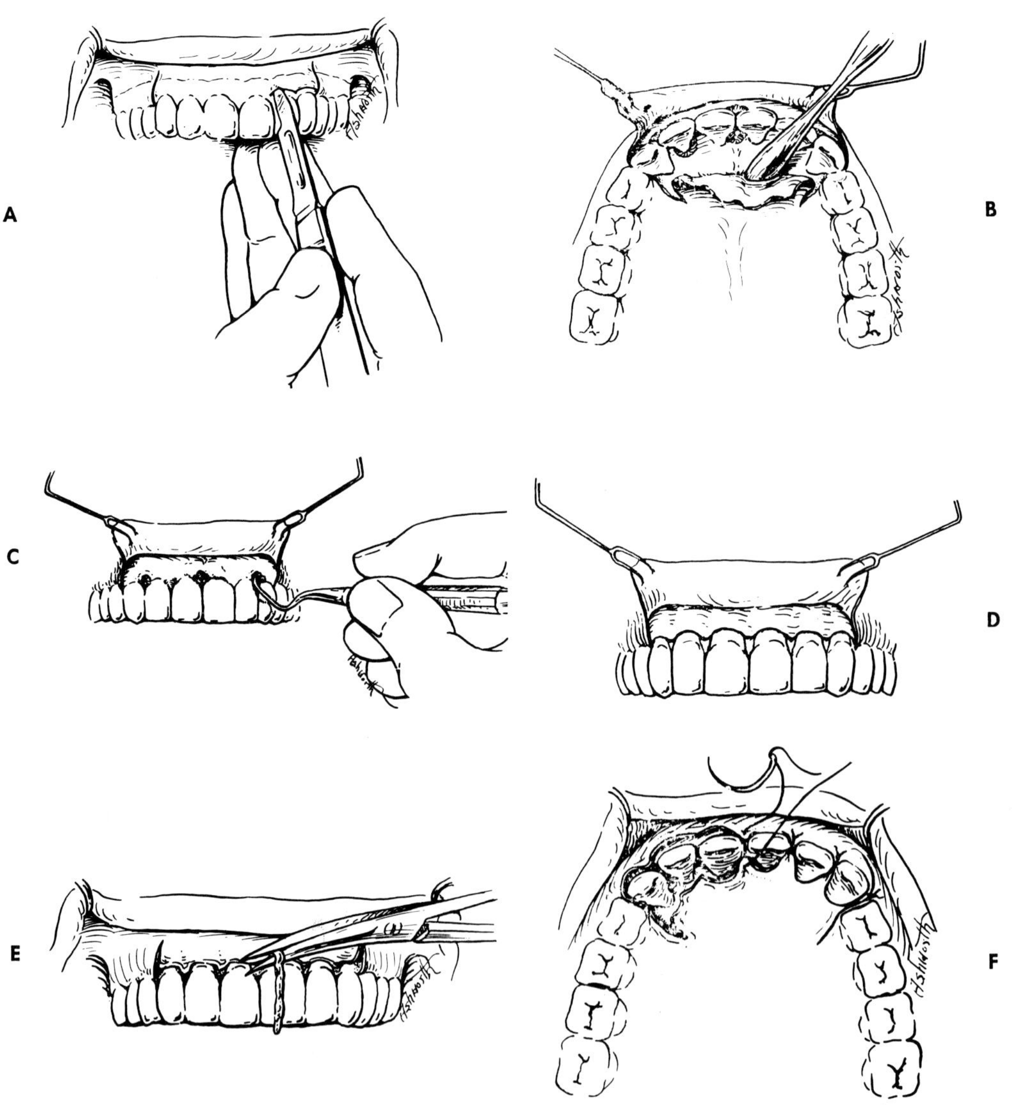


**Fig. 33-16. A,** Use a scalpel to incise the gingiva so that the flap can cover the alveolar crest. **B,** Reflect a full flap by blunt dissection with a periosteal elevator on the vestibular and oral surfaces. The bony defects resulting from periodontal disease are now exposed. **C,** Use a curette to debride the osseous margins and teeth of deposits and adherent inflammatory tissue. **D,** The conceptual ideal of alveolar form will serve as a guide in the establishment of physiologic osseous form. **E,** Do any correcting or trimming of the flap before coaptation. **F,** Suture the flap to approximate gingival and osseous margins. This will prevent displacement of flap margins during the placement of the surgical dressing. (Modified from Neumann, R.: Atlas der radicalchirurgischen Behandlung der Paradentosen, Berlin, 1926, Hermann Meusser.)

Now that the techniques for osteoectomy-osteoplasty have been discussed, the actual performance of this surgery may be followed diagrammatically in Fig. 33-16 and in clinical photographs (Figs. 33-17 and 33-18).

### Causes for failure

Failure of osseous surgery is related to reformation of pockets and/or excessive loss of bone, which are caused by the following:

1. Incomplete pocket elimination resulting from failure to create ideal bone form
2. Improper flap management
3. Sequestration or resorption of bone caused by excessive surgical trauma
4. Improper dressing management
5. Exposure of thin bony plates, alveolar dehiscences, or fenestrations during surgery
6. Postsurgical exposure of thinned bone margins
7. Infection after surgery
8. Incomplete removal of calculus
9. Poor oral hygiene after surgery
10. Root caries or pulpal problems incident to the surgery or to root exposure

## WOUND HEALING

Osseous surgery is frequently followed by further bone loss.[21] When bone is cut or left uncovered by soft connective tissue, varying amounts of bone extend-

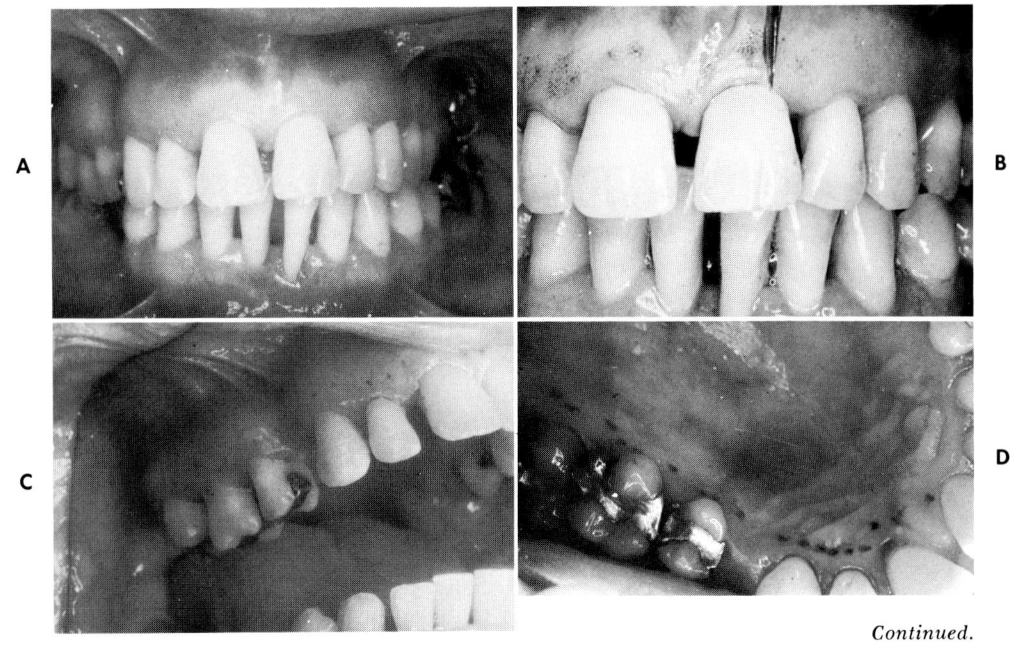


*Continued.*

**Fig. 33-17. A,** Periodontitis in a 38-year-old white woman. Her case before treatment is shown in Figs. 15-13 and 15-14. Root planing, gingival curettage, and proper oral hygiene have resolved most of the clinically evident inflammation. Pockets and osseous deformities still remain. **B** and **C,** Pocket depth has been delineated by indelible pencil on the gingiva for the purpose of illustration. A kidney-shaped scalpel is used to make an initial vertical incision preparatory to reflection of a flap. **D,** Pocket depth is delineated on the palatal gingiva.

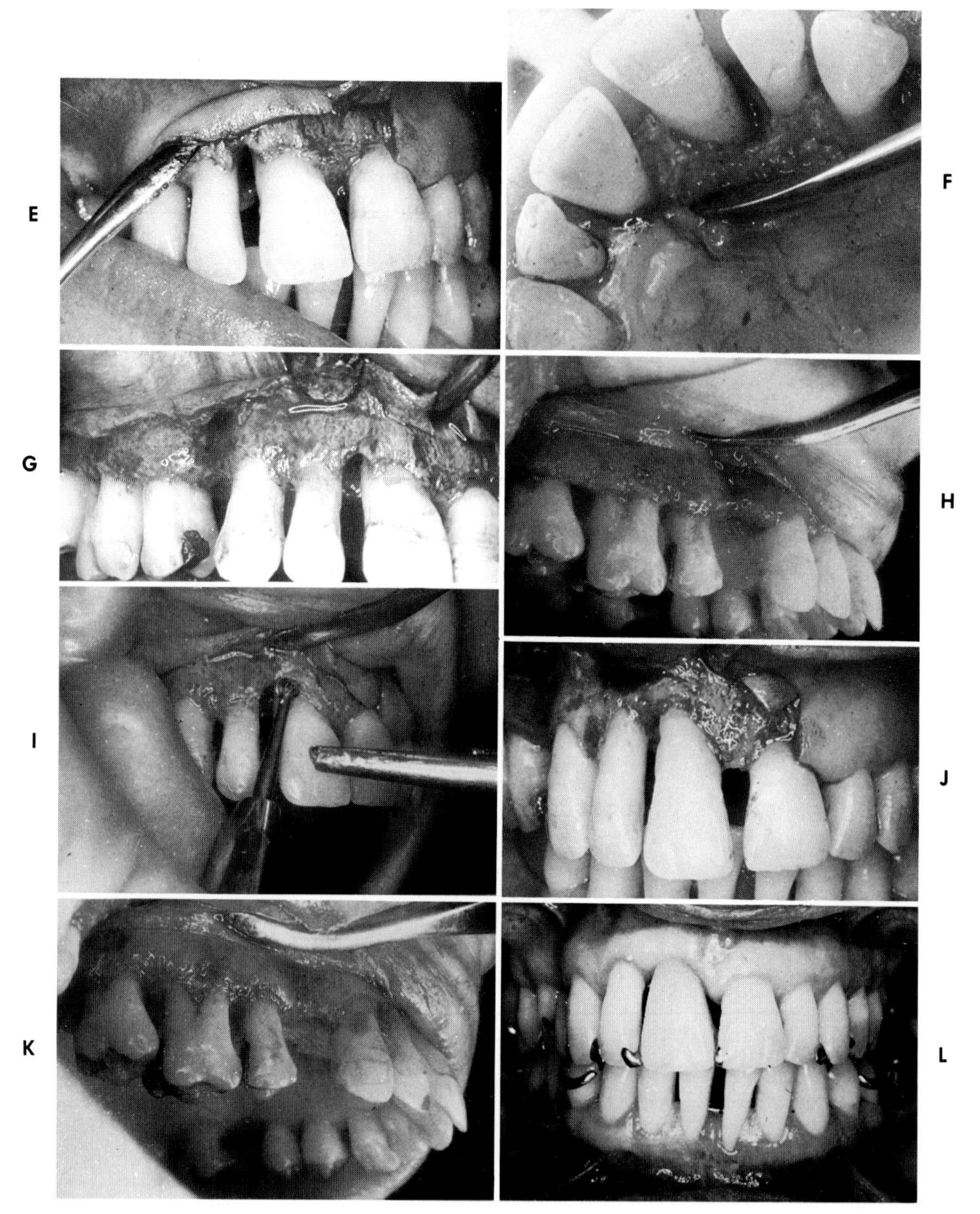


**Fig. 33-17, cont'd. E,** A full flap is reflected by blunt dissection with a periosteal elevator to expose the osseous surface deformed by disease. Note that sterile procedure, with rubber gloves, is maintained throughout the surgery. **F,** The flap is reflected on the palatal surface. Note the troughlike intra-alveolar crater on the oral surface of the maxillary incisor. **G,** The osseous surface is exposed for access. Note the deformities present. **H,** Posteriorly, blunted alveolar margins, interdental craters, and a furcation involvement on the second molar can be seen. **I,** Initial gross reductions were made with a rotary bur under saline spray. **J,** Postsurgical bone contour is evident. Reattachment was attempted on the palatal side of the central incisor. A guarded prognosis was projected for the central incisor. **K,** Posteriorly a scalloped, beveled bone form was created. Bony deformities were eliminated. **L,** Two years later a physiologic healthy periodontium is present despite occasional indifferent home care by the patient. A cast removable splint was constructed because of tooth mobility. (Restorations courtesy D. E. Erickson, El Cajon, Calif.)

A 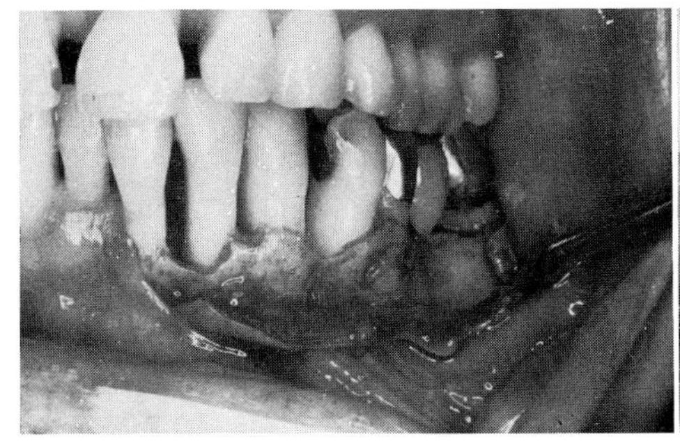 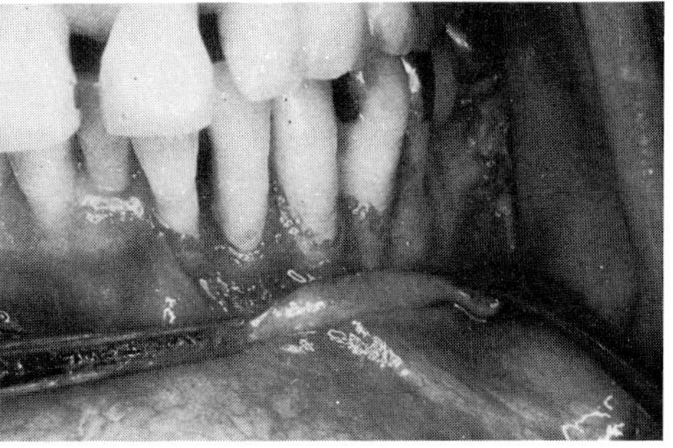 B

**Fig. 33-18.** **A,** A full flap has been reflected to reveal the bizarre pattern of bone destruction in a 28-year-old white woman. **B,** The scalloped mesiodistal outline and coronally sloping bone profile are evident after osseous surgery. This will assist the gingiva to maintain a physiologic form.

ing from the surface operated on become necrotic. This necrotic bone is resorbed by osteoclasts, which differentiate from pluripotent mesenchymal cells in adjacent marrow spaces and haversian systems. Granulation may also come from the periodontal ligament and adjacent fixed wound margins. The osseous wound thus becomes covered with a young, proliferating connective tissue. The granulation tissue is the product of a proliferation of young connective tissue from vital bone, periodontal ligament, and (to a lesser extent) soft tissue wound margins that resorbs, undermines, and removes necrotic bone as well as some vital bone.

## Phases

Experimental studies (in dogs) indicate the following phases in healing after osseous surgery[35] (Fig. 33-19).

1. Osteoclastic phase—2 to 10 days
2. Osteoblastic phase—10 to 28 days
3. Functional repair of dentoperiodontal unit and dentogingival junction—28 to 185 days

*Osteoclastic phase*

When flaps are coapted postsurgically, the earliest changes that follow the acute inflammation involve the differentiation of osteoclasts and the resorption of bone in the wound area. This is then followed by bone deposition that tends to repair the surgically created bone defect. Split-thickness flaps have been found to produce much less damage to bone.[32]

In similar experiments, when periosteum was retained, the same time intervals took place in the phases of healing but without residual deformities from the surgery.[39] Less resorption and a lesser final deformity occur when a thick layer of connective tissue is left over bone.

*Osteoblastic phase*

When flaps are reflected and then replaced, the sequence and time for bone healing are essentially the same. During the first few days there is an acute inflammatory reaction; a fibrin network is formed and begins to be replaced by collagen in 4 to 6 days. An attachment epithelium becomes evident in about a week.[30] Bone resorption begins after several days and continues for about 2 weeks unless a sequestrum is present, in which case it may continue for much longer. Repair (osteoblastic phase) then goes on for 3 to 4 weeks, at which time the resorption is almost completely repaired.[48] With the loss of thin spines and spicules and with some bone apposition, limited bone recontouring occurs.

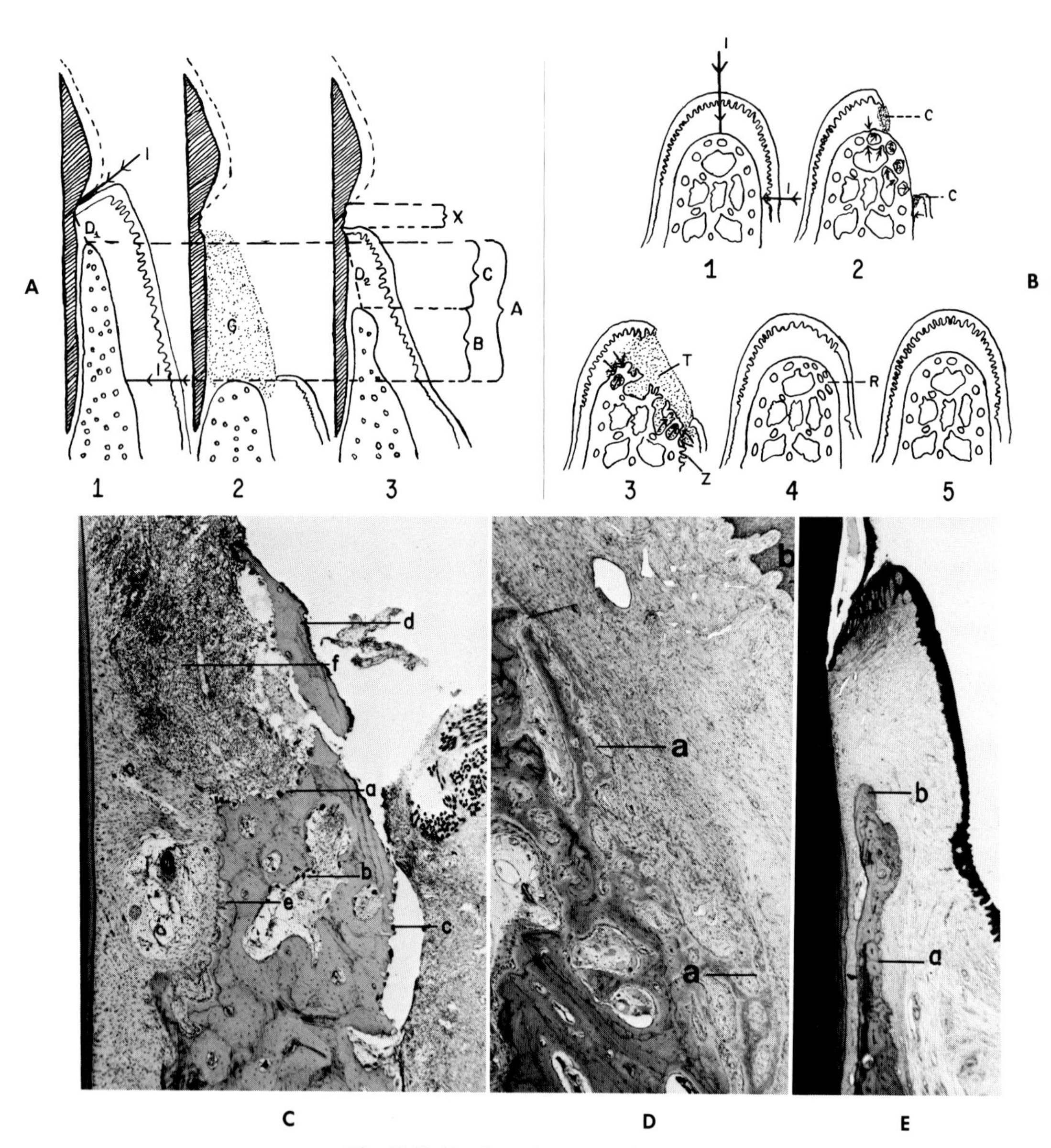


**Fig. 33-19.** For legend see opposite page.

Full maturation of the connective tissue may take as long as 6 months.[37] When flaps are loosely sutured, defects similar to those produced by bone denudation occur.

***Functional repair phase***

Reapposition of a flap to cover bone after osseous surgery undoubtedly reduces the amount of bone resorption (or sequestration) that may take place. All osseous surgery is followed by some bone loss (Fig. 33-20). In turn a period of reactive and compensatory bone deposition occurs, which may be called the repair phase (Fig. 33-21). The repair, however, rarely restores all the bone lost by surgical injury. This means that the surgeon cannot plan to cut bone like an inert clay mold and expect it to retain the precise form that he created. He must plan any necessary osseous surgery with the full knowledge of the tissue reactions that will follow surgical manipulations.[21,25-32,35-48] Furthermore, as a result of the influences of function, ultimate bone contours may differ from those established during osseous surgery.[21]

The effects of denudation of crestal alveolar bone have been observed in dogs and humans.[8,34-36,38,40] The osteoclastic phase lasts about 10 days and is followed by a repair or osteoblastic phase that lasts up to 30 days. In the interdental areas the marrow spaces contribute cellular elements that achieve a complete restoration of lost bony substance. However, part of the thin bone over the roots is lost completely. There is an ultimate loss of about 2.5 mm. of bone. The length of the junctional epithelium is relatively unchanged, and the bone lost is replaced by a long connective tissue attachment.

---

**Fig. 33-19. A,** Diagrammatic representation of healing in the area overlying the root after complete denudation of the alveolar bone (dog). ***1,*** Preoperative appearance. Between the two arrows, ***1,*** all epithelium and connective tissue, including the periosteum, were removed, baring the bone. **2,** Six to 10 days postoperative. Young connective tissue, *G,* is granulation tissue. ***3,*** Ninety-five to 185 days postoperative. *A* is the extent of complete osseous exposure and resorption (5 mm.); *B,* the extent of bone repair (2.5 mm.); *C,* the extent of final loss of alveolar bone height (2.5 mm.); $D_2$, the original length of the connective tissue attachment; *X,* the lowering of the level of the epithelial attachment below the cementoenamel junction. **B,** Diagrammatic representation of healing in the interdental area after complete denudation of alveolar bone (dog). ***1,*** Preoperative view. Arrows indicate the direction of the incision. ***2,*** Two to 4 days postoperative. Small arrows indicate the direction of osseous resorption. *C* indicates small blood clots and exposed bone. ***3,*** Six to 10 days postoperative. *T,* Young connective tissue (granulation tissue); *Z,* formation of coarse, fibrillar bone trabeculae. ***4,*** Twenty-eight days postoperative. *R,* Formation of trabecular bone at the wound site. ***5,*** Ninety-five to 185 days postoperative. Note the return to the preoperative appearance. **C,** Micrograph corresponding to **A, 2.** Undermining resorption has occurred at the crest, *a,* and in the marrow spaces facing the periodontal ligament, *b.* Frontal resorption is evident on the surface of the vestibular bony plate below the wound edge, *c.* The crest has been resorbed. An inflammatory reaction is present in the proliferating young connective tissue that occupies the former periodontal ligament area, *f,* in the bone marrow and at the edge of the incision. **D,** Micrograph corresponding to **B, *4*.** Coarse, immature trabeculae lined with osteoid and osteoblasts indicate rapid new bone formation, *a.* Surface epithelium is indicated by *b.* **E,** Micrograph corresponding to **A, *3*.** The amount of regeneration of alveolar bone 93 days after bone exposure is evident between *a* and *b.* Alveolar crest after postoperative bone loss is indicated by *a;* highest level of regeneration of the alveolar crest 93 days postoperative is indicated by *b.* The connective tissue attachment between the alveolar crest and the apical end of the attachment epithelium is twice normal length. The attachment epithelium is on cementum. The width of the periodontal ligament has returned to normal. (Courtesy M. N. Wilderman, New Orleans.[35,36,39])

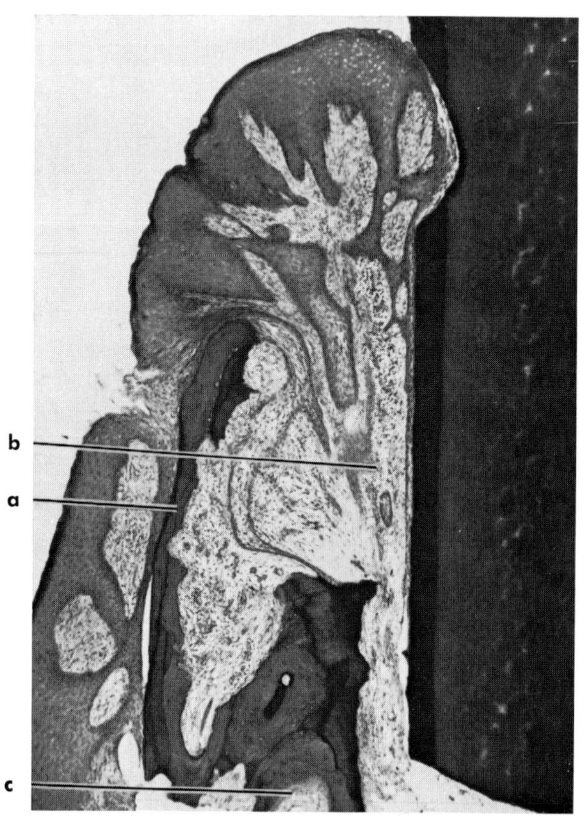


**Fig. 33-20.** Large sequestrum, *a,* in a specimen of human periodontal tissue. The notch in the tooth indicates the level of the alveolar bone at the time of surgery. At one point the necrotic bone is nearly in contact with the surface, covered by only a few degenerating epithelial cells. Extensive epithelial proliferation has taken place into the lamina propria, where the collagen fibers are being replaced by a young proliferating connective tissue, *b.* The attachment epithelium has proliferated down the root parallel to the necrotic alveolar crest. Empty lacunae are present in the bone. A few pyknotic nuclei are present in lacunae at the most apical extent of the photomicrograph, where a thin seam of osteoid, *c,* lines a marrow space. (From Grant, D. A.: J. Periodont. **38:**409, 1967.)

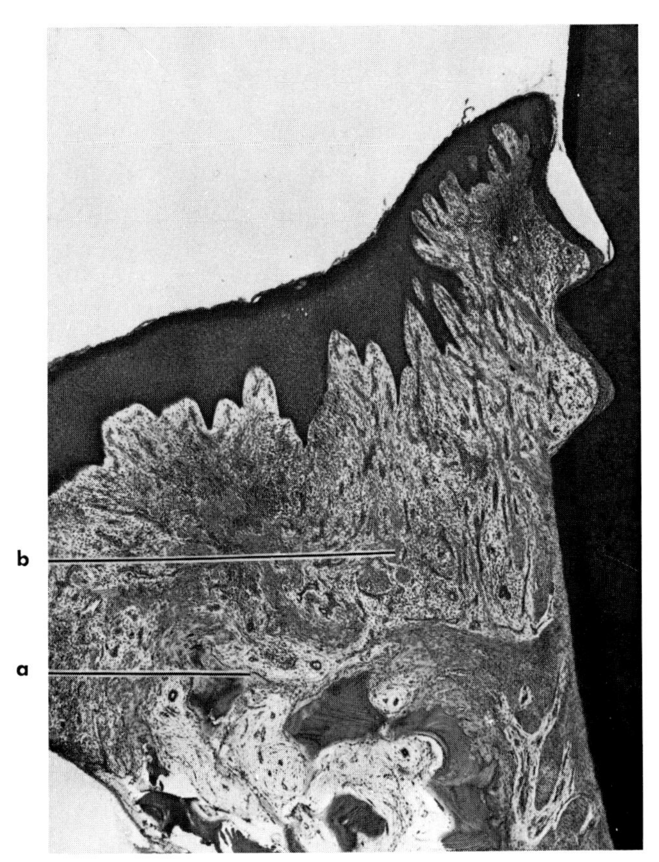


**Fig. 33-21.** Reactive and compensatory bone deposition occurs in the repair phase after osseous surgery. A large amount of osteoid, *a*, has been formed in this human specimen. The lamina propria, *b*, is filled with a highly vascular, young, proliferating connective tissue. The notches indicate the presurgical depth of the sulcus and level of the alveolar crest on the reflection of a flap.

When flaps are coapted postsurgically after osseous surgery, the amount of bone lost after reshaping is insignificant, being on the order of 0.5 to 1 mm.[6,35,37] The greater bone loss reported by some investigators could be due to the use of diamond stones.[46] The least damage, with best repair, results when high-speed engines, coolant sprays, and round carbide steel burs are used.[12,14-22,32,34,44-47]

**CHAPTER 33**

**References**


1. Ochsenbein, C., and Ross, S.: A reevaluation of osseous surgery, Dental Clinics of North America, Philadelphia, 1969, W. B. Saunders Co., vol. 13.
2. Neumann, R.: Atlas der radikal-chirurgischen Behandlung der Paradentosen, Berlin, 1926, Hermann Meusser.
3. Schluger, S.: Osseous resection—a basic principle in periodontal surgery, Oral Surg. **2**:316, 1949.
4. Carranza, F. A., and Carranza, F. A., Jr.: The management of the alveolar bone in the treatment of the periodontal pocket, J. Periodont. **27**:29, 1956.
5. Friedman, N.: Periodontal osseous surgery: osteoplasty and osteoectomy, J. Periodont. **26**: 257, 1955.
6. Heins, P. J.: Osseous surgery: an evaluation after twenty years, Dental Clinics of North America, Philadelphia, 1969, W. B. Saunders Co., vol. 13.
7. Ochsenbein, C.: Osseous resection in periodontal surgery, J. Periodont. **29**:15, 1958.
8. Glickman, I., Smulow, J. B., Tannen, R., and O'Brien, T.: Healing of the periodontium following mucogingival surgery, Oral Surg. **16**:530, 1963.
9. Prichard, J.: Advanced periodontal disease, ed. 2, Philadelphia, 1972, W. B. Saunders Co.
10. Morris, M. L.: Two approaches for interproximal osseous tapering, Periodontics **2**:259, 1964.
11. Klavan, B.: Osseous surgery, Illinois Dent. J. **34**:303, 1965.
12. O'Conner, T. W., and Biggs, N. L.: Interproximal bony contours, J. Periodont. **35**:326, 1964.
13. Easley, J. R.: Methods of determining alveolar osseous form, J. Periodont. **38**:112, 1967.
14. Heins, P. J., and Canter, S. R.: The furca involvement: a classification of deformities, J. Periodont. **6**:84, 1968.
15. Everett, F. G.: Bifurcation involvement, Oregon Dent. J. **28**:2, 1959.
16. Goldman, H. M., Shuman, A. M., and Isenberg, G. A.: Management of the partial furcation involvement, **6**:197, 1968.
17. Schallhorn, R. G.: Eradication of bifurcation defects utilizing frozen autogenous hip marrow implants, J. Ontario Dent. Ass. **45**:18, 1968.
18. Staffileno, H., Jr.: Furcation involvement in periodontics, Dent. Radiogr. Photgr. **38**:85, 1965.
19. Mann, W. A.: Autogenous transplant in the treatment of an infrabony pocket, Periodontics **2**:205, 1964.
20. Ross, S. E., Malamed, E. H., and Amsterdam, M.: Contiguous autogenous transplant, Periodontics **4**:246, 1966.
21. Grant, D. A.: Experimental periodontal surgery: sequestration of alveolar bone, J. Periodont. **38**:409, 1967.
22. Messinger, T. F., and Orban, B.: Elimination of periodontal pockets by root amputation, J. Periodont. **25**:213, 1954.
23. Bradin, M.: Precautions and hazards in periodontal surgery, J. Periodont. **33**:154, 1962.
24. Elliott, J. R., and Bowers, G. M.: Alveolar dehiscence and fenestrations, Periodontics **1**:245, 1963.
25. Grant, D. A., Friedman, N., and Orban, B.: Response of the periodontal tissues around the alveolar crest to surgical procedures. Presented before the American Academy of Periodontology, Los Angeles, 1960.
26. Giblin, J. M., Levy, S., Staffileno, H., and others: Healing of re-entry wounds in dogs, J. Periodont. **37**:238, 1966.
27. Carraro, J. J., Carranza, F. A., Jr., Albano, E. A., and Joly, G. G.: Effect of bone denudation in mucogingival surgery in humans, J. Periodont. **35**:463, 1964.
28. Weinmann, J. P., and Sicher, H.: Bone and bones, ed. 2, St. Louis, 1955, The C. V. Mosby Co.
29. West, T. L., and Bloom, A.: A histologic study of wound healing following mucogingival surgery, J. Dent. Res. **40**:675, 1961. Abstract.
30. Hiatt, W. H., Stallard, R. E., Butler, E. D., and Badgett, B.: Repair following mucoperiosteal flap surgery with full gingival retention, J. Periodont. **39**:11, 1968.

31. Pfeifer, J. S.: The reaction of alveolar bone to flap procedures in man, Periodontics 3:135, 1965.
32. Staffileno, H., Wentz, F. M., and Orban, B.: Histologic study of healing of split thickness flap surgery in dogs, J. Periodont. 33:56, 1962.
33. Everett, F. G., Waerhaug, J., and Widman, A.: Leonard Widman: surgical treatment of pyorrhea alveolaris, J. Periodont. 42:571, 1971.
34. Hoag, P. M., Wood, D. L., Donnenfeld, O. W., and Rosenfeld, L. D.: Alveolar crest reduction following full and partial thickness flaps, J. Periodont. 43:141, 1972.
35. Wilderman, M. N., Pennel, B. M., King, K., and Barron, J. M.: Histogenesis of repair following osseous surgery, J. Periodont. 41:551, 1970.
36. Wilderman, M. N., Wentz, F. M., and Orban B.: Histogenesis of repair after mucogingival surgery, J. Periodont. 31:283, 1960.
37. Donnenfeld, O. W., Hoag, P. M., and Weissman, D. P.: A clinical study on the effects of osteoplasty, J. Periodont. 41:131, 1970.
38. Carranza, F. A., Jr., and Carraro, J. J.: Effect of removal of periosteum on postoperative result of mucogingival surgery, J. Periodont. 34:223, 1963.
39. Wilderman, M. N.: Repair after a periosteal retention procedure, J. Periodont. 34:487, 1963.
40. Tavtigian, R.: The height of the facial radicular alveolar crest following apically repositioned flap operations, J. Periodont. 41:412, 1970.
41. Pennel, B. M., King, K. O., Wilderman, M. N., and Barron, J. M.: Repair of the alveolar process following osseous surgery, J. Periodont. 38:426, 1967.
42. Lobene, R. R., and Glickman, I.: The response of alveolar bone to grinding with rotary diamond stones, J. Periodont. 34:105, 1963.
43. McFall, T. A., Yamane, J. M., and Burnett, G. W.: Comparison of the cutting effect on bone of an ultrasonic cutting device and rotary burs, J. Oral Surg. Anesth. Hosp. Dent. Serv. 19:200, 1961.
44. Spatz, S.: Early reaction in bone following the use of burs rotating at conventional and ultra speeds, Oral Surg. 19:808, 1965.
45. Moss, R. W.: Histopathologic reaction of bone to surgical cutting, Oral Surg. 17:405, 1964.
46. Costich, E. R., Youngblood, P. J., and Walden, J. M.: A study of the effects of high-speed rotary instruments on bone repair in dogs, Oral Surg. 17:563, 1964.
47. Boyne, P. J.: Histologic response of bone to sectioning by high-speed rotary instruments, J. Dent. Res. 45:270, 1966.
48. Caffesse, R. J., Ramfjord, S. P., and Nasjleti, C. E.: Reverse bevel periodontal flaps in monkeys, J. Periodont. 39:219, 1968.

**Additional suggested reading**

Glickman, I., and Smulow, J. B.: Buttressing bone formation, J. Periodont. 36:365, 1965.

Goldman, H. M.: Management of the partial furcation involvement, Periodontics 6:197, 1965.

Kohler, C. A., and Ramfjord, S. P.: Healing of gingival mucoperiosteal flaps, Oral Surg. 13:89, 1960.

Larato, D. C.: Furcation involvements; incidence and distribution, J. Periodont. 41:499, 1970.

Larato, D. C.: Periodontal bone defects in the juvenile skull, J. Periodont. 41:473, 1970.

Leib, A. M., Berdon, J. K., and Sabes, W. R.: Furcation involvements correlated with enamel projections from the cemento-enamel junction, J. Periodont. 38:330, 1967.

Löe, H.: Bone tissue formation, Acta Odont. Scand. 17:325, 1959.

Marfino, N. R., Orban, B., and Wentz, F. M.: Repair of dentogingival junction following surgical intervention, J. Periodont. 30:180, 1959.

Morris, M. L.: The reattachment of human periodontal tissues following detachment, J. Periodont. 24:220, 1953.

Persson, P. A.: The regeneration of the marginal periodontium after flap operations, Acta Odont. Scand. 20:43, 1962.

Pfeifer, J. S.: The growth of gingival tissue over denuded bone, J. Periodont. 34:10, 1963.

Ramfjord, S. P., and Costich, E. R.: Healing after exposure of periosteum on the alveolar process, J. Periodont. 39:199, 1968.

Rosenberg, M. M.: Reentry of an osseous defect treated by a bone implant after a long duration, J. Periodont. 42:360, 1971.

Staffileno, H., Levy, S., and Gargiulo, A.: Histologic study of cellular mobilization and repair following a periosteal retention operation via split tissue mucogingival flap surgery, J. Periodont. 37:31, 1966.

CHAPTER THIRTY-FOUR

# Mucogingival surgery



*Definition*

Mucogingival surgery consists of procedures that are designed to (1) *create* a functionally adequate zone of attached gingiva or *retain* such a zone after a pocket has been eliminated, (2) *alter* the position of or *eliminate* a frenum, and (3) *deepen* the vestibule.

## OBJECTIVES

Although mucogingival procedures are not primarily designed to eliminate pockets or to create physiologic gingival form, they are often combined with gingivectomy-gingivoplasty, osseous surgery, or reattachment operations. Mucogingival surgery is concerned with problems that center around the relationship of the gingiva and the alveolar mucosa.[1-51]

The gingiva is structurally more able to withstand the frictional stresses of mastication and brushing than the alveolar mucosa. The gingiva is cornified and its underlying lamina propria consists of dense, well-organized fiber bundles. The attached gingiva is firmly joined to the root of the tooth and to bone. The alveolar mucosa, on the other hand, functions as a lining tissue; it has a thin, nonkeratinized epithelium, is loosely textured, has elastic fibers in the mucosa and submucosa, and is loosely bound to the periosteum of the alveolar bone. Alveolar mucosa is well adapted to permit movement.

## PROBLEMS

### Gingiva

*Pockets encroaching on the mucogingival junction*

Of the several types of mucogingival problems that have been described, the most common are those in which several millimeters of gingiva exist but pockets encroach on the mucogingival junction (Fig. 34-1, *A*). In such cases gingivectomy would leave little or no attached gingiva and the margins would be in alveolar mucosa. The resultant marginal tissue may be ill suited to withstand

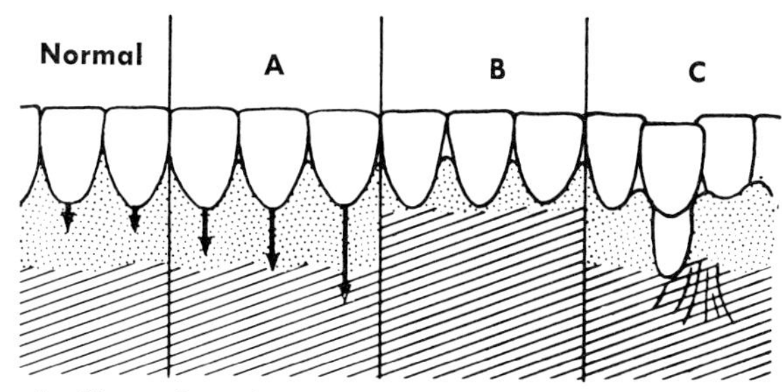


**Fig. 34-1.** Diagrammatic illustration of mucogingival problems. **A,** Adequate width of zone of attached gingiva. The bottom of the pocket (arrows) is at or beyond the mucogingival junction. **B,** Gingival width inadequate to dissipate muscle pull. The attached gingiva is too narrow or entirely absent. **C,** Extensive loss of gingiva on one tooth associated with labial malposition. Often this problem is combined with frenum pull.

**Table 34-1.** Correlation of solutions to the problems in Fig. 34-1

| **Problems** (Fig. 34-1) | **Solutions** |
|---|---|
| A | 1. Apically repositioned flap<br>2. Flap returned to original position |
| B | 1. Free gingival graft |
| C | 1. Laterally repositioned (pedicle) graft<br>2. Free gingival graft<br>3. Frenotomy (mandible)<br>4. Frenectomy (maxilla) |

the trauma of food excursions in chewing or the trauma of toothbrushing. Plaque accumulation, food impingement, and food retention can occur, resulting in further recession or pocket formation.

*Attached gingiva either narrow or absent*

When little or no gingiva exists, even shallow pockets can pose mucogingival problems (Fig. 34-1, *B*). Preconceived ideas, however, about the number of millimeters of attached gingiva that are functionally adequate should be avoided.[8,26] A functionally adequate zone of gingiva is one that will effectively dissipate muscular pull and remain in health. In some mouths 1 to 2 mm. of gingiva may be sufficient. Occasionally margins in alveolar mucosa particularly in molar regions, have been observed without clinically evident ill effects for years.

*Local recession*

A third type of problem centers about localized gingival recession involving one or two teeth (Fig. 34-1, *C*). Such defects commonly occur on labially positioned teeth and teeth with prominent roots, situations in which bony dehiscences often are noted. The absence of labial or buccal bone on these roots may predispose to gingival loss. Some problems may result in frenum pull; others appear to be caused by frenum pull.

## Frenum

*High frenum attachment*

Lesions caused by a high frenum attachment often present a mucogingival problem (Fig. 34-2). If a frenum attachment approaches the free gingiva or extends into it, any pull on the frenum may produce blanching of the gingiva and

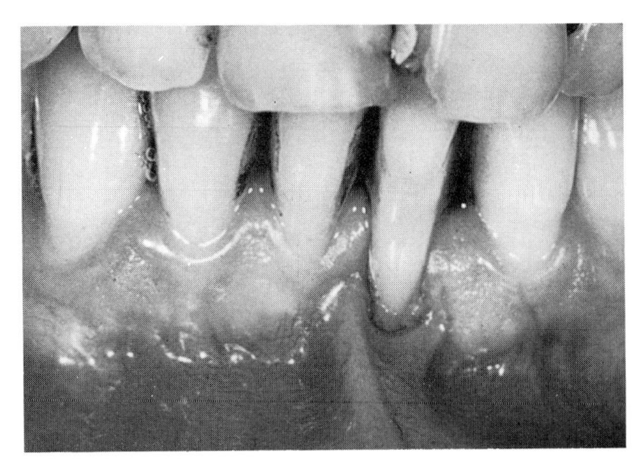

**Fig. 34-2.** Frenum pull in a lower central incisor. Note the prominence of the root.

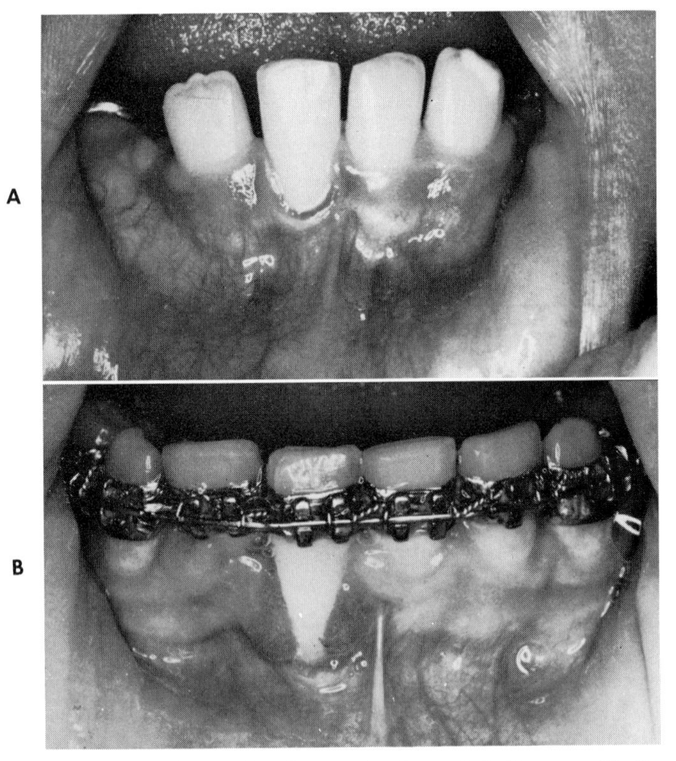

**Fig. 34-3.** Individual gingival recession in two brothers. **A** is 9 years old. Recession should be corrected at that time and requires only a simple frenotomy. **B** is 13 years old. The deformity has progressed further and now requires a laterally repositioned flap (graft) for correction. (Courtesy W. B. Hall, San Francisco.)

gaping of the gingival sulcus. Combined with minor injuries from food or toothbrush abrasion, frenum pull may result in recession, root exposure, and consequent hypersensitivity aggravated by plaque accumulation.

***Persistent mandibular labial frenum***

Persistence of the mandibular labial frenum is common.[2,22,23,27,28] The problem may first be noticed when the permanent incisors erupt. It probably should be treated when first diagnosed. If a mandibular labial frenum is allowed to persist, surgical solutions will become more complex and their success less predictable (Fig. 34-3). Maxillary labial frena in children's mouths, however, may disappear when the permanent canine teeth erupt.[23] If they persist beyond that time or if a gross maxillary frenum is attached to the incisive papilla, removal of the frenum is indicated. Other frena that are less commonly involved include the mandibular lingual frenum and buccal frena in the premolar regions.

## TREATMENT

***Terminology of mucogingival procedures***

A number of methods are available to manage the various types of mucogingival problems.[3-51] These include the following:

1. Apically repositioned flap
2. Flap replaced in its original position
   (flap curettage, flap for new attachment)
3. Laterally repositioned flap
   (sliding flap, pedicle flap)
4. Free gingival graft
5. Frenotomy, frenectomy, frenum repositioning
6. Vestibular extension

The correlation between these procedures and the problems in Fig. 34-1 is reviewed at the end of this chapter.

### Apically repositioned flap

To solve the problem shown in Fig. 34-1 under category *A,* dentists frequently use the apically repositioned flap. This procedure employs an internally beveled incision to elevate a flap consisting of free and attached gingivae (Fig. 34-4). The flap is then repositioned apically.[5-11] Such an operation was first described by Widman.[4]

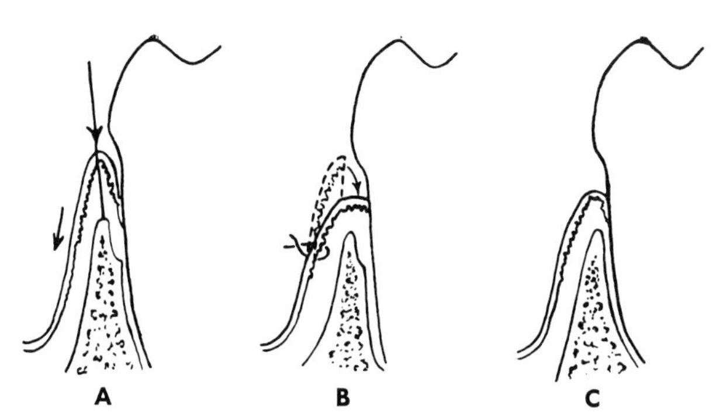


**Fig. 34-4. A,** Initial reverse bevel incision in the apically repositioned flap procedure. The attached gingiva is dissected free. **B,** Tissue adhering to the tooth is curetted away, the bony defect is exposed and treated, and the attached gingiva is repositioned and sutured in a more apical position. **C,** Postoperative result.

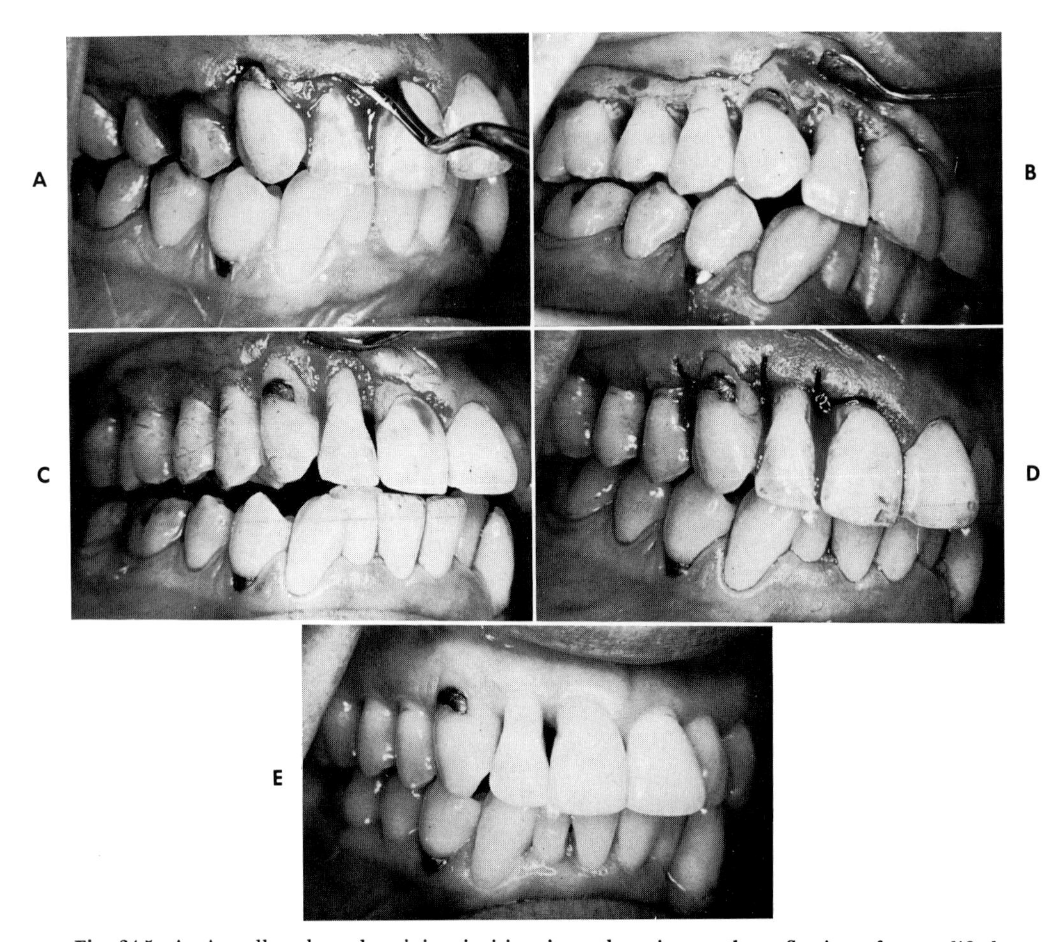


**Fig. 34-5. A,** A scalloped, undermining incision is made prior to the reflection of a modified flap. The gingiva is trimmed to the desired width, and the margin beveled via this incision. **B,** A modified flap is reflected by blunt dissection, revealing interdental craters. **C,** Osseous surgery is performed to create a physiologic alveolar form. **D,** The flap margins are approximated to the alveolar margin as the flap is positioned apically and stutured to place. **E,** The physiologic postsurgical gingival form with a functionally adequate zone of gingiva is evident. (Courtesy C. Nabers, San Antonio.)

The apically repositioned flap procedure is illustrated in Figs. 34-4 to 34-6. The initial scalloped incision,[4,8,31] employing an internal bevel, begins and terminates in an interdental area and generally is made to the alveolar bone crest. After reflection of the flap, all remaining epithelium and chronic inflammatory tissue and all interproximal soft tissue are removed. The roots, previously planed, are thoroughly planed again, after which osseous deformities may be corrected. The flap is then repositioned at a more apical level and sutured to place. The area of operation may not even require dressing when there is perfect coaptation of gingival margins and no marginal or interproximal bone has been left exposed. After healing, pockets have been eliminated and a functionally adequate zone of gingiva remains.

There is a modification of this procedure to be employed when an adequate zone of gingiva does not exist. In such a case and when there is a heavy buccal bony plate, crestal bone may be left exposed on the assumption that

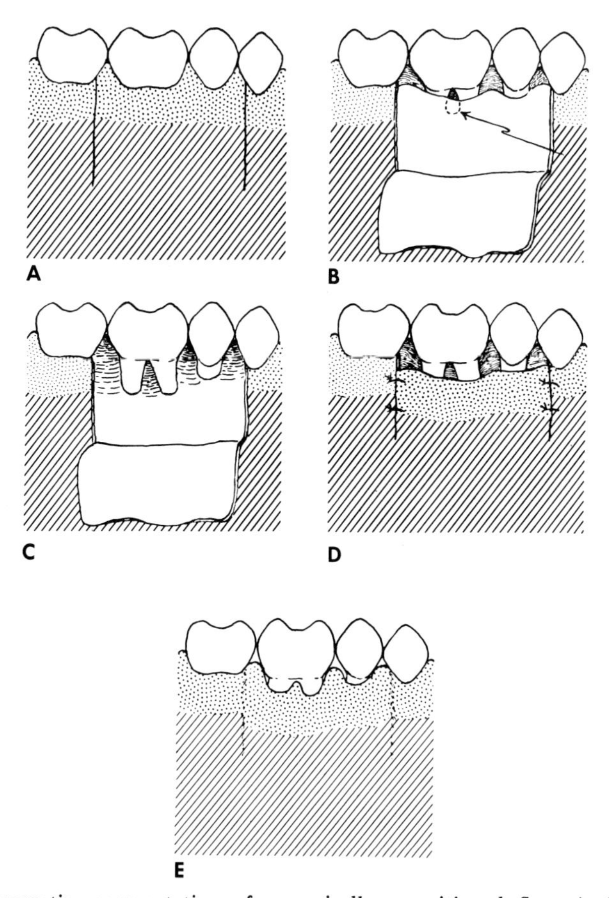


**Fig. 34-6.** Diagrammatic representation of an apically repositioned flap. **A,** Mandibular first molar with a pocket in the bifurcation area. The pocket extends below the mucogingival junction. Note that the relieving incisions are placed to the far side of the interdental spaces. **B,** Alveolar bone and interradicular crater (arrow) exposed by the flap approach. **C,** Osseous surgery has eliminated the crater. Bone ramping accomplished. **D,** Immediate postoperative view. **E,** Postoperative view approximately 1 year later.

such a procedure will result in the formation of new gingiva.[24] More commonly a free gingival graft is employed.

Histologic studies have shown that completely exposed interdental bone heals with negligible loss in height and depth.[54-58] Thin compact bone covering the root surface, on the other hand, when left completely exposed, shows a considerable loss in height at the thin crestal margin.[58] Dehiscences may also occur. Other studies have shown that this latter undesirable loss can be minimized by techniques leaving the periosteum in situ (split-thickness flap)[59-62] (Chapter 29). The dentist must thoroughly consider the great risks involved in any procedure that leaves bone exposed, especially the thin, compact bone overlying prominent roots.

## Flap replaced in original position

In selected areas in the labial maxillary anterior region, when pockets encroach on the mucogingival line, the use of an apically repositioned flap would

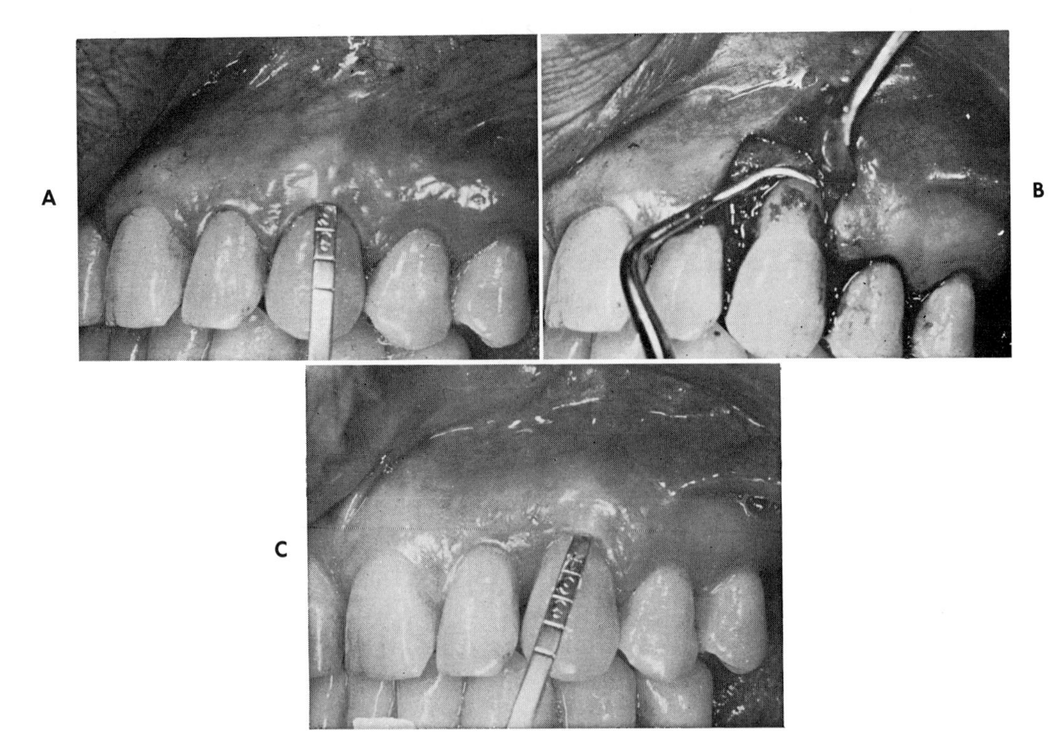


**Fig. 34-7. A,** A periodontal probe is inserted to show a pocket of 6 mm. depth on the vestibular surface of a left canine incisor. **B,** A full flap has been reflected. Note the calcified deposits (being removed). **C,** Same case 2 months later. The pocket has been eliminated. The sulcus is now 2 mm. deep. (Courtesy G. Ivancie, Denver.)

result in recession that would be cosmetically objectionable. In an attempt to create an aesthetic result via connective tissue reattachment, the dentist may replace the flap in its original position[12-14] (Fig. 34-7). The method is most successful where there is an individual deep pocket on the labial surface of a canine.

In such cases an internal bevel incision or an incision into the sulcus is used. After the flap is raised, any chronic inflammatory tissue and epithelium remaining attached to the teeth and to the inside of the flap is removed. Then the roots are curetted and the flap placed back and sutured to its original position. The operation might be considered a mucogingival procedure because it attempts to reattach the gingiva that has become detached by chronic periodontal disease. The difference between this procedure and the apically repositioned flap is that this flap is replaced as close as possible to its original position with the intent of connective tissue reattachment. (See Chapter 30.)

## Laterally repositioned flap

The laterally repositioned flap is a procedure for correcting localized recession problems when little or no gingiva remains on the labial surface of a single tooth.[15-17,61] It is also used for correcting gingival clefts. These individual gingival recessions are most often found in the area of the mandibular frenum and occasionally on the buccal aspect of other labially positioned teeth. They may be caused by or may result in frenum problems. A typical laterally repositioned flap procedure is illustrated in Fig. 34-8. A localized defect is present on a mandib-

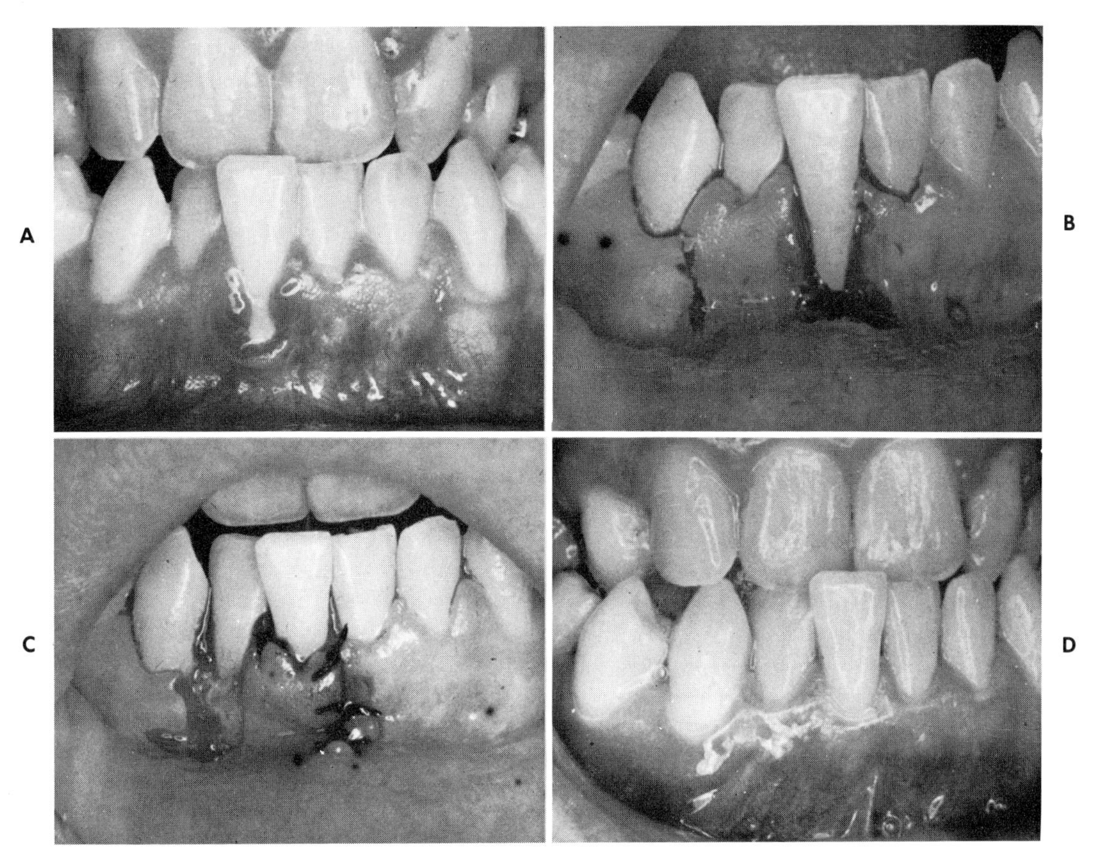


**Fig. 34-8.** Eight-year result of a laterally repositioned flap procedure. **A,** Preoperative view. **B,** Operative view. **C,** Immediate postoperative view. **D,** Eight-year postoperative view. Note that the malposition of the involved tooth was not corrected. (From the collection of H. E. Grupe.)

ular incisor. Adjacent gingiva is normal in thickness and width, adequate for use as a donor site. The tissue bordering the defect is trimmed and the root surface thoroughly planed. A prominent root may be flattened by grinding or extensive root planing. Prepare a flap at least one and one-half times as wide as the defect from the donor site and reflect it by sharp dissection, leaving the periosteum of the donor site intact.

Shift the flap to cover the exposed root surface and suture it to place without tension using silk or Ethiflex, no. 5-0 or 6-0, and an atraumatic, swaged needle. Press the flap against the tooth, using finger pressure, for 5 minutes to minimize clot formation and to encourage fibrin adherence of the flap to the tooth. Dust the operative site with an oxytetracycline adhesive powder and cover it with adhesive foil or rubber dam. Protect it with a soft periodontal pack. The exposed donor site often heals to the preoperative level. In most cases the laterally repositioned flap will attach to the denuded root surface. Probing, however, should be avoided for several months; later, inspection usually reveals a shallow sulcus.

A slightly different flap design may be used when there is an extra wide band of attached gingiva at the donor site. This procedure leaves the marginal gingival collar of the donor site intact[16] (Fig. 34-9). When an adjoining edentulous area

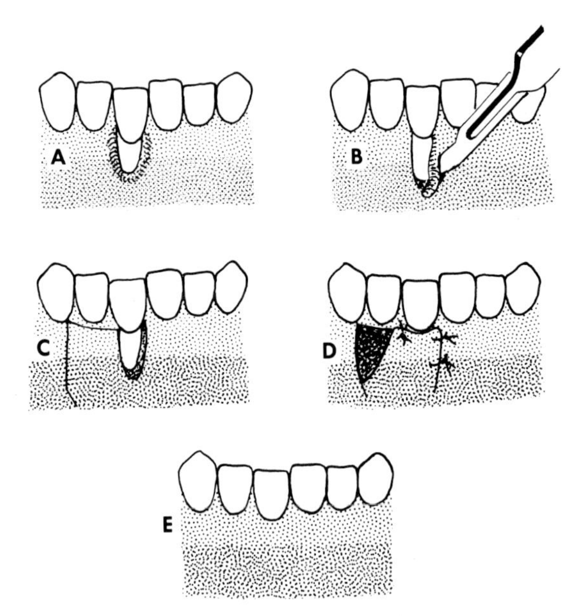


**Fig. 34-9.** Laterally repositioned flap. **A,** Severe gingival recession on the labial surface of the lower right central incisor. **B,** Excision of the margin of the lesion, including the junctional epithelium. Note that on the left side of the defect the incision is beveled externally and on the right side internally. The most prominent part of the exposed root surface to be covered is planed with a stone and very sharp curettes. **C,** Vertical incision in the donor side is one and a half tooth widths from the edge of the recession. The horizontal incision leaves a collar of gingiva on the lateral incisor. **D,** Tissue from the donor side is sharply dissected, leaving periosteum on the donor side. It is then moved over gently and sutured to the receptor side without tension, as indicated. The internal bevel of the one side and the external bevel of the other then form a lap joint, improving the chance for primary union. **E,** Appearance of the operative site after 1 year. (Modified from Grupe, H. E.: J. Periodont. **37**:491, 1966.)

with an adequate band of gingiva is available as a donor area, use the gingiva of this site to cover the exposed root surface of an adjacent tooth[20,21] (Fig. 34-10).

***Oblique rotated flap procedure***

When the gingiva of the potential donor site is unsuitable because it is finely textured or too thin and the underlying bone is thin or absent, a slightly different approach, the oblique rotated flap, may be used.[19] This procedure prevents recession of the donor site and uses as donor tissue an interdental papilla. In this area the gingiva is thicker and, most important, the underlying interdental alveolar bone is much less liable to resorption following surgery. A case with such a rotated flap is illustrated in Figs. 34-11 and 34-12. A good donor papilla is present distal to the canine. The receptor site is prepared as in the lateral repositioning technique. A papillary flap is prepared by sharp dissection, rotated 90 degrees, and sutured to position. Such flaps must be narrow to permit rotation. A 1-year postoperative result is shown in Fig. 34-11, *D.* Although some root remains exposed in most of these cases, the defect created by gingival recession has been corrected.

A variation of this operation is sometimes performed by creation of a functionally adequate band of attached gingiva when *both* papillae adjoining the cleft or individual recession are undermined and freed after the margins of the cleft have been excised.[18] Suture the two freed papillae together after either ap-

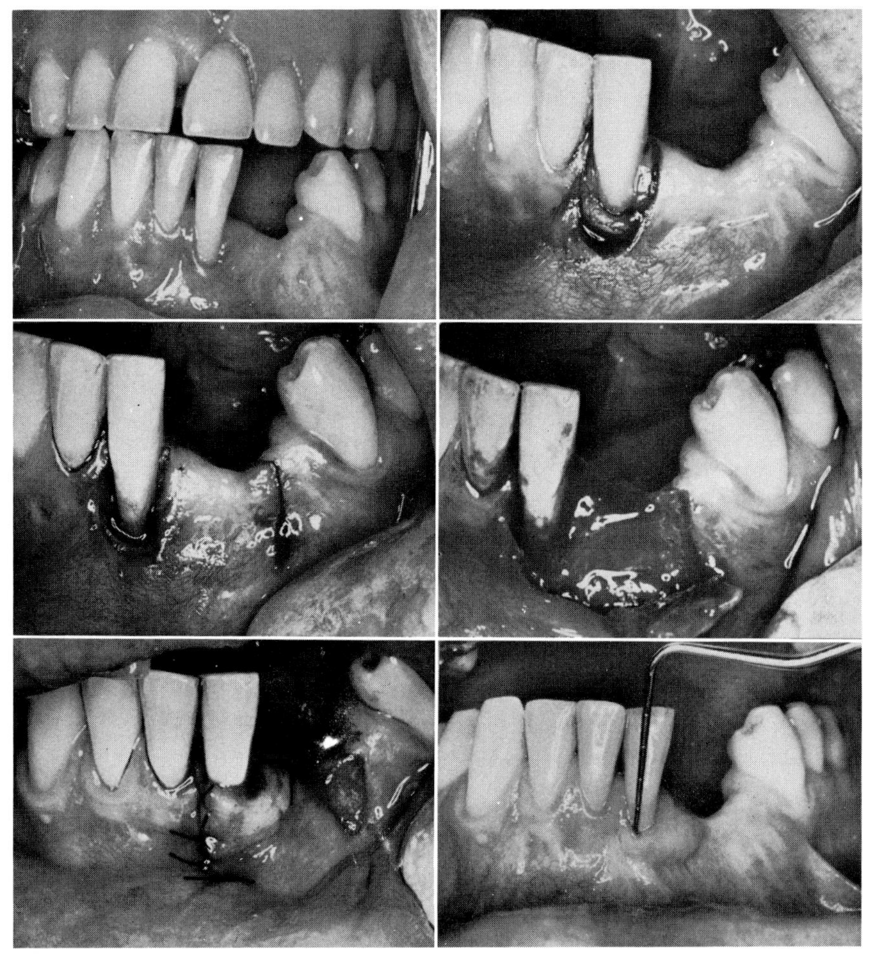

**Fig. 34-10.** The laterally repositioned sliding flap may also utilize gingiva from an adjoining edentulous donor site. The 1-year result is shown in the bottom right illustration. (From the collection of H. E. Grupe.)

posing them in a parallel fashion or rotating them toward the defect to be covered (Fig. 34-13).

Experiments on dogs have been conducted in which extensive local recession was created surgically and the defect then treated by the laterally repositioned flap technique.[61] Results showed a relatively long connective tissue attachment (2.1 mm.) and also a similarly long epithelial reattachment (2.0 mm.). However, about half (4.1 mm.) the coronal extent (8.2 mm.) of the original flap was lost. (See Fig. 33-19.)

*Wound healing*

The pedicle graft remains unchanged histologically. The coronal half of the gingival pedicle flap shrinks or atrophies possibly because of the lack of blood supply in the recipient bed. The lower half heals in the same manner as a replaced flap.

## Free gingival graft

The free gingival graft technique is one of the most versatile methods available for increasing the width of the band of attached gingiva when deep pockets

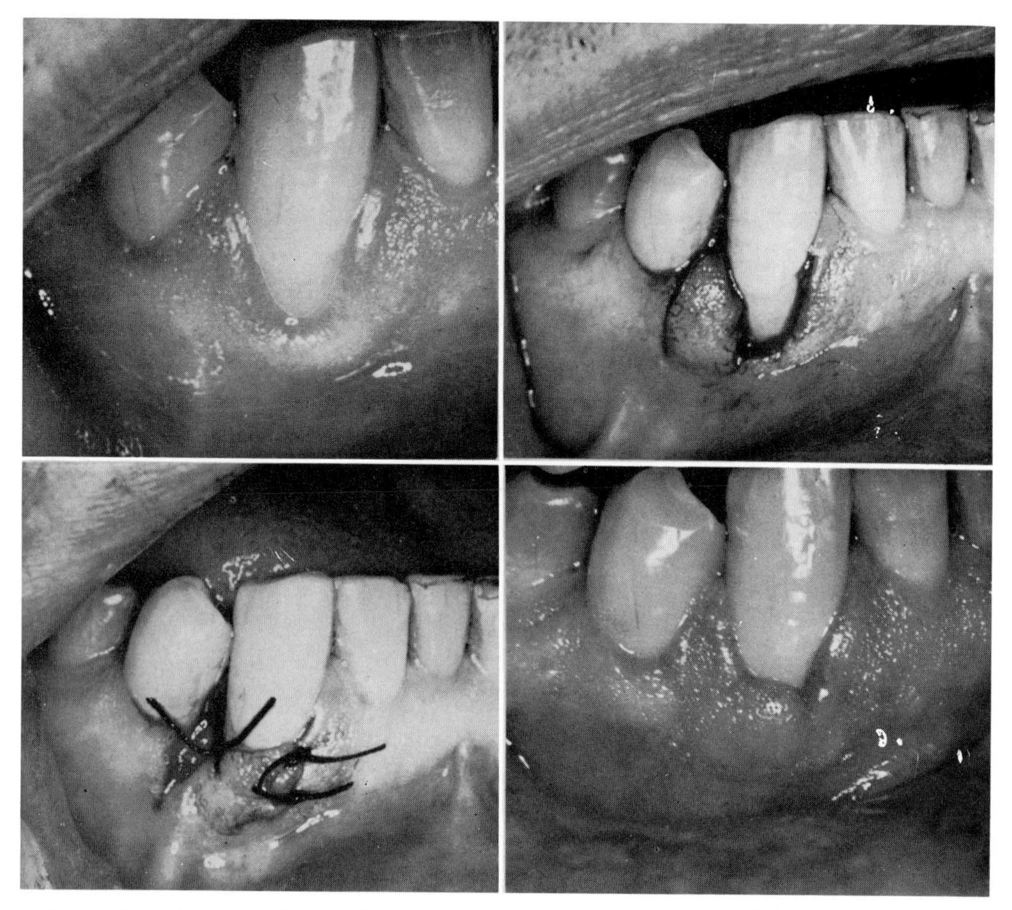

**Fig. 34-11.** Oblique rotated flap. The 1-year result is shown in the lower right illustration. (The slight remaining cleft is superficial only and does not go through to the root.) (Courtesy W. B. Hall, San Francisco.)

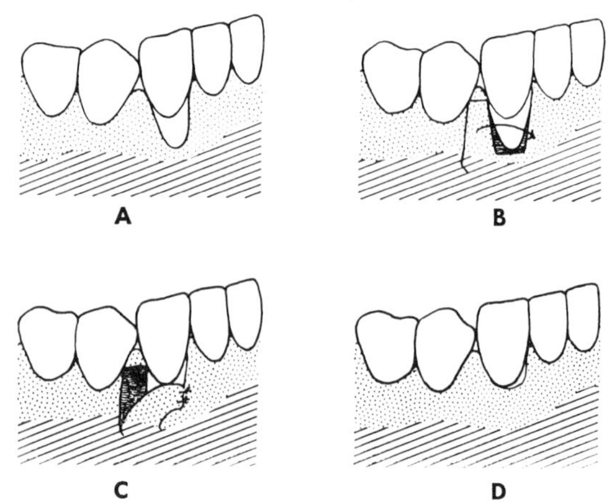


**Fig. 34-12.** Oblique rotated flap procedure. **A,** Preoperative view. Gingival recession in the lower right canine. **B,** Margin of the receded gingiva excised. The view also shows the flap being incised. **C,** Flap mobilized and sutured in its new position. **D,** Postoperative result.

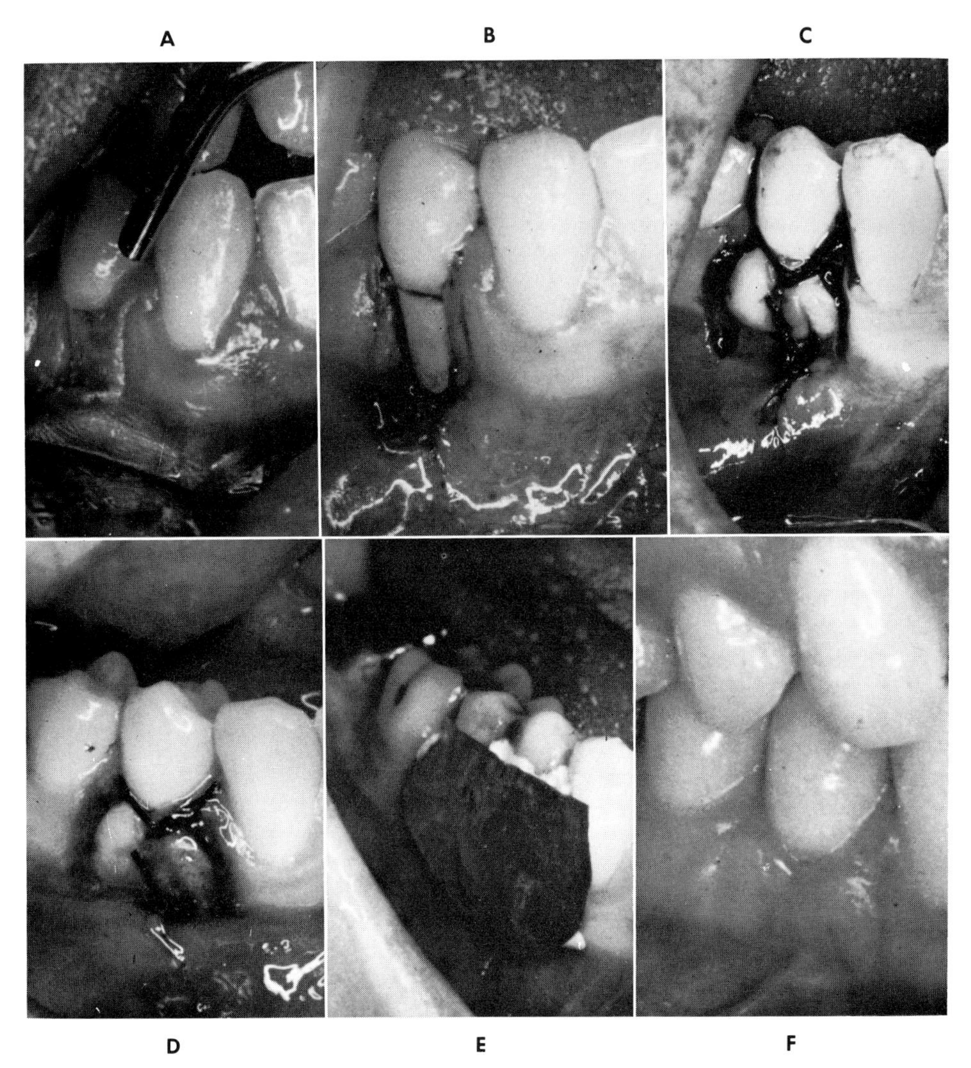


**Fig. 34-13.** Oblique rotated double papillary flap. **A,** A broad gingival cleft may be seen denuding the root of a mandibular premolar. The gingiva bordering the cleft is friable and edematous. It bleeds easily. The base of the cleft is bordered by alveolar mucosa, and a blast of air has caused the mucosa to retract, revealing a pocket. The root is planed and the friable tissue bordering the cleft is excised. **B,** The proximal gingiva mesial and distal to the cleft is not wide enough alone to cover the cleft if repositioned. **C,** Interdental gingivae and papillae mesial and distal to the cleft are repositioned laterally and sutured together in the midline of the root. Finger pressure is applied to obtain a fibrin adherence. The pedicles are ligated to the neck of the tooth by a suspensory ligature. **D,** Denture powder with Aureomycin is blown over the wound with an insufflator. **E,** Soft dressing (Coe Pak) is gently teased over the wound and the dressing is protected by a stiff adhesive foil. **F,** Postoperative result 2 years later reveals a firmly attached gingiva with less than 1 mm. sulcular depth.

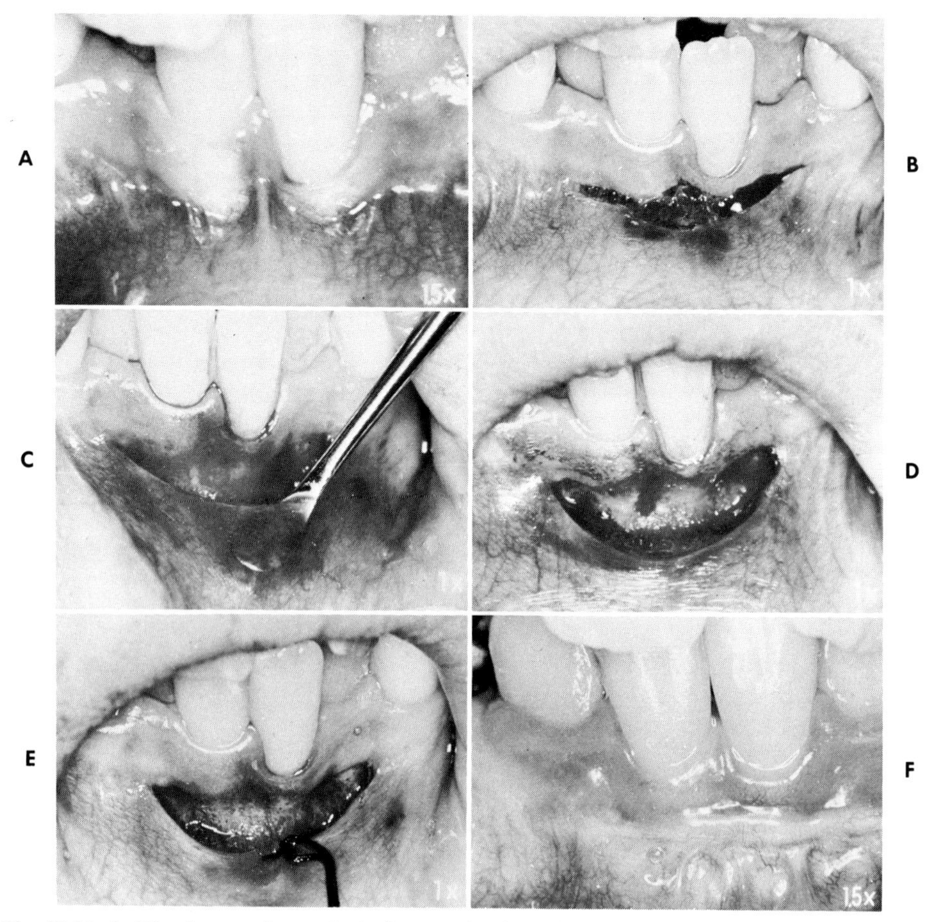


**Fig. 34-14. A,** The frenum is attached close to the free gingival margin. Considerable recession has occurred. Little gingiva remains on the mesiolabial aspect of the lower left central incisor. **B,** A horizontal incision is made at the mucogingival line. The incision must extend to include the width of at least one tooth on either side of the area to be operated on. **C,** The mucosa is dissected away and undermined. **D,** A narrow horizontal band of periosteum is scraped off at the lower end of the exposed area. **E,** The undermined mucosa is sutured to the periosteum at the lower end of the operated area. **F,** Postoperative view.

are not present[37-51] (Fig. 34-1, *B*). In the several years since the technique was introduced,[37] the indications for its use have been more clearly defined. They are as follows: (1) an absent or too narrow zone of attached gingiva and (2) a localized narrow recession or cleft. For deep, wide, localized recessions, where root coverage is the goal, and where an adequate donor site is available, the laterally repositioned flap is the technique of choice.

The optimal thickness of a free gingival graft has been investigated.[49] Both thick and thin grafts have been employed. Thicker grafts appear to be more successful when root coverage is attempted.

In performing a free gingival graft (Figs. 34-14 and 34-17), the dentist first prepares the receptor site. He makes a template of adhesive foil to the outline of the site to be covered by the graft. After anesthetizing the receptor site, he attaches the template. The coronal outline of the receptor site is then marked with a scalpel and the template removed. He next makes a shallow horizontal incision at the mucogingival junction and displaces the mucosa apically by blunt dissection. The mucosa may be undermined and sutured at a lower level. Then he trims away the epithelium of the gingiva coronal to the primary incision, leaving a receptor bed with an adequate blood supply. Root prominence may be reduced with a chisel, curette, or finishing bur.[43] Hemorrhage is controlled by the placement of a gauze sponge between the lip or cheek and the prepared receptor site.

The operator selects a donor site, usually the palate, and anesthetizes it. Then he places the template over the tissue and uses it to outline a shallow incision. He undermines the graft and frees it with a scalpel or gingivectomy knife. A thickness of approximately 1 mm. is adequate. No fatty tissue or submucosa should be included. He draws silk or Dacron suture (with swaged needle) through each corner of the graft to facilitate handling in subsequent steps. He sutures the transplant to the recipient site, applying pressure with a gauze sponge for 3 to 5 minutes to get a fibrinous adherence and to prevent blood from pooling between the graft and the recipient bed. Some operators have reported using no sutures, but relying entirely on fibrinous adherence to attach the grafted tissue. Adhesive foil or rubber dam may be placed over the site and covered with a soft pack (Coe Pak). Finally, he places Orahesive bandage over the donor site. After a week, the dressing may be removed carefully and the sutures cut and removed. Probing the root surface beneath a successful graft should be avoided for 6 weeks.

The first 2 days after a free graft is placed are probably the most critical. The graft is in contact with a fibrin net through which the plasma from the donor site must pass (Fig. 34-15, *A*). Vascularization starts at about 48 hours and continues for about a week. Collagen attachment begins at about 4 days and becomes firm by the tenth day.[62-64] Donor epithelium often sloughs and is replaced in about a week by adjacent epithelium and proliferation from surviving donor basal cells[62,64] (Fig. 34-15, *B* and *C*).

Complete healing takes from 10 to 16 weeks (Fig. 34-15, *D*), the time required being proportionate to the thickness of the graft. The free graft, like the pedicle graft, retains its morphologic characteristics even when surrounded by alveolar mucosa.[15]

## Frenotomy, frenectomy

*Frenotomy*

Mandibular frenum problems may be resolved by any of several procedures[3,6,32,38,66] (Fig. 34-1, *C*). A frequently successful, simple frenum repositioning technique is illustrated in Figs. 34-14 and 34-16. A mandibular labial frenum extends nearly to the free margin of the gingiva, and gingival recession is evident. After anesthesia is obtained, pull the lip out firmly and make an incision at the mucogingival line, extending at least one tooth to each side of the frenum bands. The incision is made parallel with the labial alveolar plate. Free the mucosal flap from the periosteum by blunt or sharp dissection until 6 to 8 mm. of periosteum have been exposed. Undermine the flap and suture it to the periosteum or muscle at a more apical level. The tissue that once was alveolar mucosa now becomes lip mucosa. After healing an area of scarification forms that prevents frenum pull. In most cases the newly bound-down tissue is covered by nonkeratinized epithelium.[67] However, a change to keratinized mucosa may occur.

After this, frenum pull will no longer be evident or constitute a problem. Frenotomy is a less traumatic approach than the apically repositioned flap and

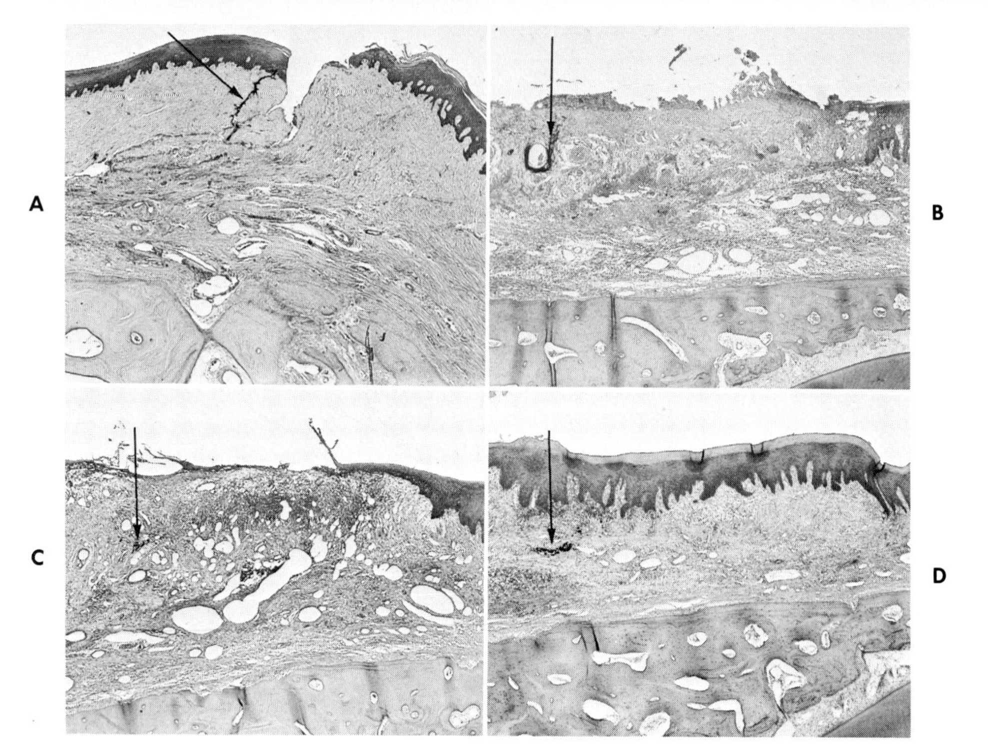


**Fig. 34-15.** **A,** Free gingival graft in a monkey at 0 hours. Note the approximation between graft tissue and receptor bed. The absence of a clot or a minimal clot is essential to retention and maturation of the graft. The donor tissue is palatal gingiva. Sometime prior to the transplant operation, the donor area was tattooed. Arrows in this series indicate the tattoo mark. **B,** Free gingival graft at 4 days. Note the necrosis of surface epithelium, the dilatation of vascular channels, and the cellular disorganization in the grafted tissue. The epithelium from the adjacent host margins is beginning to migrate over the graft. **C,** Free gingival graft at 7 days. The graft tissue is continuing to mature, and epithelium from the adjacent receptor site continues to migrate over the graft. **D,** Free gingival graft at 3 weeks. There is almost complete maturation. The surface epithelium is continuous with the adjacent receptor site and appears normal. The connective tissue also appears normal. (Courtesy W. H. Wright, Portland, Ore.)

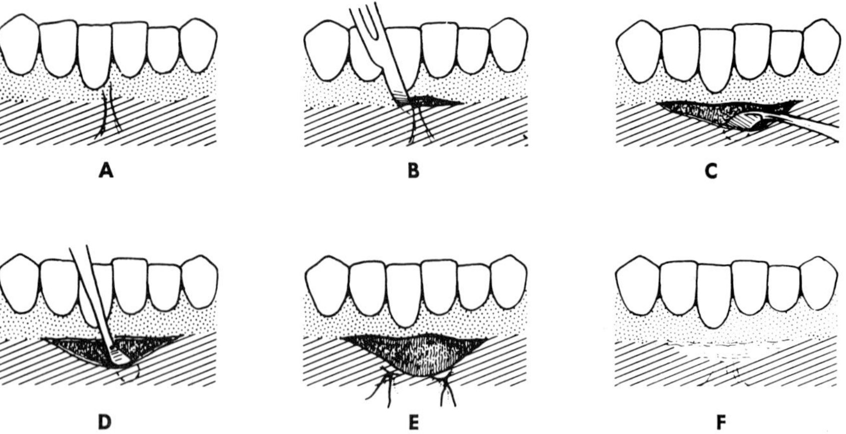


**Fig. 34-16.** Frenotomy. **A,** Preoperative appearance. Note the alignment of the lower right central incisor, which is placed outside the basal bone. The frenum inserts into the marginal gingiva. The gingiva gapes when pull is exerted on the frenum. **B,** Incision along the mucogingival line in an attempt to preserve a collar of tissue around the involved tooth. **C,** The mucosal flap is dissected from the underlying periosteum. **D,** The mucosal flap is undermined. **E,** The mucosal flap is sutured to the underlying tissue. **F,** Postoperatively a scar forms in the area operated on, separating the frenum from the gingiva. The mucosa of the scar generally has nonkeratinized epithelium.

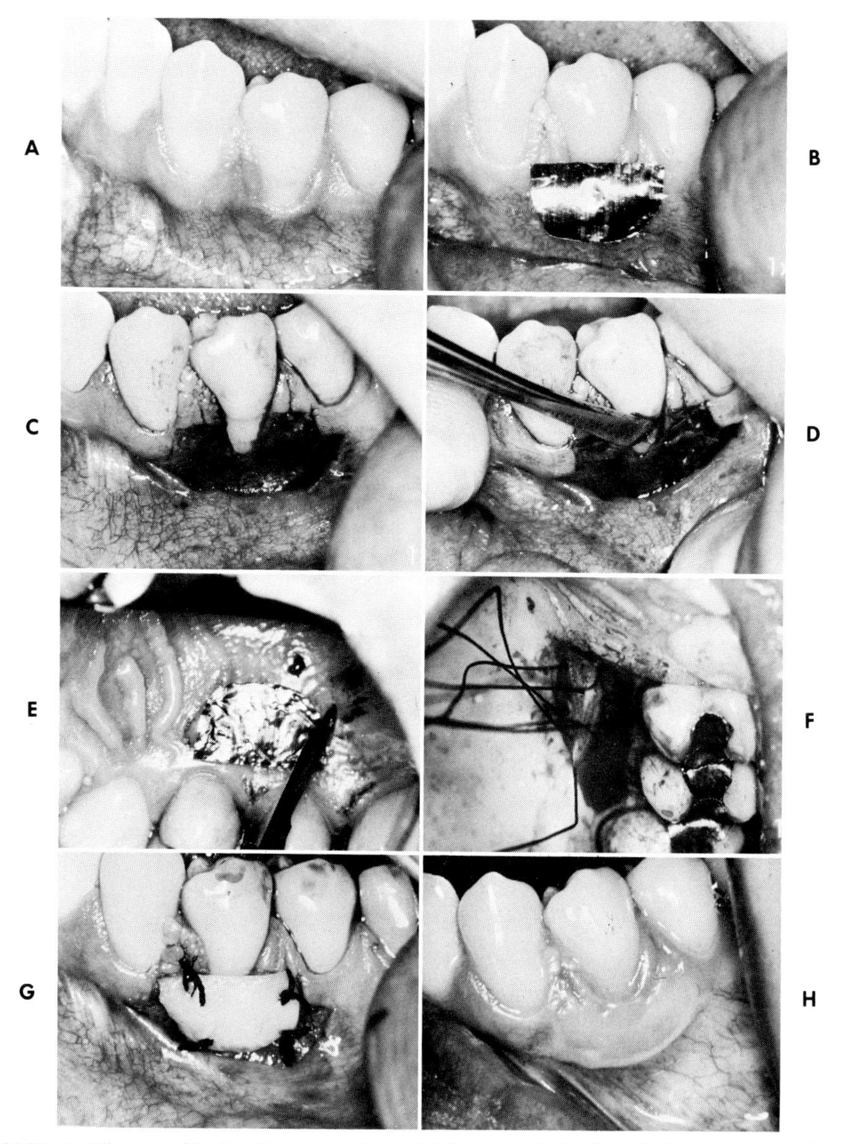


**Fig. 34-17. A,** The mandibular first premolar exhibits a partially denuded root and nearly complete absence of gingiva. **B,** A template of adhesive tinfoil is fitted over the proposed receptor site, and this area is outlined with a scalpel on its coronal (horizontal) side. **C,** The tinfoil is put aside. A shallow incision is made at the level of the mucogingival junction, and the mucosa is displaced apically by blunt dissection. The mucosa is undermined and may be sutured to the vestibule. Remove the epithelium of the gingiva coronal to the incision, leaving a receptor bed with adequate blood supply. **D,** Flatten the root prominence with chisels or finishing burs. **E,** Now move the template to a suitable donor area of palatal gingiva and make a shallow incision following the outline of the template. **F,** Free the transplant by an undermining incision. The thickness should be about 1 mm. Before completely freeing the transplant, place sutures at each end. **G,** Place the transplant in the receptor site and suture it to place. It must be held in place under mild pressure for approximately 5 minutes. **H,** Result after 1 year. (Courtesy W. B. Hall, San Francisco.)

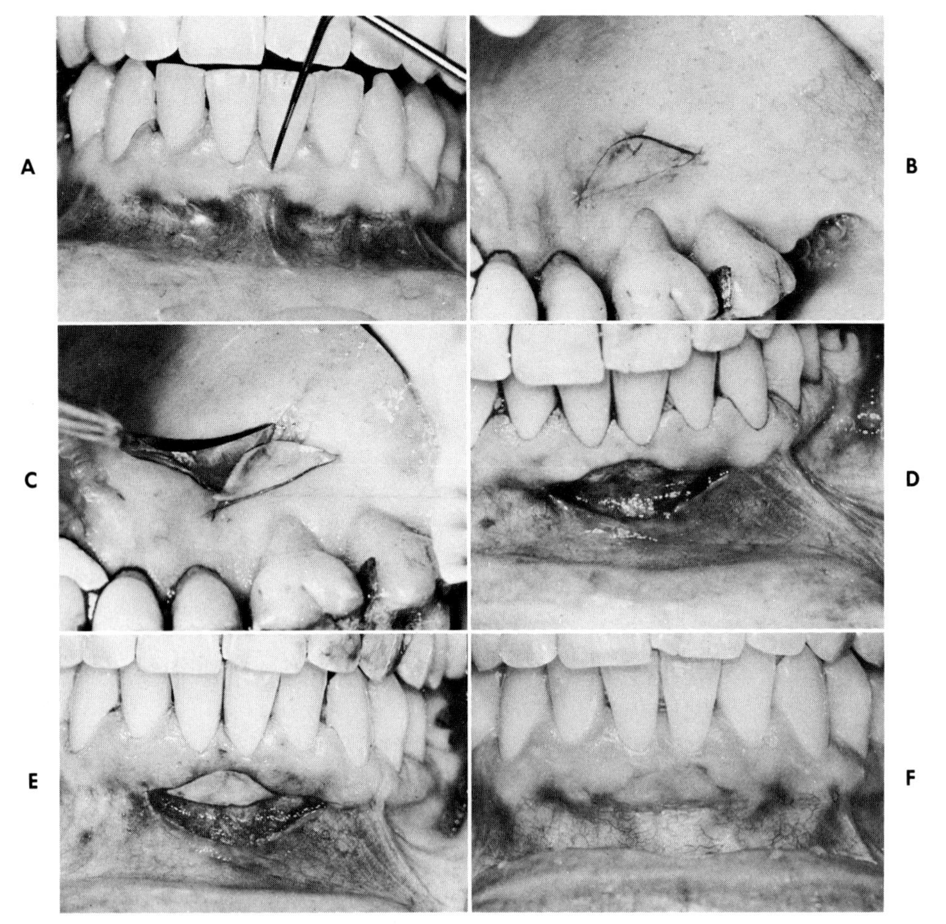


**Fig. 34-18.** Frenotomy with free gingival graft. **A,** Preoperative view. **B,** Donor tissue from the palatal gingiva. **C,** Donor tissue being dissected. **D,** Receptor site being prepared. **E,** Donor tissue inserted. **F,** Postoperative result after 1 year. (Courtesy W. B. Hall, San Francisco.)

is one of the recommended procedures when frenum-related recession, rather than pocket formation, is the cause of the mucogingival problem. Frenotomy may also be combined with a free gingival graft (Fig. 34-18).

***Frenectomy*** When the position of the maxillary frenum causes a problem, the frenum may be treated by excision at its base. The separated mucosal edges may or may not be sutured, depending on the clinical situation (Fig. 34-19).

## Vestibular extension

Procedures designed to deepen the vestibule[2] were the forerunners of many of the mucogingival procedures employed today.[3] However, the initial increased vestibular depth was not maintained with these older methods.[66] A technique called periosteal fenestration was developed to overcome the problem,[33-36a] but it met with little added success. In this procedure marginal bone remains covered by soft tissue, whereas a horizontal strip of bone apical to the mucogingival line is denuded. After healing, an area of scarification forms where the bone was bared.

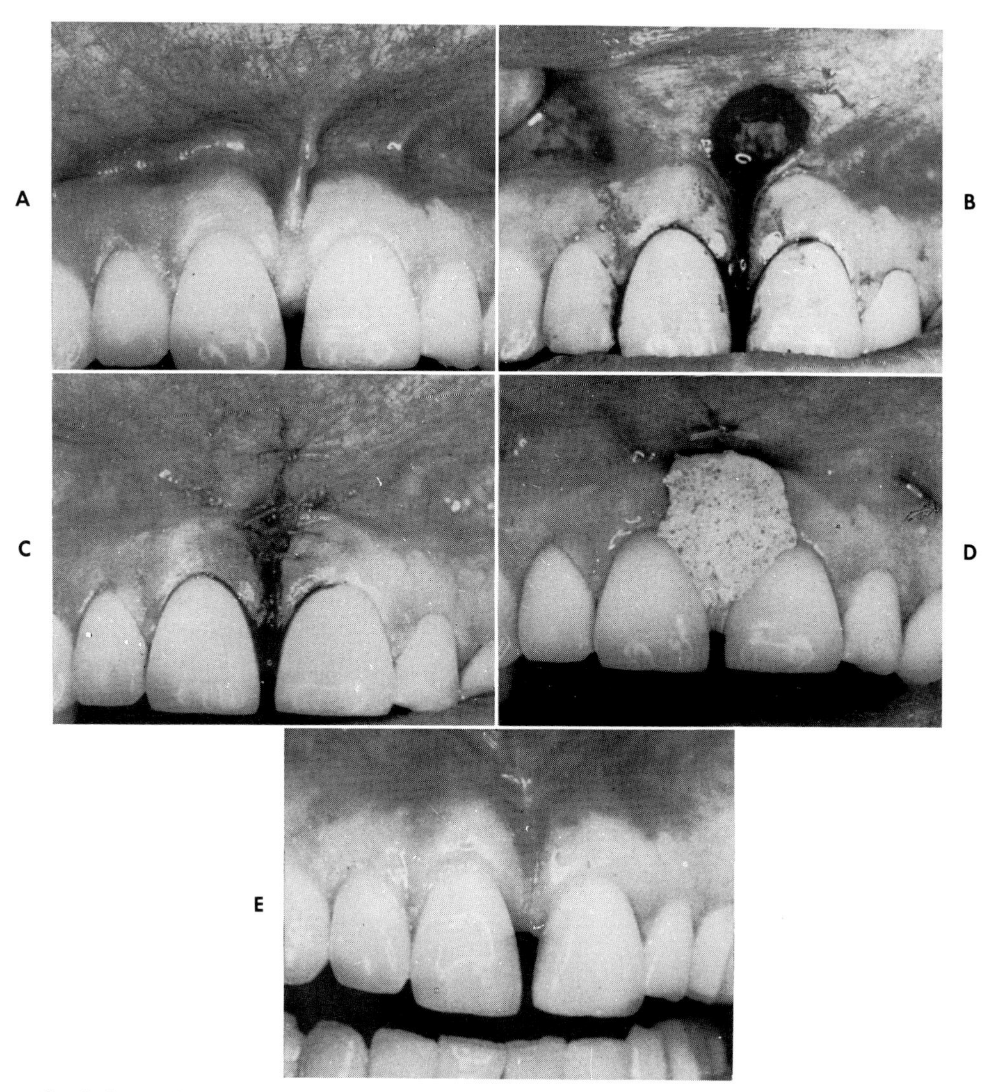


**Fig. 34-19.** **A,** Heavy maxillary frenum attached to the gingiva, extending interproximally. **B,** Excision of the frenum. Incisions are made parallel to the frenum. The heavy, fibrous interdental portion of the frenum is excised. **C,** Edges of the wound are sutured. **D,** The wound is protected by surgical dressing. **E,** Postoperative view after frenectomy.

## SELECTION OF TECHNIQUE

Clinical judgment and individual preference play a large part in the selection of techniques for treating individual mucogingival problems. In localized recession cases frenotomy may be adequate for minor problems, especially in children. If an adequate donor site is available, a laterally repositioned flap is more predictable than a free graft when root coverage is the goal. The obliquely rotated papilla and double papillary techniques may be employed when an adequate donor site for a laterally repositioned flap is not present but broad papillae are available. A free gingival graft is best when a broader band of gingiva is desired. The apically repositioned flap should be employed when deep pockets are present and the band of attached gingiva is too narrow. In every case the least traumatic procedure that will achieve the objectives of the surgery should be used. The selection of the surgical technique is based on the ease of manipulation of the tissues in a given area, the need to avoid unnecessary baring of crestal bone, the access to the surgical area, and the anticipated success in creating or retaining a functionally adequate zone of gingiva.

**CHAPTER 34**

**References**


1. Goldman, H. M.: Periodontia, ed. 3, St. Louis, 1953, The C. V. Mosby Co.
2. Hilming, F.: Om betydningen ov hojt insererende ligamenter i de marginale paradentale lidelser klinik, Odont. T. 50:602, 1942.
3. Gottsegen, R.: Frenum position and vestibule depth in relation to gingival health, Oral Surg. 7:1069, 1954.
4. Everett, F. G., Waerhaug, J., and Widman, A.: Leonard Widman: surgical treatment of pyorrhea alveolaris, J. Periodont. 42:571, 1971.
5. Nabers, C. L.: Repositioning the attached gingiva, J. Periodont. 25:38, 1954.
6. Hileman, A.: Repositioning the vestibule and frenum as adjunctive periodontal treatment procedures, Dental Clinics of North America, Philadelphia, March 1960, W. B. Saunders Co.
7. Hilming, F., and Jervoe, P.: Surgical extension of vestibular depth, Tandlaegebladet 74: 329, 1970.
8. Friedman, N.: Mucogingival surgery: the apically repositioned flap, J. Periodont. 33:328, 1962.
9. Hiatt, W. H.: The repositioned alveolar ridge mucosal flap, Periodontics 5:132, 1967.
10. Donnenfeld, O. W., Marks, R. M., and Glickman, I.: Apically repositioned flap, J. Periodont. 35:381, 1964.
11. Hiatt, W. H., Stallard, R. E., Butler, E. D., and Badgett, B.: Repair following mucoperiosteal flap surgery with full gingival retention, J. Periodont. 39:11, 1968.
12. Morris, M. L.: The unrepositioned flap, Periodontics 3:147, 1965.
13. Wade, A. B.: The flap operation, J. Periodont. 37:95, 1966.
14. Sumner, C. F.: Surgical repair of recession on the maxillary cuspid: incisally repositioning the gingival tissues, J. Periodont. 40:119, 1969.
15. Grupe, H. E., and Warren, R. F., Jr.: Repair of gingival defects by a sliding flap operation, J. Periodont. 27:92, 1956.
16. Grupe, H. E.: Modified technique for the sliding flap operation, J. Periodont. 37:491, 1966.
17. McFall, W. T.: Laterally repositioned flap—criteria for success in periodontics, Periodontics 5:89, 1968.
18. Cohen, D. W., and Ross, S. E.: The double papillae repositioned flap in periodontal therapy, J. Periodont. 39:65, 1968.
19. Pennel, B. M., Higgason, J. D., Towner, J. D., King, K. O., Fritz, B. D., and Salden, J. F.: Oblique rotated flap, J. Periodont. 36:305, 1965.
20. Robinson, R. E.: Utilizing an edentulous area as donor site in the lateral repositioned flap, Periodontics 2:79, 1964.
21. Corn, H.: Edentulous area pedicle grafts in mucogingival surgery, Periodontics 2:229, 1964.
22. Bork, K. C., and Weiler, J. F.: Frenum reduction as a treatment for periodontal atrophy, Oral Surg. 11:370, 1958.
23. Dewel, B. F.: The labial frenum, midline diastema, and palatine papilla: a clinical analysis, Dental Clinics of North America, Philadelphia, March 1966, W. B. Saunders Co.
24. Ochsenbein, C.: The double flap procedure, Periodontics 1:17, 1963.
25. Friedman, N., and Levine, H. L.: Mucogingival surgery: current status, J. Periodont. 35: 5, 1964.
26. Bowers, G. M.: A study of the width of attached gingiva, J. Periodont. 34:201, 1963.
27. Parfitt, G. J., and Mjör, I. A.: Clinical evaluation of local gingival recession in children, J. Dent. Child. 31:257, 1964.
28. Guastamacchia, C., Hofer, F., and Peccatori, G.: Studio statistico sulla frequenza di anomalie del frenulo nella popolazione scolastica (6-11 Anni) di Milano, Rass. Int. Stomat. Prat. 14: 423, 1963.
29. Spirgi, M., Corti, M., and Held, A. J.: Les vestibuloplasties dans la prophylaxie et la therapeutique des parodontolyses, Schweiz. Mschr. Zahnheilk. 73:678, 1963.

30. Edlan, A., and Mejchar, B.: Plastic surgery of the vestibulum in periodontal therapy, Int. Dent. J. **13**:593, 1963.
31. Wright, W. H.: The scalloped reverse bevel incision in mucogingival surgery, Odont. T. **73**: 515, 1965.
32. Carranza, F. A., Jr., and Carraro, J. J.: Mucogingival techniques in periodontal surgery, J. Periodont. **41**:294, 1970.
33. Robinson, R. E.: Periosteal fenestration in mucogingival surgery, J. West. Soc. Periodont. **9**:107, 1961.
34. Corn, H.: Periosteal separation—its clinical significance, J. Periodont. **33**:140, 1962.
35. Allen, D. L., and Shell, J. H.: Clinical and radiographic evaluation of a periosteal separation procedure, J. Periodont. **39**:290, 1968.
36. Carranza, F. A., Jr., Carraro, J. J., Dotto, C. A., and Cabrini, R. L.: Effect of periosteal fenestration in gingival extension operations, J. Periodont. **37**:335, 1966.
36a. Diedrich, P., Jacoby, L., and Aka, F.: Untersuchungen über die Breite der Gingiva propria nach Vestibulumplastik mit und ohne Periostfensterung, Deutsch. Zahnaerztl. Z. **27**:346, 1972.
37. Björn, H.: Free transplantation of gingiva propria, Svensk. Tandlak. T. **55**:684, 1963.
38. Nabers, J. M.: Extension of vestibular fornix utilizing a gingival graft, Periodontics **4**: 77, 1966.
39. Nabers, J. M.: Free gingival grafts, Periodontics **4**:243, 1966.
40. Brackett, R. C., and Gargiulo, A. W.: Free gingival grafts in humans, J. Periodont. **41**: 581, 1970.
41. Cowan, A.: Sulcus deepening incorporating mucosal graft, J. Periodont. **36**:188, 1965.
42. Frisch, J., and Bhaskar, S. N.: Free mucosal graft with tissue adhesives; report of 17 cases, J. Periodont. **39**:190, 1968.
43. Bressman, E., and Chasens, A. I.: Free gingival graft with periosteal fenestration, J. Periodont. **39**:298, 1968.
44. Snyder, A. J.: A technique for free autogenous grafts, J. Periodont. **40**:702, 1969.
45. Levin, M. P., Frisch, J., and Bhaskar, S. N.: Tissue conditioner dressing for free tissue grafts, J. Periodont. **40**:271, 1969.
46. Hawley, C. E., and Staffileno, H.: Clinical evaluation of free gingival grafts in periodontal surgery, J. Periodont. **41**:105, 1970.
47. Becker, N. G., Jr.: Free gingival graft utilizing a pre-suturing technique, Periodontics **5**:194, 1967.
48. Calandriello, M.: Free mucosal grafts in mucogingival surgery, Parodont. Acad. Rev. **2**:74, 1968.
49. Sullivan, H. C., and Atkins, J. H.: Free autogenous gingival grafts. I, Principles of successful grafting; II, Histology of the graft site; III, Utilization of grafts in the treatment of gingival recession, Periodontics **6**:121, 130, 152, 1968.
50. Snyder, A. J.: A technic for free autogenous gingival grafts, J. Periodont. **40**:760, 1969.
51. Pennel, B. M., Tabor, J. C., King, K. O., Towner, J. D., Fritz, B. D., and Higgason, J. D.: Free masticatory mucosa graft, J. Periodont. **40**:162, 1969.
52. Wilderman, M. N., Wentz, F. M., and Orban, B.: Histogenesis of repair after mucogingival surgery, J. Periodont. **31**:283, 1960.
53. Pfeifer, J.: The growth of gingival tissue over denuded bone, J. Periodont. **34**:10, 1963.
54. Carranza, F. A., Jr., and Carraro, J. J.: Effect of removal of periosteum on postoperative result of mucogingival surgery, J. Periodont. **34**:223, 1963.
55. Wilderman, M. N.: Repair after a periosteal retention procedure, J. Periodont. **34**:487, 1963.
56. Grant, D. A.: Experimental periodontal surgery: sequestration of alveolar bone, J. Periodont. **38**:409, 1967.
57. Pennel, B. M., King, K. O., Higgason, J. D., Towner, J. D., Fritz, B. D., and Sadler, J. F.: Retention of periosteum in mucogingival surgery, J. Periodont. **36**:39, 1965.
57a. Tavtigian, R.: The height of the facial radicular alveolar crest following apically repositioned flap operations, J. Periodont. **41**:412, 1970.
58. Staffileno, H., Wentz, F. M., and Orban, B.: Histologic study of healing of split thickness flap surgery in dogs, J. Periodont. **33**:56, 1962.
59. Staffileno, H., Levy, S., and Gargiulo, A.: Histologic study of cellular mobilization and repair following a periosteal retention via split thickness mucogingival flap surgery, J. Periodont. **37**:117, 1966.
60. Glickman, I., Smulow, J., Tanner, R., and O'Brien, T.: Healing of the periodontium following mucogingival surgery, Oral Surg. **16**:530, 1963.

61. Wilderman, M. N., and Wentz, F. M.: Repair of a dentogingival defect with a pedicle flap, J. Periodont. 35:218, 1965.
62. Janson, W. A., Ruben, M. P., Kramer, G. M., Bloom, A. A., and Turner, H.: Development of the blood supply to split-thickness free gingival autografts, J. Periodont. 40:707, 1969.
63. Oliver, R. C., Löe, H., and Karring, T.: Microscopic evaluation of the healing and revascularization of free gingival grafts, J. Periodont. Res. 3:84, 1968.
64. Gargiulo, A., and Arrocha, R.: Histo-clinical evaluation of free gingival grafts, Periodontics 5:285, 1967.
65. Sugarman, E. F.: A clinical and histological study of the attachment of grafted tissue to bone and teeth, J. Periodont. 40:381, 1969.
66. Bohannan, H. M.: Studies in the alteration of vestibular depth. I, Complete denudation; II, Periosteum retention, J. Periodont. 33:120, 354, 1962; III, Vestibular incision, J. Periodont. 34:209, 1963.
67. Ivancie, G. P.: Experimental and histologic investigation of gingival regeneration in vestibular surgery, J. Periodont. 28:259, 1957.

**Additional suggested reading**

Bhaskar, S. N., Cutright, D. E., Beasley, J. D., Perez, B., and Hunsuck, E. E.: Healing under full and partial thickness mucogingival flaps in the miniature swine, J. Periodont. 41:675, 1970.

Bradley, R. E., Grant, J. C., and Ivancie, G. P.: Histologic evaluation of mucogingival surgery, Oral Surg. 12:1184, 1959.

Erpenstein, H.: Die chirurgische Behandlung der Dehiszenz, Deutsch. Zahnaerztl. Z. 26:558, 1971.

Klavan, B.: The replaced graft, J. Periodont. 41:406, 1970.

Pfeifer, J. S.: The growth of gingival tissue over denuded bone, J. Periodont. 34:10, 1963.

Smith, R. M.: A study of the intertransplantation of alveolar mucosa, Oral Surg. 29:328, 1970.

Staffileno, H., Jr., and Levy, S.: Histologic and clinical study of mucosal transplants in dogs, J. Periodont. 40:311, 1969.

Wade, B. A.: Vestibular deepening by the technique of Edlan and Mejchar, J. Periodont. Res. 4:300, 1969.

CHAPTER THIRTY-FIVE

# Interrelated endodontics-periodontics



A close relationship exists between disease of the dental pulp and periodontal disease, and it expresses itself in several ways as follows:

1. Effect of pulpal lesions and procedures on the periodontium
2. Effect of periodontal lesions and procedures on the dental pulp
3. Endodontic failures in periodontally involved teeth

## PROBLEMS

Atrophic changes in the pulp of teeth severely involved with advanced periodontal disease are common. One third of such teeth show inflammatory pulp disease, and 10% show a pulp that is necrotic.[1] These figures pertain to teeth without caries or restorations. Exposed lateral canals and accessory apical foramina form the anatomic basis for this finding.[2,3] The frequency of such aberrant canals is considerable and continues to be underestimated by the profession.[3] When the periodontal opening of such a lateral canal or of an accessory canal or of the main apical foramen becomes exposed to the oral flora in the course of severe, advanced periodontal disease, pulpal damage may occur. In some cases the lateral or the accessory canal has become obliterated by calcification, but in most cases some entry for the microorganisms to the pulp still exists.

If pulpitis or pulp gangrene results, toxic products then infiltrate in a reverse direction from the root canal into the periodontium, aggravating and extending the periodontal lesion. This mode of aggravation of periodontal disease may also occur when the pulp disease is primary.

The floor of the pulp chamber in molars is formed of dentin, sometimes presenting numerous small vascular channels[4-6] (Fig. 35-1). Toxic breakdown products of a necrotic pulp may cause loss of the crest of the interradicular septum as seen in roentgenograms.[7]

Occasionally an apical abscess may drain via the gingival sulcus and cause the precipitous appearance of a deep pocket. In such cases root canal treatment per se can eliminate the pocket and lead to complete bone regeneration. When, on the other hand, severe pocket formation precedes the apical abscess, combined en-

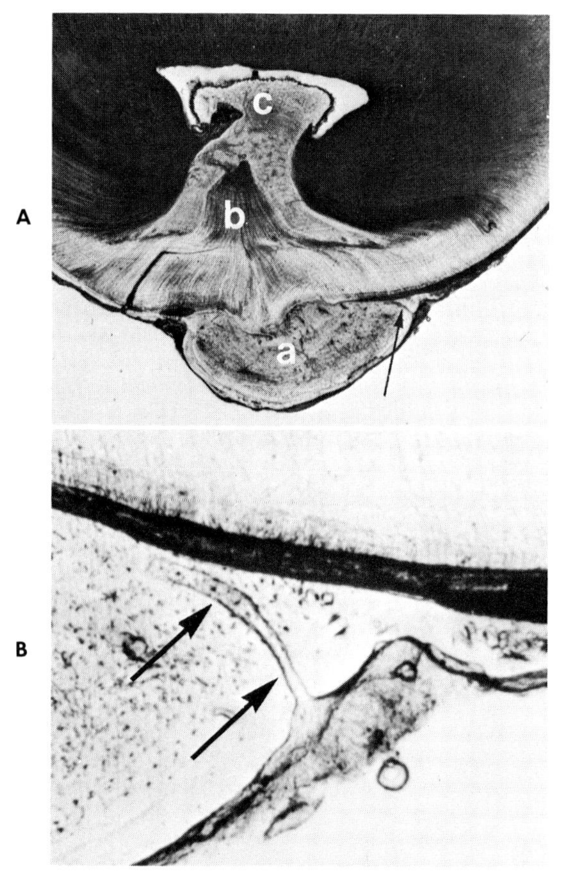


**Fig. 35-1. A,** Buccolingual section through the bifurcation of a lower first molar. Note the bifurcational ridge, *a*. A basilar cone of disturbed dentin formation, *b,* can be seen forming a dentin plug, *c,* in the pulp chamber. An accessory canal (arrow) can be seen in the intermediate ridge. **B,** Higher magnification of the accessory canal (ground sections).

dodontic-periodontal therapy (Figs. 28-8 to 28-10) is indicated. The reason for this difference lies in the fact that the root surface forming one side of a chronic deep pocket may be encrusted with calculus and coated with plaque and has been soaked in the toxic environment of the pocket. The chronicity of the periodontal lesion may have a bearing on the difference in the behaviors of these two similar lesions.[8] Accidental root perforations during endodontic therapy may also aggravate the periodontal picture, particularly if the perforation cannot be sealed quickly and the perforation is close to the bottom of the periodontal pocket.

Persistent hypersensitivity of the teeth to hot and cold at times after extensive root planing or periodontal surgery may indicate the presence of mild inflammatory pulpal changes. Clamping and clenching in drivers of trucks, buses, and road machinery may lead to a loss of vitality in the lower incisors.[10]

Periodontally diseased teeth have a somewhat greater rate of endodontic treatment failure than do teeth in good periodontal health.[1] The foramina of side canals that face the sulcus or the oral cavity, even when filled with root canal cement, may form an avenue of ingress leading to a dissolution of the root canal cement in the main canal and to reinfection.

## Diagnosis

In endodontic-periodontal problems it is important to arrive at an opinion whether the lesion is primarily endodontic or periodontal. All involved teeth must therefore be tested for vitality. The finding of a nonvital tooth in such a situation may, although not necessarily, signify primary pulpal involvement.

*Signs and symptoms*

The patient with combined endodontic-periodontal problems may present with one of the following symptoms:

1. Hypersensitivity to cold and sweet after periodontal treatment
   A mild pulpitis is found in such teeth.
2. Severe furcation involvements or exfoliation of single roots in a firm multirooted tooth
3. Periapical abscess or one located at a lateral canal draining via the gingival sulcus in a pulpless tooth
   The "pocket" is, in fact, a fistulous tract.
4. Exposure of an accessory or lateral canal or the apical foramen by a periodontal pocket, causing pulp disease (reverse pulpitis)

## Cases

In an upper anterior tooth a chronic deep pocket may exist communicating with an involved periapical area. In such a case endodontic-periodontal combined therapy may be accomplished in a single session by the use of a flap approach to gain access to the root surface and the apex (Figs. 23-8 to 23-10). A labial involvement has the best prognosis, a lingual involvement the worst.

Occasionally a periodontally involved furcation causes pulp disease through an accessory canal from the interradicular area into the pulp chamber. The floor of the pulp chamber in multirooted teeth is particularly likely to possess such vascular channels because of its embryologic history.[4,5]

There are cases that look similar on roentgenograms in which the defect in the bifurcation cannot be probed. In such cases the disease process evidently originated in the pulp and spread to the periodontium (Fig. 35-2). These patients usually respond to root canal treatment alone.

A special situation exists when one or two roots of a firm, multirooted tooth are untreatable by routine endodontic or periodontal measures. For instance, in a firm mandibular molar a single canal may be untreatable, a single root may have lost all bone, or extensive caries may almost have severed a root or involved the exposed bifurcation. The treatment of choice in such cases is root resection (removal of one or two roots in an upper molar) or hemisection (buccolingual sectioning of a mandibular molar)[11-16]; the latter procedure also involves the crown.

# THERAPY

## Hemisection

Molars with widely spread roots are better candidates for hemisection or root resection than are those with narrow root spread. Teeth with fused roots are poor candidates. After the decision for hemisection or root resection has been made, root canal treatment is performed, preferably with gutta-percha points rather than silver points. Some teeth may recover almost miraculously after only endodontic treatment, and hemisection becomes unnecessary. This usually occurs in cases in which there is no access to the lesion with a periodontal probe. However, even patients in whom the lesion can be probed sometimes recover after root canal therapy alone. Therefore it is wise to perform complete root canal therapy even

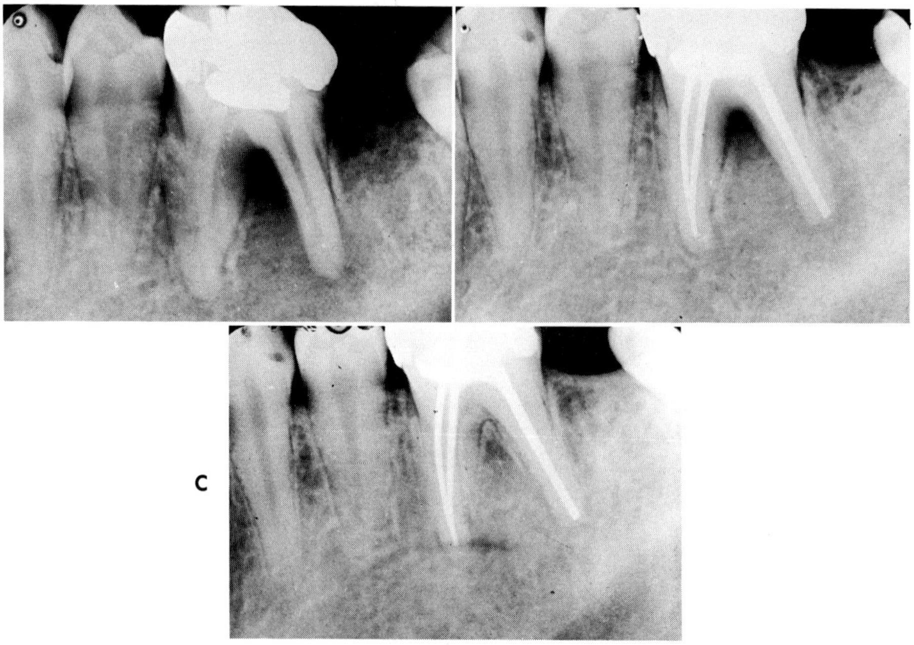

A B

C

**Fig. 35-2.** Roentgenographic progress report of the treatment of a bifurcation involvement in a mandibular first molar. **A,** Large area of rarefaction in the bifurcation involving the apex of the distal root. There was a dull, intermittent pain as well as swelling and a discharging fistula. No response to electric pulp testing could be elicited. Root canal treatment was completed on May 31, 1966. **B,** The area of rarefaction in the bifurcation and around the distal apex has decreased in size. An incipient furcation involvement on the buccal side (2 mm. deep) was noted. Routine periodontal therapy was performed in 1967. **C,** Follow-up roentgenogram taken in 1968 showed complete disappearance of the bifurcation. In this case there was little doubt to the clinician that he was dealing with an endodontic problem. Possibly, however, similar destruction might have occurred without pain or the appearance of a fistula, thus complicating the differential diagnosis. (Courtesy University of Washington School of Dentistry, Department of Endodontics.)

for roots that are to be sacrificed and then to wait a few months to see whether the lesion has healed. If there is clear indication for immediate resection, only the coronal half of the roots to be resected need be filled.

***Procedure***

After endodontic and preliminary periodontal treatment is completed, the tooth must be filled with amalgam. Remove all root canal cement and gutta-percha from the pulp chamber. This is why gutta-percha is preferred as a filling material. When silver points are cut, they may be loosened. Now prepare an undercut cavity in the pulp chamber and place an amalgam filling (Diagram 1, p. 556). In a subsequent session, do a hemisection using Carborundum disks or fissure burs (Fig. 35-3). If you proceed in this manner, the amalgam restoration will have proper retention and marginal seal and there will be no root canal cement or gutta-percha present at the margins.

The direction of the cut must be at the expense of the root to be extracted (Diagram 2, p. 556). You also wish to leave the larger part of the bifurcation with the root to be retained. During the operation of hemisection, it is good policy to take one or two roentgenograms to see whether the cut is aimed in the right direction. After complete separation, extract the diseased root, taking great

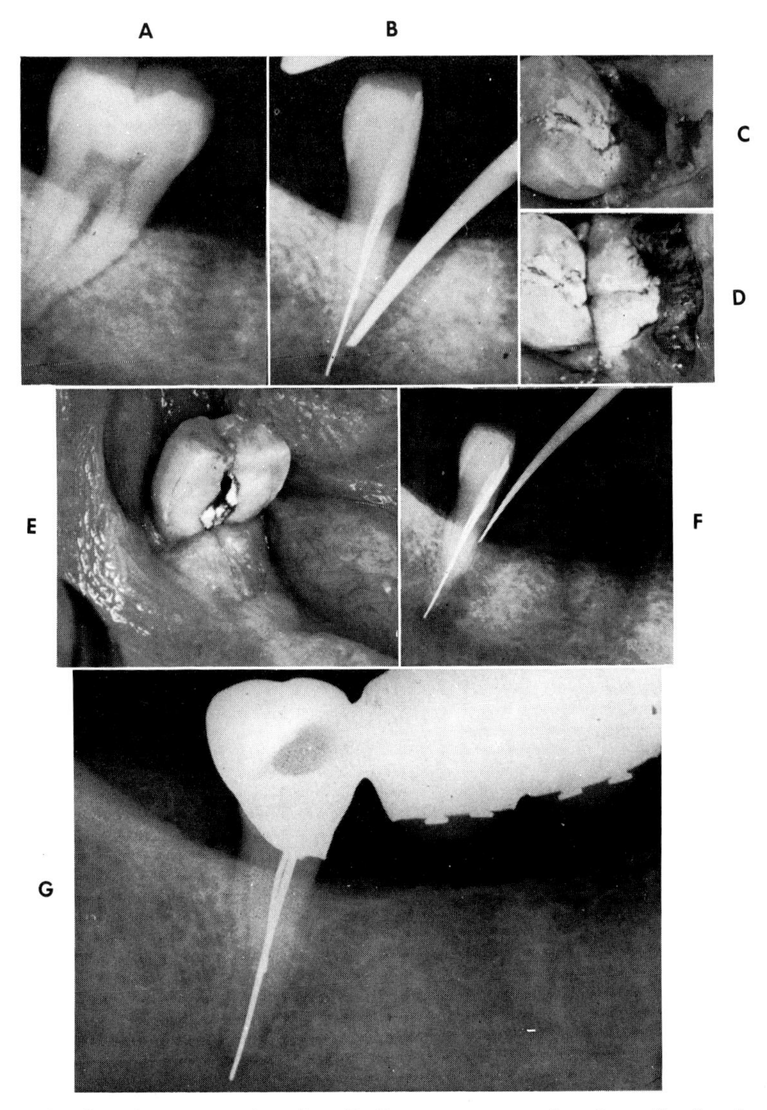


**Fig. 35-3.** Hemisection. **A,** Preoperative view. **B,** Roentgenogram taken immediately after hemisection. Chisel shows depth of the defect. **C,** Clinical view immediately after surgery. **D,** A gingival flap is placed over the surgical space left by the hemisection. **E,** Six-month postoperative view. **F,** Roentgenogram 6 months postoperative. **G,** Roentgenogram showing tooth used as a bridge abutment 3 years later. (Courtesy W. Hiatt, Denver.)

care not to loosen the remaining root, and smooth the bifurcation area to remove any bifurcational overhang. Where possible, mobilize the gingiva adjoining the socket of the extracted root, pull it toward the socket, and suture it to the remaining root with a purse string suture[13] (Fig. 35-3). Finally, contour the cut surface of the remaining half crown to make the crown resemble a premolar (Diagram 2, p. 556).

Fig. 35-4, *A,* shows the roentgenograms of a firm mandibular molar with a severely involved distal root. The premolars had been extracted by the referring dentist. The tooth was firm and had strategic importance since it was the only distal anchor. *B* shows the preserved mesial root 6 years later serving satisfactorily as distal abutment of a fixed bridge.

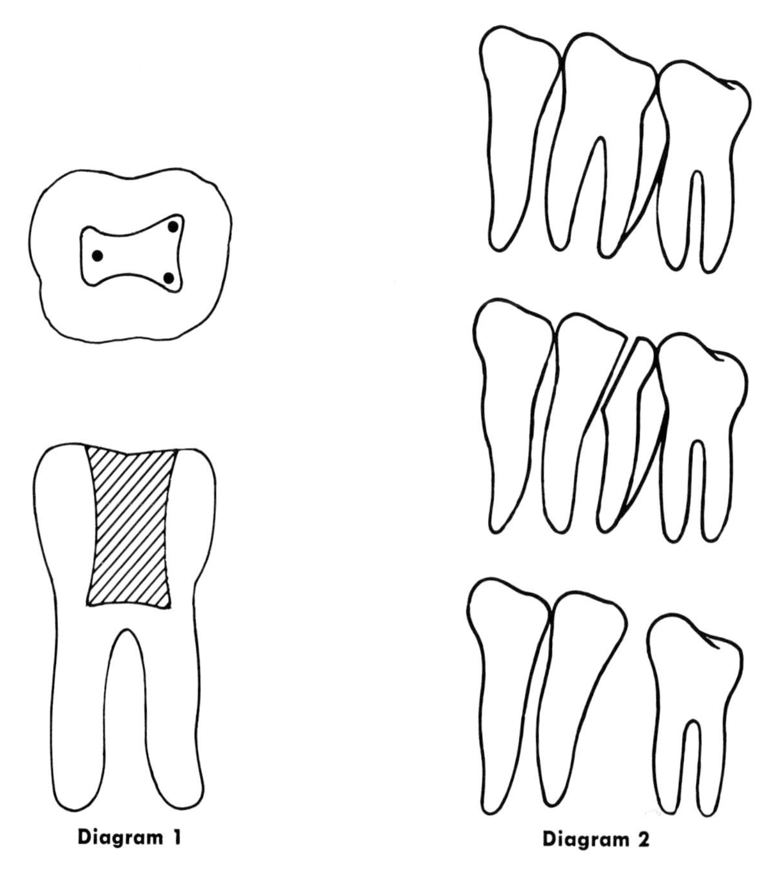


If both mesial and distal roots are to be saved, as for instance in caries of the bifurcation, make the cut vertically through the middle of the bifurcation. In most hemisections, whether one or both fragments are retained, the remaining half or halves should receive crowns. This is particularly true in cases in which both halves are retained to convert the bifurcation into an interdental area with accessible embrasure space.

**Root resection**

If a fairly firm upper molar shows severe involvement of one or both buccal roots or if both buccal roots are in good health and the lingual root is untreatable, indication for root resection may be present (Fig. 35-5). Occasionally the distobuccal root may be amputated when, because of severe curvature and distal inclination, it contacts or almost contacts the roots of the distal adjoining tooth.

After preliminary periodontal therapy, root canal treatment is completed. This is followed by toilet of the pulp chamber and preparation of an undercut amalgam restoration. At a subsequent session, resect the root or roots at fault. When the furcation is exposed, this operation does not require the raising of a flap. Then recontour the crown to make the remaining crown structure blend with the remaining root structure and to avoid leaving corners or overhangs.

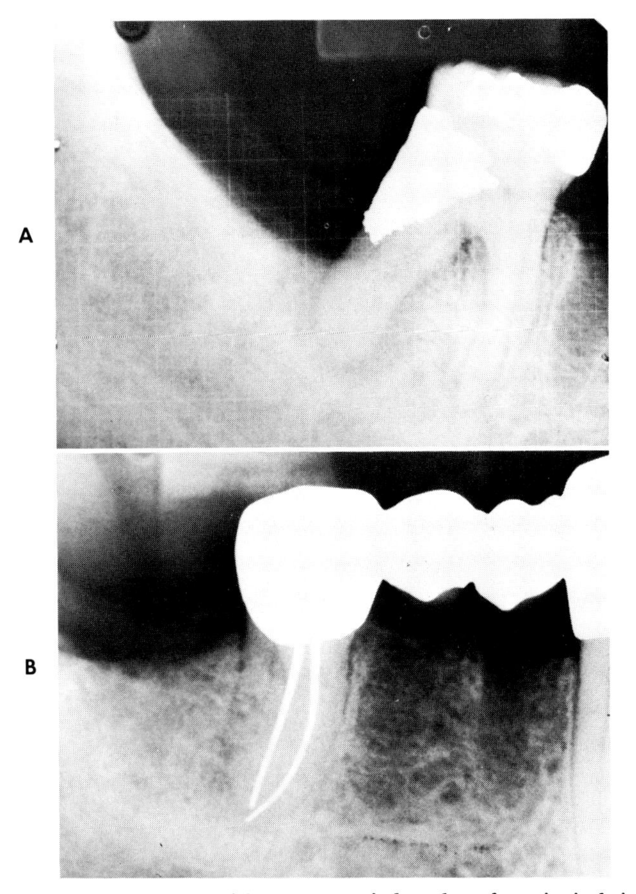


**Fig. 35-4. A,** Mandibular molar with severe periodontal and periapical involvement of the distal root. Pockets on the distal aspect measured 13 mm., indicating direct access to the periapical area. Pockets at the bifurcation measured 6 mm. on the lingual and 5 mm. on the buccal. Root canal therapy and hemisection were performed in 1965. **B,** The mesial root served as an abutment for a fixed bridge 6 years after hemisection.

At a subsequent session, prepare again a shallow cavity at the site of the resection and place a small amalgam filling over the exposed root canal filling.

Two clinical reports suggest the possibility of performing vital root resection without prior root canal therapy.[17,18] After amputation a shallow cavity is prepared at whose bottom is the pulp stump. A calcium hydroxide preparation is placed over the exposed pulp. After the preparation has set, the cavity is filled with zinc oxide–eugenol cement. At a later session a very shallow cavity is prepared and filled with amalgam. A considerable percentage of teeth so treated produce no further subjective complaint. Histologic sections through such teeth are not available. This approach must be considered unproved at present, and root canal treatment is indicated before root resection.

## Endodontic implants

Endodontic implants have been used to lengthen and thus stabilize the roots of loose teeth.[19-23] These are extra long, extra thick chrome alloy root canal points that extend beyond the apex.

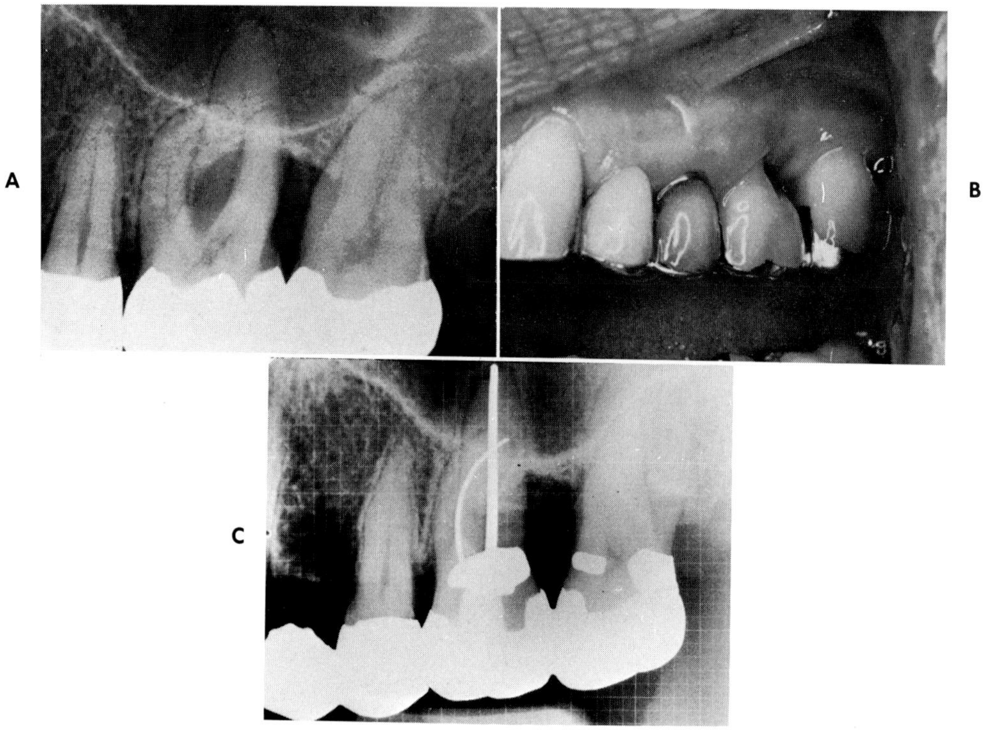

A

B

C

Fig. 35-5. **A,** Preoperative roentgenogram. Maxillary first molar with large trifurcation involvement. The distobuccal root suffers from severe alveolar bone loss. The tooth is included in an extensive fixed bridge. Root canal therapy was performed, and the distobuccal root was resected. **B,** Clinical appearance 1 year later. Note the reshaping of the crown in the area where the amputation has been performed. **C,** Roentgenogram 15 years postoperative. The tooth is firm, comfortable, and in good periapical and periodontal health.

## SUMMARY

Combined endodontic-periodontal therapy is widely used because the anatomic and clinical connections between pulp and periodontal structures are close and numerous. In most cases of this nature, endodontic procedures are performed first and when necessary are followed by periodontal measures. However, in some cases both procedures may be done at a single session.

Some rather rare pseudoperiodontal situations may, in fact, be due to *primary* pulp disease and may clear up after endodontic treatment alone: (1) the suddenly appearing deep pocket that is in reality a fistulous tract from the periapical area to the gingival sulcus of a pulpless tooth and (2) the roentgenographically diagnosed furcation involvement that cannot be probed and may be due to discharge from a necrotic pulp through a bifurcational accessory canal. Endodontic treatment alone may cure both these conditions. When advanced, chronic periodontal disease has exposed lateral canals or the apical foramen leading to *secondary* pulpitis or pulp death, the chances of curing the condition by endodontic treatment alone are slim. This is a more common situation than the two preceding. Root canal therapy and periodontal intervention (combined endodontic-periodontal therapy) is indicated.

The value of precise pocket probing and correct appraisal of the vitality of the pulp is therefore evident. In some doubtful cases the better part of wisdom is to wait until after completion of the root canal therapy to see whether spontaneous resolution (pocket closure and osseous fill-in) will occur before surgical periodontal procedures are begun. The clinical experience and acumen of the dentist must be of the highest degree to enable him to choose the procedure that will bring healing with the appropriate intervention.

**CHAPTER 35**

**References**

1. Seltzer, S.: Endodontology, New York, 1971, McGraw-Hill Book Co.
2. Sicher, H.: Ueber Pulpaerkrankungen als Folge von Paradontose, Z. Stomat. **34**:819, 1936.
2a. Simon, J. H. S., Glick, D. H., and Frank, A. L.: The relationship of endodontic-periodontic lesions, J. Periodont. **43**:202, 1972.
3. Hess, W.: The anatomy of the root canal of the teeth of the permanent dentition, London, 1925, John Bale Sons & Danielsson, Ltd.
4. Everett, F. G., and others: The intermediate bifurcational ridge, J. Dent. Res. **37**:162, 1964.
5. Kovacs, I.: Contribution à l'étude des rapports entre le development et la morphologie des racines des dents humains, Bull. Group. Int. Rech. Sci. Stomat. **7**:85, 1964.
6. Orban, B., and Mueller, E.: The development of the bifurcation of multirooted teeth, J. Amer. Dent. Ass. **16**:297, 1929.
7. Johnston, H. B., and Orban, B.: Interradicular pathology as related to accessory root canals, J. Endodont. **3**:21, 1948.
8. Hiatt, W. H.: Regeneration of the periodontium after endodontic therapy and flap operation, Oral Surg. **12**:1471, 1959.
9. Everett, F. G., Hall, W. B., and Phatak, N. M.: Treatment of hypersensitive dentin, J. Oral Ther. Pharm. **2**:300, 1966.
10. Ingle, J. I.: Occupational bruxism and its relation to periodontal disease, J. Periodont. **23**: 7, 1952.
11. Messinger, T. F., and Orban, B.: Elimination of periodontal pockets by root amputation, J. Periodont. **25**:213, 1954.
12. Amen, C. R.: Hemisection and root amputation, Periodontics **4**:197, 1966.
13. Hiatt, W. H.: The repositioned alveolar ridge mucosal flap, Periodontics **5**:132, 1967.
14. Black, G. V.: In Litch, W., editor: The American system of dentistry, Philadelphia, 1886, Lea.
15. Everett, F. G.: Bifurcation involvement, J. Oregon Dent. Ass. **28**:2, 1959.
16. Staffileno, H., Jr.: Furcation treatment in periodontics, Dent. Radiogr. Photogr. **38**:85, 1965.
17. Sternlicht, H. C.: A new approach to the management of multi-rooted teeth with advanced periodontal disease, J. Periodont. **34**:150, 1963.
18. Haskell, E. W.: Vital root resection, Oral Surg. **27**:266, 1969.
19. Orlay, H. G.: Endodontic splinting treatment in periodontal disease, Brit. Dent. J. **108**: 118, 1960.
20. Orlay, H. G.: Splinting with endodontic implant stabilizers, Dent. Pract. **14**:481, 1964.
21. Frank, A. L.: Improvement of the crown-root ratio by endosseous endodontic implants, J. Amer. Dent. Ass. **74**:451, 1967.
22. Grossman, L.: Endodontic practice, ed. 7, Philadelphia, 1970, Lea & Febiger.
23. Baumhammers, A., and Baumhammers, I.: Periodontal considerations of endosseous implants, J. Periodont, **43**:135, 1972.

**Additional suggested reading**

Hiatt, W. H., and Amen, C. R.: Periodontal pocket elimination by combined therapy, Dental Clinics of North America, Philadelphia, 1964, W. B. Saunders Co.

Rubach, W. C., and Mitchell, D. F.: Periodontal disease, accessory canals, and pulp pathosis, J. Periodont. **36**:34, 1965.

Simring, M., and Goldberg, M.: The pulpal pocket approach: retrograde periodontitis, J. Periodont. **35**:22, 1964.

Stahl, S. S.: Pathogenesis of inflammatory lesions in pulp and periodontal tissues, Periodontics **4**:190, 1966.

PART IX

# Traumatic periodontal diseases and their treatment

CHAPTER THIRTY-SIX

# Role of occlusion in periodontal disease



It has been said that when the teeth, jaws, muscles of mastication, and temporomandibular joint (components of the stomatognathic system) are in a harmonious relationship this balance will contribute to the health of the periodontium. Conversely, it has also been said that when the interrelationship is disturbed periodontal disease may follow.

More has been written, but perhaps less is known, about the precise role of occlusion in periodontal disease than about most other aspects of periodontology. The therapist is confronted with contradictory theories and methods. Therapy must depend on an understanding of the mechanisms of occlusion in both normal and pathologic physiology. The development of such an understanding is based on histologic observation of clinical material and animal experimentation. From such a base one can more meaningfully utilize the various methods of dealing with periodontal disease involving occlusion. Such disease is known as *periodontal trauma,* and this term refers to changes produced in the periodontal tissues. Some students confuse malocclusion with occlusal traumatism. To fully understand the role of occclusion in periodontal disease, one must distinguish between malocclusion, on the one hand, and occlusal traumatism, on the other.

***Definitions***

*Periodontal trauma* is a morbid condition produced by repeated mechanical forces exerted on the periodontium that exceed the physiologic limts of tissue tolerance and contribute to a breakdown of the supporting tissues of the tooth. These forces produce local circulatory disturbances in the periodontal tissues. Other tissue changes, such as those of crushing and tearing, are produced when the tooth impinges on the alveolar bone. *Trauma* refers to the precise pathologic changes occurring in the tissues, whereas *traumatism* refers to the act or acts of producing the trauma. *Occlusal traumatism* implies that the forces are occlusal.

The muscles of the cheek, tongue, and lip can also be important in the causation of periodontal trauma. This is particularly noticeable in abnormal lip and tongue actions and in abnormal swallowing patterns. In addition, habitual actions performed with the teeth, such as playing wind instruments, bobby pin opening, and pipestem biting, may contribute to traumatism.

## THE PERIODONTIUM

Preliminary to the study of periodontal trauma, a review of the normal structures of the periodontium should be undertaken (Chapter 1).

Each tooth is suspended in the alveolus by the periodontal ligament, which permits some movement of the teeth. Short-term tooth displacements are brought about by lip, tongue, and occlusal forces. When the application of the force is stopped, the tooth returns to position. There are long-term migratory movements in which growth and wear also play a role. Growth, wear, and lip-tongue-occlusal forces cause continuing changes in the position of the teeth. These movements require the supporting tissues to be constantly remodeled and adapted in response to the changing functional demands. Thus there is an ever-present functional interdependence between the teeth and the periodontium.

The periodontal ligament consists of the principal fiber bundles arranged in varying directions according to functional demands. Loose connective tissue that surrounds the blood vessels and nerve fibers is found between the bundles of the principal fibers. The cellular elements consist primarily of fibroblasts, but there are also epithelial cells (rests of Malassez) that are remnants of Hertwig's epithelial sheath. The surface of the cementum of the functioning tooth is believed to have an uncalcified layer (cementoid) along which the cementoblasts are aligned. The periodontal surface of the alveolar bone shows a similar arrangement of osteoblasts. Occasional osteoclasts may be seen within Howship's lacunae.

The osseous side of the periodontal space shows continuous change as in any other bone. The bone alongside different areas of the periodontal ligament varies in structure, depending on functional stimuli. This fact is of utmost importance for the proper understanding of periodontics and, in particular, for the proper appreciation of the role of the occlusal factor in periodontal diseases.

### Mesial migration

As has long been recognized, the teeth move continually toward the midline This is the so-called physiologic mesial migration of teeth.[1] Black estimated that the ageing dental arch becomes shorter by about 1 cm.[2,3] This shortening of the dental arch is caused by the attrition of contact points and contact planes. Despite this loss of tooth substance, the teeth remain in contact. Knowing that it takes almost a lifetime for an entire dental arch to lose 0.5 to 1 cm. in length, we should be able to realize that the physiologic mesial migration of teeth is an extremely slow process. Despite the slowness of this movement, we can distinguish the side *toward* which the teeth are moving (mesial) from the side *from* which they are moving (distal) by tissue differences in microscopic specimens. A chronologic history of some of the changes that have taken place is engraved in the calcified matrix of the alveolar bone.

The mesial and distal surfaces of a tooth are shown in Fig. 36-1. The bone and periodontal ligament of the two sides have a different structure. On the distal surface (*A*) the fiber bundles of the periodontal ligament are stretched, as if under tension. On the mesial surface (*B*) they appear wavy, as though relaxed.

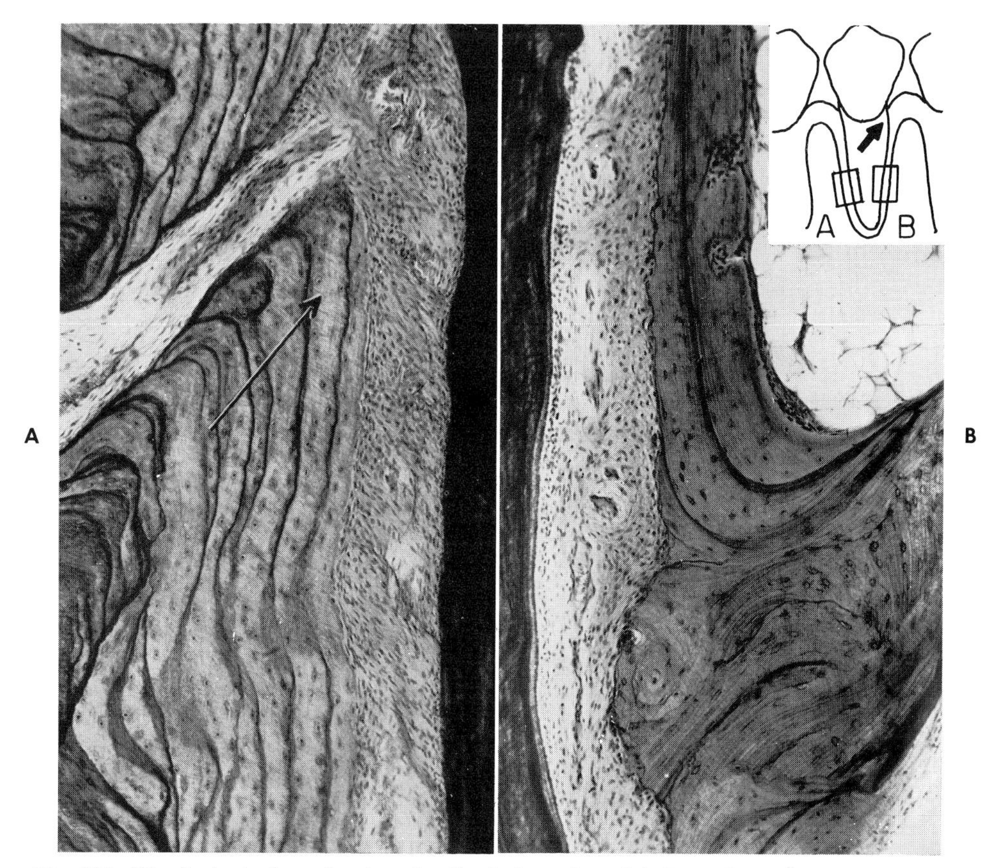


**Fig. 36-1.** Histologic sections showing the distal, **A,** and mesial, **B,** surfaces of a tooth. On the distal, **A,** the fibers are under tension. Part of the fibers are embedded in bundle bone. The bundle bone is demarcated by an irregular line containing concavities directed away from the bundle bone. These are known as reversal lines and indicate that resorption has taken place up to that line from the marrow side. The resorption stopped, the process was reversed and new lamellated bone was laid down in the form of haversian systems and parallel lamellae, replacing the bundle bone that had been resorbed. On the pressure side, **B,** the fiber bundles are relaxed. The surface of the bone has undergone resorption. (Arrow in inset shows the direction of movement of the tooth.) This bone is also lamellated, as can be seen by the tierlike arrangement, which indicates alternating periods of formation and rest. The lines between periods of bone formation are known as resting lines. (From the collection of J. P. Weinmann.)

This is not the only difference. On the distal (tension) side the alveolar bone is of bundle bone type, which signifies that coarse fiber bundles are incorporated in the bone.

Loose connective tissue areas between the principal bundles of the periodontal ligament on the distal side appear oval in shape as the result of the tension of the fiber bundles. On the mesial side of the same tooth (in the direction of migration), the fiber bundles in the perodontal ligament are rather wavy and less stretched. The loose connective tissue areas are round. No differences are perceptible in the character of the cementum. Resorption of the lamellated alveolar bone by osteoclastic activity is in progress while new bone is being laid down from the endosteum in the marrow space (Figs. 36-1, *B*, and 36-2).

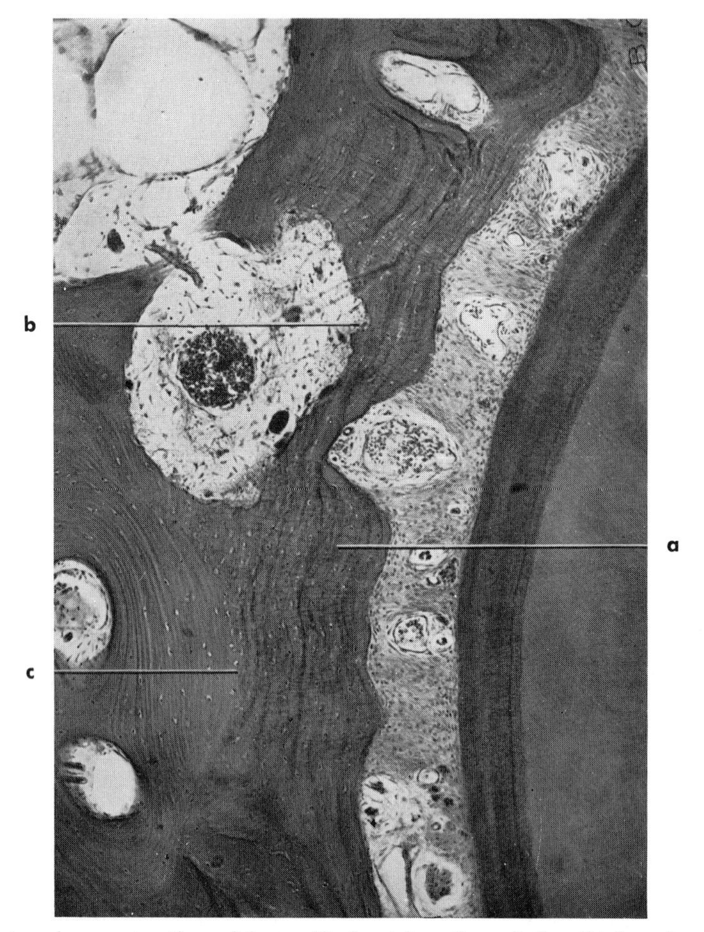


**Fig. 36-2.** Internal reconstruction of bone. Horizontal section of the distal surface of a tooth showing, *a,* formation of bundle bone on the side of tension and, *b,* resorption from the marrow spaces. Nonfunctioning parts of the bundle bone are thus eliminated, and the resorbed bone is replaced by newly formed haversian systems, *c.*

These histologic differences are a clear indication of different stimuli influencing the periodontium on the mesial and distal surfaces of the tooth as a result of this slow tooth migration. The extremely delicate mechanism of the interdependence of tissue structure and function in the periodontium is thus illustrated.

## Active eruption

Mesial migration is not the only movement of teeth. There is also movement in an occlusal direction,[4,5] which leads to eruption of the teeth into the oral cavity and brings about occlusal contact. The period of active eruption is characterized by a rather rapid movement of the teeth and is manifested in the structural arrangement of the bone trabeculae (Fig. 36-3), which are deposited in parallel layers at the fundus of the alveolus as well as at the alveolar crest. After the teeth come into occlusal contact, the active eruption process slows but never stops completely.[6] Eruption continues; and, under ideal conditions, there is a correlation between occlusal attrition and active eruption.

A few illustrations will show how active eruption affects the surrounding

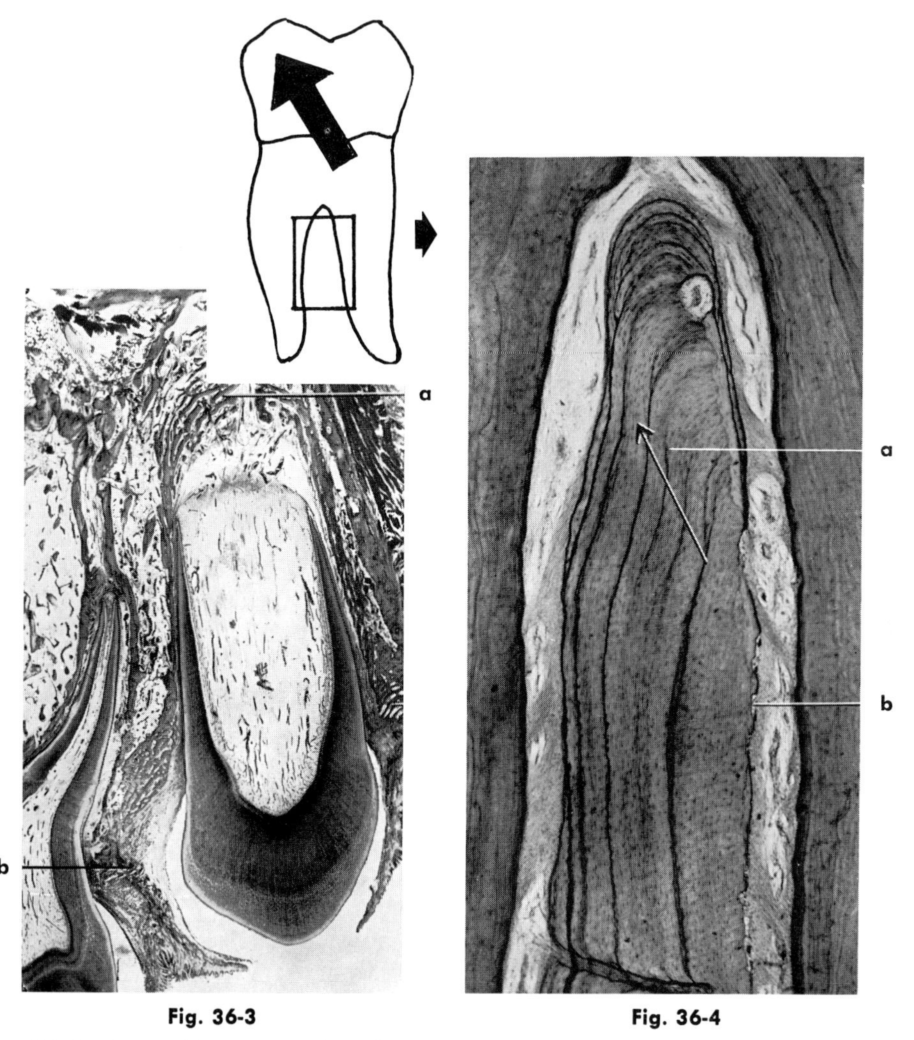


**Fig. 36-3** **Fig. 36-4**

**Fig. 36-3.** During rapid active eruption of the tooth, bone is laid down, *a,* layer by layer at the fundus of the alveolus and, *b,* as functional adaptation at the alveolar crest. Arrows show direction of the tooth eruptive movement. (From Kronfeld, R.: New York J. Dent. **6**:112, 1936.)
**Fig. 36-4.** Interradicular bone septum. Direction of tooth movement (arrow) indicated by, *a,* layer-by-layer apposition of bone and, *b,* bone resorption in pressure areas. (From Kronfeld, R.: New York J. Dent. **6**:112, 1936.)

structures. The bifurcation of a lower molar[7] is shown in Fig. 36-4. The interradicular bony septum shows layer-by-layer appositional growth in a mesio-occlusal direction. Resorption is taking place on the side of pressure. Thick cementum covers the root surface. The continuous formation of cementum is a necessary link in active eruption.

The buccal alveolar crest of a lower premolar is shown in Fig. 36-5, *A.* The bottom of the pocket is close to the cementoenamel junction and the epithelial attachment extends about 2 mm. apically along the cementum. The alveolar crest is about 1 mm. apical to the deepest penetration of the epithelium and shows layer-by-layer apposition of bone in an occlusal direction. Higher magnification (Fig. 36-5, *B*) of the alveolar crest clearly shows the arrangement of the resting lines, which indicate a predominantly occlusal growth of this alveolar crest. There

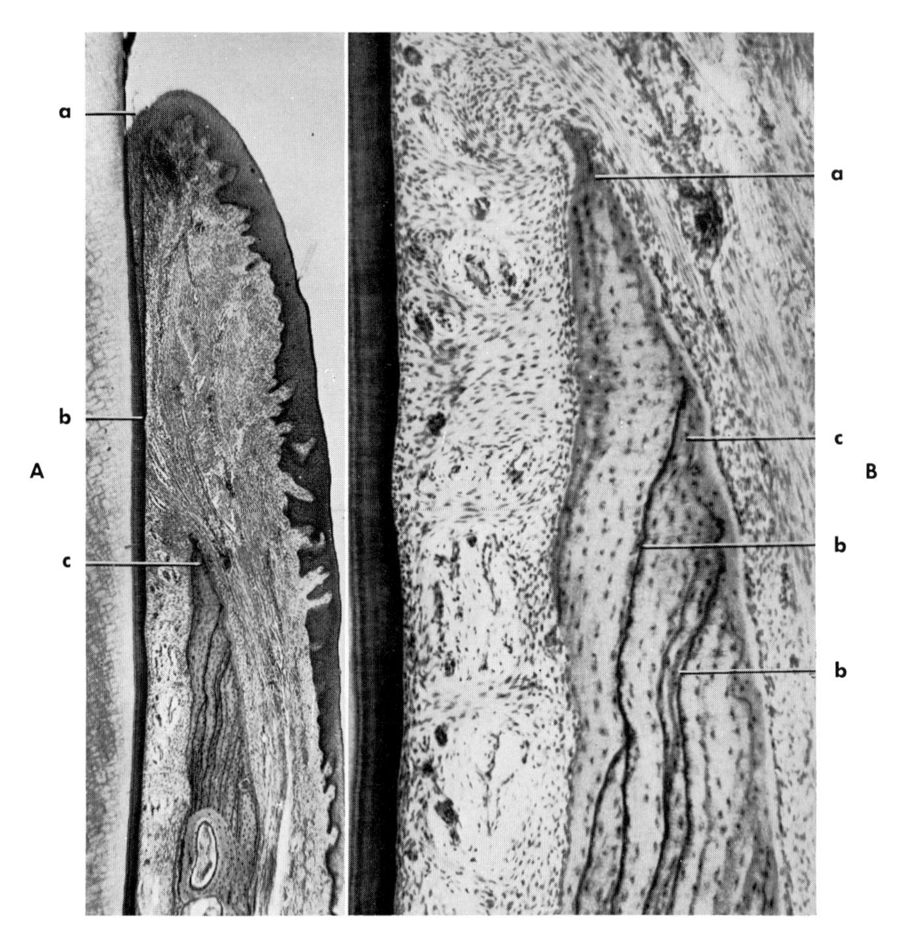


**Fig. 36-5. A,** As the result of active eruption of the tooth, bone apposition takes place at the alveolar crest. *a,* Bottom of the gingival sulcus; *b,* apical end of the epithelial attachment; *c,* tip of the alveolar crest. **B,** Higher magnification of, *a,* the tip of the alveolar crest showing, *b,* the layer-by-layer apposition of bone and, *c,* the increase in height of the alveolar crest. Bone formation is from the periosteal side, starting from a reversal line.

is a reversal line on the buccal surface of the bone below the periosteum and close to the surface. The resorption was reversed, and at the time of the patient's death active bone formation was in progress on the periosteal side of this crest. Such functionally directed tissue changes not only occur in the immediate surroundings but also have their effect deep in the supporting alveolar bone (Fig. 36-2). The bony trabeculae are rebuilt constantly in response to functional influences by a process of resorption and bone formation. This takes place constantly in the jaws, showing the interdependence between function and structure.

Active occlusal eruption of the teeth has also been observed clinically. By way of illustration, a patient complained to his dentist that a tooth was growing shorter.[8] On observation and examination the dentist noted that the seemingly shortened tooth was not actually getting shorter but was remaining fixed because of a pathologic process that stopped its eruptive movement while the other teeth erupted normally. When such teeth are removed, extensive resorption of the roots and ankylosis with the bone may be noted.[9] These processes also can affect the primary teeth. If they remain in the jaw longer than is physiologically nor-

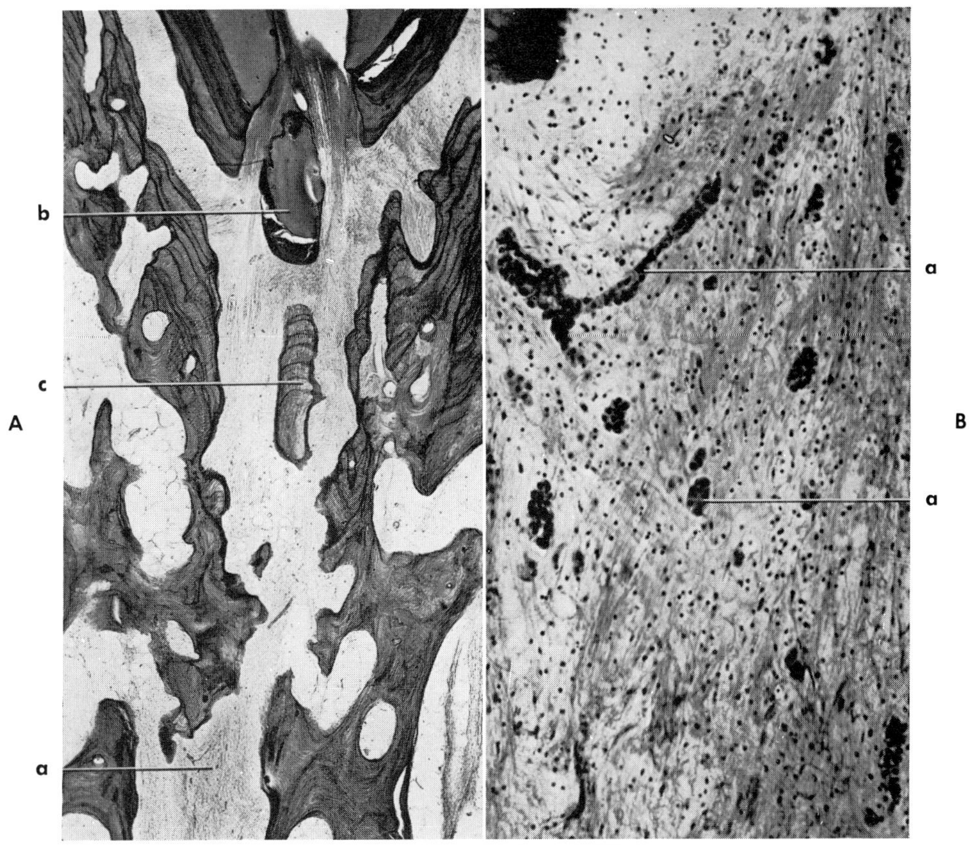


**Fig. 36-6. A,** Epithelial rests, *a,* far below the apex of the tooth, *b,* indicate that the apex once was at the level of these epithelial remnants and then actively erupted. This is also manifest by bundle bone, *c,* around the apex. **B,** Higher magnification showing the epithelial remnants, *a.*

mal, they may appear shorter than adjacent permanent teeth. In fact, they may become totally or partially submerged in the jaw, with bone and soft tissue slowly growing up around them.[10]

Other histologic findings indicate that teeth erupt actively even after they have reached the occlusal plane. Such a finding is supported by the presence of epithelial remnants far below the apex of a tooth in a nutrient canal[11] (Fig. 36-6). The epithelial rests are remnants of Hertwig's epithelial root sheath and are normally found in the periodontal ligament. If epithelial remnants remain below the apex (as in Fig. 36-6), the apex can be assumed to have been once at the place where the epithelial remnants are now seen. These epithelial structures cannot actively change their position. They have been effectively left behind by the eruption of the tooth. Deeper bony areas may contain isolated islands of bundle bone that were once alveolar bone but were left behind, unresorbed and unreplaced by lamellated bone.

Resorption and repair processes in alveolar bone take place as an adaptive physiologic mechanism so long as the natural dentition remains, although these processes are slowed in old age.[33] Whenever an endogenous or exogenous disturbance occurs, the adaptive activities of the periodontal tissues may be upset. However, tissue breakdown also takes place normally as a physiologic process be-

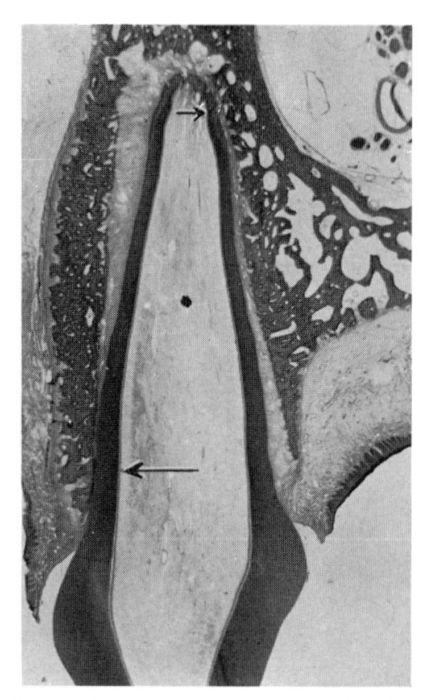

**Fig. 36-7.** Histologic section of a dog's tooth exposed to occlusal traumatism for 36 hours. The tooth was rotated around an axis in the center of the root (dot). The periodontal ligament is compressed at the alveolar margin on the buccal side and at the apex on the lingual side (arrows). The periodontal ligament is doubled in width on the corresponding areas of the opposite sides.

cause tissue elements continually die as a result of ageing. These tissues must be replaced, and the form that the rebuilding takes depends primarily on functional demands. Optimal anabolic activities depend on good health and function.

The alveolus normally has an hourglass shape, being widest at the apex and at the alveolar crest. This permits a certain amount of movement in the physiologic range. The maximum displacement of a tooth depends on the shape of the bony housing. If, for example, a severe tipping displacement brings the cervical part of the tooth into contact with the alveolar margin or the apex into contact with the alveolar bone, damage must occur. The bundles of the periodontal ligament are composed of collagen fibers that are not elastic. Therefore they can scarcely stretch under tension. The major change in these fiber bundles is from a normal, wavy state to a straightened state. That these fibers do not significantly stretch beyond their normal length provides protection against total compression of the periodontal tissues under normal functional pressure, which is one of the most important functions of the periodontal ligament.

## TISSUE CHANGES IN EXPERIMENTAL OCCLUSAL TRAUMATISM

### Occlusal traumatism in dogs

*Premature contact*

Extensive investigations in occusal traumatism have been conducted on dogs.[12] In an attempt to establish what damage could be done to the periodontal structures by occlusal traumatism, high crowns were cemented on opposing maxillary and mandibular teeth. This caused the two supraoccluding teeth to strike each time the animal closed its jaws (premature contact). The tissue changes induced in the periodontium were observed during experimental periods ranging from just a few hours to over a year and have been studied extensively. A tooth exposed to such trau-

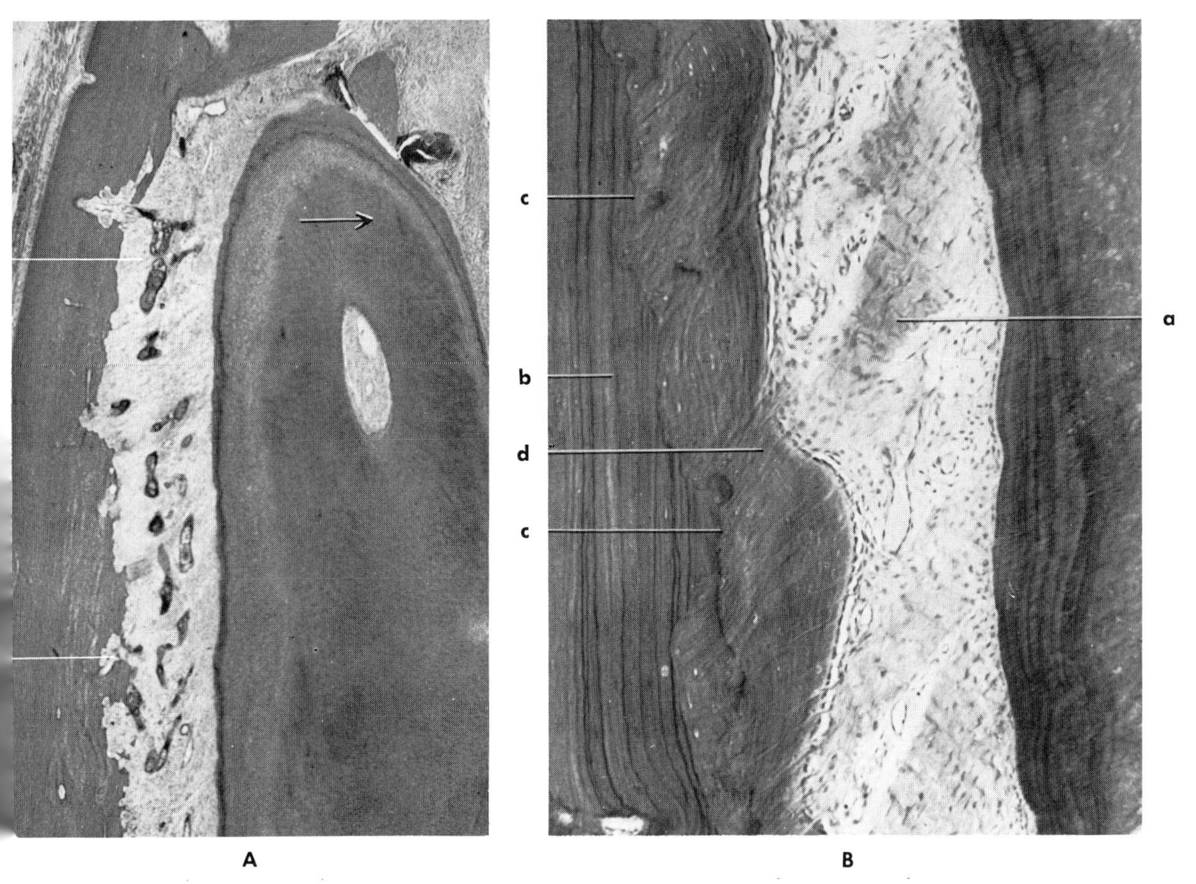


**Fig. 36-8.** Experimental occlusal traumatism in a monkey. **A,** Thrombosed blood vessels in the periodontal ligament caused by extensive tension, *a,* with resorption of bone, *b.* Movement of the apex is indicated by the arrow. **B,** Higher magnification of a tension area corresponding to that shown in **A,** 6 months after the experiment started. In **B** the periodontal ligament is completely regenerated and the resorption of alveolar bone repaired. Between the old bone, *b,* and new bone, *d,* a resorbed surface, *c* (reversal line), is evident. The new bone is of bundle bone character, forming the periodontal surface of the alveolar bone.

matic force is shown 36 hours after the crown was cemented (Fig. 36-7). The tooth was tipped around an axis close to the center of the root, as indicated by the arrows and the dot in Fig. 36-7. In these experiments small hemorrhages were noted, but no gross tears occurred at either the alveolar crest or the apex. In some more recent experiments on monkeys, thrombosis of blood vessels was noted on the tension side[13] (Fig. 36-8, *A*), leading to resorptions on the surface of the adjacent alveolar bone. Gross tears were not observed in these experiments either. Six months later the bone resorption was repaired and the periodontal ligament had regenerated (Fig. 36-8, *B*).

***Rapid collagen turnover***

A simple explanation for this repair stems from the fact that collagen fibers can be lysed, providing a pool of collagen precursors.[14] In addition, the precursors of the collagen molecules are formed in adjacent fibroblasts and pass out of the fibroblasts into the extracellular space. The precursors then combine to form new collagen fibrils. Both electron microscopic and radioautographic studies

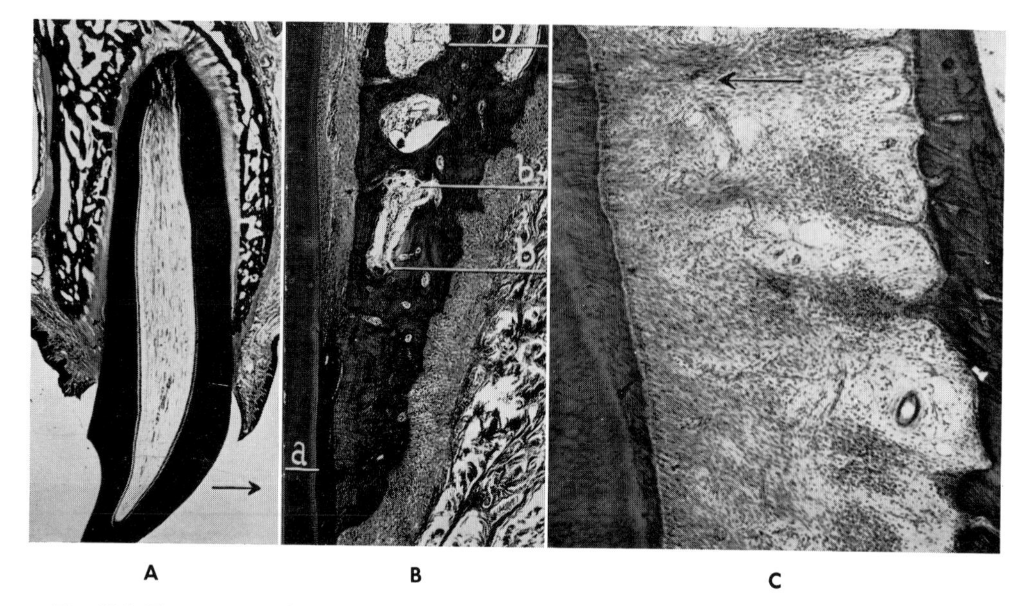


**Fig. 36-9.** Trauma experiment in a dog. **A,** The tooth was ligated to an orthodontic arch wire for 48 hours. Pressure areas occurred on the labial marginal and lingual apical aspects. Tension areas occurred in the opposite regions. **B,** Higher magnification showing, *a,* necrotic compressed periodontal ligament between the tooth and the alveolar crest and, *b,* beginning osteoclastic bone resorption in the marrow spaces. **C,** Tension side at the apex shows formation of new bone spicules and increased cellular activity to repair the damage done by the overextension. (The arrow indicates the direction of tooth movement.)

provide support for the conjecture that periodontal fibers reform in this manner.[15-17] The collagen fibers of the periodontal ligament have a much more rapid turnover than was previously believed possible.[18] Collagen synthesis occurs anywhere in the ligament, and additional collagen molecules can be fabricated and joined to preexisting fibrils. Thus the changes in width of the periodontal ligament (Fig. 36-8) are accounted for.

***Increased fibroblastic activity***

The response to this type of traumatic injury and the process of repair make a fascinating study. Fig. 36-9, *A,* shows an incisor that was ligated firmly to a labial arch wire for 48 hours. The tooth was tipped so far labially that it touched the alveolar crest. This caused a complete compression and necrosis of the periodontal ligament at the area of contact between tooth and bone (*B*). There was also a contact between tooth and bone close to the apex on the lingual side. During the 48 hours in which this intensive pressure was applied, the only tissue reaction seen in the area was in the bone marrow spaces adjacent to the pressure area; osteoclastic bone resorption was apparent. There was considerably more activity in the tension zone—at the alveolar margin on the lingual side and at the apex on the labial side; the periodontal space was double its normal width. Higher magnification (*C*) showed a tremendous increase in fibroblastic activity. The periodontal ligament was wider and more cellular than normal. Dense masses of cells had accumulated in certain areas. Osteoblasts lined the bony spicules being formed in the direction of tension. These extended toward the fiber bundles in a growth pattern. Obviously the cellular elements are of as much significance as the fibers of the periodontal ligament. Moreover, they are of prime

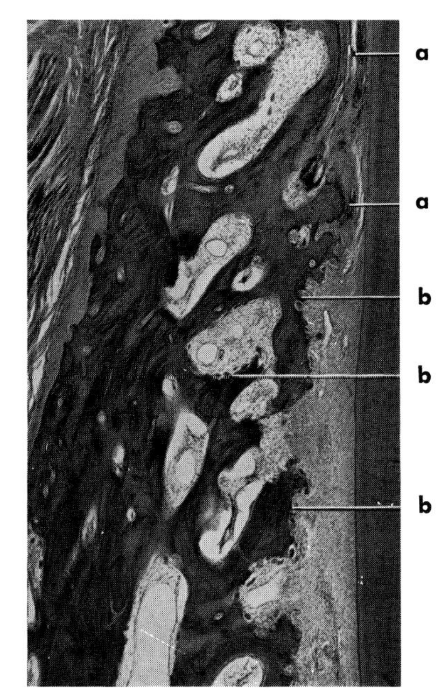


**Fig. 36-10.** Undermining bone resorption in progress 60 hours after beginning of the traumatic influence. *a,* Necrotic area without bone resorption; *b,* undermining bone resorption in progress.

importance in the processes of repair and healing. In observing the adaptive process in the pressure and the tension areas, one can see the sequence in which repair takes place.

***Undermining resorption***

The necrotic mass that is so characteristic of damage inflicted by excessive pressure is slowly eliminated by resorption of the bone adjacent to the area of pressure necrosis. This type of bone resorption has been called undermining resorption because the necrotic area is resorbed from the rear. This resorption starts in adjacent vital tissue, and the area of necrosis is thus eliminated. The process of bone resorption must proceed from the periphery since no osteoclasts or macrophages can develop in the area of maximum pressure when soft and adjacent hard tissues are dead (Fig. 36-10). The time necessary to eliminate the necrotic tissue will largely depend on the extent of the involved area. Fig. 36-11 shows an alveolar crest with a small necrotic area 14 days after application of excessive pressure. Here the necrotic area was almost entirely eliminated. Complete regeneration would have taken place in 2 or 3 more days.

***Functional adaptation***

Fig. 36-12 shows the alveolar margin of a tooth 15 days after the cementing of a high crown. Resorption proceeded considerably more slowly than in the previous case because of the greater extent of the necrotic area. Resorption was forced to progress along the boundaries of the bone marrow spaces. These appeared widened so that only a thin plate of bone lined the necrotic periodontal ligament. This specimen shows an interesting and important feature—new formation of bone on the periosteal side of the alveolar crest. This is a functional adaptation process. The progress of functional adaptation on both the pressure and the tension sides can be seen at the apex of a tooth (Fig. 36-13) exposed to traumatism for 3 weeks. The apex was moved in the direction of the arrow. Two areas of necrosis can be seen. Both were almost completely undermined and elim-

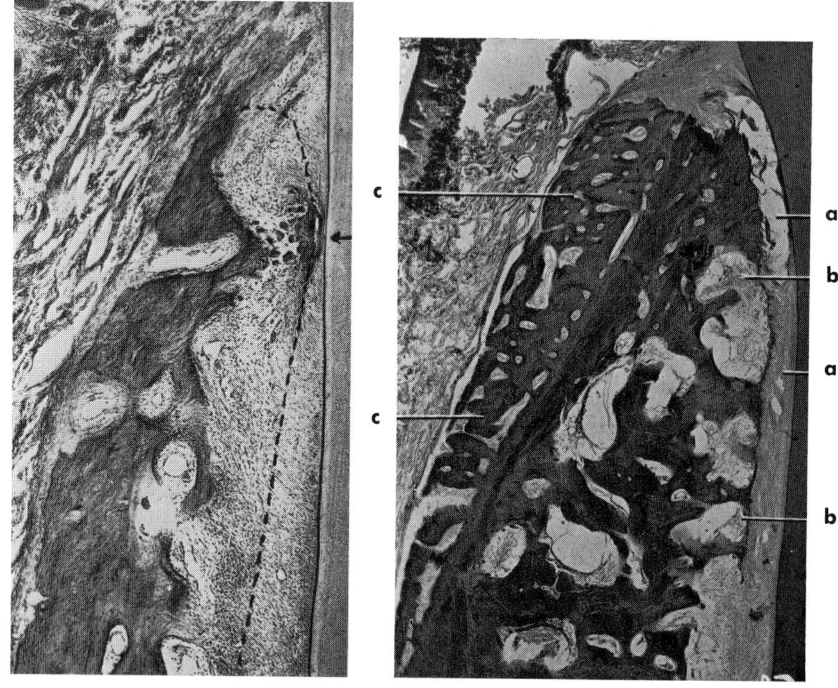


**Fig. 36-11** **Fig. 36-12**

**Fig. 36-11.** Alveolar crest with necrotic pressure area (arrow) 14 days after beginning of the trauma. The necrotic area is almost completely eliminated. The probable former shape of the alveolar bone is sketched with a dotted line.

**Fig. 36-12.** Alveolar margin 15 days after beginning of the trauma experiment. *a,* Extensive area of necrosis; *b,* undermining resorption in progress; *c,* new formation of bone on the vestibular periosteal side of the alveolar crest.

inated. The width of the periodontal ligament space was once again almost normal.

New bundle bone had been formed on the tension side, reestablishing the normal functional width of the periodontal ligament. The extent to which the apex was moved can be seen by the amount of newly formed bone. Where the two necrotic spots are present, there must originally have been bone; cementum occupies the space formerly held by the periodontal ligament. On the tension side the surface of the old alveolar bone is shown by a dark resting line, indicating the amount of bone that was produced by the stimulus of tension.

If traumatism is maintained for a long time, the processes of necrosis, resorption, and repair are repeated or continue as long as the trauma occurs. Eventually the periodontium, as well as the entire jaw, will adapt to the new functional demands. *No changes in the gingiva or the attachment epithelium were evident in any of the experiments, nor did occlusal traumatism cause pocket formation.*

***Intra-alveolar pocket***

The longest experiments conducted on a dog was of 13 months' duration. The result can be seen in Fig. 36-14. Compare the right side, *A* (traumatic side), with the left side, *B* (control side). The experimental tooth was displaced apically and lingually. The apex almost perforated the cortical plate of the mandible. No acute traumatic changes were detectable on the pressure side of the periodontal ligament. No pocket formation or migration of the epithelial attachment occurred

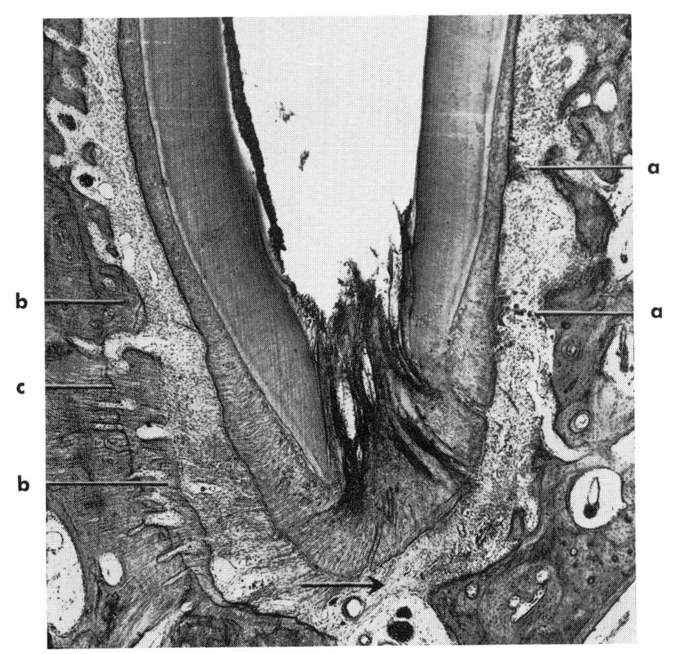


**Fig. 36-13.** Apex of a tooth exposed to trauma for 3 weeks. *a,* Necrotic areas and osteoclasts indicating the former location of the periodontal ligament and alveolar bone; *b,* newly formed bone on the tension side indicative of the amount of tooth movement; *c,* resting line showing the surface of the alveolar bone prior to trauma.

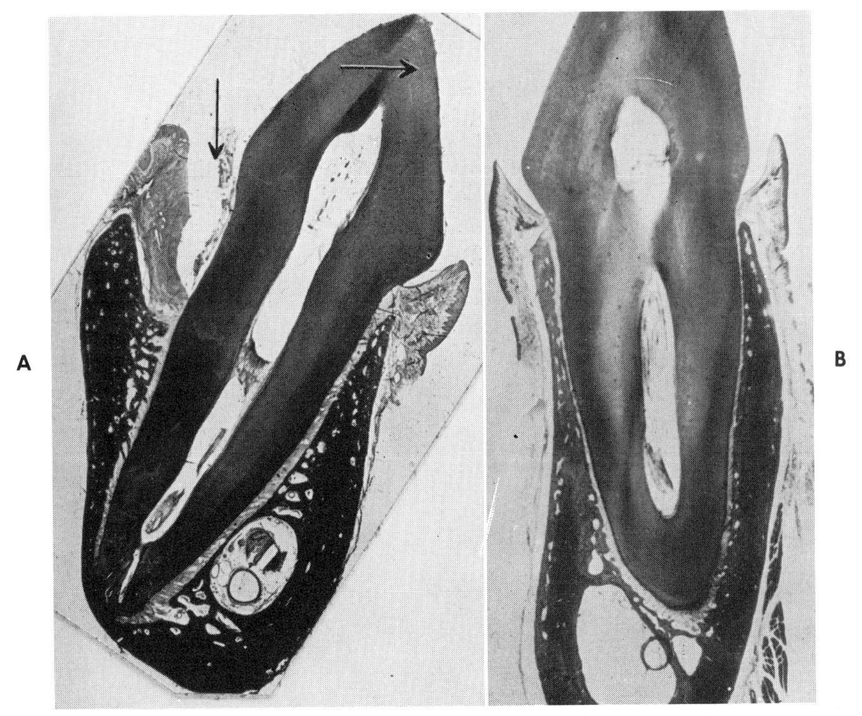


**Fig. 36-14. A,** Tooth exposed to trauma for 13 months. No traumatic tissue changes were evident in the periodontium. Intra-alveolar pocket formation on the vestibular side caused by food impaction is the result of extensive tipping of the tooth. **B,** Control tooth.

on the pressure side. On the buccal side, which was the side of tension, the development of an intra-alveolar pocket could be seen. This was the only pocket that was observed in the entire series of experiments on thirty-four dogs. The explanation for the development of this pocket is that the tooth tipped so far buccally that the crown on the opposing upper tooth caused food to be wedged into the gingival sulcus. This pocket was the result of irritation caused by food impaction resulting from the change in the position of the tooth and was not caused by occlusal traumatism.

### Occlusal traumatism in monkeys

Other investigators have confirmed these findings.[34] Experiments on monkeys have shown the same basic tissue changes that were observed in dogs. Three months after traumatism had been produced by high crowns, the traumatic injuries were completely repaired. In an experiment on monkeys, excessive occlusal forces were reported to have altered the pathway of the inflammatory infiltrate.[35] In the absence of occlusal traumatism, the inflammatory infiltrate is said to have followed the perivascular channels described by Weinmann.[18a] When occlusal traumatism was superimposed, the inflammatory infiltrate was deflected directly into the periodontal ligament.[19] Such deflection is as yet unproved.[20] If it does indeed occur, theoretically it could alter the pattern of bone destruction. (See discussion of the relation of function and structure later in this chapter.)

***Objections*** Objections have been raised that experimental occlusal traumatism as shown in dogs and monkeys does not reproduce satisfactorily the trauma observed in humans. Moreover, these experiments do not compare with periodontal traumatism in humans because in the animals the teeth were moved in one direction and the forces and movements were essentially orthodontic.

To overcome these objections, new experiments were conducted on monkeys.[20,21a] In an effort to duplicate the combined effects of inflammation and traumatism, high crowns with extensive overhangs were placed on second premolars. Mesial and distal contacts were opened to permit the mobile tooth to move mesiodistally as well as buccolingually. The animals were sacrificed at 3 days, 3 weeks, 3 months, and 6 months. The teeth had become mobile and extensively depressed. Cemental and dentinal resorption had occurred. The periodontal ligament space had widened. The direction of transseptal and principal fibers had become almost vertical. The fibers were tensely stretched (Fig. 36-15). No other new pathologic tissue reaction had occurred. *There was no pocket formation, no gingivitis, and no apical proliferation of the epithelial attachment. There was no alteration in the pathway of the inflammatory infiltrate. No vertical bone destruction had occurred.*

It is evident that all tissue changes occurring as a consequence of traumatic influences are the result of functional adaptation. The supporting tissues of the teeth adapt themselves to the requirements dictated by altered function.

## PERIODONTAL TRAUMA—HUMAN AUTOPSY FINDINGS

Does periodonal trauma also occur in humans? The answer is yes. The tissue responses to occlusal traumatism in humans are the same as those observed in experimental animals.

### Cases

The first observation of traumatic tissue changes in a human dentition was made on an autopsy specimen of a 24-year-old white man who had died of tuber-

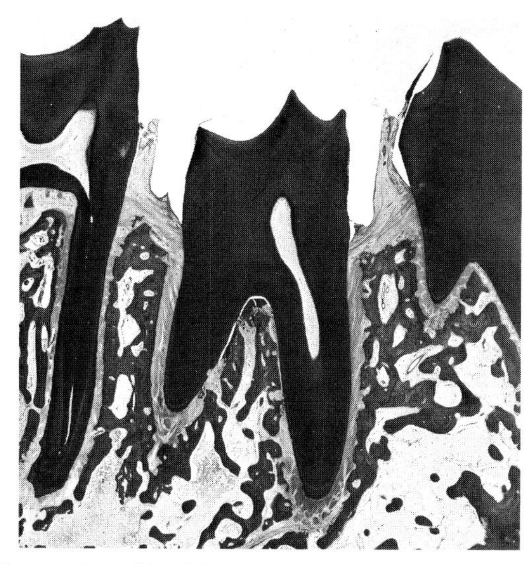

**Fig. 36-15.** Premolar of a monkey with high crown and overhang. Proximal contacts were opened. At 3 weeks the tooth was depressed and the direction of periodontal fibers changed. The periodontal ligament was widened, and the tooth was loose. Some acute traumatic changes were still present in the bifurcation. By 3 months an adaptation had taken place. No pockets or vertical bone destruction had occurred.

culosis.[22] The pertinent area of interest is shown in Fig. 36-16. The mandibular first molar was missing and the second molar had tipped mesially. In the maxilla the second premolar and second molar were missing (*A*). The first molar was present and had been restored with a gold crown. The occlusal relation was such that, on closure of the mandible, the mesiobuccal cusp of the mandibular molar came into contact with the distobuccal cusp of the maxillary molar. Microscopic examination of the specimen (*B*) revealed pressure areas, with necrosis and its consequences as found in three outlined areas. These pressure areas were present in regions where compression would be expected to have resulted from the occlusal relation of this tooth.

Necrosis was present at the mesial alveolar margin of the molar (Fig. 36-17), with undermining resorption advancing from the adjacent marrow spaces. Necrosis was also seen in the bifurcation (Fig. 36-18) and on the distal sides of both apices (Fig. 36-19). The location of pressure areas could be explained by the presence of a rotational fulcrum in the interradicular area near the bifurcation. The characteristic features of necrotic pressure areas, undermining resorption, and endosteal bone fomation behind the traumatic area were the same as those found in animal experiments. The necrotic areas had been undermined and new bone formation had taken place as a repair process. Giant cells and macrophages had been in the process of eliminating the necrotic tissue masses produced by intensive pressure.

Further information was gained from the study of an autopsy specimen of two mandibular premolars in a 64-year-old man. The two teeth presented extensive occlusal wear[23,24] (Fig. 36-20, *A*). The roentgenogram showed that the second premolar was tipped mesially and the occlusal surface was abraded obliquely to a considerable extent. The periodontal ligament space of the second premolar on

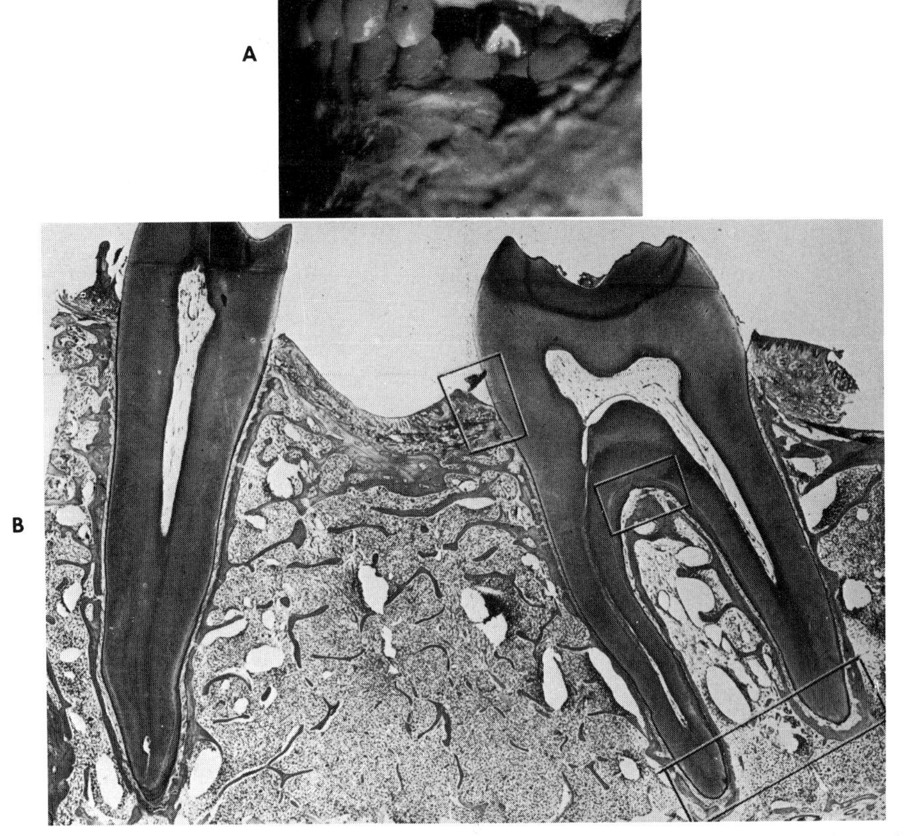


**Fig. 36-16. A,** Autopsy specimen of a human jaw (24-year-old white man). Note the occlusal relation of the maxillary first molar, mandibular second premolar, and mandibular second molar. **B,** Gross microscopic specimen of the mandibular second molar and second premolar shown in **A.** The outlined areas indicate the pressure areas produced by occlusal traumatism.

its cervical (mesiomarginal) aspects was considerably wider than normal. Judging from this evidence alone, one might suspect that an intra-alveolar (infrabony) pocket was present. The microscopic picture showed no pocket. In fact, the bottom of the sulcus was still located on enamel. Only mild papillary gingivitis was present. The periodontal ligament on the distal surface of the first premolar was of normal width. The fiber bundles were functionally arranged. A few cementum spicules were seen, probably caused by increased functional activity.[25] The periodontal ligament space of the second premolar showed a funnel-shaped widening coronally on its mesial aspect. It was bordered by numerous open marrow spaces, causing the radiolucency of this area. A higher magnification of the periodontal ligament revealed necrosis in a circumscribed area (Fig. 36-20, *B*) and an irregular pattern of root resorption extending into the dentin. The periodontal ligament did not show a regular arrangement of the principal fibers. It was rather loose and poorly organized and showed signs of compression.

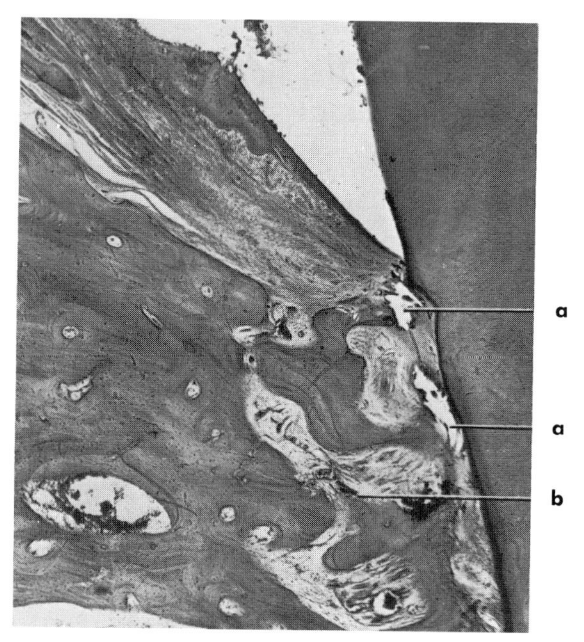


**Fig. 36-17.** Mesial alveolar marginal area of the molar shown in Fig. 36-16, *B*. Necrotic areas in the periodontal ligament are indicated by *a;* resorption of bone by *b*.

This case is of special interest because of the roentgenographic appearance of the area and because there must have been occlusal traumatism of considerable duration, as indicated by the occlusal wear and the accompanying obliteration of the pulp chamber by irregular dentin. There was no sign of injury to the gingival tissues, even though the occlusal surface was abraded and the tooth was tilted mesially. Both these factors might have favored food impaction.

The histologic findings in these human specimens are the same as those in experimental animals. Tissue changes indicative of trauma are frequently found in autopsy material.[26] In fact, in one study in which fifty human jaws were examined, moderate to extensive traumatic tissue changes were found in all specimens.

Such findings may include a necrotic area of the pressure side. A case with early bone resorption can be seen in Fig. 36-21. This specimen had many empty lacunae, indicating the presence of necrosis caused by a disturbance of the nutrition in this area. Similar findings are also shown in Fig. 36-22, an illustration of an orthodontically moved tooth.[27]

Sensitivity of teeth and pulp necrosis sometimes are related to occlusal traumatism. Such disturbances can occur whenever the anatomic relation of the apical foramen to the traumatized tissue is such that the circulation of the pulp is disturbed (Fig. 36-23).

A human specimen obtained at autopsy shows tissue changes that compare closely with those seen in the monkey experiments in which a tooth was moved forcefully to the buccal and lingual sides alternately. This tooth (Fig. 36-24, *A*) was a mandibular premolar of a 20-year-old individual who, despite previous excellent health, became ill and died suddenly. His dentition was faultless. He had thirty-two teeth in excellent alignment and occlusal relation. The gingiva appeared perfectly normal.

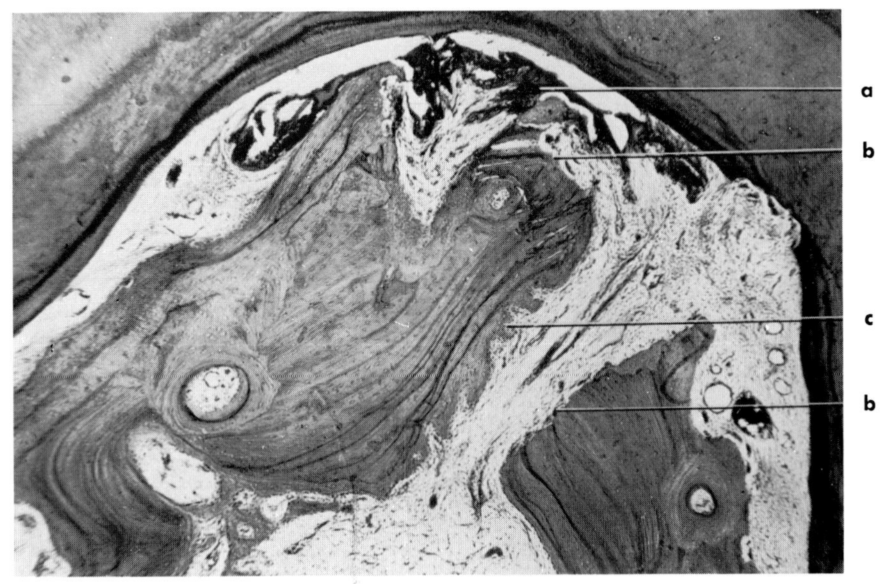


**Fig. 36-18.** Bifurcation area of molar shown in Fig. 36-16. Necrosis, *a,* and undermining bone resorption, *b,* are evident; the new formation of bone, *c,* is occurring on the endosteal side of the bone trabeculae.

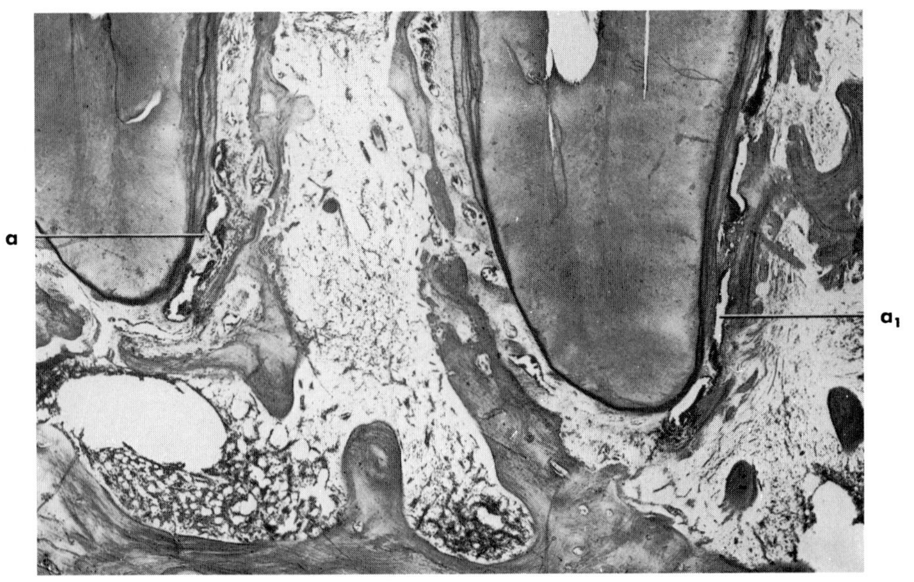


**Fig. 36-19.** Apices of the roots of the molar shown in Fig. 36-16. Necrotic areas are observed on the distal surface of both apices ($a$ an $a_1$). Undermining resorption and endosteal bone formation are also taking place.

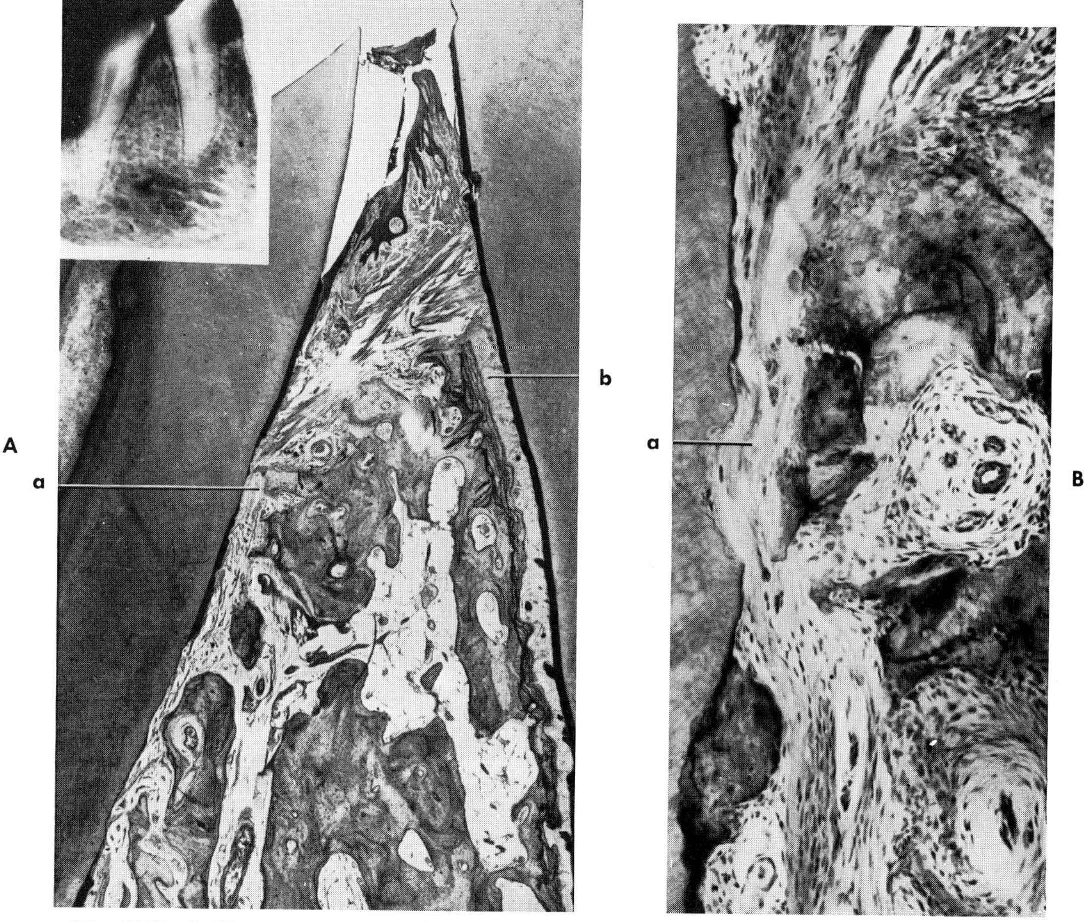


**Fig. 36-20. A, Human autopsy specimen. Two mandibular premolars show extensive occlusal** wear. The second premolar is tipped mesially. The roentgenogram (inset) shows considerable widening of the periodontal ligament space on the mesio-occlusal aspect. The microscopic specimen shows disarrangement of the lamina dura in this area, *a,* as compared to the regular outline of the lamina dura of the distal surface of the first premolar, *b.* **B,** Higher magnification of the mesial surface. Cementum resorption and the necrotic area *(a)* are indications of repeated trauma. (**A** from Kronfeld, R.: New York J. Dent. **6:**112, 1936.)

After all the teeth of this dentition had been sectioned, an unusual microscopic finding was observed on a mandibular premolar. The periodontal ligament was necrotic and contained thrombosed blood vessels at the level of the alveolar crest on both the labial and the lingual sides. There was a pressure area also on the lingual aspect close to the apex. Higher magnification of the labial and lingual alveolar crestal areas (Fig. 36-24, *B*) showed normal width of the periodontal space and a necrotic periodontal ligament. Osteoclastic resorption had started coronal as well as apical to the necrotic areas. The periodontal ligment immediately below the necrotic area was wider than normal and then became narrower toward the apex.

This person had died of a tuberculous meningitis. During the last 3 days of life, he had had muscle hypertonicity with associated spasm. Undoubtedly he clenched his jaws. Excessive force produced necrosis of the periodontal ligament.

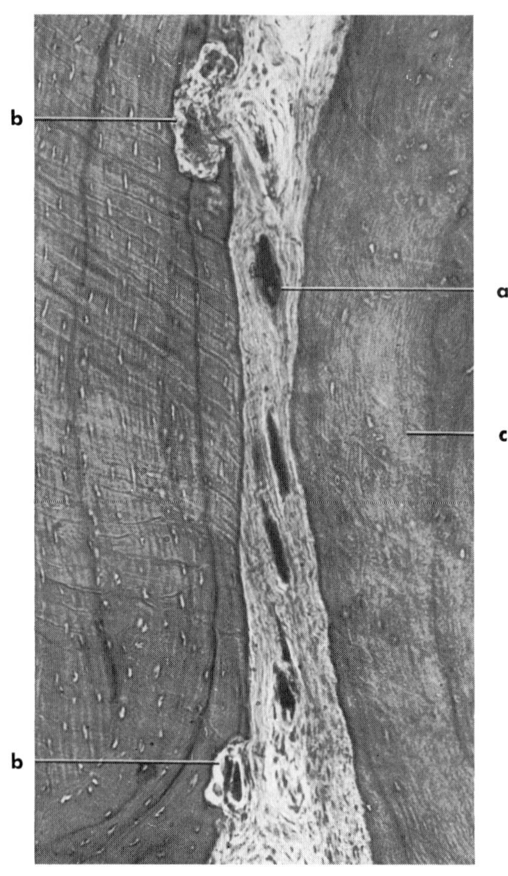


**Fig. 36-21.** Histologic section of traumatized area near the apex of a human tooth. *a,* Necrotic tissue with thrombosed blood vessels evident in the periodontal ligament; *b,* bone resorption begun; *c,* cementum.

With a little imagination we can speculate as to the results that could have occurred had the traumatism become chronic. The necrotic areas finally would have been eliminated and the periodontal ligament would have become wider. In Fig. 36-24, *A,* we can outline the inner surface of the alveolar bone to show how the bone would have been removed by osteoclastic activity (dotted line). With this widening of the periodontal ligament, the tooth would have become loose. Then the tooth could have been moved toward the buccal and lingual surfaces without undue compression of the ligament. This widening of the periodontal ligament would have occurred as an adaptation of the periodontium to excessive functional demands.

There is no reason to believe that such widening of the periodontal space would have affected the depth of the gingival sulcus. The epithelial attachment is some distance from the alveolar crest (1 to 2 mm.),[28] permitting the connective tissue to attach the gingiva to the cementum and the alveolar crest. The vascular blood supply of the marginal gingiva is derived primarily from superficial periosteal vessels. Since occlusal forces do not cause thrombosis of these periosteal vessels, the nutrition of the gingiva apparently is not adversely affected by traumatic tissue changes at the alveolar crest.

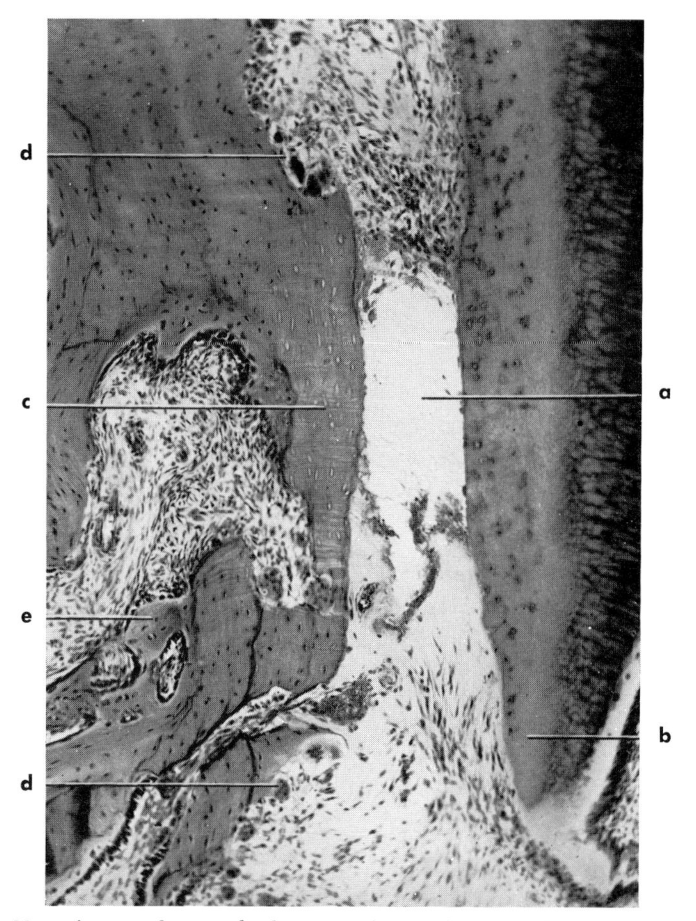


**Fig. 36-22.** *a,* Necrotic area close to, *b,* the apex of a tooth undergoing orthodontic therapy; *c,* bone adjacent to the necrotic periodontal ligament also necrotic as characterized by empty bone lacunae; *d,* undermining resorption; *e,* new formation of endosteal bone in progress. (From Oppenheim, A.: Amer. J. Orthodont. **28**:263, 1942.)

## Primary and secondary traumatism

Most of the cases discussed until now have demonstrated traumatic tissue changes in otherwise healthy periodontal structures. Under such conditions we may speak of *primary* traumatism, that is, a maldirected or excessive force exerted on a tooth with normal bone support. If prior periodontal disease has caused bone loss and weakening of the supporting tissues and occlusal trauma has caused periodontal damage, we speak of *secondary* traumatism, in other words, when the force is excessive for the diminished bone support. We can, in fact, assume that if a tooth has lost a certain amount of its periodontium even normal masticatory forces become excessive.

A condition of this type is illustrated in Fig. 36-25, *A,* which shows a maxillary lateral incisor with about half its cemental surface exposed and heavy calcified deposits present on this surface. The severely inflamed gingiva, together with pocket formation and exudation, are typical of periodontitis. The periodontal ligament is considerably widened at the crestal areas, probably because of mobility. At

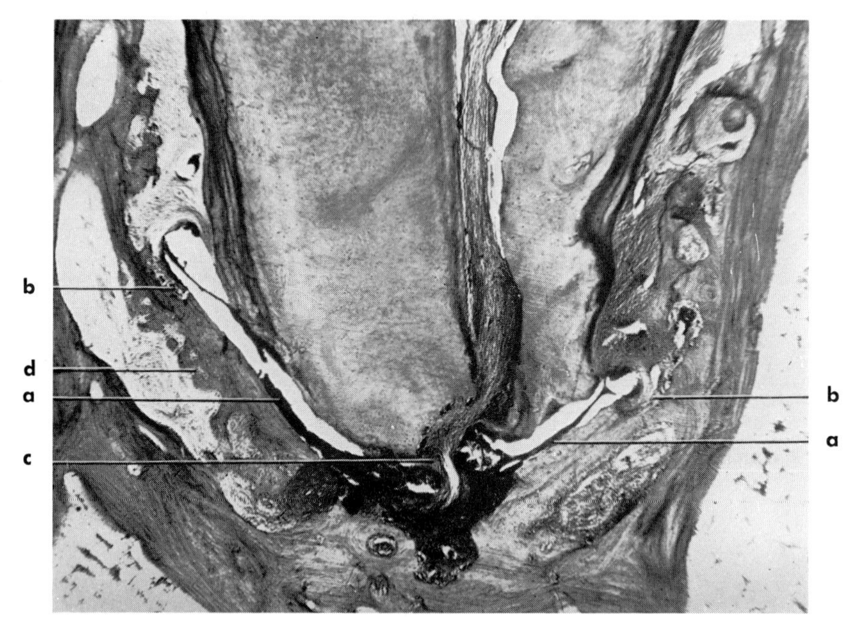


**Fig. 36-23.** Apical area of a human tooth that has been severely traumatized. *a,* Necrosis; *b,* undermining bone resorption in progress in different areas; *c,* severe necrosis directly at the apical foramen (such incidents explain occasional findings of irritation and necrosis of the pulp); *d,* endosteal bone formation.

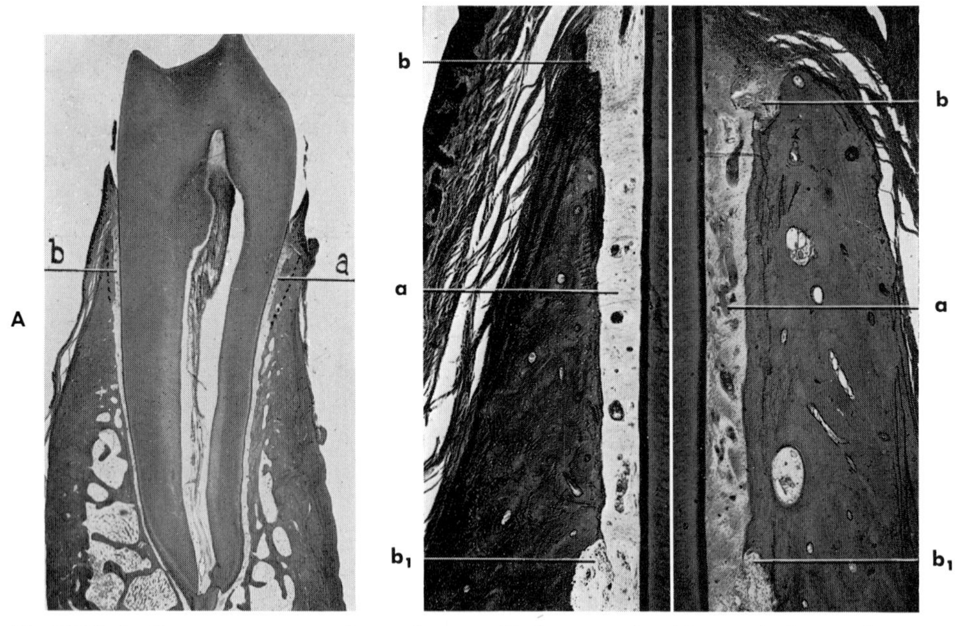


**Fig. 36-24. A,** Human autopsy specimen of a mandibular premolar. Traumatized necrotic areas are evident on the vestibular, *a,* as well as the oral, *b,* surfaces of the alveolar margin. Dotted line indicates the amount of bone resorption and widening of the periodontal ligament space that could have been expected by continued bruxism had the patient survived. **B,** Higher magnification showing the oral and vestibular margins. *a,* Hyalinization of connective tissue and thrombosed blood vessels can be observed. Undermining bone resorption is in progress on both the coronal, *b,* and the apical, $b_1$, ends of the necrotic areas.

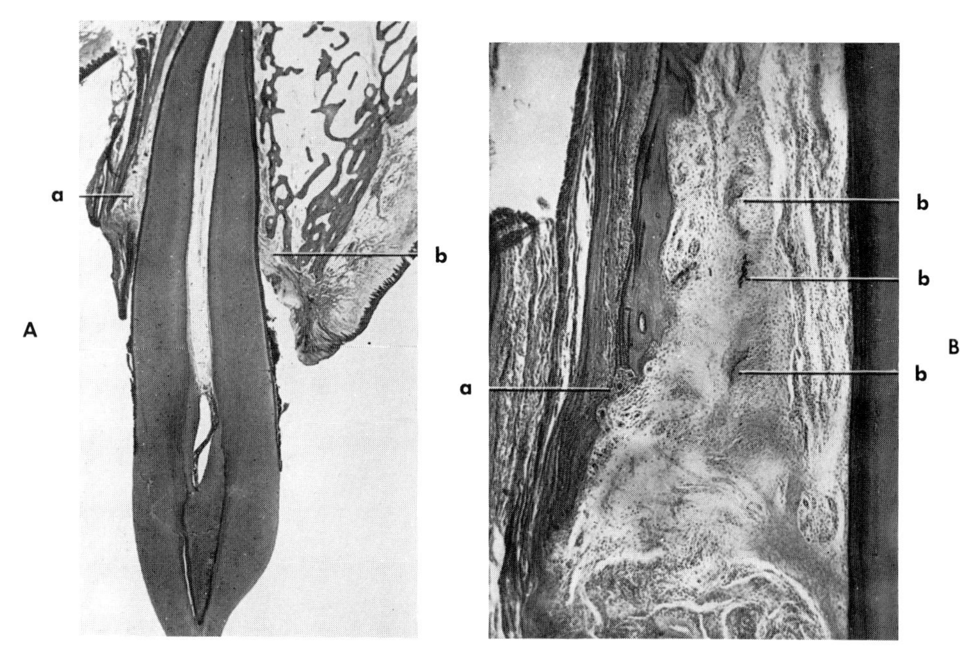


**Fig. 36-25. A,** Histologic section of a maxillary lateral incisor with severe periodontitis and extensive exposure of the root surfaces. The periodontal ligament space appears funnel shaped on both the labial, *a,* and the palatal, *b,* surfaces. **B,** Higher magnification of the marginal alveolus on the labial surface. The periodontal ligament space is wide and without any organized principal fibers. *a,* Osteoclastic activity in progress; *b,* several bone spicules apparent in the periodontal ligament, indicating what may have been the former alveolus.

higher magnification of the labial alveolar margin (Fig. 36-25, *B*), the active resorption process still in progress can be observed. There are osteoclasts in lacunae of the thin alveolar plate. The periodontal ligament consists, more or less, of loose connective tissue and barely qualifies as a ligament in this area. On close inspection a few small bone spicules are evident, remnants of the former alveolar bone proper.

Another human autopsy specimen with similar findings is shown in Fig. 36-26, *A*. The exact age of this patient is unknown, but he was apparently in his late forties to early fifties. The occlusion had been mutilated by extraction of several teeth. The second and third mandibular molars were tipped anteriorly. Microscopic examination (*B*) revealed a deep intra-alveolar (infrabony) pocket on the mesial aspect of the second molar. Below the pocket a dark body could be seen in the widened periodontal space. Higher magnification of the area (*C*) revealed a cemental tear—a piece of cementum torn from the root surface. Such cemental tears are reported in the literature, the result of sudden occlusal trauma, most often from a blow. A sudden, forceful closure might also have caused this, especially if the periodontium had been weakened, as in this case. A necrotic tissue mass lined with macrophages could be seen on the distal aspect of the distal root (*D*). This necrotic area presumably was once the periodontal ligament, destroyed by pressure from the tipping tooth. The adjacent bone showed osteoclastic activity. Such tissue changes, even though microscopic, are possible only if adjacent teeth are not in firm continuous contact. If firm continuous contact

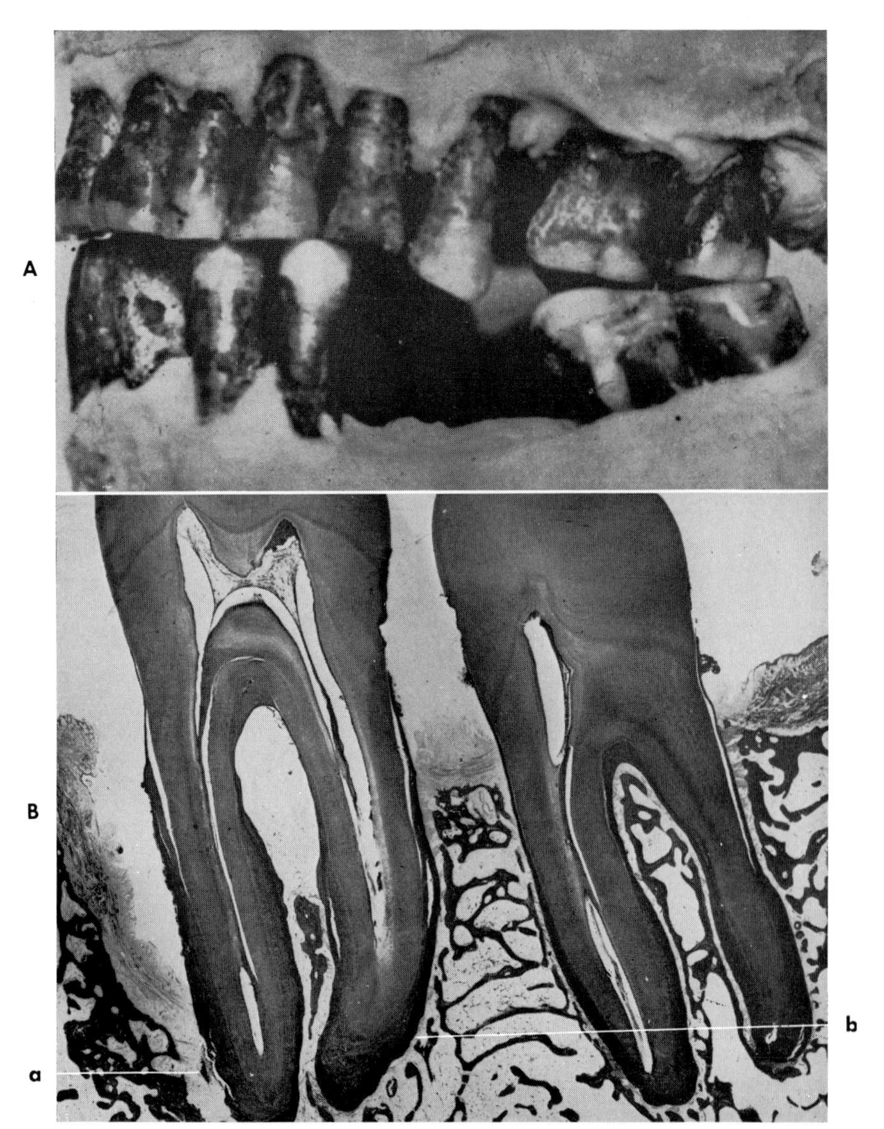


**Fig. 36-26. A,** Human autopsy specimen showing the relation of the molars to each other. The mandibular second and third molars are tipped mesially. The second premolar and first molar are missing. **B,** Microscopic section of the two mandibular molars. A deep intra-alveolar pocket is present on the mesial surface of the second molar. The bifurcation is exposed. The lamina dura of the alveolar bone at the distal aspect of the apical areas of both molars (areas of pressure) appears more discontinuous than the rest of the sockets. *a,* Cemental tear; *b,* pressure area.

exists, traumatic changes are not likely to occur on mesial or distal surfaces because the teeth brace one another in this direction.

These cases are typical of secondary traumatism, in which bone loss weakens the periodontium by reducing the alveolar surface available for the insertion of periodontal fibers and leads to a subsequent mobility of the teeth. The reduced or weakened periodontium cannot withstand occlusal forces that previously were normal and nontraumatic.

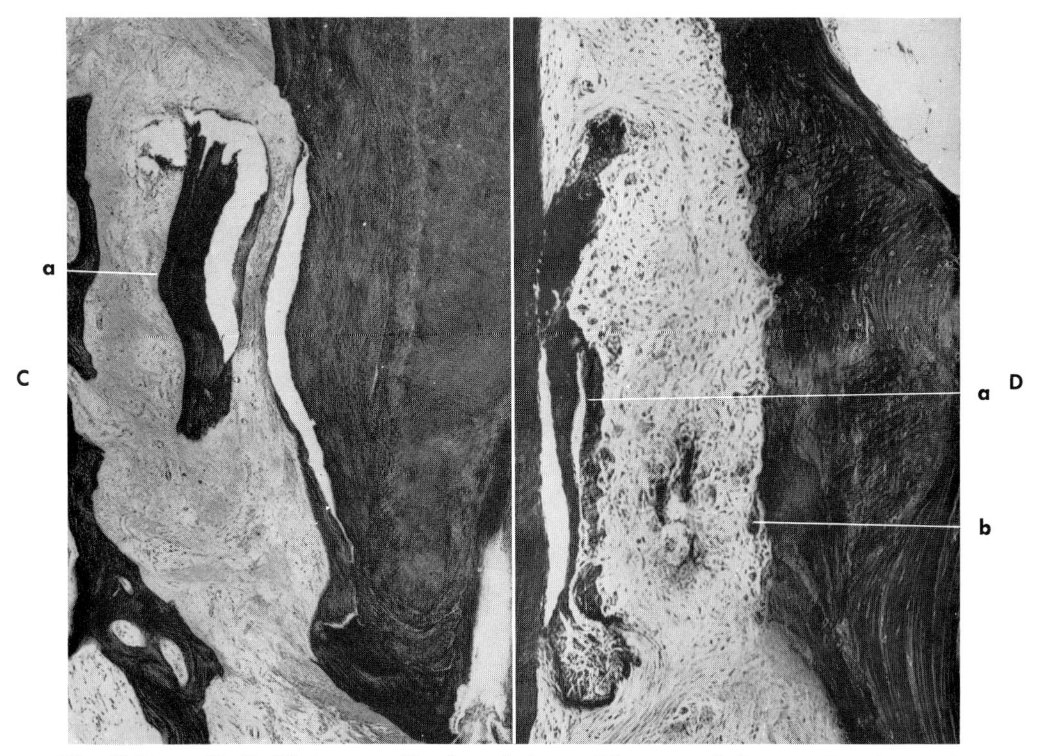


**Fig. 36-26, cont'd. C,** Higher magnification of the mesial aspect of the second molar. *a,* Cementum fragment that has been torn from the tooth. **D,** Necrotic area. *a,* Sign of the injury on the distal surface of the distal root of the second molar; *b,* resorption of the necrotic tissue and bone in progress.

*It should be reemphasized that occlusal traumatism does not cause gingivitis, periodontitis, or pocket formation.*[13] *The pathologic features of traumatism are basically different from those of inflammation.*[12,13] Traumatic tissue damage heals by formation of granulation tissue, proliferation of capillaries and fibroblasts, and activity of macrophages. This healing process need not be considered to be an inflammatory process. It will be helpful at this point to review Chapter 10, on inflammation—a basic but complex tissue response. Descriptions vary but invariably include cellular infiltration. In traumatism, of course, circulatory disturbance is present, which is created by the mechanical obstruction of blood flow in the traumatized area. Although circulatory disturbance leads ultimately to necrosis, it does not show the classical cellular signs of inflammation. There are no leukocytes, lymphocytes, or plasma cells in or around these necrotic areas or around other traumatic lesions. Elimination of such lesions starts from the periphery, when circulation is not impaired. Repair and regeneration are initiated without the classical signs of inflammation.

Whether occlusal trauma in the presence of preexisting inflammatory disease can cause the formation of pockets or typical vertical bone resorption is a hotly debated and controversial hypothesis.[19,28a,29]

Attempts have been made to classify the traumatic tissue changes as dystrophic disturbances. This designation is not entirely correct because of the transient nature of the typical traumatism lesion. These traumatic necrotic areas are not permanent lesions. They can undergo complete repair and regeneration.

The special nature and clinical importance of traumatic lesions of the periodontium make a separate classification of periodontal trauma necessary. Therefore the condition has been separated from inflammatory and dystrophic types of periodontal disorders in this text. The most important reason, however, for discussing traumatism as a separate entity is the clinical significance of the resulting tissue changes.

Periodontal trauma does not produce either gingivitis or periodontitis and cannot be held responsible for the dystrophic diseases—periodontosis, recession, and hyperplasia. Why, then, worry about occlusion in periodontal diseases, and why undertake extensive procedures to correct existing occlusal disharmonies? The answer may be found in the conclusion that structure and function are interrelated.

## RELATION OF FUNCTION AND STRUCTURE

Function and structure cannot exist without each other. This statement does not imply a mechanistic concept related to preconceived ideas of articulation derived from full denture prosthesis. Rather, it emphasizes an interrelation in the biologic sense. A good masticatory organ is one that functions comfortably and, in functioning, preserves the structural integrity of the component tissues. Pathology cannot be inferred simply because teeth do not come together as we would like them to do; nor does occlusal arrangement determine whether trauma is present. Only tissue changes can illustrate the presence of trauma.

## TISSUE CHANGES CAUSED BY PERIODONTAL TRAUMATISM

The following changes caused by occlusal traumatism may occur in the periodontal structures.

***Periodontal ligament***

In the *acute* phase of trauma, there is compression on the pressure side; crushing, hemorrhage, thrombosis, and necrosis of the periodontal ligament may occur. There is stretching on the tension side; sometimes this may cause thrombosis of the vessels and tearing of the ligament. In the *chronic* phase the periodontal ligament becomes wider; this may be reflected in clinical mobility.[31] (See discussion on experimental occlusal traumatism.) There may be hyalinization (Fig. 36-24, *B*) and a subsequent formation of fibrocartilage.[32,33] Ankylosis may occur.[33]

***Cementum***

In the *acute* phase there may be cemental tears[33] and fractures. In the chronic phase reparative changes such as cemental hyperplasia and formation of cementum spurs may occur. In addition, however, concurrent destructive changes occur (i.e., cemental resorption); and in some cases dentinal resorption may follow.

***Alveolar bone***

The physiologic reaction of alveolar bone to moderate pressure is resorption; to moderate tension, it is apposition. During the *acute* phase necrosis of bone may occur in areas of total compression of the periodontal ligament. This is followed by resorption. These mechanisms work to reestablish the normal width of the periodontal ligament. If, however, the traumatism is continued or if the reaction of the patient is poor, excessive widening of the periodontal ligament may result. This may be seen roentgenographically as a wider or funnel-shaped periodontal ligament space. Occasionally the widening appears as a rarefaction in the apical and furcation areas. Interruptions in the continuity of the lamina dura may also be seen on roentgenograms.

*Gingiva*

There is no evidence that either gingival changes or pocket formation occur as a consequence of occlusal traumatism per se; nor can festooned gingival margins or clefts be related to occlusal traumatism. The original explanation given for exaggerated marginal festooning of the gingiva and gingival clefts was that occlusal traumatism caused an impingement on the blood supply reaching the gingiva through the periodontal ligament. It has been shown, however, that the supply to the buccal and lingual gingivae is mainly through periosteal vessels coursing along the buccal and lingual surfaces of the alveolar process. Compression of the periodontal ligament will not occlude these vessels. Blanching of the gingiva can occur, however, if extremely loose teeth are luxated. In this case there will be direct impingement of the tooth against the soft tissues and the alveolar crest must have previously been resorbed to much lower levels because of periodontitis.

*Pulp*

Odontoblastic activity may be stimulated, and secondary dentin may be formed. The pulp chamber and canal may become narrower and even obliterated. Pulp stones may be formed. In some cases there may even be pulpitis and loss of pulpal vitality.

## ELECTRONIC TOOLS FOR STUDYING OCCLUSION

### Electromyography

Electromyography, the study and measurement of electric impulses generated by muscle activity, has been used for the study of occlusion. In cases of occlusal disharmonies, the electric discharges at the activation of the masticatory musculature are asynchronous, asymmetric, and hypertonic.[36] After successful therapy these return to a more normal pattern.[37]

### Telemetry

Another interesting tool for the study of periodontal occlusal relationships is intraoral telemetry, which utilizes miniaturized radio transmitters built into dental restorations. The transmitters enable the investigator to monitor and record signals at each occlusal contact.[38-41]

#### CHAPTER 36

#### References

1. Stein, G., and Weinmann, J. P.: Die physiologische Wanderung der Zähne, Z. Stomat. **23**:733, 1925.
2. Black, G. V.: Special dental pathology, Chicago, 1915, Medico-Dental Publishing Co.
3. Black, G. V.: Operative dentistry, ed. 6, revised by A. D. Black, Chicago, 1924, Medico-Dental Publishing Co., vol. 1.
4. Sicher, H.: Tooth eruption; the axial movement of teeth with limited growth, J. Dent. Res. **21**:395, 1942.
5. Weinmann, J. P.: Bone changes related to eruption of the teeth, Angle Orthodont. **11**:83, 1941.
6. Weinmann, J. P., and Sicher, H.: Correlation of active and passive eruption, Bur **46**:128, 1946.
7. Kronfeld, R.: Structure, function and pathology of the human periodontal membrane, New York J. Dent. **6**:112, 1936.
8. Gottlieb, B.: Ein Fall von scheinbarer Verkürzung eines oberen Schneidezahnes, Z. Stomat. **22**:501, 1924.
9. Kotanyi, E.: Ein weiterer klinischer Beweis des kontinuierlichen Zahndurchbruches, Z. Stomat. **28**:1055, 1930.
10. Noyes, F. B.: Submerging deciduous molars, Angle Orthodont. **2**:77, 1932.
11. Orban, B.: Ist das Paradentium eine organische Einheit? Z. Stomat. **24**:515, 1932.

12. Gottlieb, B., and Orban, B.: Die Veränderung der Gewebe bei übermässiger Beanspruchung der Zähne, Leipzig, 1931, Georg Thieme Verlag.
13. Bhaskar, S. N., and Orban, B.: Experimental occlusal trauma, J. Periodont. **26**:270, 1955.
14. Klein, L., and Weiss, P. H.: Induced connective tissue metabolism in vivo: reutilization of pre-existing collagen, Proc. Nat. Acad. Sci. **56**:277, 1966.
15. Stern, I. B.: An electron microscopic study of cementum, Sharpey's fibers and periodontal ligament in the rat incisor, Amer. J. Anat. **115**:377, 1964.
16. Stallard, R. E.: The utilization of $H^3$-proline by the connective tissue elements of the periodontium, Periodontics **1**:185, 1963.
17. Crumley, P. J.: Collagen formation in the normal and stressed periodontium, Periodontics **2**:53, 1964.
18. Carneiro, J., and Fava de Moraes, F.: Radioautographic visualization of collagen metabolism in the periodontal tissues of the mouse, Arch. Oral Biol. **10**:833, 1965.
18a. Weinmann, J. P.: Progress of gingival inflammation into the supporting structures of the teeth, J. Periodont. **12**:71, 1941.
19. Macapanpan, L. C., and Weinmann, J. P.: The influence of injury to the periodontal membrane on the spread of gingival inflammation, J. Dent. Res. **33**:263, 1954.
20. Comar, M., Kollar, J., and Gargiulo, A.: Local irritation and occlusal trauma as co-factors in the periodontal disease process, J. Periodont. **40**:193, 1969.
21. Glickman, I., and Smulow, J. B.: Alteration in the pathway of gingival inflammation into the underlying tissues induced by excessive occlusal forces, J. Periodont. **33**:7, 1962.
21a. Wentz, F. M., Jarabek, J., and Orban, B.: Experimental trauma imitating cuspal interferences, J. Periodont. **29**:117, 1958.
22. Orban, B.: Tissue changes in traumatic occlusion, J. Amer. Dent. Ass. **15**:2090, 1928.
23. Kronfeld, R.: Histologic study of the influence of function on the human periodontal membrane, J. Amer. Dent. Ass. **18**:1242, 1931.
24. Kronfeld, R.: Physiology of the human periodontal tissues under normal and abnormal occlusal conditions, Illinois Dent. J. **8**:13, 1939.
25. Bödecker, C. F.: Critical review of Gottlieb and Orban's "Die Veränderungen der Gewebe bei übermässiger Beanspruchung der Zähne," Ortho. Oral Surg. Rad. Int. J. **18**:895, 1932.
26. Orban, B., and Weinmann, J.: Signs of traumatic occlusion in average human jaws, J. Dent. Res. **13**:216, 1933.
27. Oppenheim, A.: Human tissue response to orthodontic intervention, Amer. J. Orthodont. **28**:263, 1942.
28. Gargiulo, A., Wentz, F. M., and Orban, B.: Dimensions and relations of the dentogingival junction in humans, J. Periodont. **32**:261, 1961.
28a. Glickman, I.: Role of occlusion in the etiology and treatment of periodontal disease, J. Dent. Res. **50**:199, 1971.
29. Drum, W.: Parafunktionen und Autodestruktionsprozesse, Berlin, 1969, Quintessenz.
30. Stahl, S. S.: The responses of the periodontium to combined gingival inflammation and occluso-functional stresses in four human specimens, Periodontics **6**:14, 1968.
31. Picton, D. C. A., and Slatter, J. M.: The effect on horizontal tooth mobility of experimental trauma to the periodontal membrane in regions of tension and compression in monkeys, J. Periodont. Res. **7**:35, 1972.
32. Everett, F. G., and Bruckner, R. J.: Cartilage in the periodontal ligament space, J. Periodont. **41**:165, 1970.
33. Grant, D. A., and Bernick, S.: The periodontium of ageing humans, J. Periodont. (In press.)
34. Waerhaug, J., and Hansen, E. R.: Periodontal changes incident to prolonged occlusal overload in monkeys, Acta Odont. Scand. **24**:91, 1966.
35. Glickman, I., and Smulow, J. B.: Further observations on the effects of trauma from occlusion in humans, J. Periodont. **38**:280, 1967.
36. Butler, J. H., and Stallard, R. E.: Effect of occlusal relationships on neuro-physiological pathways, J. Periodont. Res. **4**:141, 1969.
37. Ramfjord, S. P., and Ash, M. M., Jr.: Occlusion, ed. 2, Philadelphia, 1971, W. B. Saunders Co.
38. Butler, J. H.: Recent research on physiology of occlusion, Dental Clinics of North America, Philadelphia, 1969, W. B. Saunders Co., vol. 13.
39. Adams, S. H., and Zander, H. A.: Functional tooth contacts in lateral and in centric occlusion, J. Amer. Dent. Ass. **69**:465, 1964.
40. Glickman, I., Pameijer, J. H. N., Roeber, F. W., and others: Functional occlusion as re-

vealed by miniaturized radio transmitters, Dental Clinics of North America, Philadelphia, 1969, W. B. Saunders Co., vol. 13.
41. Schärer, P., and Stallard, R. E.: The use of multiple radio transmitters in studies of tooth contact patterns, Periodontics 3:5, 1965.

**Additional suggested reading**

Carranza, F. A., Jr., Simes, R. J., and Cabrini, R. L.: Effect of combined etiologic factors in experimental periodontal lesions, J. Periodont. Res., supp. 4, 1969. Abstract 28.

Dotto, C. A., Carranza, F. A., Jr., Cabrini, R. L., and others: Vascular changes in experimental trauma from occlusion, J. Periodont. **38**:183, 1967.

Geiger, A. M., Wasserman, B. H., Thompson, R. H., and others: Relationship of occlusion and periodontal disease. I, A system for evaluating periodontal status, J. Periodont. **42**:364, 1971.

Glickman, I.: Occlusion—a factor in periodontal health and disease in the circumpubertal and adolescent periods, J. Periodont. **42**:513, 1971.

Gottlieb, B., and Orban, B.: Biology and pathology of the teeth and its supporting mechanism, New York, 1938, The Macmillan Co.

Itoiz, M. E., Carranza, F. A., Jr., and Cabrini, R. I.: Histologic and histometric study of experimental occlusal trauma in rats, J. Periodont. **34**:305, 1963.

Mühlemann, H. R., and Herzog, H.: Tooth mobility and microscopic tissue changes produced by experimental occlusal trauma, Helv. Odont. Acta **5**:33, 1961.

Rateitschak, K. H., and Herzog-Specht, F. A.: Reaktion und Regeneration des Parodonts auf orthodontische Behandlung mit festsitzenden Apparaten, Schweiz. Mschr. Zahnheilk, **75**:741, 1965.

Reitan, K.: Tissue behavior during orthodontic tooth movement, Amer. J. Orthodont. **46**:881, 1960.

Stallard, R. E.: The effect of occlusal alterations on collagen formation within the periodontium, Periodontics **2**:49, 1964.

Wasserman, B. H., Thompson, R. H., Geiger, A. M., and others: Relationship of occlusion and periodontal disease. II, Periodontal status of the study population, J. Periodont. **42**:371, 1971.

Weinmann, J. P.: The adaptation of the periodontal membrane to physiologic and pathologic changes, Oral Surg. **8**:977, 1955.

Wentz, F. M., Jarabek, J., and Orban, B.: Experimental trauma imitating cuspal interferences, J. Periodont. **29**:117, 1958.

CHAPTER THIRTY-SEVEN

# Treatment of periodontal trauma



The proper management of occlusion is not merely a problem of periodontics—it is a problem of dentistry. The functional relationship of the dentition should be of paramount concern to all dentists.

To discuss occlusion from the periodontal point of view, we must have a clear understanding of the concepts and terminology that are basic to occlusion. Then we may proceed to the consideration of periodontal trauma and its treatment.

There is probably no other phase of dentistry so confused by divergence of terminology and definitions as the field of occlusion. The reader must have some insight into this problem and also a vocabulary to facilitate his learning the technique of grinding as a treatment for occlusal traumatism. Without a vocabulary, explanation of occlusion and correction of traumatism is difficult, and without a common vocabulary and defined terms, communication and understanding are impossible. Since there is no universally accepted terminology used by those who discuss occlusion,[1] it is necessary to define the terms as used in this text.

## TERMINOLOGY IN OCCLUSION

*Occlusion*

Occlusion is the relationship of the teeth when they are in contact, regardless of jaw position. Therefore the full range of jaw positions within which the teeth can make contact is included in this term.

*Rest position of the mandible*

The mandible is in rest position when the jaw is held in a relaxed state and is not being used in speech, swallowing, mastication, or parafunctional movements. Although the jaw is at rest, the muscles are not truly at rest since this position is controlled by muscle tonus. The teeth are not involved in rest position. There is an average space of 2 to 3 mm. between the upper and lower teeth, which is known as the freeway space or the interocclusal clearance.[2-5] After a person swallows or speaks, the mandible automatically assumes this position. However, since it is a postural position, it can vary with the way in which the person holds his head or body. Although rest position is considered to be relatively stable, it can be influenced by fatigue, nervous tension, or any of the physiologic or pathologic factors that influence muscle length and tonus.

***Centric***

There are a variety of definitions and usages of the term centric. Some authors think that when all the teeth are in occlusal contact the position is centric. Others believe that centric occurs with the mandible in its most retruded position. Still others believe that centric occurs slightly anterior to this point. Each group considers its defined position to be *true* centric. Terms such as false centric, acquired centric, habitual centric, or functional centric illustrate the divergence of opinions. Finally, there are some men who believe centric to be a relationship (rather than a position) of the jaws throughout the range of a certain border movement, with centric occlusion occurring at the termination in closure. These various usages are almost indelibly imprinted in our literature and language. In reading, you must try to assess which definition the author is using when he says centric.

"Centric occlusion is a tooth to tooth and jaw to jaw relationship, in which the teeth are in ideal intercuspation and all components of the masticatory system—the temporomandibular joint, the neuromuscular elements and the occlusal surfaces are in a harmonious relationship."*

To understand occlusion, you must accept centric as an *ideal* position without defining its precise location and then turn your attention to the terminal hinge relationship of the mandible.

***Terminal hinge position***

The terminal hinge position is the most retruded position of the condyle in the glenoid fossa that the patient can achieve by the activity of his own musculature (Fig. 37-1). The term refers to movement of the mandible with the head of the condyle in the most retruded position in the fossa. In this movement the mandible turns without any translating component on an arc whose axis lies in the condyle.

The importance of this movement is that the edentulous patient or the patient deprived of cuspal guidance can be trained to repeatedly go through the movement while points along the path of the movement are registered and reregistered. At a given degree of opening, a fixed reference point can be used in mounting casts on an articulator. The opening of the mandible in the terminal hinge relation is a trained movement. Humans can move their mandibles in the hinge relationship when trained to do so. Properly instructed, they can duplicate the movement. Terminal hinge relation is called *centric relation* by some authors.[5] Terminal hinge position is sometimes also called *hinge position, centric occlusion,* or *retruded position.*

***Terminal hinge occlusion***

If one closes his jaws with the lower incisors protruded beyond the upper incisors (*P* in Figs. 37-1 and 37-2) and then draws his lower jaw slowly backward, he will soon contact the maxillary incisors; then opening slightly so that the incisal edges clear each other, he will ultimately come to a point known as the terminus of the hinge relation. In this position he achieves terminal hinge occlusion (Fig. 37-2).

To review and correlate the foregoing discussion, remember that *occlusal position* is a position in which there is full contact of all teeth. This term covers

*From Ramfjord, S. P.: J. Amer. Dent. Ass. 62:21, 1961.

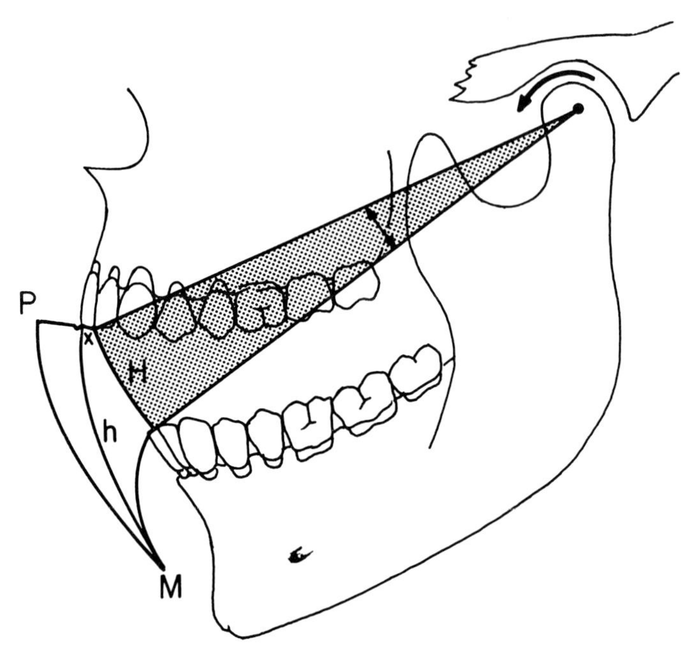


**Fig. 37-1.** The terminal hinge relation of the mandible, *H,* is the rotational path that the mandible makes about an axis in the condyles. This path is the most retruded rotational movement the patient can make under the control of his own musculature. *P,* Maximal protrusion; *M,* maximal open position; *h,* habitual closing movement.

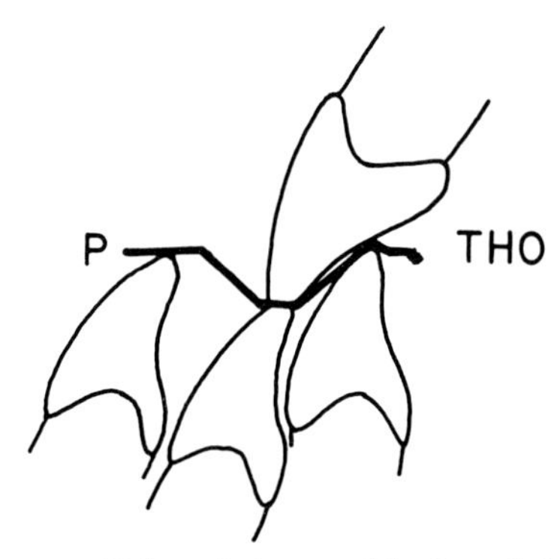


**Fig. 37-2.** Path described by the mandible as it is moved backward from its most protruded position, *P,* in full closure to the most retruded position that the patient can voluntarily assume. *THO,* Terminal hinge occlusion, which is the closure in terminal hinge relation.

any of the terms used earlier for centric (e.g., false, true, acquired, habitual, functional).

***Intercuspal position***

The intercuspal position is the firm intermeshing of a maximum number of cusps and fossae of the mandibular teeth touching tightly against the maxillary teeth. The position of the condyle in the glenoid fossa in the intercuspal position is thus determined by the maximum intercuspation of the teeth. Since the intercuspation can be altered by many factors (extractions, restorations), the position of the condyle in the glenoid fossa may not be the same as when it is determined by an ideal relationship of other components of the masticatory system (i.e., the temporomandibular joint, neuromuscular elements, and surrounding tissues).

*Median occlusal position*

When occlusal contact is made in the median plane, it is called the median occlusal position.[6] This distinction is particularly important because there are the other occlusal positions. Sicher stated, "If one opens the jaws wide and then snaps them shut, the closing muscles pull the jaw unerringly and unhesitatingly into the median occlusal position."* This is a directed movement and is not unique to the jaws. Neurologists, testing proprioceptive nerves and neural pathways, have long used a similar movement in their battery of tests. The patient is asked to touch the tip of his nose with the tip of his forefinger with his eyes closed. If there is no disease of the nervous system, he is able to do so without difficulty, although there may be some variation in many normal individuals. Proprioceptive signals play a role in guiding the shoulder, elbow, wrist, and finger into an efficient, almost precise pattern of movement. The impulses that guide this recognizable and repeatable movement arise in all the participating muscles and joints. The pattern of control (engram) is retained in the "memory banks" of the brain.

A similar memory of proprioceptive impulses also guides the mandibular muscles by reflex feedback when the jaw snaps shut. However, this movement is extraordinarily precise because neural stimuli arising in the periodontium are added to those arising in muscles and joints. The periodontal memory (engram) is subject to change with time. Eruptive and migratory tooth movements and attrition bring about changes in proprioception that, even in a completely healthy dentition, require revision of the engram to changes. Therefore the proprioceptive periodontal memory is a fleeting memory that may be recaptured or reestablished repeatedly. This occurs whenever the teeth meet in the median occlusal position.[1,7]

Edentulous people who have lost their periodontal ligaments and, consequently, the related proprioceptive nerve impulses must depend mainly on proprioceptive receptors in the capsule of the joint and the masticatory muscles.

*Protrusive and lateral occlusal positions*

An anterior occlusal position (protrusive position) and a right or left lateral occlusal position also exist. If the median occlusal position is slightly anterior to the most retruded or terminal hinge position, then we can also speak of a posterior or retrusive occlusal position. The movement into each position from median occlusal position can be termed protrusive movement, right or left lateral movement, and retrusive movement. Sometimes these movements are referred to as glides or excursive movements. The teeth also occlude in other positions intermediate between the lateral and protrusive positions and the median occlusal position.

## RANGE OF MANDIBULAR MOVEMENTS

Similar mechanisms operate when one places the incisors edge to edge (in protrusive position) or is told to touch a lower canine to an upper canine. A patient may voluntarily assume an occlusal position within the limits set by his dentition, the form of his maxilla and mandible, the mobility of his temporomandibular joints, and the ability of his musculature. In fact, he may also move the mandible with his mouth open within limits set by these same structures. You may explore these borders by opening your mouth as wide as possible, protrud-

*From Sicher, H.: J. Amer. Dent. Ass. **48**:620, 1954.

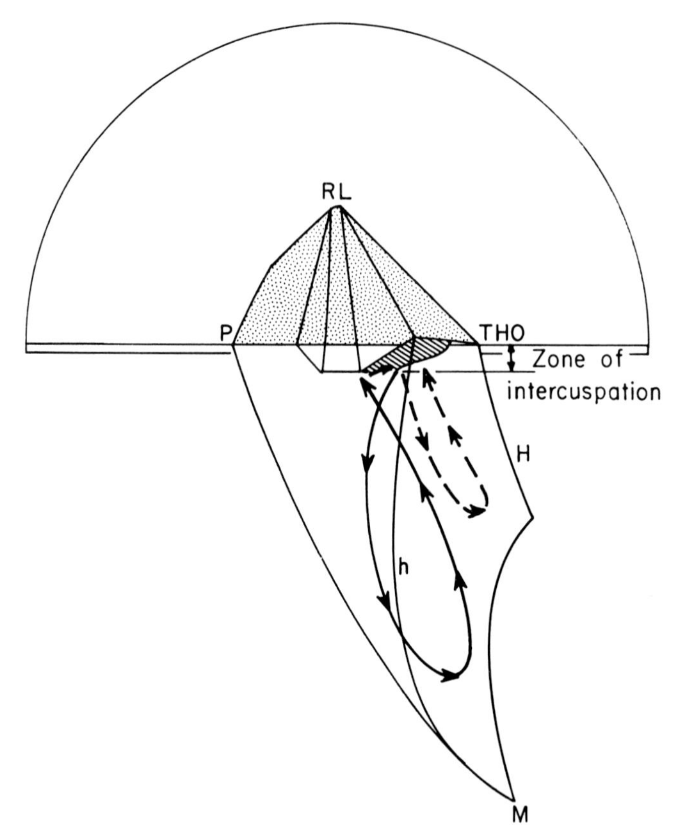


**Fig. 37-3.** A tracing plate has been used to describe the horizontal limits of mandibular movement (stippled) and the relationship to the limits of motion in a median plane. Half the plate has been removed and only those movements to the right of the median plane are shown. Arrows indicate chewing, which will be explained later in the text. *h,* Habitual closing movement; *THO,* terminal hinge occlusion; *P,* maximal protrusion; *H,* hinge movement; *M,* maximal open position.

ing the jaw as far as possible, and moving to the limits of right and left lateral excursive movements with and without the teeth in contact. If a solid reconstruction of these limits as described by the tips of the lower incisors were made, it would form a three-dimensional structure with some degree of bilateral symmetry. If it were then bisected, you could examine the range of movement in a median plane. (Reexamine Figs. 37-1 and 37-2.) The former shows the range of movement of the mandible in the median sagittal plane.

The lateral borders of movement may be noted in Fig. 37-3. A tracing plate is bisected to show the interrelationship between the horizontal and vertical borders that gives the three-dimensional extent of the envelope of motion.

***Gothic arch tracing***

The technique of using a central bearing screw and a tracing plate (Gothic arch tracing) temporarily simulates the edentulous state because tooth contact is prevented. When such a device is used, there are no coordinated nerve impulses from the periodontal ligament to guide the patient into the most retruded position. If, during hinge axis registration, a tracing (Gothic arch) is made by moving into right and left lateral position from the median occlusal position (Fig. 37-4), the apex of the angle is formed when the condyles are in the most retruded position.[9]

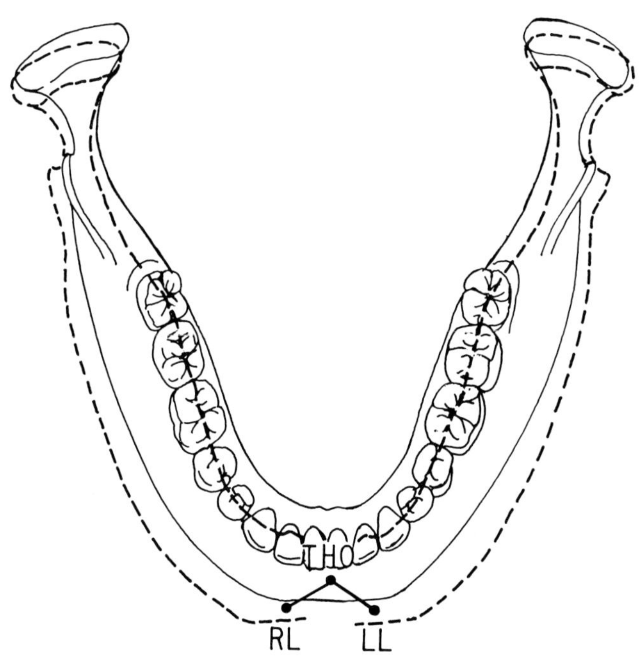


**Fig. 37-4.** Movement of the mandible from the most retruded position, *THO,* to the right lateral, *RL,* and left lateral, *LL,* positions (dotted outlines show the movement made), forming a Gothic arch tracing.

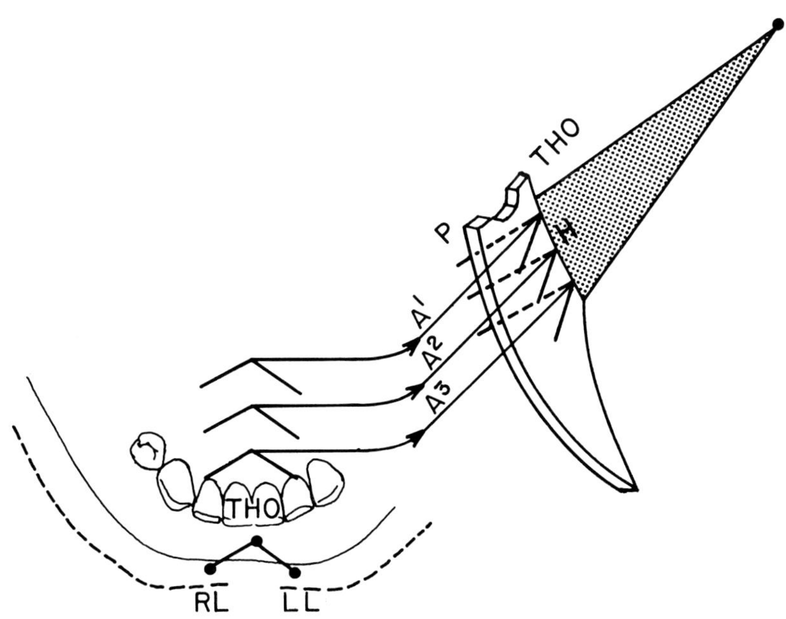


**Fig. 37-5.** Schematic drawing that relates Gothic arch tracings made in a horizontal plane with the hinge movement made in the median plane. Tracings $A^1$, $A^2$, $A^3$ can be made at different degrees of opening. Their apices contact the hinge movement or hinge relation, which is made up of an infinite number of superimposed Gothic arches. *P,* Most protruded position; *H,* hinge movement; *THO,* terminal hinge occlusion.

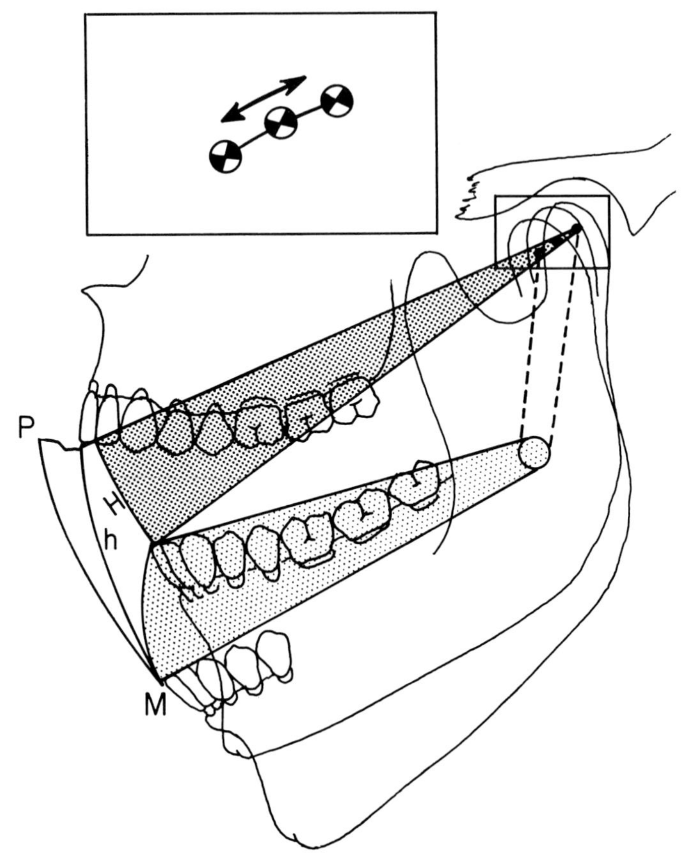


**Fig. 37-6.** Heavily stippled area represents hinge movement about a center of rotation in the condyle. The condyles continue to rotate beyond the limit of purely rotatory movement (see marking of magnified centers of rotation in inset) but also glide forward on the eminentia. These two movements, that is, further rotation and translation, have a projected center of rotation in the vicinity of the mandibular foramen. The opening beyond the limit of hinge rotation is indicated by the lightly stippled sector formed about the secondary center of rotation. The incisal point moves downward and forward and the chin point moves downward and backward as the center of rotation is carried forward by the translatory movement (see inset).

These Gothic arch tracings made at different degrees of opening can be superimposed to form part of the posterior limit of mandibular movement, that is, the terminal hinge movement (Fig. 37-5).

## Hinge movements

***Rotatory and translatory movements***

The terminal hinge movement is a limited one. The condyles are capable of a purely rotatory movement for only a short distance through a narrow arc formed by the edge of the lower incisors (*H* in Figs. 37-1 and 37-3). If the jaws continue to open, the condyles rotate further but at the same time glide forward on the articular eminences in a translatory movement (Fig. 37-6). The combined rotatory and translatory movements have a projected and more generalized center of rotation in the region of the mandibular foramen. The incisal edge moves downward and forward from the widest portion of the posterior boundary of mandibular movement (Fig. 37-6).

*Border movements*

The importance of these diagrams is that all mandibular movements must occur within their limits. The teeth may be used functionally in mastication, swallowing, and speech. They may also be used in parafunctional movements, which are discussed later. The border movements themselves are not used in mastication. Habitual mastication occurs within the borders (*h* in Figs. 37-1 and 37-3). The importance of terminal hinge movement and the interrelated terminal hinge occlusion is that they can be registered repeatedly with some degree of accuracy and can be used as a point of reference for mechanical articulators or the grinding of occlusion.

## Functional movements

*Mastication*

Consider the physiologic functional movements in mastication. These movements start with biting into food and continue with chewing, during which the food bolus is reduced in size as it is softened and moistened with saliva. The movements terminate with swallowing.

When one bites into food, arm and shoulder muscles are pitted against neck and masticatory muscles, by which means a piece of food is torn away. Considerable forces may be exerted on the teeth, yet the teeth do not make contact.

After the bite the initial chewing strokes are large and more protrusive in position (Fig. 37-3). The later strokes are smaller because the bolus is reduced, and the mandible moves toward the terminal hinge position (Fig. 37-7). The size of the bolus prevents the teeth from occluding in the early strokes, but with successive strokes the teeth come closer to each other and contact generally occurs prior to swallowing[10] (Fig. 37-7).

*Opening and closing movements*

The opening movement is performed more quickly than the closing movement, which is slower, more deliberate, and dependent on proprioceptive feedback signals.[11]

The path of movement is described as being teardrop in shape[11] (Figs. 37-7 and 37-8) and is directed from cusp incline toward the central fossa. Although there is considerable variation in the teardrop pattern, the range of movement away from the median occlusal position is limited. The border occlusal movements that you perform with articulators do not generally occur in mastication.

The opening and closing motions per se are isotonic and are not associated with strong forces. When resistance is met, isometric components develop. These are associated with greater forces but are controlled by proprioceptive impulses. Consequently heavy pressures are not generated unless the initial biting into food is especially forceful, the food is unusually coarse and resistant, the teeth are used to split hard objects (e.g., nuts), or a piece of bone or other hard material is unexpectedly encountered in the softer bolus.

## Parafunctional movements

If mastication does not generate heavy pressures, if the teeth do not contact during mastication in general, and if masticatory movements do not resemble articulator excursive glides, how then are the wear facets produced? They are distant from the median occlusal position and very common (Fig. 37-9). They are the result of parafunctional movements, which include bruxism,[12] clenching, and rocking of teeth. The term parafunction (outside or beyond function) was first suggested by Drum.[13]

*Bruxism*

Bruxism is the habit of grinding the teeth. It may occur during sleep or while awake. The patient is usually unaware of the habit which consists of rubbing the teeth in protrusive and lateral occlusal movements.

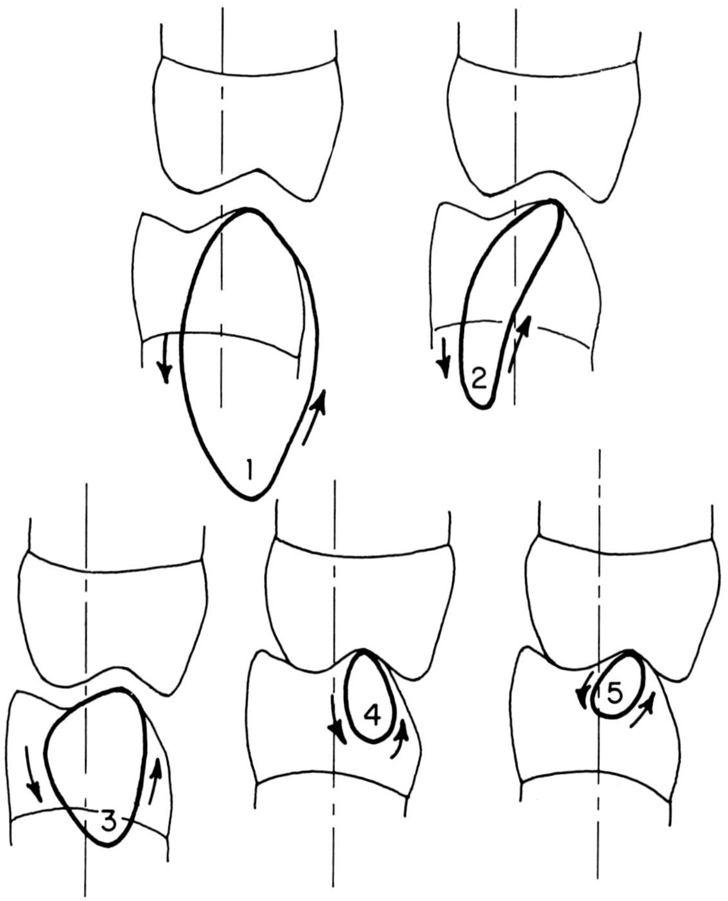


**Fig. 37-7.** Diagrams depicting five successive masticatory strokes, each made in the teardrop pattern. The first stroke is the largest, and the later strokes successively smaller. The teeth do not contact in strokes *1* through *3*, but light tooth contact is made in strokes *4* and *5* just prior to swallowing. (Adapted from Beyron, H.: Acta Odont. Scand. **22**:597, 1964.)

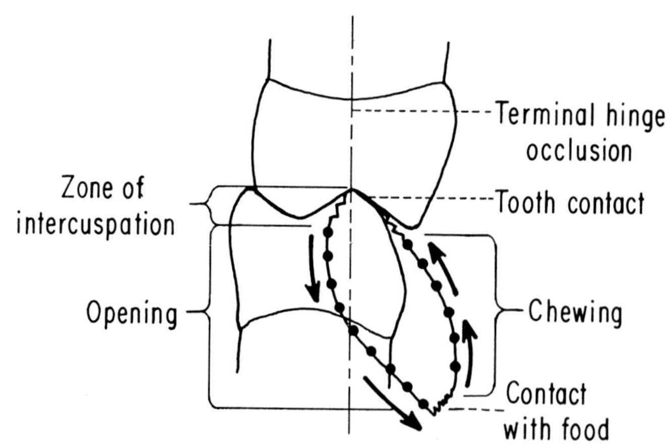


**Fig. 37-8.** Diagram depicting opening and closing movements between two opposing molars. The opening movement is performed quickly as the depressors of the mandible contract isotonically. When contact with food is made, isometric and isotonic elements combine under proprioceptive guidance and the mandible closes more slowly. Zigzag lines indicate influence of proprioceptive impulses. Chewing strokes are short of full closure. Tooth contact is made just prior to swallowing close to terminal hinge occlusion. Note the teardrop pattern and the stroke directed toward the median plane rather than toward the lateral position. The dots indicate actual recordings. (Adapted from Murphy, T. R.: Arch. Oral Biol. **10**:981, 1965.)

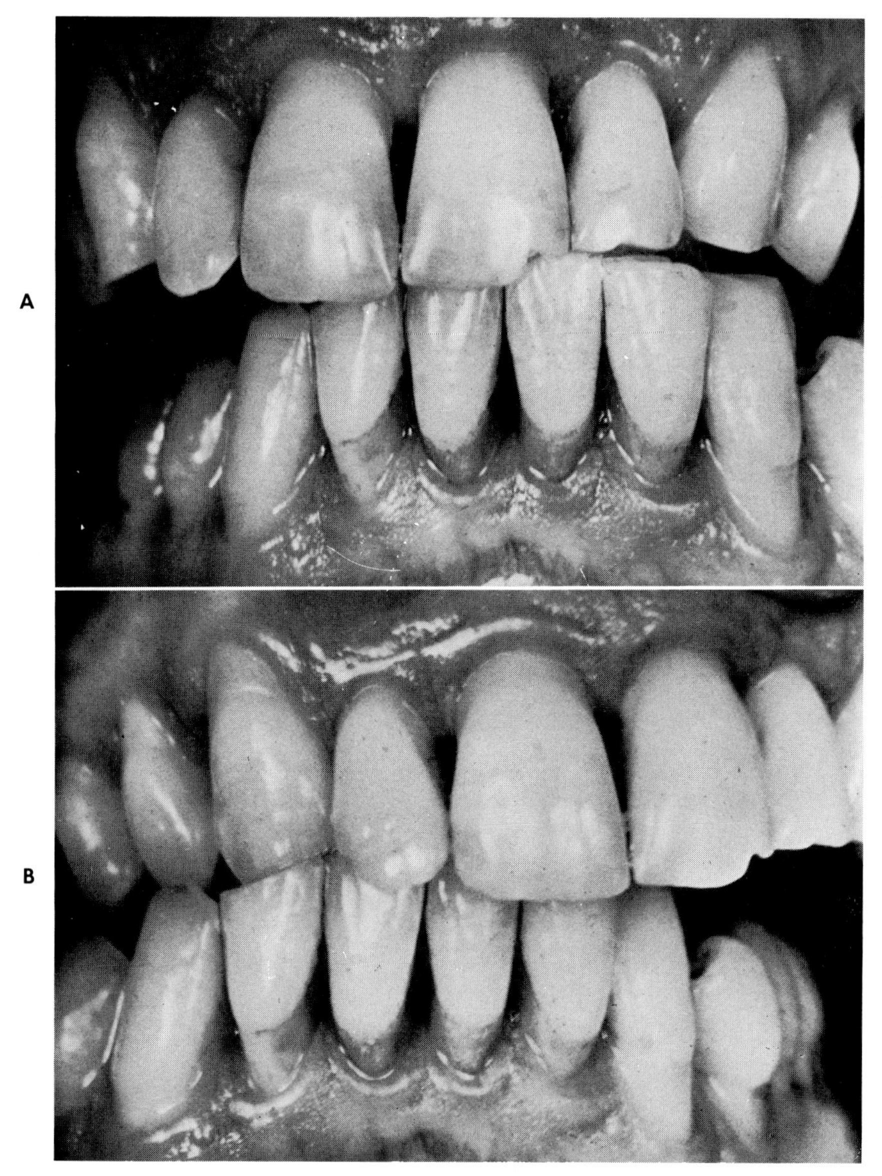


*Continued.*

**Fig. 37-9.** Dentition of a 30-year-old man in median occlusal, **A,** and protrusive, **B,** positions. The wear facets of the incisors fit the opposing teeth in extreme lateral positions, **C** and **D.** No inflammatory periodontal disease is present. Note the degree of intercuspation.

***Clenching and clamping***

Clenching and clamping are produced through isometric contraction of the masticatory muscles while the teeth are in contact, usually in median occlusal position.

***Rocking***

Rocking of the teeth, which is most deleterious, results when a slight lateral force is added to clenching.

Parafunctional movements are practically universal. They need not be abnormal or pathogenic.[14] It is not the presence of parafunctional movement but the excessive degree, frequency, and duration of these strong isometric contractions that contribute to pathology. Certainly if trauma does not result, the presence of parafunction is not pathologic. One could say that pathology results in

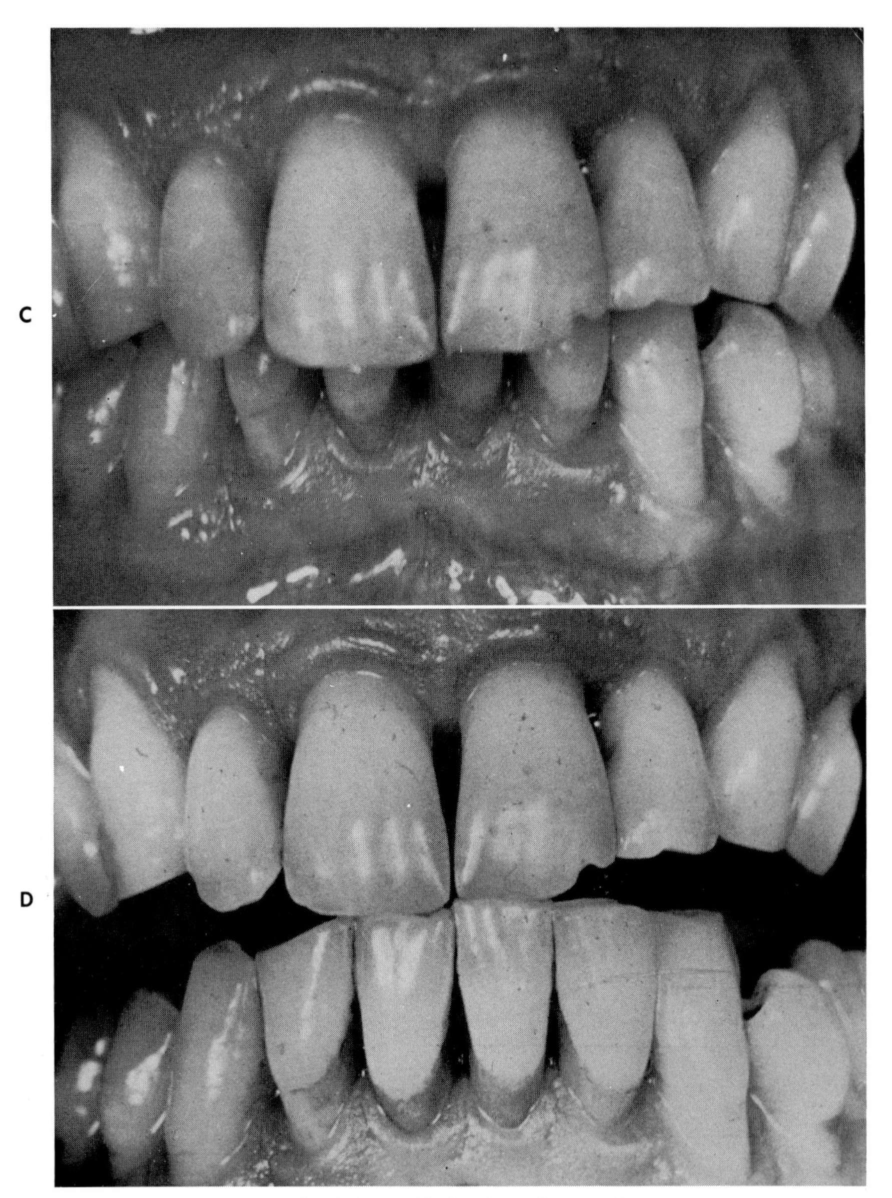


**Fig. 37-9, cont'd.** For legend see p. 601.

only a percentage of those who brux and clench. Indeed, parafunction may be useful in the dissipation of tension or of pent-up energy.

Causes for these habits are not fully known, but the habits may be psychologic, neurologic, occupational, or occlusal.[15-17] The psychologic causes may be tension or the unconscious expression of hate or displeasure.[18,19] (See the discussion on psychologic factors in Chapter 17.) When these emotions are portrayed by actors, the play of their masticatory musculature may be easily observed. Tetany (active or latent), meningitis, epilepsy, and parkinsonism constitute some of the neurologic causes for these phenomena, which may lead to hypertonicity of the masticatory musculature and to bruxism or clenching. Occupational bruxism or clenching can be seen in truck drivers[20,21] and in individuals performing feats of great strength. Sometimes bruxism may be related to stimuli from irregularities in the occlusion such as premature contacts or dental restorations that are too high; the patient tries to remove the annoying high point by compensatory parafunction.[18] Bruxism is also common in children and may permit the secondary teeth to erupt in proper position. Possibly, from a phylogenetic viewpoint, bruxism is a tooth-honing mechanism.[21a]

Persons who brux are often completely unaware of their habit and will often deny any inquiry made by the dentist. However, mates may comment about the noises produced during bruxing in sleep; and once the question is raised, the patient may then become aware of the habit. By no means, however, should the diagnosis be made in the form of an accusation implying pathology or abnormality. When some persons who brux awaken, they may feel the fatigue of the jaw muscles, pain in the temporomandibular joint, or limitation of ability to open wide. (See discussion of subjective indications of periodontal traumatism.)

Bruxism may lead to the formation of wear facets. The occlusal situation is aggravated as one tooth meets its opponent on flat planes and grips it more intimately during contact, thus contributing to the leverage and intensity of force application.

The importance of local tissue regeneration of the periodontium has been discussed. Everyday regenerative activities must go on. There is sufficient time for reparative turnover to compensate for tissue damage incident to mastication during the periods between meals when the masticatory organ is at rest. What might be significant in bruxism is that the regeneration period is reduced. When these habits occur in the presence of periodontal disease, additional stress and strain are put on the inflamed or dystrophic tissues and the chances for tissue breakdown may be increased. Koivumaa and co-workers have found a definite correlation between bruxism and temporomandibular joint and muscle disorders.[22] The relationship between bruxism and periodontal disease, although likely, has not been fully established.[23]

Prior to the treatment of traumatism by occlusal adjustment, the dentist must examine and classify the type of occlusion and tooth position relationship (intercuspation) (Figs. 37-10 to 37-13).

## OCCLUSIONS

### Ideal occlusion

A picture of ideal occlusion has been provided by orthodontic concept. This is useful in describing various occlusal relationships. The intercuspation of the teeth as defined by Angle is such that the mesiobuccal cusp of the upper first molar occludes with the mesiobuccal groove of the lower first molar.[24] The upper canine interdigitates with the distal incline of the lower canine and the mesiobuccal cusp incline of the premolar; the other premolars and molars intercuspate perfectly between and distal to these landmarks (Fig. 37-10). In addition, the occlusal plane is relatively flat; and the curve of Spee and the curve of Monson are not steep.

### Malocclusions

Deviations from this ideal occlusion are termed malocclusions. Ideal occlusion occurs only infrequently and malocclusion of one or more teeth is the rule rather than the exception. Angle classified malocclusions into class I, class II, and class III types.[24]

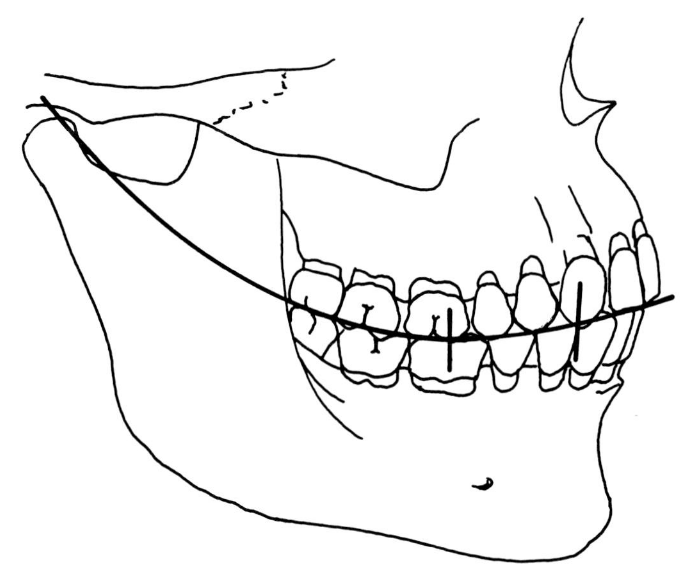

**Fig. 37-10.** Ideal occlusion. Line drawn through the occlusal plane indicates the curve of Spee. Alignment markers drawn perpendicular to this curve indicate the correct first molar and canine relationships according to Angle.

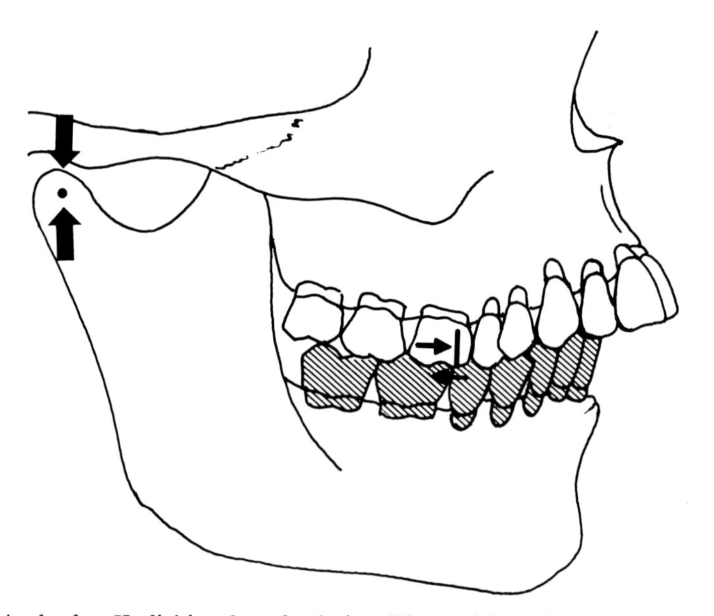

**Fig. 37-11.** Angle class II, division 1, malocclusion. The mesiobuccal cusp of the maxillary first molar intercuspates anterior to the mesiobuccal groove of the mandibular first molar. The maxillary canine is similarly anterior to the position that it occupies in the ideal occlusion. The overjet is pronounced. Large black arrows indicate that the mandible is in terminal hinge position.

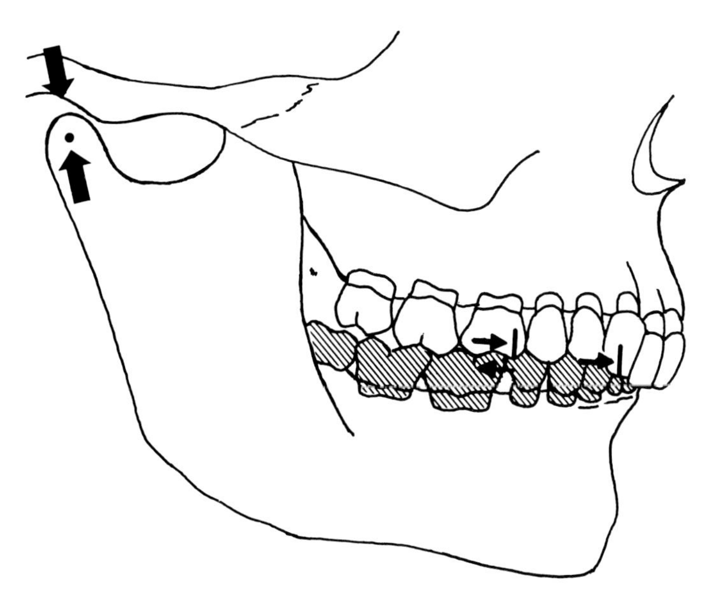

**Fig. 37-12.** Angle class II, division 2, malocclusion. The mesiobuccal cusp of the maxillary first molar intercuspates anterior to the mesiobuccal cusp of the mandibular first molar. The maxillary canine is anterior to the ideal position. Note the deep overbite. Large black arrows indicate that the mandible is in terminal hinge position.

*Angle class I and class II-1*

An Angle class I malocclusion has the correct molar relationship; however, the anterior teeth are crowded. In an Angle class II, division 1, malocclusion the mesiobuccal cusp of the maxillary molar and the maxillary canine intercuspate anterior to the position that they occupy in ideal occlusion. The overjet is pronounced, but the overbite is normal (Fig. 37-11).

*Angle class II-2*

In an Angle class II, division 2, malocclusion the maxillary teeth also occlude with the mandibular teeth anterior to their ideal position, but the overbite is pronounced (Fig. 37-12).

*Angle class III*

In the Angle class III malocclusions the mandibular teeth are in mesioversion to the maxillary teeth and the jaw is prognathic. All mandibular teeth may be in mesioversion (Fig. 37-13, *A*), or only the posterior teeth may be in mesioversion, as happens when there is a pseudoclass III malocclusion (Fig. 37-13, *B*).

Malocclusions related to major discrepancies in arch form or tooth position should be treated by the orthodontist. Malocclusions related to occlusal form discrepancies, such as premature contacts, may be treated by the periodontist or restorative dentist. In fact, many of the malocclusions that are treated by the periodontist in conjunction with the restorative dentist are actually major malocclusions. Occlusal therapy then is an important part of periodontal therapy, as difficult as the treatment of major malocclusions by conventional orthodontic methods.

This chapter discusses occlusal adjustment by grinding. The methods for occlusal adjustment can be and sometimes are applied even if traumatism is not present. For example, if many inlays are being prepared or bridgework is planned, you may want to adjust the occlusion before doing the reconstruction. On the other hand, if there is no evidence of trauma and reconstruction is not required, then there is no need to adjust an occlusion by grinding. The presence of a major or minor malocclusion does *not* necessarily mean that traumatism is present.

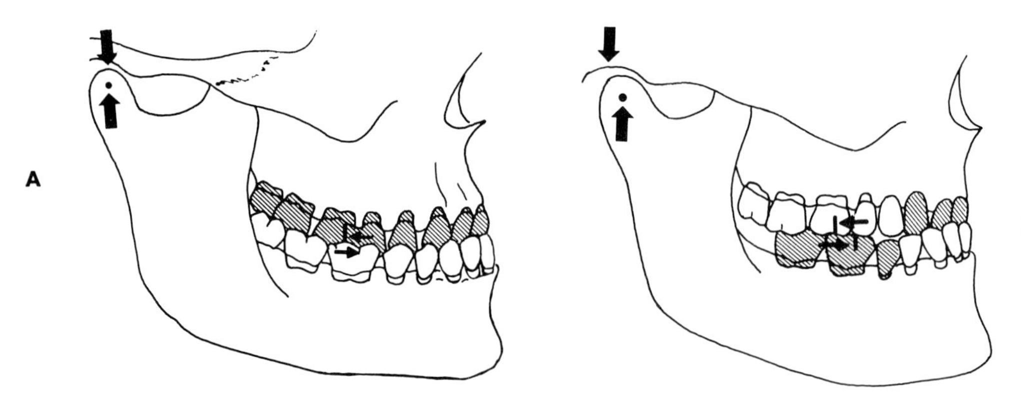


**Fig. 37-13.** Class III malocclusion. **A,** All the mandibular teeth are in mesioversion to the maxillary teeth. The jaw is prognathic. The mandibular teeth are buccal and labial to the maxillary teeth. **B,** Pseudoclass III occlusion. The anterior mandibular teeth are in mesioversion. The jaw (condyle) is brought forward to allow full intercuspation in closure. This produces a situation of habitual occlusion in class III relationship. The crossing of the posterior teeth that change from buccoversion to linguoversion is termed a crossbite.* Large black arrows indicate the terminal hinge position, **A,** and lack thereof, **B.**

*Crossbites—conditions in which the posterior arches cross relationships—with some teeth that are normally buccal now lying lingual and vice versa. This can also occur in class I and II malocclusions.

### Mutilated occlusions

An entire dentition may be maloccluded. Sometimes only one or a few teeth of an otherwise normal dentition may be in malocclusion. Such teeth may be described by the terms supraclusion, infraclusion, mesioclusion, distoclusion, tilted, or rotated. These situations frequently develop in dentitions in which teeth have been extracted and not replaced. The occlusions are then termed mutilated. There may be mutilated normal occlusions or mutilated class I, class II, or class III malocclusions. When mutilations have occurred and teeth have moved, you may have to surmise how the teeth were arranged before the extractions were performed to properly classify the occlusion.

## CLINICAL DIAGNOSIS

Just as it is necessary in the course of the examination to inspect the color, texture, and consistency of the gingival tissues, to measure the pocket depths, and to examine the teeth and occlusion, so it is necessary to examine for signs of trauma.

Since a biopsy examination of the periodontal ligament, cementum, and bone cannot be done on patients and since intraoral telemetry and electromyography are just research tools, how can you determine whether periodontal trauma is present? You must depend on clinical examination. Periodontal trauma is more easily diagnosed when a systematic and disciplined order of history and examination is used.

### Subjective indications

During the interview the patient may make one or more of the following complaints:

1. My bite seems wrong.

2. My teeth are sore when I close.
3. This tooth seems to hit before the others. It's longer.
4. My teeth and gums feel "itchy."
5. My jaws hurt (muscles of mastication).
6. My teeth are sensitive (pulpal irritation).
7. My jaw joints hurt. They make cracking noises.
8. I grind my teeth.
9. My teeth have loosened.
10. My teeth have moved.
11. I find it hard to open my mouth in the morning.

Such remarks should lead you to suspect that traumatism may have occurred. Occlusal traumatism can occur when an excessive or misdirected masticatory force is transmitted through the tooth to the periodontium, causing tissue injury. Frequently such a force arises when two opposing teeth occlude before all the other teeth meet. Such prematurities can be the direct result of malocclusions. The malocclusions may be minor (when one or two teeth are malposed) or major. However, what appears as pathologic from an orthodontic point of view (Angle class II relation, crossbite) may function physiologically without destroying periodontal tissues. On the other hand, an occlusion that appears nearly perfect from the orthodontic view may be less than perfect from the aspects of occlusion and articulation; or parafunctional habits may contribute to the breakdown of supporting structures of the tooth.

## Objective signs and tests

In the course of the examination, you should record the following data:

1. *Mobility—passive.* How loose are the teeth on palpation? Rock each tooth with instrument handles while holding the patient's head in a relatively steady position.
2. *Mobility—dynamic.* How loose are the teeth during functional and parafunctional movements? Request the patient to open and close his jaws and also to move the closed jaws into the lateral and protrusive positions. Test the teeth for mobility and heavy contacts. You may do this by holding your fingertips lightly half on the teeth and half on the gingiva. The patient should clench and rock his teeth while you carefully observe for visual signs of mobility.
3. *Migration.** Have the teeth migrated? Have some teeth elongated beyond the occlusal plane? Have others drifted forward, opening diastemas? Have teeth rotated?
4. *Palpation of the masticatory muscles.* How large and powerful are these muscles? In some cases hypertrophy of the muscles may be indicative of bruxism.
5. *Roentgenographic signs.* Have the periodontal ligament spaces widened? Is there any change in the lamina dura? Is there any radiolucency in the furcation areas? Are there periapical zones of radiolucency about vital teeth? Are there signs of root resorption? Has the pulp chamber become smaller? Remember that buccal and lingual widening of the periodontal

*Pathologic migration may also be a symptom of periodontosis. However, periodontosis is a relatively rare disease, whereas traumatism is encountered frequently.

ligament space may not be evident in the roentgenogram that represents a mesiodistal profile.

6. *Wear facets.* Are there wear facets present on the teeth beyond what you would expect for the patient's age?

Perhaps the most important signs to look for are *mobility* of teeth, *widening* of the periodontal ligament space in roentgenograms, and pathologic tooth *migration.* These are symptoms of actual damage. Wear facets indicate what the patient is doing in parafunctional movements, and they may also signify potential damage; but in the absence of other objective signs, they do not necessarily show that traumatism is occurring.

If actual damage from occlusal traumatism has been diagnosed, the source of the trauma must be determined. Examine the occlusion for disharmonies as well as to see how the force application may be contributing to the trauma. In addition, try to gain some idea of the types of mandibular movements the patient is capable of making.

#### Examination of occlusion

1. Type of occlusion
   a. Normal
   b. Angle class I
   c. Angle class II
   d. Angle class III
2. Teeth present—number and position
   a. Alignment
   b. Tilting
   c. Crowding
   d. Drifting
   e. Crossbite relationships
   f. Diastemas
   g. Relationship to occlusal plane
3. Missing teeth
4. Crown-to-root ratio of teeth
5. Buccolingual width of teeth
6. Form of the occlusal plane
   a. Type of curve of Spee (normal, exaggerated, horizontal, reverse)
   b. Mutilations caused by extrusion
   c. Double plane of occlusion (i.e., posterior teeth and anterior teeth on different planes)
7. Degree of anterior overbite and overjet
   a. Deep overbite
   b. Incisal edges contacting gingival or palatal tissue
   c. Anterior teeth in nonocclusion
8. Extent of zone of intercuspation
   a. Cusp inclination
   b. Cusp-fossa relationship
   c. Locked bite
9. Functional relations*
   a. Premature contacts in terminal hinge position
   b. Form and range of hinge movement
   c. Premature functional (working) side contacts in lateral occlusal positions and movements
   d. Nonfunctional (nonworking) side contact in lateral occlusal position and movements
   e. Premature contacts in protrusive occlusal position and movements
10. Parafunctional relations*
   a. Premature contacts in lateral occlusal positions and movements

---

*Some clinicians maintain that such observations can be made only with instruments.

   b. Nonfunctional side contact in lateral occlusal position and movements
   c. Premature contacts in protrusive occlusal position and movements
   d. Form and range of lateral and protrusive movements
11. Rest position of the mandible and extent of the freeway space*
12. Deviations in the path of opening and closing*
13. Palpation of the temporomandibular joints during functional movements

***Examination for reconstruction***

When the treatment plan includes reconstruction, other data may be needed. Some of these must be provided by an examination of well-articulated study casts, especially when missing teeth or many carious teeth are present. At times the mobility will involve so many teeth that occlusal grinding alone is not sufficient. When the treatment plan includes reconstruction as well as occlusal adjustment, additional factors need to be known:

1. Position and number of missing teeth
2. Position, number, and periodontal status of abutment teeth
3. Degree of involvement of carious teeth
4. Alignment of teeth in terms of parallelism
5. Presence of food impaction and retention areas
6. Diastemas (old or newly formed)
7. Operative quality and periodontal adequacy of existing restorations
8. Aesthetics or absence thereof

Once these factors are understood, the amount and degree of restorative dentistry necessary can be gauged and the occlusal morphology of the reconstruction planned. (See Chapters 39 and 40.)

In evaluating occlusal traumatism,, determine the direction, frequency, distribution, and intensity of functionally occurring forces (as in mastication, deglutition, and speech) and parafunctional forces (as in bruxism, clenching, tongue thrusting, and other oral habits).[5,25] Perhaps the strongest of these forces are the parafunctional when the musculature is being contracted isometrically.

Understanding occlusion is a necessary adjunct to full denture and partial denture construction, in fixed bridgework and restorative dentistry (Chapter 36), and in orthodontic therapy. Rules for adjusting occlusions have developed in some of these clinical disciplines, which are predicated on the presence of occlusal discrepancies. You will rely heavily on these rules to provide a foundation for the type of adjustment required to treat periodontal trauma.

Remember that a malocclusion does not necessarily mean that traumatism is present. Trauma is a tissue lesion. There are many instances in which tooth malpositions are present without trauma and trauma is present without tooth malpositions.

## OCCLUSAL DISHARMONIES AND THEIR TREATMENT

Therapy of occlusal trauma can be accomplished in the following ways[8]:

1. Occlusal adjustment by grinding
2. Orthodontic treatment
3. Splinting
4. Prosthetic reconstruction
5. Construction of bite guards

Often more than one of these steps must be performed. The ensuing discussion deals mainly with correction by grinding and alleviation with night guards.

*Some clinicians maintain that such observations can be made only with instruments.

## Principles

Earlier in this chapter the term *premature contact* was used. What are premature contacts? They are initial contacts of opposing tooth surfaces that are made before the remaining teeth come into contact. When do they occur? They can occur during functional and parafunctional movements. What do they do? If the premature contact occurs in centric (terminal hinge occlusion), the mandible is deflected into some other occlusal position (habitual occlusion). If the prematurity occurs during a glide movement, the adjacent teeth may be prevented from making contact during the glide. Consequently prematurities are known as interceptive or deflective contacts; and the terms *cuspal interferences* or *occlusal interferences* that prevent occlusal harmony and *occlusal disharmonies* are also used.

Prematurities often occur in conjunction with malocclusions, but malocclusion per se does not necessarily mean that premature contacts are present. Deflective contacts can and do occur in some grossly normal occlusions. Therefore, do not judge whether or not a prematurity is present on the basis of tooth arrangement, alignment, or irregularity. Rather, examine the functional and parafunctional movements of the mandible. Although trauma is not a necessary sequel of disharmony, premature contacts and trauma often exist in a cause-effect relationship. If such a cause-effect relationship exists, correct the occlusion by grinding in periodontal treatment. In the fabrication of partial dentures and fixed bridges or in the restoration of a dentition with inlays, eliminate all prematurities before the restorations are made so as not to perpetuate the disharmony. There are good and sufficient reasons for the establishment of a harmonious occlusion in such cases. Still, in the absence of trauma, prophylactic adjustment of occlusions is not a justifiable procedure.[26]

***Definition of occlusal adjustment***

Occlusal adjustment is the establishment of an occlusion according to some ideal plan by grinding the occluding and other surfaces of the teeth. In the establishment of an ideal occlusion, occlusal disharmonies are eliminated. The ideal occlusion is believed to permit function that is physiologically compatible with the periodontium, the temporomandibular joints, and the muscles of mastication. Then the stomatognathic system is said to be in harmony.

Several concepts of occlusion have been described—bilateral balance, group function, and canine protection. In addition, many dentists believe that only centric harmony is essential; yet most agree on the need for a simultaneous bilateral intercuspation of the posterior teeth in the terminal hinge position.

No matter what the articulative ideal, occlusal adjustment must obtain centric free of premature contacts. Most of the variation between the concepts occurs in the handling of eccentric movements.

***Bilateral balance***

Bilateral balance is essentially a full denture concept maintaining that occlusal forces should be equally distributed to all the teeth.[27-31] In this way each tooth carries a proportionate share of the load. In centric the cusp tip should enter the fossa to the full depth of the fossa. In lateral excursions functional and nonfunctional (working and balancing) sides are ground to make bilateral contact (equilibration). Although this method has been superseded in periodontal therapy by other methods, it is still used occasionally.

***Group function***

Clinical observations indicate that premature contacts on the nonfunctional side may be the most destructive of all premature contacts. Consequently, nonfunctional side contacts are deliberately avoided or removed. The load in lateral excursion is borne only by the functional side. The buccal slopes of mandibular buccal cusps and the lingual slopes of maxillary buccal cusps are shaped so that the load is equally distributed among these cusps at all times during lateral movment.[31-35]

However, nonfunctional side interferences are also possible on the functional side. The chewing stroke may pass beyond the median occlusal position and the lingual cusps of the functional side may come to carry the load and thus act as premature balancing contacts.[35] These must then be ground. After such corrections function is borne by groups of teeth (canines to molars of one side) in lateral excursions and by the anterior teeth in protrusive excursion.

*Canine protection*

The aim of canine-protected occlusion is that the maxillary and the mandibular canines carry the occlusal load in lateral excursions, causing the other teeth to become disoccluded.[36,37] The root length and bone support of the canines are believed to be well suited to carrying such a heavy load. Since the posterior teeth are disoccluded in excursions, they cannot be stressed by premature forces. A variant of this type of approach requires, in addition, that the posterior teeth become slightly disoccluded in protrusive glides while the anterior teeth bear the load. In centric the posterior teeth carry the load while the anterior teeth are slightly disoccluded. Such a mechanical plan is termed disocclusion.[38-40] In a disocclusion, contact on posterior teeth occurs only when the mandible is in terminal hinge occlusion (centric relation occlusion); in this position the anterior teeth are slightly out of occlusion. The canines and incisors disocclude the posterior teeth in all lateral excursive movements. Proper ridge, cusp, and groove direction must be established so that, when the cusps leave centric relation, they will be immediately disoccluded and pass without contact along shearing or escape grooves, depending on which is the functional and which the nonfunctional side.

Most dental schools teach occlusal adjustment via group function. The basic Schuyler method or some variation of it is followed. Other schools teach the methods of grinding advocated by Jankelson and others (to be discussed later).

## General objectives

Objectives in occlusal adjustment are outlined as follows[8,23,41-43b]:

1. To distribute forces in median occlusal position to the largest possible number of teeth*
2. To coordinate the median occlusal position with the terminal hinge position of the mandible either by making them coincide or by establishing freedom of movement between the two positions (long centric)*
3. To eliminate prematurities in closure and excursive movements and to gain group function so that occlusal forces are distributed to the largest number of teeth in the group

   As a corollary, premature contacts on the nonfunctional teeth should be eliminated. Chewing should be possible on the right and the left side (with equal ease). This is facilitated by the simultaneous gliding contact between the teeth on the functional side.[23]

*The question may be asked, why should the teeth be made to intercuspate well in hinge position? Although this position is not assumed often during rest or in ordinary chewing, it is apparently used during parafunctional movements such as bruxism and clenching as well as during some functional movements. The dentist's aim is not to reposition the mandible but rather to avoid premature contacts in any position in which the patient may intercuspate the teeth in functional or parafunctional activities.

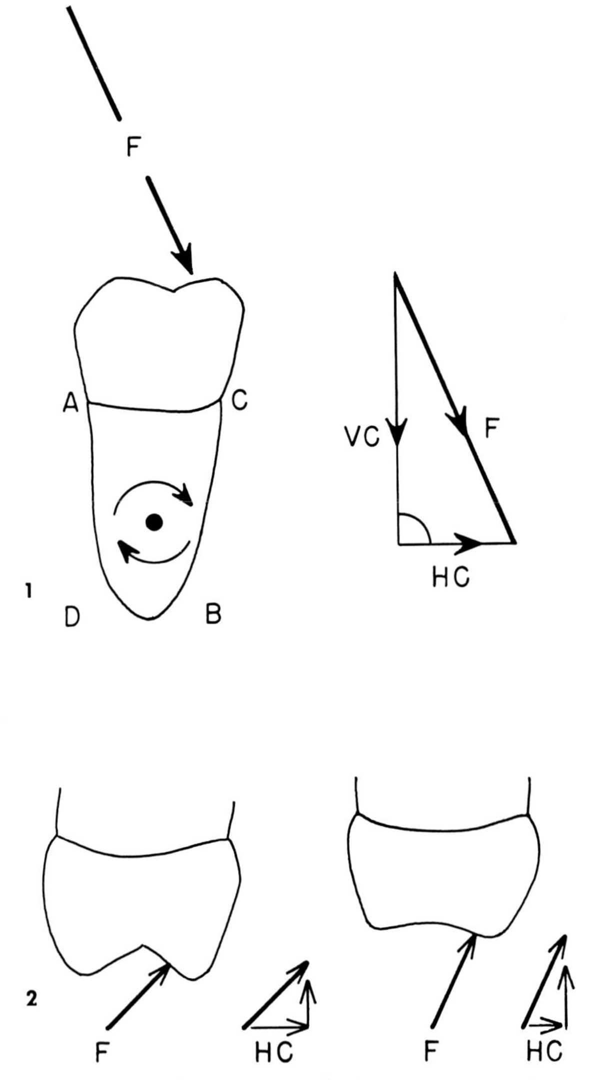


**Fig. 37-14.** **1,** A known force, *F,* directed perpendicular to a cusp surface may be divided by means of vector analysis into a vertical component, *VC,* and a horizontal component, *HC.* In the vector analysis each line represents the true magnitude of the force. The vertical component is conducted in an axial direction. The horizontal component produces a torque about the center of rotation of the tooth (dot). This causes compression at *C* and *D* and tension. **2,** Comparison of vector diagrams for forces of equal magnitude, *F,* applied to a steep-cusped tooth and a less steep-cusped (after grinding) tooth. The axial component is increased in the shallow-cusped tooth. The horizontal component, *HC,* is decreased. Consequently this tooth receives less torque.

4. To direct occlusal forces, as far as possible, centrally along the long axis of the tooth

   As a corollary, tilting or torqueing forces should be minimized.

   a. In median occlusal position the lingual cusps of the maxillary teeth and the buccal cusps of the mandibular teeth should project into the central fossae of their antagonists.
   b. Related harmonious cusp inclines should be established in all teeth of

a group and their cuspal inclinations should be reduced so that lateral vectors are minimized and long axis vectors are maximized (Fig. 37-14).

5. To improve or maintain masticatory performance since more efficient mastication is presumed to require less force
   a. Establish static relationships between cusps and fossae of opposing teeth to minimize tooth mobility during function. Then reshape plunger cusps that wedge antagonist teeth apart (Fig. 37-20).
   b. Plane-to-plane contacts do not incise and tear food efficiently and chewing therefore requires more force. Establish ball-to-plane contacts if possible.
   c. Retain cusp sharpness, establish occlusal grooves and sluiceways, and smooth tooth surfaces, for these are conducive to masticatory efficiency.
   d. When open contacts exist, reestablish proximal tooth contact since the mutual support that contact provides enhances tooth stability and avoids food impaction.
   e. When the width of the occlusal table of a tooth has been increased by wear or by grinding, narrow it.
6. To accomplish the occlusal adjustment without reducing vertical dimension and by retaining an acceptable interocclusal clearance

## Five steps in occlusal adjustment

Occlusal adjustment consists of the following five steps: (1) initial grinding, (2) harmonization in terminal hinge occlusion, (3) harmonization in protrusive position and movement, (4) harmonization in lateral occlusal position and lateral excursion, and finally, (5) reestablishment of morsal anatomy and careful polishing of all ground surfaces. These steps presume that the patient has a relatively normal occlusion or an Angle class I or class II, division 1, occlusion. Details vary for an Angle class II and a class II, division 2, occlusion and also in various crossbite and open bite relationships.

If occlusal adjustment is undertaken, it is not a simple task that can be performed hurriedly and without planning.[8,41,42] There are simple cases, to be sure, but even these should be carefully considered. Some practitioners study the occlusion in the mouth; others take study casts and mount them on an anatomic articulator. In either case a fairly complete study should be made. Some operators adjust the occlusion on articulator-mounted casts and prepare a grinding list of the corrections performed.

***Initial grinding***

Initial grinding may include the following:

1. Narrowing of buccolingual diameters
2. Shortening of extruded teeth
3. Improvement of aesthetics
4. Correction of marginal ridge relationship
5. Reduction of plunger cusps
6. Correction of rotated, malposed, or tilted teeth
7. Correction of facets and abraded teeth
8. Rounding of sharp edges when indicated

Such grinding should precede adjustment in hinge position since many interferences are eliminated during this step and often further adjustment is unnecessary. In fact, this grinding may be all that is required to remove the disharmonies.

In initial grinding, try to recarve the teeth to obtain as ideal an arch and oc-

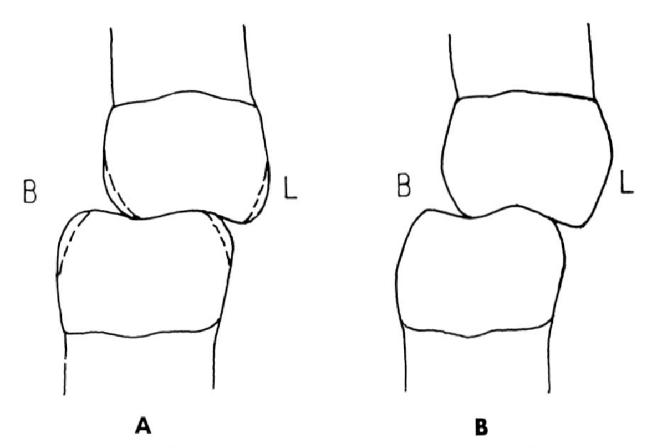


**Fig. 37-15. A,** Buccolingual narrowing. Area to be ground is outlined. **B,** Buccolingual narrowing as completed.

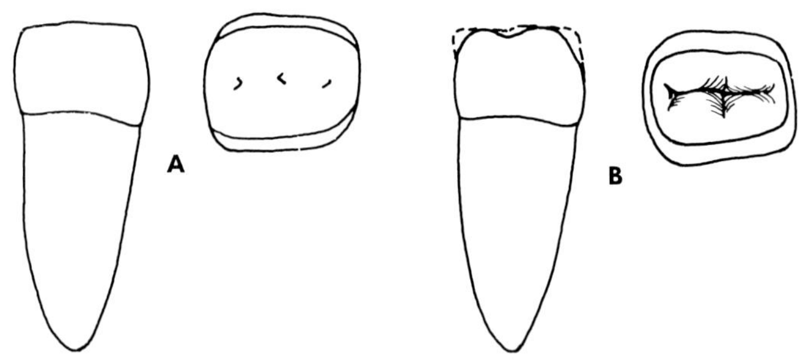


**Fig. 37-16. A,** The tooth is worn, obliterating the occlusal anatomy and making the occlusal surface broad. **B,** Reshaping narrows the occlusal table and restores the anatomy. (See also Fig. 37-19, *C*). (Modified from Miller, S. C.: Textbook of periodontia, ed. 2, Philadelphia, 1943, The Blakiston Co.)

clusal plane as possible. Once this is obtained, the steps in a definitive grinding tend to become easier.

1. *Buccolingual narrowing.* By narrowing the buccolingual diameter of the teeth you will make the occlusal table smaller and consequently the rounded extreme edges of the occlusal surface will be unable to participate in transmitting torqueing forces. Occlusal forces will become centered over the tooth and will tend to be transmitted along the long axis of the tooth (Figs. 37-15 and 37-16). This step is indicated only when such narrowing would not disturb vertical dimension by removing cusp tips that contact in centric and would not induce cheek biting.
2. *Shortening of extruded teeth.* Teeth frequently extrude after they have lost their antagonists or have migrated. The elongated tooth becomes unaesthetic and may be the premature tooth in many movements. Moreover, the plane of occlusion is disturbed and, unless the tooth is shortened, good occlusion in restorative or reconstructive dental procedures cannot be obtained. In such cases exposure of the dentin in grinding is permissible (Fig. 37-17).
3. *Improvement of aesthetics.* Although shortening of extruded teeth will improve aesthetics, there are some cases in which other factors require

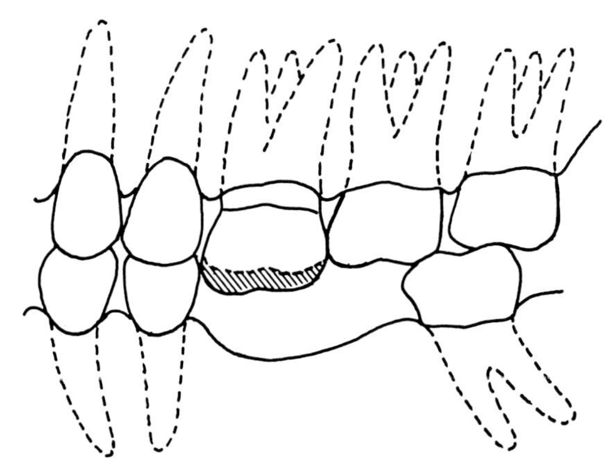

**Fig. 37-17.** An extruded tooth has been shortened (shaded area) to create a normal occlusal plane. A fixed bridge can be fabricated to restore the lower missing teeth. Had the maxillary molar been left as it was, the resultant bridge would have had a distorted occlusal plane.

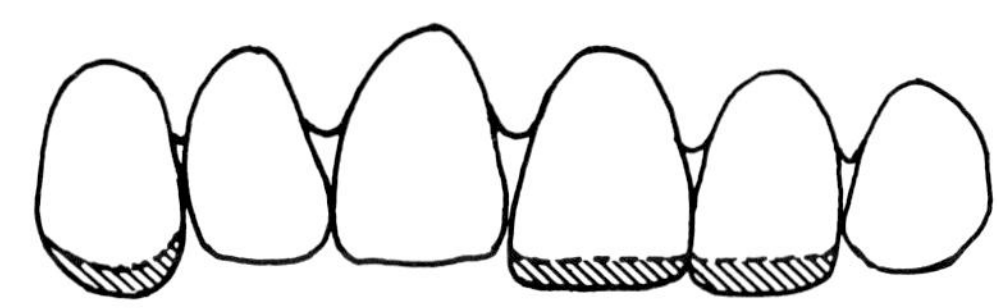

**Fig. 37-18.** When individual anterior teeth are disproportionately longer than the same teeth on the other side of the mouth, they may be ground (shaded area) to a more regular length.

attention. For instance, the anterior teeth may not be symmetric in length or may have ragged, abraded incisal surfaces. Rotate these and overlap them slightly. Such teeth can be ground to a more symmetric and regular form (Fig. 37-18).

4. *Correction of marginal ridge relationships.* Marginal ridges may exhibit three types of variation: they may be unequal in height; they may not meet at the contact area (because of rotation or malposition); or they may have faulty marginal ridge and sluiceway form (because of poor restoration or grinding). In some cases, grind these defects. When this cannot be done, correct them by restorative dentistry (Fig. 37-19).
5. *Plunger cusps and food impaction.* If a tooth has a prominent cusp that meets the marginal ridges of the pair of opposing teeth, it may wedge the opposing teeth apart. This is especially true when the opposing teeth are mobile and the antagonist is firm. Such wedging is conducive to food impaction. The wedging cusp is termed a plunger cusp. Shorten and round it without taking the tooth out of centric occlusion, for such cuspal relationships are often the sites of centric prematurity (Fig. 37-20).
6. *Rotated, malposed or tilted teeth.* Rotated teeth have been mentioned in relation to aesthetics. Careful grinding will improve the crown form of individual rotated, tilted, or malposed teeth (Fig. 37-21).
7. *Wear facets and abraded teeth.* Teeth subject to masticatory and parafunctional activity tend to wear. Such areas are known as wear facets. Abraded teeth require more force in mastication, and their wear facets should be

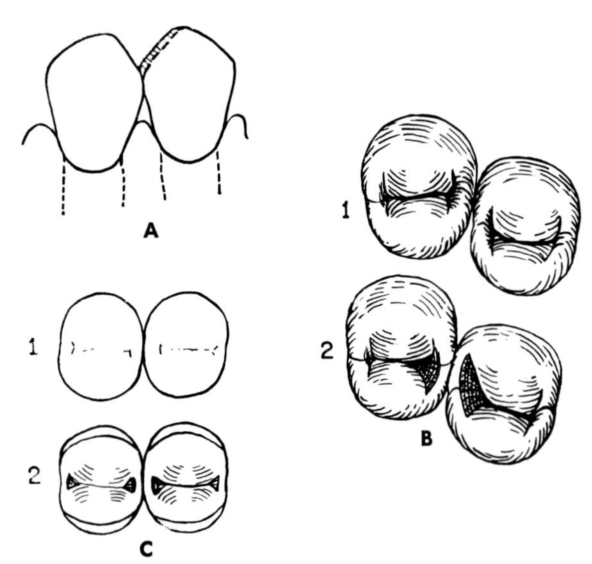


**Fig. 37-19.** Correction of marginal ridge relationships. **A,** Dotted line shows correction in teeth that are of unequal height. **B,** Rotated teeth that have, *1,* the marginal ridge of one tooth adjacent to the buccal or lingual cusp incline of the other and, *2,* the marginal ridges corrected by grinding shown by crosshatching. **C,** Worn, ground, or poorly carved tooth with faulty marginal ridge and sluiceway form, *1*; corrected, *2*.

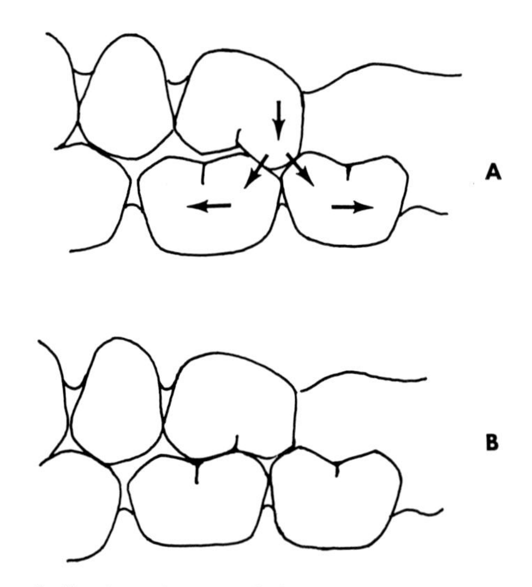


**Fig. 37-20. A,** The elongated distobuccal cusp of the maxillary molar wedges the lower molars and forces them apart. Food impaction occurs during mastication. **B,** The distobuccal cusp of the maxillary molar is rounded, and both wedging and food impaction are eliminated.

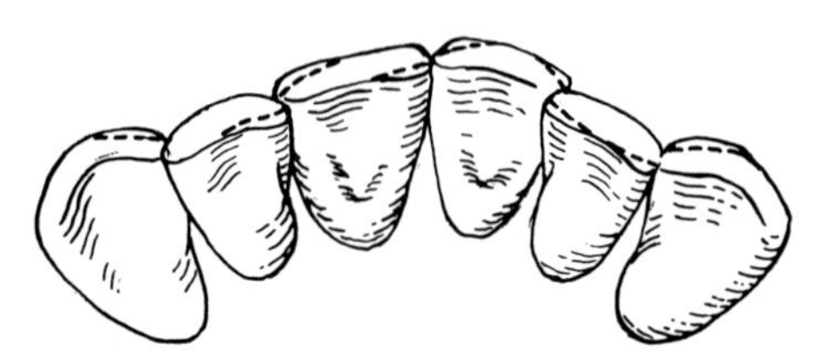

**Fig. 37-21.** Rotated lower incisors and the indicated correction (in outline) that may improve aesthetics and occlusion. (Modified from Beube, F. E.: Periodontology: diagnosis and treatment. New York, 1953, The Macmillan Co.)

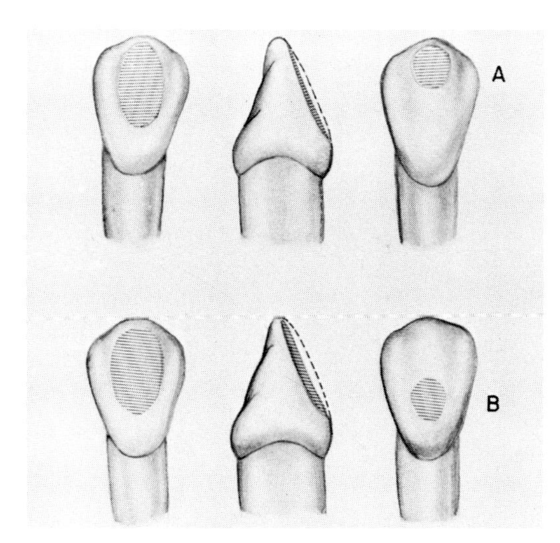


**Fig. 37-22.** A long wear facet is present, which should be reduced by recontouring the tooth. The recontouring may preserve the incisal, **A,** or cervical, **B,** region of the wear facet to preverse contact in the median occlusal position. The lower end of the wear facet is preserved in exceptional instances such as in cases of deep overbite.

reduced (Fig. 37-22). You may also recarve occlusal anatomy (Fig. 37-16) at this time, unless further steps in occlusal adjustment are planned.

8. *Sharp edges.* If the buccal surfaces of the upper teeth or the lingual surfaces of the lower teeth have worn to sharp edges, round them. Sharp edges can be irritating to the tongue and cheek. If restorations have sharp margins protruding beyond the enamel surface or if the enamel has been undermined and chipped, exposing sharp edges, round such edges and polish them smooth.

***Harmonization in terminal hinge occlusion***

The next step is to establish multiple-contact closure and to coordinate it with terminal hinge position.

1. *Disharmony between cusp inclines.* If a disharmony exists between the hinge position and the median occlusal position, the interference most frequently is between the mesial cusp inclines of the maxillary teeth (usually the lingual cusp of the first premolar) and the distal cusp inclines of the mandibular teeth. Depending on the steepness of the cuspal inclination, grind either the mesial inclines of the maxillary teeth or the distal inclines of the mandibular teeth (never both) (Figs. 37-23 and 37-24). (This is sometimes referred to as the MU-DL rule.) Reduce the steeper cusps in the direction toward which the mandible deviates.
2. *Disharmony between cusp and fossa.* If in closure of the mandible on the hinge a disharmony exists between a cusp and the opposing fossa and there is no cuspal interference in excursive movements, deepen the fossa. If cusp interference exists, reshape the cusps as noted in Fig. 37-25. Do not grind away the centric holding contact.
3. *Disharmony between the anterior teeth.* When occlusal interference exists between the anterior teeth in the hinge position (Fig. 37-26), correct the incisal edges of the mandibular incisors.

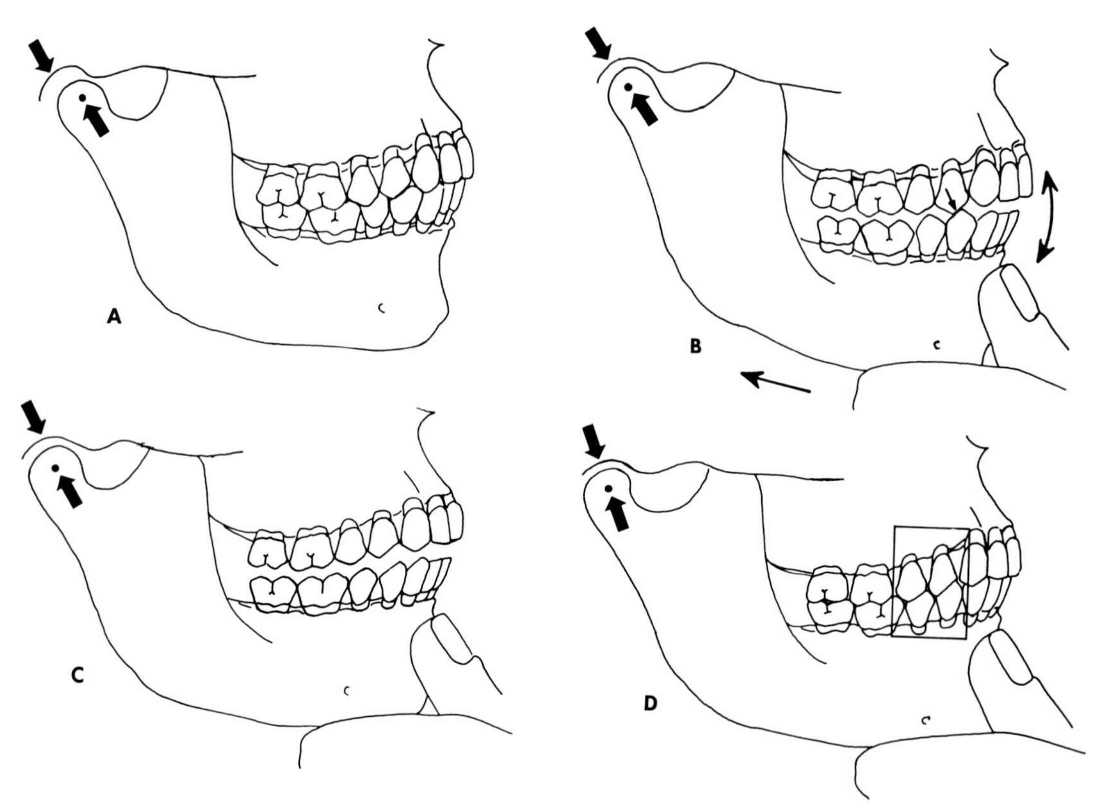


**Fig. 37-23. A,** In ordinary closure into maximum intercuspation, a premature contact causes displacement of the condyle from the fossa. **B,** The interference is located by movement in the hinge relation. **C,** Premature contact is ground away. **D,** Now maximum intercuspation occurs with the condyle in its most retruded position (arrows), as well as in habitual closure. Generally, more than one or two such interferences must be eliminated before **D** is obtained. Large black arrows show terminal hinge position, **B** to **D,** and lack thereof, **A.**

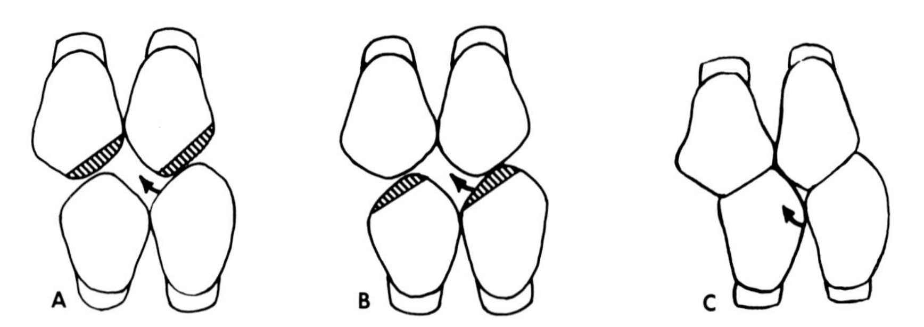


**Fig. 37-24.** Enlargement of the area in Fig. 37-23, *D,* somewhat corresponding to Fig. 37-23, *B,* before correction. Depending on cusp steepness, grind either, **A,** the mesial inclines of the maxillary teeth or, **B,** the distal inclines of the mandibular teeth, permitting the mandible to move back into terminal hinge occlusion. Area to be reshaped is shaded. **C,** After these areas are ground as indicated, round them slightly to restore their anatomy.

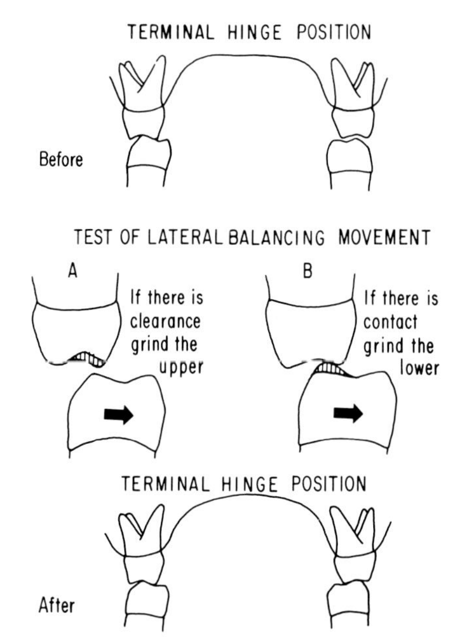


**Fig. 37-25.** If there is premature contact between a fossa and an opposing cusp in the terminal hinge position, test the excursive movement. If no cuspal interference exists in lateral excursions on the balacing side, deepen the fossa, **A.** If cuspal interference does exist on the balancing side, reshape the mandibular lingual cusp, **B,** to obtain freedom from the premature contact on closure in the terminal hinge position.

In Angle class II, division 2 (deep overbite), no grinding of posterior teeth can be performed. Such grinding will reduce vertical dimension and the anteriors will be forced into increased contact. In such cases the anterior relationship may be improved by grinding both upper and lower incisors if possible or, better, by orthodontics before other grinding steps are undertaken.

In Angle Class III habitual relationship (pseudoclass III), both upper and lower incisors may have to be ground to establish a stop in terminal hinge occlusion. The posterior teeth may still not make contact in terminal hinge position. However, you can either wait 6 to 12 months for them to erupt into position or build the teeth up with crowns or onlays to establish contact.

These steps properly performed should bring about a harmony between median occlusal and terminal hinge positions. You are now ready to consider eccentric positions and excursive movements.

Only after cuspal interferences in the hinge position have been eliminated should you proceed to correct eccentric disharmonies. Once terminal hinge position is established, be extremely careful not to disturb it in the grinding steps that follow.

***Harmonization in protrusive position and movement***

Usually protrusive position and excursion are ground before lateral excursions, but the order may be reversed. Grind the protrusive position first to deal with the special problems that relate to deep overbite cases. If the order is reversed and you inadvertently reduce vertical dimension in such a case, you may not be able to correct the resultant anterior relationship by grinding; reconstruction will then become a necessity.

1. *Establishment of incisor group contact in edge-to-edge relationship.* Bring

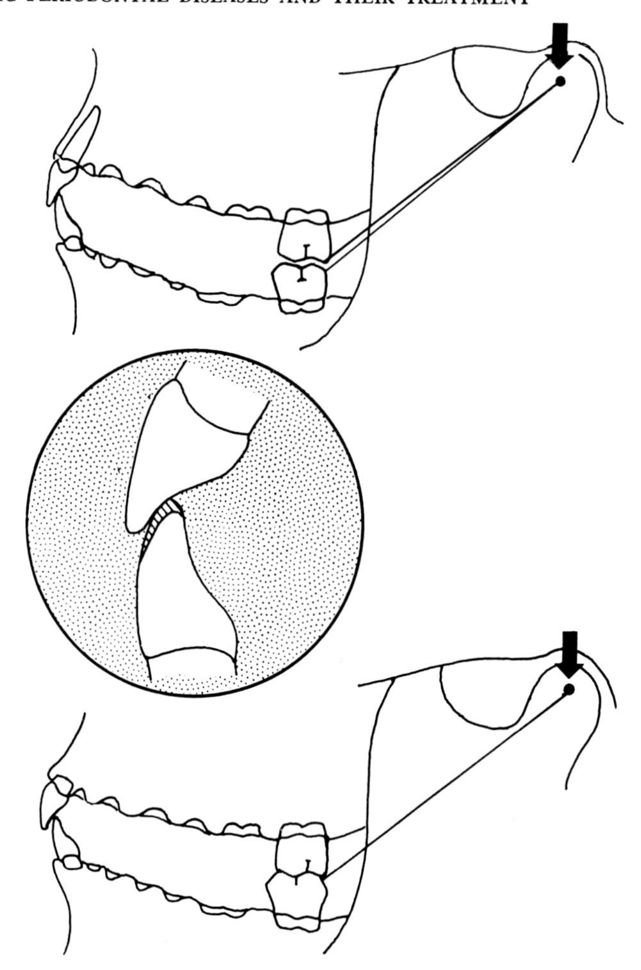

**Fig. 37-26.** Reshape the incisal edges of the mandibular incisors when there is an interference with the maxillary incisors in the hinge position.

as many incisors as possible into occlusion in edge-to-edge position. Grind the upper incisal edges to achieve this, except in class II and class III malocclusions. For these situations the lower incisors do not make contact and they (the lower incisal edges) should be ground. Another instance in which lower incisal edges may be ground is when individual incisors have extruded. No grinding of incisal edges should be done in cases of anterior open bites (Fig. 37-27).

2. *Incisor disharmony in protrusive excursion (establishment of incisal guidance).* Premature contact in protrusive movement in the anterior region may be caused by steepness of the lingual slopes of the maxillary anterior teeth. When this occurs, reduce the incisal guidance of the maxillary teeth (Fig. 37-28, *A*). If the mandibular tooth were shortened, it would lose static contact in the terminal hinge position and eventually would erupt into contact again. The mandibular incisor can be ground in protrusive interference if there is a long contact (frequently a facet is present) between the lingual surface of the maxillary tooth and the labial surface

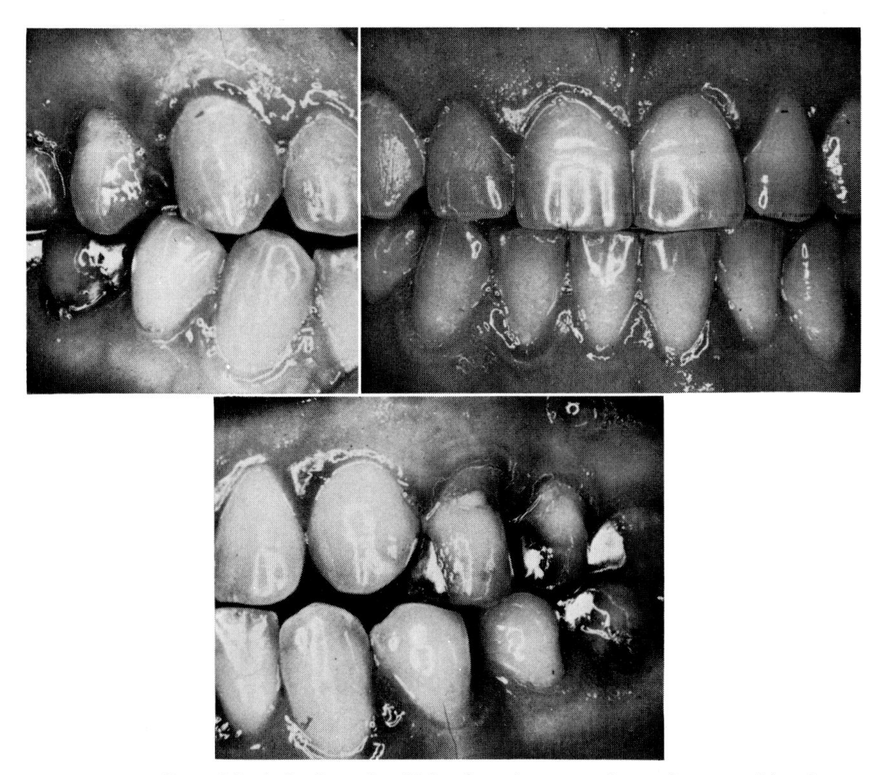

**Fig. 37-27.** No grinding of incisal edges should be done in cases of anterior open bite. Some cases are very deceptive and the anterior teeth appear to make contact. If grinding for aesthetics were done, the open bite would be increased.

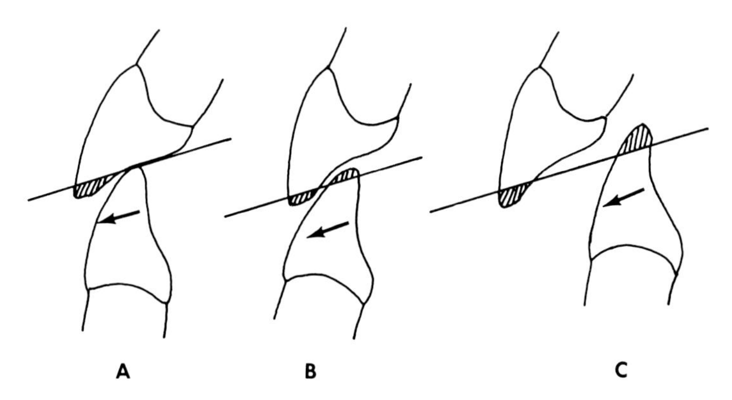


**Fig. 37-28.** Premature contacts in protrusive movement (arrows). **A,** Grind the maxillary tooth (crosshatching), unless as in **B.** If there is a long region of contact, then grind both the maxillary tooth and the mandibular tooth. If, as in **C,** the teeth do not contact in median occlusal position, grind either tooth or both teeth. The plane established by grinding should harmonize with the incisal guidance.

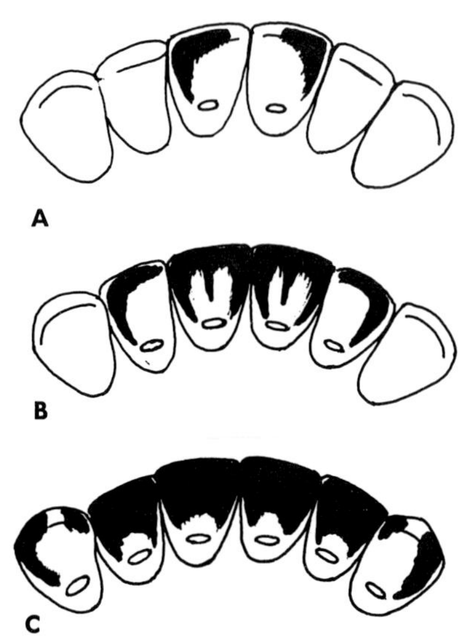


**Fig. 37-29.** The shaded area represents teeth marked during protrusive glide. In **A** only the central incisors bear the load. Grinding next brings the laterals into contact too, **B.** Finally, the canines are engaged. The distal slopes of the canines should come into functional contact during protrusive excursion, **C.**

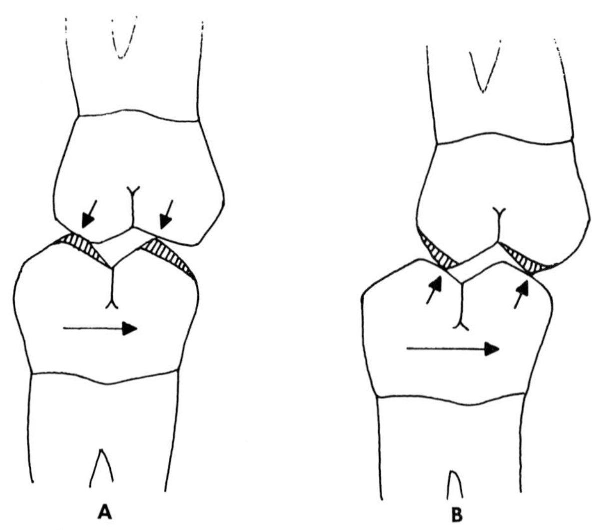


**Fig. 37-30.** If in protrusive movement premature contacts exist between opposing posterior teeth, grind either, **A,** the mesial cusp inclines of the mandibular teeth or, **B,** the distal cusp inclines of the posterior teeth, depending on which are steeper. Where possible, try to maintain cusp height and centric relations established in a previous step. Large arrows indicate direction of protrusive glide; small arrows indicate prematurities; crosshatching indicates area to be ground.

of the mandibular tooth (*B*). Tooth structure can then be reduced incisally to the most apical point of occlusal contact. The maxillary tooth may be ground for a smooth protrusive movement. When there is no contact, as in class II malocclusion, grind either maxillary or mandibular incisors, or both (*C*). As you repeat this step, gradually more and more of the anterior teeth will be brought into function during protrusive glide. The objective is to bring as many anterior teeth as possible into contact. The ideal situation is attained when the distal slope of the canine carries some of the load in protrusive excursion (Fig. 37-29).

3. *Posterior disharmony in protrusive excursion.* Premature contacts of posterior teeth in protrusive movements usually occur on the mesial inclines of the mandibular cusps (Fig. 37-30, *A*) (usually on the lingual) and on the distal inclines of the maxillary cusps (Fig. 37-30, *B*) (usually on the buccal), depending on which is the steeper incline. Eliminate these by reducing the steepest interfering inclines. The elongated third molar is often the offender in such situations.[25] When grinding these areas would result in excessive loss of tooth structure, groove the opposing inclined plane to allow cuspal freedom in protrusive excursion.
4. *Anterior open bite.* Many cases of anterior open bite caused by tongue thrust (a swallowing habit) are seen.[44] Treatment directed solely at grinding the posterior teeth to bring the anterior teeth into contact is contraindicated in such cases as long as the basic problem remains.

***Harmonization in lateral occlusal position and lateral excursion***

Group functional grinding is advocated for lateral excursions in accordance with many of Schuyler's principles. However, in healthy dentitions you may prefer to utilize canine guidance or a mutually protected occlusion. In such instances, except when the canines carry the load in lateral excursions, coordinate the inclines of the other teeth as if they were ground for group function. Then if the canine wears until the posteriors occlude, there will be no posterior disharmonies in lateral excursions. The amount of canine guidance and posterior disocclusion should be small; otherwise the torqueing force on the canine (Fig. 37-31, *A*) may be excessive.

1. *Disharmony of cuspal inclinations of opposing teeth on the working side.* It is desirable to have harmonious inclinations of the cusps of the maxillary and mandibular teeth. If in right lateral movement of the mandible the buccal cusps are in contact but the lingual cusps are out of contact (Fig. 37-31, *B*), grind the lingual incline of the buccal cusps of the maxillary tooth so that its plane will be the same as that of the buccal incline of the lingual cusp of the mandibular tooth (*C*). In this manner the cusps and fossae will remain in static relation and the buccal and lingual cusps will be in functional contact in right lateral excursive movement (*D*). If the buccal cusp of the mandibular tooth had been ground, the cutting efficiency of the tooth would have been reduced. These same rules apply when cusps of adjoining teeth have different inclinations. If you do not follow these rules, the tooth with the steeper cusps will take over the occlusal position in excursive movement and the adjoining tooth with the flatter incline will be out of contact.
2. *Disharmony of cuspal inclinations of adjacent teeth on the working side.* If the inclination of cusps of opposing teeth is the same but there is an interference in lateral excursion, you may have to reshape the buccal upper and lingual lower cusps (BU-LL, Fig. 37-32, *A*). If the buccal lower and

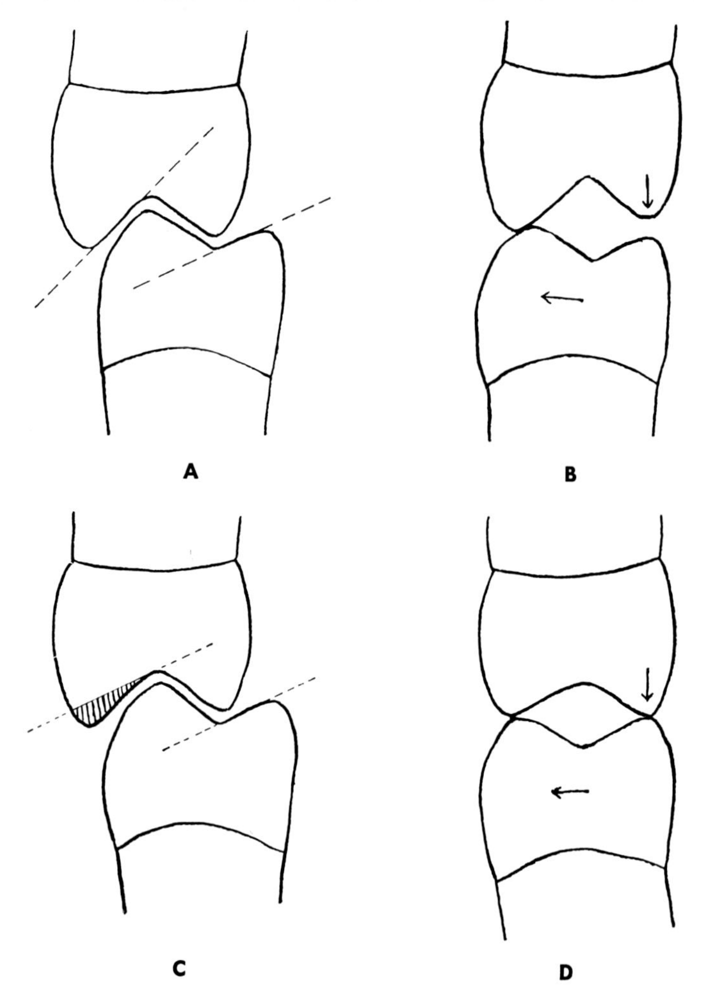


**Fig. 37-31.** If there are differences in inclination of cusps of opposing or adjacent teeth, **A,** steep inclines take cusps out of function. **B,** Reduce the steeper inclination to conform with the flatter one, **C.** This will permit good functional contact of both cusps, **D.**

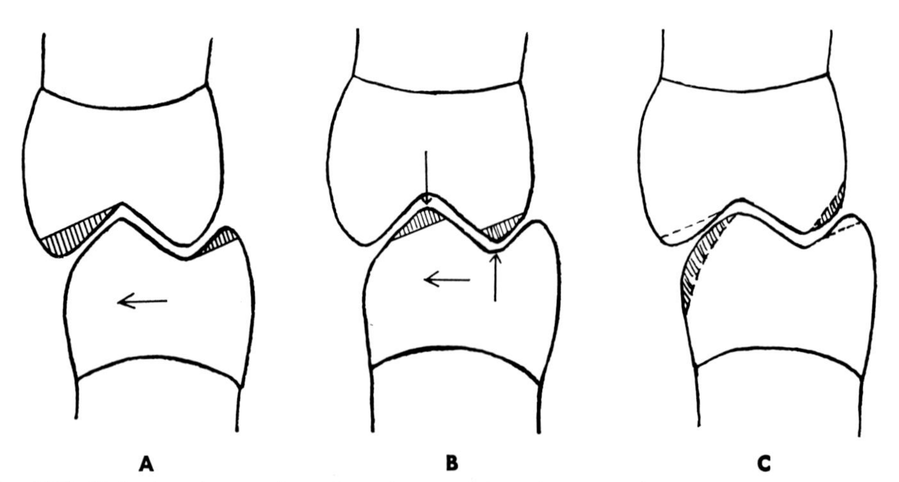


**Fig. 37-32.** If in lateral excursions there is cuspal interference, reduce the buccal upper and lingual lower cusps (BU-LL), **A.** If the buccal lower and lingual upper cusps were reduced, the tooth would be taken out of static contact, **B.** If the buccal surface of the buccal cusps of the mandibular teeth and the lingual surface of the lingual cusps of the maxillary teeth are very heavy, reduce the bulge, **C,** but do not touch the tips of the cusps.

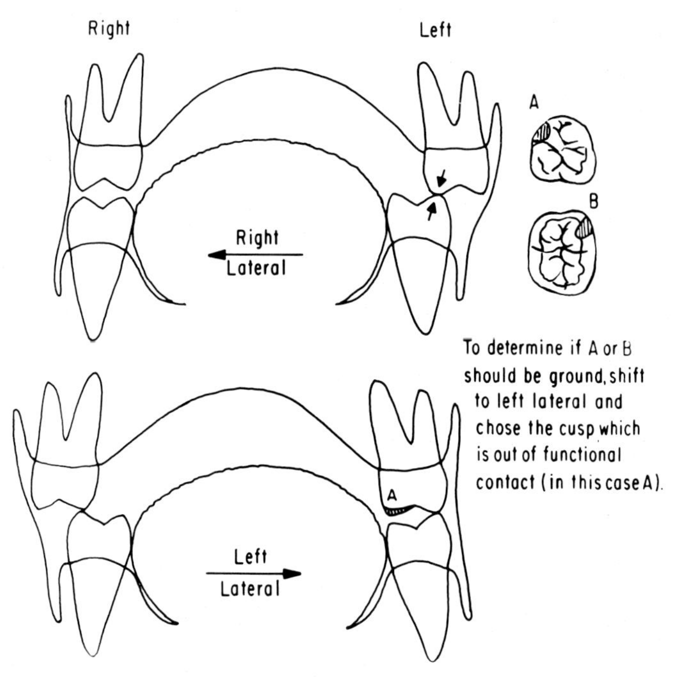


**Fig. 37-33.** In right lateral excursion a premature contact exists on the opposite, nonfunctional side (arrows), preventing tooth contact on the functional side. Note the space between the teeth of the right side. Should the upper prematurity, **A,** or the lower prematurity, **B,** be ground? To determine which, move the mandible to left lateral excursion and study the cusp relationship. Grind the cusp that is out of functional contact (in this case **A**) to correct the prematurity and permit functional contact in right lateral excursion.

lingual upper cusps were ground (*B*), the tooth would be taken out of terminal hinge occlusion and thus would be able to migrate again into a disharmonious relationship. The buccal cusps of the mandibular teeth and the lingual cusps of the maxillary teeth are responsible for keeping the teeth in their proper position and for determining the vertical dimension of the dentition. If these cusps have heavy, bulging buccal or lingual surfaces, reshape them (*C*), but be careful not to grind the respective cusp tips.

3. *Disharmonies of cuspal inclinations between the functional and nonfunctional sides (balancing side prematurities).* Proper occlusal contact may be present in the terminal hinge position; but in right lateral excursive movement, for example, a premature contact may exist on the nonworking side. In this situation the teeth do not contact on the working side (Fig. 37-33). To evaluate this situation before grinding is done, you must bring the teeth into working excursive contact at the opposite (left) side (Fig. 37-33). The decision as to which cusp will be ground is determined by the excursive position of the mandibular buccal and the maxillary lingual cusps. If the mandibular buccal cusp is in proper functional contact with the maxillary buccal cusp and the lingual cusp is out of contact, reshape the maxillary lingual cusp. If the lingual cusp is in good functional relation and the buccal cusp is out of contact, reshape the mandibular buccal cusp. If, under similar circumstances, in left lateral excursion both lingual and buccal cusps are in good functional contact,

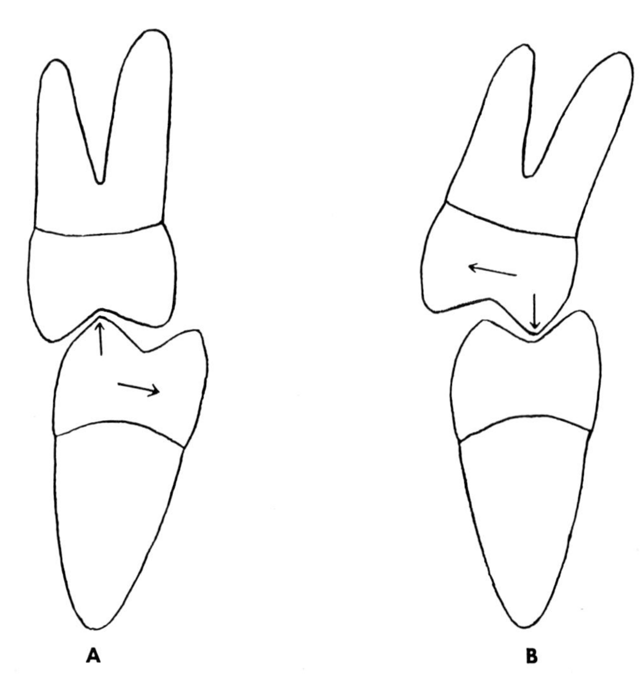


**Fig. 37-34.** **A,** If a mandibular tooth is inclined lingually and its buccal cusp is in static contact with the fossa of the maxillary tooth, grind all eccentric premature contacts by reshaping the maxillary tooth. **B,** If a maxillary tooth is inclined buccally and its lingual cusp is in static contact with the fossa of the mandibular tooth, eliminate all prematurities by reshaping the mandibular tooth.

reshape either the maxillary lingual or the mandibular buccal cusp, but never both. The cusp to be preserved is one that directs forces more closely within the long axis of the tooth. Contact on the nonfunctional side is neither necessary nor desirable in the natural dentition. Prematurities on the nonfunctional side transmit torsional forces to the periodontium that may be damaging to the temporomandibular articulation.

***Reestablishing morsal anatomy, polishing ground surfaces***

When occlusal grinding is completed, reestablish occlusal tooth anatomy. Form sluiceways and embrasures and round sharp edges slightly. Polish all tooth surfaces that were ground and make them comfortable to tongue and cheek.

## Unusual situations

***Special note concerning tipped, tilted, or rotated teeth***

When a tooth is tipped lingually or buccally, great care should be exercised in deciding on a corrective procedure. Such teeth can be very easily taken out of static contact, and migration of the tooth that has been reshaped may occur. The tooth with static cuspal contact in the hinge position should not be reshaped under any circumstances (Fig. 37-34).

***Class III malocclusions and crossbite***

Cases with class III malocclusions and crossbite require grinding in lateral excursions that is the reverse of BU-LL. In other words the lingual cusp of the upper and the buccal cusp of the lower should be ground. However, the principles of grinding are unchanged.

***Micrognathia***

In cases in which the mandible is disproportionately smaller than the maxilla, occlusion may depend on the very extreme outer tip of the occlusal surface of the mandibular teeth catching the inner tip of the maxillary teeth. Any grind-

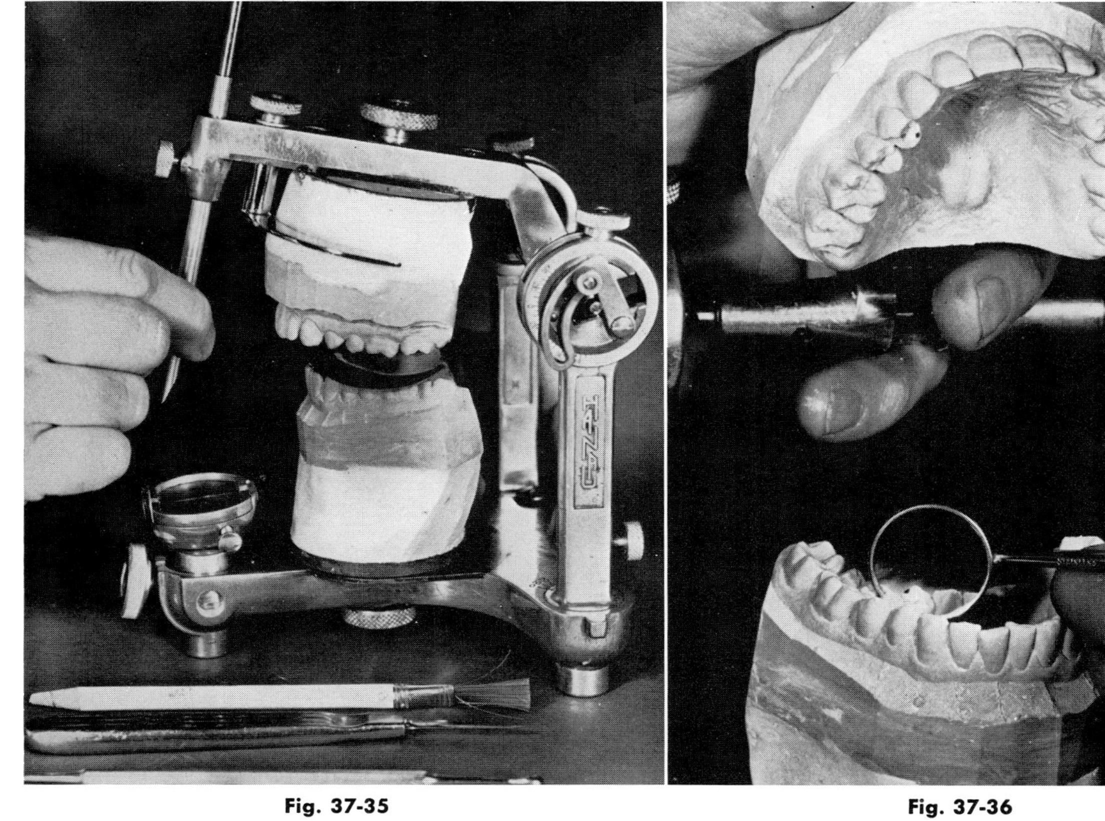


**Fig. 37-35.** Place thin, silk typewriter ribbon on the occlusal surfaces of casts in the articulator and tap the teeth gently together. (Elevate the incisal guidance pin so that it does not touch.)

**Fig. 37-36.** Mark contacts between the right maxillary first premolar, lingual cusp, and mesiobuccal incline and the mandibular first premolar, buccal cusp, and distolingual incline.

ing of these points would disocclude the teeth and cause the mandibular teeth to miss the maxillary teeth either partially or completely, collapsing the bite.

***Dual bite***

Problems arise whenever the buccolingual relation of the teeth is abnormal, the teeth are in crossbite, teeth are missing and have not been replaced, or prosthetic appliances are present that do not comply adequately with periodontal specifications. On occasion, particularly in the presence of extreme overjet, patients have trained themselves to habitually close in a second convenient protrusive position. Such patients have a dual bite. Occlusal correction may be necessary for either or both positions.

## Practical procedures

Armed with an understanding of the rules for occlusal adjustment, you are now ready to proceed with a practical case. There are two approaches. In one you will work directly in the mouth. In the other you will first do the grinding on articulator-mounted study casts; this procedure is better for students.

***Articulator procedure***

If the articulator procedure is used, good casts of the patient's dentition should be obtained. The centers of rotation (hinge) for both temporomandibular articulations should be established. Then mount the stone casts in hinge position, according to the Frankfort horizontal plane, using a face-bow. The articulator should reasonably duplicate opening-closing, protrusive, and lateral excursions.

You should now have mounted casts of the patient that can be studied and that to a certain degree can reproduce tooth-to-tooth relationships. Realize, however, that no machine, no matter how ingeniously constructed, is capable of completely reproducing the mandibular movements of an individual. Realize also that the direction, magnitude of force, and frequency of tooth contact cannot be gauged from the articulator. Many clinicians therefore prefer to correct the occlusion without any articulator mounting.

Nevertheless, those who do use the articulator correct the occlusion on the casts first, according to the rules for occlusal adjustment (Figs. 37-35 and 37-36). They then note the procedure step by step on a grinding list, which serves as a guide when the grinding is done in the mouth.

The studying, marking, and cutting of the stone casts does not ensure that the spots will be corrected to the same degree in the mouth. In fact, on the stone casts much larger portions of the teeth can and should be cut away than can be done later in the month. The grinding list is only a blueprint of what can be expected in occlusal adjustment. This procedure familiarizes the operator with the occlusion of the patient and frequently helps to avoid problems that would otherwise arise.

The procedures to be followed will be determined by the objectives for each patient. Occlusal adjustment is not an all-or-nothing measure. One patient might require only the narrowing of the buccolingual diameters of the teeth, whereas another might require more extensive adjustment. The distribution and extent of lesions present and their relation to the occlusal problem will determine the amount and type of occlusal adjustment to be done. This, however, cannot excuse crude or haphazard attempts at occlusal adjustment. The method used and the desired objectives must be precisely planned.

***Contraindications to selective grinding***

Selective grinding is contraindicated in the following situations: when pulp chambers are large, when major occlusal discrepancies may require orthodontics or reconstruction, and in patients who are poor candidates for mouth reconstruction because of psychologic factors. These patients become tooth conscious after such procedures and are unhappy with the results.

***Occlusal adjustment in the oral cavity***

After teaching the patient to close in terminal hinge position, establish the premature contacts by marking with thin articulating paper or typewriter ribbon after the teeth have been dried with cotton rolls. Encourage the patient to relax. Have him tap the teeth lightly together with the carbon paper, typewriter ribbon (special inking), or special wax in place. One or more points may be marked by the articulating paper. After consulting the grinding list, you will be able to establish easily whether the first point of contact found in the articulator is identical with the finding in the patient's mouth. If the mounting of the casts was correct and the patient closed on the hinge, there will be little question that the first points of premature contact are identical. The first premature contact can be eliminated by grinding the spot that was determined on the articulator. This will save considerable chair time and fatigue to the patient by eliminating indecision and establishing a definite goal.

After the first premature contact has thus been eliminated, dry the surfaces of the teeth once more and place the articulating paper or wax on the occlusal surfaces. The teeth are tapped together as before. Then find the next point of contact and, after consulting the grinding list, eliminate it. Previously ground spots may again come into premature contact, which indicates that insufficient tooth structure was removed.*

In this way the entire occlusion can be corrected and all premature contacts and irregularities eliminated. The rules for reshaping should be observed carefully, but exceptions can be made when necessary.

After the reshaping is finished, tapping should produce a single, resonant sound. The patient often will comment on the improvement in the occlusion—not just after it is finished but even shortly after the first prematurities have been eliminated. After the worst premature contacts have been eliminated, the patient will often be able to help in finding any remaining premature contacts by tapping his teeth lightly together on the hinge and putting his finger on the offending tooth. Most patients adapt readily to the changes in occlusion.

***Adjusting to lateral excursions***

In correcting functional occlusal disharmonies, adjust the occlusion only to the range of functional movement. In correcting for parafunctional movement, adjust the occlusion to the range of such movement as evidenced by wear facets.

***When is occlusal adjustment considered complete?***

Occlusal adjustment is not intended to relocate the mandible but rather to enable the patient to use the different jaw positions and movements with good intercuspation and to chew efficiently with comfort and without damage to the periodontium. Occlusal adjustment is complete when these aims have been accomplished.[44a]

***Jankelson's method***

Before the completion of the discussion of occlusal adjustment, consider the method of grinding advocated by Jankelson[45-48] and employed by some dentists. It is interesting because it is at variance with the previous methods.

In the Jankelson method major emphasis is placed on the cusp-fossa relationship of the teeth in terminal hinge occlusion. Deflective contacts are believed to create a physiologic instability during swallowing.

In the removal of interferences, the buccal surface of the mandibular teeth and the lingual surfaces of the maxillary teeth are ground. Excursive movements are not considered to be physiologic, and therefore no grinding of excursive movements is performed. Instead the relationship of the teeth is examined and

*Needless to say, when the grinding is done directly in the mouth, the procedure is in no way different from what it would be if the articulator-mounted procedure were used, except that there is no grinding list to consult.

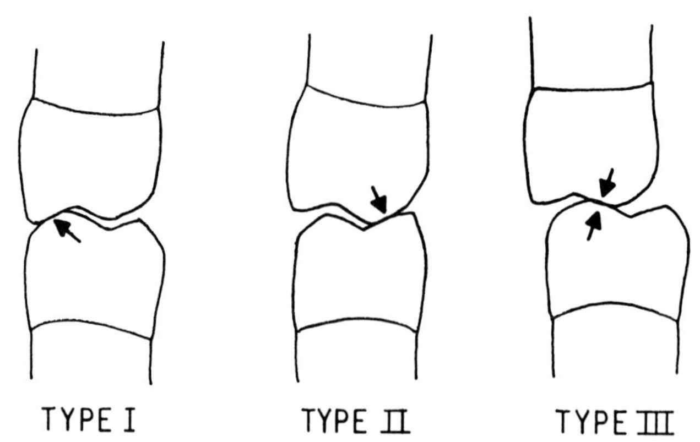


**Fig. 37-37.** Jankelson classification of prematurities. In type I the buccal surfaces of the lower teeth are in premature contact with the buccal cusps of the upper teeth. In type II the lingual surfaces of the upper teeth are in premature contact with the lingual cusps of the lower teeth. In type III the lingual cusps of the upper teeth are in premature contact with the buccal cusps of the lower teeth. Arrows indicate the areas to be corrected by grinding.

the types of prematurities are classified. Premature contacts in centric are classified as types I, II, and III (Fig. 37-37).

*Type I.* The buccal surfaces of the lower teeth are in premature contact with the buccal cusps of the upper teeth. A corresponding relationship holds for the anterior teeth.

*Type II.* The lingual surfaces of the upper posterior teeth are in premature contact with the lingual cusps of the lower teeth.

*Type III.* The lingual cusps of the upper teeth are in premature contact with the buccal cusps of the lower teeth.

These prematurities are detected by the use of 30-gauge wax strips while the mandible is moved in hinge relation by the therapist. The prematurities are evidenced by a tearing or thinning of the wax. Thin or torn wax areas are marked with a pencil; such areas are then reduced by grinding. Reduction of premature contacts produces a better cusp-fossa relationship in centric. The correction of type I and type II prematurities is in reality buccolingual narrowing (Fig. 37-15). Sometimes, as a result of these corrections, teeth that are in a poor cusp-fossa relationship are freed of restrictions and tend to shift into a better relationship. After the type I and type II prematurities are corrected, the patient is dismissed to permit this uprighting to occur.

At the next visit the patient is again tested for new type I and type II premature contacts that may have developed as a result of tooth shifting. Then type III prematurities are corrected. On completion of the correction, only the mandibular buccal cusp tips and the maxillary lingual cusp tips make registrations in the wax.

The occlusion is tested again in a week and periodically thereafter to determine whether further eruption and uprighting has produced additional prematurities.

It is possible to combine elements of Jankelson grinding with the Schuyler type of grinding (Fig. 37-32, *C*).

## OCCLUSAL ADJUSTMENT

In the discussion of function and tissue structure, a good masticatory organ was said to be one that functions comfortably and, in functioning, preserves the integrity of its component tissues. Pathology cannot be inferred simply because teeth do not come together as we would like them to do. Pathology exists only when there is a lesion in the periodontium and possibly also when there is a malfunctioning of the temporomandibular joints or the muscles of mastication accompanied by spasm and pain.[49]

Grinding to correct occlusal disharmonies is often quite useful in general and reconstructive dentistry. No positive case has been made, however, to prove that disharmonies, per se, produce periodontal disease. You cannot inspect an occlusion and decide on the basis of its arrangement that traumatism has occurred.

Correction of occlusal disharmonies is not done to prevent or cure inflammatory or dystrophic periodontal disease. No one has cured a periodontal pocket or even a gingivitis simply by grinding the occlusion or by reconstructing a bad bite. To give undue emphasis to the grinding of occlusion as a primary or exclusive treatment of periodontal disease would constitute complete neglect of the known facts of biology.

On the other hand, periodontal trauma may be a significantly aggravating factor when periodontal diseases are present.[50-54] When periodontal trauma exists with occlusal traumatism, occlusal adjustment is indicated in the treatment program because the improvement in function may permit a beneficial tissue response to occur. You must depend on clinical findings and on roentgenograms to correctly diagnose periodontal trauma. If trauma exists, it may not be adequately treated by a simple following of the rules for the grinding of the disharmonies. Such an approach, which focuses on the disharmony rather than on the periodontium, may be missing the point.

Thus, do not be surprised to find that trauma and traumatism may occur in mouths that have previously had occlusal disharmonies removed by grinding. Even when the grinding has achieved previously described norms or malocclusions have been well corrected by the orthodontist, or even in some cases in which the mouths have been well reconstructed or splinted, traumatism may still occur. How can this be? The answer is merely that trauma does not necessarily stem from disharmonies alone, that is, primarily from the influence of parafunction; nor does the treatment of disharmonies alone automatically correct parafunction and parafunctionally induced periodontal trauma.

Occlusal trauma should be treated in the absence of marginal (inflammatory) periodontal disease. Such symptoms as tooth mobility, tooth soreness, and the opening of tooth contacts should be corrected.

## Added objectives

In cases of overt, severe trauma, you may reshape the occluding surfaces of the teeth to reduce disharmonies, as in grinding; but, in addition, the following objectives become much greater in importance:

1. To immediately neutralize, minimize, or eliminate mobility
2. To reduce the zone of intercuspation, thus reducing cusp inclines so that lateral vectors of force are minimized (Figs. 37-14 to 37-16)

   In the correction of disharmonies, even when group function is gained, the resultant cusp inclination may still not be sufficiently shallow and the whole group of teeth many remain in trauma in lateral excursions. In these situations, continue to grind to reduce cusp inclination even though group function was obtained earlier.

3. To establish cusp-fossa contact that holds a tooth in position but does not lock the mandible

   In this way tooth shifting and migration are prevented; yet, since the teeth glide past each other, they cannot be pitted against each other as in rocking. Isometric parafunctional forces cannot be built up. The forces generated during movements are mostly isotonic. The isometric component of force does not build up until the mandible stops moving. Isometric forces are much stronger than isotonic forces and consequently are more damaging. If the patient cannot gain purchase (grasp) on a tooth, both shearing forces and isometric contraction will be minimized.

### Timing in relation to surgery

Occlusal adjustment for trauma must be integrated with the course of periodontal treatment. There are three times in the course of periodontal treatment when occlusal interventions may be undertaken: (1) preliminary grinding, (2) definitive grinding, and (3) check grinding.

***Preliminary grinding***

Preliminary grinding is a necessity as the first step early in treatment when the patient complains of pain or discomfort or when normal function is prevented by excessive mobility. Such complaints merit immediate attention.

If an individual tooth is involved, the grinding is referred to as spot grinding. Examples are the relieving of a tooth during endodontic treatment, the adjustment of a high spot shortly after a new restoration is placed, and the shortening of a tooth with a periodontal abscess or pericementitis.

In some instances, when an individual tooth is quite loose, the tooth may be relieved by spot grinding over many successive visits before it begins to stabilize. In other instances, as in periodontosis, successive grinding visits may result in a further eruption of the tooth, which, as it erupts, brings the bone along with it, resulting in the elimination of subcrestal defects.[55]

In general, however, preliminary grinding is a treatment of immediate need and stops short of complete occlusal adjustment.

***Definitive grinding***

Definitive grinding, or complete occlusal adjustment, is usually performed later in treatment. If the initial examination reveals tooth mobility and roentgenographic signs of trauma, the treatment plan must contain occlusal adjustment. This step will follow root scaling, for often inflammation displaces a tooth from its position at the time of examination. After scaling and the resolution of inflammation, the tooth may move back to its normal position. The decision that must be made is whether to do the adjustment before or after surgery when both steps are necessary. The timing depends on how loose the teeth are. If some teeth have mobilities of 1½ degrees or more, do the adjustment first. Fabrication of night guards may also be necessary for surgery often produces an increased looseness of teeth.[56] Postsurgical mobility is generally transient; but if it is superimposed on teeth that are already quite loose, it may become permanent. In instances when mobility is of less significance, the occlusal adjustment can be done after surgery. In this case definitive and check grinding can be done at the same time. On occasion the elimination of high spots on restorations is useful. Often bruxism is minimized after such steps.

***Check grinding***

Check grinding is generally performed as a final measure after all other therapy has been completed and prior to the dismissal of the patient. Usually a month is allowed to elapse after surgery and the mouth is checked for trauma that may have resulted from a slight shifting of the teeth. Such shifting frequently follows a total course of periodontal treatment. It can, in fact, occur because of changes in the periodontal tissues months and years after treatment.

### Reexamination and repeated occlusal adjustment

For this reason the teeth are checked for trauma and, if necessary, are adjusted at each recall visit. Teeth move, particularly periodontally involved teeth. Unless the teeth are held by fixed splints, further minor adjustments are often necessary at a later time. (See discussion on the maintenance phase in Chapter 35.) In instances of extreme malocclusion, particularly if the patient's plane of occlusion is very steep (exaggerated curve of Spee or deep overbite), orthodontics may be necessary before occlusal adjustment can be undertaken.

*Benefits*

Clinical experience has shown that after successful repeated occlusal adjustments many or all of the following benefits may be expected:

1. Loose teeth may tighten.[57]
2. Life of the dentition may be extended.
3. Food impaction, impingement, and retention may be minimized.
4. Aesthetics may be improved.
5. Bruxism and clenching may become less forceful and less frequent.
6. Reconstruction of the dentition may be facilitated.
7. Temporomandibular joint conditions may disappear.
8. Hypertonicity or spasm of facial, masticatory, or neck muscles may diminish.
9. Diastemas may close spontaneously.
10. Teeth may move into better alignment.

To repeat: complete occlusal adjustment is neither necessary nor indicated in every patient. Under certain conditions the elimination of disharmonies may not be as necessary as recontouring some of the teeth. The occlusal table can be narrowed and sluiceways can be improved. Sometimes the objective may be limited to the improvement of aesthetics.

*When occlusal adjustment for periodontal trauma is complete*

Occlusal adjustment is complete when the signs of trauma have been eliminated. If the trauma cannot be eliminated by occlusal adjustment, then resort to splinting as a sequel to treatment. In cases in which occlusal adjustment is or would be obviously unsuccessful, you may splint directly. When there is doubt, a waiting period of 6 to 12 months after occlusal adjustment should suffice to disclose whether the teeth have tightened.

*Therapy for parafunction*

Since parafunctional forces are the most common of the factors that produce trauma, a reconsideration of the treatment of trauma from the standpoint of the treatment of parafunction may be called for.

## MUSCLE THERAPY

Gottlieb believed that a patient should be taught to relax his masticatory muscles consciously and to keep his mandible in rest position at all times except when masticating.[58,59] Another approach to the treatment of bruxism is positive suggestion.[60,61] A patient may be instructed to awaken at night if he starts to grind or grit his teeth during sleep. During the day he may remind himself to keep his teeth apart. Another method is to teach the patient the habit of forcefully contracting the depressors of the mandible.[62]

## NIGHT GUARDS

Smooth-surfaced splints may also be indicated in the treatment of periodontal trauma.[63] Such horseshoe-shaped splints, which are called night guards or

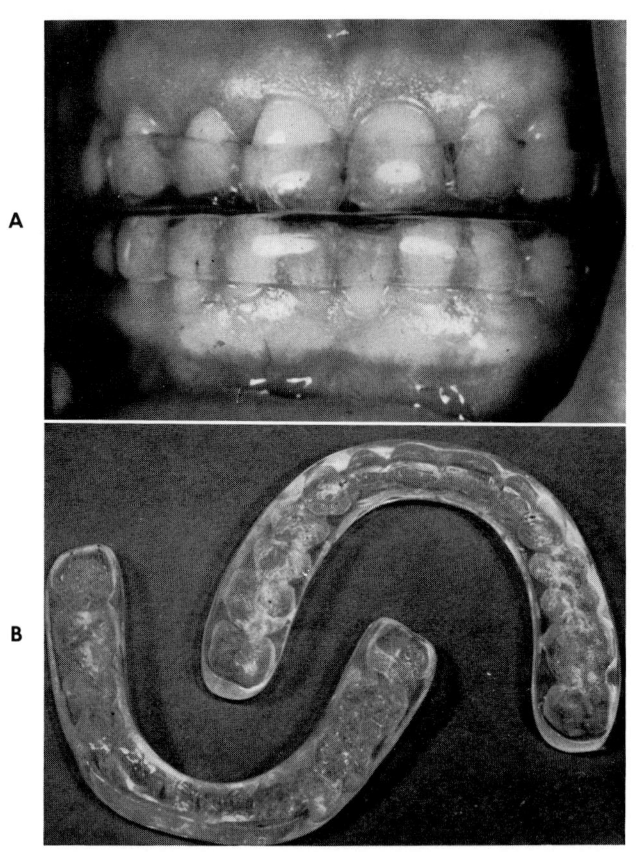


**Fig. 37-38.** Therapy for parafunction—night guard splints to prevent damage to the periodontium. **A,** In the mouth. **B,** Tooth surface view of splints.

bite stabilizers, may be constructed for one or both jaws, freeway space permitting[64-66] (Fig. 37-38). They cover all occlusal surfaces and permit the patient to move his mandible freely in all excursions. They are usually worn at night but may be worn during the day.

Many patients become so accustomed to wearing splints that they can hardly be without them. They may wear deep indentations in the acrylic material, thus giving evidence of the force and persistence of the bruxing movements. Wearing the splints may modify the nature of the habit or redirect the forces into a nontraumatic pattern. Other patients may have great difficulty in adjusting to the night guards and may give up wearing them.

The splints should be thin enough so that they are comfortable to wear, but the palate should not be covered. There must be no sharp edges to irritate the tongue or cheek, although the night guards should make complete contact in all excursions (bilateral balance). Care should be so exercised in the fitting that the splint does not encroach on the freeway space, although in many instances night guards that do this are successfully tolerated by the patient. The splints must be kept moist when not worn so that they do not warp.

Some patients do not tolerate the night guards well because they cannot fall asleep with the night guards or they object to the interference with their normal bruxing and clenching patterns. Considerable patience must be exercised in treat-

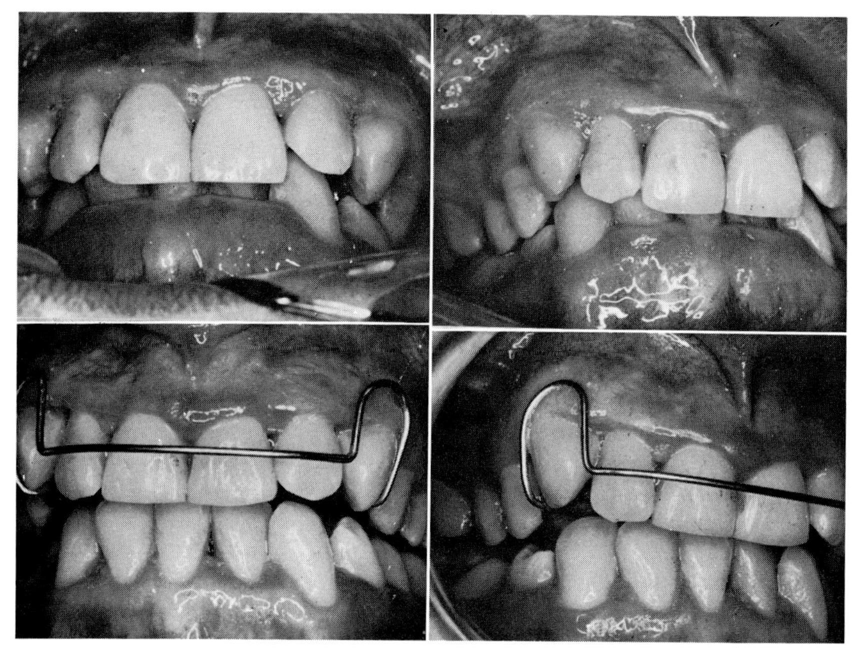

**Fig. 37-39.** When a deep overbite and an exaggerated curve of Spee exist, the patient cannot be fitted with upper and lower night guards unless the dentist opens the bite excessively. In such cases a Hawley appliance with a bite platform against which the lower incisors occlude may be used.

ing these patients. The importance of night guards must be carefully explained and, if necessary, the night guards may have to be worn during the day rather than at night. In other cases only one guard at a time can be worn.

In patients with a deep overbite or an exaggerated curve of Spee, you may not be able to prescribe night guards. In these cases a bite plane (Hawley retainer) may be used (Fig. 37-39) if the health of the lower anterior teeth permits.

**CHAPTER 37**

**References**

1. Sicher, H.: Positions and movements of the mandible, J. Amer. Dent. Ass. **48**:620, 1954.
2. Thompson, J. R.: Rest position of the mandible and its significance to dental science, J. Amer. Dent. Ass. **33**:151, 1946.
3. Thompson, J. R.: Rest position of the mandible and its application to analysis and correction of malocclusion, Angle Orthodont. **19**:162, 1949.
4. Thompson, J. R., and Craddock, F. W.: Functional analysis of occlusion, J. Amer. Dent. Ass. **39**:404, 1949.
5. Ramfjord, S. P., and Ash, M. M., Jr.: Occlusion, ed. 2, Philadelphia, 1971, W. B. Saunders Co.
6. Denton, G. B.: The vocabulary of dentistry and oral science, Chicago, 1958, American Dental Association.
7. Sicher, H., and Du Brul, L. E.: Oral anatomy, ed. 5, St. Louis, 1970, The C. V. Mosby Co.
8. Posselt, U.: Physiology of occlusion and rehabilitation, ed. 2, Philadelphia, 1968, F. A. Davis Co.
9. Orban, B.: Biologic basis for correcting occlusal disharmonies, J. Periodont. **25**:257, 1954.
10. Beyron, H.: Occlusal relations and mastication in Australian aborigines, Acta Odont. Scand. **22**:597, 1964.
11. Murphy, T. R.: The timing and mechanism of the human masticatory stroke, Arch. Oral Biol. **10**:981, 1965.

12. Nadler, S. C.: The effects of bruxism, J. Periodont. **37**:311, 1966.
13. Drum, W.: Ueber Parafunktionen, Zahnaerztl. Rundsch. **59**:257, 1950.
14. Belting, C. M., and Gupta, O. P.: The influence of psychiatric disturbances on the severity of periodontal disease, J. Periodont. **32**:219, 1961.
15. Nadler, S. C.: Detection and recognition of bruxism, J. Amer. Dent. Ass. **61**:742, 1960.
16. Ramfjord, S. P.: Bruxism, a clinical and electromyographic study, J. Amer. Dent. Ass. **62**:21, 1961.
17. Engelberger, A., Rateitschak, K. H., and Mühlemann, H. R.: Diagnostik und Therapie der funktionellen Störungen in Kausystem, Schweiz. Mschr. Zahnheilk. **70**:586, 1960.
18. Drum, W.: Parafunktionen und Autodestruktionsprozesse, Berlin, 1969, Quintessenz.
19. Nadler, S. C.: Bruxism, a classification; critical review, J. Amer. Dent. Ass. **54**:615, 1957.
20. Ingle, J. I.: Occupational bruxism and its relation to periodontal disease, J. Periodont. **23**:7, 1952.
21. Natkin, E., and Ingle, J. I.: Further report on alveolar osteoporosis and pulpal death associated with compulsive bruxism, Periodontics **1**:260, 1963.
21a. Zingeser, M. R.: Cercopithecoid canine tooth honing mechanisms, Amer. J. Phys. Anthrop. **31**:205, 1969.
22. Koivumaa, K. K., Landt, H., and Nyquist, G.: Investigations on the incidence of periodontal disease and disorders of the temporomandibular point in cases of bruxism, Tandläk. Sällsk. Förhandl. **56**:328, 1960.
23. Posselt, U.: Occlusion related to periodontics. In Ramfjord, S. P., Kerr, D. A., and Ash, M. M., editors: World workshop in periodontics, Ann Arbor, Mich., 1966, University of Michigan Press.
24. Angle, E. H.: Malocclusion of the teeth, ed. 7, Philadelphia, 1907, S. S. White Co.
25. Thielemann, K.: Die Biomechanik der Paradentose, ed. 2, Munich, 1956, Johann Ambrosius Barth.
26. Reeves, R. L.: Is prophylactic occlusal adjustment a justifiable procedure? J. Periodont. **28**:272, 1957.
27. McCollum, B. B.: Fundamentals involved in prescribing restorative dental remedies, Dent. Items Interest **61**:522, 641, 724, 852, 942, 1939.
28. Schuyler, C. H.: Fundamental principles in the correction of occlusal disharmony, natural and artificial, J. Amer. Dent. Ass. **22**:1193, 1935.
29. Schuyler, C. H.: Correction of occlusal disharmony of the natural dentition, New York Dent. J. **13**:445, 1947.
30. Miller, S. C.: Textbook of periodontia, ed. 2, Philadelphia, 1943, Blakiston Division, McGraw-Hill Book Co.
31. Schuyler, C. H.: Factors of occlusion applicable to restorative dentistry, J. Prosth. Dent. **3**:772, 1953.
32. Beyron, H.: Physio-pathologic correlations between function of the masticatory system and periodontics, Parodontologie **20**:61, 1966.
33. Schuyler, C. H.: Factors contributing to traumatic occlusion, J. Prosth. Dent. **11**:708, 1961.
34. Weinberg, L. A.: Rationale and technique for occlusal equilibration, J. Prosth. Dent. **14**:74, 1964.
35. Youdelis, R. A., and Mann, W. V.: The prevalence and possible role of nonworking contacts in periodontal disease, Periodontics **3**:219, 1965.
36. D'Amico, A.: The canine teeth-normal functional relation of the natural teeth of man, J. S. Calif. Dent. Ass. **26**:6, 49, 127, 175, 194, 239, 1958.
37. D'Amico, A.: Functional occlusion of the natural teeth of man, J. Prosth. Dent. **11**:899, 1961.
38. Stuart, C. E., and Stallard, H.: Principles involved in restoring occlusion to natural teeth, J. Prosth. Dent. **10**:304, 1960.
39. Stallard, H., and Stuart, C. E.: Eliminating tooth guidance in natural dentitions, J. Prosth. Dent. **11**:474, 1961.
40. Stallard, H., and Stuart, C. E.: Concepts of occlusion. What kind of occlusion should recusped teeth be given? Dental Clinics of North America, Philadelphia, November 1963, W. B. Saunders Co.
41. Beyeler, K.: Beschleifen der Zähne bei Paradentose, Bern, 1944, Paul Haupt.
42. Kiefer, E.: Paradentosebehandlung mit besonderer Berücksichtigung der Entlastung, Munich, 1951, Carl Hanser Verlag.
43. Schuyler, C. H.: Intra-oral methods of establishing maxillomandibular relations, J. Amer. Dent. Ass. **19**:1012, 1932.

43a. Ramfjord, S. P.: Die Voraussetzungen für eine ideale Okklusion, Deutsch. Zahnaerztl. Z. 26:106, 1971.
43b. Ross, F. I.: Occlusion, St. Louis, 1970, The C. V. Mosby Co.
44. Ray, H., and Santos, H. A.: Consideration of tongue thrusting as a factor in periodontal disease, J. Periodont. 25:250, 1954.
44a. Glickman, I., Ratcliff, P., Zander, H. A., and Sugarman, M.: When and to what extent do you adjust the occlusion during periodontal therapy? J. Periodont. 41:536, 1970.
45. Jankelson, B.: Physiology of human dental occlusion, J. Amer. Dent. Ass. 50:664, 1955.
46. Jankelson, B., Hoffman, G. M., and Hendron, J. A.: The physiology of the stomatognathic system, J. Amer. Dent. Ass. 46:386, 1953.
47. Jankelson, B.: Technique for obtaining optimum functional relationship for the natural dentition, Dental Clinics of North America, Philadelphia, March 1960, W. B. Saunders Co.
48. Jankelson, B.: Considerations in occlusion in fixed partial dentures, Dental Clinics of North America, Philadelphia, March 1959, W. B. Saunders Co.
49. Fröhlich, F.: Die okklusionbedingten Schmerzen im Kiefer-/Gesichts-Bereich, Schweiz. Mschr. Zahnheilk, 76:764, 1966.
50. Macapanpan, L. C., and Weinmann, P.: The influence of injury to the periodontal membrane on the spread of gingival inflammation, J. Dent. Res. 32:665, 1953.
51. Glickman, I.: Effect of excessive occlusal bones upon the pathway of gingival inflammation in humans, J. Periodont. 36:141, 1965.
52. Orban, B.: Traumatic occlusion and gum inflammation, J. Periodont. 10:39, 1939.
53. Glickman, I.: Inflammation and trauma from occlusion, co-destructive factors in periodontal disease, J. Periodont. 34:5, 1963.
54. Stahl, S. S.: The responses of the periodontium to combined gingival inflammation and occluso-functional stresses in four human surgical specimens, Periodontics 6:14, 1968.
55. Everett, F. G.: A preliminary report on the treatment of the osseous defect in periodontosis, J. Periodont. 35:429, 1964.
56. Glickman, I., Smulow, J. B., Vogel, G., and others: The effect of occlusal forces on healing following mucogingival surgery, J. Periodont. 37:319, 1966.
57. Mühlemann, H. R., Herzog, H., and Rateitschak, K. H.: Quantitative evaluation of the therapeutic effect of selective grinding, J. Periodont. 28:11, 1957.
58. Gottlieb, B.: Histologic considerations of the supporting tissues of the teeth, J. Amer. Dent. Ass. 30:1872, 1943.
59. Gottlieb, B.: Traumatic occlusion and the rest position of the mandible, J. Periodont. 18:7, 1947.
60. Boyens, P. J.: Value of autosuggestion in the therapy of "bruxism" and other biting habits, J. Amer. Dent. Ass. 27:1773, 1940.
61. Leof, M.: Clamping and grinding habits; their relation to periodontal disease, J. Amer. Dent. Ass. 31:184, 1944.
62. Ackerman, J. B.: A new approach to the treatment of bruxism and bruxomania, New York Dent. J. 32:259, 1966.
63. Karolyi, M.: Beobachtungen über Alveolarpyorrhoe, Oest.-Ungar. Vjschr. Zahnheilk. 17:259, 1901.
64. Gottlieb, B.: Schmutzpyorrhoe, Paradentalpyorrhoe und Alveolaratrophie, Berlin, 1925, Urban & Schwarzenberg.
65. Allen, D. L.: Accurate occlusal bite guards, Periodontics 5:93, 1967.
66. Berliner, A.: Ligatures, splints, bite planes and pyramids, Philadelphia, 1964, J. B. Lippincott Co.

#### Additional suggested reading

Anderson, D. J., and Picton, D. C. A.: Tooth contact during chewing, J. Dent. Res. 36:21, 1957.
Beyeler, K.: Bruxismus und Prothetik, Parodontopathies 17:320, 1963.
Bien, S. M.: Hydrodynamic damping of tooth movement, J. Dent. Res. 45:907, 1966.
Butler, J. H., and Zander, H. A.: Evaluation of two occlusal concepts, Parodont. Acad. Rev. 2:5, 1968.
Courant, P.: Use of removable acrylic splints in general practice, J. Canad. Dent. Ass. 33:494, 1967.
De Boever, J.: Experimental occlusal balancing-contact interference and muscle activity. An electromyographic study with permanently applied electrodes, Parodont. Acad. Rev. 23:59, 1969.

Dempster, W. T., and Duddles, R. A.: Tooth statics; equilibrium of a free-body, J. Amer. Dent. Ass. **68**:651, 1964.

Eschler, J.: Bruxism and function of the masticatory muscles, Parodontologie **15**:109, 1961.

Eschler, J.: Das Verhalten der Kiefergelenke bei pathologischen Okklusionen, Parodontologie **18**:200, 1964.

Frisch, J., Katz, L., and Ferreira, A. J.: A study on the relationship between bruxism and aggression, J. Periodont. **31**:409, 1960.

Fröhlich, E.: Die Parafunktionen, Symptomatologie, Aetiologie und Therapie, Deutsch. Zahnaerztl. Z. **21**:536, 1966.

Geiger, A.: Occlusion in periodontal disease, J. Periodont. **36**:387, 1965.

Giordano, J. V., editor: Symposium on occlusion, Dental Clinics of North America, Philadelphia, March 1962, W. B. Saunders Co.

Glickman, I.: Clinical significance of trauma from occlusion, J. Amer. Dent. Ass. **70**:607, 1965.

Glickman, I., and Smulow, J. B.: Further observations on the effects of trauma from occlusion, J. Periodont. **38**:280, 1967.

Graber, G.: Psychisch motivierte Parafunktionen auf Grund von Aggressionen und Myoarthropathien des Kauorgans, Schweiz. Mschr. Zahnheilk. **81**:713, 1971.

Grupe, H. E., and Gromek, J. J.: Bruxism splint, J. Periodont. **30**:156, 1959.

Guggenheim, P., and Cohen, L.: The nature of masseteric hypertrophy, Arch. Otolaryng. **73**:15, 1961.

Hofman, M., and Diemer, R.: Die physiologische Zahnbewegung, Deutsch. Zahnaerztl. Z. **12**:707, 1966.

Isaacson, J. D., and Ledley, R. S.: Tooth statics, J. Amer. Dent. Ass. **69**:805, 1964.

Kawamura, Y., Tsukamoto, S., and Miyoshi, K.: Gnashing induced by electrical stimulation of rabbit brain cortex, Amer. J. Physiol. **200**:916, 1961.

Lipke, D., and Posselt, U.: Parafunctions of the masticatory system (bruxism), J. West. Soc. Periodont. **8**:133, 1960.

Mühlemann, H. R.: Ten years of tooth mobility measurements, J. Periodont. **31**:110, 1960.

Murphy, T. R.: The progressive reduction of tooth cusps as it occurs in natural attrition, Dent. Pract. **19**:8, 1968.

Natkin, E., and Ingle, J. I.: A further report on osteoporosis and pulpal death associated with compulsive bruxism, Periodontics **1**:260, 1963.

O'Leary, T. J., Rudd, K. D., and Nabers, C. L.: Factors affecting horizontal tooth mobility, Periodontics **4**:308, 1966.

O'Leary, T. J., Rudd, K. D., and Nabers, C. L., and others: The effect of mastication and deglutition on tooth mobility, Periodontics **5**:26, 1967.

Parfitt, G. J.: The dynamics of a tooth in function, J. Periodont. **32**:102, 1961.

Perry, H. T., Lammie, G. A., Main, J., and Teuscher, G. W.: Occlusion in a stress situation, J. Amer. Dent. Ass. **60**:626, 1960.

Picton, D. C. A.: A study of normal tooth mobility and the changes with periodontal disease, Dent. Pract. **12**:167, 1962.

Powell, R. N.: Tooth contact during sleep; association with other events, J. Dent. Res. **44**:959, 1965.

Posselt, U.: Occlusion related to periodontics. In Ramfjord, S. P., Kerr, D. A., and Ash, M. M., editors: World workshop in periodontics, Ann Arbor, Mich., 1966, University of Michigan Press.

Posselt, U.: The physiology of mastication, J. West Soc. Periodont. **9**:40, 1961.

Posselt, U.: Studies in the mobility of the human mandible, Acta Odont. Scand., vol. 10, supp., p. 19, 1952.

Posselt, U., and Emslie, R. D.: Occlusal disharmonies and their effect on periodontal diseases, Int. Dent. J. **9**:367, 1959.

Posselt, U., and Wolff, I. B.: Treatment of bruxism by bite guards and bite plates, J. Canad. Dent. Ass. **29**:773, 1963.

Rateitschak, K. H.: Reaction of periodontal tissue to artificial (orthodontic) forces. In Eastoe, J. E., Picton, D. C. A., and Alexander, A. G., editors: The prevention of periodontal disease, London, 1971, Henry Kimpton.

Rateitschak, K. H., Fistarol, A. F., and Wolf, H. F.: Parafunctionen, Schweiz. Mschr. Zahnheilk. **76**:289, 1966.

Reding, G. R., Rubright, W. C., and Rechtschaffen, A.: Sleep pattern of tooth grinding; its relationship to dreaming, Science **145**:725, 1964.

Rivera, A. N., Lozano, R., and Aguilar, P.: Glucosa ensangre en relación con movilidad dentaria, Rev. Asoc. Dent. Mex. **18**:529, 1961.

Schaerer, P., and Stallard, R. E.: The effect of an occlusal interference on tooth contact occurrence during mastication, Helv. Odont. Acta **10**:49, 1966.

Schireson, S.: Grinding teeth for masticatory efficiency and gingival health, J. Prosth. Dent. **13**:337, 1963.

Shapiro, S., and Shanon, J.: Bruxism as an emotional reactive disturbance, Psychosomatics **6**:427, 1965.

Sheppard, I. M., and Markus, N.: Total time of tooth contacts during mastication, J. Prosth. Dent. **12**:460, 1962.

Shore, N. A.: Occlusal equilibration, Philadelphia, 1959, J. B. Lippincott Co.

Smith, R.: Periodontal conditions associated with buckling of the lower anterior teeth; etiology, diagnosis and treatment, J. Amer. Dent. Ass. **34**:303, 1947.

Spengeman, W. G.: The curve of Spee leveling appliance (COSA), Amer. J. Orthodont. **54**:202, 1968.

CHAPTER THIRTY-EIGHT

# Orthodontic measures in periodontal therapy



## INDICATIONS

Orthodontic procedures are often incorporated as part of the therapeutic management of the periodontal patient. When the disease increases in severity, there is a tendency for teeth to loosen and to migrate. These migrations may range from slight to extensive. Periodontics has traditionally included measures for the treatment of tooth migrations.[1] It would be an oversimplification, however, to limit treatment to such migrations. Periodontal and orthodontic techniques and concepts can be correlated,[2] for example, in the elimination of bony defects and pockets incident to tilting of teeth, in the correction of malpositions that might predispose to periodontal disease,[2a] in the treatment of pathology arising during orthodontic therapy, in the preparation of the mouth for reconstruction, and in the improvement of aesthetics as well as the repositioning of periodontally involved teeth.

Orthodontic treatment for individuals with periodontal disease may be indicated in the following situations[3-4b]:

1. Existing tooth malpositions promoting the incidence of periodontal disease or affecting its course
   a. Mouths with crowded teeth
   b. Deep overbites
2. Tooth migrations caused by disease, parafunction, or mutilation of the dentition
   a. Tooth migration caused by oral parafunctions such as tongue thrusting
   b. Tooth migrations seen in inflammation or encountered in periodontosis
   c. Tooth migrations resulting from trauma, loss of teeth, or other mutilation of the dentition

When a combined approach is indicated, problems may develop in the responsibility for treatment. Although many orthodontists will accept adult patients for full treatment, some are unwilling to treat patients whose periodontal structures have been damaged by disease. Since some orthodontists may not be familiar with periodontal disease and therapy, they are reluctant to become involved in treatment. Therefore periodontists have assumed some responsibility for adult orthodontic treatment.

## Pathologic and physiologic factors

When migration is caused by periodontal disease, it is accelerated with the loss of alveolar bone. Teeth drift away from the pocket side and move toward areas of greatest attachment. Chronic inflammatory connective tissue is found in the area from which the tooth has migrated. The presence of inflammation, edema, exudate, and capillary proliferation tends to increase tooth mobility and migration.

Physical forces can act on the tooth in a manner similar to that of an orthodontic appliance. These pressures may be exerted by the actions of the tongue, lips, and cheeks,[5,6] by various habits (Fig. 38-1), by newly placed fillings, by rocking partial dentures, etc. Final tooth position is dependent on the balance of forces acting upon the tooth. Drifting occurs only when the forces are unbalanced. Mesial migration, continuous eruption, and other physiologic tooth movements occur in all dentitions throughout life. Although these factors may influence the migration of periodontally involved teeth, they are responsible for the drifting of otherwise uninvolved teeth as well. Examples of nonphysiologic tooth movements are those caused by thumbsucking, collapse about an extracted molar, and tongue thrusting.

Finally, changes in the metabolism of the patient may influence the periodontium.[7,8] Pregnancy, scurvy, and altered carbohydrate metabolism have been associated with increased tooth mobility; these effects have not been adequately studied, however.[9] In acromegaly, diphenylhydantoin-induced hyperplasia, Paget's disease, and tumors the growth of tissues can move teeth. Such aberrations may contribute to migrations caused by periodontal pathology.

## Malpositions predisposing to periodontal disease

Tooth migration can contribute to further periodontal breakdown by producing alterations in occlusion. Contacts between teeth may open and permit food impaction. The buccal and lingual plates may become perforated or completely resorbed. Craters or infrabony defects may occur where thick bony ledges are present. Buckling may result in gingivae with bulbous or unphysiologic form, which encourages food impingement. Moreover the migrating tooth may alter patterns of mastication and parafunction, thus bringing about periodontal traumatism. The reverse is also true, for traumatism may be responsible for migration.

Not all malpositions are caused by migration. Some are produced during the development and eruption of the teeth. Repositioning such malposed teeth is indicated if a relationship to periodontal disease can be demonstrated. It may also be warranted in the absence of periodontal disease when aesthetic needs or reconstructive requirements dictate or conditions potentially hazardous to the periodontal health of the patient become apparent.

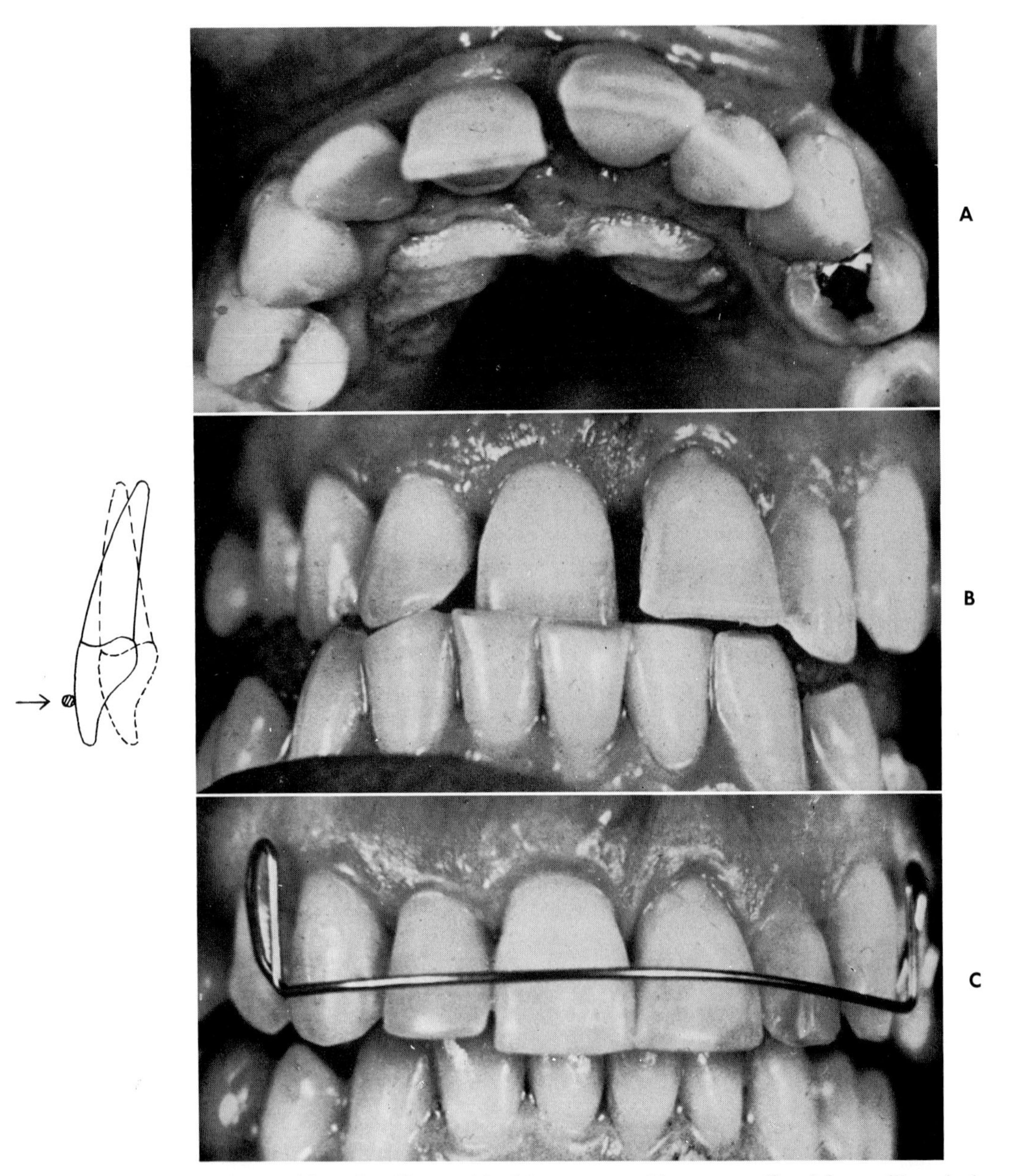


**Fig. 38-1. A,** Dentition of a 40-year-old white woman with a protruding left maxillary incisor. The referring dentist mistakenly thought that this malposition was caused by periodontosis. No pocket could be demonstrated on this tooth. **B,** On examination in the right lateral protrusive position, the misalignment was found to have been caused probably by forces incident to parafunctional movement. This movement forced the upper right central and left lateral incisors labially. **C,** After orthodontic repositioning of the teeth and occlusal correction. Once teeth have been moved into correct position, such an appliance is often worn at night indefinitely as a passive retainer to eliminate the need for further splinting. If this were not done, the teeth might move back into their former protruded position.

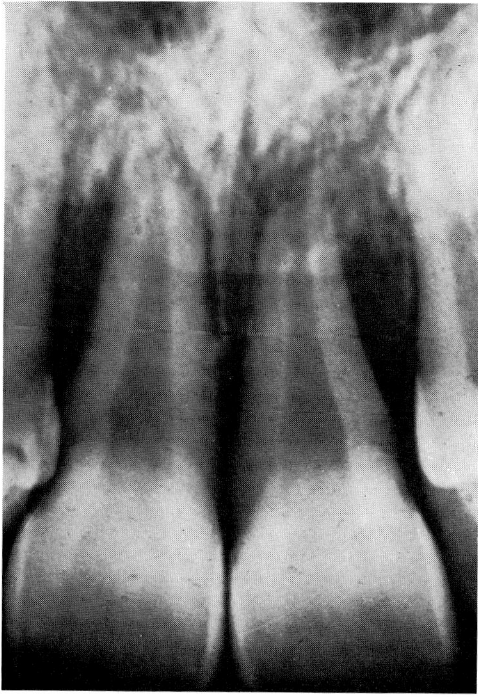

**Fig. 38-2.** Extensive resorption of bone around two maxillary central incisors of a 10-year-old girl. The tissue had been traumatized by a slipped-off rubber band used in orthodontic treatment.

## Lesions incident to orthodontic treatment

Periodontal lesions may be produced as a consequence of treatment during the course of orthodontic tooth movement.[9a,9b,18,19] Such lesions are commonly related to the appliance per se. However, periodontal trauma may be the result of orthodontic forces exerted on the teeth, or occlusal traumatism may occur during the tooth movement (jiggling, Chapter 36).

Fixed appliances tend to promote inflammation because food retention and deposit formation are increased and proper performance of oral hygiene procedures is hindered. An appliance may directly traumatize the tissues when wires bend or settle into the gingiva. Ill-fitting bands are irritating, and, when bands are forced under the gingiva, pockets may be formed.

Removable appliances may compress the gingiva against the teeth, and clasps may impinge on the gingiva. Wires that are occlusal to the contact point may settle and separate the teeth. Rubber bands may slip and be lost under the gingiva, causing exfoliation of teeth (Fig. 38-2). Thus appliances may initiate and perpetuate periodontal disease.

Orthodontic forces produce movement by causing bone and connective tissue to resorb and reform. A small amount of tooth resorption and bone loss may occur in the most properly managed case. When excessive (unphysiologic) pressures are used, bone loss tends to increase. Dramatic bone loss and root resorption can occur in such cases.

Occlusal traumatism may result from orthodontic tooth movement. To re-

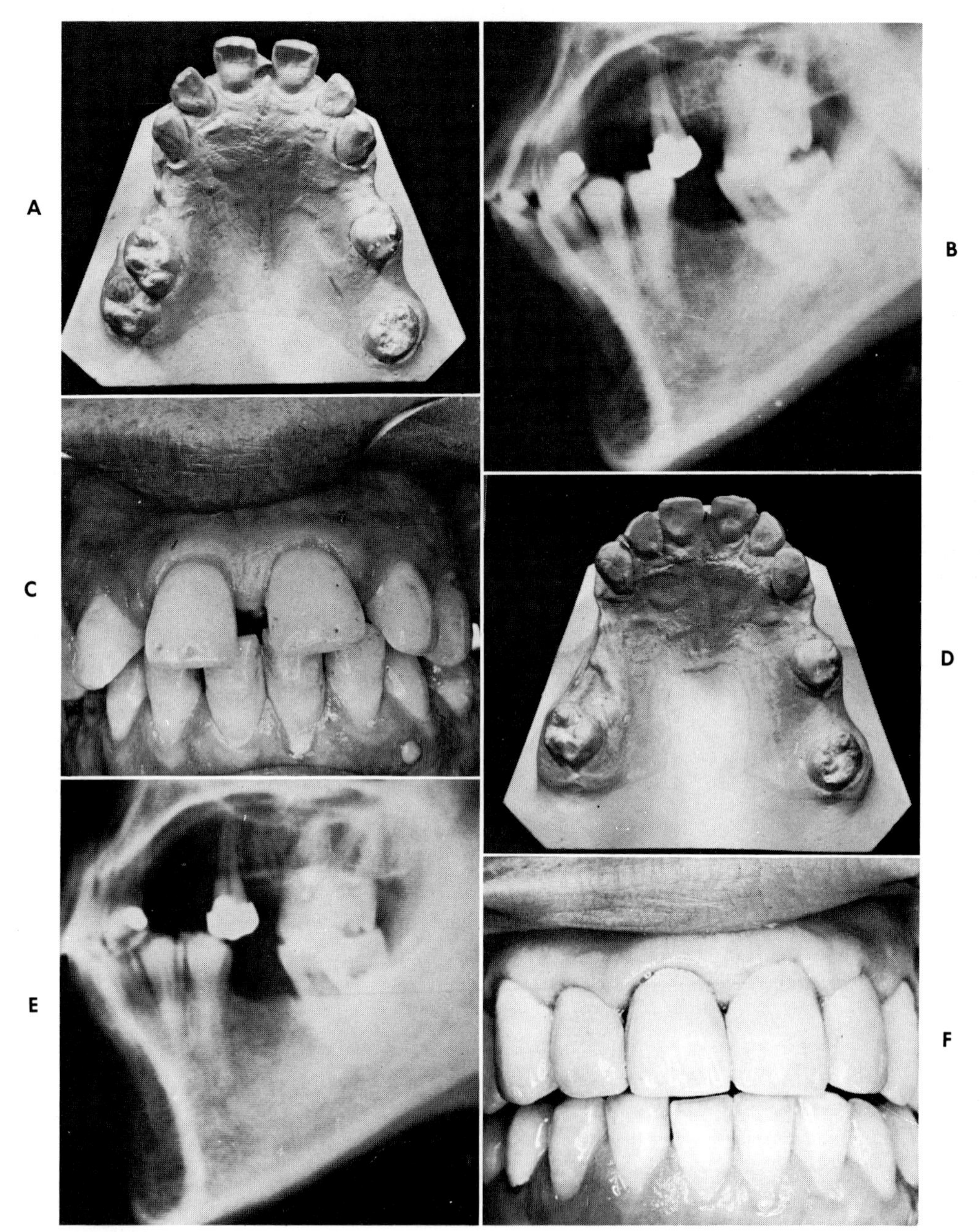


**Fig. 38-3. A** to **C,** Preoperative views. **D** and **E,** After orthodontic tooth movement. **F,** After reconstruction.

position teeth, you will sometimes have to move them counter to the forces of occlusion. Traumatism tends to occur, particularly when teeth are moving through cusp-to-cusp relationships. Jiggling, a situation in which orthodontic forces move the tooth in one direction and occlusal forces move the tooth in the opposite direction, is especially damaging.

At the completion of therapy, even when ideal intercuspation is achieved,

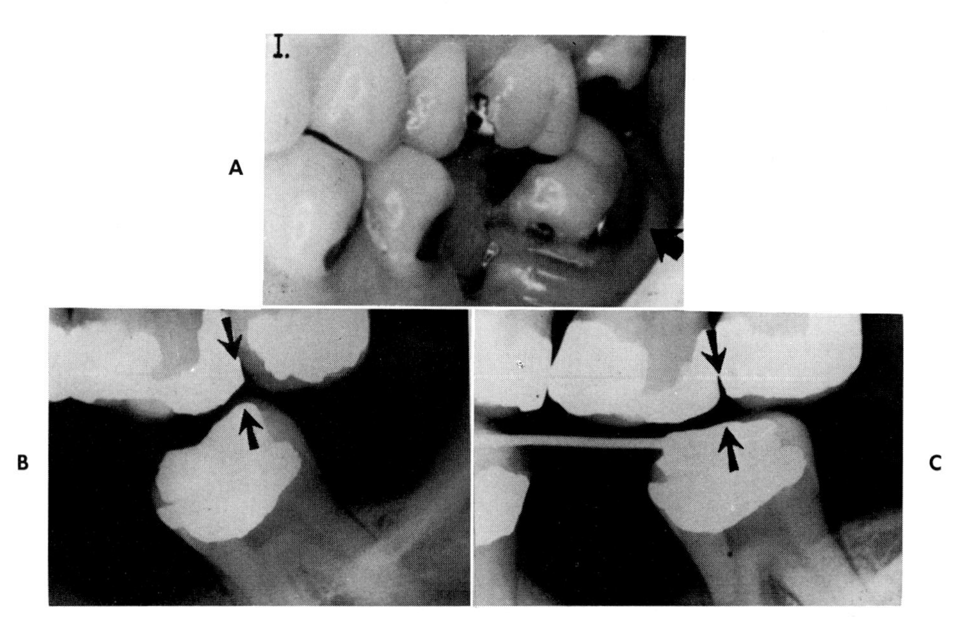


**Fig. 38-4.** Early loss of the mandibular first molar resulted in the mesial tipping of the second molar. Tooth movement to upright and parallel the abutment teeth was needed. **A,** Preoperative clinical view. **B,** Original bitewing film demonstrating the mesial tipping of the mandibular left second molar in relation to the maxillary left first and second molars. **C,** After tooth movement. Note the second molar in a more favorable position. (Courtesy M. H. Marks and G. Wisor, Levittown, Pa.)

minute occlusal discrepancies may exist. Moreover, maximal intercuspation may occur in an eccentric position (i.e., away from terminal hinge occlusion). These premature contacts should be corrected by occlusal adjustment. Standard periodontal procedures may be used in the treatment of other lesions that develop during orthodontic treatment.

### Aesthetic improvement

Migration, which is often the first sign of periodontal disease evident to the patient, tends to be unsightly. Embarrassment and a sense of impending tooth loss may compel the patient to seek treatment. We are all familiar with the patient who screens her teeth with her hand or who draws her upper lip over protruding teeth. The correction of such conditions (Fig. 38-3) is of considerable emotional value. A positive mental attitude may lead to a better maintenance of oral health by more diligent oral hygiene.

## PREPARATION FOR RECONSTRUCTION

Dentitions that have been mutilated by missing and migrated teeth frequently require extensive reconstruction.[2a] The more complex the reconstruction needed, the greater is the likelihood that some preliminary orthodontic treatment will be needed (Fig. 38-4). The reasons for this are that fixed splinting requires parallel abutments, pontic spaces of sufficient width, open embrasures, and an aesthetic and harmonious occlusion. To bring about these conditions, the dentist must upright tilted and protruded teeth. When teeth are properly positioned, torque is minimized and forces are transmitted in the long axis of the tooth. In

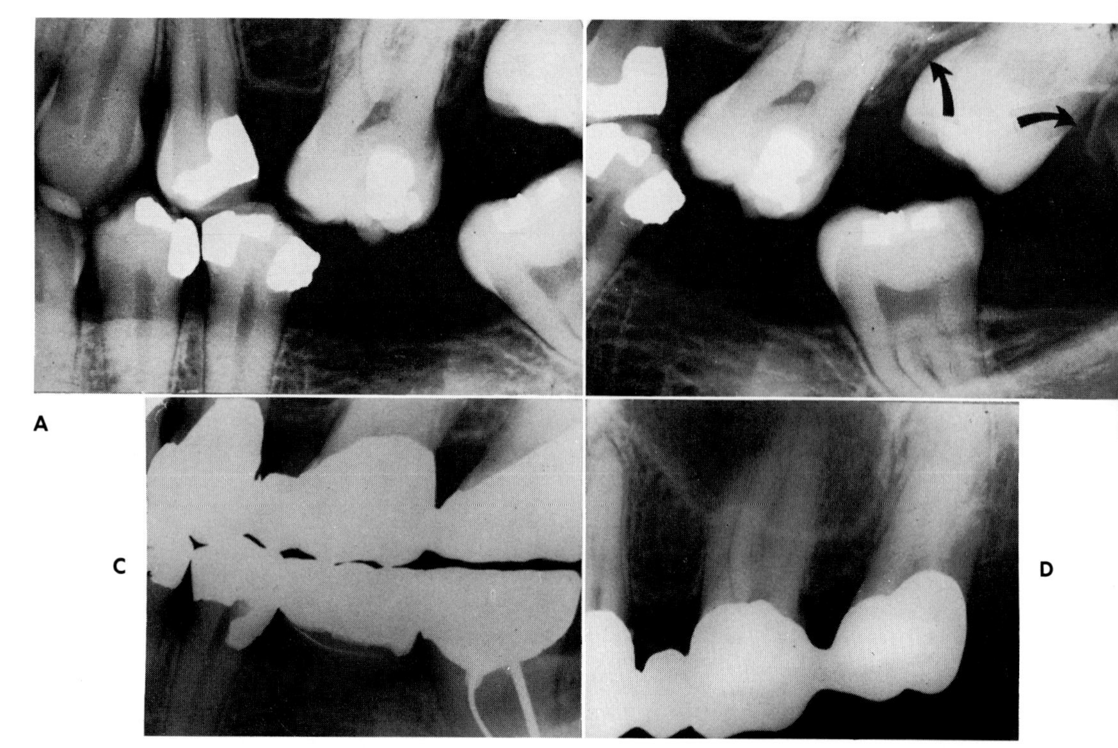


**Fig. 38-5. A and B, Preoperative bitewing films of an occlusion mutilated by extractions.** The molars have drifted forward. There are deep pockets mesial and distal of the maxillary molar (arrows). **C** and **D,** After orthodontics, parallelism for bridgework has been obtained and the occlusal plane is more normal. The maxillary alveolar bone has become level and the pocket has thus been eliminated.

addition, parallel preparations are obtained with more ease and there is less chance of pulp exposure. The repositioning of grossly malposed teeth may permit the retention of these teeth in the restorative plan, whereas the teeth might otherwise have to be extracted.[10] Moreover, the uprighting of tilted teeth may eliminate pockets brought about by the relationship of the tilted tooth to the adjacent alveolar ridge (Figs. 38-5 and 38-6).

*Minor tooth movement*

Periodontal orthodontics generally utilizes simplified techniques compared with those utilized in full orthodontic therapy. The distances through which the teeth are moved are usually small. The objective of treatment is limited to securing a functional and aesthetic occlusion, but not necessarily an ideal one. The orthodontic intervention is minimal and has been termed minor tooth movement.[16]

*Adult orthodontics*

Generally, however, the public and the profession at large do not fully recognize the possibilities of such treatment in adults. The majority of malposed periodontally involved teeth in adult patients can be treated by a combination of orthodontic and periodontal measures.

Reitan showed that the adult periodontium is capable of responding to orthodontic forces after an initial lag of 8 days.[11] Therefore age is not a contraindication for tooth movement. Moreover, a tooth with some bone loss is as suitable a candidate for movement as is a tooth without bone loss. On the

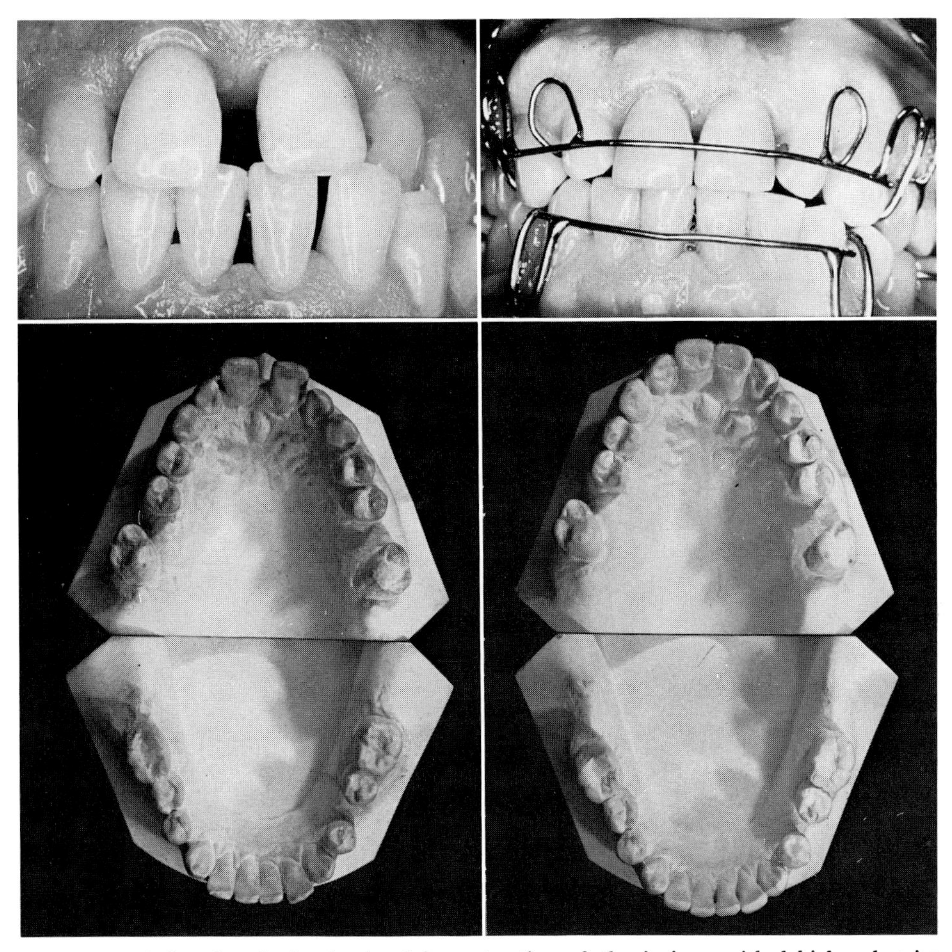

**Fig. 38-6.** Periodontal orthodontics involving retraction of the incisors with labial arch wire (note the lower left lateral and upper central incisors), mesial movement of the upper incisors with finger springs, and correction of the crossbite of the upper left lateral incisor and canine. Retention is necessary after active treatment.

other hand, most authorities are agreed that inflammation is a hindrance to orthodontic progress and should be resolved before orthodontic therapy.[4]

When periodontal fibers are moderately stressed, a physiologic adaptation of the inner alveolar wall results, with bone formation occurring in areas of tension and bone resorption in areas of compression. The remodeling of bone brings about a new positioning of the tooth as long as the periodontium is maintained in health. Since all tooth movements, migratory or orthodontic, are mediated by the periodontium, an understanding of the biology of the periodontium is essential.[12-14,18] The reader is referred to the section on experimental occlusal traumatism in Chapter 36.

## APPLIANCES

Teeth can be repositioned by the creation of a controlled disbalance of forces acting on the tooth, which is the essence of orthodontics. Although spontaneous repositioning of migrated teeth sometimes follows periodontal therapy,[15] tooth

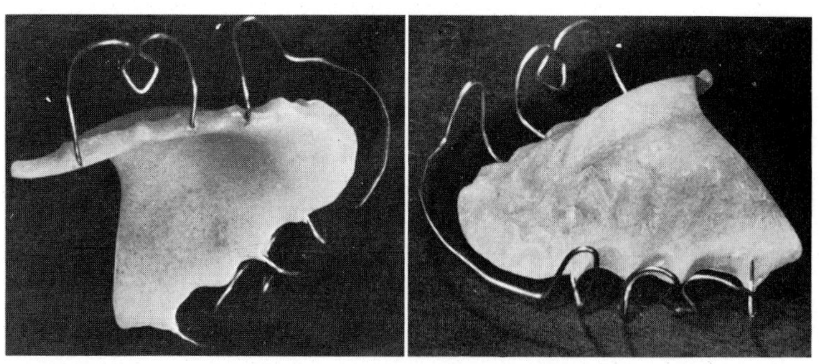

**Fig. 38-7.** Schwarz appliance (labial wire, 21 gauge; lugs, 19 gauge; arrowhead clasps, 24 gauge). The appliance is held in place by the arrowhead clasps, which engage the tooth interproximally below its greatest convexity to allow for continuous eruption.

movement generally requires the use of appliances. These specialized implements must be carefully controlled to do the work for which they are intended.

An orthodontic appliance is an implement designed to place pressure against a tooth to produce movement. There are two types of appliance, removable and fixed, with numerous variations of each. An intermittent force is produced by removable appliances, whereas a continuous application of force is provided by the fixed type. Although a majority of orthodontists in the United States used the fixed appliances, some orthodontists and many periodontists and general practitioners favor the removable kind, which are effective in a cooperative patient (Figs. 38-6 and 38-7). Either type may be used with success. Occasionally the patient's fixed bridgework or partial denture can be adapted as an appliance by the addition of springs, etc.

## Removable appliances

Since the scope of tooth movement is limited and special training is necessary for the use of fixed appliances, the removable appliances have become more commonly used. These have their advantages: they afford ease in case management, are not very irritating, and do not interfere with oral hygiene. Adults who feel conspicuous and uncomfortable with fixed appliances find removable appliances, which can be taken out at work and for social engagements, more to their liking. Furthermore, they have sufficient motivation and maturity to cooperate by replacing the appliance regularly (Fig. 38-1).

One such appliance is simple, consisting of a tissue-borne palatal or lingual acrylic base that is festooned to accommodate the teeth and that supports various springs, hooks, arch wires, spurs, etc.[6,17] (Fig. 38-7). The device is held in place by two to four clasps. Occasionally the patient's fixed bridgework or partial denture can be adapted as an appliance by the addition of springs, etc.

*Hawley appliance and Schwarz appliance*

Such appliances as well as the Schwarz appliance resemble a Hawley retainer and are often referred to as such (Figs. 38-1, 38-3, 38-7, and 38-8). Nevertheless, they are active appliances, as is the all-wire Crozat appliance,[22] whereas the retainer used after orthodontic treatment is a passive appliance.

*Elastics*

Rubber dam elastics may be used in conjunction with appliances. The rubber resembles the tooth in color and for aesthetic reasons is often substituted for wire. Elastics are stretched between hooks and the teeth to be moved and may even be used in place of an arch wire.

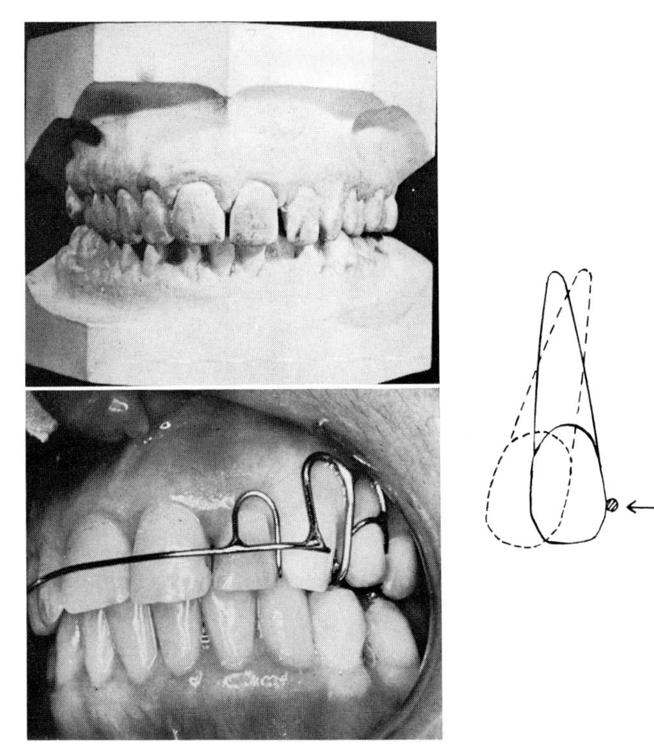

**Fig. 38-8.** Mesial movement of the left central and lateral incisors utilizing finger springs. The clasp and arch wire are separated in this appliance to provide ease in the adjustment of each. The arch wire may be made of 36-gauge gold wire, and the finger spring may be of 22-gauge or 25-gauge gold wire. The device can also be fabricated of steel wires.

## Management

*Activation*

Movement is produced by the activation of springs, rubber bands, and the arch wire. Activation means the flexing of some elastic material against the tooth, which prevents the flexed material from springing back to shape. The force is exerted until the tooth has slowly moved and the activated part is again in a resting state. Such appliances are termed active appliances and may be used to move teeth in buccolingul or mesiodistal directions and also to rotate, intrude, or extrude teeth. Appliances that are activated by the orofacial musculature are called functional appliances. The orthodontic school based on their concept is called functional jaw orthopedics.[20]

*Bite plate and bite plane*

When alteration of cusp relationships or the plane of occlusion of a posterior tooth is planned, the teeth must be freed of occlusal contact. This is usually done with a bite plate, which is a platform added to the anterior palatal portion of the Hawley device (Fig. 38-1). If the platform is inclined, the occluding teeth will migrate along its slope and the device may be termed an inclined bite plane. Some appliances may be split and have expansion screws incorporated for the expansion of the arch. An adequate freeway space should be present, and mandibular anterior teeth should be firm when bite plates and bite planes are used.

*Adjusting the appliance*

Loops that connect the treatment wires to the base of the appliance are used to activate these wires. Activation is produced when the loops are opened and closed. The proper position of the wires can be maintained only if compensa-

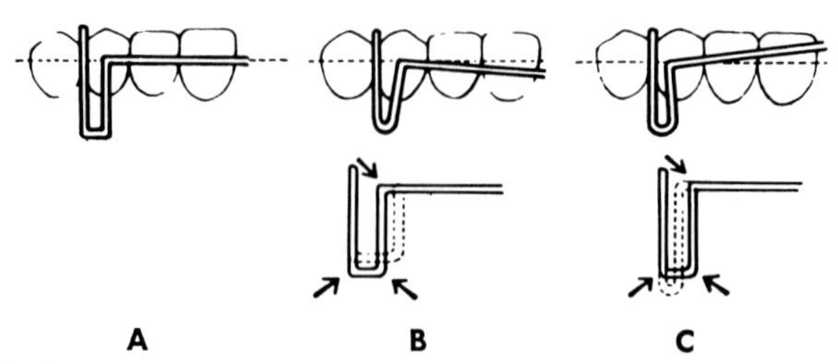


**Fig. 38-9. A,** Loop before adjustment. **B,** Loop opened and arch wire displaced. Proper position can be maintained only if compensating bends are made at arrows. **C,** Loop closed and arch wire displaced. Position of the arch wire can be maintained by compensating bends made at the arrows.

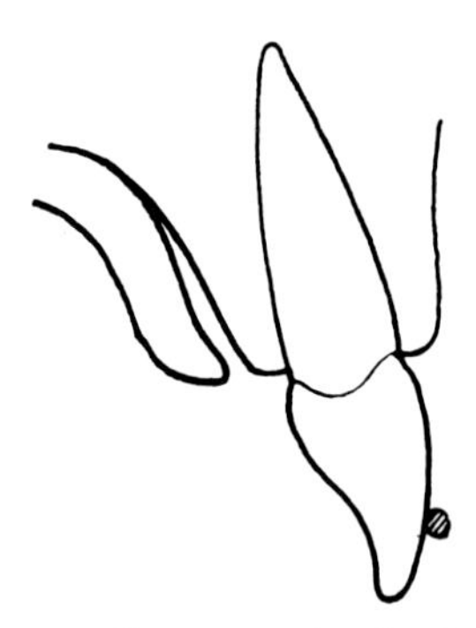

**Fig. 38-10.** Undermining of appliance adjacent to alveolar bone to provide room for movement of tooth and apposition of palatal bone as the tooth is moved.

ting bends are made in the horizontal portion of the loop during adjustments, as indicated in Fig. 38-9.

Of course, the acrylic base must be trimmed so that it does not prevent movement by its contact with the tooth. Generally only 1 mm. at a time is trimmed, and the base thus serves to limit the movement. The festooned margin of the base acts as a stop and should be relieved wherever necessary to free a tooth so that the tooth may be moved. In addition, the acrylic should be undermined adjacent to the area of movement to permit space for the gingiva and for apposition of bone on the palatal surface of the maxillary alveolar plate (Fig. 38-10).

*Anchorage*

Appliances are designed to provide both anchorage and orthodontic force. A force pitted against a tooth will be transmitted equally in the opposite direction, the appliance distributing the force to the tooth to be moved and to the anchorage teeth. The resultant movement is proportionate to the relative strength of attachment of each tooth. Therefore the anchorage should be strong and stable to ensure movement of the proper tooth. Theoretically some reciprocal movement of the anchorage, however slight, must occur even when a minimal force is applied.

*Tipping movement*

Removable appliances generally produce tipping movements in which the crown is moved a greater distance than the apex (Figs. 38-1 and 38-8). Although the apex may remain in place when very gentle forces are used, usually the crown and apex move in opposite directions about the center of rotation of the tooth. In teeth with undamaged alveolar support, this center is located near the cervical

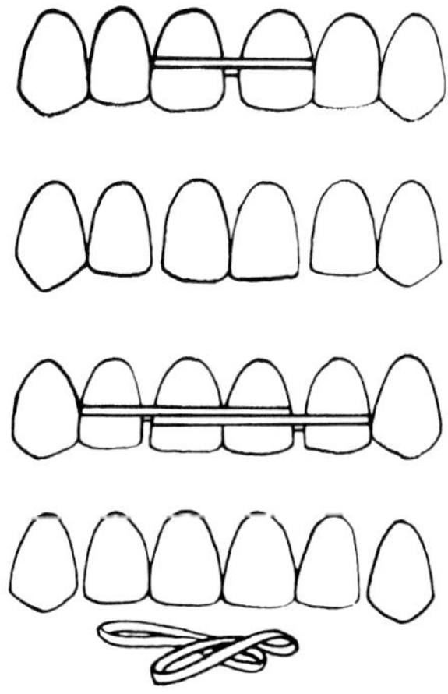

**Fig. 38-11.** Place rubber dam elastic or orthodontic rubber band around two central incisors to draw them together. Then use two rubber bands to draw the lateral incisors toward the central incisors, which are used for anchorage.

third of the root. As alveolar bone is lost in periodontal disease, the center moves closer to the apex, thus facilitating tipping or tilting of the tooth.

***Bodily movement***

Bodily movement implies the movement of crown and apex in the same direction and generally requires the use of a fixed appliance. The tooth is fastened to the arch wire by means of a bracketed band. Tooth movement of a very limited scope, such as the closing of a diastema or the rotation of an individual tooth, sometimes can be achieved without fabricated appliances. In these instances rubber dam elastics, elastic ligature, grassline ligature, wire ligation, tongue depressors, and even finger pressure may be used. Such methods do not afford precision in control, and close observation is necesary. However, they appeal to the operator for the following reasons: they require no preparation; they take seemingly little chair time; and, should they fail, appliances can always be used.

## Ligatures

***Rubber dam elastics***

Rubber dam elastics, which come in various widths, are stretched around teeth for repositioning (Fig. 38-11). The elastic is removed by the patient at mealtime and replaced with a new one afterward, which maneuvers require cooperation and dexterity. If the bands slip apically, they may cause severe damage (Fig. 38-2); therefore the dentist and patient must be alert and perceptive. Slipping may be prevented if ligature wire loops are placed on the teeth and the twisted ends used as guards (Fig. 38-12). Notches cut into the tooth will serve the same purpose; but this can be done only when the tooth is part of a subsequent restorative plan. Orthodontic bands with soldered spurs can also be used. Since the force of the elastic acts equally, two teeth with similar support can be drawn together (Fig. 38-11). If movement is intended for only one tooth, the anchorage tooth and the malposed tooth must have disproportionate support. This can be arranged by pitting the tooth to be moved against several other teeth by means of elastic wrapped about the anchoring teeth (Fig. 38-11) or by the splinting of several anchor teeth with ligature wire (Fig. 38-12) or welded bands.[16]

***Elastic nylon thread***

Elastic nylon thread is available in light, medium, and heavy.[21] Medium thread is used as the arch wire, and light thread is used interproximally in the

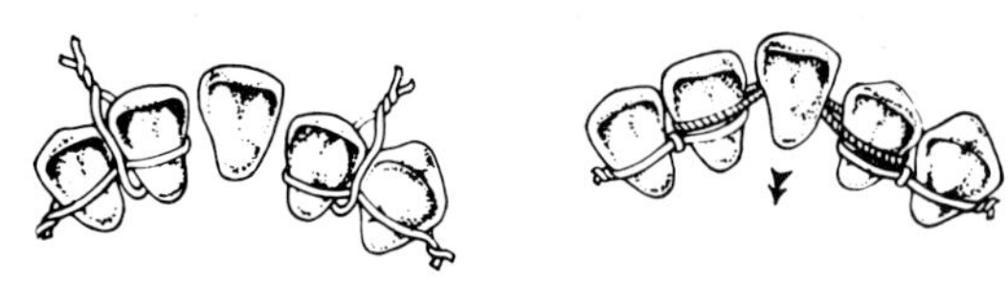

**Fig. 38-12.** Central incisor moved into alignment with rubber dam elastic (crosshatched) while the two adjacent teeth on each side are ligated with wire ligature to provide anchorage.

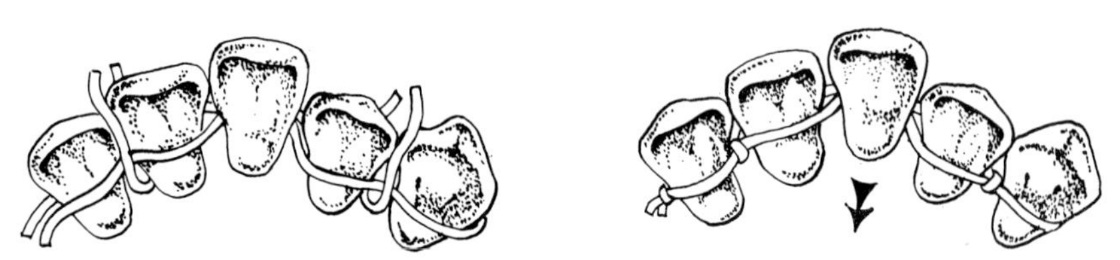

**Fig. 38-13.** Application of elastic nylon thread for minor tooth movement.

manner of wire ligation (Fig. 38-13). The thread is placed by the dentist, not the patient. Its management in all other respects is similar to that of rubber dam elastics since it forms a large elastic band once the ends are tied together. It has the advantage of being aesthetic, but it has many of the disadvantages of the fixed appliance.

***Grassline ligature***

Grassline ligatures are twisted threads of unwaxed silk that shrink approximately 25% when wet. Their mode of action differs from elastic deformation. The grassline is knotted about several contiguous anchor teeth, which serve to counteract the forces of shrinkage on them, and a long unknotted strand is placed about the tooth to be moved, which therefore receives the full effect of the shrinkage. (Fig. 38-14). Although grassline may be effective, precise control is not possible and care must be exercised. Grassline may become foul smelling, and the ligatures must be replaced frequently because they loosen after shrinking.[16]

***Wire ligature***

Wire ligatures can be used to produce an almost immediate movement if the teeth are sufficiently loose. The wire is dead soft and therefore is practically inelastic. Movement is obtained by digital pressure while the interproximal loops are being tightened. Wire ligature improperly applied during temporary splinting to immobilize teeth may result in an unexpected movement of teeth. Rubber dam elastics, elastic nylon thread, grassline, and wire ligatures all give a rather limited control and require great care in their use.

## PREREQUISITES FOR ORTHODONTIC MOVEMENT

Among the prerequisites for orthodontic movement, two are of prime importance: (1) there must be adequate space in the arch for the movement and (2) the orthodontic forces must be of small magnitude. Desired space can be created by occlusal grinding, interproximal stripping, extraction, or orthodontic movement. Orthodontic forces, according to A. M. Schwarz, should be no greater than 17 gm. (½ oz.).[9a] More than this amount will cause necrosis, which will delay movement until undermining resorption has been completed. Other undesirable consequences of excessive force are root resorption, bone loss, mobility, and discomfort.

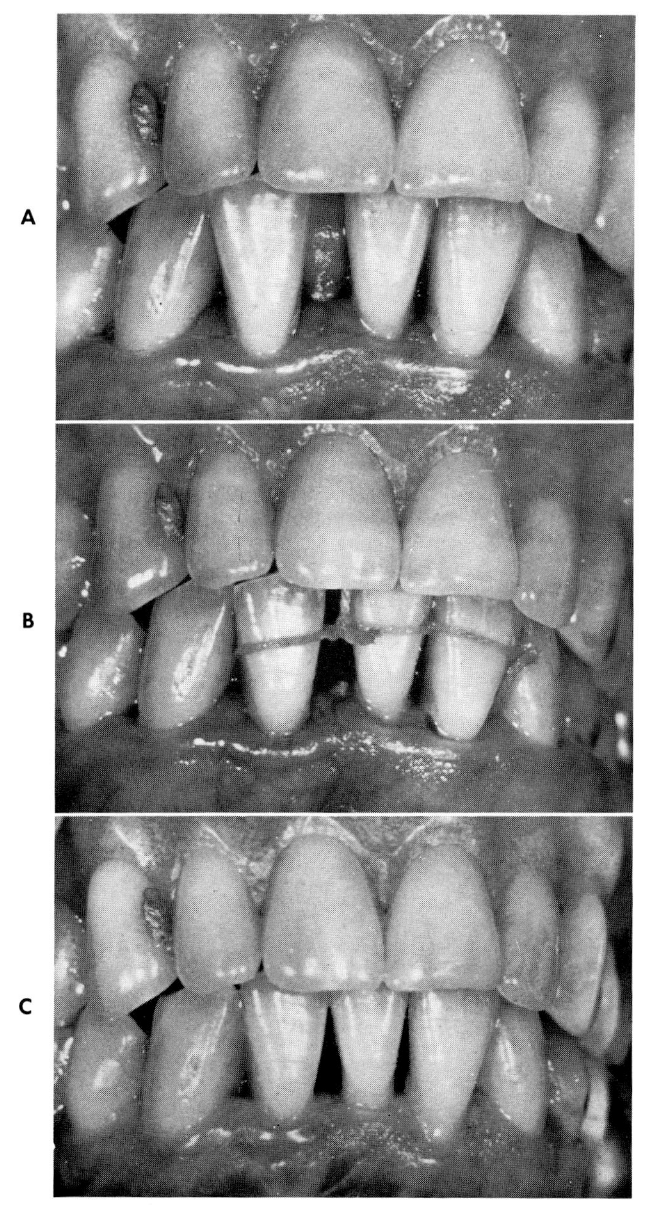


**Fig. 38-14. A,** Buckling of the mandibular anterior teeth and lingual displacement of the mandibular central incisor. **B,** The malaligned tooth was extracted and the remaining teeth were moved by grassline ligature. **C,** There is good alignment of three incisors.

***Order of treatment***

Orthodontic treatment may precede or follow initial periodontal therapy.[3] Occlusal adjustments are generaly performed after the tooth movement has been completed.

***Retention***

Movement may loosen teeth, and there is a tendency for them to return to their old positions. They should therefore be held in position long enough to preclude relapse.[23] In those cases in which splinting is part of the treatment plan, there is no further problem. In other instances, wire ligation, welded bands, Hawley retainers, and night guards may be needed for retention (Figs. 38-1, 38-8,

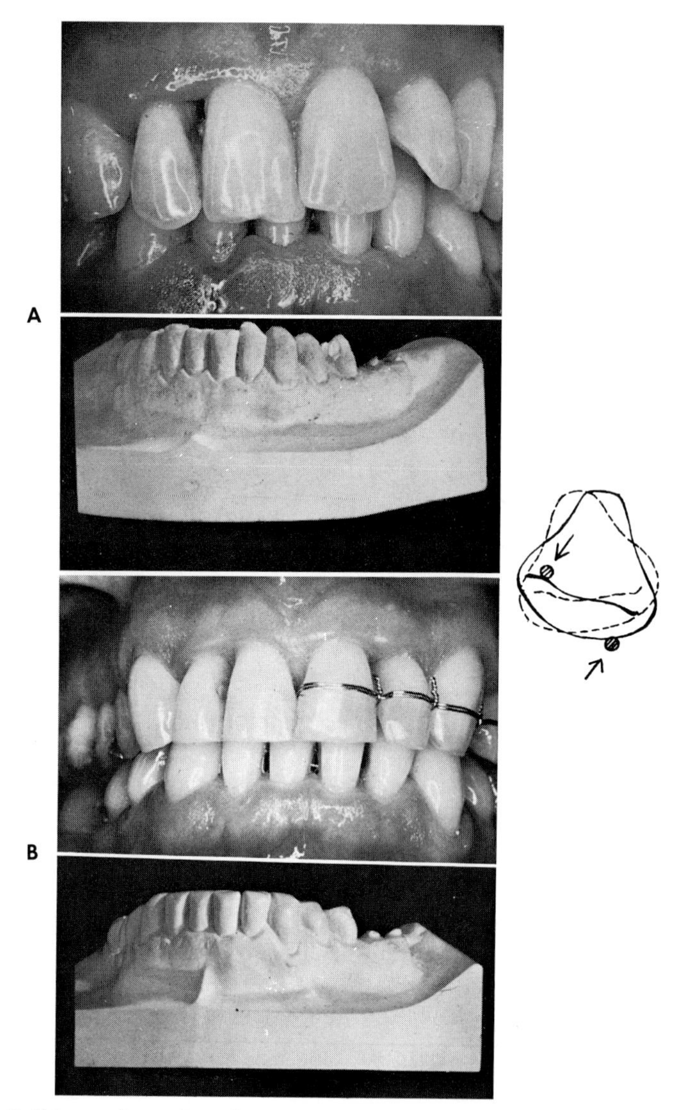


**Fig. 38-15. A,** Drifting and rotation of an upper left lateral incisor that occluded with the projecting lower left canine. **B,** The lower canine was shortened, the lateral and central incisors were stripped to provide space, and the lateral incisor was rotated back into position. After treatment, wire ligation served as a temporary retainer during the retention period. Such corrections of rotations in adult patients may require permanent retention.

and 38-15). Occlusal adjustment and habit-breaking procedures are often necessary to maintain the newly gained positions.

## RESULTS OF TREATMENT

Kronfeld repositioned the teeth of a patient with periodontosis, and the teeth became firm and the condition improved.[24] Similar results have been noted by others. Gottlieb explained such improvement as being caused by the replacement of degenerating tissue by newly formed tissues.

When migrated teeth are repositioned, beneficial changes may result from the improved relationship of teeth to each other and to the alveolar bone. When tilted teeth are uprighted, pockets may disappear (Figs. 38-4 and 38-5). Occlusal traumatism may be reduced. Reestablished mesiodistal contact relationships minimize food impaction and provide intrinsic support. Improved tooth and gingival contour combine to prevent food impingement and provide functional stimulation of the attached gingiva. Reconstruction may be aided, and aesthetics can be improved. In all, such tooth movements can be of decided therapeutic value.

On the other hand, injudicious treatment may inadvertently lead to pathology. Perception, dexterity, and knowledge of the biology of the tissues involved are basic to the use of orthodontics for the periodontal patient.

**CHAPTER 38**

**References**

1. Stern, I. B.: Tooth malpositions and periodontal pathosis: an evaluation of etiology and considerations in treatment, J. Periodont. **29**:253, 1958.
2. Morris, M. L.: Orthodontic-periodontic relationship. In Horowitz, S. L., and Hixon, E. H., editors: The nature of orthodontic diagnosis, St. Louis, 1966, The C. V. Mosby Co.

2a. Marks, M. H., and Corn, H.: The role of tooth movement in periodontal therapy, Dental Clinics of North America, Philadelphia, 1969, W. B. Saunders Co., vol. 13.

3. Rateitschak, K. H.: Orthodontics and periodontology, Int. Dent. J. **18**:108, 1968.
4. Rateitschak, K. H.: Möglichkeiten und Grenzen der orthodontischen Therapie im parodontal geschwächten Gebiss, Deutsch. Zahnaerztl. Z. **21**:32, 1966.

4a. Gianelli, A. A.: Orthodontic considerations in periodontal therapy, J. Periodont. **41**:119, 1970.

4b. Alexander, P. C.: Orthodontic procedures in periodontal therapy, J. Periodont. **28**:46, 1957.

5. Breitner, C.: Tooth-supporting apparatus under occlusal changes, J. Periodont. **13**:72, 1942.
6. Schwarz, A. M., and Gratzinger, M.: Removable orthodontic appliances, Philadelphia, 1966, W. B. Saunders Co.
7. Cheraskin, E., Ringsdorf, W. M., Jr., Sety, A. D., and others: Resistance and susceptibility to oral disease. III. A study in clinical tooth mobility and carbohydrate metabolism, J. Calif. Dent. Ass. **41**:416, 1965.
8. Priester, E. S.: Die endogenen Ursachen der Zahnlockerung, Deutsch. Zahnaerztebl. **15**:132, 1961.
9. Mühlemann, H. R.: Tooth mobility, J. Periodont. **38**:686, 1967.

9a. Schwarz, A. M.: Tissue changes incidental to orthodontic tooth movement, Int. J. Orthodont. **18**:331, 1932.

9b. Atherton, J. D., and Kerr, N. W.: Effect of orthodontic tooth movement on the gingivae, Brit. Dent. J. **124**:555, 1968.

10. Bernstein, M.: Orthodontics in periodontal and prosthetic therapy, J. Periodont. **40**:577, 1969.
11. Reitan, K.: The initial tissue reaction incident to orthodontic tooth movement as related to the influence of function, Acta Odont. Scand., vol. 9, supp., 1951.
12. Oppenheim, A.: Die Veränderungen der Gewebe inbesondere des Knochens bei der Verschiebung der Zähne, Oest.-Ungar. Vjschr. Zahnheilk. **27**:302, 1911.
13. Reitan, K.: Tissue behavior during orthodontic tooth movement, Amer. J. Orthodont. **46**:881, 1960.
14. Orban, B.: Biologic problems in orthodontia, J. Amer. Dent. Ass. **23**:1849, 1936.
15. Ross, I. F.: Endogenous tooth movement, J. Amer. Dent. Ass. **60**:738, 1960.
16. Hirschfeld, L., and Geiger, A.: Minor tooth movement in general practice, ed. 2, St. Louis, 1966, The C. V. Mosby Co.
17. Adams, C. P.: The design and construction of removable orthodontic appliances, Baltimore, 1964, The Williams and Wilkins Co.
18. Edwards, J. G.: A study of the periodontium during orthodontic rotation of teeth, Amer. J. Orthodont. **54**:441, 1968.
19. Tirk, T. M., Guzman, C. A., and Nalchajian, R.: Periodontal tissue response to orthodontic treatment studied by panoramix, Angle Orthodont. **37**:94, 1967.

20. Andresen, V., Häupl, K., and Petrik, L.: Funktions-Kieferorthopädie, ed. 6, Munich, 1957, Johann Ambrosius Barth.
21. Goldstein, M. C.: Adult orthodontics and the general practitioner, J. Canad. Dent. Ass. **24**:261, 1958.
22. Wiebrecht, A. T.: Crozat appliances in interceptive maxillofacial orthopedics, Milwaukee, 1969, E. F. Schmidt Co.
23. Riedel, R. A.: A review of the retention problem, Angle Orthodont. **30**:179, 1960.
24. Kronfeld, R.: Zur Therapie der pathologischen Wanderung, Z. Stomat. **27**:765, 1929.

#### Additional suggested reading

Baer, P. N., and Coccaro, P. J.: Gingival enlargement coincident with orthodontic therapy, J. Periodont. **35**:436, 1964.

Bekeny, A. R., and DeMarco, T. J.: The effects of the rubber tooth positioner on the gingiva of orthodontic patients during retention, J. Periodont. **42**:300, 1971.

Brender, P.: Major orthodontics in periodontia, Parodontologie **17**:95, 1963.

Ertinger, H.: Die kieferorthopädische Behandlung Erwachsener und ihre Lösung in Einzelfällen, Fortschr. Kieferorthop. **16**:284, 1956.

Gryson, J. A.: Changes in the periodontal ligament incident to orthodontic therapy, Periodont. Abstr. **13**:14, 1965.

Hoover, D. R.: Looking at orthodontics through the critical eye of the periodontist, Amer. J. Orthodont. **53**:532, 1967.

Iyer, V. S.: Biting platforms in orthodontic appliances, Dent. Pract. **15**:194, 1965.

Jacobson, A.: Biomechanics of orthodontic forces, J. Dent. Ass. S. Afr. **21**:211, 1966.

Kessler, S. J., and Zweig, J. M.: Adult orthodontics and mouth reconstruction, J. Amer. Dent. Ass. **69**:572, 1964.

Lamons, F. F.: The Crozat removable appliance, Amer. J. Orthodont. **50**:265, 1964.

Macapanpan, L. C., Weinmann, J. P., and Brodie, A. G.: Early tissue changes following tooth movement in rats, Angle Orthodont. **24**:79, 1954.

Rateitschak, K. H.: Reaction of periodontal tissue to artificial (orthodontic) forces. In Eastoe, J. E., Picton, D. C. A., and Alexander, A. G., editors: The prevention of periodontal disease, London, 1971, Henry Kimpton.

Reitan, K.: Effects of force magnitude and direction of tooth movement on different alveolar bone types, Angle Orthodont. **34**:244, 1964.

Ross, I. F.: Reactive positioning and improved gingival architecture. J. Periodont. **34**:444, 1963.

Ross, I. F.: Reactive positioning of the teeth; a reappraisal, Periodontics **2**:172, 1964.

Rothenberg S., and Shapiro, E.: The orthodontic management of functional problems in periodontal therapy, Dental Clinics of North America, Philadelphia, March 1960, W. B. Saunders Co.

Schluger, S.: Periodontal aspects of orthodontic treatment, Pract. Orthodont. **2**:111, 1968.

Stallard, H.: Survival of the periodontium before and after orthodontic treatment, Amer. J. Orthodont. **50**:583, 1964.

Thielemann, K.: Zur kieferorthopädischen Versorgung von Paradentosekranken, Paradentium **15**:29, 1943.

Zaki, A. E., and Van Huysen, G.: Histology of the periodontium following tooth movement, J. Dent. Res. **42**:1373, 1963.

Zamet, S.: Combined periodontal surgery and orthodontic movement in the treatment of an isolated palatal intrabony pocket, Dent. Pract. **17**:314, 1967.

CHAPTER THIRTY-NINE

# Splinting



Periodontal disease impairs tooth support and permits secondary traumatism to occur. As a consequence, teeth may loosen. Thus the reduction of mobility is an important objective of periodontal therapy. Root planing, curettage, oral hygiene, and surgery* may cause teeth to tighten as inflammation is resolved.[1] Occlusal adjustment, periodontal orthodontics, and restorative dentistry may alter occlusal relationships and redirect forces, thereby reducing traumatism. Increasing the support of loose teeth may also increase their firmness. The device used for such treatment is the splint.[1a-6,42]

*Definition*

A splint is any appliance that joins two or more teeth to provide support. Splints, like bridges, may be fixed or removable or a combination of both. They may be temporary, provisional, or permanent according to the type of material and duration of use. They may be internal or external depending on whether tooth preparation is required. Permanent splints are also referred to as periodontal prostheses.

## THEORETICAL AIMS

The theoretical aims of splinting are as follows[7]:

1. Rest is created for the supporting tissues, giving them a favorable climate for repair of trauma.
2. Mobility is reduced immediately and, hopefully, permanently.[8] In particular, jiggling movements are reduced or eliminated.
3. Forces received by one tooth are distributed to a number of teeth.
4. Proximal contacts are stabilized and food impaction is prevented.
5. Migration and overeruption are prevented.
6. Masticatory function is improved.
7. Discomfort and pain are eliminated.

Certain qualifications identify the ideal splint.[9] It should be (1) simple, (2) economic, (3) stable and efficient, (4) hygienic, (5) nonirritating, (6) not interfering with treatment, and (7) aesthetically acceptable.

*There may be an increase in mobility immediately after surgery. This is usually transient.

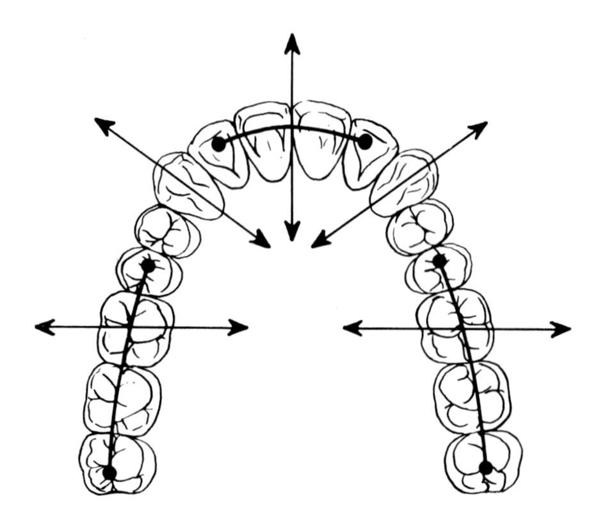

**Fig. 39-1.** Lines with arrows indicate direction of mobility in loosened teeth. Lines with dots at each end indicate points of stability of the same teeth. Splinting should include at least two groups of teeth so that the groups will reciprocally stabilize their mobilities by their points of firmness. (Adapted from Roy, M.: Dent. Cosmos **72**:390, 1930.)

## MODE OF ACTION

A loose tooth splinted to adjacent firm teeth is stabilized. When many teeth are loose, adjacent quadrants should be included in the splint. Teeth tend to loosen buccolingually yet may remain firm mesiodistally. Adjacent quadrants therefore have complimentary strengths and weaknesses. Cross-arch splinting (Fig. 39-1) reduces mobility to the least common denominator. Teeth are thus immobilized and occlusal forces are distributed over a broader area.[10,11] Traumatism is minimized, repair is enhanced, and teeth may be made firm again. Even when teeth do not tighten, the splint may serve as a sort of orthopedic brace that permits the retention of loose teeth in useful function.[12]

## INDICATIONS

When moderate to advanced mobilities (1½ or more) are present and cannot be treated by any other means, splinting is indicated.[13] There is no reason for splinting nonmobile teeth as a preventive measure. Splinting is only one measure that is sometimes used in the treatment of periodontal disease. It should not be used without other measures that may be necessary such as root planing, oral hygiene instruction, and procedures for pocket elimination.

## TEMPORARY SPLINTING

Temporary splinting is a useful adjunct in many areas of treatment.[1a,14] If you intend to use such a device until the teeth tighten, external splints are in order because they are disposable. They may be used to facilitate instrumentation (root planing, curettage, occlusal corrections) that might be difficult on loose teeth. They are of benefit in periodontal surgery. They may serve as anchorage or provide retention after orthodontic movement.

### Choice of splint

Since there are several types of splints available, once the decision has been made to proceed with temporary splinting, a type must be selected. The choice depends on the severity of mobility, the stage of treatment involved, and the anticipated outcome. Other considerations, such as the location and distribution of missing and carious teeth, the functional and aesthetic needs, and the cost, may also be important. Any splint may be chosen as long as it is equal to the task. The specific advantages and disadvantages of the method and material must be weighed against the needs of the patient.

***Internal splints***

Internal temporary splints should be used when permanent splinting is to follow. Such splints are useful in the transition to permanent splinting. They may also be used on a provisional basis when the prognosis is guarded. Thus treatment is possible while final judgment is being deferred. Even when splinting cannot save teeth, it can make for a gradual and less distressing transition to full dentures.

A point of caution is in order. Once an internal device has been used, the patient may be committed to periodontal prosthesis. You must advise him of this commitment before undertaking treatment.

***External splints***

External temporary splints include the following: ligatures, welded band splints, continuous clasps, and night guards.

***Ligatures***

Ligatures are a satisfactory means of stabilizing the anterior teeth.[15-17] Fig. 39-2 demonstrates the fabrication and use of a wire ligature splint. Dead-soft stainless steel wire 0.007 to 0.010 inch thick is used. Brass or silk ligatures are not as adequate. Double a 12-inch length for use as an arch wire and bend it about the six anterior teeth. Position it apical to the contact points and incisal to the cingula and then loosely twist one end (*A*). Provide for edentulous spaces by twisting the buccal and lingual strands of the arch wire together. Place single strands (*B*) interdentally around the arch wires and below the contact points. Tighten them by twisting clockwise with a hemostat, needle holder, or Howe pliers. The interdental strands (*C*) should not be so tight that they bring the arch wires into contact or produce tooth movement. To properly distribute force, tighten the last interdental ligature after all the other interdental ligatures and the arch wire are tightened. Clip the ends of the wires (*D, E,* and *G*) short (2 to 3 mm.) and bend them into the interdental space to minimize catching food or injuring soft tissues (*E*). When the wires are properly positioned, both splint and teeth are held fast. However, be careful that the splint does not slip incisally or gingivally. Slippage can be controlled by additional cervical loops (below the cingulum) (*F* and *H*) or incisal loops (above the contact points). These oppose the direction of slippage and keep the splint in place.

Check the occlusion for interferences before dismissing the patient. Instruct him in oral hygiene procedures to prevent accumulation or deposition of material around the splinted teeth.[18] In addition, brush self-cure acrylic over the wires. This will improve aesthetics, reduce irritation, and tend to prevent displacement (*I*).

Although ligation is a form of temporary splinting, ligatures may be used for several months provided they are tightened and replaced periodically.

***Welded band splints***

Welded band splints are useful for the temporary stabilization of posterior teeth[13,18a] (Fig. 39-3). Adapt a strip of stainless steel 0.003 to 0.005 inch thick to a tooth and weld it to form a band. Weld the next strip to the mesial surface of the first band. Seat the two pieces while adapting the second strip to the tooth. Then weld the second strip to form a band. Several strips can be added and formed into bands for successive teeth. The contact points must permit the band material to slip between the teeth. If necessary, you can separate the teeth by placing brass wire ligatures interdentally for 24 hours prior to splinting.

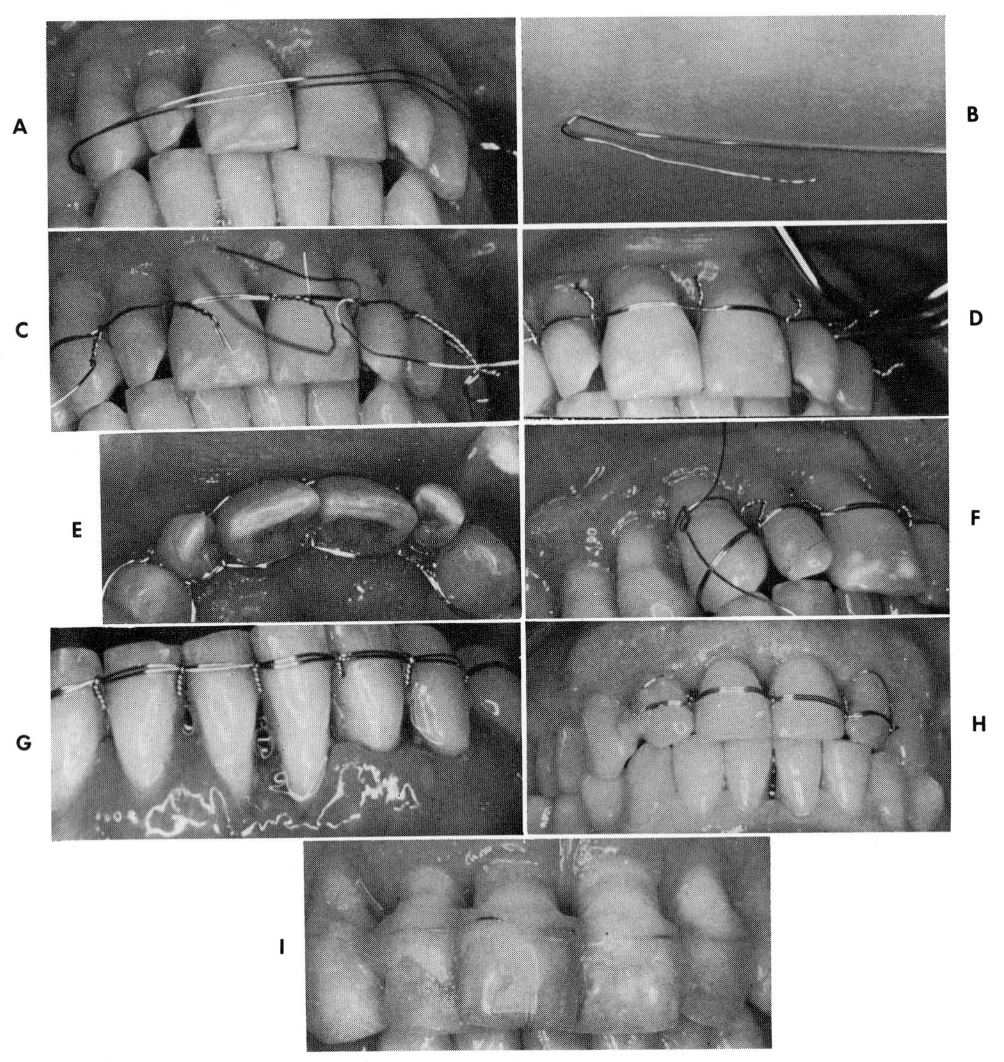


**Fig. 39-2.** Steps in wire ligation for temporary splinting. (See text for explanation.)

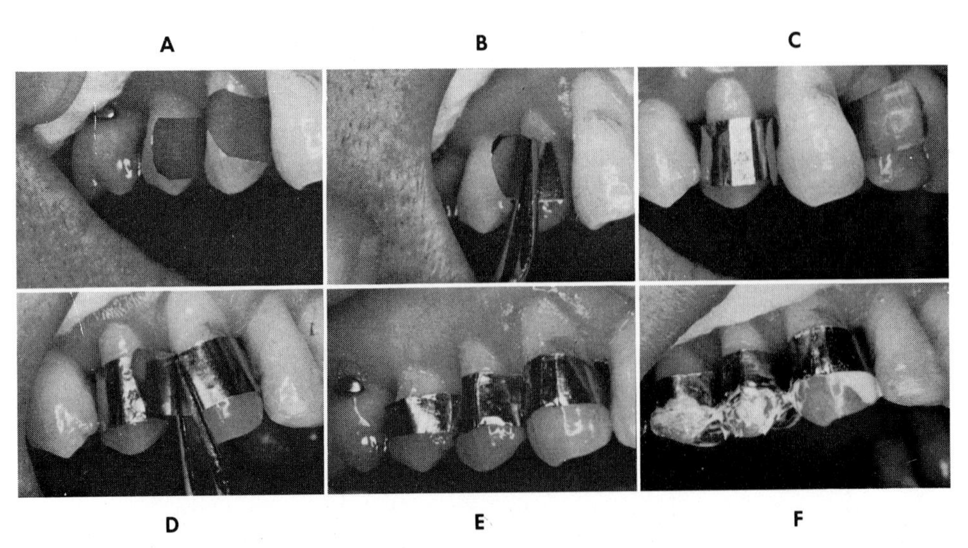


**Fig. 39-3.** Fabrication of a welded splint. (See text for explanation.)

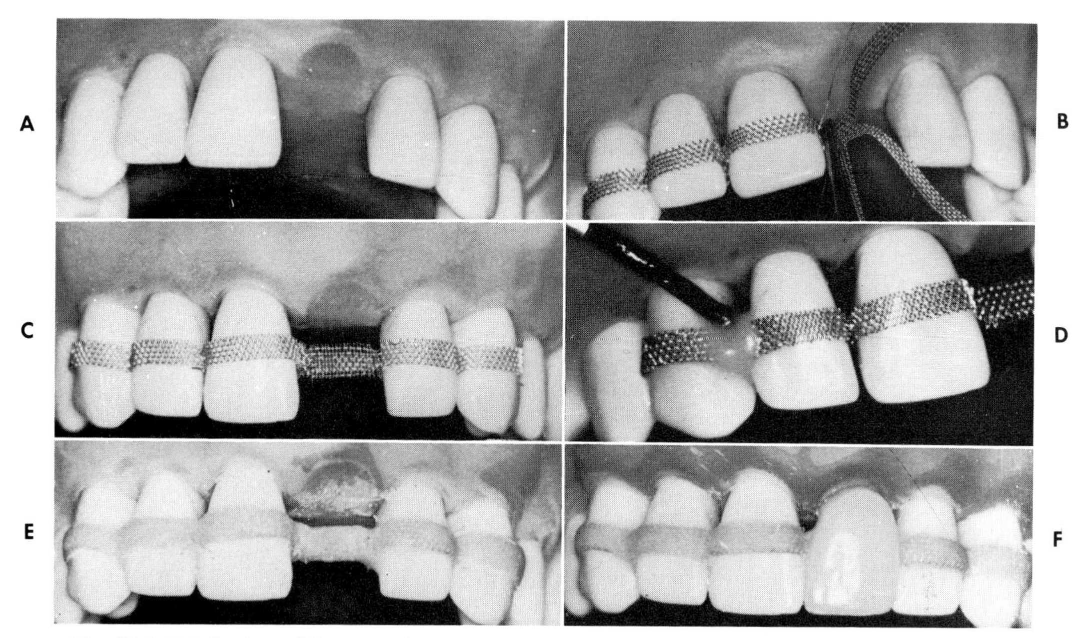


**Fig. 39-4.** Fabrication of brass mesh temporary splint. (See text for explanation.) (Courtesy W. Johnson, Carlsbad, Calif.)

A modification of the welded band splint permits a single-band thickness in the contact area by the welding of a second band to the distobuccal and distolingual line angles of the first band, and so on. Another modification uses a combination of the welded band with a wire splint.[19]

Be careful that the bands do not impinge on the gingiva. Also, check the occlusion for interferences. Sometimes adaptation can be improved by the use of contouring pliers and burnishers. It is possible to coat the splint with acrylic for aesthetic appearance. Be additionally careful not to perform minor tooth movements with the splint. Special attention should be given to home dental care procedures.

A provisional splint made of brass mesh, interdental wire, and fast-setting acrylic is useful in splinting both anterior and posterior teeth.[20] It may be used to splint mobile teeth that are separated by edentulous spaces (Fig. 39-4, *A*). Bend a strip of 80-gauge brass mesh as a continuous ribbon around the buccal and lingual surfaces of the teeth to be splinted *(B)* or as two separate strips. Adapt the brass mesh to the teeth and guide it into the interproximal spaces with a plastic instrument. Use light ligature wire for interdental ties (*B* and *C*). When the mesh crosses an edentulous space, make proximal ties with the ligature wire, bordering the edentulous area (*C*). Then paint quickcure acrylic over the splint (*D*). Pontics may be applied for aesthetics (*E* and *F*).

***Continuous clasps***

Continuous clasps may be made of acrylic, gold, or stainless cast[21-23] (Fig. 39-5). These simple splints may be seated and removed in the fashion of a partial denture, or they can be ligated or cemented to place. Using them as freely removable appliances is advantageous since adequate oral hygiene is permitted. They afford protracted temporary stabilization, yet they can be removed for social engagements. They may also be used at night on a part-time basis. They are not aesthetic and may impede speech. Care should be taken to avoid irritat-

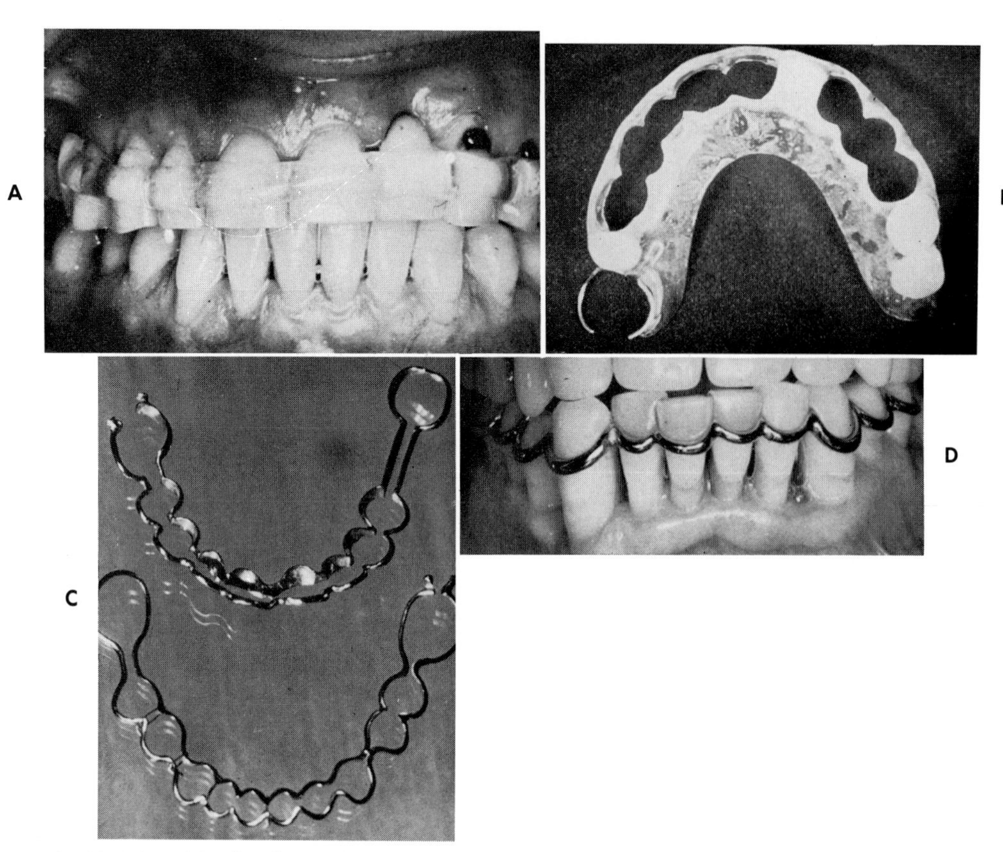


**Fig. 39-5.** **A** and **B,** Acrylic continuous clasp splint. **C,** Stainless steel continuous clasp with studs for wire ligatures. **D,** Gold continuous clasp. (**A** and **B** courtesy A. Krause, Leipzig; **D** courtesy A. Gargiulo, Chicago.)

ing sharp edges and occlusal interferences. More elaborate continuous clasps can be used as permanent splinting devices, although removable splints may not contribute to a permanent decrease in mobility.[24]

***Night guards***

Night guards are special splints used for the alleviation of bruxism and clenching and the deleterious influence that these habits may have on the teeth and periodontium[25-27a] (Fig. 39-6). They are made of acrylic, and they completely cover the occlusal surfaces of the teeth. They can be constructed for one or both jaws. If freeway space permits, both arches can be covered. These splints can be made thin enough to be quite comfortable while being worn. When a single splint is to be worn, fabricate it and adjust the occlusal contact so that a smooth maximal contact in gliding movement is attained. The same contact should be sought for upper and lower splints when both are to be worn. The acrylic should extend just over the height of tooth contact and be finished with a thin edge for ease of insertion and removal and for retention when worn. Many patients have become so accustomed to wearing night guards that they cannot sleep without them.

In general, the night guard splint tends to stabilize mobile teeth. Care must be taken that the night guard splint does not rock and is not flexible. When single guards are used, the patient may pit the occlusal edge of the guard against one or more opposing teeth and cause them to loosen.

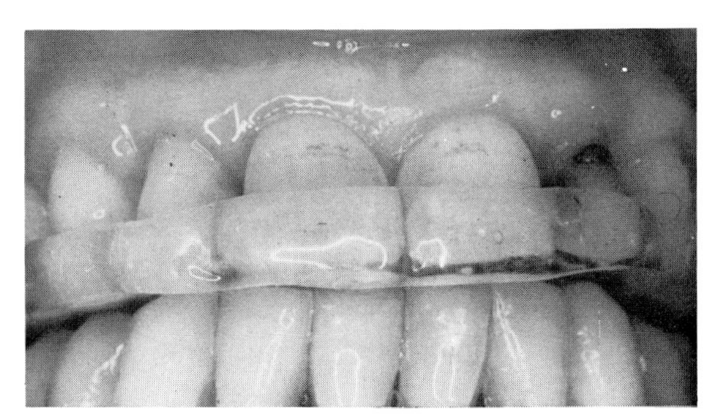

**Fig. 39-6.** Acrylic night guard used as a splint.

## Evaluation

*External temporary splints*

Somes external temporary devices tend to be unaesthetic or unhygienic. They lack durability, rigidity, dimensional stability, and/or fit. The materials of other devices may stretch, warp, or loosen, and retention is poor. These conditions may permit decay or, on occasion, cause the teeth to shift. Some splints tend to break and may not last long. On the other hand, external splints are prepared easily and economically. They can be removed and replaced readily. Some may cause gingival irritation but not pulpal damage. Tooth structure is not removed and, if the teeth become firm, the device may be discarded. Temporary splints have a definite place in the periodontal therapeutic armamentarium.

*Internal temporary splints*

Internal temporary splints include acrylic (A splints), amalgam, and pin and acrylic splints* (Fig. 39-7). (These splints require cavity preparations in the teeth to be stabilized.) They tend to be more serviceable than the external temporary splints, yet they have many of the same shortcomings. Their value varies with their rigidity, accuracy of fit, and the patient's susceptibility to caries. The materials tend to wear and break and are dependent on the strength of the bonding medium. The position of the splint, marginal adaptation, and interproximal joints tend to promote caries, calculus deposition, and inflammation. Moreover, maintenance needs are increased as oral hygiene procedures are made more difficult. When only part of the occlusal surface is covered by the splint, occlusal contacts may displace individual teeth from the splint. Extensive gingival recession, root indentations, and furcations make tooth preparation more difficult and may incur pulp involvement. Nevertheless, internal temporary splints have a definite place in periodontal treatment, provided they are used in situations for which they are suited. When the need for temporizing ceases, there should be no hesitation about conversion to definitive splinting. A delay may serve only to magnify the hazards involved in temporary splinting. A major cause of failure in periodontal treatment is the lack of, or delay in executing, adjunctive prosthesis or splinting in the patient who requires it.

*Acrylic splints (A splints)*

Internal temporary acrylic splints require the preparation of a channel approximately 3 mm. wide and 2 mm. deep in several teeth. The preparations should be slightly undercut for retention. The pulpal surfaces should be coated with a protectant.

*See references 1b, 13, 18, 18a, 22, 23, 27a-31, 35, 35a.

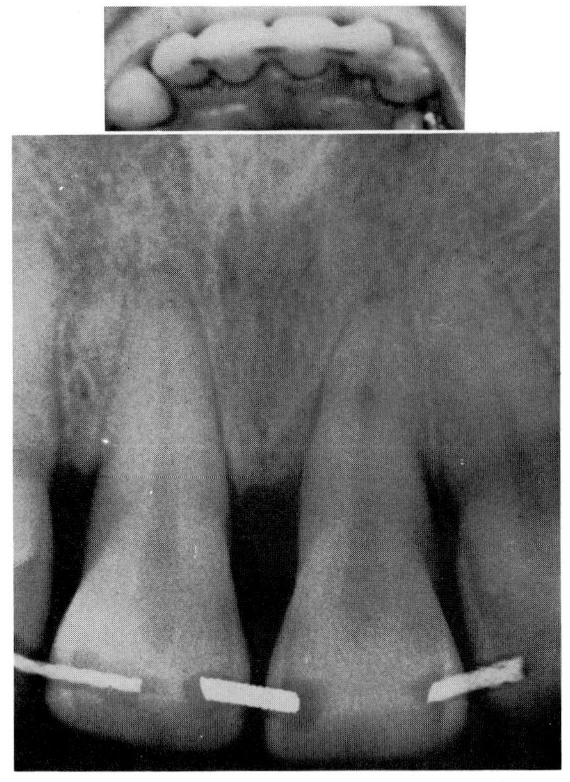

Fig. 39-7. Roentgenogram of maxillary incisors splinted together by the insertion of short lengths of wire into class III preparations. (Courtesy A. Gargiulo, Chicago; from the collection of A. Berliner.)

Lay a piece of platinized knurled wire (16 to 22 gauge) in the channel, flow in self-cure acrylic, and allow the wire to set in the acrylic in the channel (Fig. 39-7). Adjust the occlusion and polish the splint. Sometimes proper interproximal contour and marginal adaptation can be ensured by the use of a plaster or compound matrix.[27a,28,29,35]

***Amalgam splints***

The amalgam splint is similar to the A splint (Fig. 39-8).[30] It is, in some ways, superior to the A splint; but it lacks the strength of cast gold. Its use is limited to the posterior teeth. Prepare the teeth in accordance with sound operative principles. Make a matrix of self-cure acrylic and return the matrix to the mouth. Condense the amalgam in one unit. From two to five teeth may be splinted in this fashion.

***Acrylic full crowns***

Fixed temporary bridges with acrylic crowns and pontics may also serve as temporary splints (Fig. 39-9).[31] They should be used when permanent fixed splints made of gold, etc. will ultimately replace them. There are many ways to make acrylic splints. One simple method utilizes duplicates of the patient's study models. The temporary acrylic splint is then made on the models of the prepared teeth and is rebased in the mouth after the teeth are prepared.

With time, acrylic wears and breakage becomes a problem. Consequently some clinicians prefer cast occlusals; others are concerned with the cervical relationship of the acrylic and prefer metal copings, which they believe are less irritating to the gingiva and less likely to permit caries because of washout of the cement.

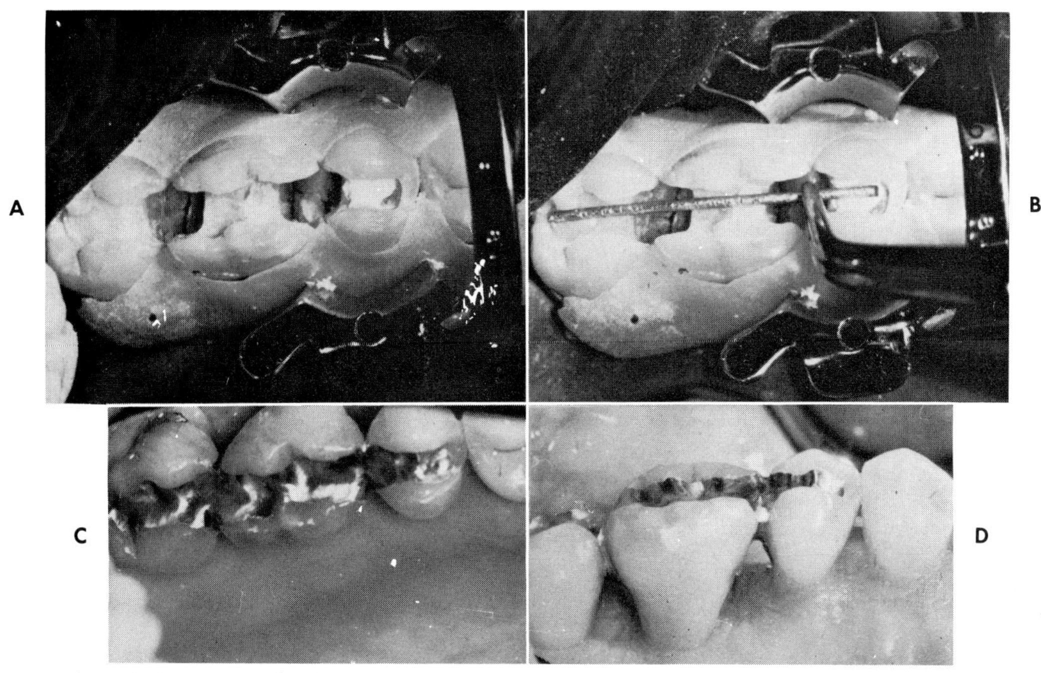


**Fig. 39-8.** Steps in the fabrication of an amalgam splint. **A,** Cavity preparation. **B,** Placement of supporting bar or wire. **C,** Finished splint, occlusal view. **D,** Lateral view to show the marginal finish and open embrasures. (Courtesy J. Atkins, Los Angeles.)

## PERMANENT SPLINTING—PERIODONTAL PROSTHESIS

Complete dental treatment includes periodontal and restorative aspects, which are extensively interrelated. Successful treatment most often requires both types of therapy. There are many instances in which one cannot succeed without the other. This interdependence applies as much to a single tooth as it does to the whole dentition. The importance of stabilizing loose teeth has been discussed. Permanent splinting is indicated whenever periodontal treatment does not reduce mobility to the point at which the teeth can function without added support. Such devices serve *to stabilize loose teeth, to redistribute occlusal forces, to reduce traumatism,* and *to aid in the repair of the periodontal tissues.* They are fabricated after periodontal treatment has been completed when their use will extend the functional lifetime of the teeth. Such appliances must be constructed according to specifications that will be discussed in the following section.

### Classification

Permanent splints may be classified as follows:

1. Removable—external
   a. Continuous clasp partial dentures
   b. Swing-lock devices
2. Fixed—internal
   a. Gold crowns and inlays
   b. Posts in root canals
3. Combined
   a. Partial dentures and splinted abutments
   b. Removable—fixed splints
4. Endodontic

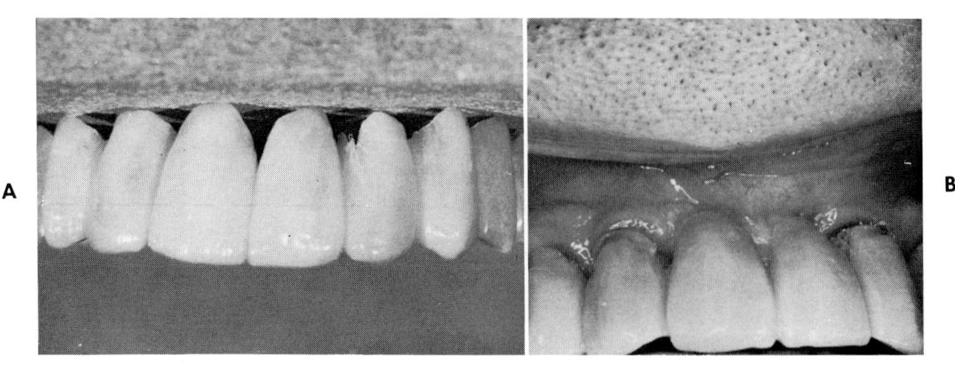


**Fig. 39-9.** Temporary acrylic splint made from the patient's model. **A,** Prior to insertion. **B,** After insertion on the prepared teeth but prior to rebasing with self-cure acrylic.

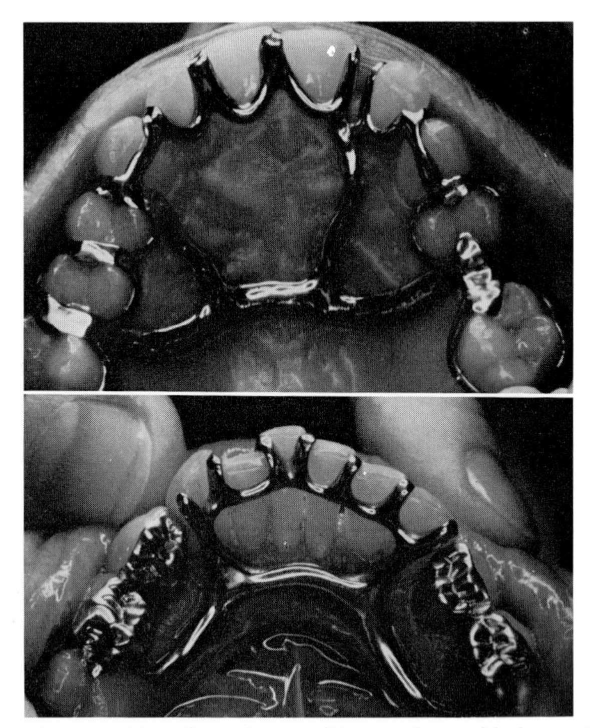

**Fig. 39-10.** Permanent removable splints for maxillary and mandibular arches. Finger clasps extended over incisal or occlusal contacts to the vestibular surfaces fix the teeth in place. (Maxillary splint courtesy C. Hoffman; mandibular splint courtesy H. E. Greenlee, La Mesa, Calif.)

***Removable permanent splints—external***

Removable permanent devices incorporate continuous clasps and fingers that brace loose teeth[1b,3,32-34] (Fig. 39-10). They strongly resemble partial dentures, and their features may be included in partial dentures. They support the teeth from the lingual surface and may incorporate additional support from the labial surface or use intracoronal rests. Palatal bars may also be added to provide a cross-arch splinting effect. Some partial dentures use pins that fit into grooves or holes in inlays[36,42a] (Fig. 39-11, *A*).

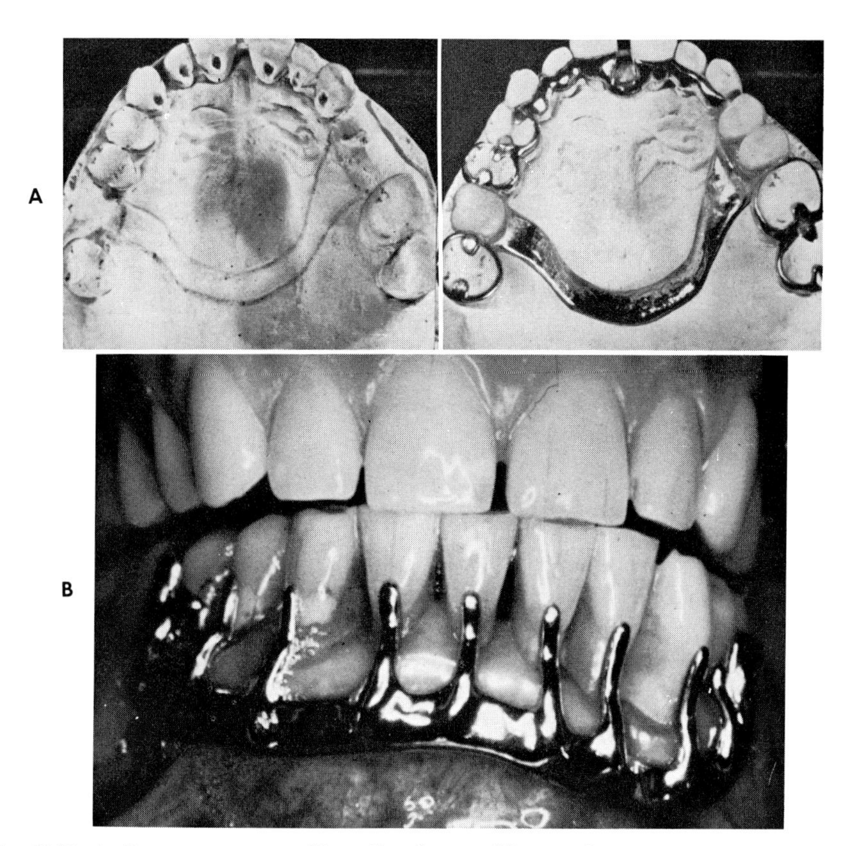


**Fig. 39-11. A,** Permanent removable splint for maxillary arch employing gold tubes (hollow inlays) cemented in the anterior teeth and pins that are part of the partial denture for support of the mobile teeth. **B,** Swing-lock partial denture. Mobile anterior teeth are fixed by the labial and lingual bars. A distal extension partial denture is attached to the splint by a stress breaker. (**A** courtesy E. Munch-Hansen, Virum, Denmark; **B** courtesy C. Miller, San Diego.)

The cosmetic disadvantages of labial continuous clasping can be overcome by use of the swing-lock appliance. In addition, periodontal trauma that may occur in the insertion and removal of a rigid splint can be avoided (Fig. 39-11, *B* and *C*). Swing-lock appliances may be useful in situations in which fixed splinting is not possible or feasible, for example, in advanced age, poor physical or mental status, and advanced mobility (Figs. 39-10 and 39-11).

***Fixed permanent splints—internal***

Fixed permanent devices may incorporate a series of soldered castings (crowns, three-quarter crowns, inlays, horizontal pin splints, pin ledges, or root canal posts).[1b,3,5,37-42] The splint is cemented to place. Full coverage is simple to perform if recession is not extensive and teeth are parallel. Otherwise, inlays or pin ledges may be more conserving of tooth structure and simpler to use. It is important that these splints be rigid. They should be of narrow buccolingual diameter. The occlusal relationships should be harmonious. The teeth and splint should be reciprocally stabilized in all directions (mesial, distal, orovestibular, apical). Otherwise the splint may still move about some fulcrum point and traumatism may result.[43] Traumatism can also occur when a tooth is in improper occlusion.[44] Finally, the teeth must be capable of supporting a splint. The fixed splint, properly made, is one of the most effective dental restorations for the stabilization of teeth. It is comfortable and aesthetic (Fig. 39-12).

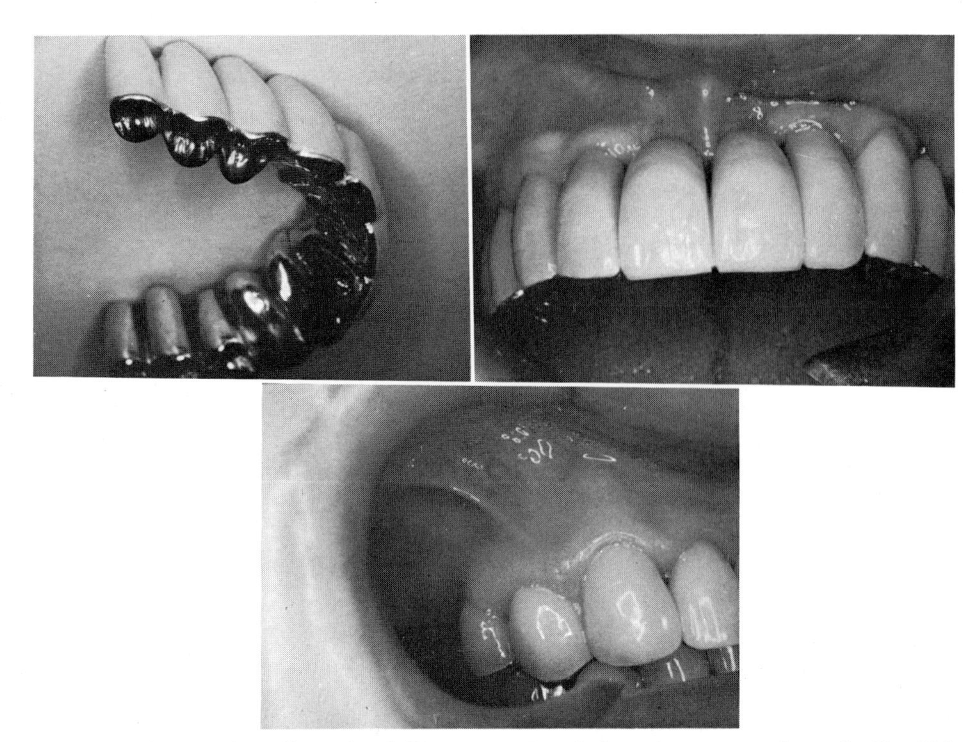

**Fig. 39-12.** Fixed bridge splint using full coverage. Completion of treatment shown in Fig. 39-9. (Courtesy H. Schwartz, Seattle.)

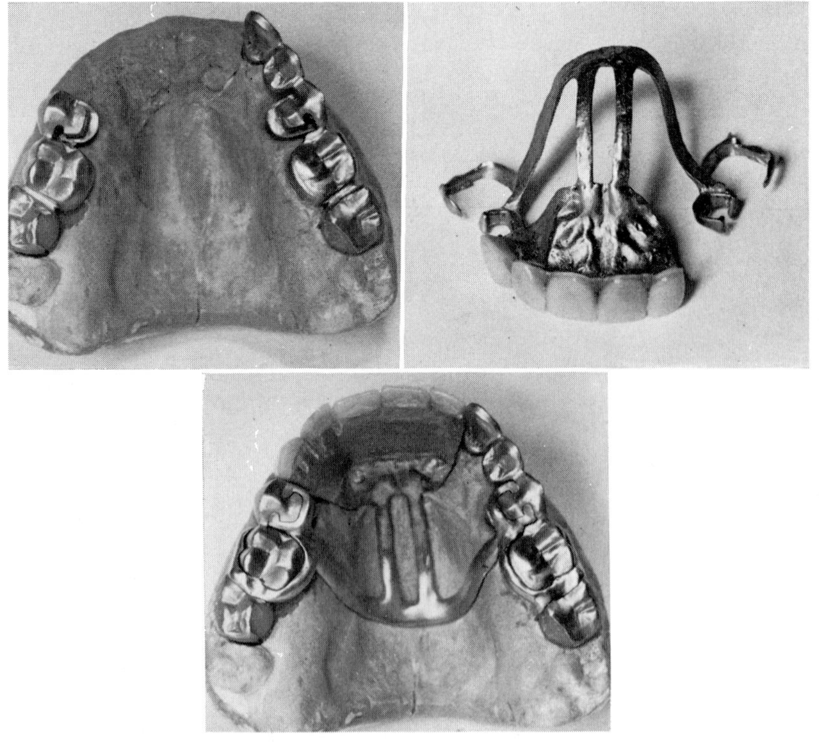

**Fig. 39-13.** Partial denture with splinted abutments. (Courtesy J. Rotzler, Basel.)

*Combinations*

Despite the advantages inherent in fixed splinting, there are many instances in which partial dentures are necessary in a periodontally weakened dentition.[45] These instances are governed by the distribution of remaining teeth. When partial dentures are used, the abutment teeth should be splinted[46] and the clasps and rests placed so that stabilization is afforded in all directions (Fig. 39-13). Recessed retainers and precision attachments are extremely useful in this ragard. When the teeth are mobile, they may be jeopardized if the partial denture is completely dependent on the abutments. In these instances stress breakers may be used. On occasion, tissue-borne appliances may be necessary. Partial dentures can cause extensive damage if they impinge on the marginal gingiva. They should be designed to avoid such damage and should be remade or relined when settling is evident. When possible, distal extention partial dentures should be avoided by the use of cantilever fixed splints. However, a palatal bar may be incorporated into a full-arch fixed splint to provide cross-arch stabilization. When all segments cannot be paralleled, jewelers screws or internal attachments may be used to combine the segments of the splint (Fig. 39-14). Such sectional splinting is sometimes indicated when there are only a few remaining abutments or when some teeth have a guarded prognosis. Telescope crowns are sometimes used in the making of removable fixed splints.

*Endodontic splinting*

Interest has been focused on the use of endodontic chrome-cobalt implants as a splinting device.[47,48] Such implants are, in fact, overlong, extra-thick chrome alloy root canal points. When seated, they extrude beyond the apex by as much as 5 to 10 mm. into the maxillary or mandibular bone. This splinting does not comply with the definition of splinting given herein since the tooth gains support not by being connected with another tooth but by lengthening the root as if it were.

## Evaluation

*Periodontal prosthesis*

There is considerable confusion over the need for periodontal prosthesis. Many popular indications for rehabilitation do not depend on existing lesions but are based on deviation from theoretical standards rather than on basic biologic norms. This sometimes encourages a degree of reconstruction when reconstruction is not really indicated. Splinting should not be performed unless indicated by clinical or roentgenographic manifestations (mobility, migration, loss of bone). On the other hand, there may be a tendency to undersplint when actual pathology is present. We have all seen one mobile tooth splinted to one firm tooth and find that, before long, mobility has developed in the sound tooth.

Splinting is generally effective therapeutically and generally achieves the objectives set for it. In addition, there are the mental and emotional values that relate to the tightening of loose teeth.

*Splinting and functional stresses*

The question often is asked whether splinting interferes with the physiologic functional movements of the teeth and ultimately leads to some damage. Remember: splinting frequently is used when considerable loss of supporting structure has occurred and when even normal stresses might be too much for the supporting tissues. The movement of mobile teeth is not physiologic. Under such conditions the teeth should be relieved of excessive stress. Splinting should not be visualized as causing a complete elimination of functional movement, however. Lateral stresses might be eliminated largely by splinting, but stresses in the direction of the long axes of the teeth are not eliminated by even the longest and most rigid splint. These functional stimuli exerted in the long axes of the

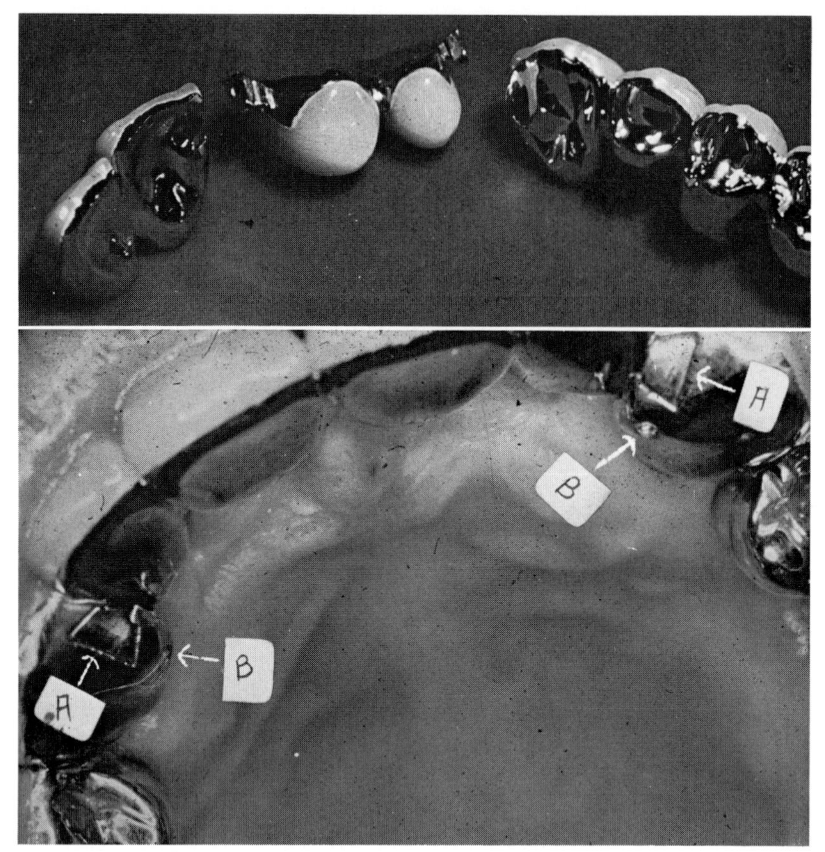


**Fig. 39-14.** Fixed removable splint. When problems of tooth alignment are present or a guarded prognosis for a tooth is held, a splint utilizing precision attachments, *A,* fixed by means of a screw, *B,* may be used. The unit is preformed so that it may be incorporated in the wax-up. (Courtesy D. E. Erickson, El Cajon, Calif.)

teeth in a splint usually are enough to keep supporting tissues in good functional condition. The purpose of a splint is to distribute and to redirect functional and afunctional forces to bring them within the tolerance of the supporting tissues and to eliminate any mobility that might be present.

Almost all splints demand an extra measure of motivation and diligence from the patient in the execution of oral hygiene measures. Therefore splinting should be undertaken only in such patients who have proved their will and ability to cooperate in these measures.[49]

**CHAPTER 39**

**References**

1. Rateitschak, K. H.: The therapeutic effect of local treatment on periodontal disease assessed upon evaluation of different diagnostic criteria, J. Periodont. 34:540, 1963.

1a. Baumhammers, A.: Temporary and semi-permanent splinting, Springfield, Ill., 1971, Charles C Thomas, Publisher.

1b. Böttger, H., Drum, W., Elbrecht, H. J., and others: Die prothetische Behandlung des parodontal-geschädigten Gebisses (Parodontoseschienen), Munich, 1968, Banaschewski.

1c. Posselt, U.: Physiology of occlusion and rehabilitation, ed. 2, Philadelphia, 1969, F. A. Davis Co.

2. Simring, M.: Splinting; theory and practice, J. Amer. Dent. Ass. 45:402, 1952.

3. Witkowski, O.: The tightening of loose teeth (translated by Neumann, E., and Gabriel, W. H.), London, 1912, Bailliere, Tyndall & Cox.
4. Kluczka, J.: Ueberblick über die Parodontose-Schienen, Zahnaerztl. Welt **59**:656, 1958.
5. Gottlieb, B., and Orban, B.: Zahnfleischentzündung und Zahnlockerung, ed. 2, Berlin, 1936, Berlinische Verlagsanstalt.
6. Ratcliff, P. A.: Periodontal therapy. In Ramfjord, S. P., Kerr, D. A., and Ash, M. M., editors: World workshop in periodontics, Ann Arbor, Mich., 1966, University of Michigan Press.
7. Posselt, U.: Occlusion related to periodontics. In Ramfjord, S. P., Kerr, D. A., and Ash, M. M., editors: World workshop in periodontics, Ann Arbor, Mich., 1966, University of Michigan Press.
8. Cross, W. G.: The importance of immobilization in periodontology, Parodontologie **8**:119, 1954.
9. Simring, M., and Thaller, J. L.: Temporary splinting for mobile teeth, J. Amer. Dent. Ass. **53**:429, 1956.
10. Weinberg, L. A.: Force distribution in splinted anterior teeth, Oral Surg. **10**:484, 1957.
11. Weinberg, L. A.: Force distribution in splinted posterior teeth, Oral Surg. **10**:1268, 1957.
12. Ward, H. L., and Weinberg, L. A.: An evaluation of periodontal splints, J. Amer. Dent. Ass. **63**:48, 1961.
13. Stern, I. B.: The status of temporary fixed-splinting procedures in the treatment of periodontally involved teeth, J. Periodont. **31**:217, 1960.
14. Amsterdam, M., and Fox, L.: Provisional splinting; principles and technics, Dental Clinics of North America, Philadelphia, March 1959, W. B. Saunders Co.
15. Hirschfeld, L.: The use of wire and silk ligatures, J. Amer. Dent. Ass. **41**:647, 1950.
16. Rothner, J. T.: Non-buckling metal ligation, J. Periodont. **34**:437, 1963.
17. Puckett, J.: Wire ligature, a feasible form of temporary splinting, J. Periodont. **32**:254, 1961.
18. Ehrlich, P., Frisch, J., and Nedelman, C.: Hygienic esthetic anterior splinting, J. S. Calif. Dent. Ass. **36**:225, 1968.
18a. Goldman, H., and Cohen, W.: Periodontal therapy, ed. 4, St. Louis, 1968, The C. V. Mosby Co.
19. Block, P. L.: Wire-band splint for immobilizing loose posterior teeth, J. Periodont. **39**:17, 1968.
20. Johnson, W. N., and Groat, J. E.: A new fixed temporary dental splint, Periodont. Abstr. **14**:153, 1966.
21. Friedman, N.: Temporary splinting, an adjunct to periodontal therapy, J. Periodont. **24**:229, 1953.
22. Baer, P. N., Malone, F. J., and Boyd, C. R.: A removable-fixed periodontal splint, Oral Surg. **9**:1057, 1956.
23. Krause, A.: Beitrag zur Behandlung des parodontal geschädigten Gebisses mit Kunststoffschienen, Deutsch. Stomat. **11**:904, 1961.
24. Waerhaug, J.: Periodontology and partial prosthesis, Int. Dent. J. **18**:101, 1968.
25. Gottlieb, B.: Schmutzpyorrhoe, Paradentalpyorrhoe und Alveolaratrophie, Berlin, 1925, Urban & Schwarzenberg.
26. Grupe, H. E., and Gromek, J. J.: Bruxism split, J. Periodont. **30**:156, 1959.
27. Posselt, U., and Wolff, I.-B.: Bite guards and bite plates: follow-up examination of their effect on bruxism and temporomandibular symptoms, Parodontopathies, p. 326, 1963.
27a. Berliner, A.: Ligatures, splints, bite planes and pyramids, Philadelphia, 1964, J. B. Lippincott Co.
28. Obin, J. N., and Arvins, A. N.: The use of self-curing resin for temporary stabilization of mobile teeth due to periodontal involvement, J. Amer. Dent. Ass. **42**:320, 1951.
29. Kothe, J., and Taatz, H.: Die intrakoronale Kunststoffdraht-Schiene, Zahnaerztl. Welt **65**:426, 1964.
30. Lloyd, R. S., and Baer, P. N.: The amalgam splint, Dental Clinics of North America, Philadelphia, March 1964, W. B. Saunders Co.
31. Talkov, L.: Temporary acrylic fixed bridgework and splint, J. Prosth. Dent. **2**:693, 1952.
32. Heintz, U.: A new type of periodontal splint to be attached to partial dentures, Dent. Abstr. **3**:425, 1958.
33. Grohs, R.: Die abnehmbare Greiferschiene, Z. Stomat. **23**:99, 1937.
34. Loos, S.: Die Bedeutung der Teilprothetik für die Behandlung der Parodontose, Z. Stomat. **45**:513, 1948.

35. Kessler, M.: A variation of the "A" splint, J. Periodont. **41**:268, 1970.
35a. Liatukas, E. L.: The amalgam splint, J. Periodont. **38**:392, 1967; **41**:272, 1970.
36. Munch-Hansen, E.: The pinsplint, a removable splint fixation; a modification of von Weissenfluh's "Hülsen-Stiftschiene," J. Periodont. **32**:322, 1961.
37. Burgess, J. K.: Modern attachments for bridgework and stabilizers for loose teeth, Dent. Cosmos **57**:1335, 1915.
38. Singer, H.: Der festsitzende Zahnersatz im parodontal geschädigten Lückengebiss, Deutsch. Stomat. **11**:767, 1961.
39. Mamlock, H. J.: Die Befestigungsschiene, Berlin, 1912, Hermann Meusser.
40. Baumhammers, A.: Fixed permanent splints, J. Prosth. Dent. **15**:351, 1965.
41. Sanell, C., and Feldman, A. J.: Horizontal pin splint for lower anterior teeth, J. Prosth. Dent. **12**:138, 1962.
42. Grieder, A., and Cinotti, W. B.: Periodontal prosthesis, St. Louis, 1968, The C. V. Mosby Co.
42a. Weissenfluh, H. V.: Die Hülsenstift-Verankerung für abnehmbare Parodontoseschienen und partielle Prothesen. In Böttger, H., Drum, W., and Elbrecht, H. J.: Die prothetische Behandlung des parodontal-geschädigten Gebisses (Parodontoseschienen), Munich, 1968, Banaschewski.
43. Rotzler, J.: Periodontometrische Untersuchungen über die Immobilisierungs-Möglichkeit gelockerter Zähne, Schweiz. Mschr. Zahnheilk. **69**:885, 1959.
44. Glickman, I., Stein, R. S., and Smulow, J. B.: The effect of increased functional forces upon the periodontium of splinted and non-splinted teeth, J. Periodont. **32**:290, 1961.
45. Stewart, K. L., and Rudd, K. D.: Stabilizing periodontally weakened teeth with removable partial dentures, J. Prosth. Dent. **19**:475, 1968.
46. Schär, E.: Die Eingliederung von Kronenschienen in Verbindung mit partiellen Prothesen bei parodontalen Erkrankungen, Parodontopathies, p. 335, 1966.
47. Orlay, H. G.: Endodontic splinting treatment in periodontal disease, Brit. Dent. J. **108**:118, 1960.
48. Orlay, H. G.: Splinting with endodontic implant stabilizers, Dent. Pract. **14**:481, 1964.
49. Schärer, P.: Patient motivation in periodontal prosthesis, Parodontologie **25**:60, 1971.

### Additional suggested reading

Budtz-Jorgensen, E.: Die prothetische Behandlung der Paradentose, ed. 3, Leipzig, 1944, Hermann Meusser.

Chacker, F. M., and Serota, B.: Provisional periodontal prosthesis, Periodontics **4**:265, 1966.

Coulomb, A.: Intraosseous fixation, Rev. Stomat.-Odont. Nord France **21**:177, 1966.

Falck, K.: Ueber Befestigungsschienen. In Kranz, P., and Falck, K.: Alveolar-pyorrhoe, Berlin, 1922, Hermann Meusser.

Fuchs, P.: Experimentelle Untersuchungen zur Behandlung von funktionellen Kiefergelenks-beschwerden mit Aufbissplatten, Deutsch. Zahnaerztl. Z. **27**:383, 1972.

Heiman, G. R., Biven, G. M., Kahn, H., and others: Temporary splinting using an adhesive system, Oral Surg. **31**:819, 1971.

Held, A. J., and Chaput, A.: Les parodontolyses, Paris, 1959, Prelat. (This book contains excellent references of the European literature.)

Kiefer, E.: Paradentosebehandlung mit besonderer Berücksichtigung der Entlastung, ed. 2, Munich, 1951, Carl Hanser Verlag.

Koivumaa, K. K.: Changes in periodontal tissues and supporting structures connected with partial dentures, Helsinki, 1956, Kirjapaino oy Libris.

Lindgren, B.: Full coverage or pinledge—their indications from a periodontal view point, Sverige Tandläkärforb. Tidn. **58**:287, 1966.

Moffa, J. P.: Retentive properties of parallel pin restorations, J. Prosth. Dent. **17**:387, 1967.

Overby, G. E.: Intracoronal splinting of mobile teeth by use of screws and sleeves, J. Periodont. **33**:270, 1962.

Surber, J. V., and Duboff, P.: Provisional intracoronal splinting: an improved technique, J. Periodont. **42**:592, 1971.

Weissmann, B.: Non-parallel universal horizontal pin splint, J. Prosth. Dent. **15**:339, 1965.

Weski, O.: Ueber Zahnschienen, Deutsch. Med. Wschr. **40**:2082, 1914.

Wolf, H. F., and Rateitschak, K. H.: Einfache temporäre Schienungsmöglichkeiten, Deutsch. Zahnaerztebl. **19**:525, 1965.

Wolff, W., and Stock, G.: Die Wiederbefestigung lockerer Zähne, ed. 2, Berlin, 1927, Berlinische Verlagsanstalt.

CHAPTER FORTY

# Periodontal considerations in restorative dentistry



Prosthetic dentistry and operative dentistry have an important role in periodontal treatment. Improperly constructed restorations, carious lesions, and their sequelae can become etiologic factors in periodontal disease. Properly constructed restorations are of therapeutic value.

From the periodontal viewpoint the outer surface of a restoration is of significance.[1] Proper contact area, contour, occlusion, marginal adaptation, and surface finish are as important to periodontics as they are to restorative dentistry.[2-4,13-15] These factors influence the course and direction of masticatory forces, the deflection of the food bolus, and the collection and retention of deposits and debris.

## INDIVIDUAL RESTORATIONS

When preparing for individual restorations, you should have a clear understanding of the anatomic features of the area in which you will be working. Damage to the periodontium may occur during cavity and crown preparation[13] and impression taking, through careless use of separating disks, and from overfilled or overextended temporary fillings and crowns. Injudicious use of Adrenalin string packs and of electrocautery to expose the margins of preparations must be avoided.[16,17]

*Contact areas*

The interdental space has the shape of a sagging pup tent and is occupied by the interdental papilla (Fig. 40-1). The papilla covers the alveolar bone, which may be considered the floor. The proximal surfaces of the teeth form the sides, and the contact area forms the peak. The embrasure spaces are the diverging tooth surfaces that open toward the vestibule, the oral cavity, and the occlusal surface. If the contact area is improperly restored, pathologic manifestations may follow. Open contacts lead to food impingement, and obliterated contacts may cause inflammation of the papilla by tending to retain food or plaques in areas that are difficult to reach.

*Contour*

Buccal and lingual contours of restorations are equally important. They should protect the gingival margin from injury caused by food particle retention, but they should not deprive the gingiva of stimulation by food excursion. The

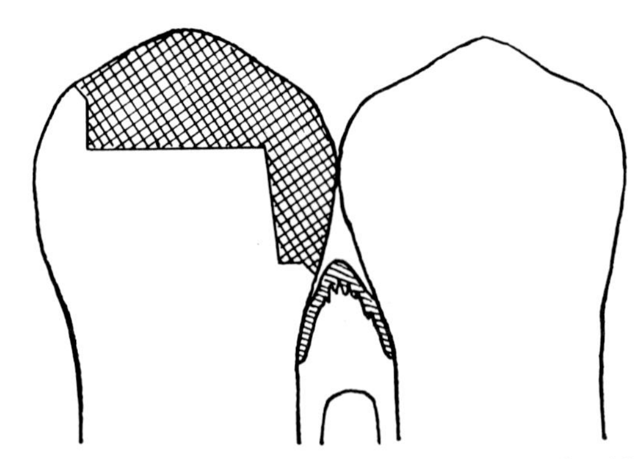

**Fig. 40-1.** Diagrammatic illustration of restored contact in a young dentition with sharp contact point. (Courtesy C. M. Stebner, Laramie.)

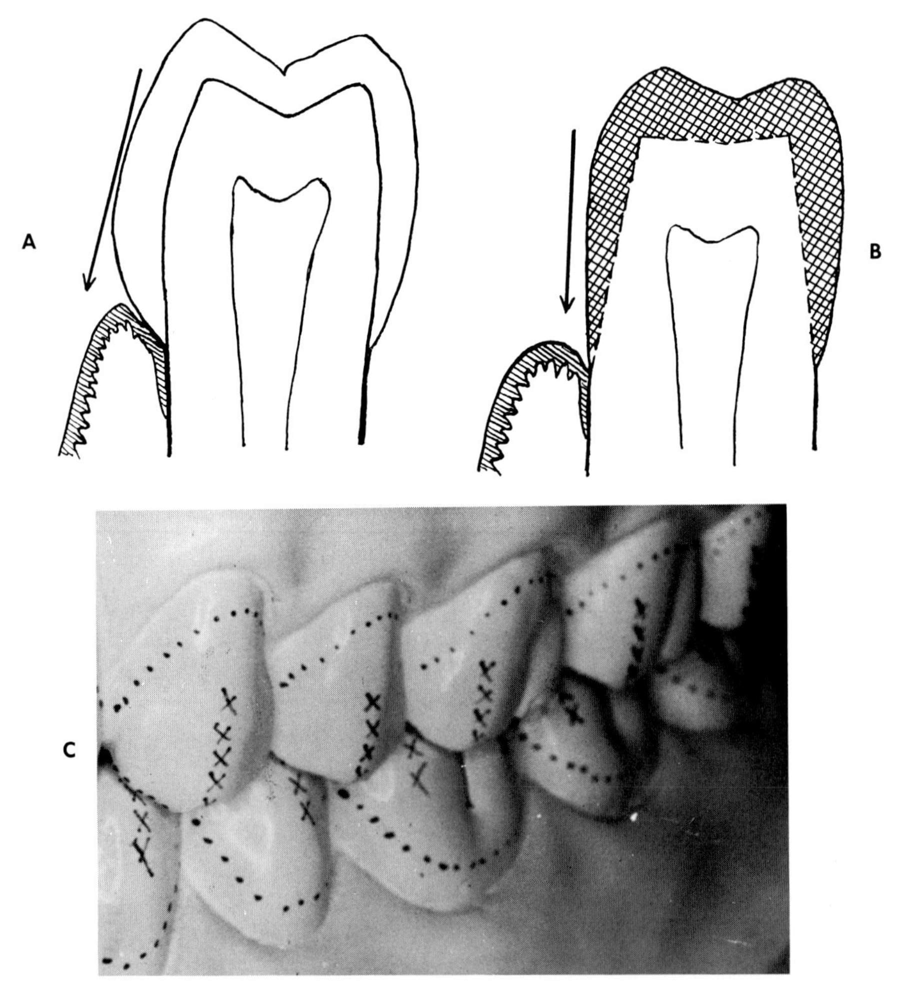


**Fig. 40-2.** Diagrammatic illustrations of, **A,** overcontoured margin that tends to accumulate plaque below the height of contour and, **B,** undercontoured crown with the deflecting contours missing. Injury to the gingiva can occur. **C,** Model of the ideal tooth-to-tissue (gingiva) relationship. Dotted lines show proper height of contour.

cervical margins should not, however, direct food into the gingival sulcus (Fig. 40-2).

*Occlusion*

The newly developed occlusal surfaces of restorations should be in good occlusal relationship.[18] They should not predispose to occlusal traumatism. The rules that apply to occlusal adjustment also apply to the restoration. Strive for occlusal relationships that are within the range of physiologic tolerance of the periodontium. Narrow the buccolingual diameters. Design sluiceways and marginal ridges to carry the bolus off the occlusal table so that food impaction is prevented. Each restoration must conform with the physiologic and topographic relations of the natural dentition. Natural dentitions that require occlusal adjustment, however, should be corrected before the tooth is restored. Complete reconstructions are best performed after some preplanning of the desired occlusion. You may use any appropriate anatomic articulator as an aid to the planning and development of the occlusion. An occlusion devoid of interferences should be developed. Grasping contacts or balancing side interference should be avoided. Interferences should be eliminated before reconstruction is attempted. There should be a harmony between hinge position, median occlusal position, and excursive positions of the mandible. In young persons the cuspal height may be steeper than in older persons who exhibit occlusal wear.

*Margins*

The restoration must blend at its margin into the tooth structure without any noticeable ledge, step, or overhang.[5,19] If you guide a periodontal explorer over the margin of a restoration, you should barely be aware of passing from tooth surface to the surface of the restoration. There should be no cement margins exposed. Silicate cement or plastic fillings seldom permit satisfactory gingival margins. These materials are not satisfactory for contact points on occlusal surfaces either.

Gottlieb believed that gingival floors of dental restorations in caries-resistant people should not be placed below the gingival margin.[6] This opinion has been supported in numerous studies showing that margins placed below the gingival sulcus can lead to a gingival irritation.[7-9,20-23] Silicate cement and plastic self-cure fillings make the poorest subgingival margins.[7,8,20] Well-condensed and well-polished amalgam, gold foil, and expertly constructed porcelain are preferable. All periodontists have had the experience of having a patient referred for treatment of gingivitis around a porcelain jacket crown whose gingival margins did not fit perfectly. True, some patients can tolerate a considerable amount of irritation; however, others can tolerate no amount without responding with an overt gingivitis. Gingival margins of restorations in caries-resistant, middle-aged, or older people might be better placed at, rather than below, the gingival margin, except when cosmetic considerations dictate otherwise. Under no circumstances should any subgingival overhangs or deficiencies be permitted.

*Surface finish and texture*

Another important factor is the surface texture—the polish of the restoration. The higher the polish and the less porous the material, the healthier will be the surrounding tissues. Smooth surfaces are better tolerated than rough ones, and bacterial deposits cannot attach themselves as easily to highly polished surfaces.

## PERIODONTAL PROSTHESIS

*Pontic form and solder joints*

Pontics should fulfill form requirements similar to those of the abutments. They should be shaped to permit proper hygienic measures. The space between the abutment and a pontic must be constructed so that the interdental embrasure

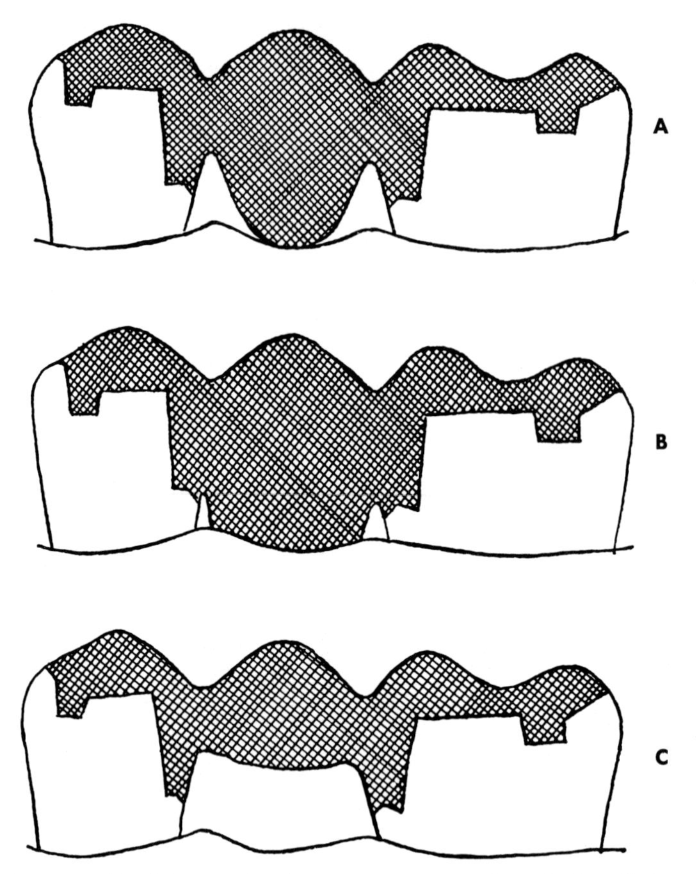


**Fig. 40-3. A,** Proper solder joints and embrasure spaces in a fixed bridge. **B,** Improper solder joints and embrasures in a fixed bridge. **C,** So-called "hygienic" pontic, which is, in fact, difficult to keep clean. (Courtesy C. M. Stebner, Laramie.)

space can be kept clean easily by the patient* (Fig. 40-3, *A*). These principles also apply in splinted abutments. Fig. 40-4 shows a case in which this rule has been carried out. The margins of the fillings are flush with the tooth surfaces. The solder joints and embrasure forms are constructed to permit good oral hygiene. These rules may be violated if solder joints are placed too close to the margins of the abutments. The gingival embrasure space between abutment and pontic may become so narrow that it cannot be cleansed (Fig. 40-3, *B*). Such construction not only is harmful to the gingiva but also predisposes to caries.

The so-called hygienic bridge (Fig. 40-3, *C*) is difficult to keep clean, and plaque adheres easily to its undersurface. When an ill-constructed pontic is placed next to a periodontally treated tooth, keeping the abutment clean becomes difficult. The best arrangement is to have the pontic touch the ridge with a rounded tip (Fig. 40-5, *A*) and not with a saddle (Fig. 40-5, *B*). The patient should be able to use interdental stimulators, Stim-U-Dents, or plastic bridge cleaners (Zon, Explac), to pass dental tape or cotton yarn between the abutment and pontic,

*Commercial laboratories frequently violate this cardinal rule. The dentist must therefore be certain that his technician is instructed in the design of cleansible, accessible embrasures.

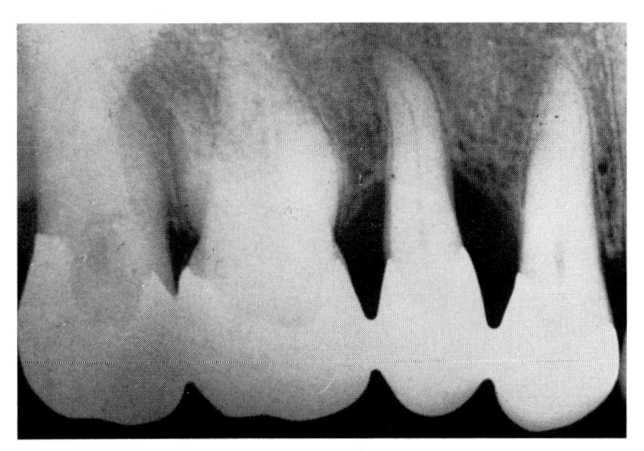

**Fig. 40-4.** Roentgenogram of proper contour, good solder joint, and good embrasure form in a fixed periodontal splint. (Courtesy M. Cattoni, Houston.)

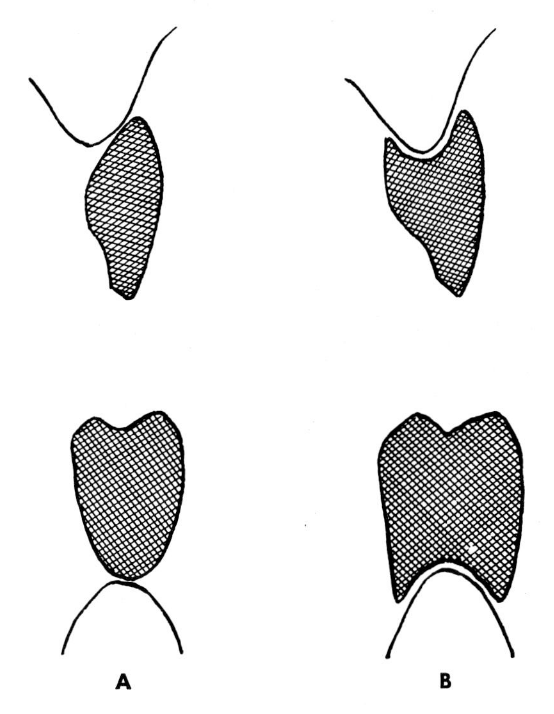


**Fig. 40-5. A,** Proper construction of pontics. Note the convex form against the ridge. **B,** Improper construction of pontics, contacting the ridge like a saddle, which makes cleansing impossible.

and to cleanse under the pontic. Rinsing devices such as the Water Pik are often helpful around complicated bridgework and orthodontic appliances.

## Precision attachments

When design factors demand, you may be forced to make a sectional fixed bridge. This can be done by a dovetail occlusal rest, a ball-socket arrangement, a fixed solderless joint, or a precision attachment. The negative part can be

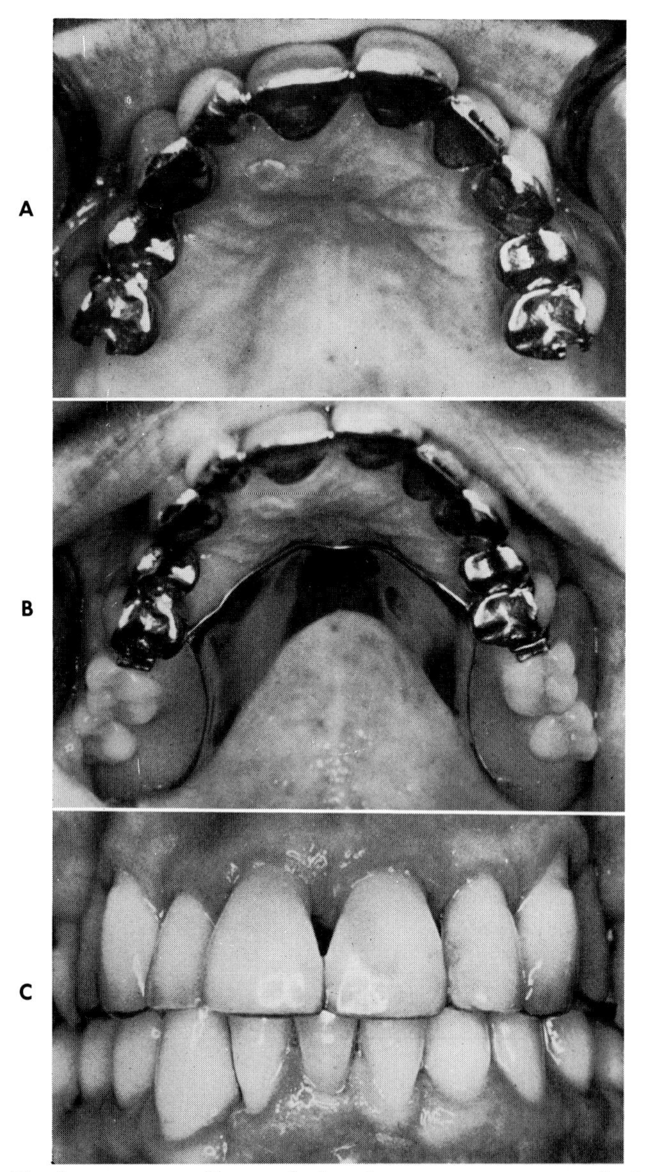


**Fig. 40-6. A,** Fixed permanent splint employing three-quarter crowns and pin ledges. **B,** Construction of a partial denture with stress breakers and wide palatal bar. **C,** Satisfactory aesthetic appearance. Embrasures are sufficiently broad to permit proper cleansing.

placed in one of the abutments and the positive part on the pontic or on an abutment, according to specific conditions (Chapter 39).

## Stress breakers

One of the most important considerations in partial denture construction is the method of securing the denture to the teeth. Those teeth with a history of periodontal disease may be weakened and of questionable value as single abutments. Splinting them to create multiple abutments is of great benefit. Broken stress arrangement between the abutment and the partial denture may also be useful. Whatever construction is used, remember that stress should be distributed and abutments should not be overloaded (Chapter 39).

## PARTIAL DENTURE DESIGN

Lingual bars as well as plastic or metal plates, can do extensive damage to the gingiva (Fig. 16-11). If a lingual bar is too close to the lingual surface of the gingiva, the lower margin of the bar can cut into the tissue. Be careful to avoid impingement of the settling denture.

Maxillary metal or plastic plates that cover the gingiva and extend to the teeth can also cause severe damage. Palatal bars (Fig. 40-6) probably are the safest design, and the horseshoe-shaped denture probably the most dangerous.

For years there has been controversy regarding the superiority of fixed or removable prosthesis.[10-12,24] Most operators prefer fixed bridgework because of the superior splinting effect that can be achieved. Moreover, some mouths can be kept cleaner. It may seem paradoxical, but a common observation is that single abutment teeth are most difficult to keep clean. Conversely, well-constructed bridges are cleansed as easily as natural teeth. Some operators prefer removable partial dentures. Partial dentures are also used when fixed bridgework is not possible or practical.

The final choice of prosthesis requires the evaluation of (1) the number and position of the remaining teeth, (2) the periodontal status of these teeth, (3) the clinical crown and root length, and (4) the patient. The personal preferences and abilities of the operator are also involved in this choice.

In recent years reconstruction has been advocated and supported by a number of philosophic rationalizations (occlusal rehabilitation, full-mouth splinting, bite-opening, oral dynamics, oral orthopedics). Sometimes well-intentioned but misguided zeal has been expended in these directions.[10] In the final analysis, prosthetic interventions should be chosen on the basis of their biologic value for treatment of patients demonstrating pathology.

**CHAPTER 40**

**References**

1. Romine, E. R.: Relation of operative and prosthetic dentistry to periodontal disease, J. Amer. Dent. Ass. **44**:742, 1952.
2. Terkla, L. G.: Crown morphology in relation to operative and crown and bridge dentistry, Oregon Dent. J. **25**:2, Dec., 1955.
3. Cripps, S.: Periodontal disease and restorative dentistry, Dent. Pract. **18**:199, 1968.
4. Ivancie, G. P.: Interrelationship between restorative dentistry and periodontics, J. Prosth. Dent. **8**:819, 1958.
5. Ogilvie, A. L.: Vital factors interrelating periodontology and restorative dentistry, J. Amer. Acad. Gold Foil Oper. **4**:15, 1961. (This article has an excellent bibliography.)
6. Gottlieb, B.: Schmutzpyorrhoe, Paradentalpyorrhoe und Alveolaratrophie, Berlin, 1925, Urban & Schwarzenberg.
7. Waerhaug, J., and Zander, H. A.: Reaction of gingival tissues to self-curing acrylic restorations, J. Amer. Dent. Ass. **54**:760, 1957.
8. Zander, H. A.: Effects of silicate cement and amalgam on the gingiva, J. Amer. Dent. Ass. **55**:11, 1957.
9. Waerhaug, J.: Histologic considerations which govern where the margins of restorations should be located in relation to the gingiva, Dental Clinics of North America, Philadelphia, March 1960, W. B. Saunders Co.
10. Waerhaug, J.: Periodontology and partial prosthesis, Int. Dent. J. **18**:101, 1968.
11. Cohn, L. A.: Physiologic basis for tooth fixation in precision-attached partial dentures, J. Prosth. Dent. **6**:220, 1956.
12. Posselt, U.: Physiology of occlusion and rehabilitation, Philadelphia, 1962, F. A. Davis Co.

13. Motsch, A.: Parodontale Gesichtspunkte bei der konservierenden und prothetischen Planung und Behandlung, Parodontologie **24:**109, 1970.
14. Ross, I. F.: The relation between periodontal therapy and fixed restorative care, J. Periodont. **42:**13, 1971.
15. Gottlieb, B., and Orban, B.: Zahnfleischentzündung und Zahnlockerung, ed. 2, Berlin, 1936, Berlinische Verlagsanstalt.
16. Löe, H., and Silness, J.: Tissue reaction to string packs used in fixed restorations, J. Prosth. Dent. **13:**318, 1963.
17. Knolle, G.: Gefahren bei der Anwendung des Adrenalinfadens, Deutsch. Zahnaerztebl. **21:**348, 1967.
18. Patur, B.: The role of occlusion and the periodontium in restorative procedures, J. Prosth. Dent. **21:**371, 1969.
19. Gilmore, N., and Sheiham, A.: Overhanging dental restorations and periodontal disease, J. Periodont. **42:**8, 1971.
20. App, G. R.: Effect of silicate, amalgam and cast gold on the gingiva, J. Prosth. Dent. **11:**3, 1961.
21. Eichner, K.: Der Kronenrand und das marginale Parodontium, Deutsch. Zahnaerztl. Z. **24:**741, 1969.
22. Fröhlich, E.: Zahnfleischrand und künstliche Krone in pathologisch-anatomischer Sicht, Deutsch. Zahnaerztl. Z. **22:**1252, 1967.
23. Silness, J.: Periodontal conditions in patients treated with dental bridges, J. Periodont. Res. **5:**225, 1970.
24. Grieder, A., and Cinotti, W. R.: Periodontal prosthesis, St. Louis, 1968, The C. V. Mosby Co.

#### Additional suggested reading

Burman, L. R., and Tang, C.: The abutment tooth, J. Dent. Med. **18:**83, 1963.

Carlsonn, G. E., Hedegard, B., and Koivumaa, K. K.: Studies in partial denture prosthesis. III. A longitudinal study of mandibular partial dentures with double extension saddles, Acta Odont. Scand. **20:**95, 1962.

Cohn, L. A.: Intergrating treatment procedures in occluso-rehabilitation, J. Prosth. Dent. **7:**511, 1957.

Frechette, A. R.: The influence of partial denture design on distribution of force to abutment teeth, J. Prosth. Dent. **6:**195, 1956.

Fröhlich, E.: Pathologic-anatomical aspects of the relationship between gingival margin and artificial crowns, Deutsch. Mschr. Zahnheilk. **22:**1258, 1967.

Gade, E.: Hygienic problems of fixed restorations, Int. Dent. J. **13:**318, 1963.

Gordon, I.: The danger zone. Use and abuse of full coverage, Alpha Omegan **54:**126, 1961.

Held, A. J.: Progress in the treatment of periodontal diseases, Int. Dent. J. **13:**46, 1963.

Koivumaa, K. K.: Changes in periodontal tissues and supporting structures connected with partial dentures, Suom. Hammaslääk. Toim. vol. 52, supp., 1956.

Koivumaa, K. K., Hedegard, B., and Carlsson, G. E.: Studies in partial denture prosthesis. I. An investigation into dentogingivally supported partial dentures, Suom. Hammaslääk. Toim. **56:**248, 1960.

Kramer, G. M.: Reconstruction first, or periodontal treatment first, J. Amer. Dent. Ass. **64:**199, 1962.

Long, A. C.: Acrylic resin veneered crowns: the effect of tooth preparation and crown fabrication on periodontal health, J. Prosth. Dent. **19:**370, 1968.

Marcum, J. S.: The effect of crown marginal depth on gingival tissues, J. Prosth. Dent. **17:**479, 1967.

Sorrin, S.: Relationship of periodontia to operative and preventive dentistry, New York Dent. J. **23:**398, 1953.

Stibbs, G. D.: The role of operative dentistry in the prevention of periodontal disease, J. Amer. Dent. Ass. **45:**645, 1952.

Thomas, B. O. A.: Relationship of operative procedures to the health of the periodontal tissues, J. Amer. Dent. Ass. **39:**522, 1949.

Veldkamp, D. F. A.: The relationship between tooth form and gingival health, Dent. Pract. **14:**158, 1963.

Wupper, H.: Die parodontal abgestützte prothese, Heidelberg, 1967, Dr. Alfred Hüthig Verlag GMBH.

PART X

# The treated case

CHAPTER FORTY-ONE

# Criteria for successful maintenance



## REEVALUATION

On the completion of periodontal treatment, the patient should be reexamined and reevaluated. Do this prior to proceeding with sequential dental treatment or discharge. The reexamination should include recharting for measurement of pocket depth and tooth mobility, notation of tissue color, texture, form, and tooth hypersensitivity, and evaluation of the patient's ability to perform oral hygiene procedures adequately. Roentgenograms and pulp testing may also be included. Record the findings on the initial examination chart in a different-colored ink. A comparison of pretreatment and posttreatment chartings will permit you to evaluate the effectiveness of treatment. The status of the patient's periodontal health can be estimated by comparison with accepted norms, and an impression of long-term prognosis and the results of treatment can be gained. In addition, when other forms of dentistry are to follow, the restorative treatment plan can be finalized.

### Pocket depth

Posttreatment sulcular depth should not exceed 3 mm. If there is any evidence of residual pocket depth, the involved areas should be retreated. Exceptions to this rule may be made in patients in whom physical or emotional status, advanced age, or extrinsic anatomic considerations make complete pocket elimination unfeasible. In advanced cases of periodontal disease, the objective of treatment might be to prolong the life of the dentition even though all pockets cannot be eliminated. In these instances, however, other criteria for gingival health should be met.

### Mobility

Tooth mobility is often, but not always, reduced by treatment. Sometimes moderate or advanced looseness may remain unchanged.[1] Note the extent of mobility with due regard for the transient mobility that sometimes follows surgery. Continuing mobility of class 1½ or more may be an indication for splinting

(Chapter 39). Advise the patient of the possible need for splinting at the time the original treatment plan is presented to him. There is rarely justification for such a need to come as a surprise to the patient since the indications for splinting are usually evident at the time of the initial examination. Moreover, the patient has a right to understand the total extent of possible treatment before it is started. On the other hand, if the properly informed patient procrastinates when the time for splinting arrives, you may be required to assume a firm role so that the results of treatment are not forfeited.

### Tissue, color, texture, and form

After the completion of periodontal therapy, the gingiva should be pink, firm, and securely attached to the teeth. Stippling, which varies between individuals and in its distribution in the gingiva, may be lost following surgery and then gradually reappear over a period of several months. The gingival margins should be thin and should taper to the teeth. The interdental papillae should be cone shaped and the gingiva festooned when viewed from the facial or buccal aspect of the teeth. Thick and irregular margins and poor papillary contour tend to promote food impingement and plaque retention and thus favor pocket formation. Examine the proximity of the frenum, muscle attachments, vestibular fornix, and sublingual space to the gingival margin since marginal surgery may inadvertently create positional relationships that are potentially harmful.

### Oral hygiene

Determine the effectiveness of the patient's oral hygiene by examining the teeth and tissues for debris, inflammation, and exudate, by taking a plaque index, and by observing the patient's routine. Some patients lack digital dexterity and others lack motivation.[6,16a] In addition, gingival margins may have been positioned apically and embrasure spaces opened. Splints or other forms of prostheses may be present. These factors all tend to make oral hygiene more difficult to perform as the need for it is increased. If any part of the oral hygiene procedure is not performed well, further instruction or a change in the prescribed procedures may be advisable. A patient who has not demonstrated proficiency in oral hygiene should not be dismissed if improvement is practical.[2] On the other hand, when he is fastidious in his home care, less than ideal results such as reverse architecture or residual pockets[3] may often be maintained in periodontal health without surgical retreatment.

### Roentgenograms and pulp testing

When, on the one hand, periodontal treatment is to be followed by other forms of dentistry or the treatment period has been unusually long, retake some roentgenograms. Observation of caries status and bone levels is then possible. In addition, test the vitality of the pulps. The findings of these procedures can be compared with earlier findings to determine prognosis and to finalize the restorative treatment plan. The findings also serve as a record against which future changes can be measured.

If, on the other hand, the patient is to be discharged without further treatment, roentgenograms need not be taken for at least 2 years, since some time is necessary before new bone can be seen. Thereafter, full-mouth roentgenograms should be taken at regular intervals.

### Conclusions

The posttreatment examination will usually indicate that the treatment has been carried to a successful completion. Explain to the patient the gains of treatment and the importance of maintaining these gains.[4] Then dismiss the patient from active treatment and enter his record in the recall system.

On occasion the examiation will reveal areas that have not been resolved to your complete satisfaction. These areas should be retreated if further treatment can remedy the situation. If, because of local anatomic factors or the physical or mental status of the patient, retreatment would be fruitless or possibly damaging, you may have to regard the case as complete. Treatment is complete when a result that is optimal for the patient has been reached.

If periodontal retreatment or other forms of dentistry are undertaken, another reevalution should be performed after their completion.

## MAINTENANCE PHASE

With the completion of all dental treatment, the state of dental health is at an optimum for that patient.[5] The expectation that the patient will continue at this level, however, is not completely realistic. The state of health can be modified with the passage of time by the various extrinsic and intrinsic changes that occur during a lifetime. You and the patient should, by continued cooperative effort, seek to minimize these detrimental changes to provide the patient with a healthy, functional dentition for life. The importance of excellent oral hygiene cannot be overemphasized. By diligent and successful plaque control patients may retain teeth in good health that once had a doubtful prognosis. This requires proper and diligent habits on the part of the patient and his seeking out and obtaining proper and adequate dental health care that is periodontally oriented.[7-10] Such care consists of periodic reexamination, preventive maintenance, and treatment. The arrangement that provides for notification and appointment of the patient for such purposes is known as the *recall system.*

Treatment therefore consists of two phases—active treatment for the interception and cure of the disease process and periodic observation, supervision, and treatment calculated to prevent recurrence. The latter phase, often called *preventive maintenance,* will now be discussed.[2,5,11]

The first year after treatment is a most critical period since the patient has already demonstrated his susceptibility to periodontal disease, the causes of which tend to be persistent and recurrent. Moreover oral hygiene habits are difficult to learn and unlearn. After periodontal treatment the first recall visit should be scheduled at 3 or 4 months. Thereafter, the interval may be lengthened to 4 or 6 months or occasionally longer. The frequency of visits should depend on the rate of calculus deposition, the patient's ability and resolution in home dental care, the clinical condition of the tissues, and the presence or absence of pathology. Examine the patient frequently enough to prevent or intercept disease processes before they cause irreversible damage. In time, changes in the dental, psychologic, or intrinsic status of the patient may occur and completely alter the established equilibrium. In this regard, old etiologic factors may recur or new ones may develop. Caries, particularly root caries, can be a vexing problem. There may be alterations in bone level, tooth mobility, pocket depth, or number of teeth remaining in the mouth. Finally, acute conditions such as necrotizing ulcerative gingivitis, pericoronitis, periodontal abscess, pulpitis, or traumatic injury can occur with sudden rapidity. The patient, of course, should return for treatment if any sign of disease becomes apparent. However, since many signs of disease are not obvious to the patient, your careful observation and supervision are a necessity.

## Recall examination

Reexamine the patient at every recall. Make dated notations with a different-colored ink on the same chart, or make a new chart. You will then be able to compare chartings with ease. Unless the patient presents with an acute problem, first attention at the recall should be given to the status of oral hygiene. If improvement is needed, give new instruction as indicated (Chapter 24).

The recall examination should include the following:

1. Inspection of the oral cavity for neoplasms
2. Thorough examination for caries
3. Reappraisal of tooth mobility
4. Examination of pocket depth (recharting at least every 5 years)
5. Check of tissue color, consistency, and architecture
6. Evaluation of oral hygiene procedures
7. Review of the occlusion
8. Examination of pulp vitality
9. Check of bone levels

You will need roentgenograms to properly perform the examination. A full-mouth series may be taken every second or third year, and bitewing films at shorter intervals to avoid excessive exposure to radiation. In addition, remember to remove all temporary splints (i.e., wire splints) and all temporarily cemented permanent splints to fully examine the covered teeth.

Every recall examination results in a diagnosis and reappraisal of the patient's condition, from which you may draw conclusions concerning the prognosis of the patient's dental health.

When a dental hygienist is available, she may instruct in oral hygiene, perform root planing, and treat root sensitivity. However, you must make the initial examination, reexamine for deposits, and perform corrective occlusal adjustment or surgical retreatment where indicated.

The recall findings will frequently indicate that the patient's condition has been maintained satisfactorily. Then all that is required of you is to remove deposits, smooth root surfaces, and polish the clinical crowns of the teeth. Cleanse and reinsert, as indicated, splints that have been removed. On occasion, minor alterations in the occlusion may require attention.

When these procedures have been accomplished, inform the patient of his current dental health status. This reappraisal, which concludes the appointment, serves to remind the patient of the necessity of continued supervision, and it stimulates dental cooperation in plaque control in the interim until the next recall.[2,7,10] Then dismiss the patient and enter his record in the recall system.

## Retreatment

From time to time, findings of special significance will be made during the recall examination. These may indicate the presence of new lesions or extensions of the original disease. For example, bone may not regenerate in an intra-alveolar defect after a reattachment procedure, or there may be new areas of pocket formation and bone resorption. Mobility may be increased. There may be tissue changes induced by the presence of fixed or removable prostheses. Caries or pulpal disease may occur. Changes in the patient's systemic status may alter his capacity to withstand insults to the periodontium that were previously well tolerated. In these instances, develop a treatment plan based on the findings and render treatment to extend the useful life of the dentition.

## CONCEPT OF CURE

At times the results of treatment may fall short of the projected goal. The failure to obtain optimal treatment effects or to maintain periodontal health after successful treatment may be assigned to occurrences during treatment or after it.

### Failure

A failure to obtain satisfactory results during active periodontal treatment may be caused by any of the following[8,9]: (1) a wrong diagnosis, incomplete examination, or inadequate record,[15] (2) inappropriate or incomplete treatment,[16] and (3) deficient oral hygiene by the patient.

The recurrence of periodontal disease after apparently successful treatment may be caused by any of the following:

1. Inadequate oral hygiene by the patient
2. Incomplete scaling and root planing in the maintenance program
3. Incomplete treatment or the wrong diagnosis
4. Inappropriate or improper dental restorations or prosthesis
5. Failure to carry out associated prosthetic or restorative procedures
6. Intrinsic or other factors beyond your or the patient's control

### Degree of success

Occasionally the situation becomes hopeless and some teeth must be extracted or full dentures made. In periodontics, as in all healing arts, the degree of success is variable. It depends on your diagnostic and manipulative ability,[13] the severity of the disease, the cooperation of the patient, the objectives of treatment, the intrinsic status of the patient, and the advancing state of the basic biologic principles and operative procedures on which all therapy rests.[11] If the useful life of the dentition has been prolonged significantly and there are no signs of pathology present, then treatment is successful. There can be no blameworthy failures unless you have ignored present-day concepts and techniques. There may be unsuccessful results, however, even in the most properly managed cases. Continued inflammation and loss of attachment apparatus or increased mobility in one or more areas are indicative of an unsuccessful result.

*Poor home dental care*

Although some unsuccessful results might have been avoided, others could not. Failures are sometimes caused by a lack of cooperation by the patient.[10,14] Figs. 41-1 and 41-2 illustrate a recurrence of localized breakdown because of poor oral hygiene and undiagnosed diabetes. (See Chapter 17, on the psychologic aspects of periodontics, and Chapter 25, on home dental care.)

*Questionable teeth*

You will not always be able to be completely accurate in your diagnosis, and treatment plans may not provide for all eventualities. If you attempt to treat teeth with a questionable prognosis, you cannot be successful in every case. The area of distinction between a questionable and a hopeless tooth may not be very apparent.[17] Moreover, the treatment of questionable teeth is a high-risk situation and the patient should be apprised of this at the start of therapy.

*Therapeutic judgment*

Therapeutic judgment rests on clincal experience and a knowledge of biologic principles. In some instances the objectives of treatment for a specific pa-

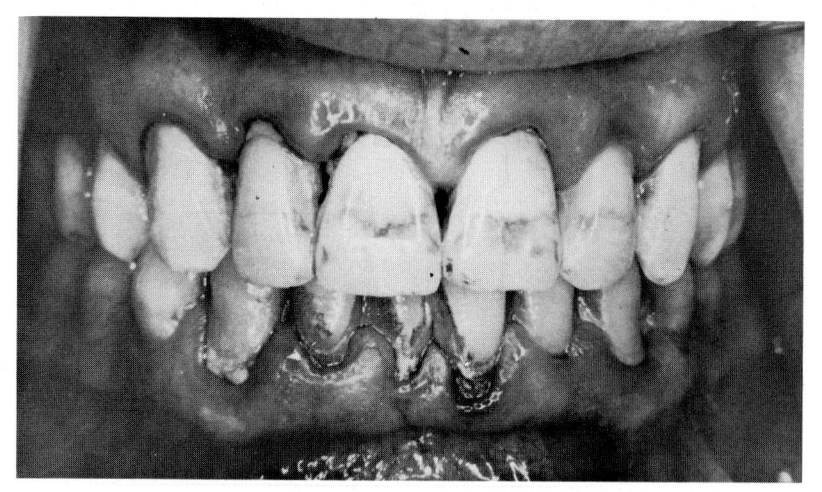

**Fig. 41-1.** Case of moderate periodontitis at the time of examination.

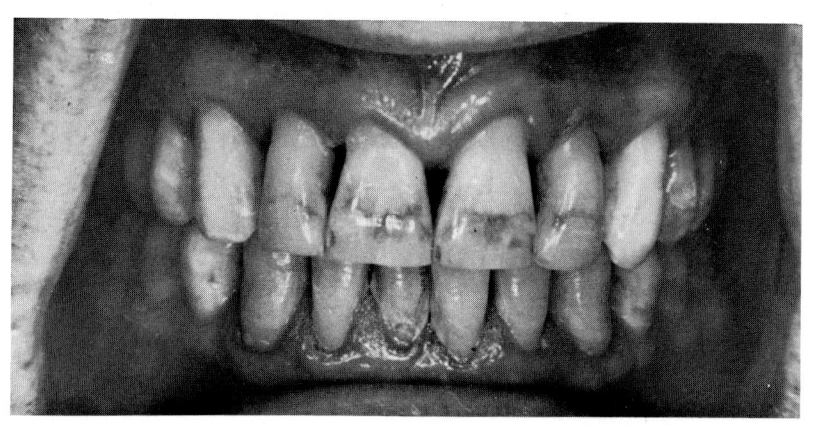

**Fig. 41-2.** Same case 2 years after treatment. Some localized inflammation is present. The patient practiced irregular and incomplete plaque removal. Later he was found to have diabetes.

tient are not achievable. In other instances your feel for the total situation and the patient is inexact. On the other hand, there are many situations in which procedural tactics are secondary and insight and empathy are primary. If these are not brought into play, expertise in technique is unavailing and somehow each operation is performed at a maladroit time in a maladroit manner. The results in such cases can be quite devastating.

## Intrinsic factors

Periodontal treatment frequently does not take intrinsic factors sufficiently into account. Knowledge concerning the intrinsic factor in the etiology of periodontal disease is vague. Errors in the proper evaluation of the intrinsic factor can occur. This may happen even with the cooperation of competent physicians.

## Basic knowledge

We still know very little about the etiology of periodontosis and desquamative gingivitis. In fact, on rare occasions, gingivitis or periodontitis may not respond. However, when further knowledge is developed, these patients may be successfully managed.

*Cure*

When is periodontal disease cured and what constitutes a cure?[5] When the signs and symptoms of periodontal disease have been removed and have been replaced by the signs of periodontal health, a cure can be considered achieved. Although the integrity of the tissues may be completely restored without any evidence of recession beyond the normal levels for bone and gingiva, more often the margins of these tissues will be found positioned somewhat apically. Whereas this may constitute a deformity in the architectural sense, it does not represent any manifestation of disease. Cure, then, is the attainment of a functional and healthy periodontal and dental status, with or without some impairment of structural supports.

## Case presentations

Periodontal disease can be cured, and periodontal health can be maintained. However, every dentist experiences occasional failure or partial failure. At other times the destructive lesions of periodontal disease may be so severe or so irregular in distribution that an ideal result cannot be achieved. This final section of the book shows some results that may be less than ideal so that you can gain a realistic and balanced view of therapy.

*Failure*

The appearance of a patient's mouth before treatment is shown in Fig. 41-1. After the completion of treatment, the criteria for periodontal health were met and the patient was placed on a maintenance program. Over a 5-year period the patient suffered repeated relapses; a few were acute in nature (periodontal abscesses); some could be attributed to errors or omissions in oral hygiene; others could be explained only by the possible effects of intrinsic causes since the extrinsic insult was minimal when compared to the severity of the inflammatory response. Repeated intrinsic evaluations yielded no evidence of disease until diabetes was lately discovered. Undoubtedly the diabetes predisposed this patient to exaggerated tissue responses to extrinsic irritants because of lessened resistance. The appearance of the patient's mouth 2 years after treatment (at the time of a recall appointment) can be seen in Fig. 41-2. Marginal inflammation and some fibrosis appear evident. Maintenance of periodontal health in such a patient requires regular monitoring and even frequent retreatment in localized areas.

The dentition of a 26-year-old white woman is shown in Fig. 41-3. The roentgenograms are shown in Fig. 41-4. The patient had been twice divorced and supported four children by working as a waitress. She appeared for treatment with a recurrent necrotizing ulcerative gingivitis. She had a history of dental neglect and had lost all but eight mandibular teeth. Initial treatment to reduce the acute phase of the disease was given. After this the nature of the disease was described to the patient and treatment to eradicate the tissue deformities was suggested. The patient requested treatment which was performed. The course of treatment was marked by broken appointments and irregular, inadequate oral hygiene. The patient changed jobs several times and finally left the city. Prognosis for this patient was poor. The possible emotional etiology of the disease remained, and, in addition, poor oral hygiene and an indifferent attitude might well have predisposed the patient to eventual loss of the remaining teeth.

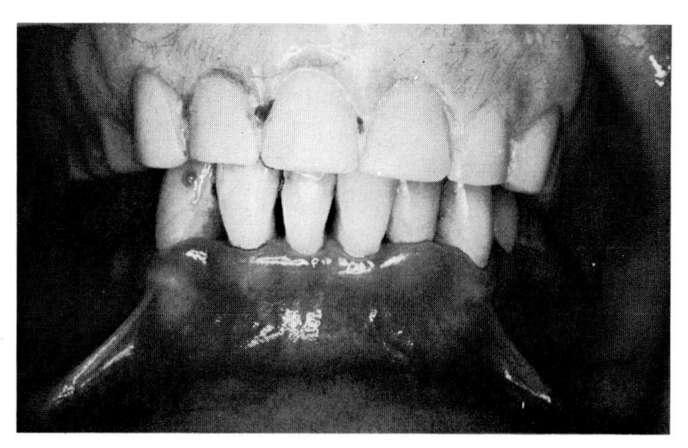

**Fig. 41-3.** Recurrent necrotizing ulcerative gingivitis in a 26-year-old woman.

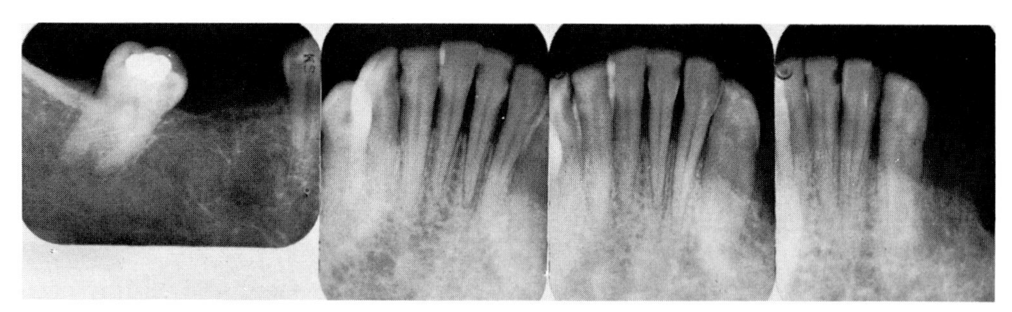

**Fig. 41-4.** Roentgenograms showing loss of all but seven teeth because of neglect and lack of dental awareness. Alveolar bone destruction was horizontal in character and of a mild to moderate degree.

*Success*

A 36-year-old white man with advanced periodontitis is shown in Fig. 41-5. Roentgenograms before treatment are shown in *A*. Pocket depths ranged up to 10 mm., and significant mobility patterns were present in many teeth. Extraction was advised for the mandibular right first premolar and the mandibular left second premolar because of tortuous complex pocket formation, up to 10 mm. in depth, and because of the class 3 mobility of these teeth. Poor prognosis was held for the mandibular right second premolar and the maxillary right first molar. A guarded prognosis was projected for the rest of the dentition because of the severity of the disease, the complexity of the pocket formation and bone destruction (*B*), and the variety of etiologic factors present. The patient had visited his dentist regularly and had been unaware of the presence of periodontal disease. He was informed of his condition and of the prognosis. His desire to keep his teeth was so great that he requested treatment. Extensive treatment consisting of prolonged root planing, intensive oral hygiene coaching, provisional splinting, occlusal adjustment, and advanced surgical procedures, including reattachment attempts, was performed. Exacting attention was given to instruction in home dental care and to the reduction of tooth mobility. A cast removable splint was constructed to control tooth mobility. Depending on further response and maintenance of periodontal health, this would be replaced by fixed splinting.

Two years later the periodontal tissues were in good clinical condition (Fig.

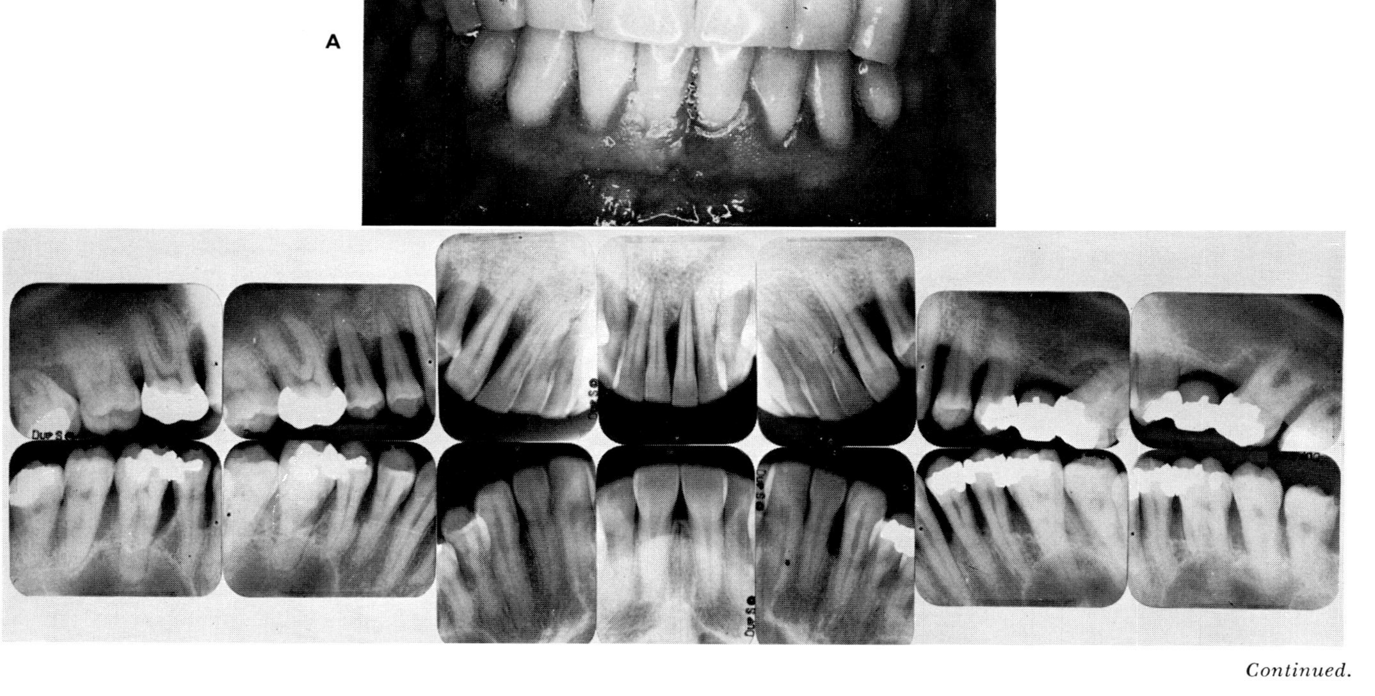

*Continued.*

**Fig. 41-5. A,** Advanced bone destruction caused by periodontitis in a 36-year-old man. Despite regular visits to the dentist, the patient was unaware that he had periodontal disease. **B,** Roentgenograms at the time of examination showing severe generalized bone destruction that is irregular in form and distribution. There are both horizontal and vertical patterns. Significant tooth mobility was also present.

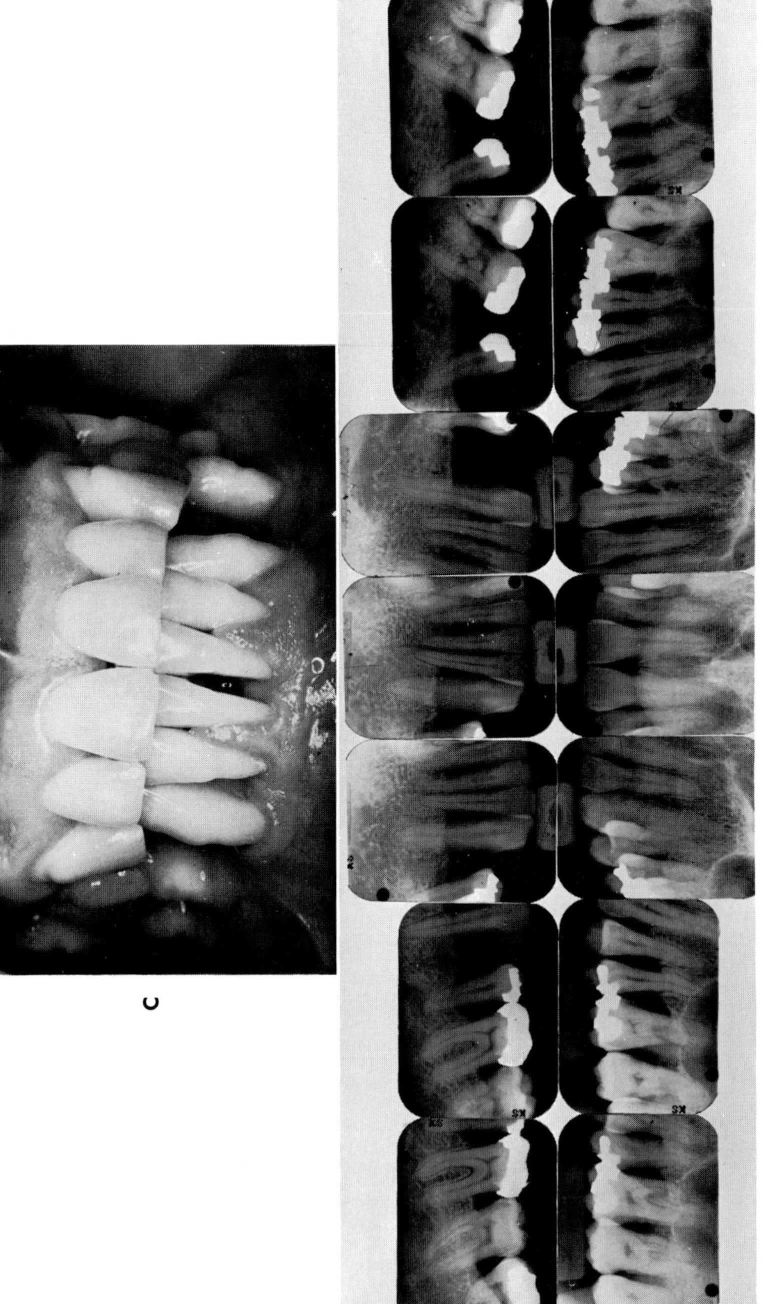

**Fig. 41-5, cont'd. C,** Two years after treatment the gingiva is generally firm, pink, and stippled. No pockets are present, but there are localized areas of redness of one marginal gingiva. Tooth mobility is controlled by two cast removable splints. **D,** Roentgenograms 2 years after treatment showing a more regular bony profile. The effects of past bone destruction can be seen in the missing alveolar bone.

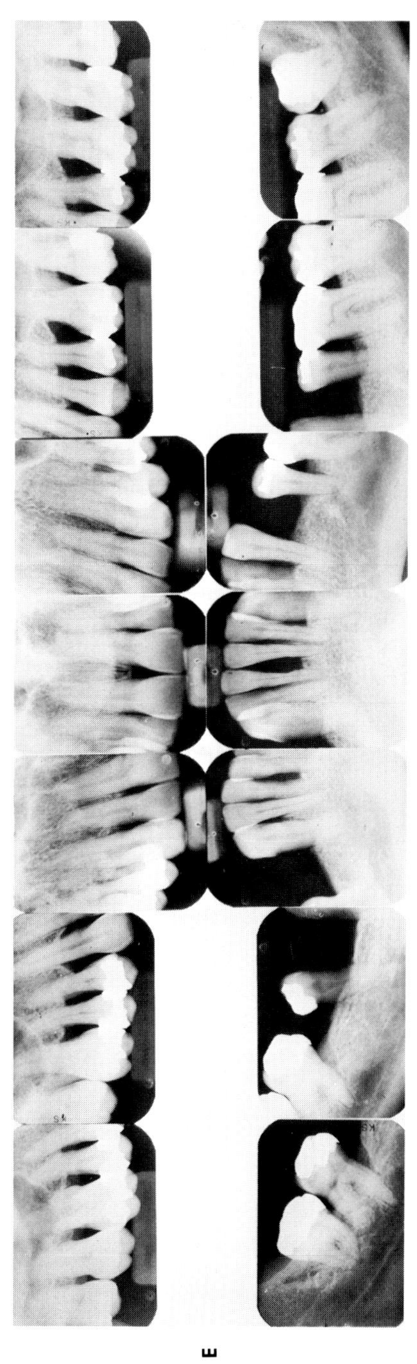


**Fig. 41-5, cont'd. E,** Roentgenograms 8 years after treatment with continued maintenance. Note that the bone levels have been maintained.

41-5, *C* and *D*). The gingivae were generally pink, firm, and stippled. The patient was conscientious in home dental care and regularly followed a maintenance program. The initial guarded prognosis was changed to a good prognosis, despite the considerable loss of tooth support. Eight years later, gingival health was present. Roentgenograms indicated that bone levels had been maintained (*D* and *E*).

## SUMMARY

Notwithstanding the occasional negative result, periodontal treatment usually meets with predictable success. The period of preventive maintenance, including occasional instances of retreatment, serves to extend the success of treatment and the useful life of the natural dentition.[3] Moreover, the recall examination and re-evaluation serve to unify all dental therapy around a common preventive goal—*to preserve the patient's natural dentition in a state of health, comfort, and good appearance.*

**CHAPTER 41**

**References**

1. Everett, F. G., and Stern, I. B.: When is tooth mobility an indication for extraction? Dental Clinics of North America, Philadelphia, 1969, W. B. Saunders Co., vol. 13.
2. Parks, S. R.: The responsibility of the patient in the treatment of periodontal disease, J. Amer. Dent. Ass. **55**:230, 1957.
3. Oliver, R. C.: Tooth loss with and without periodontal therapy, Periodont. Abstr. **17**:8, 1969.
4. Sorrin, S.: Success or failure in periodontal therapy, New York Dent. J. **29**:271, 1959.
5. Wentz, F. M.: What is known in periodontology? J. Periodont. **29**:232, 1958.
6. Wade, A. B., Lobene, R. R., Schärer, P., and Guldener, P. H.: Current concepts: How do I motivate my patients towards good and permanent oral hygiene? Parodontologie **25**:56, 58, 60, 61, 1971.

6a. Derbyshire, J. C.: Patient motivation in periodontics, J. Periodont. **41**:630, 1970.

7. Gallagher, J. W.: Periodontics in general practice, J. Amer. Dent. Ass. **49**:533, 1954.
8. Ogilvie, A. L.: Recall and maintenance of the periodontal patient, Periodontics **3**:198, 1967.
9. Chace, R.: The maintenance phase of periodontal therapy, J. Periodont. **22**:234, 1951.
10. Thomas, B. O. A.: What is periodontal maintenance care and whose responsibility is it? J. West. Soc. Periodont. **11**:8, 1963.
11. Cross, W. G.: Some causes of failure in periodontal treatment, Parodontopathies **18**:127, 1966.
12. Rateitschak, K. H.: Misserfolge bei der Parodontaltherapie und ihre Ursachen, Parodontopathies **18**:149, 1966.
13. Ward, H. L., and Kirsch, S.: Factors influencing negative tissue response after periodontal therapy, J. Periodont. **33**:379, 1962.
14. Trott, J. R.: Biological approach to dental practice: periodontics, J. Canad. Dent. Ass. **28**:687, 1962.
15. Bradley, R. E.: Periodontal failure related to improper prognosis and treatment planning, Dental Clinics of North America, Philadelphia, 1972, W. B. Saunders Co., vol. 16.
16. Kramer, G. M.: Dental failures associated with periodontal surgery, Dental Clinics of North America, Philadelphia, 1972, W. B. Saunders Co., vol. 16.
17. Everett, F. G., and Hall, W. B.: Grenzen der Behandlung parodontotischer Zahne, Deutscher Zahnärztekalender, 1973, Munich, Urban & Schwarzenberg. (In press.)

# Index*



*Boldface numbers refer to pages with illustrations and tables.

**E**

**H**

## N